THE ENCYCLOPEDIA OF

Natural Medicine

THIRD EDITION

Selected titles also by Michael T. Murray

What the Drug Companies Won't Tell You and Your Doctor Doesn't Know

Hunger Free Forever

The Encyclopedia of Healing Foods

THE ENCYCLOPEDIA OF
Natural Medicine

THIRD EDITION

MICHAEL T. MURRAY, N.D.
JOSEPH E. PIZZORNO, N.D.

ATRIA PAPERBACK

NEW YORK   LONDON   TORONTO   SYDNEY   NEW DELHI

The ideas, procedures, and suggestions in this book are not intended as a substitute for the medical advice of your trained health professional. All matters regarding your health require medical supervision. Consult your physician before adopting the suggestions in this book, as well as about any condition that may require diagnosis or medical attention. The authors and publisher disclaim any liability arising directly or indirectly from the use of this book.

ATRIA PAPERBACK
A Division of Simon & Schuster, Inc.
1230 Avenue of the Americas
New York, NY 10020

Copyright © 1998, 2012 by Joseph E. Pizzorno and Michael T. Murray

All rights reserved, including the right to reproduce this book
or portions thereof in any form whatsoever. For information
address Atria Books Subsidiary Rights Department,
1230 Avenue of the Americas, New York, NY 10020.

First Atria Paperback edition July 2012

ATRIA PAPERBACK and colophon are trademarks of Simon & Schuster, Inc.

For information about special discounts for bulk purchases,
please contact Simon & Schuster Special Sales at 1-866-506-1949
or business@simonandschuster.com.

The Simon & Schuster Speakers Bureau can bring authors to
your live event. For more information or to book an event
contact the Simon & Schuster Speakers Bureau at 1-866-248-3049
or visit our website at www.simonspeakers.com.

Designed by Joe Rutt/Level C

Manufactured in the United States of America

20 19 18 17 16 15 14 13 12 11

Library of Congress Cataloging-in-Publication Data is available.

ISBN 978-1-4516-6300-6
ISBN 978-1-4516-6301-3 (ebook)

To the beauty, truth, and wisdom of naturopathic medicine
This book is dedicated to naturopathic medicine and to those physicians and healers who have bestowed the virtues of the "healing power of nature" throughout history, and to those who will do so in the future.

ACKNOWLEDGMENTS

Most of all, I would like to acknowledge the inner voice that has guided me in my life, providing me with inspiration, strength, and humility at the most appropriate times.

I was blessed to have wonderful parents whose support and faith never waned. If every child were loved as much as I was, it would truly be a wonderful world. I have tried to carry on this legacy with my own wonderful children, Lexi, Zach, and Addison. My beautiful wife, Gina, thank you. Your love has been a constant source of comfort and inspiration. I am a lucky man to have you!

This work represents a great deal of things to me, including commitment and dedication. Over the now 25 years that this book as been a part of my life, there have been many people who have played a role in its creation and continued success. Foremost among these are the entire naturopathic community, as well as other members of the natural health movement, including the health food industry, and their respective patients and customers, who are the primary supporters of my work. Thank you so very much.

Finally, I am deeply honored to have Dr. Joseph Pizzorno not only as my coauthor but also as a truly valued friend and inspiration. Thank you for everything, Joe!

Michael T. Murray, N.D.

As Dr. John Bastyr said to me as a doubting student 40 years ago during the dark ages of natural medicine, "The truth of our medicine will come out." So many times while laboring on this update I was reminded of the remarkable wisdom of the pioneers whose insights again and again are being validated by modern research. I hope this work will serve as a tribute to these remarkable and courageous men and women who suffered so much for daring to speak the truth.

I know of no greater validation for a teacher than to learn from his students and see them make a real difference in the world. Dr. Michael Murray has had a remarkable impact on decreasing disease and suffering through his research, teaching, and writing, and his advocacy of science-based natural medicine. Thank you, my dear friend.

The greatest joys in my life are my dear wife, Lara, and children, Raven and Galen. Lara, dear, thank you for your bountiful love and nurturing. Congratulations on your burgeoning career as an inspiring author (*Your Bones*) on your own. Love you.

Raven, dear daughter, I am so proud of you! Achieving your M.S. in nutrition and R.D. from Bastyr University and now serving as supervising nutritionists at a clinic for eating disorders—you are such a gift to your patients. Son Galen, I watch in amazement as you excel at everything you do and at every level of education. The future is yours to create, and I wait with anticipation to see the impact you will make on the world. Raven and Galen, thank you for your love—I am blessed to have such wonderful children.

Joseph E. Pizzorno, N.D.

CONTENTS

Acknowledgments   vii
Preface   xi

SECTION I

INTRODUCTION TO NATURAL
MEDICINE   1

What Is Natural Medicine?   3
The Healing Power Within   18

SECTION II

THE FOUR CORNERSTONES
OF GOOD HEALTH   27

A Positive Mental Attitude   29
A Health-Promoting Lifestyle   39
A Health-Promoting Diet   48
Supplementary Measures   68

SECTION III

SPECIAL TOPICS   83

A Cellular Approach to Health   85
Cancer Prevention   95
Detoxification and Internal Cleansing   109
Digestion and Elimination   131
Heart and Cardiovascular Health   146
Immune System Support   169
Longevity and Life Extension   183
Silent Inflammation   198
Stress Management   204
Obesity and Weight Management   220

SECTION IV

SPECIFIC HEALTH PROBLEMS   243

Acne   245
Acquired Immunodeficiency Syndrome
    (AIDS) and HIV Infection   253

Alcohol Dependence   265
Alzheimer's Disease   276
Anemia   292
Angina   301
Anxiety   313
Asthma   322
Attention-Deficit/Hyperactivity
    Disorder   340
Autism Spectrum Disorder   348
Boils   353
Breast Cancer (Prevention)   356
Bronchitis and Pneumonia   367
Candidiasis, Chronic   376
Canker Sores   389
Carpal Tunnel Syndrome   392
Cataracts   396
Celiac Disease   402
Cerebral Vascular Insufficiency   408
Cervical Dysplasia   412
Chronic Fatigue Syndrome   420
Chronic Obstructive Pulmonary
    Disease   431
Common Cold   435
Congestive Heart Failure   442
Constipation   451
Crohn's Disease and Ulcerative Colitis
    (Inflammatory Bowel Disease)   456
Cystitis and Interstitial Cystitis/
    Painful Bladder   471
Depression   478
Diabetes   503
Diarrhea   548
Ear Infection (Otitis Media)   557
Endometriosis   565
Erectile Dysfunction   570
Eczema (Atopic Dermatitis)   582
Fibrocystic Breast Disease   587
Food Allergy   592
Gallstones   605

Glaucoma	615
Gout	622
Hair Loss in Women	630
Hay Fever	635
Headache, Nonmigraine	639
Heart Arrhythmias	643
Hemorrhoids	647
Hepatitis	652
Herpes	660
High Blood Pressure	666
High Cholesterol and/or Triglycerides	680
Hives (Urticaria)	692
Hyperthyroidism	702
Hypoglycemia	707
Hypothyroidism	716
Infertility (Female)	724
Infertility (Male)	731
Insomnia	748
Irritable Bowel Syndrome	757
Kidney Stones	764
Macular Degeneration	774
Menopause	781
Menstrual Blood Loss, Excessive (Menorrhagia)	796
Migraine Headache	800
Multiple Sclerosis	812
Nonalcoholic Fatty Liver Disease (NAFLD)/Nonalcoholic Steatohepatitis (NASH)	822
Osteoarthritis	827
Osteoporosis	844

Parkinson's Disease	868
Peptic Ulcer	876
Periodontal Disease	883
Premenstrual Syndrome	890
Prostate Cancer (Prevention)	903
Prostate Enlargement (BPH)	915
Psoriasis	923
Rheumatoid Arthritis	932
Rosacea	948
Seborrheic Dermatitis	954
Sinus Infections	957
Sports Injuries, Tendinitis, and Bursitis	962
Strep Throat (Streptococcal Pharyngitis)	967
Stroke (Recovery From)	971
Systemic Lupus Erythematosus	976
Uterine Fibroids	980
Vaginitis	984
Varicose Veins	992
Glossary	999
Appendix A: Are You an Optimist?	1007
Appendix B: Glycemic Index, Carbohydrate Content, and Glycemic Load of Selected Foods	1013
Appendix C: Acid-Base Values of Selected Foods	1021
References	1029
Index	1181

PREFACE

This book was written in an effort to update the public's knowledge about the use of natural medicines in the maintenance of health and treatment of disease. It dispels a common myth about the use of natural remedies—that natural medicine is "unscientific." This book contains information based on firm scientific inquiry and represents an evidence-based approach to wellness. This encyclopedia is without question the most thoroughly researched and referenced book on the use of natural medicines ever written for the public.

The book must not be used in place of consulting a physician or other qualified health care practitioner. It is designed for use in conjunction with the services provided by physicians practicing natural medicine. Readers are strongly urged to develop a good relationship with a physician knowledgeable in the art and science of natural and preventive medicine, such as a naturopathic physician. In all cases involving a medical complaint, ailment, or therapy, please consult a physician. Proper medical care and advice can significantly improve the quality of your life and extend your life span.

Although this book discusses numerous natural approaches to various health conditions, it is not intended as a substitute for appropriate medical care. Please keep the following in mind as you read:

- Do not self-diagnose. If you have concerns about any subject discussed in this book, please consult a physician, preferably a naturopathic doctor (N.D.), nutritionally oriented medical doctor (M.D.) or doctor of osteopathy (D.O.), chiropractor (D.C.), or other natural health care specialist.

- Make your physician aware of all the prescription medications, over-the-counter medications, nutritional supplements, or herbal products you are currently taking, in order to avoid any negative interactions.

- If you are currently taking a prescription medication, you absolutely must work with your doctor before discontinuing any drug or altering any drug regimen.

- Many health conditions require a multifactorial solution: medical, nutritional, and lifestyle changes. Do not rely solely on a single area of focus. You can't just take pills and not change your diet, or do the diet and the pills but ignore the lifestyle issues. Any truly effective approach to health must be fully integrated.

We believe that if you commit to following the guidelines of natural health care described in this book, you will be rewarded with a life full of health, vitality, and vigor.

Michael T. Murray, N.D.
Joseph E. Pizzorno, N.D.

INTRODUCTION TO NATURAL MEDICINE

What Is Natural Medicine?

··

The doctor of the future will give no medicine, but will interest his patient in the care of the human frame, in diet and in the cause and prevention of disease.

—THOMAS EDISON

Introduction

An evolution in the core principles of health care has been occurring over the last few decades. At the forefront of this change is naturopathic medicine—a system of medicine based on the belief that the human body has a remarkable innate healing ability. Naturopathic doctors (N.D.'s) view the patient as a complex, interrelated system—a whole person—and focus on promoting health through natural, nontoxic therapies such as nutrition, lifestyle modification, herbal remedies, psychological measures, and many others.

Naturopathic medicine is helping to usher in the emerging paradigm in medicine. A *paradigm* is a model used to explain events. As our understanding of the environment and the human body evolves, new paradigms are developed. For example, in physics the cause-and-effect views of Descartes and Newton were replaced by Einstein's theory of relativity, quantum mechanics, and approaches in theoretical physics that take into considerations the tremendous interconnectedness of the universe.

The new paradigm in medicine also focuses on the interconnectedness of body, mind, emotions, social factors, and the environment. While the old paradigm viewed the body basically as a machine that can be fixed best with drugs and surgery, the emerging new model considers these measures secondary to natural, noninvasive techniques that promote health by supporting the body's own healing processes. The relationship between the physician and patient is also evolving. The era of the physician as a demigod is over. The era of self-empowerment is beginning.

Naturopathic Medicine: A Brief History

Naturopathy (the word means "nature cure") is a method of healing that employs various natural means to empower an individual to achieve the highest level of health possible. Despite its philosophical links to many cultures, modern naturopathic medicine grew out of natural healing systems in 18th- and 19th-century Europe and the United States. The European tradition of "taking the cure" at natural springs or spas had gained a foothold in America by the middle of the 18th century. The custom helped make Germany and the United States especially receptive to the ideas of naturopathy. Among the movement's earliest promoters were Sebastian

Kneipp, a priest who credited his recovery from tuberculosis to bathing in the Danube; and Benedict Lust, a physician who trained at the water-cure clinic that Kneipp had founded in Europe. Lust arrived in the United States in the 1890s and began using the term *naturopathy* to describe an eclectic compilation of doctrines of natural healing.

In 1902, Lust founded the first naturopathic college of medicine in the United States in New York City. It taught a system of medicine that included the best of what was then known about nutritional therapy, natural diet, herbal medicine, homeopathy, spinal manipulation, exercise therapy, hydrotherapy, electrotherapy, stress reduction, and other natural therapies. The basic tenets of Lust's view of naturopathy are summarized in his article "The Principles, Aim and Program of the Nature Cure":[1]

> The natural system for curing disease is based on a return to nature in regulating the diet, breathing, exercising, bathing and the employment of various forces to eliminate the poisonous products in the system, and so raise the vitality of the patient to a proper standard of health. . . .

THE PROGRAM OF NATUROPATHIC CURE

1. ELIMINATION OF EVIL HABITS, or the weeds of life, such as over-eating, alcoholic drinks, drugs, the use of tea, coffee and cocoa that contain poisons, meat eating, improper hours of living, waste of vital forces, lowered vitality, sexual and social aberrations, worry, etc.

2. CORRECTIVE HABITS. Correct breathing, correct exercise, right mental attitude. Moderation in the pursuit of health and wealth.

3. NEW PRINCIPLES OF LIVING. Proper fasting, selection of food, hydropathy, light and air baths, mud baths, osteopathy, chiropractic and other forms of mechano-therapy, mineral salts obtained in organic from, electropathy, heliopathy, steam or Turkish baths, sitz baths, etc. . . .

> There is really but one healing force in existence and that is Nature herself, which means the inherent restorative power of the organism to overcome disease. Now the question is, can this power be appropriated and guided more readily by extrinsic or intrinsic methods? That is to say, is it more amenable to combat disease by irritating drugs, vaccines and serums employed by superstitious moderns, or by the bland intrinsic congenial forces of Natural Therapeutics, that are employed by this new school of medicine, that is Naturopathy, which is the only orthodox school of medicine? Are not these natural forces much more orthodox than the artificial resources of the druggist? The practical application of these natural agencies, duly suited to the individual case, are true signs that the art of healing has been elaborated by the aid of absolutely harmless, congenial treatments.

The early naturopaths, including Lust, attached great importance to a natural, healthful diet. So did many of their contemporaries. John Kellogg, a physician, Seventh-day Adventist, and vegetarian, ran the Battle Creek Sanitarium, which utilized natural therapies; his brother, Will, built and ran a factory in Battle Creek, Michigan, to produce health foods such as shredded wheat and granola biscuits. Driven both by personal convictions about the benefits of cereal fibers and by commercial interests, the Kellogg brothers, along with a former employee, C. W. Post, helped popularize naturopathic ideas about food.

Naturopathic medicine grew and flourished in the early part of the 20th century.

However, in the mid-1930s several factors led to the medical profession's establishing the foundation for its current virtual monopoly on health care: (1) the medical profession finally stopped using therapies such as bloodletting and mercury dosing, replacing them with new therapies that were more effective for treating symptoms and much less toxic; (2) foundations supported by the drug industry began heavily subsidizing medical schools and drug research; and (3) the medical profession became much more of a political force, resulting in the passing of legislation that severely restricted the viability of other health care systems.[2]

Naturopathy has experienced a tremendous resurgence since the mid-1970s when the profession was nearly extinct. This resurgence is largely related to increased public awareness about the role of diet and lifestyle in chronic diseases and the failure of modern medicine to deal effectively with these disorders. In addition, the 1978 founding of Bastyr University, with its focus on teaching science-based natural medicine and its landmark achievement of accreditation, played a major role.

The Philosophy of Naturopathic Medicine

Although the term *naturopathy* or *naturopathic medicine* was not used until the late 19th century, the philosophical roots of this medical system go back thousands of years. Drawing on the healing wisdom of many cultures, including India's ayurveda, China's Taoism, and Greece's Hippocratic school of medicine, naturopathic medicine is a system founded on seven time-tested principles:

Principle 1: The healing power of nature (*vis medicatrix naturae*). Naturopathic physicians believe that the body has considerable power to heal itself. It is the role of the physician to facilitate and enhance this process with the aid of natural nontoxic therapies.

Principle 2: Identify and treat the cause (*tolle causam*). The naturopathic physician is trained to seek the underlying causes of a disease rather than simply suppress the symptoms, which are viewed as expressions of the body's attempt to heal. The causes of disease can arise at the physical, mental-emotional, and spiritual levels.

Principle 3: First, do no harm (*primum non nocere*). The naturopathic physician seeks to do no harm with medical treatment by employing safe and effective natural therapies.

Principle 4: Treat the whole person (holism). Naturopathic physicians are trained to view an individual as a whole, a complex interaction of physical, mental-emotional, spiritual, social, and other factors.

Principle 5: The physician as teacher (*docere*). The naturopathic physician is foremost a teacher, educating, empowering, and motivating the patients to assume more personal responsibility for their health by adopting a healthful attitude, lifestyle, and diet.

Principle 6: Prevention is the best cure. Naturopathic physicians are specialists in preventive medicine. Prevention of disease and support of health are accomplished through education and life habits.

Principle 7: Establishing health and wellness. Establishing and maintaining optimal health and promoting wellness are the primary goals of the naturopathic physician. While health is defined as the state of optimal physical, mental, emotional, and spiritual well-being, wellness is defined as a state of health characterized by a positive emotional state. The naturopathic physician strives to increase the level of wellness regardless of the disease or level of health. Even in cases of severe disease, a high level of wellness can often be achieved.

Naturopathic Therapy

Naturopathic physicians' primary focus is on promoting health and preventing disease. In addition to providing recommendations on lifestyle, diet, and exercise, naturopathic physicians may elect to utilize a variety of therapeutic modalities to promote health. Some naturopathic physicians choose to emphasize a particular therapeutic modality, while others are more eclectic and utilize a number of modalities; some naturopaths elect to focus on particular medical fields such as pediatrics, natural childbirth, physical medicine, and so on.

Naturopathic medicine is inclusive, in that it incorporates a variety of healing techniques. The current treatments naturopathic physicians are trained in include clinical nutrition, botanical medicine, homeopathy, Oriental medicine and acupuncture, hydrotherapy, physical medicine including massage and therapeutic manipulation, counseling and other psychotherapies, and minor surgery. In addition, in many states licensed naturopathic physicians can prescribe pharmaceutical drugs.

Clinical Nutrition

Clinical nutrition, or the use of diet as a therapy, serves as the foundation of naturopathic medicine. There is an ever-increasing body of knowledge that supports the use of whole foods and nutritional supplements in the maintenance of health and treatment of disease.

Botanical Medicine

Plants have been used as medicines since antiquity. Naturopathic physicians are professionally trained in herbal medicine and know both the historical uses of plants and modern pharmacological mechanisms.

Homeopathy

The term *homeopathy* is derived from the Greek words *homeo*, meaning "similar," and *pathos*, meaning "disease." Homeopathy is a system of medicine that treats a disease with a dilute, potentized agent, or drug, that will produce the same symptoms as the disease when given to a healthy individual, the fundamental principle being that like cures like. Homeopathic medicines are derived from a variety of plant, mineral, and chemical substances.

Traditional Chinese Medicine and Acupuncture

Traditional Chinese medicine and acupuncture are part of an ancient system of medicine involving techniques used to enhance the flow of vital energy (chi). Acupuncture involves the stimulation of certain specific points on the body along chi pathways called meridians. Acupuncture points can be stimulated by the insertion and withdrawing of needles, by the application of heat (moxibustion), by massage, by the application of laser light or electrical current, or by a combination of these methods.

Hydrotherapy

Hydrotherapy may be defined as the use of water in any of its forms (hot, cold, ice, steam, etc.) and methods of application (sitz bath, douche, spa or hot tub, whirlpool, sauna, shower, immersion bath, pack, poultice, foot-bath, fomentation, wrap, colonic irrigation, etc.) in the maintenance of health or treatment of disease. It is one of the ancient methods of treatment. Hydrotherapy has been used by many different peoples, including the Egyptians, Assyrians, Persians, Greeks, Hebrews, Hindus, and Chinese.

Physical Medicine

Physical medicine refers to the use of physical measures in the treatment of an individual. This includes the use of physiotherapy equipment such as ultrasound, diathermy, and other electromagnetic energy agents; therapeutic exercise; massage; joint mobilization (manipulative) and immobilization techniques; and hydrotherapy.

Counseling and Lifestyle Modification

Counseling and lifestyle modification techniques are essential to the naturopathic physician. A naturopath is formally trained in the following counseling areas:

1. Interviewing and responding skills, active listening, the assessment of body language, and other contact skills necessary for the therapeutic relationship

2. Recognition and understanding of prevalent psychological issues, including developmental problems, abnormal behavior, addictions, stress, problematic sexuality, etc.

3. Various treatment measures, including hypnosis and guided imagery, counseling techniques, correction of underlying organic factors, and family therapy

Naturopathic Primary Care

The modern naturopathic physician provides all phases of primary health care. That is, naturopathic physicians are trained to be the doctor first seen by the patient for general (nonemergency) health care. Clinical assessment generally follows the conventional medical model, with a medical history, physical exam, laboratory evaluation, and other well-accepted diagnostic procedures, but the clinical assessment may be influenced by nonconventional diagnostic techniques such as tests for nutrient deficiencies, toxin load, and physiological function.

A typical first office visit with a naturopathic doctor often takes one hour. Since naturopathic physicians consider one of their primary goals to be teaching the patient how to live healthfully, the time devoted to discussing and explaining principles of health maintenance and medical aspects is one of the aspects that set naturopaths apart from many other health care providers.

The patient-physician relationship begins with a thorough medical history and interview process designed to explore all aspects of a patient's lifestyle. The physician will perform standard diagnostic procedures if these are needed, including physical exam and blood and urine analysis. Once a good understanding of the patient's health and disease status is established (making a diagnosis of a disease is only one part of this process), the doctor and patient work together to establish a treatment and health-promotion program.

Because many naturopathic physicians function as primary health care providers, standard medical monitoring, follow-up, and exams are critical to good patient care. Patients are encouraged to receive regular yearly checkups, including a full physical.

When therapies are used, outcomes are assessed using conventional tools (e.g., patient interview, physical exam, laboratory tests, radiological imaging, etc.).

Contrasting Naturopathy to Allopathy

You may be asking how naturopathic physicians view health differently from conventional medical doctors. First of all, by definition and philosophy most conventional medical doctors practice *allopathic* medicine. *Allopathy* refers to conventional medicine as practiced by a graduate of a medical school or college granting the degree of doctor of medicine (M.D.). It is a system of medicine that focuses primarily on treating disease rather than on promoting health.

The fundamental difference between naturopathy and allopathy is that the allopathic physician tends to view good health primarily as a physical state in which there is no obvious disease present. In contrast, naturopathic physicians recognize true health as the state of optimal physical, mental, emotional, and spiritual well-being. The key difference between naturopathic and allopathic physicians is apparent if we look at how each type of doctor views not only health but also disease.

To illustrate the differences, let's take a look at how each views and addresses the "infection equation." The infection equation is like a mathematical equation, such as $1 + 2 = 3$. In the infection equation, what determines the outcome is the interaction of the host's immune system with the infecting organism. A naturopathic doctor tends to use treatments designed to enhance the immune system, while most conventional doctors tend to use treatments designed to kill the invading organism. Conventional medicine has been obsessed with infective agents rather than host defense factors. This obsession really began with Louis Pasteur, the 19th-century physician and researcher who played a major role in the development of the germ theory. This theory holds that different diseases are caused by different infectious organisms, with the patient as a passive victim. Much of Pasteur's life was dedicated to finding substances that would kill the infecting organisms. Pasteur and others since him who pioneered effective treatments of infectious diseases have given us a great deal, for which we all should be thankful. However, there is more to the infection equation.

Another 19th-century French scientist, Claude Bernard, also made major contributions to medical understanding. Bernard, however, had a different view of health and disease. Bernard believed that the state of a person's internal environment was more important in determining disease than the pathogen itself. In other words, Bernard believed that the person's internal "terrain," or susceptibility to infection, was more important than the germ. Physicians, he believed, should focus more attention on making this internal terrain a very inhospitable place for disease to flourish.

Bernard's theory led to some rather interesting studies. In fact, a firm advocate of the germ theory would find some of these studies to be absolutely crazy. One of the most interesting studies was conducted by a Russian scientist named Élie Metchnikoff, the discover of white blood cells. He and his research associates consumed cultures containing millions of cholera bacteria, yet none of them developed cholera. The reason: their immune systems were not compromised. Metchnikoff believed, like Bernard, that the correct way to deal with infectious disease was to focus on enhancing the body's own defenses.

During the last part of their lives, Pasteur and Bernard engaged in scientific discussions on the virtues of the germ theory and Bernard's perspective on the internal terrain. On his deathbed, Pasteur supposedly said: "Bernard was right. The pathogen is nothing. The terrain is everything." Unfortunately, Pasteur's legacy is the obsession with the pathogen, and modern medicine has largely forgotten the importance of the "terrain."

Now, we want to make it very clear that advances in conventional medicine can produce lifesaving results when used appropriately. There is little argument, for example, that when used appropriately, antibiotics save lives. However, there is also little argument that antibiotics are grossly overprescribed. While the appropriate use of antibiotics makes good medical sense, what does not make sense is the reliance on antibiotics for such conditions as acne, recurrent bladder infections, chronic ear infections, chronic sinusitis, chronic bronchitis, and nonbacterial sore throats. The antibiotics rarely provide a substantial benefit, and these conditions are effectively treated with natural measures.

The widespread use and abuse of antibiotics is increasingly alarming for many reasons, including the near epidemic of chronic candidiasis as well as the development of "superbugs" that are resistant to currently available antibiotics. We are coming dangerously close to a "post-antibiotic era" in which many infectious diseases will once again become almost impossible to treat.[3,4]

Since there is evidence that resistance to antibiotics is less of a problem when these medications are used sparingly, a reduction in antibiotic prescriptions may be the only significant way to address the problem. The consensus of medical experts as well as the World Health Organization is that antibiotic use must be restricted and inappropriate use halted if the growing trend toward bacterial resistance to antibiotics is to be halted and reversed.

Our interpretation of this challenge is that it is going to force conventional medical thinkers to take a closer look at ways to enhance resistance against infection. Our belief is that as they do so they will discover the healing power of nature. There is an ever-increasing body of knowledge that supports the use of whole foods, nutritional supplements, and a healthful lifestyle and attitude in enhancing resistance to infection. For example, children deficient in any of a large number of nutrients, such as vitamin A, vitamin C, and zinc, are far more susceptible to a wide range of infectious agents. While in the short term antibiotics may be critically important, in the long run they do nothing to improve an impaired immune system, so infections continue to recur.

Using Naturopathic Medicine as a Treatment

In addition to promoting good health, natural medicines such as herbal products and nutritional supplements are often used as direct substitutes for conventional drugs. However, an important distinction must be made: in most cases the use of these natural medicines involves promoting the healing process rather than suppressing symptoms. To illustrate this point, let's look at osteoarthritis (the most common form of arthritis) and consider the natural approach vs. the drug approach.

Osteoarthritis is characterized by a breakdown of cartilage. Cartilage serves an important role in joint function. Its gel-like nature provides protection to the ends of joints by acting as a shock absorber. Degeneration of the cartilage is the hallmark feature of osteoarthritis. This degeneration causes inflammation, pain, deformity, and limitation of motion in the joint.

The primary drugs used in the treatment of osteoarthritis are the nonsteroidal anti-inflammatory drugs, or NSAIDs. These include, for example, aspirin, ibuprofen (Motrin), naproxen (Aleve), piroxicam (Feldene), diclofenac (Voltaren), and the newer COX-2 inhibitor drugs such as celecoxib (Celebrex). Although NSAIDs are extensively used in the United States, these drugs are associated with side effects such as gastrointestinal upset, headaches, and dizziness, and are therefore recommended for only short periods of time. In addition, about 7,000 Americans die each year from ulcers produced by the older NSAIDs.[5] Newer versions such as rofecoxib (Vioxx, withdrawn from the market in 2004) and celecoxib are now known to increase the risk of death due to heart damage, and they still carry a significant risk of gastrointestinal bleeding. It is estimated that in the first five years after these drugs were approved, more than 60,000 people in the United States may have lost their lives from side effects.[6]

Not widely known is that while these drugs may suppress the symptoms of osteoarthritis in the short term, clinical studies have shown that in the long run they may actually accelerate joint destruction and block cartilage repair by inhibiting the formation of key compounds in cartilage known as glycosaminoglycans (GAGs). These compounds are responsible for maintaining the proper water content in the cartilage matrix, thereby helping cartilage keep its gel-like nature and shock-absorbing qualities. Simply stated, aspirin and other NSAIDs are designed to fight disease rather than promote health.[7–13]

In contrast, the natural approach to the treatment of osteoarthritis facilitates the body's natural healing process. For example,

glucosamine sulfate appears to address one of the underlying factors that can cause osteoarthritis: the reduced manufacture of cartilage components (specifically GAGs). By getting at the root of the problem—not only increasing the rate of cartilage formation but also improving the health of the cartilage—glucosamine sulfate both reduces symptoms, including pain, and helps the body repair damaged joints.[14–16] In head-to head comparison studies with NSAIDs such as ibuprofen, piroxicam, and celecoxib, glucosamine has been shown to provide comparable or greater benefit.[17–20] While side effects are common and even expected with pharmaceutical drugs, glucosamine sulfate does not cause side effects. The only advantage of the drugs is that symptom relief occurs more quickly than with the natural therapies, but this advantage lasts for only a few weeks. Within a few months, glucosamine sulfate results in greater symptom relief. For more information, see the chapter "Osteoarthritis."

Complementary Aspects of Naturopathic Medicine

In addition to being used as primary therapy, naturopathic medicine is valuable as a complementary approach to conventional medicine, especially in severe illnesses that require pharmacological and/or surgical intervention, such as cancer, angina, congestive heart failure, Parkinson's disease, and trauma. For example, a patient with severe congestive heart failure who requires drugs such as digoxin and furosemide can benefit from the appropriate use of thiamine, carnitine, and coenzyme Q_{10} supplementation. Although there are double-blind studies demonstrating the value of these agents as complementary therapies in congestive heart failure, they are rarely prescribed by conventional medical doctors in the United States. For more information, see the chapter "Congestive Heart Failure."

Using Naturopathic Medicine as Prevention

Ultimately, naturopathic medicine may prove most useful in the prevention of disease. Naturopathic physicians are trained to spend considerable time and effort in teaching patients the importance of adhering to a health-promoting lifestyle, diet, and attitude. True primary prevention involves addressing a patient's risk for disease (especially for heart disease, cancer, stroke, diabetes, and osteoporosis) and instituting a course of action designed to reduce controllable risk factors.

The health benefits and cost-effectiveness of disease prevention programs have been clearly demonstrated. Studies have consistently found that participants in wellness-oriented programs had a reduced number of days of disability (a 43% reduction in one study), a lower number of days spent in a hospital (a 54% drop in one study), and a lower amount spent on health care (a remarkable 76% decrease in one study).[21]

The Need for Naturopathic Medicine

There is a tremendous need for naturopathic medicine to become the dominant method of medicine in practice. Each year in the United States we spend more than $2 trillion on health care—or, more accurately, we are spending the majority of these dollars on "disease care." Health care costs now consume 17% of the gross national product (GNP), with the percentage of GNP spent on health care continuing to increase at twice the rate of inflation. We cannot afford to continue to go in this direction.

If naturopathic medicine, with its focus on promoting health and preventing disease, became the dominant medical model, not only would health care costs be dramatically reduced, but the health of Americans would improve dramatically. It is a sad fact that while we are grossly outspending every other nation in the world on health care, as a nation we are not healthy. Almost half of adults suffer from one or more chronic diseases (such as cancer, diabetes, arthritis, and heart disease) as well as obesity. What's especially alarming about these statistics is that these apply to adults supposedly in their prime.

Definitions of Prevention	
DEFINITION	**DESCRIPTION**
Primary prevention	Lifestyle modification, decreased intake of dietary fat, increased dietary fiber intake, increased intake of plant foods, nutritional supplementation, smoking cessation, alcohol abuse cessation, counseling, immunization
Secondary prevention	Early detection of subclinical disease to prevent further disability: screening for hypertension, hearing impairment, visual acuity, osteoporosis, high cholesterol, cancer
Tertiary prevention	Minimizing disability and handicap from established disease

The numbers are far worse for the elderly, virtually all of whom suffer from one or more chronic degenerative diseases

Health Status of Americans Ages 18 to 64 [22]

One chronic disease: 29%

Two chronic diseases: 18%

Three or more chronic diseases: 7%

Wellness-Oriented Medicine Is the Solution

Wellness-oriented medicine, such as naturopathic medicine, provides a practical solution to escalating health care costs and poor health status. Equally important is that this orientation can increase patient satisfaction. Studies have observed that patients utilizing the natural-medicine/health-promotion approach are more satisfied with the results of their treatment than they are with the results of conventional treatments like drugs and surgeries. A few studies have directly compared the satisfaction of patients using natural medicine with that of patients using conventional medicine. The largest study was done in the Netherlands, where natural medicine practitioners are an integral part of the health care system. [24] This extensive study compared satisfaction in 3,782 patients seeing either a conventional physician or a complementary practitioner. The patients seeing the natural medicine practitioner reported better results for almost every condition. Of particular interest was the observation that the patients seeing a complementary practitioner were somewhat sicker at the start of therapy, and that in only 4 of the 23 conditions did the conventional medical patients report better results.

Percentage of Adult Americans Suffering from the 10 Most Common Chronic Diseases [23]						
CONDITION	**MEN (%)**			**WOMEN (%)**		
	Ages 18–44	Ages 45–64	Age 65+	Ages 18–44	Ages 45–64	Age 65+
Arthritis	4.1	21.4	38.3	6.4	33.9	54.4
Respiratory disease (asthma, emphysema, chronic bronchitis)	5.5	8.8	16.7	9.3	11.4	12.6
Cancer	0.2	2.3	5.2	0.5	2.2	3.8
Chronic sinusitis	13.6	16.3	14.1	18.3	19.9	17.0
Diabetes	0.8	5.1	9.1	1.0	5.7	9.9
Hay fever	10.3	7.9	NA	12.1	9.8	NA
Hearing impairment	6.3	19.6	36.2	4.0	10.6	26.8
High blood pressure	6.6	25.4	32.7	5.7	27.4	45.6
Ischemic heart disease	0.3	8.7	17.9	0.3	4.3	12.1
Visual impairment	4.3	6.2	10.4	1.7	3.2	18.8

NA = data not available

Patient Satisfaction with Complementary Practitioners Compared with Medical Specialists[24]		
SYMPTOM	**COMPLEMENTARY PRACTITIONER PATIENTS, % IMPROVED**	**MEDICAL PATIENTS, % IMPROVED**
Palpitations	63	59
Stiffness	67	54
Feeling very ill	75	78
Itching or burning	71	50
Tiredness or lethargy	70	60
Fever	86	100
Pain	70	58
Tension or depression	69	65
Coughing	76	50
Blood loss	100	100
Tingling, numbness	59	40
Shortness of breath	77	53
Nausea or vomiting	71	67
Diarrhea or constipation	67	50
Poor vision or hearing	31	47
Paralysis	80	67
Insomnia	58	45
Dizziness and fainting	80	53
Anxiety	65	64
Skin rash	58	50
Emotional instability	56	63
Sexual problems	57	57
Other	75	56

Why Is There a Bias Against Natural Medicine on the Part of Medical Doctors?

The simple answer to this important question is that many doctors are simply not educated in the value of nutrition and other natural therapies. In fact, most were told during their education that alternative medicines are worthless. Many doctors are not aware of, or choose to ignore, data on beneficial natural therapies such as diet, exercise, and dietary supplements, even if the data are overwhelmingly positive. Rather than admit they don't know whether natural therapies might be valid, most doctors have a knee-jerk reaction that such treatments can't be helpful. They often suffer from what we refer to as the "tomato effect," alluding to the widely held belief in North America in the 18th century that tomatoes were poisonous, even though they were a dietary staple in Europe. It wasn't until 1820, when Robert Gibbon Johnson ate a tomato on the courthouse steps in Salem, Indiana, that the "poisonous tomato" barrier was broken in the minds of many Americans.

In medicine, many physicians have an attitude regarding alternative therapies that is quite similar to this "tomato effect." For example, though diet is a critical foundation of health, when patients ask their doctor about dietary therapy or a nutritional supplement for a particular condition, even if the nutritional approach has considerable support in the scientific literature that proves its safety and effectiveness, most doctors will caution patients against going the natural route or tell them that while it won't hurt them, it won't help them either. The truth is that in many cases, the doctor just doesn't know anything about it. Keep in mind that it took the medical community more than 40 years to accept the link between low folic acid levels during pregnancy and crippling birth defects of the spinal cord (neural tube defects such as spina bifida). It is estimated that 70 to 85% of the more than 100,000 children born with neural tube defects during that time could have been born healthy if doctors had not been so biased against scientific data on nutritional supplements.[25] The good news is that in the two decades since the publication of the first edition of this book, the medical community has become more receptive to natural therapies. Unfortunately, its political organizations continue to work at the local, state, and federal levels to prevent licensing of naturopaths, insurance equality, and critical research.

Naturopathic Training

A licensed naturopathic physician (N.D.) attends an accredited four-year graduate-level naturopathic medical school. Admission requirements are similar to those required for conventional medical school. Specifically, applicants must have a bachelor's degree or a higher degree from an accredited college or university, and must have taken courses in general chemistry, organic chemistry, physics, algebra, general biology, psychology, and English composition.

Curriculum

The curriculum is divided into two primary categories, academic and clinical. The first academic year is primarily composed of the study of the normal structure and function of the body (anatomy, physiology, biochemistry, histology, embryology, etc.). The second year focuses on the pathological transitions to disease, along with clinical recognition of these processes using physical, clinical, radiological, and laboratory diagnostics.

The third and fourth academic years focus on conventional and naturopathic perspectives in clinical diagnostics for pediatrics, gynecology, obstetrics, dermatology, neurology, endocrinology, cardiology, gastroenterology, and geriatrics. During the third and fourth years there is also a focus on naturopathic therapies. Students are required to take core classes (usually two or three quarters) in botanical medicine, homeopathy, counseling, diet, therapeutic nutrition, and physical medicine. Students are then able to choose which modality to focus on in elective advanced courses or may choose courses in other areas such as acupuncture and ayurvedic medicine to meet elective requirements.

The clinical curriculum begins first with students assisting in patient care and/or in the pharmacy and laboratory. Although no naturopathic medical school currently has inpatient facilities, all schools have extensive clinical facilities where students work under the direction of supervising naturopathic physicians and conduct complete patient evaluation, treatment, and monitoring, and perform other aspects of patient care. Students are also required to observe or work under the direction of licensed primary care physicians.

Accredited Schools

The Council on Naturopathic Medical Education (CNME) was created in 1978 to establish and administer educational programs and colleges of naturopathic medicine. Currently, there are seven schools in the United States and Canada that train naturopathic physicians with accreditation:

Bastyr University
14500 Juanita Drive NE
Kenmore, WA 98028-4966
Phone: (425) 823-1300
Fax: (425) 823-6222
www.bastyr.edu

National College of Natural Medicine
049 SW Porter Street
Portland, OR 97201
Phone: (503) 552-1555
www.ncnm.edu

National University of Health Sciences
200 E Roosevelt
Lombard, IL 60148
Phone: (630) 629-2000
Fax: (630) 889-6499
www.nuhs.edu

Southwest College of Naturopathic
  Medicine
2140 E Broadway Road
Tempe, AZ 85282
Phone: (480) 858-9100
Fax (480) 858-9116
www.scnm.edu

University of Bridgeport—College of
  Naturopathic Medicine
Health Science Center
60 Lafayette Street
Bridgeport, CT 06604
Phone: (800) EXCEL UB ext. 4108
www.bridgeport.edu/naturopathy

Canadian College of Naturopathic
  Medicine
1255 Sheppard Avenue E
Toronto, ON M2K 1E2
Phone: (416) 498-1255,
  toll-free (866) 241-2266
www.ccnm.edu

Boucher Institute of Naturopathic
  Medicine
Boucher Centre, 300-435 Columbia
  Street
New Westminster, BC V3L 5N8
Phone: (604) 777-9981
Fax: (604) 777-9982
www.binm.org

Professional Licensure

Currently, 16 states, the District of Columbia, and the United States territories of Puerto Rico and the United States Virgin Islands have licensing laws for naturopathic doctors. In these states, naturopathic doctors are required to graduate from an accredited four-year residential naturopathic medical school and pass an extensive postdoctoral board examination (NPLEX) in order to receive a license. Legal provisions allow the practice of naturopathic medicine in several other states, and efforts to gain licensure elsewhere are currently under way. Naturopathic physicians are also recognized throughout all provinces in Canada.

Licensed naturopathic physicians must fulfill state-mandated continuing education requirements annually, and will have a specific scope of practice defined by their state's law. Currently there are licensing laws for naturopathic physicians in:

Alaska

Arizona

California

Connecticut

District of Columbia

Hawaii

Idaho

Kansas

Maine

Minnesota

Montana

New Hampshire

North Dakota

Oregon

Utah

Vermont

Washington

United States territories: Puerto Rico and Virgin Islands

Professional Organizations

The American Association of Naturopathic Physicians (AANP) is the national professional organization of licensed naturopathic physicians. The organization is also seeking to differentiate professional trained naturopaths from unscrupulous individuals claiming to be naturopaths because they received a "mail-order" degree. In states that license naturopaths, it is apparent who is a qualified naturopathic physician. In other states, since there is no licensing board overseeing the profession, people receiving mail-order diplomas from nonaccredited correspondence schools may call themselves N.D.'s, but there is a major difference in the quality of education and training between a licensable N.D. who graduated from an accredited school and a mail-order N.D. In states that do not license naturopaths, the best criteria for legitimacy are that a doctor is a graduate of one of the schools listed above and that he or she is a member of the AANP, which restricts membership to only those N.D.'s who are graduates of accredited institutions. For more information contact:

American Association of Naturopathic Physicians
4435 Wisconsin Avenue, NW, Suite 403
Washington, DC 20016
Phone: (202) 237-8150,
    toll-free (866) 538-2267
Fax: (202) 237-8152
www.naturopathic.org

The Future of Naturopathic Medicine

To some, naturopathic medicine, as well as the entire concept of natural medicine, appears to be a fad that will soon pass. However, when the subject is considered with an open mind, it is quite clear that naturopathic medicine is at the forefront of the future. It is obvious that an evolution is occurring in health care and that as a result more natural therapies are gaining acceptance even in mainstream medical circles.

One of the pervasive myths about naturopathic medicine has been the belief there is no firm scientific evidence for the use of the natural therapies naturopathic physicians employ. However, as this book attests, scientific studies and observations have upheld the validity not only of diet, nutritional supplements, and herbal medicines but also of some of the more esoteric natural healing treatments, including acupuncture, biofeedback, meditation, and homeopathy. In many instances, scientific investigation has not only validated the natural measure but also led to significant improvements and greater understanding. In the past 30 or so years there have been tremendous advances in the understanding of the ways in which many natural therapies and compounds work to promote health or treat disease.

Even in mainstream medicine there is a growing trend toward using substances found in nature, including compounds naturally found in the human body such as interferon, interleukin, insulin, and human growth hormone, in place of synthetic drugs. Add to this the growing popularity of nutritional supplements and herbal products and it is quite obvious that a trend is emerging toward natural medicine. Suffice it to say that it appears that the concepts and philosophy of naturopathic medicine will persist and be a major part of the medicine of the future.

. . . .

QUICK REVIEW

- **Naturopathic medicine is a system of medicine that focuses on prevention and the use of nontoxic, natural therapies to treat and reverse disease.**

- **Naturopathic medicine is built upon seven underlying principles.**

  Principle 1: The healing power of nature (*vis medicatrix naturae*).

  Principle 2: Identify and treat the cause (*tolle causam*).

  Principle 3: First, do no harm (*primum non nocere*).

  Principle 4: Treat the whole person (holism).

  Principle 5: The physician as teacher (*docere*).

  Principle 6: Prevention is the best cure.

  Principle 7: Establishing health and wellness.

- **As health care costs skyrocket, there is a tremendous need for naturopathic medicine.**

The Healing Power Within

· ·

Nature is doing her best each moment to make us well. She exists for no other end. Do not resist. With the least inclination to be well, we should not be sick.

—HENRY DAVID THOREAU

Introduction

One of the fundamental principles of naturopathic medicine is the body's innate ability to spontaneously heal itself. Evidence that this ability exists can be found by examining the *placebo response*. Undoubtedly you have heard this term. A placebo supposedly does not have a medicinal effect, yet these "sugar pills" and sham treatments often produce tremendous effects.

One of the more dramatic examples of the placebo effect reported in medical literature involves a patient of Dr. Bruno Klopfer, a researcher involved in the testing of the drug Krebiozen back in 1950.[1] Krebiozen had received sensational national publicity as a "cure" for cancer. These reports caught the eye of a man with advanced cancer—a lymphosarcoma. The patient, Mr. Wright, had huge tumor masses throughout his body and was in such desperate physical condition that he frequently had to take oxygen by mask, and fluid had to be removed from his chest every two days. When the patient discovered that Dr. Klopfer was involved in research on Krebiozen, he begged to be given Krebiozen treatments. Dr Klopfer gave them, and the patient's recovery was startling: "The tumor masses had melted like snowballs on a hot stove, and in only a few days, they were half their original size!" The injections were continued until Mr. Wright was discharged from the hospital and had regained a full and normal life, a complete reversal of his disease and its grim prognosis.

However, within two months of his recovery, a report that Krebiozen was not effective was leaked to the press. Learning of this report, Mr. Wright quickly began to revert to his former condition. Suspicious of the patient's relapse, his doctors decided to take advantage of the opportunity to test the dramatic regenerative capabilities of the mind. The patient was told that a new version of Krebiozen had been developed that overcame the difficulties described in the press, and some of the drug was promised to him as soon as it could be procured.

With much pomp and ceremony a saline water placebo was injected, increasing the patient's expectations to a fevered pitch. Recovery from his second near terminal state was even more dramatic than the first. Mr. Wright's tumor masses melted, his chest fluid vanished, and he became a true picture of health. The saline water injections were continued, since they worked such wonders. He then remained symptom-free for over two months. Then a definitive announcement appeared in the press: "Nationwide tests show Krebiozen to be a worthless drug in the treatment of cancer." Within a few days of this report, Mr. Wright was readmitted to the hospital in dire straits. His faith now gone, his last hope vanished, he died two days later.

What is the placebo response? Is it all in a person's mind? Absolutely not! Recent research demonstrates that the placebo response is a complex phenomenon, initiated by the mind and leading to a cascade of real, measurable effects. In brief, the placebo response is the activation of the healing centers of our being in a way that produces profound physiological changes. The body has two internal mechanisms to maintain health. The first is the inherent internal healing mechanism, vital force, chi, or primitive life support and repair mechanism that operates even in a person who is asleep, unconscious, or comatose. The second mechanism involves the power of the mind and emotions to intervene and affect the course of health and disease in a way that enhances or supersedes the body's innate vital force. The placebo response seems to involve activation of the higher control center, but that is not to say that its effects are solely in the mind.

One of the leading researchers of the placebo response is Dr. Fabrizio Benedetti of the University of Turin in Italy. He has conducted some very detailed studies trying to discover the underlying features of the placebo response.[2] For example, numerous studies have documented that the pain-relieving effects of a placebo are mediated by endorphins, the body's own morphine-like substances. In roughly 56% of patients in clinical studies, a placebo saline injection is as effective as morphine for severe pain; furthermore, this pain relief can be completely nullified by adding naloxone, a drug that blocks the effects of morphine, to the saline. As a result of these sorts of experiments, a great deal of the credit for the placebo response has been given to endorphins, but Dr. Benedetti's research has shown that a placebo can produce much more profound changes than simply increasing endorphin levels. For example, he has shown that a saline placebo can reduce tremors and muscle stiffness in people with Parkinson's disease. That is not surprising, perhaps, but what is very interesting is that researchers found that at the same time that the placebo produced noticeable improvements in symptoms, there was a significant change in the measured activity of neurons in the patients' brains as shown by a brain scan. In particular, as they administered the saline they found that individual neurons in the subthalamic nucleus (a common target for surgical attempts to relieve Parkinson's symptoms) began to fire less often and with fewer "bursts"—a characteristic feature associated with Parkinson's tremors. Somehow the saline placebo resulted in the processing of the information by healing centers in the brain to specifically target an effect that would reduce the dysfunction in the areas of the brain affected by Parkinson's disease.

Other studies have shown that both the placebo response and the experience of particular emotions produce demonstrable changes in brain activity visible through modern imaging techniques (e.g., CAT scans and MRIs). For example, one study showed that expectation or hope is able to stimulate the part of the brain that is activated by pain medications and associated with pain relief. In addition, numerous changes in chemical mediators of pain, inflammation, and mood have also been demonstrated with the placebo response. The bottom line here is that there is tremendous evidence that the placebo response is a highly specific and targeted healing effect that is triggered by both conscious and unconscious activity in the brain. Rather than discounting and trying to avoid a placebo response, modern medicine should be more intent on developing techniques and practices designed to stimulate the same healing centers within patients as noted in these studies with placebos.[3]

The Placebo Response in Medical Research

The development of the drug industry is based largely upon the perceived value of the placebo-controlled trial. In order for a drug to be approved it must show a therapeutic effect greater than that of a placebo. Because the outcome of a trial can be affected by both doctors' and patients' beliefs about the value of a treatment, most placebo-controlled trials are usually conducted in double-blind fashion: that is, not only are the patients unaware when they are receiving a placebo; the doctors are unaware as well. Nearly all studies conducted this way show some benefit in the placebo group. For example, in 1955 researcher H. K. Beecher published his groundbreaking paper "The Powerful Placebo," in which he concluded that across the 26 studies he analyzed, an average of 32% of patients responded to a placebo.[4] This is a generally accepted figure, although there is evidence that under some conditions in real-life clinical practice, placebo response may be as high as 80 to 90%. The reason is that in the real world the placebo response is enhanced by both the doctor's and the patient's expectations.

Conditions That Respond Significantly to Placebo

Angina

Anxiety

Arthritis

Asthma

Behavioral problems

Claudication, intermittent

Common cold

Cough, chronic

Depression

Diabetes (type 2)

Drug dependence

Dyspepsia

Gastric ulcers

Hay fever

Headaches

Hypertension

Insomnia

Labor and postpartum pain

Ménière's disease

Menstrual cramps

Nausea of pregnancy

Pain

Premenstrual syndrome

Psychoneuroses

Tremor

The Holy Trinity of the Placebo Response

Noted Harvard psychologist Herbert Benson, M.D., has described three basic components to heightening a placebo response: the belief and expectation of the patient, the belief and expectation of the physician, and the interaction between the physician and the patient. When these three are in concert, the placebo effect is greatly magnified. Benson believes that the placebo effect yields beneficial clinical results in 60 to 90% of diseases. He states that the placebo "has been one of medicine's most potent assets and it should not be belittled or ridiculed. Unlike most other treatments, it is safe and inexpensive and has withstood the test of time."[5] We agree with him completely.

As powerful as the placebo response is, it still requires activation. If the therapeutic interaction between the physician and the patient does not stimulate the patient's hope, faith, and belief, the chances of success are measurably diminished no matter how strong or effective a medication may be. It has been repeatedly demonstrated in clinical trials designed to better understand the placebo effect that the beliefs of both the patient and the doctor, as well as their trust in each other and the process, generate a significant portion of the therapeutic results.

Conventional medicine often criticizes and belittles therapies that have not been stringently tested using the double-blind, placebo-controlled trial, but in doing so it is arguing against something that is time-tested—the art of healing. The bottom line here is that patients of a compassionate, warm, and caring physician will experience better outcomes and fewer medication-related side effects than patients of an uninterested, cold, and uncaring physician.

The Opposite of a Placebo

The word *placebo* comes from the Latin term for "I will please." Its polar opposite is *nocebo*, Latin for "I will harm." The nocebo effect is just the opposite of the placebo effect. It describes the experience of having a side effect from an apparently inert treatment or substance. Healthy individuals have adverse effects from placebos about 25% of the time, but if patients are specifically asked about adverse effects, this figure can rise to 70%. While a nocebo response is usually used to

describe an adverse reaction to a placebo, it could also be applied to describe an unusual or exaggerated response to a medication. Does that mean that a nocebo effect is not real? Not at all.[6]

Symptoms and Side Effects Produced by Placebos

Anger

Anorexia

Behavioral changes

Depression

Dermatitis

Diarrhea

Drowsiness

Hallucinations

Headache

Lightheadedness

Pain

Palpitation

Pupillary dilation

Rash

Weakness

The Power of Expectations

Just as the placebo response is influenced by a patient's attitude, so too is the nocebo response. It is another example of the power of expectations. The classic example given is the fact that in the Framingham Heart Study, women were four times more likely to die from a heart attack if they believed they were prone to heart disease, compared with women with similar risk profiles who did not have that belief.[7] Expectations are influenced by a lot of factors, all of which play a role in establishing the level of faith in the patient.

Definitions of Some Expectation Effects Behind the Placebo Response	
Hawthorne effect	Subjects respond to knowledge of being evaluated and observed
Jastrow effect	Subjects respond to explicit expectations about outcome
Pygmalion effect	Evaluators expect therapeutic benefit, so they see it
John Henry effect	Control subjects attempt to emulate expected outcomes
Halo effect	Subjects respond to treatment novelty (i.e., new technology)
Experimenter effect	Evaluators consciously (or not) interpret outcomes differently
Socialization effect	Others reporting benefit influence outcomes
Value effect	The price of treatment influences expected outcomes

The Role of Faith and Spirituality in Medicine

Most physicians as well as patients ignore one of the most powerful healing techniques known. Prayer costs nothing, has no negative side effects, and fits perfectly into any treatment plan. No matter what faith you embrace, you can use the power of prayer to lead you to better health—of body, mind, and soul.

Most physicians are taught that any consideration of religious commitment is beyond the legitimate interest and scope of medical care. It should not be this way, but the reality is that many believe faith and medical science are mutually exclusive despite the fact that numerous scientific studies have now fully validated the efficacy of faith, prayer, and religion in healing.[8,9]

In addition, patients know that prayer works. In a poll of 1,000 U.S. adults, 79% endorsed the belief that spiritual faith and prayer can help people recover from disease, and 63% agreed that physicians should talk to patients about spiritual faith and prayer. Indeed, many medical experts feel that *not* to include a spiritual dimension in a patient's plan for treatment and recovery is to be medically irresponsible.[10]

One of the leaders in bringing the healing power of prayer to the forefront is Larry Dossey, M.D., author of best-selling books such as *Healing Words: The Power of Prayer and the Practice of Medicine* (HarperCollins, 1993), *Prayer Is Good Medicine* (Harper-Collins, 1996), and *The Extraordinary Healing Power of Ordinary Things* (Harmony/Random House, 2006). In these books, Dr. Dossey provides a thorough review of the scientific evidence. Not surprisingly, he found that prayer has received relatively little attention from the research community. His systematic analysis of more than 4.3 million published reports indexed on Medline (a bibliographic database compiled by the U.S. National Library of Medicine) from 1980 to 1996 revealed only 364 studies that included faith, religion, or prayer as part of the treatment. The numbers are small, but the conclusion is huge: the data show that prayer and religious commitment promote good health and healing.

Scientific investigation into the healing power of prayer has shown that prayer can affect physical processes in a variety of organisms. Specifically, studies have explored the effects of prayer on humans and on nonhuman subjects, including water, enzymes, bacteria, fungi, yeast, red blood cells, cancer cells, pacemaker cells, seeds, plants, algae, moth larvae, mice, and chicks. In these studies, prayer affected the manner in which these organisms grew or functioned. What scientists discovered—no doubt to their amazement—is that prayer affected a number of biological process, including

- Enzyme activity
- The growth rates of leukemic white blood cells
- Mutation rates of bacteria
- Germination and growth rates of various seeds
- The firing rate of the heart's natural pacemaker cells
- Healing rates of wounds
- Size of goiters and tumors
- Time required to awaken from anesthesia
- Autonomic effects such as electrical activity of the skin
- Hemoglobin levels

Given the scientific support for prayer's beneficial effects, *not* praying for the best possible outcome may be the equivalent of deliberately withholding an effective drug or surgical procedure.

If praying is good for others, can we do it for ourselves? Absolutely. Dr. Benson of Harvard found that patients who prayed or meditated evoked their body's relaxation response. This response—the exact opposite of the stress response, the "fight-or-flight" reaction that we feel during tense situations—includes decreases in heart rate, breathing rate, muscle tension, and sometimes even blood pressure. The medical implications of the relaxation response are enormous and may serve as the underlying basis for most mind-body techniques, such as guided imagery (discussed below) and meditation. The relaxation response has been shown to produce useful effects in a variety of different disease states. For example, cancer patients who undergo chemotherapy and learn to evoke the relaxation response are significantly less likely to experience nausea and fatigue.[11]

CREATING THE RELAXATION RESPONSE

Here is a simple exercise that will improve your ability to breathe from the diaphragm, achieve the relaxation response, and reduce stress. Practice the following for at least five minutes, twice a day.

- Find a quiet, comfortable place to sit or lie down.
- Place your feet slightly apart and find a comfortable position for your arms.
- Inhale through your nose and exhale through your mouth.
- Concentrate on your breathing.
- Inhale while slowly counting to four. Notice with each breath you take that you are breathing effortlessly by using your diaphragm. You should feel as if the air is first expanding into your abdomen and up into your lungs, then expanding warmth to all parts of your body.
- Pause for 1 second, then slowly exhale to a count of four. As you exhale, your abdomen should move inward. As the air flows out, feel the tension and stress leave your body.
- As you begin to relax, clear your mind of any distractions by imagining a peaceful, healing environment.
- Repeat the process for 5 to 10 minutes or until you achieve a sense of deep relaxation.

If you find yourself having trouble learning how to relax or perform visualization exercises, find a practitioner who specializes in guided imagery by contacting the Academy for Guided Imagery at (800) 726-2070 or www.acadgi.com, or you can ask your doctor for a referral. Taking a yoga class is also a great way to learn how to breathe with your diaphragm and learn how to relax.

Religion and the Heart

Jeff Levin, Ph.D., the author of *God, Faith and Health*, is recognized as one of the leading researchers in the field of spirituality and health. As a first-year graduate student in the School of Public Health at the University of North Carolina in Chapel Hill, Levin became intrigued by two articles that found a surprising and significant connection between spirituality and heart disease, a connection that remains one of the best-researched areas of the positive effects of religious behavior on health. His curiosity led to an in-depth evaluation and pioneering research on the impact of religious practices on disease.[12] In *God, Faith and Health*, Dr. Levin notes that there are more than 50 studies in which religious practices were found to be protective against heart disease, decreasing the risk of death from heart attacks and strokes as well as reducing the incidence of numerous risk factors including high blood pressure and elevated cholesterol and triglyceride levels. In particular, Dr. Levin highlights the strong inverse correlation between religious commitment and blood pressure that was evident no matter what religion an individual chose to practice or his or her geographical location or ancestry.

Final Comments

Often practitioners of natural medicine are asked for a blueprint for good health and effective healing. Most people are looking for a simple answer, but our feeling is that living healthfully requires a truly comprehensive commitment in all aspects of being. Here are what we consider the critical steps to living with vibrant health:

QUICK REVIEW

The placebo response provides significant evidence of an innate healing ability.

- **A great deal of the credit for the placebo response has been ascribed to its ability to increase endorphin levels.**
- **Placebos have been shown to have an impact on centers of the brain that stimulate healing.**
- **The placebo response produces numerous changes in chemical mediators of pain, inflammation, and mood.**
- **The overall placebo response is about 32% in clinical trials, but in some real-life clinical circumstances it may be as high as 80 to 90%.**

- **Patients of a compassionate, warm, and caring physician will experience better outcomes and fewer medication-related side effects than patients of an uninterested, cold, and uncaring physician.**
- **Numerous scientific studies have now fully validated the efficacy of faith, prayer, and religion in healing.**
- **There are more than 50 studies in which religious practices were found to be protective against heart disease, decreasing the risk of death from heart attacks and strokes as well as reducing the incidence of numerous risk factors including high blood pressure and elevated cholesterol and triglyceride levels.**

- Step 1: Incorporate spirituality into your life.
- Step 2: Develop a positive mental attitude.
- Step 3: Focus on establishing positive relationships.
- Step 4: Follow a healthful lifestyle.
- Step 5: Be active and get regular physical exercise.
- Step 6: Eat a health-promoting diet.
- Step 7. Support your body through proper nutritional supplementation and body work.

The next section discusses these steps fully.

Last, one of the fundamental principles of naturopathic medicine as well as other time-tested systems of medicine is to first remove obstacles to a cure. What do we mean by obstacles to a cure? Well, a nutrient deficiency is often a major obstacle to true healing, as are things such as habitual expression of anger, contamination with heavy metals or environmental toxins, genetic predispositions and metabolic abnormalities, and obesity. These obstacles often make even the most powerful medicines—whether natural or man-made—ineffective. Establishing a relationship with a naturopathic physician or other wellness-oriented professional is often a valuable step toward identifying and eliminating obstacles to a cure. Removing such obstacles allows the healing power within the best opportunity for success.

THE FOUR CORNERSTONES OF GOOD HEALTH

· ·

*H*ealth is a term that is difficult to define; a definition somehow tends to place unnecessary boundaries on its meaning. While health is often viewed as simply the absence of disease, the World Health Organization defines it as "a state of complete physical, mental, and social well-being, not merely the absence of disease or infirmity." This definition provides for a positive range of health well beyond the absence of sickness.

The question of health or disease often comes down to individual responsibility. In this context, responsibility means choosing a healthful alternative over a less healthful one. If you want to be healthy, simply make healthful choices and take the appropriate action to achieve the results you desire.

Achieving and maintaining health will usually be quite easy if you focus on strengthening what we refer to as the four cornerstones of good health. You can liken these cornerstones to the four legs on a chair or table. If you want that chair or table to remain upright when stress is placed upon it, the four legs must be intact and strong. Likewise, if you want to have good—or, better yet, ideal—health, it is essential that the following four areas be strong:

- A positive mental attitude
- A healthful lifestyle: exercise, sleep, and health habits
- A health-promoting diet
- Supplementary measures

The principles and recommendations given in Section II are absolutely essential to incorporate into your life if you desire ideal health.

A Positive Mental Attitude

....

Introduction

Optimal health begins with a positive mental attitude. There is a growing body of evidence that the thoughts and emotions you experience on a regular basis determine to a very large extent the level of health you experience as well as the quality of your life. Life is full of events that are beyond our control, but we do have full control over our response to these events. Our attitude goes a long way in determining how we view and respond to all of the challenges of life. You will be much happier, much healthier, and much more successful if you can adopt a positive mental attitude rather than a pessimistic view.

Studies using various scales to assess attitude have shown that individuals with a pessimistic attitude have poorer health, are prone to depression, are more frequent users of medical and mental health care, exhibit more decline in memory and brain function with aging, and have a lower survival rate compared with optimists.[1-8] One of the most recent studies involved a study of 5,566 people who completed a survey at two time points: between ages 51 and 56 and then again between ages 63 and 67. The results showed that people with negative attitudes were 7.16 times more likely to be depressed 10 years later.[8]

Determine Your Level of Optimism

Attitude is reflected by *explanatory style*, a term developed by noted psychologist Martin Seligman to describe the way we habitually explain the events in our lives.[7] To determine your level of optimism, take the Attributional Style Questionnaire developed by Seligman, provided in Appendix A. Techniques to help you learn to be more optimistic are given later in this chapter.

Attitude, Personality, Emotions, and Immune Function

The importance of attitude to human health has been demonstrated in the links between the brain, emotions, and immune system. Research in the field of psychoneuroimmunology indicates that every part of the immune system is connected to the brain in some way, either via a direct nervous tissue connection or through the complex language of chemical messengers and hormones. What scientists are discovering is that every thought, emotion, and experience sends a message to the immune system that either enhances or impairs its ability to function. A simplistic view is that positive emotions, such as joy, happiness, and optimism, tend to boost immune system function, whereas negative emotions, such as depression, sadness, and pessimism, tend to suppress it.

Studies examining immune function in optimists vs. pessimists have demonstrated significantly better immune function in the optimists.[5,9–12] The immune system is so critical to preventing cancer that if emotions and attitude were risk factors for cancer, one would expect to see an increased risk of cancer in people who have long-standing depression or a pessimistic attitude. Research supports this association.[13,14]

Just as research has identified attitude traits that are associated with impaired immune function, it has also identified a collection of "immune power" traits. These include a positive mental attitude, an effective strategy for dealing with stress, and a capacity to effectively deal with life's traumas and challenges.[14,15]

Attitude and Cardiovascular Health

In addition to the brain and immune system, the body's cardiovascular system is intricately tied to emotions and attitude. The relationship of explanatory style (optimistic or pessimistic) to incidence of coronary heart disease was examined as part of the Veterans Affairs Normative Aging Study, an ongoing cohort study of older men.[6] Men reporting high levels of optimism had a 45% lower risk for angina pectoris, nonfatal myocardial infarction, and death from coronary heart disease than men reporting high levels of pessimism. Interestingly, a clear dose-response relationship was found between levels of optimism and each outcome.

To illustrate how closely the cardiovascular system is linked to attitude, one study showed that measures of optimism and pessimism affected something as simple as ambula-

tory blood pressure.[16] Pessimistic adults had higher blood pressure levels and felt more negative and less positive than optimistic adults. These results suggest that pessimism has broad physiological consequences.

Excessive anger, worrying, and other negative emotions have also been shown to be associated with an increased risk for cardiovascular disease; however, these emotions may simply reflect a pessimistic explanatory style.

Attitude and Self-Actualization

A positive mental attitude is absolutely essential for us to really live life to the fullest. It also helps propel us to be the best that we can be. There appears to be an innate drive within each of us to achieve the experience of self-actualization in our lives. Self-actualization is a concept developed by Abraham Maslow, the founding father of humanistic psychology. His theories were the result of intense research on psychologically healthy people over a period of more than 30 years. Maslow was really the first psychologist to study healthy people, as he strongly believed such research would create a firm foundation for the theories and values of a new psychotherapy.[17]

Maslow discovered that healthy individuals are motivated toward self-actualization, a process of "ongoing actualization of potentials, capacities, talents, as fulfillment of a mission (or call, fate, destiny, or vocation), as a fuller knowledge of, and acceptance of, the person's own intrinsic nature, as an increasing trend toward unity, integration, or synergy within the person."[17] In other words, healthy people strive and are actually driven to be all that they can be.

Maslow developed a five-step pyramid of

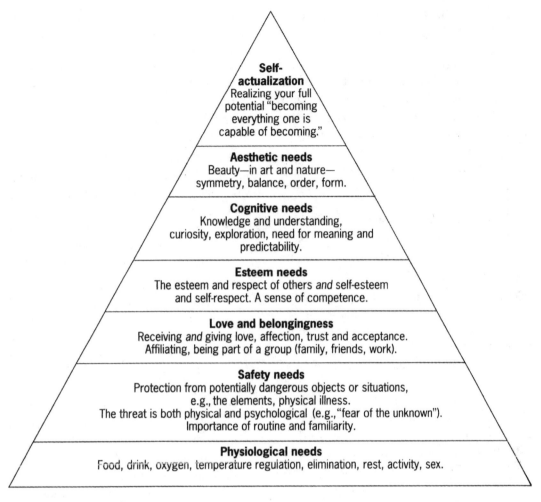

Self-actualization
Realizing your full potential "becoming everything one is capable of becoming."

Aesthetic needs
Beauty—in art and nature—symmetry, balance, order, form.

Cognitive needs
Knowledge and understanding, curiosity, exploration, need for meaning and predictability.

Esteem needs
The esteem and respect of others *and* self-esteem and self-respect. A sense of competence.

Love and belongingness
Receiving *and* giving love, affection, trust and acceptance. Affiliating, being part of a group (family, friends, work).

Safety needs
Protection from potentially dangerous objects or situations, e.g., the elements, physical illness. The threat is both physical and psychological (e.g.,"fear of the unknown"). Importance of routine and familiarity.

Physiological needs
Food, drink, oxygen, temperature regulation, elimination, rest, activity, sex.

Maslow's Hierarchy of Needs

human needs in which personality development progresses from one step to the next. The needs at the lower levels must be satisfied before the next level can be achieved. When needs are met, the individual moves toward well-being. The figure above displays Maslow's hierarchy of needs.

The primary needs that form the base of the pyramid are basic survival or physiological needs—the satisfaction of hunger, thirst, sexual desire, and the need for shelter. These are essential biological needs. The next step consists of needs for safety—security, order,

and stability. These feelings are essential in dealing with the world. If these needs are satisfied, the individual can progress to the next step, love. This level refers to the ability to love and be loved. The following step, self-esteem, requires approval, recognition, and acceptance. These elements contribute strongly to high self-esteem and self-respect. The final step is self-actualization—the utilization of one's creative potential for self-fulfillment.

Maslow studied self-actualized people and noted that they had strikingly similar characteristics. Here in abbreviated form are some of Maslow's findings:

1. Self-actualized people perceive reality more accurately and effectively than others and are more comfortable with it. They have an unusual ability to detect the spurious, the fake, and the dishonest. They judge experiences, people, and things correctly and efficiently. They possess an ability to be objective about their own strengths, possibilities, and limitations. This self-awareness enables them to clearly define their values, goals, desires, and feelings. They are not frightened by uncertainty.

2. Self-actualized people have an acceptance of self, others, and nature. They can accept their own human shortcomings without condemnation. They do not have an absolute lack of guilt, shame, sadness, anxiety, or defensiveness, but they do not experience these feelings to unnecessary or unrealistic degrees. When they do feel guilty or regretful, they do something about it. Generally, they will feel bad about discrepancies between what is and what ought to be.

3. Self-actualized people are relatively spontaneous in their behavior, and far more spontaneous than that in their inner life, thoughts, and impulses. They seldom allow convention to keep them from doing anything they consider important or basic.

4. Self-actualized people have a problem-solving orientation toward life instead of an orientation centered on self. They commonly have a mission in life, some problem outside themselves that enlists much of their energies. In general, this mission is unselfish and is involved with the philosophical and the ethical.

5. Self-actualized people have a quality of detachment and a need for privacy. It is often possible for them to remain above the battle, to be undisturbed by things that upset others. The meaning of their life is self-decision, self-governing, and being an active, responsible, self-disciplined, deciding person rather than a helpless pawn ruled by others.

6. Self-actualized people have a wonderful capacity to appreciate again and again the basic pleasures of life such as nature, children, music, and sexual experience. They approach these basic experiences with awe, pleasure, wonder, and even ecstasy.

7. Self-actualized people commonly have mystic or "peak" experiences, times of intense emotion in which they transcend self. During a peak experience they have feelings of limitless horizons, feelings of unlimited power, and at the same time feelings of being more helpless than ever before. There is a loss of place and time, and feelings of great ecstasy, wonder, and awe. The experience ends with the conviction that something extremely important and valuable has happened, and the person is to some extent transformed and strengthened by the experience.

8. Self-actualized people have deep feelings of identification with, sympathy toward, and affection for other people in spite of occasional anger, impatience, or disgust.

9. Self-actualized people have deeper and more profound interpersonal relationships than most other adults, but not necessarily deeper than children. They are capable of more closeness, greater love, more perfect identification, and more erasing of ego boundaries than other people would consider possible. One consequence is that self-actualized people have especially deep ties with

rather few individuals and their circle of friends is small. They tend to be kind to or at least patient with almost everyone, yet they speak realistically and harshly of those who they feel deserve it, especially individuals who are hypocritical, pretentious, pompous, or self-inflated.

10. Self-actualized people are democratic in the deepest possible sense. They are friendly toward everyone regardless of class, education, political beliefs, race, or color. They believe it is possible to learn something from everyone. They are humble in the sense of being aware of how little they know in comparison with what could be known and what is known by others.

11. Self-actualized people are strongly ethical and moral. However, their notions of right and wrong and of good and evil are often not conventional ones.

12. Self-actualized people have a keen, unhostile sense of humor. They don't laugh at jokes that hurt other people or are aimed at others' inferiority. They can make fun of others in general, or of themselves, when they are foolish or when they try to appear big despite being small. They are inclined toward thoughtful humor that elicits a smile, is intrinsic to the situation, and arises spontaneously.

13. Self-actualized people are highly imaginative and creative. The creativeness of a self-actualized individual is not of the special-talent type such as Mozart's, but rather is similar to the naive and universal creativeness of unspoiled children.

Practical Application of Maslow's Hierarchy of Needs		
LEVEL OF NEED	**GENERAL REWARDS**	**OCCUPATIONAL FACTORS**
Self-actualization	Growth Achievement Advancement Creativity	Challenging job Opportunities for creativity Achievement in work Promotion
Self-esteem	Self-respect Status Prestige	Social recognition Job title High status of job Feedback from the job itself
Belonging	Love Friendship Belongingness	Work groups or teams Supervision Professional associations
Safety	Security Stability Protection	Health and safety Job security Contract of employment
Physiological Water Sleep Sex	Food Working conditions	Pay

The Road to Self-Actualization

Self-actualization doesn't happen all at once. It happens by degrees, subtle changes accumulating one by one. Self-actualization begins when you take personal responsibility for your own positive mental state, your life, your current situation, and your health. Once you take on this responsibility, it is up to you to direct your life. You must commit yourself to being the best you can be at whatever you do in life. For motivation, here is an all-time favorite quote from Goethe:

> Until one is committed there is hesitancy, the chance to draw back, always ineffectiveness. Concerning all acts of initiative (and creation), there is one elementary truth, the ignorance of which kills countless ideas and splendid plans: that the moment one definitely commits oneself, then Providence moves too. All sorts of things occur to help one that would never have otherwise occurred. A whole stream of events issues from the decision raising in one's favor all manner of unforeseen incidents and meetings and material assistance which no man could have dreamed would have come his way. Whatever you can do, or dream you can, begin it. Boldness has genius, power and magic in it. Begin it now!

The Seven Steps to a Positive Mental Attitude

In an effort to help you develop a positive mental attitude as well as attain self-actualization, we offer the following seven key steps:

Step 1: Become an Optimist

The first step in developing a positive mental attitude is to become an optimist rather than a pessimist. Fortunately, according to Dr. Seligman, we are, by nature, optimists.[18] Optimism is a vital component of good health and an ally in the healing process. Focus on the positives even in challenging situations.

Step 2: Become Aware of Self-Talk

We all talk to ourselves. There is a constant dialogue taking place in our heads. Our self-talk makes an impression on our subconscious mind. In order to develop or maintain a positive mental attitude you must guard against negative self-talk. Become aware of your self-talk and then consciously work to imprint positive self-talk on the subconscious mind. Two powerful tools in creating positive self-talk are questions (Step 3) and affirmations (Step 4).

Step 3: Ask Better Questions

One of the most powerful tools that Dr. Murray has found useful in improving the quality of his self-talk and, hence, the quality of his life is a series of questions originally given to him by Anthony Robbins, author of the best sellers *Unlimited Power* and *Awaken the Giant Within*. According to Tony, the quality of your life is equal to the quality of the questions you habitually ask yourself. Tony's belief is based on the idea that you will get an answer to whatever question you ask your brain.

Let's look at an example. An individual is met with a particular challenge or problem. He can ask a number of questions when in this situation. Questions many people may ask in this circumstance include "Why does this always happen to me?" and "Why am

I always so stupid?" Do they get answers to these questions? Do the answers build self-esteem? Does the problem keep reappearing? What would be a higher-quality question? How about "This is a very interesting situation. What do I need to learn from this situation so that it never happens again?" Or how about "What can I do to make this situation better?"

In another example, let's look at an individual who suffers from depression. Questions she might ask herself that may not be helping her situation include "Why am I *always* so depressed?" "Why do things *always* seem to go wrong for me?" and "Why am I so unhappy?" Better questions she might ask herself include "What do I need to do to gain more enjoyment and happiness in my life?" "What do I need to commit to doing in order to have more happiness and energy in my life?" After she has answered these questions, she might ask, "If I had happiness and high energy levels right now, what would it feel like?" You will be amazed at how powerful questions can be in your life. Changing the questions she asks reprograms her subconscious into believing she has an abundance of energy. Unless there is a physiological reason for the chronic fatigue (e.g., see the chapter "Chronic Fatigue Syndrome"), it won't take long before the subconscious believes.

Regardless of the situation, asking better questions is bound to improve your attitude. If you want to have a better life, simply ask better questions. It sounds simple because it is. If you want more energy, excitement, and/or happiness in your life, simply ask yourself the following questions on a consistent basis:

1. What am I most happy about in my life right now?

   Why does that make me happy?

   How does that make me feel?

2. What am I most excited about in my life right now?

   Why does that make me excited?

   How does that make me feel?

3. What am I most grateful about in my life right now?

   Why does that make me grateful?

   How does that make me feel?

4. What am I enjoying most about in my life right now?

   What about that do I enjoy?

   How does that make me feel?

5. What am I committed to in my life right now?

   Why am I committed to that?

   How does that make me feel?

6. Whom do I love? (Start close and move out.)

   Who loves me?

7. What must I do today to achieve my long-term goal?

Step 4: Employ Positive Affirmations

An affirmation is a statement with some emotional intensity behind it. Positive affirmations can make imprints on the subconscious mind to create a healthy, positive self-image. In addition, affirmations can actually fuel the changes you desire. You may want to have the following affirmations in plain sight to recite them over the course of the day:

I am blessed with an abundance of energy!

Love, joy, and happiness flow through me with every heartbeat.

I am thankful to God for all of my good fortune!

YES I CAN!

Here are some very simple guidelines for creating your own affirmations. Have fun with it! Positive affirmations can make you feel really good if you follow these guidelines.

1. Always phrase an affirmation in the present tense. Imagine that it has already come to pass.

2. Always phrase the affirmation as a positive statement. Do not use the words *not* and *never.*

3. Do your best to totally associate with the positive feelings that are generated by the affirmation.

4. Keep the affirmation short and simple but full of feeling. Be creative.

5. Imagine yourself really experiencing what you are affirming.

6. Make the affirmation personal to you and full of meaning.

Using the above guidelines and examples, write down five affirmations that apply to you. State these affirmations aloud while you are taking your shower, driving, or praying.

Step 5: Set Positive Goals

Learning to set goals in a way that results in a positive experience is another powerful method for building a positive attitude and raising self-esteem. Goals can be used to create a "success cycle." Achieving goals helps you feel better about yourself, and the better you feel about yourself, the more likely you are to achieve your goals. Here are some guidelines to use in setting goals.

1. State the goal in positive terms; do not use any negative words in your goal statement. For example, it is better to say "I enjoy eating healthful, low-calorie, nutritious foods" than to say "I will not eat

sugar, candy, ice cream, and other fattening foods."

2. Make your goal attainable and realistic. Again, goals can be used to create a success cycle and positive self-image. Little things add up to make a major difference in the way you feel about yourself.

3. Be specific. The more clearly your goal is defined, the more likely you are to reach it. For example, if you want to lose weight, what is the weight you desire? What is the body fat percentage or measurements you desire? Clearly define what it is you want to achieve.

4. State the goal in the present tense, not the future tense. In order to reach your goal, you have to believe you have already attained it. You must program yourself to achieve the goal. See and feel yourself having already achieved the goal.

Any voyage begins with one step and is followed by many other steps. Remember to set short-term goals that can be used to help you achieve your long-term goals. Get into the habit of asking yourself the following question each morning and evening: "What must I do today to achieve my long-term goal?"

Step 6: Practice Positive Visualization

Positive visualization or imagery is another powerful tool in creating health, happiness, and success. We have to be able to see our life the way we want it to be before this can happen. In terms of ideal health, you absolutely must picture yourself in ideal health if you truly want to experience this state. You can use visualization in all areas of your life, but especially when it comes to your health; in fact, some of the most promising research on the power of visualization involves enhancing the immune system in the treatment of cancer. Be creative and have fun with positive visualizations, and you will soon find yourself living your dreams.

Step 7: Laugh Long and Often

When you laugh frequently and take a lighter view of life, you will find that life is much more enjoyable. Researchers are discovering that laughter enhances the immune system and promotes improved physiology. Recent medical research has also confirmed that laughter:

- Enhances the blood flow to the body's extremities and improves cardiovascular function.
- Plays an active part in the body's release of endorphins and other natural mood-elevating and painkilling chemicals.
- Improves the transfer of oxygen and nutrients to internal organs.

Here are eight tips to help you get more laughter in your life.

1. **Learn to laugh at yourself.** Recognize how funny some of your behavior really is—especially your shortcomings or mistakes. We all have little idiosyncrasies or behaviors that are unique to us that we can recognize and enjoy. Do not take yourself too seriously.

2. **Inject humor anytime it is appropriate.** People love to laugh. Get a joke book and learn how to tell a good joke. Humor and laughter really make life enjoyable.

3. **Read the comics to find a strip that you find funny and follow it.** Humor is very individual: what one person may find funny, another may not. But the funny papers have something for everybody. Find a comic strip that you think is particularly funny and look for it every day or week.

4. **Watch comedies on the small screen.** With modern technology, it is amazingly easy to find something funny on television or the Internet. When you are in need of a good laugh, try to find something that you can laugh at on TV or YouTube. Some favorites are the old-time classics such as *The Andy Griffith Show, Gilligan's Island, The Mary Tyler Moore Show,* and so on.

5. **Go to comedies at the movie theater.** Most people love to go to the movies and especially enjoy a good comedy. When people see a funny movie together, they find themselves laughing harder and longer than if they had seen the same scene by themselves. We all feed off each other's laughter during and after the movie. Also, laughing together helps build good relationships.

6. **Listen to comedy audiotapes in your car while commuting.** Check your local record store, bookstore, video store, or library for recorded routines by your favorite comedian. If you haven't heard or seen many comedians, go to your library first. You'll find an abundance of tapes to investigate, and you can check them out free.

7. **Play with kids.** Kids really know how to laugh and play. If you do not have kids of your own, spend time with your nieces, your nephews, or neighborhood children with whose families you are friendly. Become a Big Brother or Sister. Investigate local Little Leagues. Help out at your church's Sunday school and children's events.

8. **Ask yourself, "What is funny about this situation?"** Many times we find ourselves in seemingly impossible situations, but if we can laugh about them, somehow they become enjoyable, or at

least tolerable. We have all heard people say, "This is something that you will look back on and laugh about." Well, why wait? Find the humor in the situation and enjoy a good laugh immediately.

Final Comments

Our attitude is just like our physical body in that it requires constant conditioning to stay fit. Just as you do not find yourself in excellent physical condition after one exercise session, you may not find yourself with a positive mental attitude after reading this book.

We want to encourage you to really work at staying positive and optimistic through life. We all will have our fair share of challenges, and many of them will feel unfair and undeserved—bad things do happen to good people. However, what really determines our life's direction is not what happens in our lives but how we respond to the challenges. Hardship, heartbreak, disappointments, and failures are often the fuel for joy, ecstasy, compassion, and success. By conditioning your attitude to be positive, you will experience a higher level of health and happiness in your life. One of the best ways to condition your attitude is to regularly read or listen to inspiring books.

QUICK REVIEW

- **A positive mental attitude is the real foundation for optimal health.**
- **There is an innate drive in all living things to be the best that they can be.**
- **Achieving self-actualization begins by taking personal responsibility for your own positive mental state, your life, your current situation, and your health.**
- **The seven key steps to developing and maintaining a positive mental attitude are:**

Step 1: Become an optimist.
Step 2: Become aware of self-talk.
Step 3: Ask better questions.
Step 4: Employ positive affirmations.
Step 5: Set positive goals.
Step 6: Practice positive visualization.
Step 7: Laugh long and often.

- **Read or listen to inspiring messages.**

A Health-Promoting Lifestyle

Introduction

Without question, a healthful lifestyle improves longevity and the quality of life. The key components of a healthful lifestyle discussed in this chapter are avoiding cigarette smoking, engaging in a regular exercise program, and practicing good sleep habits.

Smoking Is Deadly

A large body of research reveals that smokers have a three- to fivefold increase in the risk of cancer and heart disease compared with nonsmokers. The more cigarettes smoked and the longer the period of years a person has smoked, the greater the risk of dying from cancer, a heart attack, or a stroke. Overall, the average smoker dies seven to eight years sooner than the nonsmoker and has a greater burden of disease.

Tobacco smoke contains more than 4,000 chemicals, of which more than 50 have been identified as carcinogens. If you want good health, you absolutely must stop smoking! And here's some good news: if you quit smoking now, it's possible for you to reduce your risk of cancer to the same level as that of people who never smoked. Studies have found that 10 years after quitting, an ex-smoker's risk of dying from lung cancer is 30% to 50%

less than the risk for those who continue to smoke. After 15 years, an ex-smoker's risk is almost the same as that of a person who never smoked. Quitting smoking also reduces the risk for developing heart disease, emphysema, and other cancers. You'll live longer—and you'll live better.[1]

Various measures, including nicotine-containing skin patches or chewing gum, acupuncture, and hypnosis, have all been shown to provide some benefit, but not much. In a systematic review of the efficacy of interventions intended to help people stop smoking, data were analyzed from 188 randomized controlled trials.[2] Encouragement to stop smoking by a physician during a routine office visit resulted in a 2% cessation rate after one year. Supplementary measures such as follow-up letters or visits had an additional effect. Behavioral modification techniques such as relaxation, rewards and punishment, and avoiding trigger situations, taught in groups or individual sessions led by a psychologist, had no greater effect than the 2% rate achieved by simple advice from a physician. Eight studies of acupuncture showed an overall effectiveness rate of roughly 3%. Hypnosis was judged to be ineffective even though trials have shown a success rate of 23%; the reason is that in these studies no biochemical marker such as breakdown products of nicotine in the urine was used to accurately determine effectiveness. Nicotine replacement therapy (gum or patch) was effective in about 13% of smokers who sought help in quitting. All together these results are not very encouraging.

No matter what strategy you choose, it appears the best results occur when people quit cold turkey rather than trying to taper down. If you smoke, quit now! Here are 10 tips to help you.

1. List all the reasons you want to quit smoking, and review them every day.

2. Set a specific day to quit, tell at least 10 friends that you are going to quit smoking, and then do it!

3. Throw away all cigarettes, butts, matches, and ashtrays. If you feel the need to have something in your mouth, chew on raw vegetables, fruits, or gum. If your fingers seem empty, play with a pencil.

4. Take one day at a time.

5. Realize that 40 million Americans have quit. If they can do it, so can you!

6. Visualize yourself as a nonsmoker with a fatter pocketbook, pleasant breath, unstained teeth, and the satisfaction that comes from being in control of your life.

7. Join an online support group. While research on this is still in its early stages, doing so appears to double or even triple success rates.

8. When you need to relax, perform deep breathing exercises rather than reaching for a cigarette.

9. Avoid situations that you associate with smoking.

10. Each day you don't smoke, reward yourself. Buy yourself something with the money you've saved, or plan a special reward as a celebration for quitting.

The Importance of Regular Exercise

Regular physical exercise is obviously vital to good health. We all know this, yet less than 50% of Americans exercise on a regular basis. While the immediate effect of exercise is stress on the body, with regular exercise the body adapts—it becomes stronger, functions more efficiently, and has greater endurance. The entire body benefits from regular exercise, largely as a result of improved cardiovascular and respiratory function. Exercise enhances the transport of oxygen and nutrients into cells at the same time as it enhances the transport of carbon dioxide and other waste products out of cells. You will find that exercise increases your overall energy levels.

Physical inactivity is a major reason so many Americans are overweight. This is especially true for children—research indicates that childhood obesity is associated more with inactivity than with overeating.[3] There is also strong evidence suggesting that 80 to 86% of adult obesity begins in childhood. If you have kids, get them active. If you are not active yourself, make a change and get active, especially if you have weight to lose. Adults who are physically active tend to have less of a problem with weight loss for the following reasons:

- When weight loss is achieved by dieting without exercise, a substantial portion of the total weight loss comes from the lean tissue, primarily as water loss.

- When exercise (especially strength training) is included in a weight loss program, there is usually an improvement in body composition: an increase in muscle mass and a decrease in body fat.

- Exercise helps counter the reduction in basal metabolic rate (BMR) that usually accompanies dieting alone.

- Exercise increases the BMR for an extended period of time following the exercise session.
  - Moderate to intense exercise may help suppress the appetite.
  - People who exercise while on a weight loss program are better able to maintain the weight loss than those who do not exercise.

Exercise promotes the efficient burning of fat. Muscle tissue is the primary user of fat calories in the body, so the greater your muscle mass, the greater your fat-burning capacity. If you want to be healthy and achieve your ideal body weight, you *must* exercise.

Exercise and Mood

Regular exercise exerts a powerful positive effect on mood. Tension, restlessness, depression, feelings of inadequacy, and worrying diminish greatly with regular exercise. Exercise alone has been demonstrated to have a tremendous impact on improving mood and the ability to handle stressful life situations.[4]

Regular exercise has been shown to increase powerful mood-elevating substances in the brain known as endorphins.[5] These compounds have effects similar to those of morphine, although much milder. There is a clear association between exercise and endorphin elevation, and when endorphins go up, mood follows.[6]

If the benefits of exercise could be put in a pill, you would have the most powerful health-promoting medication available. Take a look at this long list of health benefits produced by regular exercise:

Musculoskeletal System

Increases muscle strength

Increases flexibility of muscles and range of joint motion

Produces stronger bones, ligaments, and tendons

Lessens chance of injury

Enhances posture, poise, and physique

Improves balance

Heart and Blood Vessels

Lowers resting heart rate

Strengthens heart function

Lowers blood pressure

Improves oxygen delivery throughout the body

Increases blood supply to muscles

Enlarges the arteries to the heart

Bodily Processes

Improves the way the body handles dietary fat

Reduces heart disease risk

Helps lower total blood cholesterol and triglycerides

Raises HDL, the "good" cholesterol

Helps improve calcium deposition in bones

Prevents osteoporosis

Improves immune function

Aids digestion and elimination

Increases endurance and energy levels

Promotes lean body mass, burns fat

Mental Processes

Provides a natural release for pent-up feelings

Helps reduce tension and anxiety

Improves mental outlook and self-esteem

Helps relieve moderate depression

Improves the ability to handle stress

Stimulates improved mental function

Relaxes and improves sleep

Increases self-esteem

Physical Fitness and Longevity

The better shape you are in physically, the greater your odds of enjoying a long and healthy life. Most studies have showed that someone who is not fit has an eightfold greater risk of having a heart attack or stroke than a physically fit individual. Researchers have estimated that for every hour of exercise, there is a two-hour increase in longevity. That is quite a return on investment.

The Aerobics Center Longitudinal Study involved 9,777 men ranging in age from 20 to 82 who had completed at least two preventive medical examinations (on average 4.9 years apart) at the Cooper Clinic in Dallas, Texas, from December 1970 through December 1989. All study subjects achieved at least 85% of their age-predicted maximal heart rate (220 minus their age) during the treadmill tests at both exams. The men were further categorized by their level of fitness based on their exercise tolerance on a standard treadmill test. This measure is a sound objective indicator of physical fitness, as it has been shown to correlate positively with maximal oxygen uptake. The men were divided into five groups, with the first group categorized as unfit and groups two through five being categorized as fit. The higher the group number, the higher level of fitness.

The highest age-adjusted death rate (all causes) was observed in men who were unfit at both exams (122.0 deaths per 10,000 man-years); the lowest death rate was in men who were physically fit at both examinations (39.6 deaths per 10,000 man-years). Furthermore, men who improved from unfit to fit between the first and subsequent examinations had an age-adjusted death rate of 67.7 per 10,000 man-years, representing a reduction in mortality of 44% relative to men who remained unfit at both exams. Improvement in fitness was associated with lower death rates after adjusting for age, health status, and other risk factors for premature mortality. For each 1-minute increase in exercise tolerance between examinations, there was a corresponding 7.9% decrease in risk of mortality.[7]

Creating an Effective Exercise Routine

The time you spend exercising is a valuable investment in good health. To help you develop a successful exercise program, here are seven steps to follow.

Step 1: Realize the Importance of Physical Exercise

The first step is realizing just how important it is to get regular exercise. We cannot stress enough how vital regular exercise is to your health, but what we say means absolutely nothing unless it really sinks in and you accept it as well. You must make regular exercise a top priority in your life.

Step 2: Consult Your Physician

If you are not currently on a regular exercise program, get medical clearance if you have health problems or if you are over 40. The main concern is the functioning of your heart. Exercise can be quite harmful (and even fatal) if your heart is not able to meet the increased demands placed on it.

It is especially important to see a physician if any of the following applies to you:

Heart disease

Smoking

High blood pressure

Extreme breathlessness with physical exertion

Pain or pressure in chest, arm, teeth, jaw, or neck with exercise

Dizziness or fainting

Abnormal heart action (palpitations or irregular beat)

Step 3: Select an Activity You Can Enjoy

If you are healthy enough to begin an exercise program, select an activity that you feel you would enjoy. Choose activities from the list below, or come up with some on your own. Make a commitment to do one activity a day for at least 20 minutes and preferably 1 hour. Make your goal the enjoyment of the activity. The important thing is to move your body enough to raise your pulse a bit above its resting rate. Try:

Bicycling

Bowling

Dancing

Gardening

Golfing

Heavy housecleaning

Jazzercise

Jogging

Stair climbing

Stationary bike

Swimming

Tennis

Treadmill

Walking

Weight lifting

The best exercises are the kind that elevate your heart rate the most. Aerobic activities such as walking briskly, jogging, bicycling, cross-country skiing, swimming, aerobic dance, and racquet sports are good examples. Brisk walking (5 miles an hour) for approximately 30 minutes may be the very best form of exercise for weight loss. Walking can be done anywhere; it requires no expensive equipment, just comfortable clothing and well-fitting shoes; and the risk for injury is extremely low. If you are going to walk on a regular basis, we strongly urge you to purchase a pair of high-quality walking or jogging shoes.

Step 4: Monitor Exercise Intensity

Exercise intensity is determined by measuring your heart rate (the number of times your heart beats per minute). This can be determined quickly by placing the index and middle fingers of one hand on the side of the neck just below the angle of the jaw or on the opposite wrist. Count the number of heartbeats for 6 seconds. Simply add a zero to this number and you have your pulse. For example, if you counted 14 beats, your heart rate would be 140. Would this be a good number? It depends upon your "training zone."

A quick and easy way to determine your maximum training heart rate is to simply subtract your age from 185. For example, if you are 40 years old, your maximum heart rate would be 145. To determine the bottom of the training zone, simply subtract 20 from this number. In the case of a 40-year-old this would be 125. So the training range would be between 125 and 145 beats per minute. For maximum health benefits you must stay in this range and never exceed it.

Step 5: Do It Often

You don't get in good physical condition by exercising once; you have to do it on a regular basis. A minimum of 15 to 20 minutes of exercising at your training heart rate at least three times a week is necessary to gain any significant cardiovascular benefits from exercise.

Step 6: Make It Fun

The key to getting the maximum benefit from exercise is to make it enjoyable. Choose something you have fun doing. If you can find enjoyment in exercise, you are much more likely to exercise regularly.

One way to make exercise fun is to get a workout partner. For example, if you choose walking as your activity, find one or two people in your neighborhood you would enjoy walking with. An added plus is that if you have plans to walk together, you will be more likely to actually get out there than if you depended solely on your own willpower. Commit to walking three to five mornings or afternoons each week, and increase the exercise duration from an initial 10 minutes to at least 30 minutes.

Step 7: Stay Motivated

No matter how committed you are to regular exercise, at some point in time you are going to be faced with a loss of enthusiasm for working out. Our suggestion is to take a break. Not a long break; just skip one or two workouts. This gives your enthusiasm and motivation a chance to recoup so that you can come back with an even stronger commitment.

Here are some other things to help you to stay motivated:

- **Thumb through fitness magazines.** Try ones such as like *Men's Health*, *Muscle and Fitness*, or *Runner's World*. Looking at pictures of people in fantastic shape can be inspiring. In addition, these types of magazines typically feature articles on new exercise routines that you may find interesting.

- **Set exercise goals.** Being goal-oriented helps keep us motivated. Success breeds success, so set a lot of small goals that can easily be achieved. Write down your daily exercise goal and check it off when you complete it.

- **Vary your routine.** Variety is very important to help you stay interested in exercise. Doing the same thing every day becomes monotonous and drains motivation. Continually find new ways to enjoy working out.

- **Keep a record of your activities and progress.** Sometimes it is hard to see the progress you are making, but if you write in a journal, you'll have a permanent record of your progress. Keeping track of your progress will motivate you to continued improvement.

Strength Training

We also recommend that everyone engage in strength training (such as lifting weights or performing resistance exercises) at least three times a week. Strength training is especially valuable, as it not only increases muscle strength but also stabilizes blood sugar, promotes fat loss, and protects against age-related muscle loss.

The Importance of Sleep

Sleep is perhaps one of the least understood physiological processes. Its value to human health and proper functioning is without question. Sleep is absolutely essential to both the body and the mind. Impaired sleep, altered sleep patterns, and sleep deprivation wreak havoc on mental and physical function. Many health conditions, particularly depression, chronic fatigue syndrome, and fibromyalgia, are either entirely or partially related to sleep deprivation or disturbed sleep.

Over the course of a year, more than half of the U.S. population will have difficulty falling asleep. About 33% of Americans experience insomnia on a regular basis, with 17% of the population claiming that insomnia is a major problem in their lives. Many use over-the-counter sedatives to combat insomnia, while others seek stronger prescription medications from their physicians. Each year up to 10 million people in the United States receive prescriptions for drugs to help them go to sleep. (The natural treatment of insomnia is described in the chapter "Insomnia.")

As with other health conditions, the most effective treatment of insomnia is based upon identifying and addressing causative factors. The most common causes of insomnia are psychological—depression, anxiety, and tension. If psychological factors do not seem to be the cause, various foods, drinks, and medications may be responsible. There are numerous compounds in food and drink and well over 300 drugs that can interfere with normal sleep.

Some of the benefits of sleep are probably mediated through growth hormone (GH). An anabolic hormone, GH has been called by some the "antiaging" hormone. Several research projects are now studying its rejuvenating effects when it is injected. The reason for the excitement is that GH stimulates tissue regeneration, liver regeneration, muscle building, breakdown of fat stores, normalization of blood sugar regulation, and a whole host of other beneficial processes in the body. In other words, it helps convert fat to muscle. Small amounts of GH are secreted at various times during the day, but most GH secretion occurs during sleep.

Sleep functions as an antioxidant for the brain: free radicals that can damage neurons are removed as you snooze. Most people can tolerate a few days without sleep and fully recover. However, chronic sleep deprivation appears to accelerate aging of the brain, causes neuronal damage, and leads to night-time elevations in the stress hormone cortisol (see the chapter "Insomnia" for improving sleep quality).

How Much Sleep Do You Need?

Exactly how much sleep is required by an individual varies from one person to the next and from one stage of life to another. A one-year-old baby requires about 14 hours of sleep a day, a five-year-old about 12, and adults about 7 to 8. In addition, women tend to require more sleep than men. As people age their sleep needs may decline (the research is not clear), but so does their ability to sustain sleep, probably as a result of decreased levels of important brain chemicals such as serotonin and melatonin. The elderly tend to sleep less at night but doze more during the day than younger adults.

Normal Sleep Patterns

From observation of eye movement and electroencephalographic (EEG) recordings, we know that there are two distinct types of sleep: REM (rapid eye movement) sleep, which is when dreaming takes place; and non-REM sleep.

Non-REM sleep is divided into stages 1 through 4 according to level of EEG activity and ease of arousal. As sleep progresses there is a deepening of sleep and slower brain wave activity until REM sleep, when suddenly the brain becomes much more active. In adults, the first REM sleep cycle is usually triggered 90 minutes after going to sleep and lasts about 5 to 10 minutes. After the flurry of activity, brain wave patterns return to those of non-REM sleep for another 90-minute sleep cycle.

Each night most adults experience five or more sleep cycles. REM sleep periods grow progressively longer as sleep continues; the

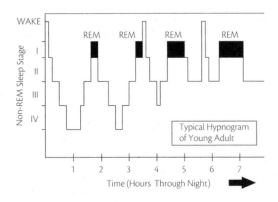

Normal Sleep Architecture

last sleep cycle may produce an REM sleep period that can last about an hour. Non-REM sleep accounts for approximately 50% of this 90-minute sleep cycle in infants and about 80% in adults. As people age, in addition to getting less REM sleep, they tend to awaken at the transition from non-REM to REM sleep.

The Importance of Dreams

Dreams are very important to our physical and mental well-being. A dream is a sequence of sensations, images, and thoughts passing through a sleeping person's mind. We also use the word *dream* to refer to a wish, fantasy, desire, or fanciful vision. It is our dreams that propel us as we roll through this life. They are powerful, inspirational, and potentially healing. The famous author Anatole France said something about dreams and life that we think really hits home: "Existence would be intolerable if we were never to dream."

The importance of dreams to mental health is obvious if you examine what happens to people who are deprived of REM sleep. In the early 1960s, the pioneering dream researcher William C. Dement conducted several interesting studies in which

subjects sleeping in a laboratory setting were awakened the moment REM began to occur and then allowed to go back to sleep. The experiment continued for one week. During this time the test group reported increased irritability, anxiety, and appetite. In other studies people deprived of REM sleep exhibited profound personality changes—extreme irritability, depression, anxiety, and so on—that disappeared when they were allowed to dream again.[8]

Humans have been attempting to answer the question "Where do dreams come from and what do they mean?" since the dawn of civilization. Some ancient cultures considered the content of dreams to be more significant than the events of their waking lives, but the modern view of dreams was initially swayed a bit by fears that dreams might undermine moral conduct or that they are meaningless, the result of random nerve firings or physical discomfort. The emerging view is a more holistic one, as it recognizes that dreams have both physiological and psychological causes.

Modern psychology became fascinated with dreams through the work of Sigmund Freud, who saw dreams as the window to the soul. Freud's classic view was that dreams were safe expressions of impulses and desires buried in the subconscious mind.

Other scientists in the early 1900s also began looking into dreams. Carl Jung, Alfred Adler, and William Stekel, as well as other psychologists who followed them, developed their own theories on the meanings and interpretations of dreams.

We believe that some dreams can aid us in working out issues in our waking lives. Dreams allow us an opportunity to view what is being imprinted on our subconscious mind. They are often symbolic attempts to sort out the options we can choose in life. Obviously, there are times when dreams are not psychologically meaningful. For example, if you are suffering from indigestion or a peptic ulcer and experience a violent dream where you are getting stabbed in the stomach, we would not recommend trying to uncover some deep psychological issue. The problem with trying to interpret every dream is that not every dream will be meaningful. Nonetheless, we think it is important to examine every dream for possible clues for personal growth.

If you are interested in learning more about dreams, we recommend going to the website of the International Association for the Study of Dreams (asdreams.org). This organization is "dedicated to the pure and applied investigation of dreams and dreaming." Its purposes are to "promote an awareness and appreciation of dreams in both professional and public arenas; to encourage research into the nature, function, and significance of dreaming; to advance the application of the study of dreams; and to provide a forum for the exchange of ideas and information on dreams," as its website notes.

Final Comments

Just like the other four cornerstones of good health, the importance of a health-promoting lifestyle cannot be overstated. Lifestyle definitely comes down to choices. If you want to be healthy, simply make healthful choices. Choose to not smoke. Choose to find physical activities that you enjoy and do them often. Make getting a good night's sleep a priority and have fun with your dreams. These simple lifestyle choices will have a profound effect on your health and the quality of your life.

QUICK REVIEW

- **Breathe clean air. Smoking is still a major contributor to an early death.**
- **Be physically fit. Physical inactivity is a major reason so many are overweight.**
- **Sleep well. Many health conditions are either entirely or partially related to sleep deprivation or disturbed sleep.**

A Health-Promoting Diet

Let your food be your medicine and let your medicine be your food.
—HIPPOCRATES

Introduction

The purpose of this chapter is to initiate the reader into the growing field of nutritional medicine by focusing on key dietary recommendations for a health-promoting diet. Most naturopathic physicians utilize these principles to help educate and inspire their patients to attain a higher level of wellness. The critical importance to health of a whole-foods diet cannot be overstated.

It is now well established that certain dietary practices can either cause or prevent a wide range of diseases, particularly chronic degenerative diseases such as heart disease, cancer, and other conditions associated with aging. In addition, more and more research indicates that certain diets and foods offer immediate therapeutic benefit.

There are two basic facts underlying the diet-disease connection: (1) a diet rich in plant foods (whole grains, legumes, nuts and seeds, fruits, and vegetables) is protective against many diseases that are extremely common in Western society, and (2) a low intake of plant foods is a causative factor in the development of these diseases and provides conditions under which other causative factors are more active.

The Importance of a Plant-Based Diet

Although the human gastrointestinal tract is capable of digesting both animal and plant foods, a number of physical characteristics indicate that *Homo sapiens* evolved to digest primarily plant foods. Specifically, our 32 teeth include 20 molars, which are perfect for crushing and grinding plant foods, along with 8 front incisors, which are well suited for biting into fruits and vegetables. Only our front four canine teeth are specifically designed for meat eating. Our jaws swing both vertically to tear and laterally to crush, but carnivores' jaws swing only vertically. Additional evidence that supports the body's preference for plant foods is the long length of the human intestinal tract. Carnivores typically have a short bowel, whereas herbivores have a bowel length proportionally comparable to that of humans. Thus the human bowel length favors plant foods.[1]

Nonhuman wild primates such as chimpanzees, monkeys, and gorillas are also omnivores or, as often described, herbivores and opportunistic carnivores. They eat mainly fruits and vegetables but may also eat small animals, lizards, and eggs if given the opportunity. Only 1% and 2%, respectively, of the total calories consumed by gorillas and orangutans are animal foods. The remainder of their diet is from plant foods. Because humans are between the weights of the gorilla and orangutan, it has been suggested that humans are designed to eat around 1.5% of their diet as animal foods.[2] Most Americans, however, derive well over 50% of their calories from animal foods.

Although most primates eat a considerable amount of fruit, it is critical to point out that the cultivated fruit in American supermarkets is far different from the highly nutritious wild fruits these animals rely on. Wild fruits have a slightly higher protein content and a higher content of certain essential vitamins and minerals, but cultivated fruits tend to be higher in sugars. Cultivated fruits are therefore very tasty to humans, but because they have a higher sugar composition and also lack the fibrous pulp and multiple seeds found in wild fruit that slow down the digestion and absorption of sugars, cultivated fruits raise blood sugar levels much more quickly than their wild counterparts.

Wild primates fill up not only on fruit but also on other highly nutritious plant foods. As a result, wild primates weighing 1/10th as much as a typical human ingest nearly 10 times the level of vitamin C and much higher amounts of many other vitamins and minerals. Other differences in the wild primate diet are also important to point out, such as a higher ratio of alpha-linolenic acid (an essential omega-3 fatty acid) to linoleic acid (an essential omega-6 fatty acid).[2]

Determining what foods humans are best suited for may not be as simple as looking at the diet of wild primates. There are some structural and physiological differences between humans and apes. The key difference may be the larger, more metabolically active human brain. In fact, it has been theorized that a shift in dietary intake to more animal foods may have been the stimulus for brain growth. The shift itself was probably the result of limited food availability that forced early humans to hunt grazing mammals such as antelope and gazelles. Archaeological data support this association: the brains of humans started to grow and become more developed at about the same time as evidence shows an increase in bones of animals butchered with stone tools at sites of early villages.

Improved dietary quality alone cannot fully explain why human brains grew, but it definitely appears to have played a critical role. With a bigger brain, early humans were able to engage in more complex social behavior, which led to improved foraging and hunting tactics, which in turn led to even higher-quality food intake, fostering additional brain evolution.

Data from anthropologists looking at hunter-gatherer cultures are providing much insight as to what humans are designed to eat; however, it is very important to point out that these groups were not entirely free to determine their diets. Instead, their diets were molded by what was available to them. Regardless of whether hunter-gatherer communities relied on animal or plant foods, the incidence of diseases of civilization, such as heart disease and cancer, is extremely low in such communities.[3]

It should also be pointed out that the meat that our ancestors consumed was much different from the meat found in supermarkets today. Domesticated animals have always had higher fat levels than their wild counterparts, but the desire for tender meat has led to the breeding of cattle that produce meat with a fat content of 25 to 30% or more, compared with less than 4% for free-living animals and wild game. In addition, the type of fat is considerably different. Domestic beef contains primarily saturated fats and is very low in omega-3 fatty acids. In contrast, the fat of wild animals contains more than five times as much polyunsaturated fat per gram and has good amounts of beneficial omega-3 fatty acids (approximately 4 to 8%).[4]

The Pioneering Work of Burkitt and Trowell

Much of the link between diet and chronic disease originated from the work of two medical pioneers: Denis Burkitt, M.D., and Hugh Trowell, M.D., authors of *Western Diseases: Their Emergence and Prevention*, first published in 1981.[5] Although now extremely well recognized, their work is actually a continuation of the landmark work of Weston A. Price, a dentist and author of *Nutrition and Physical Degeneration*. In the early 1900s, Dr. Price traveled the world observing changes in the structure of the teeth and palate as various cultures discarded traditional dietary practices in favor of a more "civilized" diet. Price was able to follow individuals as well as cultures over periods of 20 to 40 years and carefully documented the onset of degenerative diseases as their diets changed. On the basis of extensive studies examining the incidence of diseases in various populations and his own observations of primitive cultures, Burkitt formulated the following sequence of events:

- **First stage.** In cultures consuming a traditional diet consisting of whole, unprocessed foods, the incidence of chronic diseases such as heart disease, diabetes, and cancer is quite low.

- **Second stage.** As the culture moves toward eating a more Western-style diet, there is a sharp rise in the number of individuals with obesity and diabetes.

- **Third stage.** As more and more people abandon their traditional diet, conditions that were once quite rare become extremely common. Examples are constipa-

tion, hemorrhoids, varicose veins, and appendicitis.

- **Fourth stage.** Finally, with full westernization of the diet, other chronic degenerative or potentially lethal diseases, such as heart disease, cancer, osteoarthritis, rheumatoid arthritis, and gout, become extremely common.

Since Burkitt and Trowell's pioneering research, a virtual landslide of data has continually emphasized the Western diet as the key factor in virtually every chronic disease, especially obesity and diabetes. The following table lists diseases with convincing links to a diet low in plant foods. Many of these now common diseases were extremely rare before the 20th century.

Diseases Strongly Associated with a Low-Fiber Diet	
TYPE OF DISEASE	**SPECIFIC DISEASES**
Metabolic	Obesity, gout, diabetes, kidney stones, gallstones
Cardiovascular	High blood pressure, strokes, heart disease, varicose veins, deep vein thrombosis, pulmonary embolism
Colonic	Constipation, appendicitis, diverticulitis, diverticulosis, hemorrhoids, colon cancer, irritable bowel syndrome, ulcerative colitis, Crohn's disease
Other	Dental caries, autoimmune disorders, pernicious anemia, multiple sclerosis, thyrotoxicosis, psoriasis, acne

Trends in U.S. Food Consumption

During the 20th century, food consumption patterns changed dramatically. Total dietary fat intake rose from 32% of calories in 1909 to 43% by the end of the century. Overall carbohydrate intake dropped from 57% to 46%; and protein intake remained fairly stable at about 11%.

Compounding these detrimental patterns are the individual food choices people make. The biggest changes were significant rises

Trends in Quantities of Foods Consumed per Capita (Pounds per Year)				
FOODS	**1909**	**1967**	**1985**	**1999**
Meat, Poultry, and Fish				
Beef	54	81	73	66
Pork	62	61	62	50
Poultry	18	46	70	68
Fish	12	15	19	15
Total	146	203	224	199
Eggs	37	40	32	32
Dairy Products				
Whole milk	223	232	122	112
Low-fat milk	64	44	112	101
Cheese	5	15	26	30
Other	47	159	190	210
Total	339	450	450	453
Fats and Oils				
Butter	18	6	5	5
Margarine	1	10	11	8
Shortening	8	16	23	22
Lard and tallow	12	5	4	6
Salad and cooking oil	2	16	25	29
Total	41	53	68	70
Fruits				
Citrus	17	60	72	79
Noncitrus, fresh	154	73	87	115
Noncitrus, processed	8	35	34	37
Total	179	168	193	231

(continued on next page)

Trends in Quantities of Foods Consumed per Capita (Pounds per Year)				
FOODS	**1909**	**1967**	**1985**	**1999**
Vegetables, Excluding Potatoes				
Tomatoes	46	36	38	55
Dark green and yellow	34	25	31	39
Other, fresh	136	87	96	126
Other, processed	8	35	34	39
Total	224	183	199	259
Potatoes, White				
Fresh	182	67	55	49
Processed	0	19	28	91
Total	182	86	83	140
Legumes				
Dry beans, peas, nuts, and soybeans	16	16	18	22
Grain Products				
Wheat products	216	116	122	150
Corn	56	15	17	28
Other grains	19	13	26	24
Total	291	144	165	202
Sugar and Sweeteners				
Refined sugar	77	100	63	68
Syrups and other sweeteners	14	22	90	91
Total	91	122	153	159

Modified from United States Department of Agriculture, *Food Review* 2000, 23:8–15

in the consumption of meat, fats and oils, and sugars and sweeteners in conjunction with the decreased consumption of noncitrus fruits, vegetables, and whole-grain products. The largest change was the switch from a diet with a high level of complex carbohydrates, which naturally occur in grains and vegetables, to a tremendous and dramatic increase in the number of calories consumed from simple sugars. Currently, more than half of the carbohydrates being consumed are in the form of sugars (sucrose, corn syrup, etc.)

being added to foods as sweetening agents. High consumption of refined sugars is linked to many chronic diseases, including obesity, diabetes, heart disease, and cancer.

The Government and Nutrition Education

Throughout the years, various governmental organizations have published dietary guidelines, but the recommendations of the United

States Department of Agriculture (USDA) have become the most widely known. In 1956, the USDA published *Food for Fitness: A Daily Food Guide.* This became popularly known as the Basic Four Food Groups. The Basic Four were:

Milk group (milk, cheese, ice cream, and other milk-based foods)

Meat group (meat, fish, poultry, and eggs, with dried legumes and nuts as alternatives)

Fruit and vegetable group

Breads and cereals group

One of the major problems with the Basic Four Food Groups model was that graphically, it suggested that the food groups are equal in health value. The result was overconsumption of animal products, dietary fat,

and refined carbohydrates, and insufficient consumption of fiber-rich foods such as fruits, vegetables, and legumes. This in turn has resulted in many premature deaths, chronic diseases, and increased health care costs.

As the Basic Four Food Groups became outdated, various other governmental as well as medical organizations developed guidelines of their own designed to reduce the risk of either a specific chronic degenerative disease, such as cancer or heart disease, or all chronic diseases.

In an attempt to create a new model in nutrition education, the USDA first published the Eating Right Pyramid in 1992. That resulted in harsh criticisms from numerous experts and other organizations. One big question was "Is it appropriate to have the USDA making these recommendations?" After all, the USDA serves two somewhat

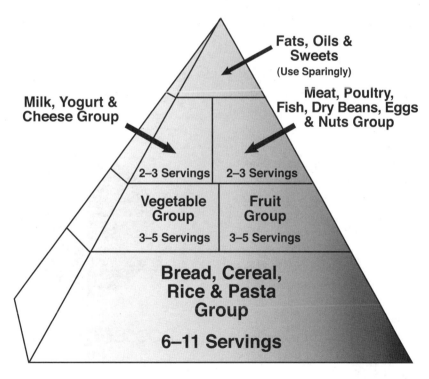

U.S. Department of Agriculture Food Pyramid

conflicting roles: (1) it represents the food industry and (2) it is in charge of educating consumers about nutrition. Many people believe that the pyramid was weighted more toward dairy products, red meat, and grains because of influence from the dairy, beef, and grain farming and processing industries. In other words, the pyramid was designed not to improve the health of Americans but rather to promote the USDA agenda of supporting multinational agrifoods giants.

One of the main criticisms of the Eating Right Pyramid was that it did not stress strongly enough the importance of high-quality food choices. For example, the bottom of the pyramid represented the foods that should make up the bulk of a healthful diet: the Bread, Cereal, Rice, and Pasta Group. Eating 6 to 11 servings a day from this group was supposedly the path to a healthier life. But the Eating Right Pyramid did not take into consideration how quickly blood glucose levels rise after certain types of food are eaten—an effect referred to as the foods' glycemic index (GI). The GI is a numerical scale used to indicate how fast and how high a particular food raises blood glucose (blood sugar) levels. Foods with a lower GI create a slower rise in blood sugar, whereas foods with a higher GI create a faster rise in blood sugar. Some of the foods that the pyramid was directing Americans to eat more of, such as breads, cereals, rice, and pasta, can greatly stress blood sugar control, especially if derived from refined grains, and are now being linked to an increased risk for obesity, diabetes, and cancer. The pyramid did not stress that individuals need to choose whole, unrefined foods in this category.

In June 2011 the USDA unveiled a new food icon, MyPlate, to replace the food pyramid. This simplified illustration is designed to help Americans make healthier food choices. MyPlate is the first step in a multiyear effort to raise consumers' awareness and educate them about eating more healthfully. The initial launch came with some simple recommendations:

Balancing Calories

- Enjoy your food, but eat less.
- Avoid oversize portions.

Foods to Increase

- Make half your plate fruits and vegetables.
- Make at least half your grains whole grains.
- Switch to fat-free or low-fat (1%) milk.

Foods to Reduce

- Compare sodium in foods like soup, bread, and frozen meals—and choose the foods with lower numbers.
- Drink water instead of sugary drinks.

We hope this new campaign will be more successful than prior efforts—and that the program will focus on communicating important nutritional guidance and not yield to political pressure.

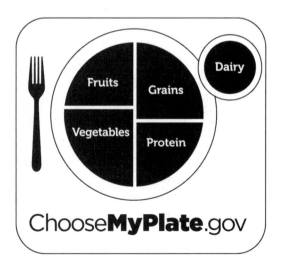

USDA MyPlate

The Optimal Health Food Pyramid

On the basis of existing evidence we have created the Optimal Health Food Pyramid, which incorporates the best of two of the most healthful diets ever studied—the traditional Mediterranean diet and the traditional Asian diet. In addition, the Optimal Health Food Pyramid more clearly defines healthful choices within the categories and stresses the importance of vegetable oils and regular fish consumption as part of a healthful diet. We based the Optimal Health Food Diet on the following nine principles:

1. Eat a rainbow assortment of fruits and vegetables.
2. Reduce exposure to pesticides, heavy metals, and food additives.
3. Eat to support blood sugar control.
4. Do not overconsume animal foods.
5. Eat the right types of fats.
6. Keep salt intake low, potassium intake high.
7. Avoid food additives.
8. Take measures to reduce foodborne illness.
9. Drink sufficient amounts of water each day.

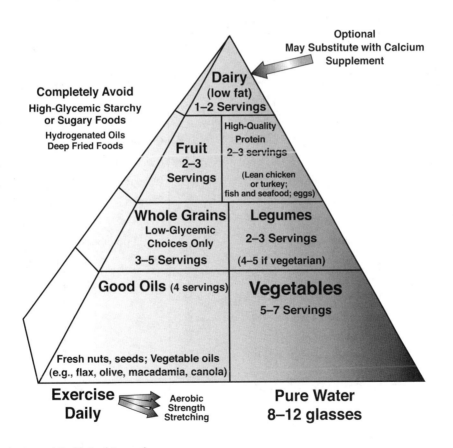

The Optimal Health Food Pyramid

1. Eat a Rainbow Assortment of Fruits and Vegetables

A diet rich in fruits and vegetables is the best bet for preventing virtually every chronic disease. That fact has been established time and again in scientific studies on large numbers of people. The evidence in support of this recommendation is so strong that it has been endorsed by U.S. government health agencies and by virtually every major medical organization, including the American Cancer Society. "Rainbow" simply means that selecting colorful foods—red, orange, yellow, green, blue, and purple—provides the body with powerful antioxidants as well as the nutrients it needs for optimal function and protection against disease.

Fruits and vegetables are so important in the battle against cancer that some experts have said, and we believe, that cancer is a result of a "maladaptation" over time to a reduced level of intake of fruits and vegetables. As a study published in the medical journal *Cancer Causes and Control* put it, "Vegetables and fruit contain the anticarcinogenic cocktail to which we are adapted. We abandon it at our peril."[6] A vast number

The Rainbow Assortment of Foods				
RED	**DARK GREEN**	**YELLOW AND LIGHT GREEN**	**ORANGE**	**PURPLE**
Apples (red)	Artichoke	Apples (green or yellow)	Apricots	Beets
Bell peppers (red)	Asparagus	Avocado	Bell peppers (orange)	Blueberries
Cherries	Bell peppers (green)	Banana	Butternut squash	Blackberries
Cranberries	Broccoli	Bell peppers (yellow)	Cantaloupe	Currants
Grapefruit	Brussels sprouts	Bok choy	Carrots	Cabbage (purple)
Grapes (red)	Chard	Cabbage	Mangoes	Cherries
Radishes	Collard greens	Cauliflower	Oranges	Eggplant
Raspberries	Cucumbers	Celery	Papaya	Onions (red)
Plums (red)	Green beans	Fennel	Pumpkin	Grapes (purple)
Strawberries	Grapes (green)	Kiwi fruits	Sweet potatoes	Pears (red)
Tomatoes	Honeydew melon	Lemons	Yams	Plums (purple)
Watermelon	Kale	Lettuce (light green types)		Radishes
	Leeks	Limes		
	Lettuce (dark green types)	Onions		
	Mustard greens	Pears (green) or yellow)		
	Peas	Pineapple		
	Spinach	Squash (yellow)		
	Turnip greens	Zucchini		

of substances found in fruits and vegetables are known to protect against cancer.[7-9] Some experts refer to these as "chemopreventers," but they are better known to many as phytochemicals. Phytochemicals include pigments such as carotenes, chlorophyll, and flavonoids; dietary fiber; enzymes; vitamin-like compounds; and other minor dietary constituents. Although they work in harmony with antioxidants such as vitamin C, vitamin E, and selenium, phytochemicals exert considerably greater protection against cancer than these simple nutrients.

Examples of Anticancer Phytochemicals

PHYTOCHEMICAL	ACTIONS	SOURCES
Carotenes	Antioxidants Enhance immune functions	Dark-colored vegetables such as carrots, squash, spinach, kale, tomatoes, yams, and sweet potatoes; fruits such as cantaloupe, apricots, and citrus
Coumarins	Antitumor properties Enhance immune functions Stimulate antioxidant mechanisms	Carrots, celery, fennel, beets, citrus fruit
Dithiolthiones, glucosinolates, and thiocyanates	Block cancer-causing compounds from damaging cells Enhance detoxification	Vegetables in the brassica family—cabbage, broccoli, brussels sprouts, kale, etc.
Flavonoids	Antioxidants Direct antitumor effects Immune-enhancing properties	Fruits, particularly darker fruits such as berries, cherries, and citrus fruits; also tomatoes, peppers, and greens
Isoflavonoids	Block estrogen receptors	Soy and other legumes
Lignans	Antioxidants Modulate hormone receptors	Flaxseed and flaxseed oil; whole grains, nuts, and seeds.
Limonoids	Enhance detoxification Block carcinogens	Citrus fruits, celery
Polyphenols	Antioxidants Block carcinogen formation Modulate hormone receptors	Green tea, chocolate, red wine
Sterols	Block production of carcinogens Modulate hormone receptors	Soy, nuts, seeds

---

EASY TIPS TO REACH YOUR FIVE-A-DAY GOAL

- Buy many kinds of fruits and vegetables when you shop, so you have plenty of choices.
- Stock up on frozen vegetables for easy cooking so that you always have a vegetable dish with dinner.
- Use the fruits and vegetables that go bad quickly (peaches, asparagus) first. Save hardier varieties (apples, acorn squash) or frozen goods for later in the week.
- Keep fruits and vegetables where you can see them. The more often you see them, the more likely you are to eat them.
- Keep a bowl of cut-up vegetables on the top shelf of the refrigerator.
- Make up a big tossed salad with several kinds of greens, cherry tomatoes, cut-up carrots, red pepper, broccoli, scallions, and sprouts. Refrigerate in a large glass bowl with an airtight lid, so a delicious mixed salad will be ready to enjoy for several days.
- Keep a fruit bowl on your kitchen counter, table, or desk at work.
- Treat yourself to a fruit sundae. Top a bowl of your favorite cut-up fruits with vanilla yogurt, shredded coconut, and a handful of nuts.

- Pack a piece of fruit or some cut-up vegetables in your briefcase or backpack; carry moist towelettes for easy cleanup.
- Add fruits and vegetables to lunch by having them in soup, salad, or cut-up raw.
- Use thinly sliced pears or apples in your next omelet.
- At dinner, serve steamed or microwaved vegetables.
- Increase portions when you serve vegetables. One easy way of doing so is adding fresh greens such as Swiss chard, collards, or beet greens to stir-fries.
- Choose fresh fruit for dessert. For a special dessert, try a fruit parfait with low-fat yogurt or sherbet topped with lots of berries.
- Add extra varieties of vegetables when you prepare soups, sauces, and casseroles (for example, add grated carrots and zucchinis to spaghetti sauce).
- Take advantage of salad bars, which offer ready-to-eat raw vegetables and fruits and prepared salads.
- Use vegetable-based sauces such as marinara sauce and juices such as low-sodium V-8 or tomato juice.
- Freeze lots of blueberries. They make a great summer replacement for ice cream, ice pops, and other sugary foods.

---

2. Reduce Exposure to Pesticides, Heavy Metals, and Food Additives

In the United States, more than 1.2 billion lb of pesticides and herbicides are sprayed on or added to food crops each year. That is roughly 5 lb of pesticides for each man, woman, and child. There is a growing concern that in addition to the significant number of cancers caused by the pesticides directly, exposure to these chemicals damages the body's detoxification mechanisms, thereby raising the risk of cancer and other diseases. To illustrate just how problematic pesticides can be, take a quick look at the health problems of the farmer. The lifestyle of farmers is generally healthy: compared with city dwellers, farmers have access to lots of fresh food; they breathe clean air, work hard, and have a lower rate of cigarette smoking and alcohol use. Yet studies show that farmers have a higher risk of lymphomas, leukemias, and cancers of the stomach, prostate, brain, and skin.[10–12] Exposure to pesticides may explain this.

Perhaps the most problematic pesticides are the halogenated hydrocarbons such as DDE, PCB, PCP, dieldrin, and chlordane. These chemicals persist almost indefinitely in the environment. For example, a similar pesticide, DDT, has been banned for nearly 30 years, yet it can still be found in the soil and root vegetables such as carrots and potatoes.

Our bodies have a tough time detoxifying and eliminating these compounds. Instead, they end up being stored in our fat cells. What's more, inside the body these chemicals can act like the hormone estrogen. They are thus suspected as a major cause of the growing epidemic of estrogen-related health problems, including breast cancer.[13] Some evidence also suggests that that these chemicals increase the risk of lymphomas, leukemia, and pancreatic cancer, as well as play a role in low sperm count and reduced fertility in men.[14]

Avoiding pesticides is especially important for children of preschool age. Children are at greater risk for two reasons: they eat more food relative to body mass, and they consume more foods higher in pesticide residues, such as juices, fresh fruits, and vegetables. A recent University of Washington study that analyzed levels of breakdown products of organophosphorus pesticides (a class of insecticides that disrupt the nervous system) in the urine of 39 urban and suburban children two to four years old found that concentrations of pesticide metabolites were six times lower in the children who ate organic fruits and vegetables than in those who ate conventional produce.[15]

After conducting an analysis of USDA pesticide residue data for all pesticides for 1999 and 2000, Consumers Union warned parents of small children to limit or avoid conventionally grown foods known to have high pesticide residues, such as cantaloupe, green beans (canned or frozen), pears, strawberries, tomatoes (Mexican-grown), and winter squash.[16] The University of Washington study added apples to this list.

Unfortunately, not only pesticides have entered our food supply. The EPA now maintains a list of the levels of herbicides, toxic metals (arsenic, cadmium, lead, and mercury), and even radionuclides in the foods we eat. It is beyond the scope of this book to address all of these. The bottom line is that just like pesticides, all these toxins increase our risk of almost every disease.

How to Avoid Toxins in the Diet

- Do not overconsume foods that have a tendency to concentrate pesticides, such as animal fat, meat, eggs, cheese, and milk.

- Buy organic produce, which is grown without the aid of synthetic pesticides and fertilizers. Although less than 3% of the total produce in the United States is grown without pesticides, organic produce is widely available.

- Develop a good relationship with your local grocery store produce manager. Explain your desire to reduce your exposure to pesticides, heavy metals, and waxes. Ask what measures the store takes to ensure that toxin residues are within approved limits. Ask where the store obtains its produce; make sure the store is aware that foreign produce is much more likely to contain excessive levels of pesticides as well as pesticides that have been banned in the United States.

- Try to buy local produce in season.

- Peeling off the skin or removing the outer layer of leaves of some produce may be all you need to do reduce pesticide levels. The downside is that many of the nutritional benefits of fruits and vegetables are concentrated in the skin and outer layers. An alternative measure is to remove surface pesticide residues, waxes, fungicides, and fertilizers by soaking the item in a mild solution of additive-free soap such as Ivory or pure castile soap. All-natural, biodegradable vegetable cleansers are also available at most health food stores. To use, spray the food with the cleanser, gently scrub, and rinse.

- Eat smaller, wild-caught fish rich in omega-3 fatty acids and avoid eating larger species and farmed fish with the exception of tilapia. Best choices are sardines, anchovies, small mackerel, salmon, and small tuna.

3. Eat to Support Blood Sugar Control

Concentrated sugars, refined grains, and other sources of simple carbohydrates are quickly absorbed into the bloodstream, causing a rapid rise in blood sugar. In response, the body boosts secretion of insulin by the pancreas. High-sugar junk-food diets definitely lead to poor blood sugar regulation, obesity, and ultimately type 2 diabetes and heart disease.[17–19] The stress on the body that these diets cause can promote the growth of cancer as well.

As already discussed, the glycemic index of a food refers to how quickly blood sugar levels will rise after it is eaten. However, the GI does not indicate how much carbohydrate is in a typical serving of a particular food, so another tool is needed. The glycemic load (GL) is a way to assess the effect of carbohydrate consumption that takes the GI into account but gives a fuller picture of the effect that a food has on blood sugar levels. A GL of 20 or more is high, a GL of 11 to 19 inclusive is medium, and a GL of 10 or less is low. For example, beets have a high GI but a low GL. Although the carbohydrate in beets has a high GI, the amount of carbohydrate is low, so a typical serving of cooked beets has a relatively low GI (about 5). Thus, as long as you eat a reasonable portion of a low-GL food, the impact on blood sugar is acceptable and the food will not cause blood sugar instability. For example, a diabetic can enjoy some watermelon (GI 72) as long as he or she keeps the serving size reasonable; the GL for 120 g watermelon is only 4.

In essence, foods that are mostly water (such as apples and watermelon), fiber (for example, beets and carrots), or air (such as popcorn) will not cause a steep rise in blood sugar even if their GIs are high as long as portion sizes are moderate. To help you design a healthful diet, we provide a list of the GI, fiber content, and GL of common foods in Appendix B.

4. Do Not Overconsume Animal Foods

Considerable evidence indicates that a high intake of red or processed meat increases the risk of an early death. For example, in a cohort study of half a million people age 50 to 71 at the start of the study, men and women who ate the most red and processed meat had an elevated risk for overall mortality compared with those who ate the least.[20]

Study after study seems to indicate that the higher the intake of meat and other animal products, the higher the risk of heart disease and cancer, especially cancers of the colon, breast, prostate, and lung, whereas a diet focusing on plant foods has the opposite effect.[21,22]

There are many reasons for this association. Meat lacks the antioxidants and phytochemicals that protect against cancer. At the same time, it contains lots of saturated fat and other potentially carcinogenic compounds, including pesticide residues, heterocyclic amines, and polycyclic aromatic hydrocarbons, the last two of which form when meat is cooked at high temperatures (grilled, fried, or broiled). The more well-done the meat, the higher level of amines as well.[23]

Some proponents of a diet high in meats claim that people should eat the way their "caveman" ancestors did. That argument does not really hold up. As already discussed, the meat of wild animals that early humans consumed had a fat content of less than 4%.

The demand for tender meat has led to the breeding of cattle whose meat contains 25 to 30% or more fat. Corn-fed domestic beef contains primarily saturated fats and virtually no beneficial omega-3 fatty acids (discussed later), whereas the fat of wild animals contains more than five times the polyunsaturated fat per gram and has substantial amounts (about 4–8%) of omega-3 fatty acids.

Particularly harmful to human health are cured or smoked meats, such as ham, hot dogs, bacon, and jerky, that contain sodium nitrate and/or sodium nitrite—compounds that keep the food from spoiling but dramatically raise the risk of cancer. These chemicals react with amino acids in foods in the stomach to form highly carcinogenic compounds known as nitrosamines.

Research in adults makes a convincing argument for avoiding these foods. Even more compelling is the evidence linking consumption of nitrates to a significantly increased risk of the major childhood cancers (leukemias, lymphomas, and brain cancers):

- Children who eat 12 hot dogs per month have nearly 10 times the risk of leukemia compared with children who do not eat hot dogs.[24]
- Children who eat hot dogs once a week double their chances of brain tumors; eating hot dogs twice a week triples the risk.[24]
- Pregnant women who eat two servings per day of any cured meat have more than double the risk of bearing children who will eventually develop brain cancer.[25]
- Kids who eat the most ham, bacon, and sausage have three times the risk of lymphoma.[24]

In addition, kids who eat ground meat once a week have twice the risk of acute lymphocytic leukemia compared with those who eat none; eating two or more hamburgers weekly triples the risk.[24]

Healthier Food Choices	
REDUCE YOUR INTAKE OF:	**SUBSTITUTE:**
Red meat	Fish and white meat or poultry
Hamburgers and hot dogs	Soy-based or vegetarian alternatives
Eggs	Egg Beaters and similar reduced-cholesterol products
	Tofu
High-fat dairy products	Low-fat or nonfat products
Butter, lard, other saturated fats	Olive oil
Ice cream, pies, cake, cookies, etc.	Fruits
Fried foods, fatty snacks	Vegetables, fresh salads
Salt and salty foods	Low-sodium foods, salt substitute
Coffee, soft drinks	Herbal teas, green tea, fresh fruit and vegetable juices
Margarine, shortening, and other source of trans-fatty acids or partially hydrogenated oils	Olive, macadamia nut, or coconut oil; vegetable spreads that contain no trans-fatty acids (available at most health food stores)

Fortunately, vegetarian alternatives to these standard components of the American diet are now widely available, and many of them actually taste quite good. Consumers can find soy hot dogs, soy sausage, soy bacon, and even soy pastrami at their local health food stores as well as in many mainstream grocery stores. Those who must have red meat are encouraged to eat only lean cuts of meat, preferably from animals raised on grass rather than corn or soy.

5. Eat the Right Types of Fats

There is no longer any debate: the evidence is overwhelming that a diet high in fat, particularly saturated fat, trans fatty acids, and cholesterol, is linked to heart disease and numerous cancers. Both the American Cancer Society and the National Cancer Institute recommend a diet that supplies less than 30% of calories as fat. However, just as important as the amount of fat is the type of fat consumed. The goal is to decrease total fat intake (especially intake of saturated fats, trans-fatty acids, and omega-6 fats) while increasing intake of omega-3 fatty acids and monounsaturated fatty acids.

What makes a fat "bad" or "good" has a lot to do with the function of fats in the body. Cellular membranes are made mostly of fatty acids. The type of fat consumed determines the type of fatty acid present in the cell membrane. A diet high in saturated fat (primarily from animal fats), trans-fatty acids (from margarine, shortening, and other products that contain hydrogenated vegetable oils), and cholesterol results in unhealthy cell membranes. Without a healthy membrane, cells lose their ability to hold water, vital nutrients, and electrolytes. They also lose their ability to communicate with other cells and to be controlled by regulating hormones, including insulin. Without the right type of

fats in cell membranes, cells simply do not function properly. Considerable evidence indicates that cell membrane dysfunction is a critical factor in the development of many diseases.[26–29]

One diet that provides an optimal intake of the right types of fat is the traditional Mediterranean diet—food patterns typical of some Mediterranean regions in the early 1960s, such as Crete, parts of the rest of Greece, and southern Italy. The traditional Mediterranean diet has shown tremendous benefit in preventing and even reversing heart disease and cancer as well as diabetes.[30] It has the following characteristics:

- Olive oil is the principal source of fat.
- It features an abundance of plant-based foods (fruit, vegetables, breads, pasta, potatoes, beans, nuts, and seeds).
- Foods are minimally processed, and there is a focus on seasonal and locally grown foods.
- Fresh fruit is the typical everyday dessert, sweets containing concentrated sugars or honey being consumed a few times per week at most.
- Dairy products (principally cheese and yogurt) are consumed in low to moderate amounts.
- Fish is consumed on a regular basis.
- Poultry and eggs are consumed in moderate amounts (1–4 times weekly) or not at all.
- Red meat is consumed in low amounts.
- Wine is consumed in low to moderate amounts, normally with meals.

Olive oil contains not only the monounsaturated fatty acid oleic acid but also several antioxidant agents that may account for some of its health benefits. Olive oil is particularly valued for its protection against heart disease.

It lowers the harmful low-density lipoprotein (LDL) cholesterol and increases the level of protective high-density lipoprotein (HDL) cholesterol. It also helps prevent circulating LDL cholesterol from becoming damaged by free radicals, and it has been proved to help control the elevated blood triglycerides so common in diabetes.[30]

6. Keep Salt Intake Low, Potassium Intake High

Electrolytes—potassium, sodium, chloride, calcium, and magnesium—are mineral salts that can conduct electricity when dissolved in water. For optimal health, it is important to consume these nutrients in the proper balance. For example, too much sodium in the diet from salt can disrupt this balance. Many people know that a high-sodium, low-potassium diet can cause high blood pressure and that the opposite can lower blood pressure,[31,32] but not as many are aware that the former diet also raises the risk of cancer.[33]

In the United States, only 5% of sodium intake comes from the natural ingredients in food. Prepared foods contribute 45% of our sodium intake; 45% is added in cooking, and another 5% is added at the table. You can reduce your salt intake by following these tips:

- Take the salt shaker off the table.
- Omit added salt from recipes and food preparation.
- If you absolutely must have the taste of salt, try salt substitutes such as No Salt and Nu-Salt. These products are made with potassium chloride and taste very similar to regular salt (sodium chloride).
- Learn to enjoy the flavors of unsalted foods.
- Try flavoring foods with herbs, spices, and lemon juice.

- Read food labels carefully to determine the amounts of sodium. Learn to recognize ingredients that contain sodium. Salt, soy sauce, salt brine, baking soda (sodium bicarbonate), and any ingredient with *sodium* in its name (such as monosodium glutamate) contain sodium.
- In reading labels and menus, look for words that often signal high sodium content, such as *smoked, barbecued, pickled, broth, soy sauce, teriyaki, Creole sauce, marinated, cocktail sauce, tomato base, Parmesan,* and *mustard sauce.*
- Do not eat canned vegetables or soups, which are often extremely high in sodium.
- Choose low-salt (reduced-sodium) products when available.

Most Americans' diets have a potassium-to-sodium (K:Na) ratio of less than 1:2. In other words, they ingest twice as much sodium as potassium. But experts believe that the optimal dietary K:Na ratio is greater than 5:1, which means we should be getting about ten times more potassium than we currently do. However, even this may not be optimal. A natural diet rich in fruits and vegetables can easily produce much higher K:Na ratios, because most fruits and vegetables have a K:Na ratio of at least 50:1. The average K:Na ratios for several common fresh fruits and vegetables are as follows:

Carrots	75:1
Potatoes	110:1
Apples	90:1
Bananas	440:1
Oranges	260:1

7. Avoid Food Additives

Food additives are used to prevent spoiling, add color, or enhance flavor; they include such substances as preservatives, artificial flavorings, and acidifiers. Although the government has banned many synthetic food additives, it should not be assumed that all the additives currently used in the U.S. food supply are safe. A great number of food additives remain in use that are being linked to such diseases as depression, asthma or other allergy, hyperactivity or learning disabilities in children, and migraine headaches.[34–37]

The U.S. Food and Drug Administration (FDA) has approved the use of more than 2,000 different food additives. It is estimated that the per capita daily consumption of these food additives is approximately 13 to 15 g, with the result that each of us takes in an astounding 10 to 12 lb of these chemicals every year. This leads to many questions: Which food additives are safe? Which should be avoided? An extremist might argue that no food additive is safe. However, many food additives fulfill important functions in the modern food supply. And while some are synthetic compounds with known cancer-causing effects, many substances approved as additives are natural in origin and possess health-promoting properties. Obviously, the most sensible approach is to focus on whole, natural foods and avoid foods that are highly processed.

An illustration of the problem with food additives involves one of the most widely used synthetic food colors, FD&C yellow no. 5, or tartrazine. Tartrazine is added to almost every packaged food as well as to many drugs, including some antihistamines, antibiotics, steroids, and sedatives. In the United States, the average daily per capita consumption of certified dyes is 40 mg, of which 25 to 40% is tartrazine; among children, consumption is usually much higher.

Although the overall rate of allergic reactions to tartrazine is quite low in the general population, such reactions are extremely common (20 to 50%) in individuals sensitive to aspirin as well as in other allergic individuals. Like aspirin, tartrazine is a known inducer of asthma, hives, and other allergic conditions, particularly in children. In addition, tartrazine, as well as benzoate (a preservative) and aspirin, increases the production of a compound that raises the number of mast cells in the body. Mast cells are involved in producing histamine and other allergic compounds. A person with more mast cells in the body is typically more prone to allergies. For example, more than 95% of patients with hives have a higher than normal number of mast cells.

In studies using provocation tests in patients with hives, the proportion of those with sensitivities to tartrazine and other food additives has ranged from 5 to 46%. Diets eliminating tartrazine as well as other food additives have in many cases been shown to be of great benefit to patients with hives and other allergic conditions, such as asthma and eczema.

8. Take Measures to Reduce Foodborne Illness

Foodborne illness is caused by consumption of contaminated foods or beverages. Although the food supply in the United States is one of the safest in the world, the Centers for Disease Control and Prevention estimates that 76 million people get sick in the United States each year from foodborne illness; more than 300,000 are hospitalized, and 5,000 die.[38] The microbe or toxin enters the body through the gastrointestinal tract and often causes the first symptoms there, so nausea, vomiting, abdominal cramps, and diarrhea are common symptoms in many foodborne diseases. Most cases of foodborne illness are mild, but serious diarrheal disease or other complications may occur.

More than 250 different organisms have

been documented as being capable of causing foodborne illness.[39] Most of these cases are infections by a variety of bacteria, viruses, and parasites, but poisonings can also occur as a result of ingestion of harmful toxins from organisms that have contaminated the food; for example, botulism occurs when the bacterium *Clostridium botulinum* grows and produces a powerful paralytic toxin in foods. The botulism toxin can produce illness even if the bacteria are no longer present.

Most of the common causes of foodborne infections are microorganisms frequently present in the intestinal tracts of healthy animals. Meat and poultry can become contaminated during slaughter by contact with small amounts of intestinal contents, and fresh fruits and vegetables can be contaminated if they are washed or irrigated with water that is tainted with animal manure or human sewage.

The most common causes of foodborne infections are the bacteria *Campylobacter*, *Salmonella*, and *Escherichia coli* species O157:H7 and a group of viruses called caliciviruses, also known as the Norwalk and Norwalk-like viruses. Undercooked meat and poultry, raw eggs, unpasteurized milk, and raw shellfish are the most common sources of these organisms.

The foremost measure to reduce the risk of foodborne illness is to cook meat, poultry, and eggs thoroughly. Using a thermometer to measure the internal temperature of meat is a good way to be sure that it is cooked sufficiently to kill bacteria. For example, ground beef should be cooked to an internal temperature of 160°F, poultry should reach a temperature of 185°F, and an egg should be cooked until the yolk is firm.

Also take care to avoid contaminating foods by making sure to wash hands, utensils, and cutting boards after they have been in contact with raw meat or poultry and before they touch another food. Cooked meat should be served on a clean platter, rather than put back on the one that held the raw meat. Wash fresh fruits and vegetables in running tap water. A soft-bristle brush with a little mild soap can be used. Greens can be swished in cold water as many times as needed to get them clean.

9. Drink Sufficient Amounts of Water Each Day

Water is essential for life. The average amount of water in the human body is about 10 gallons. We recommend that you drink at least 48 fl oz water per day to replace the water that is lost through urination, sweat, and breathing. Even mild dehydration impairs physiological and performance responses.[40] Many nutrients dissolve in water so they can be absorbed more easily in the digestive tract. Similarly, many metabolic processes need to occur in water. Water is a component of blood and thus is important for transporting chemicals and nutrients to cells and tissues and removing waste products. Each cell is constantly bathed in a watery fluid. Water absorbs and transports heat. For example, heat produced by muscle cells during exercise is carried by water in the blood to the surface, helping to maintain the right temperature balance. The skin cells also release water as perspiration, which helps maintain body temperature.

Several factors are thought to increase the likelihood of chronic mild dehydration: a faulty thirst "alarm" in the brain; dissatisfaction with the taste of water; regular exercise that increases the amount of water lost through sweat; living in a hot, dry climate; and consumption of caffeine and alcohol, both of which have a diuretic effect.

There is currently great concern over the U.S. water supply. It is becoming increasingly difficult to find pure water. Most of the water supply is full of chemicals, including not only chlorine and fluoride, which are routinely added, but also a wide range of toxic organic compounds and chemicals, such as PCBs, pesticide residues, and nitrates, and heavy metals such as lead, mercury, and cadmium. It is estimated that lead alone may contaminate the water of more than 40 million Americans. You can determine the safety of your tap or well water by contacting your local water company; most cities have quality assurance programs that perform routine analyses.

Nutritional Supplementation

Nutritional supplementation—the use of vitamins, minerals, and other food factors to support good health as well as to prevent or treat illness—is an important component of nutritional medicine. The key functions of nutrients such as vitamins and minerals in the human body revolve around their role as essential components in enzymes and coenzymes. One of the key concepts in nutritional

medicine is to supply the necessary support or nutrients to allow the enzymes of a particular tissue to work at optimal levels. The concept of "biochemical individuality" was developed by nutritional biochemist Roger Williams in the 1970s to recognize the wide range in humans' enzymatic activity and nutritional needs. These observations also provided the basis for *orthomolecular medicine*, as envisioned by two-time Nobel laureate Linus Pauling who coined the term to mean "the right molecules in the right amounts" (*ortho* is Greek for "right"). Orthomolecular medicine seeks to maintain health and prevent or treat diseases by optimizing nutritional intake and/or prescribing supplements.

In addition to serving as necessary components in enzymes and coenzymes, many nutrients seem to exert pharmacologic effects. Most of these effects appear to be the result of enzyme induction or inhibition. In other words, when used at levels above those required for normal physiology, nutrients can induce the manufacture of enzymes, induce enzymes to become more active, or even inhibit enzyme action. For example, the B vitamin niacin (nicotinic acid) is well known as a lipid-lowering agent when given at high

QUICK REVIEW

Follow these guidelines:

1. **Eat a "rainbow" assortment of fruits and vegetables.**
2. **Reduce exposure to pesticides, heavy metals, and food additives.**
3. **Eat to support blood sugar control.**
4. **Do not overconsume animal foods.**
5. **Eat the right types of fats.**
6. **Keep salt intake low, potassium intake high.**
7. **Reduce exposure to pesticides, heavy metals, and food additives.**
8. **Take measures to reduce foodborne illnesses.**
9. **Drink sufficient amounts of water each day.**

dosages (2–6 g per day in divided doses). Its mechanism of action appears to be inhibition of enzymes that manufacture very-low-density lipoprotein (VLDL) while stimulating the production or activity of enzymes that take up LDL in the liver. The advantage of using nutrients at pharmacological dosages is that they are more recognizable to the body and better metabolized than synthetic drugs, as evidenced by a better safety profile. Even so, the use of nutrients as pharmacological agents is closely akin to drug therapy. That being the case, it is imperative that they be used and monitored appropriately.

Final Comments

The dietary guidelines and principles that are detailed in this chapter represent our answer to the hotly debated question "What is the best diet?" After a review of every popular diet in detail as well as thousands of scientific articles on the role of diet in human health, our offering here is based on the evolutionary understanding of what constitutes the optimal diet. The bottom line for a health-promoting diet is to reduce the intake of potentially harmful substances—foods laden with empty calories, additives, and artificial sweeteners—and replace them with natural foods, preferably organically grown.

Supplementary Measures

···

Introduction

In this chapter we will explore the use of supplementary measures to support and achieve good health. We intend these to be used in conjunction with a health-promoting attitude, diet, and lifestyle. Examples of supplementary measures include pharmaceutical medications, surgeries, nutritional supplements, herbal medicines, physical therapies (chiropractic care, massage, and other bodywork), acupuncture, homeopathy, and any other treatment measure designed to support or improve health.

We divide supplementary measures into two categories: essential and adjunctive. An example of an essential supplementary measure is the use of insulin in the treatment of insulin-dependent diabetes. Without it, diabetics would either die or suffer greatly. There are numerous other examples where an appropriately used medication or surgery is absolutely essential to support good health.

Very few natural approaches are considered essential in the strict sense. Most would be classified as adjunctive. What this means is that they complement, complete, or support other therapies. For example, Saint-John's-wort extract has shown very good results in the treatment of depression. However, it is not an essential medication. We view it as an important adjunctive tool to support psychological therapies, lifestyle modification, and dietary recommendations used in the treatment of depression. You can view these adjunctive therapies as temporary crutches to be discarded when and if function is restored.

There are two supplementary measures that, while not strictly essential, could be viewed as critical based upon their tremendous impact on health—nutritional supplementation and physical care.

Nutritional Supplementation

Nutritional supplementation encompasses the use of vitamins, minerals, other food factors, and botanicals to support good health as well as prevent or treat illness. The very term *nutritional supplementation* denotes that these compounds are supplementary measures. A person cannot make up for poor dietary habits, a negative attitude, and a lack of exercise by taking pills, whether the pills are drugs or nutritional supplements. Although many nutritional supplements are effective in improving health, for the long term it is absolutely essential that attention be devoted to developing a positive mental attitude, a regular exercise program, and a healthful, whole-foods diet.

The functions of nutrients such as vitamins and minerals in the human body revolve around their role as essential components in enzymes and coenzymes. Enzymes are molecules involved in speeding up chemical reactions necessary for human bodily function. Coenzymes are molecules that help the enzymes in their chemical reactions.

Enzymes and coenzymes work to either join molecules together or split them apart by making or breaking the chemical bonds that join molecules together. One of the key concepts in nutritional medicine is to supply the necessary support or nutrients to allow all the enzymes of a particular tissue to work at optimal levels.

Most enzymes are composed of a protein along with a cofactor that is typically an essential mineral and/or vitamin. If the essential mineral or vitamin is lacking, the enzyme cannot function properly. When we provide the necessary mineral or vitamin through diet or a nutritional formula, the enzyme is then able to perform its vital function. For example, zinc is necessary for the enzyme that activates vitamin A in the visual process. Without zinc, vitamin A cannot be converted to its active form. This deficiency can result in what is known as night blindness. By supplying the body with zinc, we are performing enzyme therapy—allowing the enzyme to perform its vital function.

Many enzymes require additional support in order to perform their function. The support is in the form of a coenzyme, a molecule that functions along with the enzyme. Most coenzymes are composed of vitamins and/or minerals. Without the coenzyme, the enzyme is powerless. For example, vitamin C functions as a coenzyme to the enzyme proline hydroxylase, which is involved in collagen synthesis. Without vitamin C, collagen synthesis is impaired, resulting in failure of wounds to heal, bleeding gums, and easy bruising. There may be plenty of proline hydroxylase (the enzyme), but in order for it to function it needs vitamin C.

The Growing Popularity of Nutritional Supplementation

In the last few decades more Americans than ever are taking nutritional supplements. Research shows that over half of all Americans take some form of dietary supplement on a regular basis.[1] Why are so many Americans taking supplements? They know they are not getting all that they need from their diets and realize that supplements make them feel healthier. Numerous studies have demonstrated that most Americans consume a diet that is nutritionally inadequate. Comprehensive studies sponsored by the U.S. government (NHANES I, II, III, and 2007–8; 10-State Nutrition Survey; USDA nationwide food consumption studies; etc.) have revealed that marginal nutrient deficiencies exist in a substantial portion of the U.S. population (approximately 50%) and that for some selected nutrients more than 80% of people in certain age groups consumed less than the Reference Daily Intake or Recommended Daily Intake (RDI).

These studies indicate that most Americans are extremely unlikely to consume a diet meeting the RDI for all nutrients. In other words, while it is theoretically possible that a healthy individual can get all the nutrition he or she needs from foods, the fact is that most Americans do not even come close to meeting all their nutritional needs through diet alone. In an effort to increase their intake of essential nutrients, many Americans look to vitamin and mineral supplements. Multivitamin products—defined as dietary supplements that contain at least three vitamins (some may also contain minerals)—were the most frequently reported supplement in all the NHANES surveys.[1]

While most Americans are deficient in a

vitamin or mineral, the level of deficiency is usually not so great that obvious nutrient deficiencies are apparent. A severe deficiency disease such as scurvy (severe lack of vitamin C) is extremely rare, but marginal vitamin C deficiency is thought to be relatively common. The term *subclinical deficiency* is often used to describe marginal nutrient deficiencies. In many instances the only clue to a subclinical nutrient deficiency may be fatigue, lethargy, difficulty in concentration, a lack of well-being, or some other vague symptom. Worse, however, is that—as we extensively document in this book—chronic, long-term marginal deficiencies are an underlying cause of most of the disease we suffer in Western societies. Diagnosis of subclinical deficiencies is an extremely difficult process that involves detailed dietary or laboratory analysis. It's not worth the cost to perform these tests because they are usually far more expensive than taking a year's supply of the vitamin being tested for.

The RDI Is Not Enough

Recommended Dietary Allowances (RDAs) for vitamins and minerals were first prepared by the Food and Nutrition Board of the National Research Council in 1941. These guidelines were originally developed to reduce the rates of severe nutritional deficiency diseases such as scurvy (deficiency of vitamin C), pellagra (deficiency of niacin), and beriberi (deficiency of vitamin B_1). In the mid-1990s these guidelines were replaced with the RDIs. The RDIs show no more promise than the RDAs did in providing the public with useful information on the intake of nutrients needed for the prevention, mitigation, and treatment of a wide range of conditions and diseases.

A tremendous amount of scientific research indicates that the optimal level for many nutrients, especially the antioxidant nutrients vitamins C and E, beta-carotene, and selenium, may be much higher than the current RDIs. The RDIs focus only on the prevention of overt nutritional deficiencies in population groups; they do not define optimal intake for an individual.

The RDIs also do not adequately take into consideration environmental and lifestyle factors that can destroy vitamins and bind minerals in a way that makes them unavailable to the body. For example, even the Food and Nutrition Board acknowledges that smokers require at least twice as much vitamin C compared with nonsmokers. But what about other nutrients and smoking? And what about the effects of alcohol consumption, food additives, heavy metals, carbon monoxide, and other chemicals associated with our modern society that are known to interfere with nutrient function? The hazards of modern living may be another reason many people take supplements.

While the RDIs have done a good job of defining nutrient intake levels to prevent nutritional deficiencies, there is still much to be learned regarding the optimal intake of nutrients.

The Vitamin and Mineral Content of Conventionally Grown Foods Has Decreased Dramatically in the Past Century

Even if you are conscientiously working to eat more whole foods, it is very difficult if not impossible to get all the required nutrients from food alone. A sad fact is that conventionally grown foods do not contain as high a concentration of nutrients today as they did in the past. For example, one study showed that vitamin levels have decreased by as much as 37% from 1950 to 1999,[2] and another found that trace minerals have dropped by as much as 77% from 1940 to 1991.[3] While the researchers are arguing whether this is due to synthetic fertilizers or different types of seeds, the bottom line is that even supposedly "good" foods are depleted. Eating more organically grown foods will help, but we see no alternative to smart supplementation.

Conditionally Essential Nutrients

In addition to essential nutrients, there are a number of food components and natural physiological agents discussed in this book that have demonstrated impressive health-promoting effects. Examples include flavonoids, probiotics, carnitine, and coenzyme Q_{10}. These compounds exert significant therapeutic effects with little, if any, toxicity. More and more research indicates that these accessory nutrients, although not considered "essential" in the classical sense, play a major role in preventing illness as well as exerting specific therapeutic effects and promoting healthy aging. We refer to these compounds as "conditionally essential" to indicate that there are certain conditions where their use becomes essential in order for the body to function properly.

Some Practical Recommendations

There are four primary recommendations we make to people to help them design a foundation nutritional supplement program:

1. Take a high-quality multiple vitamin and mineral supplement.
2. Take extra plant-based antioxidants such as flavonoid extracts or "green foods."
3. Take a high-quality fish oil product to provide 1,000 mg EPA + DHA per day.
4. Take enough vitamin D (typically 2,000 to 4,000 IU per day) to elevate your blood levels to the optimal range.

Recommendation 1: Take a High-Quality Multiple Vitamin and Mineral Supplement

Taking a high-quality multiple vitamin and mineral supplement providing all of the known vitamins and minerals serves as a foundation upon which to build. Dr. Roger Williams, one of the premier biochemists of our time, states that healthy people should use multiple vitamin and mineral supplements as an "insurance formula" against possible deficiency. This does not mean that a deficiency will occur in the absence of the vitamin and mineral supplement, any more than not having fire insurance means that your house is going to burn down. But given the enormous potential for individual differences from person to person and the varied mechanisms of vitamin and mineral actions, supplementation with a multiple formula seems to make sense. The following recommendations provide an optimal intake range to guide you in selecting a high-quality multiple. (Note that vitamins and minerals are usually measured in one of three different units: IU = International Units, mg = milligrams, or mcg = micrograms.) For children up to two years of age, the dosage should be the low end of the range listed, multiplied by 20% (0.20). For example, the recommended low-end dosage for vitamin B_1 (thiamine) is 10 mg, so the daily dosage for children up to two years would be 10 mg × 0.20 = 2 mg. For

Recommendations for a Daily Multiple Vitamin and Mineral Supplement	
VITAMIN	**DAILY DOSE FOR ADULTS AND CHILDREN 9 YEARS AND OLDER**
Vitamin A (retinol)[a]	2,500–5,000 IU
Vitamin A (from beta-carotene)	5,000–25,000 IU
Vitamin B$_1$ (thiamine)	10–100 mg
Vitamin B$_2$ (riboflavin)	10–50 mg
Vitamin B$_3$ (niacin)	10–100 mg
Vitamin B$_5$ (pantothenic acid)	25–100 mg
Vitamin B$_6$ (pyridoxine)	25–100 mg
Vitamin B$_{12}$ (methylcobalamin)	400 mcg
Vitamin C (ascorbic acid)[b]	250–1,000 mg
Vitamin D[c]	1,000–2,000 IU
Vitamin E (mixed tocopherols)[d]	100–200 IU
Vitamin K$_1$ or K$_2$	60–300 mcg
Niacinamide	10–30 mg
Biotin	100–300 mcg
Folic acid	400 mcg
Choline	10–100 mg
Inositol	10–100 mg
MINERAL	**RANGE FOR ADULTS AND CHILDREN 4 YEARS AND OLDER**
Boron	1–6 mg
Calcium[e]	600–1,000 mg
Chromium[f]	200–400 mcg
Copper	1–2 mg
Iodine	50–150 mcg
Iron[g]	15–30 mg
Magnesium	250–500 mg
Manganese	3–5 mg
Molybdenum	10–25 mcg
Potassium	NA[h]
Selenium	100–200 mcg
Silica	1–25 mg
Vanadium	50–100 mcg
Zinc	15–30 mg

a. Women of childbearing age who may become pregnant should not take more than 2,500 IU of retinol per day owing to the possible risk of birth defects.

b. It may be easier to take vitamin C separately.

c. Elderly people living in nursing homes or at northern latitudes should supplement at the high range.

d. It may be more cost-effective to take vitamin E separately rather than as a component of a multiple vitamin.

e. Women who have or who are at risk of developing osteoporosis may need to take a separate calcium supplement to achieve the recommended level of 1,000 mg per day.

f. For diabetes and weight loss, doses of 600 mcg of chromium can be used.

g. Most women who have gone through menopause and most men rarely need supplemental iron.

h. The FDA restricts the amount of potassium in supplements to no more than 99 mg. Potassium needs are best met through diet and the use of potassium salts used as salt substitutes.

children two to four years old, the dosage is 40% of the low end of the range given; for children four to eight years old, the dosage is 60% of the low-end adult dosage; and for children nine years old or older the full adult dosage is sufficient.

Read labels carefully to find multiple vitamin/mineral formulas that contain doses in these ranges. Be aware that you will not find a formula that provides all of these nutrients at these levels in one single pill—it would be too big. Usually you'll need to take at least three to six tablets per day to meet these levels. While many once-daily supplements provide good levels of vitamins, they tend to be insufficient in the amount of some of the minerals they provide. Your body needs the minerals as much as the vitamins—the two work hand in hand.

WHEN TO TAKE YOUR SUPPLEMENTS

- Multiple vitamin and mineral supplements are best taken with meals. Whether you take them at the beginning or end of a meal is up to you. If you are taking more than a couple of pills, you may find that taking them at the beginning of a meal is more comfortable. Taking a handful of pills on a full stomach may cause a little stomach upset.
- Flavonoid-rich herbal extracts can be taken with meals or at any other time desired.
- "Green food" drinks make great between-meal snacks (especially if you are trying to lose a little weight, as they can quell an overactive appetite).
- Fish oil supplements are best taken at or near the beginning of a meal to avoid any fishy aftertaste—some people burp up a little of the oil if they take it at the end of the meal on a full stomach.
- Vitamin D$_3$ is best taken with meals.

Recommendation 2: Take Extra Plant-Based Antioxidants Such as Flavonoid Extracts or "Green Foods"

The terms *free radical* and *antioxidant* are becoming familiar to most health-minded individuals. Loosely defined, a free radical is a highly reactive molecule that can bind to and destroy cellular structures and blood components. Free radical (oxidative) damage is what makes us age. Free radicals have also been shown to be responsible for the initiation of many diseases, including the two biggest killers of Americans—heart disease and cancer.

Antioxidants, in contrast, are compounds that help protect against free radical damage. Antioxidant nutrients such as beta-carotene, selenium, vitamin E, and vitamin C have been shown to be very important in protecting against the development of heart disease, cancer, and other chronic degenerative diseases. In addition, antioxidants are also thought to slow down the aging process.

Based on extensive data, it appears that a combination of antioxidants will provide greater protection than a large dosage of any single antioxidant. Therefore, in addition to consuming a diet rich in plant foods (especially fruits and vegetables) and taking a high-potency multiple vitamin and mineral formula as detailed above in Recommendation 1, we recommend using some form of plant-based antioxidant to ensure broader antioxidant protection. Look to either flavonoid-rich extracts or green foods. Flavonoids are plant pigments that exert antioxidant activity and have effects that are more potent and more effective against a broader range of oxidants than the traditional antioxidant nutrients vitamins C and E, beta-carotene, selenium, and zinc. Besides lending color to fruits and flowers, flavonoids are responsible for many of the medicinal properties of foods, juices, herbs, and bee pollen.

More than 8,000 flavonoid compounds have been characterized and classified according to their chemical structure. Flavonoids are sometimes called "nature's biological response modifiers" because of their anti-inflammatory, antiallergenic, antiviral, and anticancer properties.[4]

Because certain flavonoids concentrate in specific tissues, it is possible to take flavonoids that target specific conditions. For example, one of the most beneficial groups of tissue-specific plant flavonoids are the proanthocyanidins (also referred to as *procyanidins*). These molecules are found in high concentrations (up to 95%) in grape seed and pine bark extracts. We recommend either grape seed or pine bark extract for most people under the age of 50 for general antioxidant support, as each appears to be especially useful in protecting against heart disease. For those over 50, ginkgo biloba extract is generally the best choice. If there is a strong family history of cancer, however, the best choice is clearly green tea extract (see below). Identify which flavonoid or flavonoid-rich extract is most appropriate for you and take it according to the recommended dosage. There is tremendous overlap among the mechanisms of action and benefits of flavonoid-rich extracts; the key point here is to take the one that is most specific to your personal needs.

The term *green food* refers to green tea and a number of commercially available products containing dehydrated barley grass, wheatgrass, or algae sources such as chlo-

Selecting a Flavonoid Supplement		
FLAVONOID-RICH EXTRACT	**DAILY DOSE FOR ANTIOXIDANT SUPPORT**	**INDICATION**
Green tea extract (60–70% total polyphenols)	150 to 300 mg	Systemic antioxidant. May provide the best protection against cancer; best choice if there is a family history of cancer. Also protects against damage to cholesterol molecules.
Grape seed extract or pine bark extract (95% procyanidolic oligomers)	100 to 300 mg	Systemic antioxidant; best choice for most people under age 50. Also specific for the lungs, diabetes, varicose veins, and protection against heart disease.
Ginkgo biloba extract (24% ginkgo flavonglycosides)	240 to 320 mg	Best choice for most people over the age of 50. Protects brain and vascular lining.
Milk thistle extract (70% silymarin)	200 to 300 mg	Best choice for additional antioxidant protection of liver or skin needs.
Bilberry extract (25% anthocyanidins)	160 to 320 mg	Best choice to protect the eyes.
Hawthorn extract (10% proanthocyanidins)	300 to 600 mg	Best choice in heart disease or high blood pressure

BENEFITS OF GRAPE SEED AND PINE BARK EXTRACT

The proanthocyanidins are one of the most beneficial groups of plant flavonoids. The most active proanthocyanidins are those bound to other proanthocyanidins in compounds referred to as procyanidolic oligomers (PCOs) or oligomeric proanthocyanidins (OPCs). Although PCOs exist in many foods, supplemental sources such as extracts from grape seeds (*Vitis vinifera*) and the bark of the French maritime (Landes) pine have shown significant benefits in clinical studies for the following health conditions:

Asthma
Atherosclerosis, hypertension, metabolic syndrome, and type 2 diabetes
Attention-deficit/hyperactivity disorder
Male infertility
Osteoarthritis
Periodontal disease
Varicose veins, venous insufficiency, and capillary fragility
Visual function, retinopathy, and macular degeneration

PCOs exert broad-spectrum antioxidant activity and are clinically useful in many other health conditions because of this action. A great deal of clinical research shows that supplementation with PCOs for six weeks at dosages of 150 to 300 mg considerably improves the serum (blood) total antioxidant capacity and ORAC score. Because of this effect (and others), throughout this book we recommend using grape seed extract or pine bark extract.

rella or spirulina. Mixing with water or juice rehydrates such formulas. These products—packed full of phytochemicals, especially carotenes and chlorophyll—are more convenient than trying to sprout and grow your own source of greens. An added advantage is that they tend to taste better than, for example, straight wheatgrass juice.

The green foods are particularly rich in natural fat-soluble chlorophyll—the green pigment that converts sunlight to chemical energy in plants, algae, and some microorganisms. Like the other plant pigments, chlorophyll also possesses significant antioxidant and anticancer effects. It has been suggested that chlorophyll be added to certain beverages, foods, chewing tobacco, and snuff to reduce cancer risk. A better recommendation would be to include green food products and fresh green vegetable juices regularly in the diet.

As far as product selection and dosage goes, we recommend looking at a product's stated ORAC (oxygen radical absorbance capacity) value. Although there are many categories of antioxidants, researchers often measure antioxidant activity according to its ORAC value. In general, the higher the ORAC value of a food, the more capable that food is of exerting antioxidant protection against age-related conditions. The average North American diet provides less than 1,000 ORAC units per day. However, nutritional experts recommend an intake of 3,000 to 6,000 ORAC units per day, from a variety of sources. Many of the commercially available green food products are able to deliver this high ORAC value in one or two servings. Read labels carefully and choose respected brands. There are many excellent super green food products out there.

Recommendation 3: Take a High-Quality Fish Oil Product to Provide 1,000 mg EPA + DHA per Day

One of the major advances in nutritional medicine has been the ability to produce a fish oil supplement that is a highly concentrated source of long-chain omega-3 fatty acids and also free from damaged fats (lipid peroxides), heavy metals, environmental contaminants, and other harmful compounds. These pharmaceutical-grade fish oil concentrates are so superior to earlier fish oil products that they are revolutionizing nutritional medicine. Alternatively, vegetarian sources of long-chain omega-3 fatty acids produced from algae are now available.

While most Americans eat way too much of the omega-6 oils found in meats and most vegetable oils, they suffer a relative deficiency of the omega-3 oils—a situation that is associated with an increased risk for heart disease and about 60 other conditions including cancer, arthritis, stroke, high blood pressure, skin diseases, and diabetes. Particularly important to good health are the longer-chain omega-3 fatty acids such as eicosapentaenoic acid (EPA) and docosahexaenoic acid (DHA) found in fish, especially cold-water fish such as salmon, mackerel, herring, and halibut. Although the body can convert alpha-linolenic acid (a short-chain omega-3 fatty acid found in flaxseed oil, walnuts, chia, and many other nuts and seeds) to the longer-chain omega-3s, it is not a very efficient process.[5]

Some Conditions Benefited by Fish Oil Supplementation

Allergies

Alzheimer's disease

Arthritis

Asthma

Attention-deficit/hyperactivity disorder

Autoimmune diseases (rheumatoid arthritis, lupus, MS, etc.)

Cancer (prevention and treatment adjunct)

Depression

Diabetes

Eczema

Elevated triglyceride levels

Heart disease (prevention and treatment)

High blood pressure

Inflammatory conditions (e.g., ulcerative colitis, Crohn's disease)

Macular degeneration

Menopause

Osteoporosis

Pregnancy

Psoriasis

Why are the long-chain omega-3 fatty acids so important? The answer has to do with the function of these fatty substances in cellular membranes and inflammation. A diet that is deficient in omega-3 fatty acids, particularly EPA and DHA, results in altered cell membranes. Without a healthy membrane, cells lose their ability to hold water, vital nutrients, and electrolytes. They also lose their ability to communicate with other cells and be controlled by regulating hormones. They simply do not function properly. Cell membrane dysfunction is a critical factor in the development of virtually every chronic disease, especially cancer, diabetes, arthritis, and heart disease. Not surprisingly, long-chain omega-3 fatty acids have shown tremendous protective effects against all of these diseases.[5]

Long-chain omega-3 fatty acids are also transformed into regulatory compounds known as prostaglandins. These compounds carry out many important tasks in the body. They regulate inflammation, pain, and swelling; they play a role in maintaining blood pressure; and they regulate heart, digestive, and kidney function. Prostaglandins also participate in the response to allergies, help control transmission of signals along the nerves, and help regulate the production of steroids and other hormones. Through their effects on prostaglandins and related compounds, long-chain omega-3 fatty acids can mediate many physiological processes, so they are useful in virtually every disease state as well. Eating a diet rich in omega-6 and low in omega-3 fatty acids strongly promotes inflammation, which underlies many diseases and is associated with a significantly increased risk for many cancers—most notably breast and prostate cancer.

In selecting a fish oil supplement, it is essential to use a brand that you trust. Quality control is an absolute must to ensure that the product is free from heavy metals such as lead and mercury, pesticides, lipid peroxides, and other contaminants. For general health, the recommended dosage is 1,000 mg EPA + DHA per day. Read the label carefully, as it is not 1,000 mg fish oil, but 1,000 mg EPA + DHA. For therapeutic purposes such as reducing inflammation or lowering triglyceride levels, the dosage recommendation is usually 3,000 mg EPA + DHA per day.

In addition to taking a high-quality fish oil, we think it is also a good idea to take 1 tbsp flaxseed oil per day. Flaxseed oil is unique because it contains the essential fatty acids alpha-linolenic acid (an omega-3 fatty acid) and linoleic acid (an omega-6 fatty acid) in appreciable amounts. The best way to take flaxseed oil is by adding it to foods. Do not cook with flaxseed oil, because it is easily damaged by heat and light; add it to foods after they have been cooked, or use it as a salad dressing. You can also try dipping bread into it, adding it to hot or cold cereal, or spraying it over popcorn. Here is a sample salad dressing featuring flaxseed oil:

Flaxseed Oil Basic Salad Dressing
4 tbsp organic flaxseed oil
1½ tbsp lemon juice
1 medium garlic clove, crushed
Pinch of seasoned salt or salt-free seasoning
Freshly ground pepper to taste

Place all ingredients in a salad bowl and whisk together until smooth and creamy. Jazz up this basic recipe to your own personal taste by using your favorite herbs and spices.

Recommendation 4: Take Enough Vitamin D (Typically 2,000 to 4,000 IU per Day) to Elevate Your Blood Levels to the Optimal Range

A huge and growing amount of research has now shown that vitamin D deficiency is very common (at least 50% of the general population and 80% of infants are deficient) and plays a major role in the development of many of the chronic degenerative diseases.[6–8] In fact, vitamin D deficiency may be the most common medical condition in the world, and vitamin D supplementation may be the most cost-effective strategy to improve health, reduce disease, and increase longevity. Those deficient in vitamin D have twice the rate of death and a doubling of risk for many diseases, such as cancer, cardiovascular disease, diabetes, asthma, and autoimmune diseases such as multiple sclerosis.[8,9] Vitamin D deficiency syndrome (VDDS) is a newly designated disorder linked to a myriad of health issues.

Vitamin D Deficiency Syndrome (VDDS)

- Low blood level of 25-hydroxyvitamin D (<25 ng/ml)

- Presence of at least two of the following conditions:

  o Osteoporosis

  o Heart disease

  o High blood pressure

  o Autoimmune disease

  o Chronic fatigue

  o Cancer

  o Allergies

  o Asthma

  o Psoriasis or eczema

  o Recurrent infections

Vitamin D is actually more of a prohormone than a vitamin. We produce vitamin

D_3 (cholecalciferol) in our body by the reaction of a chemical in our skin in response to sunlight. This vitamin D_3 is converted by the liver and then the kidneys to its active hormonal form, 1,25-dihydroxyvitamin D [calcitriol, or 1,25-$(OH)_2D$], which acts as a vital key to unlock binding sites on the human genome for the expression of the genetic code. The human genome contains more than 2,700 binding sites for calcitriol; those binding sites are near genes involved in virtually every known major disease.

There are two primary forms of supplemental vitamin D: D_3 (cholecalciferol) and D_2 (ergocalciferol). Supplemental vitamin D_3 is derived from either lanolin or cod liver oil extract and is the form of vitamin D that most effectively treats vitamin D deficiency. Vitamin D_2 is derived from fungal sources, so

---

RISK FACTORS FOR VITAMIN D DEFICIENCY

- **Insufficient exposure to sunlight.** Working and playing indoors, covering up with clothes or sunscreen when outside, or residing at a high latitude can make it likely that individual gets insufficient exposure to sunlight.
- **Aging.** Seniors are at greater risk due to lack of mobility (which means they may be less likely to be outside) and skin that is less responsive to ultraviolet light.
- **Darker skin.** A high incidence of vitamin D deficiency and its associated conditions in darker-skinned individuals is widely documented.
- **Breastfeeding.** Breastfeeding will result in vitamin D deficiency in the baby if the mother fails to ensure her own levels are high enough to provide for her baby's needs. When the mother is deficient, the breast-fed child will be deficient due to the low vitamin D content of the mother's breast milk.
- **Obesity.** Fat-soluble vitamin D gets trapped in fat tissue, preventing its utilization by the body.

WARNING: People with the following conditions should take vitamin D only with the guidance of a knowledgeable physician:

- Primary hyperparathyroidism
- Sarcoidosis
- Granulomatous tuberculosis
- Some cancers

---

it is sometimes referred to as vegetarian vitamin D. Unfortunately, vitamin D_2 is not naturally present in the human body and may have actions within the body different from those of vitamin D_3. So most experts prefer D_3.

The ideal method for determining the optimal dosage requires a readily available blood test for 25-hydroxyvitamin D [calcidiol, or 25-(OH)D]. While some people can achieve an optimal level with just 600 IU per day (or 20 minutes per day of sunlight exposure), others have a genetic requirement for as much 10,000 IU per day. The only way to determine where you fall is by testing. Many doctors are now routinely checking vitamin D status in their patients. You can also order a test from www.vitamindcouncil.org: you collect a small blood sample by skin prick and send it in to the lab. For optimal health, 25-(OH)D blood levels should be around 50–80 ng/ml (125–200 nmol/L).

Physical Care

A critical component of overall good health is the physical status of the body. The physical care of the human body involves addressing the following four areas:

Breathing

Posture

Bodywork

Aerobics and strength training

WHAT ABOUT PREGNANCY?

Pregnancy obviously results in an increased need for nutrients, including vitamins and minerals. Deficiency or excess of any of a number of nutrients can lead to birth defects in the baby and/or complications during pregnancy for the mother. What is a mother-to-be to do? In addition to eating a highly nutritious diet that focuses on whole, unprocessed foods, it is very important to take the following supplements:

1. A high-potency, full-spectrum prenatal multiple vitamin and mineral
2. Additional iron if needed
3. A fish oil supplement
4. Vitamin D$_3$: 2,000 to 4,000 IU per day
5. A plant-based antioxidant formula

HIGH-POTENCY MULTIPLE VITAMIN
AND MINERAL FORMULA

The discovery that folic acid supplementation in early pregnancy can reduce the incidence of neural tube defects in babies by as much as 80% has been referred to as one of the greatest discoveries of the last part of the 20th century. But folic acid is just one of many essential nutrients. What about the others? Are they less important than folic acid? Absolutely not! A deficiency of virtually any nutrient during pregnancy is going to have serious repercussions for mother and baby. Furthermore, adequate levels of key nutrients such as antioxidants, calcium, magnesium, and other B vitamins may help ensure a healthy pregnancy and delivery by preventing complications of pregnancy such as gestational diabetes and the potentially life-threatening condition preeclampsia (also known as toxemia of pregnancy).

Simply stated, taking a multiple vitamin and mineral supplement designed specifically for pregnant and lactating women makes perfectly good sense. The only caveat is to make sure that the vitamin A content is provided by beta-carotene rather than retinol. Do not take more than 3,000 IU of vitamin A per day if you are pregnant unless it is provided in the form of beta-carotene rather than as retinol. Unlike retinol, beta-carotene carries with it no toxic effects on the fetus.

ADDITIONAL IRON IF NEEDED

The dramatic increase in the need for iron during pregnancy usually cannot be met through diet alone. Supplementation is often warranted. Usually the amount of iron contained in a prenatal multiple is sufficient, but if a mother-to-be develops anemia or has evidence of low iron stores (serum ferritin is the best determination), then additional supplementation is required. Ferrous sulfate is the most popular iron supplement, but it is certainly less than ideal, as it often causes constipation or other gastrointestinal disturbance. The best forms of iron supplements are ferrous succinate, ferrous glycinate, ferrous fumarate, and ferrous pyrophosphate. Of these, we prefer ferrous pyrophosphate that is micronized (very small particle size) and then microencapsulated. The advantages of this form are that it is extremely stable, has no taste or flavor, is free from gastrointestinal side effects, and provides a sustained-release form of iron (up to 12 hours) with a high relative bioavailability, especially if it is taken on an empty stomach.

For iron deficiency during pregnancy, a woman will need to take an additional 30 mg iron twice per day between meals for best absorption. If this recommendation results in abdominal discomfort, then try the pyrophosphate form, or the supplement can be taken with meals three times per day.

FISH OIL SUPPLEMENT

Take a high-quality fish oil supplement to increase the level of omega-3 fatty acids available to the growing fetus. One of the more important omega-3 fatty acids for fetal development is DHA. In fact, DHA is essential for proper brain and eye development, as it is the primary structural fatty acid in the gray matter of the brain and retina of the eye. Take 1,000 mg EPA+DHA per day.

VITAMIN D: 2,000 TO 4,000 IU PER DAY

Maternal vitamin D deficiency is associated with a higher risk of a number of complications of pregnancy, including preeclampsia, gestational diabetes, preterm birth, fetal growth restriction, low birth weight, and maternal muscle weakness. In a double-blind trial, pregnant women in Canada were randomly assigned during their first trimester to receive 400 IU, 2,000 IU, or 4,000 IU of vitamin D$_3$ per day until delivery.[10] The percentage of women who achieved sufficient blood levels of vitamin D was significantly higher in the group that received 4,000 IU per day, and these women and their babies were less likely to have deficient or insufficient vitamin D serum levels. There were no adverse events related to the dose of vitamin D. Women with adequate levels of vitamin D have children with a significantly reduced risk of autism, allergies, asthma, and diabetes type 1.

PLANT-BASED ANTIOXIDANT FORMULA

Grape seed extract, pine bark extract, bilberry extract, green tea extract, and/or super green foods can be consumed safely at recommended dosages and offer significant health benefits for the mother and developing child.

Since the importance of regular aerobic exercise and strength training was discussed in the chapter "The Healing Power Within," the other three components are discussed here.

Breathing

Have you ever noticed how a sleeping baby breathes? With each breath the baby's abdomen rises and falls because the baby is breathing with its diaphragm. If you are like most adults, you tend to fill only your upper chest because you do not utilize the diaphragm. Shallow breathing tends to produce tension and fatigue. One of the most important methods of maintaining health as well as producing more energy and less stress in the body is breathing with the diaphragm. Try it. Take a deep, natural breath in by using your diaphragm and let it out slowly. Learn what it feels like to breathe easily and naturally using your diaphragm; you will definitely notice improved energy levels, reduced tension, and improved mental alertness.

Posture

Posture, the manner in which the body is held, is extremely important to good health. First of all, when the body is slouched, with shoulders slumped and head down, diaphrag-

matic breathing is more difficult. As a result, poor posture promotes shallow breathing and low energy levels, not to mention possible physical repercussions due to misalignment of vertebrae and/or muscle spasms. Have you noticed that when you breathe with the diaphragm, the spine becomes more erect, the shoulders are pushed back, and the head is pulled up? Energetic posture and good diaphragmatic breathing usually go hand in hand.

One of the keys to gaining more energy in your body is to assume a more energetic posture. It sends a message to the subconscious that you are energized and ready to go. Become aware of how you are holding your body as well as how you are breathing. You will probably notice that when you have low energy levels, you tend to hold your body in a tight posture with your head slightly down and shoulders slouched. When you find yourself in this position, just start breathing with your diaphragm and pull your head up by imagining a cord affixed to the top of your head gently pulling your spine and neck straight and into alignment.

By becoming aware of your breathing and your posture, you may notice a great deal of muscular tension or stress in certain areas of your body. That is where the next phase of physical care of the body comes into play—bodywork.

Bodywork

The need to touch and be touched is universal. In other countries around the world, bodywork practitioners are relied upon much more than in the United States. However, there is a growing trend among Americans toward increased popularity of bodywork treatments.

There are many different types of bodywork to choose from, including various massage techniques, chiropractic spinal adjustment and manipulation, Rolfing, reflexology, shiatsu, and many more. Fortunately, all of these techniques can provide benefits, so it is really a matter of personal preference. Find a technique or practitioner that you really like and incorporate bodywork into your routine.

Both of this book's authors are fortunate to have experienced a broad range of bodywork, from Rolfing and deep tissue massage (often referred to as sports massage) to more gentle techniques such as Trager massage, Feldenkrais, and craniosacral therapy. Our experience has led us to the conclusion that the therapist is more critical to the outcome than the technique. The technique is only a tool. The result is largely dependent upon the person using the tool. If your physical body (as well as your attitude) is in need of a tune-up, begin looking for a good chiropractor or body worker. How do you find such a person? Word of mouth is probably the best method. Ask around.

Our own personal belief is that the most effective techniques are those that teach body awareness and address underlying structural problems. We have divided these techniques into two major classifications: deep tissue work and light touch therapies. The techniques we discuss below require a practitioner to undertake extensive education and training before calling himself or herself a certified therapist.

Deep tissue work such as Rolfing and Hellerwork are probably the most powerful bodywork techniques, able to quickly create change in body posture and energy levels. Unlike massage and spinal adjustment, Rolfing and Hellerwork are focused not on the muscles and spine but rather on the fascia, the network of elastic sheathing that helps support the body, keeping bones, muscles, and organs in place. According to Rolfers and Hellerwork practitioners, the fascia can be damaged by physical injury, emotional trauma, and bad postural habits, throwing the body out of alignment. Rolfing, Hellerwork, and other deep tissue treatments attempt to bring the body back into balance, restore efficiency of movement, and increase mobility by stretching and lengthening the fascia to bring it back it to its natural form and pliability.

Rolfing or Hellerwork treatments consist of 10 or 11 sessions, each lasting between 60 and 90 minutes. Treatments are sequential, beginning with more superficial treatments and ending with deeper massage. Deep tissue treatment can be quite painful, but the rewards are worth it. Deep tissue therapies can be quite remarkable in their ability to improve breathing, posture, tolerance of stress, and energy levels. In addition, many people going through deep tissue therapy report resolution of emotional conflicts. It seems that many painful or traumatic experiences are stored in the fascia and muscles as tension. Releasing the tension and restoring freedom in the fascia can produce remarkable increases in energy levels.

If Rolfing or Hellerwork is too painful for you, there are three light touch therapies that can produce similar but more gradual results and feel incredibly pleasurable. The first technique is called Tragerwork or Trager massage. Tragerwork was the innovation of Milton Trager, M.D. According to Trager, we all develop mental and physical patterns that may limit our movements or contribute to fatigue as well as pain and tension. During a typical session, the practitioner gently and rhythmically rocks, cradles, and moves the client's body so as to encourage the client to see that freedom of movement and relaxation are entirely possible. The aim of the treatment is not so much to massage or manipulate, but rather to promote feelings of lightness, freedom, and well-being. Clients are also taught a series of exercises to do at home. Called Mentastics, these simple, dance-like movements are designed to help clients maintain and enhance the feelings of flexibility and freedom they may have experienced during the sessions.

The other "light touch" therapies that we recommend are two similar techniques: Alexander and Feldenkrais. In these methods the practitioner guides the patient to become aware of habitual and limited movement patterns and replace them with more optimal movements. Like many bodywork techniques, these techniques are difficult to describe. Basically, what these techniques teach is body awareness. The participant learns the difference between muscular tension and relaxation, and how different postures feel—restricted or free.

Final Comments

Supplementary measures can make a dramatic impact on a person's quality of health and quality of life. In some cases a supplementary measure is a primary therapy; in other situations it may be simply supporting or promoting good health. We highly recommend incorporating nutritional supplementation and physical care as essential supplementary measures to support or attain good health.

QUICK REVIEW

- **Supplementary measures are either essential or adjunctive to good health.**
- **Two supplementary measures that could be viewed as essential, based upon their tremendous impact on health, are nutritional supplementation and physical care.**
- **The components of a foundational nutritional supplement program are:**

  1. **Take a high-quality multiple vitamin and mineral supplement.**
  2. **Take extra plant-based antioxidants such as flavonoid extracts or "green foods."**
  3. **Take a high-quality fish oil product to provide 1,000 mg EPA + DHA per day.**

  4. **Take enough vitamin D_3 (typically 2,000 to 4,000 IU per day) to elevate your blood levels to the optimal range.**
- **The physical care of the human body involves the following four areas:**
  - **Breathing with the diaphragm promotes good health, higher energy levels, and feelings of less stress.**
  - **Posture is extremely important to the physical care of the body.**
  - **Bodywork can provide enormous benefits.**
  - **Exercise should include both aerobic and strength training.**

SPECIAL TOPICS

A Cellular Approach
to Health

· ·

Introduction

The underlying cause of fatigue and many diseases, especially chronic degenerative diseases, is basic cellular dysfunction. A cellular approach to health reflects the recognition that the external and internal environment of a cell and its membrane composition, communication and signaling pathways, enzymatic activity, and cellular energy production all affect the function of that cell and, in turn, the human body's tissues and organs.

A basic cellular approach to health involves supplying both nutrients essential to cellular function and key protective antioxidants to protect cellular structures from being damaged by high blood sugar levels, toxins, and inflammation. The basic dietary and nutritional supplementation guidelines given in Section II are absolutely critical in these goals. This chapter will discuss in more detail their effects on basic cellular function.

Homeostasis and Cell Membranes

One of the basic functions of a cell is to create homeostasis—the ability to maintain a constant and steady internal environment. The cell accomplishes this goal by constantly adjusting its physiological processes, much

the way a thermostat in a house will turn the heat or air-conditioning on and off. Every organism on the planet, from the simplest single-celled amoeba to the human being, relies on cellular homeostasis to sustain life.

The first step in achieving a constant internal environment is creating a healthy cell membrane—the wall between the internal cell and its external environment. Without a healthy membrane, cells lose their ability to hold water, vital nutrients, and electrolytes. They also lose their ability to communicate with other cells and be controlled by regulating hormones. They simply do not function properly. An alteration in cell membrane function can result in cell injury and death, which contribute to a number of chronic diseases. Cell membranes are composed chiefly of fatty acids derived from the diet. As a result, the composition of cell membranes and the resulting structure, function, and integrity can be influenced by dietary changes. A diet high in saturated fat (mostly from animal fats) and trans-fatty acids produces cell membranes that are much less fluid in nature than the membranes of people who eat optimal levels of monounsaturated fats (from nuts, seeds, and olive oil) and essential fatty acids, especially the omega-3 fatty acids.

Cell membranes also act as a "pool" from which fatty acids are transformed into hormone-like compounds called eicosanoids.

These compounds are responsible for regulating a wide variety of cellular processes, including inflammation, platelet aggregation, and constriction and dilation of blood vessels, as well as cardiovascular, digestive, and kidney function. Changing the type or ratio of dietary fat can produce significant changes in physiology. For example, a higher ratio of omega-3 to omega-6 fatty acids in cell membranes leads to a greater production of anti-inflammatory and brain-protective compounds known as resolvins and protectins.[1]

Research has documented that the type of fat within cell membranes plays a huge role in the risk of certain diseases. For example, several studies have shown that subjects who had a higher levels of the long-chain omega-3 fatty acids EPA + DHA in their red blood cell membranes had a 70% reduction in the risk of having a heart attack, compared with those with lower omega-3 content.[2,3] The total trans-fatty acid content of cell membranes has also been found to affect risk of cardiovascular disease: those with higher levels of trans-fatty acids in their red blood cells had a threefold increase in the risk of having a heart attack.[4]

The type of fatty acids in cell membranes also is a significant factor in how hormones affect cells. For example, long-chain omega-3 fatty acids and monounsaturated fats appear to improve the response to the hormone insulin, while saturated fats, trans-fatty acids, and too much cholesterol in cell membranes have the opposite effect.[5–9] Insulin not only facilitates the proper utilization of glucose (sugar) but also plays a role in other aspects of cellular function and nutrition: the transport of vitamin C into cells requires insulin,[10] and insulin has been shown to affect protein metabolism as well as the transport of a number of amino acids, neurotransmitters, nutrients, and other molecules across the cell membrane.[11–16]

A system called the sodium-potassium pump is one of the key mechanisms for achieving cellular homeostasis. This system pumps three sodium ions out of the cell for every two potassium ions that it pumps in. In doing so, it helps maintain three important cell characteristics—resting electrical potential, pH, and cellular volume. It also plays a role in many more cellular functions, including cell communication, antioxidant protection, and regulation of other important cellular ions such as calcium. This simple pump utilizes about 33% of a cell's daily energy production. For nerve cells, it is even more critical, and is responsible for nearly 70% of the nerve cell's energy expenditure. Obviously, impairment of the sodium-potassium pump is severely detrimental to the health of the cell.

The sodium-potassium pump can get damaged in several ways. For example, an elevation in blood sugar (hyperglycemia, as occurs in diabetes or after a large intake of high-sugar foods) is known to induce the production of inflammatory proteins, increase oxidative damage, and lead to the binding of glucose to cellular proteins (glycosylation), and any one of these potential mechanisms can lead to damage of the sodium-potassium pump. Other ways the pump can be damaged include oxidative damage and lack of oxygen (hypoxia). Oxygen is required for normal cellular function. When oxygen is lacking, significant tissue damage occurs—that is what happens in a heart attack or stroke. On the other side of the sword, highly reactive oxygen-containing molecules lead to free radical or oxidative damage. That is where antioxidants come into play.

Antioxidants

Antioxidants are compounds that protect against cellular damage caused by free radicals and other toxins. Loosely defined, a free radical is a highly reactive oxygen-containing molecule that can destroy body tissues, especially cell membranes. All atoms contain small particles, called electrons, that rotate around the atom's nucleus (center). Normally electrons come in pairs, but sometimes molecules will lose an electron. During the production of cellular energy, for example, it is common for one of the electrons of an oxygen atom to get stripped away. Because of this unpaired electron, the oxygen atom—now a free radical—becomes unstable and goes on a frantic search to find another electron to complete the set. In the process, though, it can destroy the molecule it has robbed of an electron. This process is known as oxidation, and it is responsible for a cut apple's turning brown or a car's becoming rusty. Damage by free radicals is what makes us age, and free radicals are partly responsible for many diseases, including the two leading killers of Americans, heart disease and cancer.

Antioxidants, in contrast, are compounds that protect against free radical damage. They work by "calming down" the free radical, lending it one of its own electrons and thus putting an end to its rampage. By mopping up free radicals, antioxidants prevent damage to cell structures and DNA (the genetic material in the nucleus of the cell).

There are three main points to keep in mind in seeking to increase antioxidant protection:

- The antioxidant system of the body relies on a complex interplay of many different dietary antioxidants.
- Taking any single antioxidant nutrient is not enough. Total protection requires a strategic, comprehensive dietary and supplement program.
- Although dietary supplements are important, they cannot replace a diet rich in antioxidants.

Mitochondrial Function and Energy Production

Mitochondria are among the most important compartments (organelles) within a cell. They are miniature energy factories, responsible for producing 97% of the body's chemical energy. Mitochondria also play an essential role in other cellular processes. On average there are 300 to 400 mitochondria per cell, but very active cells, such as those in the brain, muscle tissue, and liver, have hundreds of thousands of mitochondria per cell.[17]

Mitochondria also have their own DNA (mtDNA), which is inherited from the mother only. In other words, while the DNA that resides in the nucleus of cells in your body is composed of strands from both your mother and your father, the mitochondria in your cells also have DNA, which comes only from your mother. Mitochondria will grow and multiply to meet increased energy requirements. Sometimes, however, mitochondrial energy production appears to be insufficient to meet energy demands. There is a growing list of health conditions thought to be the result of impaired mitochondrial function.

Because mitochondria are the energy-producing part of the cell, mitochondrial DNA and mitochondrial membranes are particularly exposed to damage from reactive oxygen-containing molecules: mtDNA is damaged at a frequency nearly 20 times greater than that for nuclear DNA.[18] This increased damage, combined with a lack of protective molecules known as histones as well as a lack of DNA repair activity, leads to a 17-fold higher mutation rate in mtDNA than in nuclear DNA. The progressive accumulation of mutations over a lifetime is thought to lead to a decline in mitochondrial energy production, and has been proposed as a theory behind the aging process.[19]

When the accumulation of damage to mitochondrial tissue and mtDNA leads to loss of mitochondrial energy production efficiency, the stage is set for a vicious circle. Oxidative damage causes mutations in mtDNA, alterations in cell signaling pathways, and increased leakage of high-energy intermediate molecules, resulting in decreased energy production. Energy depletion, with consequent cellular dysfunction and inflammation, leads to tissue dysfunction, aging, and degenerative disease, as well as an increase in reactive oxygen-containing molecules and a depletion of cellular antioxidants such as glutathione. And because there are now fewer cellular antioxidants available to combat oxidative stress, further cell damage occurs. Many diseases have been associated with mitochondrial damage, including Alzheimer's disease and other types of dementia, Parkinson's disease, epilepsy, autism, chronic fatigue syndrome, cardiovascular disease, diabetes, and migraine headache.[20–24]

Mitochondrial Optimization Strategies

To optimize cellular function, it is critical to promote proper mitochondrial function and maintain energy production. To accomplish this goal, a three-part strategy is recommended: provide nutrients needed for optimal mitochondrial function, increase intake of the antioxidants that best protect the mitochondria, and reduce exposure to factors that damage mitochondria. The first two goals are achieved in most situations by following the guidelines for foundational nutritional supple-

ments given in the chapter "Supplementary Measures." When it comes to reducing exposure to factors that damage mitochondria, unfortunately, the task is a bit harder. There is a long list of factors that can damage the mitochondria. Aging, cigarette smoke, and elevated blood sugar levels all contribute to mitochondrial damage, as do a long list of environmental toxins, including cyanide, carbon monoxide, ozone, heavy metals such as cadmium and mercury, and various herbicides and pesticides.[25–27] Additionally, many drugs are known to poison the mitochondria, including various antibiotics, beta-blockers, migraine medications, L-dopa, and statins.[28,29]

Of these drugs, the most commonly used by far are the statins. Statins work to lower cholesterol by blocking an enzyme (HMG-CoA reductase) that produces a compound (mevalonate) that is the direct precursor to cholesterol (see the figure on page 89). The problem is that statins inhibit the production of not only cholesterol but a whole host of other substances that have important bodily biochemical functions, including coenzyme Q_{10}.

Coenzyme Q_{10} (CoQ_{10}) is a critical component in the manufacture of energy within the cells. Although the body makes some of its own CoQ_{10}, considerable research shows significant benefits from supplementation, especially in people with any sort of heart disease, including high cholesterol levels, congestive heart failure, angina, and high blood pressure.

Since statin drugs reduce the production of CoQ_{10}, they have the potential to produce some serious consequences in organs such as the heart, liver, muscles, and brain, which require large amounts of CoQ_{10} to function properly. The research seems to support this observation, since the serious side effects of statin drugs (muscle, brain, pancreatic, liver, and sexual dysfunction) appear to be related

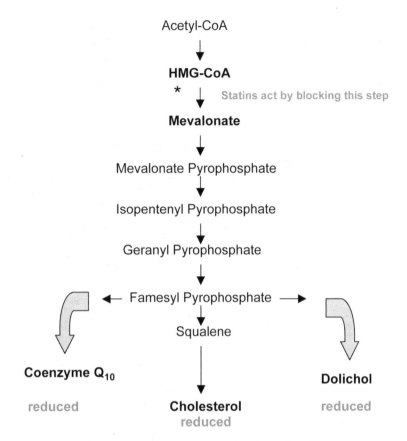

Acetyl-CoA

↓

HMG-CoA

*   ↓   Statins act by blocking this step

Mevalonate

↓

Mevalonate Pyrophosphate

↓

Isopentenyl Pyrophosphate

↓

Geranyl Pyrophosphate

↓

← Famesyl Pyrophosphate →

Squalene

Coenzyme Q$_{10}$ **Dolichol**

reduced   **Cholesterol**   reduced

reduced

Cholesterol Manufacture in the Liver Showing the End Products Affected by Statin Drugs

to lowering CoQ$_{10}$ levels and reducing mitochondrial function.[30]

Interestingly, deaths attributed to heart failure have nearly doubled since 1989—a year after statins first hit the market in a big way. If you are taking a statin drug or any of the other drugs known to impair mitochondrial function, you definitely need to supplement with CoQ$_{10}$.

A Closer Look at CoQ$_{10}$

CoQ$_{10}$ is an essential component of the mitochondria and plays a critical role in the production of energy within the body's cells. A good analogy for the role of CoQ$_{10}$ in the body is the role of a spark plug in a car engine. Just as the car cannot function without that initial spark, the human body cannot function without CoQ$_{10}$. Coq$_{10}$ is also a very important antioxidant that protects against mitochondrial and cellular damage.

Although CoQ$_{10}$ can be synthesized within the body, there are a number of circumstances where the body simply does not make sufficient amounts. As the brain, heart, and muscles are among the most metabolically active tissues in the body, a CoQ$_{10}$ deficiency affects these tissues the most and can lead to serious problems there. Deficiency could be a result of impaired CoQ$_{10}$ synthesis caused by nutritional deficiencies, environmental exposure, taking various prescription drugs, a genetic or acquired defect in CoQ$_{10}$ synthesis, or increased tissue needs. Diseases that increase the need for CoQ_{10} are primarily heart and vascular diseases, including high cholesterol levels and high blood pressure. In addition, people over the age of 50 may have increased CoQ_{10} requirements, as levels are known to decline with advancing age.[31–35]

Given the central role of CoQ_{10} in mitochondrial function and cellular antioxidant protection, its clinical applications are extensive. There are many conditions where CoQ_{10} may offer benefit, so there is no question that it should be considered a conditionally essential nutrient required to restore health. Specific clinical contexts for the use of CoQ_{10} include:

- General antioxidant
- Cardiovascular disease
  - High blood pressure
  - Congestive heart failure
  - Cardiomyopathy
  - Protection during cardiac surgery
  - High cholesterol being treated by drugs, especially statins
- Cancer (to boost immune function and/or offset chemotherapy side effects)
- Diabetes
- Male infertility
- Alzheimer's (prevention)
- Parkinson's disease (prevention and treatment)
- Periodontal disease
- Macular degeneration
- Migraine headache

The therapeutic use of CoQ_{10} has been clearly documented in both animal studies and human trials for the conditions listed above, especially cardiovascular disease.[36,37] Biopsy results from heart tissue in patients with various cardiovascular diseases showed a CoQ_{10} deficiency in 50 to 75% of cases. Correction of a CoQ_{10} deficiency can often produce dramatic clinical results in patients with any kind of heart disease, but most often it takes some time to see benefit. For example, the effect of CoQ_{10} on lowering blood pressure is usually not seen until after 4 to 12 weeks of therapy, and the typical reductions in both systolic and diastolic blood pressure with CoQ_{10} therapy in patients with high blood pressure are modest, in the 10% range.[38]

Commercially, CoQ_{10} is primarily produced by a yeast fermentation process. CoQ_{10} exists in two interchangeable chemical forms, ubiquinone and ubiquinol. About 95% of the CoQ_{10} in the body is in the ubiquinol form. However, ubiquinone can be easily converted to ubiquinol.

Until recently CoQ_{10} as a dietary supplement has been available as only ubiquinone. Ubiquinone is insoluble in water and is difficult to absorb when given on an empty stomach. However, when ubiquinone is given with food (especially with oils), it is absorbed at least twice as well as on an empty stomach.[39] Ubiquinol became available as a dietary supplement in the United States in 2007. There is no question that ubiquinol has greater solubility and as a result greater bioavailability than ubiquinone, but exactly how much better it is absorbed remains to be answered.[40,41] In the only published study at this point that looked at ubiquinol absorption, it was always given in a total of 10 capsules a day that included the emulsification agents diglycerol monooleate, canola oil, soy lecithin, and beeswax.[41] It is possible that ubiquinone may have fared almost as well as the ubiquinol given the significant amount of oil and emulsifiers consumed along with the ubiquinol. Curiously, the study did not directly compare ubiquinol with ubiquinone by having a group take ubiquinone in the exact same capsules.

Estimated Daily Dosage Requirements for Different Popular Forms of CoQ_{10}				
TARGET	**COQ_{10} SOFTGELS**	**Q-GEL**	**BIOQ10 SA**	**UBIQUINOL**
Normal blood levels (0.7–1.0 mcg/ml)	50–100 mg	50–75 mg	25–50 mg	25–50 mg
General support for the body (2.5 mcg/ml)	150–200 mg	125–175 mg	100–150 mg	100–150 mg
Brain support (3.5 mcg/ml)	300–400 mg	250–300 mg	150–200 mg	150–200 mg
Price per 100 mg*	$0.20	$0.50	$0.40	$0.80

*Approximate price in 2012.

Before jumping on the ubiquinol bandwagon, realize that ubiquinone has an extensive history of successful use, particularly in oil-based soft gelatin capsules (softgels). Furthermore, several technologies are now used to enhance the bioavailability of ubiquinone, such as particle size reduction (nanonization) and solubility enhancement by use of emulsifying agents (as in Q-Gel), carriers, and self-emulsifying systems.[42] For example, complexing ubiquinone to a soy peptide (as in BioQ10 SA) provides exceptional bioavailability, as the soy peptide emulsifies the CoQ_{10} and helps usher it into the bloodstream.[43]

Based upon existing data from published clinical studies, it is possible to calculate the approximate blood levels of CoQ_{10} produced by different commercial forms. This helps in calculating the dosage of CoQ_{10} needed to achieve targeted blood levels. For example, with people who are taking a statin drug or those seeking general antioxidant support, the goal is to achieve a blood level of CoQ_{10} slightly above the normal level, which is 0.7–1.0 mcg/ml. For people with cardiovascular disease, periodontal disease, or other conditions not involving the brain, the target is 2.5 mcg/ml. And for brain conditions such

CONDITIONALLY ESSENTIAL NUTRIENTS

There is a growing list of compounds that we typically make in sufficient quantities, but situations exist where because of either a health issue, genetics, a drug, or some other factor a person may not be able to manufacture enough to keep up with demand. Since an essential nutrient is a nutrient required for normal body functioning that either cannot be synthesized by the body or cannot be made in amounts adequate for good health, we have come up with the term *conditionally essential nutrients* to describe these situations. The long-chain omega-3 fatty acids, CoQ_{10}, and glucosamine are classic examples of conditionally essential nutrients. Here is a list of others:

GLUCOSAMINE	COENZYME Q10	CARNITINE	SAME
Lutein	Glutamine	Melatonin	Phosphatidylserine
Glutathione	5-HTP	Arginine	Hyaluronic acid
Ribose	Beta-alanine	GABA	Glycerophosphocholine
Choline	Inositol	Betaine	Nucelotides
Tocotrienols	Carnosine	Alpha-lipoic acid	Beta-alanine

as Parkinson's disease, the dosage target is at least 3.5 mcg/ml. The chart on page 91 provides the dosage recommendations for the various forms. Keep in mind that divided dosages (taking the CoQ_{10} two to three times per day) with meals will result in higher blood levels compared with a single dose, especially at higher dosage levels.

Acid-Base Values and Human Health

For the body to function properly, it must maintain the proper balance of acidity and alkalinity (pH) in the blood and other body fluids. There is accumulating evidence that certain disease states, such as osteoporosis, rheumatoid arthritis, gout, and many others, are influenced considerably by dietary acid-alkaline balance. For example, osteoporosis may be the result of a chronic intake of acid-forming foods consistently outweighing the intake of alkali-producing foods, with the result that the bones are constantly forced to give up their alkaline minerals (calcium and magnesium) in order to buffer the excess acid.

For most people, the achievement of proper pH balance is quite simple: make sure that you have a higher intake of alkali-producing foods than of acid-producing foods. Basically, an alkaline diet is one that focuses on vegetables, fruit, and legumes while avoiding overconsumption of grains, meat, dairy, and most nuts except hazelnuts (filberts). Keep in mind that there is a difference between acidic foods and acid-forming foods. For example, while foods such as lemons and other citrus fruits are acidic, they actually have an alkalizing effect on the body. What is important is the pH of the metabolic end products after the food has been digested. For example, the citric acid in citrus fruit is metabolized in the body to its alkaline

form (citrate) and may even be converted to bicarbonate, another alkaline compound. Appendix C provides a brief table on the acid or alkaline effect of common foods.

In addition to diet, mineral supplements in which the minerals are bound to citrate, carbonate, and other alkaline compounds can also be used to promote an alkaline pH. In one study, supplementation with alkaline minerals was shown to influence symptoms in patients with low back pain.[44] Eighty-two patients with chronic low back pain received a daily alkaline multimineral supplement over a period of four weeks in addition to their usual medication. Pain symptoms were quantified with a standard pain rating scale. After four weeks of supplementation, the mean pain rating dropped by 49%, and 76 out of 82 patients showed a significant reduction in low back pain. Improvements paralleled increases in total blood pH, though blood pH rose only slightly, from 7.456 to 7.470 (this was not surprising, as the body works extremely hard to maintain blood pH within a very narrow range). Interestingly, only intracellular magnesium increased (by 11%), while the levels of other minerals were not significantly changed, and the level of serum magnesium was actually slightly reduced after the supplementation (−3%).

Supplementation with alkaline mineral compounds may help with many other minor aches or pains. Think about all of the people who may be putting their health at risk by taking various pain relievers and anti-inflammatory drugs for these aches and pains. Eliminating their pain may be as simple as restoring proper pH control.

In addition to alkaline mineral supplements, green foods are exceptional in their ability to promote proper pH control. Perhaps the best method to take advantage of this action is to consume green food products—commercially available products containing dehydrated barley grass, wheatgrass, or algae sources such as chorella or spirulina. Mixing with water or juice rehydrates such formulas. These products not only promote proper pH but are packed full of phytochemicals, especially carotenes and chlorophyll, and are more convenient than trying to sprout and grow your own source of greens.

QUICK REVIEW

- A basic cellular approach to health involves first supplying essential critical nutrients required for cellular function and then supplying key antioxidants to protect cellular structures from damage by high blood sugar levels, toxins, and inflammation.

- One of the basic functions of a cell is to create homeostasis—the ability to maintain a constant and steady internal environment.

- Without a healthy membrane, cells lose their ability to hold water, vital nutrients, and electrolytes.

- Research has documented that the type of fat within cell membranes plays a huge role in the risk of certain diseases.

- Long-chain omega-3 fatty acids and monounsaturated fats in cell membranes appear to improve the response to the hormone insulin, while saturated fats, trans-fatty acids, and too much cholesterol in cell membranes have the opposite effect.

- The sodium-potassium pump is an important mechanism for achieving cellular homeostasis.

- An elevation in blood sugar (hyperglycemia) induces the production of inflammatory proteins, increases oxida-tive damage, and leads to the binding of glucose to cellular proteins (glycosylation), any one of which can damage the sodium-potassium pump.

- The antioxidant system of the body relies on a complex interplay of many different dietary antioxidants.

- Taking any single antioxidant nutrient is not enough. Total protection requires a strategic, comprehensive dietary and supplement program.

- Although dietary supplements are important, they cannot replace a diet rich in antioxidants.

- Mitochondria are the energy factories of the body, responsible for producing 97% of the body's chemical energy.

- Many diseases have been associated with mitochondrial damage: Alzheimer's disease and other types of dementia, Parkinson's disease, autism, chronic fatigue syndrome, cardiovascular disease, diabetes, and migraine headache.

- To optimize mitochondrial function, a three-part strategy is recommended: provide nutrients needed for optimal mitochondrial function, increase antioxidant intake, and reduce exposure to factors that damage mitochondria.

- CoQ_{10} is an essential component of the

mitochondria and plays a critical role in the cellular production of energy.

- Although the body makes some of its own CoQ_{10}, considerable research shows significant benefits from supplementation, especially in people with any sort of heart disease, including high cholesterol levels, congestive heart failure, angina, and high blood pressure.

- Achieving optimal pH balance through diet and supplementation is an important health goal.

Cancer Prevention

Introduction

No other disease strikes as much fear deep within our souls as cancer. The reason? Almost all of us have witnessed firsthand the ravaging effects of cancer, as well as chemotherapy and radiation, on a loved one. Cancer statistics in the United States present us with some sobering facts:

- More than 1.25 million new cases of invasive cancer will be diagnosed each year.

- An additional 1.5 million new cases of noninvasive cancers will be diagnosed each year.

- More than 500,000 people will die from cancer each year.

- Cancer causes one in five of all deaths.

- Cancer will affect one out of every three people alive today.

- Of those diagnosed with cancer, 50% will die of their disease.

- The annual economic toll of cancer is more than $110 billion.[1]

Despite dedicating significant resources to the battle against cancer, conventional medicine alone has had very limited success against this disease. Granted, there have been some tremendous advances for a few of the less common cancers, but for the most part we are losing the war on cancer—more people are dying of cancer today in America than ever before.

We've all heard it said: "An ounce of prevention is worth a pound of cure." When it comes to cancer, that old saying carries a ton of truth. There is no guarantee, but the basic strategy for cancer prevention is reducing or eliminating as many risk factors associated with cancer as possible while at the same time focusing on those health habits, dietary factors, lifestyle components, and attitudes that are linked to a reduced risk of getting cancer.

Understanding and Preventing Cancer

To understand how natural prevention strategies are effective in preventing cancer, it helps to know some basic facts about the cells in your body and cancer. Your body contains trillions of cells. Within each cell is a central core known as the nucleus. Inside the nucleus lies the key to life itself: a long, twisted molecule of deoxyribonucleic acid, better known as DNA. Put simply, DNA contains the instructions (the genes) that the cell needs to make its vital proteins as well as replicate itself. Abnormal changes in a cell's DNA are called *mutations*. Usually cells with mutations recognize they are damaged and simply die—a process called apoptosis. But sometimes they continue to divide at a rapid, uncontrolled rate to form clumps of cells that grow into the mass of tissue we call a tumor. There are two types of tumors: benign and malignant.

- Benign tumors are not cancerous because the cells are normal (they have not mutated) and do not usually pose a threat to life. They can usually be surgically removed or treated with drugs. Cells from benign tumors do not spread to other parts of the body.

- Malignant tumors are cancerous. Their mutated cells divide without control or order, and they can invade and damage nearby tissues and organs. Also, cancer cells can break away from a malignant tumor and enter the bloodstream or the lymphatic system, forming new tumors in other organs.

Mutations are usually the result of DNA molecules coming into contact with free radicals—highly reactive atoms that can destroy or alter body structures, including DNA. Free radicals assault us from all directions. Some of these come from our environment, in pollutants such as chemicals or cigarette smoke; others come from our diet, in the form of fats damaged by frying or nitrates in smoked or cured meats. Even sunlight produces free radical damage. But free radicals also result from the cell's own metabolic activity. Most carcinogens (cancer-causing compounds) are dangerous because they cause severe free radical or oxidative damage to DNA.

Fortunately, nature counteracts free radicals and the oxidation they cause by neutralizing them with other molecules known as *antioxidants*. By mopping up free radicals, antioxidants are powerful weapons in the fight against cancer and other degenerative diseases. So if you want to reduce your risk of cancer, it's important to:

- Reduce free radical formation in the body.

- Limit exposure to dietary and environmental sources of free radicals.

- Increase your intake of antioxidant nutrients and other substances that support immune function.

Identifying Risk Factors

Cancer risk factors fall into two main categories: inherited and environmental. There's not a lot we can do to eliminate genetic risk factors, because they're passed on from generation to generation and are present at birth. However, inherited genetic defects are responsible for only about 15% of all cancers. This statistic means that approximately 85% of all cancers result from environmental risk factors, such as diet, lifestyle, and exposure to harmful substances.

In assessing the likelihood that an individual will develop a certain disease, specialists in epidemiology (observational and statistical studies of people and diseases) use a concept known as *relative risk*. Relative risk (abbreviated RR) is a number that shows how much more likely it is that individuals who possess a certain trait will develop a condition, compared with individuals who do not share that trait. For example, someone whose RR is 1.5 is 50% more likely to develop a condition than someone whose RR is 1. A relative risk of 2 means you are twice as likely (100% more likely), and so on.

Here's one dramatic statistic that should make the point. Compared with nonsmokers, cigarette smokers are said to have a relative cancer risk of 10—in other words, they are 10 times, or 1,000%, more likely to get lung cancer than someone who never smoked.

A few words of caution: relative risk is a statistic that's used to compare large numbers of people. So we cannot with any certainty predict your specific (absolute) risk as an individual. Some nonsmokers get lung cancer, while some smokers never develop the disease. If you are a nonsmoker, we have no idea if you will be, among every 10 people who develop lung cancer, the 1 who doesn't smoke. If you are a smoker, we cannot accurately predict if you will be the rare smoker who evades the disease.

This chapter discusses the main cancer risk factors and then offers a self-assessment survey. By completing that survey, you'll be able to evaluate your risk of developing certain cancers. The higher the rating, the more aggressive your primary prevention strategies will need to be.

Genetic Factors

Studies on identical twins (who share the exact same DNA) confirm the point we made above, that most cancers do not arise from genetic defects. Instead, diet and lifestyle play a more significant role. Surprisingly, that's true even for cancers that tend to run in families. Still, researchers have identified about 30 genetic defects that increase the risk

for certain cancers. Some of these cancers are rare; they also tend to be types that develop more often in childhood.

Age

It's a fact of life: the older you are, the more likely you are to develop cancer. As we age, our cells become less proficient at repairing damage to our DNA. As a result, there are more cells present in the body that possess mutations and that are prone to develop cancer. In the year 2000, more than 60% of new cancer cases and more than 70% of all cancer-related deaths occurred in people over the age of 65.

Family History

Some (but not most) cancers seem to run in families. For example, if a woman has two first-degree relatives (mother, aunt, or sister) who developed breast cancer, her risk for breast cancer is two to five times greater

---

SHOULD YOU HAVE GENETIC TESTING?

Perhaps the best-known example of cancer with a genetic basis is an inherited mutation in two genes whose function is to suppress the development of breast cancer. Overall, these mutated genes (known as BRCA1 and BRCA2) are responsible for about 10% of all cases of the disease. A little more than half of women who inherit mutations in these genes will develop breast cancer by age 70. These women also have a greater risk of ovarian cancer.

If you have a strong family history of cancer, it's worthwhile to talk to your doctor about blood tests that can identify genetic mutations. It's important to understand and weigh the benefits and risks of genetic testing before these tests are done. Testing is expensive, and some health plans do not cover the costs. There is concern that people with abnormal genetic test results will not be able to get

life insurance, or coverage may be available only at a much higher cost.

We do not recommend genetic testing as a cancer screening method. This advice is especially true with respect to identifying the mutated BRCA genes, since only about one woman out of 850 carries these mutations. From the public health perspective, not enough women at risk would be identified to justify the enormous cost of widespread testing. In addition, even if you have the BRCA1 or BRCA2 mutation, you still have only about a 50/50 chance of developing breast cancer before the age of 70.

If you elect to undergo genetic testing and a mutated gene is found, you will need to be more aggressive in your prevention plan and schedule more frequent exams to monitor for early signs of cancer.

than that of a woman without such a family history. The same sort of relationship exists concerning prostate cancer in men.

Race

Overall, black Americans are more likely to develop cancer than persons of other racial and ethnic groups (see the table below). The incidence of certain types of cancers also varies by race. Compared with other groups, black men are more likely to have cancers of the prostate, colon and rectum, and lung. In fact, black men have at least a 50% higher rate of prostate cancer than any other group. In contrast, breast cancer rates are highest among white women (114 per 100,000) and lowest among Native American women (33.4 per 100,000).

Overall Incidence of Cancer Among Ethnic/ Racial Groups[2]	
GROUP	**RATE (PER 100,000)**
Blacks	445
Whites	402
Asians/Pacific Islanders	280
Hispanics	273
Native Americans	153

Some of the differences in cancer rates among racial and ethnic groups may be due to factors associated with social class rather than race or ethnicity. Such factors include education, access to health care, occupation, income, and exposure to harmful substances in the environment. Diet is also critical to look at in evaluating data on race and cancer.

Medical History

Sometimes, having one disease can increase your risk for developing another. Diseases known to increase the risk of certain cancers include alcoholism, chronic hepatitis, diabetes, history of genital warts, HIV infection, inflammatory bowel disease (Crohn's disease and ulcerative colitis), and peptic ulcer. The presence of any of these conditions requires a more concerted effort to reduce cancer risk.

Hormonal Factors

Certain cancers, most notably prostate and breast cancer, are affected by hormonal factors. In prostate cancer, the primary hormonal factor is testosterone, while in breast cancer the hormone of concern is estrogen. For more information, see the chapter "Breast Cancer (Prevention)," or the chapter "Prostate Cancer (Prevention)."

Environmental Factors

As described above, exposure to tobacco smoke is a leading cause of cancer, especially lung cancer. A long and growing list of other environmental factors linked to certain cancers includes pesticides, herbicides, heavy metals, asbestos, solvents, and possibly exposure to electrical power lines. The risk depends on the concentration, intensity, and duration of exposure. Substantial increases in risk have been demonstrated in occupational settings where workers have been exposed to high concentrations of certain chemicals, metals, and other substances.

Certain Medical Treatments

Sometimes medical treatment increases the risk of certain cancers. For example, radiation therapy and many chemotherapy drugs carry with them an increased risk for producing new cancers later on. Estrogen and oral contraceptives have been linked to an increased risk of breast cancer. The term *iatrogenic* refers to diseases that arise inadvertently as a result of medical or surgical treatment.

Lifestyle Factors

The importance of a healthful lifestyle in cancer prevention cannot be overstated. The key components are avoiding tobacco use and exposure to cigarette smoke; exercising regularly; and avoiding alcohol or drinking only moderate amounts.

Smoking

The evidence is overwhelming that smoking is the most preventable cause of cancer and premature death in the United States. Smoking is responsible for nearly 90% of all lung cancers. Lung cancer mortality rates are more than 20 times higher for current male smokers and 12 times higher for current female smokers compared with people who have never smoked. Smoking is also associated with an increased risk for virtually every other cancer and accounts for at least 30% of all cancer deaths. Smoking is also a major cause of heart disease (the leading cause of death in the United States), strokes, chronic bronchitis, and emphysema.

Passive smoking—exposure to secondhand smoke—is an important risk for cancer (particularly lung and breast cancer) and is an even greater risk for causing heart disease. People who don't smoke but who inhale smoke from the environment may be even more susceptible to the free radical damage the chemicals in smoke cause to their heart and arteries, because their bodies just aren't used to dealing with such a heavy toxic load. One study found that a woman who has never smoked has an estimated 24% greater risk of getting lung cancer if she lives with a smoker.[3] The U.S. Environmental Protection Agency estimates that passive smoking causes 3,000 lung cancer deaths each year.

Exercise

A number of studies have found a link between low physical activity levels and an increased cancer risk. On the other hand, increased physical activity, whether from structured exercise or physical labor, has been found to cut the overall cancer risk nearly in half. The greater the activity level, the lower the risk. The association is strongest for colon and breast cancers. The preventive effects of exercise are seen even in people who have other risk factors, such as poor diet, excess body weight, and smoking.[4,5]

Alcohol Consumption

There is a clear association between alcohol consumption and many forms of cancer. The higher the dose (amount of alcohol), the greater the risk. While moderate consumption (that is, one glass of wine, one beer, or 1 fl oz hard liquor per day) poses little risk, drinking alcohol beyond this amount greatly increases the chance of getting cancer of the throat, liver, colon, or breast. Alcohol is metabolized into highly reactive compounds such as acetaldehyde that act as free radicals and damage DNA repair mechanisms, further raising the risk.

Psychological Factors

Stress, personality, attitude, and emotional state are thought to predict the development of many diseases, including cancer. Although this idea is somewhat controversial, personality stereotypes have emerged that reflect an increased risk for certain diseases. For example, the so-called type A personality—easily angered, competitive, and hard-driving—is associated with an increased risk for heart disease. The typical cancer personality is type C, associated with the denial and suppression of emotions, in particular anger. Other features of this pattern are "pathological niceness," avoidance of conflicts, exaggerated social desirability, harmonizing behavior, overcompliance, excessive patience, high rationality, and a tendency toward feelings of helplessness. What the type C personality displays on the outside is a facade of pleasantness. However, this outward expression quickly dissolves during times of stress. Typically the type C personality deals with stress through excessive denial, avoidance, and suppression and repression of emotions.[6] This internalization is thought to contribute to the development of cancer by amplifying the negative effects that stress produces on the immune system.

What research continues to tell us is that how a person handles stress is more crucial than the stressor itself and that the response to stress is highly individualized. Two people might have the same stressful experience, but they may react to it in entirely different ways; as a result, some may develop cancer, while others may not.[7]

It is our belief that helping a person develop an effective method to deal with stress is more important than identifying a particular "cancer personality." Put simply, dealing with stress in a positive manner through exercise, relaxation techniques, and counseling appears to offer protection against cancer and boost immune function regardless of personality type. In contrast, inappropriate ways of dealing with stress such as suppression of emotion, denial, drinking alcohol, using drugs, or overeating will have a negative effect.

Two chapters—"A Positive Mental Attitude," and "Stress Management"—provide general recommendations that have also been shown to fight cancer and boost immune function.

Diet

Dietary factors are the major cause of cancer in the United States. There are two main reasons. One is that a poor diet fails to supply the body with the nutrients and other dietary factors it needs to maintain healthy cells and tissues. A poor diet means the immune system is less able to defend against foreign invaders that can trigger the onset of cancer.

Another reason poor diet is a concern is that it promotes obesity. A report by RAND Corporation researchers found that obesity contributes at least as much to the development of chronic degenerative disease—including cancer—as smoking does.[8] Obesity severely disturbs the body's ability to regulate the complex interactions among diet, metabolism, physical activity, hormones, and growth factors. Women who are obese after menopause have a 50% higher relative risk of breast cancer. Obese men have a 40% higher relative risk of colon cancer. Gallbladder and endometrial cancer risks are five times higher among obese individuals, and obesity appears to raise the risk of cancers of the kidney, pancreas, rectum, esophagus, and liver.

In the chapter "A Health-Promoting Diet," we focus on general dietary recommendations for good health that overlap with specific dietary recommendations for cancer prevention. The recommendations in the chapter "Supplementary Measures" provide a strong level of additional cancer-fighting support. The goal of these recommendations is to reduce dietary factors that increase cancer risk while increasing the intake of substances that protect against cancer.

Dietary Factors That Increase Cancer Risk

Meats

Dairy products

Total fat	Legumes
Saturated fats	Cabbage
Refined sugar	Other vegetables
Total calories	Nuts
Alcohol	Fruit

Dietary Factors That Decrease Cancer Risk

Fish

Whole grains

SELF-ASSESSMENT OF CANCER RISK

By completing this self-assessment, you'll generate a score that indicates your relative risk of cancer. Reading the information in the "Rationale" column will provide you with a quick summary of the scientific data explaining why these variables are important.

Our solution to the difficult task of determining cancer risk was to insert as many variables as we possibly could into a single self-assessment questionnaire. For example, we know from our research that smokers who eat a diet rich in the brassica vegetables—those in the cabbage family, such as broccoli, cauliflower, cabbage, watercress, bok choy, kale, and so on—have a lower relative risk of developing lung cancer. So the smoker who does not eat brassica vegetables would have a relative risk for developing lung cancer of 10, while the smoker who eats these foods would have a lower RR. By adding up two scores, one for factors that increase risk and another for factors that decrease risk, and then multiplying them together, you'll get a general sense of where you stand on the cancer risk continuum compared with other people in this country.

Another caveat: This survey is for guidance only. It has not been scientifically validated in large clinical trials. Still, the information it provides may be useful as a guide to understanding your relative risk of developing cancer, and may help inspire you to take certain steps to reduce that risk through natural strategies, diet, and nutritional support, as described in the following chapters.

INSTRUCTIONS

For each of the following, please enter 1 if the cancer risk factor does *not* apply to you. Otherwise, enter the appropriate risk number as shown. (Note: insert only one number for each factor 1 through 14.)

SECTION 1: FACTORS THAT INCREASE CANCER RISK

FACTOR	RISK	SCORE	RATIONALE
Smoking			More than 30% of all cancer deaths are attributable to smoking. Quitting smoking dramatically reduces risk. For breast cancer, people who smoked at some time in their lives have a RR of 2.0 compared with people who never smoked or who were never exposed to high levels of passive smoke; for individuals exposed to passive smoke before age 12, the RR for breast cancer is 4.5.[9]
Active (currently smoking)	10.0		
Ever active (ever smoked, but have not smoked in at least one year)	2.0		
High exposure to passive smoke (especially as a child)	4.5		

(*continued on next page*)

FACTOR	RISK	SCORE	RATIONALE
Immediate family member with cancer: grandparent(s), parent(s), or sibling(s)	2.5		Family members have a two- to threefold increased risk of developing the same type of cancer.
Electromagnetic radiation exposure (telephone installers, line workers, etc.)	2.0		Significant electromagnetic radiation from any source increases the risk of cancer. Certain occupations associated with electromagnetic radiation increase risk. In one study, RR was 2.17 in those who worked as telephone installers, repairers, and line workers; and in another 1.65 for system analysts/programmers.[10]
Not eating fish or not taking a fish oil supplement	2.0		During 30 years of follow-up, men who ate no fish had a two- to threefold higher frequency of prostate cancer than did those who ate moderate or high amounts.[11]
Red meat consumption			Researchers at the National Cancer Institute have found that those who ate their beef medium-well or well-done had more than three times the risk of stomach cancer compared with those who ate their beef rare or medium-rare. They also found that people who ate beef four or more times a week had more than twice the risk of stomach cancer than compared with consuming beef less frequently. Eating meat one or more times a week carries with it a relative risk for colon cancer of 1.90 compared with eating no meat.[12] Well-done meats increased the risk of developing breast cancer by a factor of 4.6.[13]
1 time per week or less	1.5		
>4 times per week	2.0		
If you usually eat meat well-done or smoked	3.0		
Low consumption of fruits and vegetables (<1.5 servings/day)	1.65		Fruits and vegetables contain an array of cancer-fighting compounds. Individuals who consumed less than 1.5 servings of fruit and vegetables per day had a relative risk for developing colorectal cancer of 1.65.[14]
Obesity/total calories	1.5		Obesity was associated with a statistically significant 50–60% increased risk of pancreatic cancer.[15] People who rank in the highest third of body mass index have a 1.9-fold higher risk of dying from breast cancer than those in the lowest third.[16]
Above-average consumption of sugar (American average is about 5 oz/day)	1.6		High levels of sucrose intake were associated with a 1.59 relative risk of colon cancer.[17] High refined sugar consumption had a relative risk for colorectal cancer of 1.4.[18] Foods that produce sharper elevations in blood sugar levels were associated with a relative colorectal cancer risk of 1.8.[19]
Depression	1.4		Depression is associated with an increased cancer risk, probably through its effects on suppressing immune function.[20]
Diesel emissions (heavy equipment operators, tractor drivers)	1.4		30 years of working on a job with exposure to diesel motor emissions increased RR to 1.43.[21]

FACTOR	RISK	SCORE	RATIONALE
Dairy (>1 serving per day)	1.4		Women who consumed the highest amount of lactose (1 or more servings of dairy per day) had a 44% greater risk for all types of invasive ovarian cancer compared with those who ate less than 3 servings monthly.[22] Men who consume 2.5 servings a day of dairy products had a 50% increased risk of prostate cancer.[23]
Refined flour intake	1.3		The RR of colon cancer increased 1.32 for an increase of 1 serving per day of refined flour products (e.g., white bread, pasta).[24]
Using omega-6 polyunsaturated oils (corn, safflower, sunflower, and soy oil), especially for cooking	1.4		Women who consumed the most polyunsaturated fats were 20% more likely to develop breast cancer.[25] Heating cooking oil to high temperatures was associated with a 1.64-fold increased risk of lung cancer.[26]
Alcohol Men > 21 drinks/week Women > 10/week	 1.2 1.2		Men who consumed 21–41 drinks per week or more than 41 drinks per week had relative risks of 1.23 and 1.57, respectively. Those who drank beer had a relative risk of 1.09 and 1.36, respectively. For spirits, the risk was 1.21 and 1.46, respectively.[27] Excessive alcohol poses a relative risk of 1.28 for colon cancer.[28] Consumption of more than 20 g per day of alcohol (approximately 10 drinks per week) led to a relative risk breast cancer of 1.23.[29] One to three drinks per week, on average, did not increase the risk of breast cancer in this study.
Avoid the sun and don't take vitamin D	2.5		Those with low levels of vitamin D have a two- to threefold increased risk of most cancers—2.63 relative risk for colon cancer and 2.33 relative risk for breast cancer.[30–32]
TOTAL SCORE FOR SECTION 1:		____	

SECTION 2: FACTORS THAT DECREASE CANCER RISK

FACTOR	RISK	SCORE	RATIONALE
Taking a multivitamin with folate For 14 years or more For 5 to 14 years	 0.25 0.80		Women who took multivitamin supplements containing folic acid for more than 15 years were 75% less likely to develop colon cancer than women who did not use supplements. Women who took a folic-acid-containing multivitamin for 5 to 14 years were about 20% less likely to develop cancer.[33]

(continued on next page)

FACTOR	RISK	SCORE	RATIONALE
Fluid consumption (>2.5 1/day)	0.50		Consuming >2.5 liters of fluid per day resulted in a 49% lower incidence of bladder cancer than consuming less than 1.3 liters per day.[34]
Selenium supplement (200 mcg per day)	0.50		Selenium supplementation is associated with reductions in incidence of all cancers, especially lung, colorectal, and prostate cancer, and is associated with a 50% decreased risk of mortality from cancer.[35]
Fish consumption 3 times/week	0.50		During 30 years of follow-up, men who ate no fish had a two- to threefold higher frequency of prostate cancer than did those who ate moderate or high amounts.[10] Similar results have been seen in other cancers.
Vegetables in the brassica family, including cabbages, kale, broccoli, brussels sprouts, and cauliflower (>5 servings/week)	0.50		Protective effect against lung, stomach, colon and rectal cancers have been noted with vegetables in the brassica family.[36,37]
Legume or soy milk consumption >5 servings/week	0.50		Soy milk (more than once a day) was associated with a 70% reduction in risk of prostate cancer,[38] while a relative risk of 0.53 was seen for all cancers with a legume intake of >2 times/week vs. <1 time/week.[39]
Zinc supplement	0.55		Zinc supplementation reduced relative risk of prostate cancer to 0.55.[40]
Regular exercise, equal to or greater than 5 hours per week	0.45		Risk for many cancers (e.g., colon and breast cancer) is reduced by 40–50% among the most active individuals, compared with the least active.[41]
Vegetable consumption >4 servings/day or >28 servings/week	0.70		Colon cancer risk with frequent raw and cooked vegetable consumption was 0.85 and 0.69, respectively.[14] In a study comparing those who ate more than 28 servings of vegetables/week with those who ate <14 servings per week, the relative risk for prostate cancer was 0.65 among the higher-consumption group.[42]
Vitamin E supplement (400 IU/day)	0.70		Consumption of vitamin E showed a reduction in the rate of prostate cancer by 32%.[43] After 12 years of follow-up, bladder cancer risk was reduced by 30%.[44]
Green tea consumption of ≥3 cups per day or the use of green tea extract (300 mg per day)	0.70		A decreased recurrence of breast cancer was observed with consumption of more than 3 cups of green tea.[45] Green tea drinking decreased RR to 0.52 for stomach cancer.[46,47] Consumption of 10 cups per day decreased incidence of all cancers to 0.55. However, this level produces caffeine side effects.
Garlic consumption of >20 g (5 cloves)/week	0.60		Garlic consumption reduces colorectal cancer risk to 0.69 and stomach cancer to 0.53.[48]

FACTOR	RISK	SCORE	RATIONALE
Olive oil consumption >1 tbsp/day	0.75		Women who consumed olive oil had a 25% lower risk of breast cancer.[25]
Wine consumption (1–13 glasses/week)	0.80		Drinkers of 1–13 glasses of wine per week had a relative risk of 0.78 compared with nondrinkers of wine.[49]
Whole grains	0.85		Colon cancer risk was reduced to 0.85 with consumption of whole grains vs. refined flour products.[24]
Fruit, 2 servings/day	0.85		Citrus consumption reduced colon cancer relative risk to 0.86, other fruits to 0.85.[12]
Vitamin D$_3$ supplementation 2,000 to 4,000 IU per day	0.3		Vitamin D has been shown to reduce the relative risk of all cancer by 0.30.[30–32]
TOTAL SCORE FOR SECTION 2:		_____	

DETERMINING YOUR CANCER RISK

To determine your relative risk, add up your scores in Section 1 and place the sum on the line indicated. Remember that if a factor does not apply to you, then enter a 1 in the "Score" column. After adding all of the scores, divide the sum by 14. Indicate the result here:

Total score (section 1) = _____ divided by 14 = _____
Repeat that process for Section 2, only this time divide the result by 16.

Total score (section 2) = _____ divided by 16 = _____
Now take those two results and multiply them together.
Section 1 result _____ × Section 2 result _____ = RR _____

The result is an approximate guideline that indicates your risk of developing cancer. Remember, a relative risk of 2 means you are twice as likely to develop cancer as someone with a RR of 1. If your RR is 0.75, you are 25% *less* likely to develop cancer.

Putting It All Together

Constructing your own personal daily plan for preventing cancer involves strategies for strengthening the four cornerstones of good health detailed in Section II of this book:

- A positive mental attitude
- A healthful lifestyle
- A health-promoting diet
- Supplementary measures

Focusing on these foundations provides the strongest general protection against cancer.

For additional and more specific recommendations for preventing breast or prostate cancer, please go to the chapter "Breast Cancer (Prevention)," or the chapter "Prostate Cancer (Prevention)." For an even more extensive resource on cancer and natural medicine, see our book *How to Prevent and Treat Cancer with Natural Medicine* (Atria, 2002).

VITAMIN D AND CANCER

The connection between vitamin D deficiency and cancer was first made by Drs. Frank and Cedric Garland of the University of California, San Diego. After finding that the incidence of colon cancer was nearly three times higher in New York than in New Mexico, the Garland brothers hypothesized that lack of sun exposure (resulting in a lack of vitamin D) played a role. They published their hypothesis in 1980.[30]

Research now indicates that being deficient in vitamin D increases the risk of death and cancer almost as much as cigarette smoking.[31,32] According to Michael Holick, M.D., Ph.D., a noted vitamin D researcher, avoiding sun exposure to prevent skin cancer resulted in such a drop in vitamin D levels that for every life saved from skin cancer, 55 women died from breast cancer and 55 to 60 men died from prostate cancer. While his assertion is controversial, the research is very clear that vitamin D deficiency dramatically increases risk of many cancers, especially breast and colon.

A four-year placebo-controlled study that investigated the effects of 1,100 IU vitamin D_3 and/or 1,400 mg calcium on cancer risk in 1,179 postmenopausal women over age 55 showed that vitamin D supplementation produced a dramatic 60% drop in the risk of developing any form of cancer.[50]

Final Comments

One key strategy in the prevention of cancer is periodic screening. Screening means getting a regular checkup to look for cancer. Screening is especially important for people who have certain risk factors, such as a family history of certain cancers or exposure to environmental toxins.

The major benefit with regular screening examinations by a health care professional is that it can lead to early detection of cancer. Screening-accessible cancers—especially cancers of the breast, colon, rectum, cervix, prostate, testicles, oral cavity, and skin—account for about half of all new cancer cases. In general, the earlier a cancer is discovered, the more likely it is that treatment will be successful. Self-examination for cancers of the breast and skin may also result in detection of tumors at earlier stages. We can't stress enough the importance of having a complete regular physical exam. Your life may depend on it!

American Cancer Society Recommendations for the Early Detection of Cancer	
SITE	**RECOMMENDATION**
Cancer-related checkup	A cancer-related checkup is recommended every three years for people ages 20 to 40 and every year for people 40 or older. This exam should include health counseling and, depending on a person's age and gender, might include examinations for cancers of the thyroid, oral cavity, skin, lymph nodes, and testes or ovaries, as well as for some nonmalignant diseases.
Breast	Women 40 and older should have a mammogram every two years and an annual clinical breast examination (CBE) by a health care professional. They also should perform monthly breast self-examination. Women ages 20–39 should have a CBE by a health care professional every three years and should perform monthly breast self-examination.
Colon and rectum	Beginning at age 50, men and women should follow one of the examination schedules below: • A fecal occult blood test every year and a flexible sigmoidoscopy every 5 years • A colonoscopy every 10 years • A double-contrast barium enema every 5 to 10 years A digital rectal exam should be done at the same time as sigmoidoscopy, colonoscopy, or double-contrast barium enema. People who have a family history of colon cancer should talk with a doctor about a different testing schedule.
Prostate	The American Cancer Society recommends that both the prostate-specific antigen (PSA) blood test and the digital rectal examination be offered annually, beginning at age 50, to men who have a life expectancy of at least 10 years and to younger men who are at high risk. Men in high-risk groups, such as blacks and those with a strong familial predisposition (i.e., two or more affected first-degree relatives), may begin at a younger age (i.e., 45 years).
Uterus	Cervix: All women who are or have been sexually active or who are 18 and older should have an annual Pap test and pelvic examination. After three or more consecutive satisfactory examinations with normal findings, the Pap test may be performed less frequently. Discuss the matter with your physician. Endometrium: Women with a family history of cancer of the uterus should have a sample of endometrial tissue examined when menopause begins.

Source: Modified from information from the American Cancer Society, Inc.

QUICK REVIEW

- Cancer is the result of mutations in a cell's DNA.
- To reduce your risk of cancer, it's important to:
  - Reduce free radical formation in the body.
  - Limit exposure to dietary and environmental sources of free radicals.
  - Increase your intake of antioxidant nutrients and other substances that support immune function.
- In assessing the likelihood that an individual will develop a certain disease, specialists in epidemiology (observational and statistical studies of people and diseases) use a concept known as *relative risk*.
- Compared with nonsmokers, cigarette smokers are said to have a relative cancer risk of 10—in other words, they are 10 times, or 1,000%, more likely to get lung cancer than someone who never smoked.
- The key components of a cancer-preventing lifestyle are avoiding tobacco use and exposure to cigarette smoke; exercising regularly; and avoiding alcohol or drinking only moderate amounts.
- The typical cancer personality is type C, associated with the denial and suppression of emotions, in particular anger.
- Dietary factors are the major cause of cancer in the United States.
- A report by RAND Corporation researchers found that obesity contributes at least as much to the development of chronic degenerative disease—including cancer—as smoking does.
- Constructing your own personal daily plan for preventing cancer involves strategies for strengthening the four cornerstones of good health detailed in Section II of this book.
- In general, the earlier a cancer is discovered, the more likely it is that treatment will be successful.

Detoxification and
Internal Cleansing

Introduction

Have you ever noticed that many people treat their cars better than their bodies? They wouldn't dream of ignoring a warning light on the dash letting them know that it is time to change the oil, but they often ignore the telltale signs that their body is in dire need of cleanup or critical support. To see if you need a tune-up, answer the following questions. If you answer yes to any of them, you definitely need to pay attention to detoxification.

- Do you feel that you are not as healthy and vibrant as other people your age?

- Do you have low energy levels?

- Do you often have difficulty thinking clearly?

- Do you often feel blue or depressed?

- Do you get more than one or two colds a year?

- Do you suffer from premenstrual syndrome, fibrocystic breast disease, or uterine fibroids?

- Do you have sore, achy muscles for no particular reason?

- Do you have bad breath or stinky stools?

Is improving detoxification really an effective solution to help with all of these symptoms? In most cases, the answer is absolutely yes. Toxins can damage the body in an insidious and cumulative way. Once the body's detoxification system becomes overloaded, toxic metabolites accumulate, and we become progressively more sensitive to other chemicals, some of which are not normally toxic.

The concepts of internal cleansing and detoxifying have been around for quite some time. In modern times, as society has increasingly been exposed to toxic compounds in air, water, and food, it has become apparent that an individual's ability to detoxify substances to which he or she is exposed is of critical importance for overall health.

When you reduce the toxic load on the body and give the body proper nutritional support, in most cases these bothersome symptoms will disappear. Even more important, by addressing these warning signs now we can ensure better long-term health and avoid the progression of minor problems to more serious conditions.

What Are Toxins?

A toxin is defined as any compound that has a detrimental effect of cell function or structure. Obviously, some toxins cause minimal negative effects, while others can be fatal. In this chapter we address the following categories of toxins:

Heavy metals

Persistent organic pollutants (POPs)

Microbial compounds

Breakdown products of protein metabolism

This chapter will focus on enhancing detoxification primarily by promoting improved liver function. Our modern environment seriously overloads the liver, resulting in increased levels of circulating toxins in the blood, which damage most of our body's systems. A toxic liver sends out alarm signals, which are manifested as psoriasis, acne, chronic headaches, inflammatory and autoimmune diseases, and chronic fatigue.

Just a Few of the Thousands of Chemicals Detectable in Every Living Human Being

Toxic metals (lead, cadmium, mercury, arsenic, others)

Polycyclic aromatic hydrocarbons

Volatile organic compounds

Tobacco smoke by-products (including more than 500 chemicals)

Phthalates

Acrylamides

Dioxins, furans, PBDEs (fire retardants), and polychlorinated biphenyls (PCBs)

Organochlorine by-products from chlorination of water

Organophosphate pesticides

Organochlorine pesticides

Carbamate pesticides

Herbicides

Pest repellents

Disinfectants

Types of Toxins

Heavy Metals

The toxic metals aluminum, arsenic, cadmium, lead, mercury, and nickel are often referred to as "heavy metals," to distinguish them from nutritional minerals such as calcium and magnesium (technically, aluminum is not a heavy metal, but it is definitely toxic). Heavy metals tend to accumulate within the brain, kidneys, liver, immune system, and other body tissues, where they can severely disrupt normal function.[1-6]

The typical person living in the United States has more heavy metals in his or her body than are compatible with good health. It is conservatively estimated that up to 25% of the U.S. population suffers from heavy metal poisoning to some extent.

Most of the heavy metals in the body are a result of environmental contamination from industry. In the United States alone, industrial sources dump more than 600,000 tons of lead into the atmosphere, to be inhaled or—after being deposited on food crops, in fresh water, and in soil—to be ingested. Although we are no longer using leaded gasoline in cars (it is still used in piston engine airplanes and helicopters, however), its use for so many decades added a large amount of lead to the environment, from which it is only very slowly cleared. Other common sources of heavy metals include lead from the solder in tin cans, pesticide spray cans, and cooking utensils; cadmium and lead from cigarette smoke; mercury from dental fillings, contaminated fish, and cosmetics; and aluminum from antacids and cookware. Some professions with extremely high exposure include battery makers, gasoline station attendants, printers, roofers, solderers, dentists, and jewelers.

Toxic metals cause damage in three main

Sources of Heavy Metals and Symptoms Associated with Toxicity		
HEAVY METAL	**PRIMARY SOURCES**	**LINKED TO THESE DISEASES**
Aluminum	Aluminum-containing antacids; aluminum cookware; drinking water	Alzheimer's disease; dementia; behavioral disorders; impaired brain function
Arsenic	Drinking water	Fatigue; headaches; heart disease and strokes; nerve disorders; anemia; Raynaud's phenomenon
Cadmium	Cigarette smoke; drinking water	Fatigue; impaired concentration and memory; high blood pressure; loss of smell; anemia; dry skin; prostate cancer; kidney problems
Lead	Cigarette smoke; car exhaust; dolomite, bonemeal, and oyster shell calcium supplements; drinking water	Fatigue; headache; insomnia; nerve disorders; high blood pressure; attention-deficit/hyperactivity disorder; learning disabilities; anemia
Mercury	Dental amalgams (silver fillings); drinking water; fish and shellfish; air in places where coal is burned to produce electricity	Fatigue; headache; insomnia; nerve disorders; high blood pressure; impaired memory and concentration
Nickel	Air and water	Heart disease; immune system dysfunction; allergies

ways: by blocking the activity of enzymes (for example, mercury blocks the enzyme that converts the thyroid hormone T4 to the more active T3, resulting in functional hypothyroidism), by displacing minerals (such as lead replacing calcium in bones, making them weaker), and by increasing oxidative stress, which negatively affects virtually all tissues and functions in the body.

Early signs of heavy metal poisoning are usually vague. They also depend upon the level of toxicity. Mild cases of toxicity may be associated with headache, fatigue, and impaired ability to think or concentrate. As toxicity increases, so does the severity of signs and symptoms. A person with severe toxicity may experience muscle pains, indigestion, tremors, constipation, anemia, pallor, dizziness, and poor coordination.

Heavy metals have a very strong affinity for body tissues composed largely of fat, such as the brain, nerves, and kidneys. As a result, heavy metals are almost always linked to disturbances in mood and brain function as well as neurological problems (including multiple sclerosis) and high blood pressure (the kidneys regulate blood pressure). Numerous studies have demonstrated a strong relationship between intelligence, childhood learning disabilities, and body stores of lead, aluminum, cadmium, and mercury.[7–12] Basically, the higher a child's level of heavy metals, the lower the child's IQ.

Determination of Heavy Metal Toxicity
Determining the body load of toxic metals can be difficult and is controversial. Measuring blood levels of mercury, lead, cadmium, and arsenic is good for determining current exposure. However, it is not very good for determining total body load, which better correlates with toxicity.

In the past, hair mineral analysis was considered a useful tool for measuring toxic heavy metals. Unfortunately, more recent research shows that some people have trouble eliminating heavy metals from the body, so they can show low levels in the hair even when the body levels are high.

At this time, the best way of determining body load is with challenge testing. This involves taking drugs that chelate heavy metals in the body; the resulting chelation products are then excreted in the urine. The level of toxic metals in the urine after chelation correlates with the body load.

Anyone who is interested in optimal health should be evaluated for heavy metal load. This recommendation is particularly true if you have been exposed to heavy metals or have symptoms associated with heavy metal toxicity (see the table on page 111).

Persistent Organic Pollutants

This category of toxins is primarily dealt with by the liver and includes drugs, alcohol, solvents, formaldehyde, pesticides, herbicides, and food additives. It is staggering to contemplate the tremendous load placed on the liver as it detoxifies the incredible quantity of toxic chemicals it is constantly exposed to.

Symptoms of exposure to or toxicity from POPs can vary. Most common are psychological and neurological symptoms such as depression, headaches, mental confusion, mental illness, tingling in the hands and feet, abnormal nerve reflexes, and other signs of impaired nervous system function. The nervous system is extremely sensitive to these chemicals. Respiratory tract allergies and increased rates for many cancers are also noted in people chronically exposed to chemical toxins.[13-19] Research also shows that POPs are also especially damaging to the endocrine system. Surprisingly, high levels of POPs are more predictive of diabetes than overweight is.

Microbial Compounds

Toxins produced by bacteria and yeast in the gut can be absorbed by the body, causing significant disruption of body functions. Examples of these types of toxins include endotoxins, exotoxins, toxic amines, toxic derivatives of bile, and various carcinogenic substances.

Gut-derived microbial toxins have been implicated in a wide variety of diseases, including liver diseases, Crohn's disease, ulcerative colitis, thyroid disease, psoriasis, lupus erythematosus, pancreatitis, allergies, asthma, and immune disorders.

In addition to toxic substances being produced by microorganisms, antibodies formed against microbial antigens can cross-react with the body's own tissues, thereby causing autoimmune diseases. Diseases that have been linked to cross-reacting antibodies include rheumatoid arthritis, myasthenia gravis, diabetes, and autoimmune thyroiditis.

To reduce the absorption of toxic substances, we recommended a diet rich in fiber, particularly soluble fiber, such as that found in vegetables, guar gum, pectin, and oat bran. Fiber has an ability to bind to toxins within the gut and promote their excretion.

The immune system as well as the liver is responsible for dealing with the toxic substances that are absorbed from the gut.

Breakdown Products of Protein Metabolism

The kidneys are largely responsible for the elimination of toxic waste products of protein breakdown (ammonia, urea, etc.). You can support this important function by drinking adequate amounts of water and avoiding excessive protein intake.

Diagnosis of Toxicity

In addition to directly measuring toxin levels in the blood or urine, or by biopsy of fat, there are a number of special laboratory techniques useful in assessing how well we detoxify the chemicals we are exposed to. Clearance tests measure the levels of caffeine, acetaminophen, benzoic acid, and other compounds after ingestion of a specified amount. Other tests for liver function (serum bilirubin and liver enzymes) are also important but are less sensitive. Genetic testing is a newer option that can determine which detoxification enzymes are not optimal. Perhaps the best way to help determine if your liver is functioning up to par is to look over the following list. If any factor applies to you, we recommend following the guidelines for improving liver function given below:

- More than 20 pounds overweight
- Diabetes
- Presence of gallstones
- History of heavy alcohol use
- Psoriasis
- Natural and synthetic steroid hormone use
  - Anabolic steroids
  - Estrogens
  - Oral contraceptives
- High exposure to certain chemicals or drugs:
  - Cleaning solvents
  - Pesticides
  - Antibiotics
  - Diuretics
  - Nonsteroidal anti-inflammatory drugs
  - Thyroid hormone
- History of viral hepatitis

Naturopathic physicians use a number of special laboratory techniques to determine the presence of microbial compounds, including tests for the presence of abnormal microbial concentrations and disease-causing organisms (stool culture); microbial by-products (urinary indican test); and endotoxins (erythrocyte sedimentation rate is a rough estimator).

The determination of the presence of high levels of breakdown products of protein metabolism and kidney function involves both blood and urine measurement of these compounds.

How the Body's Detoxification System Works

The body eliminates toxins either by directly neutralizing them or by excreting them in the urine or feces (and to a lesser degree through the hair, lungs, and skin). Toxins that the body is unable to eliminate build up in the tissues, typically in our fat stores. The liver, intestines, and kidneys are the primary organs of detoxification.

The Liver

The liver is a complex organ that plays a key role in most metabolic processes, especially detoxification. The liver is constantly bombarded with toxic chemicals, both those produced internally and those coming from the environment. The metabolic processes that make our bodies run normally produce a wide range of toxins for which the liver has evolved efficient neutralizing mechanisms. However, the level and type of internally produced toxins increase greatly when metabolic processes go awry, typically as a result of nutritional deficiencies.

Major Detoxification Systems		
ORGAN	**METHOD**	**TYPICAL TOXIN NEUTRALIZED**
Skin	Excretion through sweat	Fat-soluble toxins such as DDT, heavy metals such as lead and cadmium
Liver	Filtering of the blood	Bacteria and bacterial products, immune complexes
	Bile secretion	Cholesterol, hemoglobin breakdown products, extra calcium
	Phase I detoxification	Many prescription drugs (e.g., amphetamine, digitalis, pentobarbital), many over-the-counter drugs (acetaminophen, ibuprofen), caffeine, histamine, hormones (both internally produced and externally supplied), benzopyrene (carcinogen from charcoal-broiled meat), aniline dyes, carbon tetrachloride, insecticides (e.g., aldrin, heptachlor), arachidonic acid
	Phase II detoxification	
	Glutathione conjugation	Acetaminophen, nicotine from cigarette smoke, organophosphates (insecticides), epoxides (carcinogens)
	Amino acid conjugation	Benzoate (a common food preservative), aspirin
	Methylation	Dopamine (neurotransmitter), epinephrine (hormone from adrenal glands), histamine, thiouracil (cancer drug), arsenic
	Sulfation	Estrogen, aniline dyes, coumarin (blood thinner), acetaminophen, methyl-dopa (used for Parkinson's disease)
	Acetylation	Sulfonamides (antibiotics), mescaline
	Glucuronidation	Acetaminophen, morphine, diazepam (sedative, muscle relaxant), digitalis
	Sulfoxidation	Sulfites, garlic compounds
Intestines	Mucosal detoxification	Toxins from bowel bacteria
	Excretion through feces	Fat-soluble toxins excreted in the bile
		Mercury and lead
Kidneys	Excretion through urine	Many toxins after they are made water-soluble by the liver
		Cadmium, mercury, and lead

Many of the chemicals the liver must detoxify come from our environment: the content of our bowel, the food we eat, the water we drink, and the air we breathe. The polycyclic hydrocarbons (e.g., DDT; dioxin; 2,4,5-T; 2,4-D; PCBs; and PCP), which are components of various herbicides and pesticides, are one example. Yet even those

eating unprocessed organic foods need an effective detoxification system, because even organically grown foods contain naturally occurring toxic constituents.

The liver plays several roles in detoxification. It filters the blood to remove large toxins, synthesizes and secretes bile full of cholesterol and other fat-soluble toxins, and

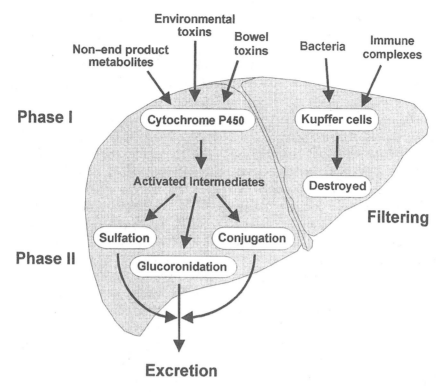

The Liver's Detoxification Pathways

enzymatically disassembles unwanted chemicals. This enzymatic process usually occurs in two steps referred to as Phase I and Phase II, with Phase I chemically modifying the chemicals to make them an easier target for one or more of the Phase II enzyme systems. The liver also plays a critical role in the excretion of metal toxins such as mercury.

Proper functioning of the liver's detoxification systems is especially important for the prevention of cancer. Up to 90% of all cancers are thought to be due to the effects of environmental carcinogens, such as those in cigarette smoke, food, water, and air, combined with deficiencies of the nutrients the body needs for proper functioning of the detoxification and immune systems. Our exposure to environmental carcinogens varies widely, as does the efficiency of our detoxification enzymes. High levels of exposure to

carcinogens coupled with sluggish detoxification enzymes significantly increase our susceptibility to cancer.

The link between our detoxification system's effectiveness and our susceptibility to environmental toxins, such as carcinogens, is exemplified in a study of chemical plant workers in Turin, Italy, who had an unusually high rate of bladder cancer. When the liver detoxification enzyme activity of all the workers was tested, those with the poorest detoxification system were the ones who developed bladder cancer.[20] In other words, all were exposed to the same level of carcinogens, but those with poor liver function were the ones who developed the cancer.

Fortunately, the detoxification efficiency of the liver can be improved with dietary measures, special nutrients, and herbs. Ultimately, your best protection from cancer is to avoid carcinogens and make sure your detoxification system is working well in order to eliminate those you can't avoid.

Filtering the Blood

One of the liver's primary functions is filtering the blood. Almost two quarts of blood pass through the liver every minute for detoxification. Filtration of toxins is absolutely critical for the blood that is coming from the intestines, because it is loaded with bacteria, endotoxins (toxins released when bacteria die and are broken down), antigen-antibody complexes (large molecules produced when the immune system latches on to an invader to neutralize it), and various other toxic substances.

When working properly, the liver clear 99% of the bacteria and other toxins from the blood before it is allowed to reenter the general circulation. However, when the liver is damaged, this filtration system breaks down.

The Bile

The liver's second detoxification process involves the synthesis and secretion of bile. Each day the liver manufactures approximately one quart of bile, which serves as a carrier in which many toxic substances are effectively eliminated from the body. Sent to the intestines, the bile and its toxic load are absorbed by fiber and excreted. However, a diet low in fiber means these toxins are not bound in the feces very well and are reabsorbed. Even worse, bacteria in the intestine often modify these toxins so that they become even more damaging. Another example of the problem with a low-fiber diet is toxic metal excretion. The liver normally clears through the bile about 1% of the body load of mercury every day. However, 99% of what is excreted in the bile is often reabsorbed, due to insufficient dietary fiber intake. Besides eliminating unwanted toxins, the bile emulsi-

fies fats and fat-soluble vitamins, improving their absorption in the intestine.

Phase I Detoxification

The liver's third role in detoxification involves a two-step enzymatic process for the neutralization of unwanted chemical compounds. These include not only drugs, pesticides, and toxins from the gut but also normal body chemicals such as hormones and inflammatory chemicals (such as histamine) that would become toxic if allowed to build up. Phase I enzymes directly neutralize some chemicals, but many other toxins are converted to intermediate forms that are then processed by Phase II enzymes. Unfortunately, these intermediate forms are often much more chemically active and therefore more toxic, so if the Phase II detoxification systems aren't working adequately, these intermediates hang around and are far more damaging.

Phase I detoxification of most chemical toxins involves a group of enzymes that collectively have been named cytochrome P450. Some 50 to 100 enzymes make up the cytochrome P450 system. Each enzyme works best in detoxifying certain types of chemicals, but with considerable overlap in activity among the enzymes. In other words, some may metabolize the same chemicals, but with differing levels of efficiency. This fail-safe system ensures maximum detoxification.

The activity of the various cytochrome P450 enzymes varies significantly from one individual to another based on genetics, the individual's level of exposure to chemical toxins, and nutritional status. Since the activity of cytochrome P450 varies so much, so does an individual's risk for various diseases. For example, as highlighted in the study of chemical plant workers in Turin, Italy, discussed above, those with underactive cytochrome P450 are more susceptible to cancer.[20] This variability of cytochrome P450 enzymes is also seen in differences in people's ability to detoxify the carcinogens found in cigarette smoke and helps to explain why some people can smoke without too much damage to their lungs, while others develop lung cancer after only a few decades of smoking. Those who develop cancer are typically those who are exposed to a lot of carcinogens and/or those whose cytochrome P450 isn't working very well.[21]

Even among healthy adults, the level of activity of Phase I detoxification varies greatly. One way of determining the activity of Phase I is to measure how efficiently a person detoxifies caffeine. Using this test, researchers have found a surprising 5- to 15-fold difference in the detoxification rates of apparently healthy adults.[22]

When cytochrome P450 metabolizes a toxin, it tries to either chemically transform it into a less toxic form, make it water-soluble, or convert it to a more chemically active form. The best result is the first option, that is, simply neutralizing the toxin. This is what happens to caffeine. Making a toxin water-soluble is also effective because this makes it easier for the kidneys to excrete it in the urine. The final option is to transform the toxin to more chemically reactive forms, which are more easily conjugated by the Phase II enzymes and made water-soluble.

While ultimately very important for our health, this transformation of toxins into more chemically active toxins can cause several problems. One is the production of free radicals as the toxins are transformed. For each toxin metabolized by Phase I, a free radical is generated. Without adequate free radical defenses, every time the liver neutralizes a toxin to protect the body, it itself is damaged by the free radicals produced.

The most important antioxidant for neutralizing the free radicals produced as Phase I by-products is glutathione, a small molecule composed of three amino acids—cysteine, glutamic acid, and glycine. In the process of neutralizing free radicals, however, glutathione is oxidized to glutathione disulfide. Glutathione is also required for one of the key Phase II detoxification processes, and so when high levels of toxin exposure produce so many free radicals from Phase I detoxification that all the glutathione is used up, Phase II processes dependent upon glutathione stop.

Another potential problem occurs because the toxins transformed into activated intermediates by Phase I are even more toxic than before. Unless quickly removed from the body by Phase II detoxification mechanisms, they can cause widespread problems. Therefore, the rate at which Phase I produces activated intermediates must be balanced by the rate at which Phase II finishes their processing. Unfortunately, due to genetic variations or nutritional deficiencies, some people have a very active Phase I detoxification system but very slow or inactive Phase II enzymes. The end result is that these people suffer severe toxic reactions to environmental poisons.

An imbalance between Phase I and Phase II can also occur when a person is exposed to large amounts of toxins in a short period or lower levels of toxins for a long period. In these situations, so many toxins are being neutralized that the critical nutrients needed for Phase II detoxification get used up, allowing the highly toxic activated intermediates to build up.

Recent research shows that cytochrome P450 enzyme systems are found in other parts of the body, especially the brain cells. Inadequate antioxidants and nutrients in the brain result in an increased rate of neuron damage, such as that seen in Alzheimer's and Parkinson's patients.

As with all enzymes, the cytochrome P450 enzymes require several nutrients for proper functioning. A deficiency of any of these means more toxins floating around doing damage.

Inducers of Phase I Detoxification. Cytochrome P450 is induced (that is, activated) by some toxins and also by some foods and nutrients. Obviously, it is beneficial to improve Phase I detoxification in order to get rid of the toxins as soon as possible. This is best accomplished by providing the needed nutrients and nontoxic stimulants while avoiding those substances that are toxic. However, stimulation of Phase I is *not* a good idea if your Phase II systems are not functioning properly.

Substances That Activate Phase I Detoxification

Drugs

- Alcohol
- Nicotine in cigarette smoke
- Phenobarbital
- Sulfonamides
- Steroids

Foods

- Cabbage, broccoli, and brussels sprouts
- Charcoal-broiled meats (due to their high levels of toxic compounds)
- High-protein diet
- Oranges and tangerines (but not grapefruits)

Nutrients

- Niacin
- Vitamin B_1 (thiamine)
- Vitamin C

Herbs

- Caraway seeds
- Dill seeds

Environmental toxins

- Carbon tetrachloride
- Exhaust fumes
- Paint fumes
- Dioxin
- Pesticides

All of the drugs and environmental toxins listed above activate P450 to combat their destructive effects, and in so doing, not only use up compounds needed for this detoxification system but contribute significantly to free radical formation and oxidative stress.

Among foods, those in the brassica family (for example, cabbage, broccoli, and brussels sprouts) contain chemical constituents that stimulate both Phase I and Phase II detoxification enzymes. One such compound is a powerful anticancer chemical called indole-3-carbinol. It exerts a strong stimulant effect on detoxifying enzymes in the gut as well as the liver.[23] The net result is significant protection against several toxins, especially carcinogens. This helps explain why consumption of brassica vegetables protects against cancer.

Oranges and tangerines as well as the seeds of caraway and dill contain limonene, a phytochemical that has been found to prevent and even treat cancer in animal models.[24] Limonene's protective effects are probably due to the fact that it is a strong inducer of both Phase I and Phase II detoxification enzymes that neutralize carcinogens.

Inhibitors of Phase I Detoxification. Many substances inhibit cytochrome P450. This situation is perilous, as it makes toxins potentially more damaging because they remain in the body longer before detoxification. For example, if you are taking statin drugs or others metabolized by phase I enzymes, or you are exposed to elevated levels of toxins, *don't* eat grapefruits or drink grapefruit juice. Grapefruit contains a flavonoid called naringenin that can decrease cytochrome P450 activity by 30%, slowing the elimination of many drugs and toxins from the blood.[25]

Inhibitors of Phase I Detoxification
Drugs

- Benzodiazepines (e.g., Halcion, Centrax, Librium, Valium, etc.)
- Antihistamines (used for allergies)
- Cimetidine and other stomach-acid-secretion blocking drugs (used for stomach ulcers)
- Ketoconazole
- Sulfaphenazole

Foods

- Naringenin from grapefruit juice
- Curcumin from the spice turmeric
- Capsaicin from red chili pepper
- Eugenol from clove oil

Other

- Aging
- Toxins from inappropriate bacteria in the intestines

Curcumin, the compound that gives turmeric its yellow color, is interesting because it inhibits Phase I while stimulating Phase II. This effect is also very useful in preventing cancer. Curcumin has been found to inhibit carcinogens such as benzopyrene (the carcinogen found in charcoal-broiled meat) from inducing cancer in several animal models. It appears that the curcumin exerts its anticarcinogenic activity by lowering the activation of carcinogens while increasing the detoxification of those that are activated. Curcumin has also been shown to directly inhibit the growth of cancer cells.[26]

In particular, if you smoke or are regularly exposed to secondhand smoke, we recommend eating a lot of curries (turmeric is the key component of curry). Most of the cancer-inducing chemicals in cigarette smoke are carcinogenic only during the period between activation by Phase I and final detoxification by Phase II, and so the curcumin in turmeric can have a dramatic impact. In one human study, 16 chronic smokers were given 1.5 g turmeric per day while six nonsmokers served as a control group.[27] At the end of the 30-day trial, the smokers receiving the turmeric demonstrated a significant reduction in the level of mutagens excreted in the urine. This result is quite significant, as the level of urinary mutagens is thought to correlate with the systemic load of carcinogens and the efficacy of detoxification mechanisms.

The Phase I detoxification enzymes are less active in old age. Aging also decreases blood flow though the liver, further aggravating the problem. Combined with lack of the physical activity necessary for good circulation and the poor nutrition commonly seen in the elderly, these factors add up to a significant impairment of detoxification capacity. This helps to explain why toxic reactions to drugs are seen so commonly in the elderly—they are unable to eliminate drugs fast enough, so toxic levels build up. Another reason is that many elderly people take so many drugs that they are overloading their detoxification systems.

To ensure Phase I is working well, we recommend that you eat plenty of foods from the brassica family (cabbage, broccoli, and brussels sprouts), foods rich in B vitamins (nutritional yeast, whole grains), foods high in vitamin C (peppers, cabbage, and tomatoes), and citrus fruits (oranges and tangerines, but not grapefruits).

Phase II Detoxification

Phase II detoxification involves a process called conjugation, in which a protective compound binds a toxin by adding a small chemical to it. This conjugation reaction either neutralizes the toxin or makes the toxin more easily excreted through the urine or bile. Phase II enzymes act on some toxins directly, while others must first be activated by the Phase I enzymes. There are essentially six Phase II detoxification pathways: glutathione conjugation, amino acid conjugation, methylation, sulfation, acetylation, and glucuroni-

dation. Some toxins are neutralized through more than one pathway.

In order to work, these enzyme systems need nutrients both for their activation and to provide the small molecules they add to the toxins to bind them. In addition, they need metabolic energy to function and to synthesize some of the small conjugating molecules. If the liver cells' energy-producing structures, the mitochondria, are not functioning properly (malfunctioning can be caused by aging, magnesium deficiency, or lack of exercise), Phase II detoxification slows down, allowing the buildup of toxic intermediates. The first table below lists the key nutrients needed by each of the six Phase II detoxification systems. The second table lists the activators, and the third lists the inhibitors of Phase II enzymes.

Nutrients Needed by Phase II Detoxification Enzymes	
PHASE II SYSTEM	**REQUIRED NUTRIENTS**
Glutathione conjugation	Glutathione, vitamin B_6
Amino acid conjugation	Glycine
Methylation	S-adenosyl-methionine
Sulfation	Cysteine, methionine, molybdenum
Acetylation	Acetyl coenzyme A
Glucuronidation	Glucuronic acid

Inducers of Phase II Detoxification Enzymes	
PHASE II SYSTEM	**INDUCER**
Glutathione conjugation	Foods in the brassica family (cabbage, broccoli, brussels sprouts), limonene-containing foods (citrus peel, dill weed seed, caraway seeds)
Amino acid conjugation	Glycine
Methylation	Lipotropic nutrients (choline, methionine, betaine, folic acid, vitamin B_{12})
Sulfation	Cysteine, methionine, taurine
Acetylation	None found
Glucuronidation	Fish oils, cigarette smoking, birth control pills, phenobarbital, limonene-containing foods

Inhibitors of Phase II Detoxification Enzymes	
PHASE II SYSTEM	**INHIBITOR**
Glutathione conjugation	Deficiency of selenium, vitamin B_2, glutathione, or zinc
Amino acid conjugation	Low-protein diet
Methylation	Deficiency of folic acid or vitamin B_{12}
Sulfation	Nonsteroidal anti-inflammatory drugs (e.g., aspirin), tartrazine (yellow food dye), molybdenum deficiency
Acetylation	Deficiency of vitamin B_2, vitamin B_5, or vitamin C
Glucuronidation	Aspirin, probenecid

Glutathione Conjugation. Many toxic chemicals, including heavy metals, solvents, and pesticides, are fat-soluble. This situation makes it very difficult for the body to eliminate them. The primary way the body eliminates fat-soluble compounds is by excreting them in the bile. Remember that the problem with excreting toxins in the bile is that as much as 99% of the bile-excreted toxins can be reabsorbed due to inadequate fiber in the diet. Fortunately, with the help of glutathione the body is able to convert the fat-soluble toxins into a water-soluble form, allowing more efficient excretion via the kidneys. The elimination of fat-soluble compounds, especially heavy metals like mercury and lead, is dependent upon an adequate level of glutathione, which in turn is dependent upon adequate levels of methionine and cysteine. When increased amounts of toxic compounds are present, the body draws upon its stores of methionine and cysteine to produce more glutathione, thus protecting the liver.

Glutathione is also an important antioxidant. This combination of detoxification and free radical protection means that glutathione is one of the most important anticarcinogens and antioxidants in our cells. Consequently, a deficiency of glutathione can be devastating. When glutathione is used up faster than it can be produced by the body or absorbed from the diet, we become much more susceptible to toxin-induced diseases, such as cancer, especially if our Phase I detoxification system is highly active.

A deficiency can be induced either by diseases that increase the need for glutathione, by deficiencies of the nutrients needed for synthesis, or by diseases that inhibit its formation. For example, people with idiopathic pulmonary fibrosis, adult respiratory distress syndrome, HIV infection, hepatic cirrhosis, cataracts, or advanced AIDS have been found to have a deficiency of glutathione, probably due to their greatly increased need for glutathione, both as an antioxidant and for detoxification. Smoking increases the rate of utilization of glutathione, both in the detoxification of nicotine and in the neutralization of free radicals produced by the toxins in the smoke. The same is true of alcohol, with glutathione production directly proportional to the amount of alcohol consumed.

Glutathione is available through two routes: diet and synthesis. Dietary glutathione (found in fresh fruits and vegetables, cooked fish, and meat) is absorbed well by the intestines and does not appear to be affected by the digestive processes.[28] However, the same is probably not true for glutathione supplements.[29]

There are other ways to increase glutathione. For example, in healthy individuals, a daily dosage of 500 mg vitamin C may be sufficient to elevate and maintain good tissue glutathione levels.[30] In one double-blind study, the average red blood cell glutathione concentration rose nearly 50% with 500 mg per day of vitamin C.[30] (However, increasing the dosage to 2,000 mg raised RBC glutathione levels by only another 5%.) Other substances that can help increase glutathione synthesis include N-acetylcysteine (NAC), whey protein (which is high in cysteine), glycine, and methionine, but vitamin C appears to offer greater benefit in raising glutathione levels at the least cost even in severe glutathione deficiency.[31]

Over the past 5 to 10 years the use of NAC and glutathione products as antioxidants has become increasingly popular among nutritionally oriented physicians and the public, but is this use valid?

There is a biochemical rationale for this practice. It is thought that NAC acts as a precursor for glutathione, and that taking extra glutathione should raise tissue glutathione levels. While supplementing the diet with high doses of NAC may be beneficial in cases of extreme oxidative stress (e.g., AIDS, cancer patients going through chemotherapy, or drug overdose), it may be an unwise practice in healthy individuals. The reason? One study indicated that when NAC was given orally to six healthy volunteers at a dosage of 1.2 g per day for four weeks, followed by 2.4 g per day for an additional two weeks, it actually increased oxidative damage by acting as a pro-oxidant.[32] On the other hand, many studies have shown NAC to effectively raise blood cell levels of glutathione, and long-term safety studies, some lasting several years and enrolling thousands of patients, show that it is very safe.

To ensure that glutathione conjugation is working well, eat plenty of glutathione-rich foods (asparagus, avocado, and walnuts), vegetables in the brassica family (such as cabbage and broccoli), and limonene-rich foods, which stimulate glutathione conjugation (orange peel oil, dill and caraway seeds). In addition, we recommend taking extra vitamin C (1,000 to 3,000 mg per day in divided dosages). Those with exposure to toxic metals such as mercury will find NAC particularly beneficial, as it both increases glutathione levels and directly chelates methyl mercury out of the body.

Amino Acid Conjugation. The body uses several amino acids (glycine, taurine, glutamine, arginine, and ornithine) to combine with and neutralize toxins. Of these, glycine is the most commonly utilized in Phase II amino acid detoxification. People suffering from hepatitis, alcoholic liver disorders, carcinomas, chronic arthritis, hypothyroidism, toxemia of pregnancy, and excessive chemical exposure are commonly found to have a poorly functioning amino acid conjugation system. For example, using the benzoate clearance test (a measure of the rate at which the body detoxifies benzoate by conjugating it with glycine to form hippuric acid, which is excreted by the kidneys), the rate of clearance is half in those with liver disease compared with healthy adults, so in these people all the toxins requiring this pathway stay in the body doing damage almost twice as long.[33]

Even in apparently normal adults, a wide variation exists in the activity of the glycine conjugation pathway. This is due not only to genetic variation but also to the availability of glycine in the liver. Glycine and the other amino acids used for conjugation become deficient on a low-protein diet and when chronic exposure to toxins results in depletion.

To ensure that amino acid conjugation is working well, simply make sure that you are eating adequate amounts of protein-rich foods. When additional protein is required, whey protein has the highest biological value.

Methylation. Methylation involves conjugating methyl groups to toxins. Most of the methyl groups used for detoxification come from S-adenosyl-methionine (SAM-e). SAM-e is synthesized from the amino acid methionine. This synthesis requires the nutrients choline, vitamin B_{12}, and folic acid.

SAM-e is able to inactivate estrogens through methylation, a fact that supports the use of methionine in conditions of estrogen excess, such as PMS. Its effects in preventing estrogen-induced cholestasis (stagnation of bile in the gallbladder) have been demonstrated in pregnant women and those on oral contraceptives.[34] In addition to its role in promoting estrogen excretion, methionine has been shown to increase membrane fluidity, which is typically decreased by estrogens, thereby restoring several factors that promote bile flow. Methionine also promotes the flow of lipids to and from the liver in humans. Methionine is a major source of numerous sulfur-containing compounds, including the amino acids cysteine and taurine.

To ensure that methylation is working adequately, eat foods rich in folic acid (green leafy vegetables), vitamin B_6 (whole grains and legumes), and vitamin B_{12} (animal products or supplements). Methionine deficiency is not likely to be a problem because methionine is widely available in the diet.

Methylation also has other very important functions in the body. For example, it is used to detoxify homocysteine, an intermediate metabolite that damages the brain and heart if not eliminated, and it binds to arsenic, helping excrete it in the urine.

Sulfation. Sulfation is the conjugation of toxins with sulfur-containing compounds. The sulfation system is important for detoxifying several drugs, food additives, and toxins.

Sulfation, like the other Phase II detoxification systems, results in decreased toxicity and increased water solubility of toxins, making it easier for them to be excreted in the urine or sometimes the bile. Sulfation is also used to detoxify some normal body chemicals and is the main way we eliminate steroid hormones (such as estrogen) and thyroid hormones so that they don't build up to damaging levels. Since sulfation is the primary route for the elimination of neurotransmitters as well, dysfunction in this system may contribute to the development of some nervous system disorders.

Many factors influence the activity of sulfate conjugation. For example, the diet needs to contain adequate amounts of methionine and cysteine. A diet low in these amino acids has been shown to reduce sulfation.[35] Sulfation is also reduced by excessive levels of molybdenum or vitamin B_6 (over about 100 mg per day).[36] In some cases, sulfation can be increased by supplemental sulfate, extra amounts of sulfur-containing foods in the diet, and the amino acids taurine and glutathione. Another key nutrient is the trace mineral molybdenum, which is required for most of the enzymes involved in sulfur metabolism.

To ensure that sulfation is working adequately, consume adequate amounts of sulfur-containing foods, such as whey protein, eggs, red peppers, garlic, onions, broccoli, and brussels sprouts.

Acetylation. Conjugation of toxins with acetyl coenzyme A (acetyl-CoA) is the method by which the body eliminates sulfa drugs (antibiotics commonly used for urinary tract infections). This system appears to be especially sensitive to genetic variation, with those having a poor acetylation system being far more susceptible to sulfa drugs and other antibiotics. While not much is known about how to directly improve activity of this system, it is known that acetylation is dependent on thiamine (vitamin B$_2$), pantothenic acid (B$_5$), and vitamin C.[37]

To ensure that acetylation is working adequately, eat foods rich in B vitamins (nutritional yeast, whole grains) and vitamin C (peppers, cabbage, citrus fruits).

Glucuronidation. Glucuronidation, the combining of glucuronic acid with toxins, requires the enzyme UDP-glucuronyl transferase (UDPGT). Many commonly prescribed drugs are detoxified through this important pathway. It also helps to detoxify aspirin, menthol, vanillin (synthetic vanilla), food additives such as benzoates, and some hormones. Glucuronidation appears to work well in most of us and doesn't seem to require special attention, except for those with Gilbert's syndrome—a relatively common syndrome characterized by a chronically elevated serum bilirubin level (1.2 to 3.0 mg/dl). Previously considered rare, this disorder is now known to affect as much as 5% of the general population. The condition is usually without symptoms, although some patients do complain about loss of appetite, malaise, and fatigue (typical symptoms of impaired liver function). The main way this condition is recognized is by a slight yellowish tinge to the skin and white of the eye due to inadequate metabolism of bilirubin, a breakdown product of hemoglobin.

The activity of UDPGT is increased by foods rich in limonene (citrus fruits and the seeds of dill and caraway). Eating these foods not only improves glucuronidation but also has been shown to protect us from chemical carcinogens.

To ensure that glucuronidation is working properly, eat sulfur-rich foods (see above) and citrus fruit (but not grapefruit). If you have Gilbert's syndrome, be sure to drink at least 48 fl oz water per day. Also, methionine administered as SAM-e has been shown to be quite beneficial in treating Gilbert's syndrome.[38]

Sulfoxidation. Sulfoxidation is the process by which the sulfur-containing molecules in drugs (such as chlorpromazine, a tranquilizer) and foods (such as garlic) are metabolized. It is also the process by which the body eliminates sulfite food additives used to preserve foods and drugs. Various sulfites are widely used in potato salad (as a preservative), salad bars (to keep the vegetables looking fresh), dried fruits (sulfites keep dried apricots orange), and some drugs (such as those used for asthma). Normally, the enzyme sulfite oxidase metabolizes sulfites to safer sulfates, which are then excreted in the urine. Those with a poorly functioning sulfoxidation system have an increased ratio of sulfite to sulfate in their urine.

When the sulfoxidation detoxification pathway isn't working very well, people become sensitive to sulfur-containing drugs and foods containing sulfur or sulfite additives. This is especially important for asthmatics, who can react to these additives with life-threatening attacks.

Dr. Jonathan Wright, one of the leading holistic medical doctors in the country, discovered several years ago that providing molybdenum to asthmatics with an elevated ratio of sulfites to sulfates in their urine resulted in a significant improvement in their condition. Molybdenum helps because sulfite oxidase is dependent upon this trace mineral. Although most nutrition textbooks believe molybdenum deficiency to be uncommon, an Austrian study of 1,750 patients found that 41.5% were molybdenum deficient.[39]

To ensure that sulfoxidation is working adequately, eat foods rich in molybdenum such as legumes (beans) and whole grains.

Practical Applications

The activity of and interplay between Phase I and Phase II reactions is possibly the single most important factor that determines our biochemical individuality. Genetic factors are clearly important. One illustration of this is the strong odor in the urine that some people experience after eating asparagus (the odor is a function of variability in liver detoxification). While this phenomenon is virtually unheard of in China, it is estimated that almost 100% of the French experience such an odor; about 50% of adults in the United States notice this effect).

While sophisticated laboratory tests are necessary to prove that a specific liver detoxification system is dysfunctional, several signs and symptoms can give us a good idea of when the liver's detoxification systems are not functioning well or are overloaded. In general, anytime you have a bad reaction to a drug or environmental toxin you can be pretty sure there is a detoxification problem. The table below lists symptoms that are directly tied to a particular dysfunction.

The Importance of Bile Flow

Once the liver has modified a toxin, it needs to be eliminated from the body as quickly as possible. One of the primary routes of elimination is through the bile. However, when the excretion of bile is inhibited (a condition called cholestasis), toxins stay in the liver longer. Cholestasis has several causes, including obstruction of the bile ducts and impairment of bile flow within the liver. The most common cause of obstruction of the bile ducts is the presence of gallstones. Currently, it is conservatively estimated that 20 million people in the United States have gallstones. Nearly 20% of women over 40 and 8% of men over 40 are found to have gallstones on biopsy, and approximately 500,000 gallblad-

Dysfunctional Liver Detoxification Systems	
SITUATION	**SYSTEM MOST LIKELY DYSFUNCTIONAL**
Adverse reactions to sulfite food additives (such as in commercial potato salad or salad bars)	Sulfoxidation
Asthma reactions after eating at a restaurant	Sulfoxidation
Caffeine intolerance (even small amounts keep you awake at night)	Phase I
Chronic exposure to toxins	Phase II glutathione conjugation
Eating asparagus results in a strong urine odor	Sulfoxidation
Garlic makes you sick	Sulfoxidation
Gilbert's disease	Phase II glucuronidation
Intestinal toxicity	Phase II sulfation and amino acid conjugation
Liver disease	Phase I and Phase II dysfunction
Perfumes and other environmental chemicals make you feel ill	Phase I
Toxemia of pregnancy	Phase II amino acid conjugation
Yellow discoloration of eyes and skin, not due to hepatitis	Phase II glucuronidation

ders are removed in the United States each year because of gallstones. The prevalence of gallstones in this country has been linked to the high-fat, low-fiber diet consumed by the majority of Americans.

Impairment of bile flow within the liver can be caused by a variety of agents and conditions (listed below). These conditions are often associated with alterations of liver function in laboratory tests (serum bilirubin, alkaline phosphatase, SGOT, LDH, GGTP, etc.), signifying cellular damage. However, relying on these tests alone to evaluate liver function is not adequate, since laboratory values may remain normal in the initial or subclinical stages of many problems. Among the symptoms people with cellular damage to the liver may complain of are fatigue, general malaise, digestive disturbances, allergies and chemical sensitivities, premenstrual syndrome, and constipation.

Causes of Cholestasis

- Presence of gallstones
- Alcohol
- Endotoxins
- Hereditary disorders such as Gilbert's syndrome
- Hyperthyroidism or thyroxine supplementation
- Viral hepatitis
- Pregnancy
- Natural and synthetic steroidal hormones
  - Anabolic steroids
  - Estrogens
  - Oral contraceptives
- Certain drugs
  - Aminosalicylic acid
  - Chlorothiazide
  - Erythromycin estolate
  - Mepazine
  - Phenylbutazone
  - Sulfadiazine
  - Thiouracil

Perhaps the most common cause of cholestasis and impaired liver function is alcohol. In some especially sensitive individuals, as little as 1 fl oz alcohol can produce damage to the liver, in the form of fatty deposits. All active alcoholics demonstrate this fatty infiltration of the liver.

SAM-e has been shown to be quite beneficial in treating two common causes of stagnation of bile in the liver: estrogen excess (due to either oral contraceptive use or pregnancy) and Gilbert's syndrome.[40]

Putting It All Together

A rational approach to aiding the body's detoxification involves (1) decreasing exposure to toxins; (2) eating a diet that focuses on fresh fruits and vegetables, whole grains, legumes, nuts, and seeds; (3) adopting a healthful lifestyle, including avoiding alcohol and exercising regularly; (4) taking a high-potency multiple vitamin and mineral supplement; (5) using special nutritional and herbal supplements to protect the liver and enhance liver function; and (6) going on a 3- to 7-day nutritional cleansing at the change of each season.

Diet and Liver Function

The first step in supporting proper liver function is following the dietary recommendations given in the chapter "A Health-Promoting Diet." Such a diet will provide a wide range of essential nutrients the liver needs to carry out its important functions. If you want to have a healthy liver, there are three things you definitely want to stay away from: saturated fats, refined sugar, and alcohol. A diet high in saturated fat increases the risk of developing fatty infiltration and/or cholestasis. In contrast, a diet rich in dietary fiber, particularly soluble fiber, promotes increased bile secretion.

Special foods rich in factors that help protect the liver from damage and improve liver function include high-sulfur foods such as garlic, legumes, onions, and eggs; good sources of soluble fiber, such as pears, oat bran, apples, and legumes; vegetables in the brassica family, especially broccoli, brussels sprouts, and cabbage; artichokes, beets, carrots, and dandelion; and many herbs and spices such as turmeric, cinnamon, and licorice.

Drink alcohol in moderation (no more than two glasses of wine or beer or 2 fl oz hard liquor per day for men, half that for women), and avoid alcohol altogether if you suffer from impaired liver function. Alcohol overloads detoxification processes and can lead to liver damage and immune suppression.

Follow the Recommendations for Nutritional Supplementation

The recommendations given in the chapter "Supplementary Measures" for nutritional supplementation are quite useful in promoting detoxification. A high-potency multiple vitamin and mineral supplement is a must in trying to deal with all the toxic chemicals we are constantly exposed to. Antioxidant vitamins such as vitamin C, beta-carotene, and vitamin E are obviously quite important in protecting the liver from damage as well as helping in detoxification mechanisms, but even simple nutrients such as B vitamins, calcium, and trace minerals are critical in the elimination of heavy metals and other toxic compounds from the body.[41–43]

DRINK WATER!

Low fluid consumption in general and low water consumption in particular make it difficult for the body to eliminate toxins. As a result, low water consumption increases the risk for cancer and many other diseases. Drinking enough water is another basic axiom for good health that you've probably heard a thousand times. But it's true: you need to drink at least six to eight glasses of water (48 to 64 fl oz) each day. That means having a glass of water every two waking hours. Don't wait until you're thirsty; schedule regular water breaks throughout the day instead.

Special Nutritional Factors

Choline, betaine, methionine,[44,45,46] vitamin B_6, folic acid, and vitamin B_{12} are important. These nutrients are *lipotropic agents*, compounds that promote the flow of fat and bile to and from the liver. In essence, they have a decongesting effect on the liver and promote improved liver function and fat metabolism. Lipotropic formulas appear to increase the levels of two important liver substances, SAM-e and glutathione.

Formulas containing lipotropic agents are very useful in enhancing detoxification reactions and other liver functions. Nutrition-oriented physicians recommend lipotropic formulas for a wide variety of conditions, including a number of liver disorders such as hepatitis, cirrhosis, and chemical-induced liver disease.

Most major manufacturers of nutritional supplements offer lipotropic formulas. In taking a lipotropic formula, the important thing is to take enough of the formula to provide a daily dose of 1,000 mg choline and 1,000 mg methionine and/or cysteine. Alternatively, SAM-e can be used at a dosage of 200 to 400 mg per day.

Plant-Based Medicines and Liver Function

There is a long list of plants that exert beneficial effects on liver function. However, the most impressive research has been done on the extract of milk thistle (*Silybum marianum*), known as silymarin. Silymarin contains a group of flavonoid compounds that have a tremendous protective effect on the liver and also enhance detoxification processes.

Silymarin prevents damage to the liver by acting as an antioxidant as well as by other important mechanisms demonstrated in a number of experimental studies. In animal research, silymarin has been shown to protect against liver damage from extremely toxic chemicals such as carbon tetrachloride, amanita toxin, galactosamine, and praseodymium nitrate.[47,48]

One of the key ways in which silymarin enhances detoxification reaction is by preventing the depletion of glutathione. As discussed above, glutathione protects the liver from oxidative damage and is critically linked to the liver's ability to detoxify. The higher the glutathione level, the greater the liver's capacity to detoxify harmful chemicals. Typically, when we are exposed to chemicals that can damage the liver, including alcohol, the concentration of glutathione in the liver is substantially reduced. This reduction in glutathione makes liver cells susceptible to damage. Silymarin not only prevents the depletion of glutathione induced by alcohol and other toxic chemicals but also has been shown to increase the level of glutathione in the liver by up to 35%.[49] Since the ability of the liver to detoxify is largely related to the level of glutathione in the liver, the results of this study seem to indicate that silymarin can increase detoxification reactions by up to 35%.

In human studies, silymarin has been shown to have positive effects in treating liver diseases of various kinds, including cirrhosis, chronic hepatitis, fatty infiltration of the liver (from chemicals or alcohol), and inflammation of the bile duct.[50-54] The standard dosage for silymarin is 70–210 mg three times per day.

Fasting

Fasting is often used as a detoxification method, as it is one of the quickest ways to increase elimination of wastes and enhance the body's healing processes. Fasting is defined as abstinence from all food and drink except water for a specific period of time, usually for a therapeutic or religious purpose.

Although therapeutic fasting is probably one of the oldest known therapies, it has been largely ignored by the medical community despite the fact that significant scientific research on fasting exists in the medical literature. Numerous medical journals have carried articles on the use of fasting in the treatment of obesity, chemical poisoning, rheumatoid arthritis, allergies, psoriasis, eczema, thrombophlebitis, leg ulcers, irritable bowel syndrome, impaired or deranged appetite, bronchial asthma, depression, neurosis, and schizophrenia.

One of the most significant studies regarding fasting and detoxification appeared in the *American Journal of Industrial Medicine* in 1984.[55] This study involved patients who had ingested rice oil contaminated with polychlorinated biphenyls (PCBs). All patients reported improvement in symptoms, and some observed "dramatic" relief, after undergoing 7- to 10-day fasts. This research supports past studies of PCB-poisoned patients and indicates the therapeutic effects of fasting as an aid to detoxification.

It is important to point out that caution must be used when fasting. Please consult a physician before going on any unsupervised fast.

If you elect to try a fast, we strongly advise supporting detoxification reactions while fasting, especially if you are carrying a particularly heavy toxic load or have a long history of exposure to fat-soluble toxins like pesticides. The reason is that during a fast, stored toxins in our fat cells are released into the system. For example, the pesticide DDT has been shown to be released from body fat during a fast and may reach blood levels toxic to the nervous system.[56]

The best way to support detoxification during a fast is to choose a 3-day fresh vegetable juice fast (instead of a water fast or a longer fast). Longer fasts require strict medical supervision at an inpatient facility, while a short fast can usually be conducted at home.

For a three-day juice fast, each day you will consume three or four 8–12-fl-oz juice meals spread throughout the day. During this period your body will begin ridding itself of stored toxins. Drinking fresh juice for cleansing reduces some of the side effects associated with a water fast such as light-headedness, tiredness, and headaches. While on a fresh juice fast, individuals typically experience an increased sense of well-being, renewed energy, clearer thought, and a sense of purity. Be sure to use vegetable juices (preferably fresh and organic), not fruit juice, as the high level of sugars in fruit juice can cause widely fluctuating blood sugar levels.

To further aid in detoxification, follow these guidelines:

1. Take a high-potency multiple vitamin and mineral formula to provide general support.

2. Take a lipotropic formula to provide a daily dose of 1,000 mg choline and 1,000 mg methionine and/or cysteine. Alternatively, SAM-e can be used at a dosage of 200 to 400 mg per day.

3. Take 1,000 mg vitamin C three times per day.

4. Take 1–2 tbsp of a fiber supplement at night before retiring, preferably a soluble fiber such as powdered psyllium seed husks, guar gum, or oat bran.

5. If you are carrying a particularly heavy toxic load, take silymarin at a dosage of 70 to 210 mg three times per day.

Other Tips on Fasting

Although a short juice fast can be started at any time, it is best to begin on a weekend or during a period when adequate rest can be ensured. The more rest, the better the results, as energy can be directed toward healing instead of other body functions.

Prepare for a fast by having only fresh fruits and vegetables as the last meal on the day before the fast begins. (Some authorities recommend a full day of raw food to start a fast, even a juice fast.)

Only fresh vegetable juices (ideally prepared from organic produce) should be consumed for the next three to five days. As noted above, have four 8- to 12-fl-oz glasses of fresh juice throughout the day. In addition to the fresh juice, drink pure water. The quantity of water should be dictated by thirst, but it should be at least four 8-fl-oz glasses every day during the fast.

Do not drink coffee; bottled, canned, or frozen juice; or soft drinks. Herbal teas can be quite supportive of a fast, but they should not be sweetened.

Exercise is not usually encouraged during fasting. It is a good idea to conserve energy and allow maximal healing. Short walks and light stretching are useful, but heavy workouts tax the system and inhibit repair and elimination.

Rest is one of the most important aspects of a fast. A nap or two during the day is recommended. Less sleep will usually be required at night, since daily activity is lower. Body temperature usually drops during a fast, as do blood pressure, pulse, and respiratory rate—all measures of the slowing of the body's metabolic rate. It is important, therefore, to stay warm.

When it is time to break your fast, reintroduce solid foods gradually by limiting portions. Do not overeat. It is also a good idea to eat slowly, chew thoroughly, and eat foods at room temperature.

QUICK REVIEW

- **The ability to detoxify is a major determinant of a person's level of health.**
- **It is conservatively estimated that up to 25% of the U.S. population suffers from heavy metal poisoning to some extent.**
- **Exposure or toxicity to food additives, solvents (cleaning products, formaldehyde, toluene, benzene, etc.), pesticides, herbicides, plasticizers, and other toxic chemicals can give rise to a number of psychological and neurological symptoms.**
- **Toxins produced by bacteria and yeast in the gut can be absorbed, causing significant disruption of body functions.**
- **The liver is a complex organ that plays a key role in most metabolic processes, especially detoxification.**
- **The liver's detoxification mechanisms include:**
  - **Filtration of the blood**
  - **Formation of bile**

  - **Phase I detoxification reactions**
  - **Phase II detoxification reactions**
- **Glutathione is an important detoxification compound; vitamin C supplementation is the most cost-effective method to raise glutathione levels.**
- **Silymarin, the flavonoid complex from milk thistle, is a well-researched way to improve liver function.**
- **Fasting is one of the quickest ways to increase elimination of wastes and enhance the healing processes of the body.**
- **We strongly advise support of detoxification reactions during fasting, especially if you are carrying a particularly heavy toxic load or have a long history of exposure to fat-soluble toxins such as pesticides.**

Digestion and Elimination

Introduction

If we are to gain the nutritional benefits from foods, they must be properly digested, absorbed, and eliminated. The best food in the world will go to waste if the body is unable to process it. Fortunately, the human digestive system is quite efficient in extracting the necessary nutrients from foods.

The major functions of the gastrointestinal system are to break down and absorb nutrients. The digestive system extends from the mouth to the anus. It consists of the gastrointestinal tract and its appendage organs, such as salivary glands, the liver and gallbladder, and the pancreas.

Digestion occurs as a result of both mechanical and chemical processes. The mechanical processes of digestion are brought about by grinding and crushing the food mass and mixing it with digestive juices during propulsion through the digestive tract. The digestive juices are responsible for the chemical breakdown of food. The active compounds in the digestive juices are primarily hydrochloric acid and enzymes.

The Digestive Process

The digestive process begins in the mouth. Chewing food thoroughly is the first step toward getting the most from the food you eat. Chewing signals other components of the digestive system to get ready to go to work; it also allows food to mix with saliva. Saliva contains the enzyme salivary amylase to break down starch molecules into smaller sugars. Once the food has been chewed, it is transported through the esophagus into the stomach.

Food is broken down in the stomach by mechanical as well as chemical means. The stomach churns and gyrates to promote the mixing of the food with its digestive secretions, including hydrochloric acid and the enzyme pepsin. These factors are critical to proper protein digestion and mineral absorption. If hydrochloric acid secretion is insufficient or inhibited, proper protein digestion will not occur. Food remains in the stomach until it is reduced to a semiliquid consistency. In general, this process takes anywhere from 45 minutes to four hours. Once the food material leaves the stomach it is referred to as chyme.

It takes chyme approximately two to four hours to make its way through the 21-foot-long small intestine. The small intestine is divided into three segments: the duodenum is the first 10 to 12 inches, the jejunum is the middle portion and is about 8 feet long, and the ileum is about 12 feet long. The small intestine participates in all aspects of digestion, absorption, and transport of ingested materials. It secretes a variety of digestive and protective substances as well as receives the secretions of the pancreas, liver, and gallbladder.

Absorption of minerals occurs predomi-

131

nately in the duodenum; absorption of water-soluble vitamins, carbohydrates, and protein occurs primarily in the jejunum; and the ileum absorbs fat-soluble vitamins, fat, cholesterol, and bile salts.

Diseases involving the small intestine often result in malabsorption syndromes characterized by multiple nutrient deficiencies. Examples of common causes of malabsorption include celiac disease (gluten intolerance), food allergy or intolerance, intestinal infections, and Crohn's disease.

The Pancreas

The pancreas produces enzymes that are required for the digestion and absorption of food. Each day the pancreas secretes about 1.5 quarts of pancreatic juice in the small intestine. Enzymes secreted include lipases, proteases, and amylases.

Lipases, along with bile, function in the digestion of fats. Deficiency of lipase results in malabsorption of fats and fat-soluble vitamins. Amylases break down starch molecules into smaller sugars. The salivary glands as well as the pancreas secrete amylase. The proteases secreted by the pancreas (trypsin, chymotrypsin, and carboxypeptidase) function in digestion by breaking down protein molecules into single amino acids. Incomplete digestion of proteins creates a number of problems for the body, including the development of allergies and formation of toxic substances during putrefaction (the breakdown of protein by bacteria).

As well as being necessary for protein digestion, proteases serve several other important functions. The proteases are largely responsible for keeping the small intestine free from bacteria, yeast, and parasites such as protozoa and worms. A lack of proteases or other digestive secretions greatly increases an individual's risk of having an intestinal infection, including chronic candida infections of the gastrointestinal tract. The proteases also are important in the prevention of tissue damage during inflammation, the formation of fibrin clots, and the deposition of immune complexes in body tissues.

The Liver and Biliary System

The liver manufactures bile, an extremely important substance in the absorption of fatty acids and fat-soluble vitamins. Bile produced by the liver is either secreted into the small intestine or stored in the gallbladder. Bile also plays an important role in making the stool soft by promoting the incorporation of water into the stool. Without enough bile, the stool can become quite hard and difficult to pass.

Like pancreatic enzymes, bile also serves to keep the small intestine free from microorganisms. Each day about one quart of bile is secreted into the small intestine. About 99% of what is excreted in the bile is reabsorbed in people who consume a low-fiber diet.

When additional bile acids are ingested, usually as ursodeoxycholic acid or ox bile salts, they are known to increase the output of bile and help promote a mild laxative effect. Another method of increasing the output of bile (a choleretic effect) is using herbal compounds such as milk thistle or artichoke extract.

The Colon

The colon is about five feet in length and functions in the absorption of water, electrolytes (salts), and, in limited amounts, some of the final products of digestion. The large

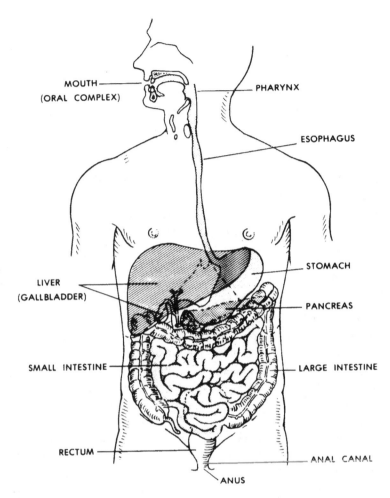

The Digestive System

intestine also provides temporary storage for waste products, which serve as a medium for bacteria. The health of the colon is largely determined by the types of foods that are eaten. In particular, dietary fiber is of critical importance in maintaining the health of the colon.

As important as proper digestion is the effective elimination of waste products. A bowel movement every 12 to 24 hours is critical to good health. This frequency of elimination requires eating foods high in dietary fiber. Such a diet is rich in fruits, vegetables, whole grains, legumes, nuts, and seeds. A high-fiber diet increases both the frequency and the quantity of bowel movements, decreases the transit time of stools, decreases the absorption of toxins from the stool, and appears to be a preventive factor in several diseases that affect the colon, including constipation, colon cancer, diverticulitis, hemorrhoids, and irritable bowel syndrome.

Stress and Digestion

The autonomic nervous system controls all unconscious nervous activity. One part of it, the sympathetic nervous system, stimulates the fight-or-flight response; the other part, the parasympathetic nervous system, is responsible for the processes of digestion, repair, restoration, and rejuvenation. During stressful periods the sympathetic system dominates over the parasympathetic, directing the body to shunt blood and energy away from the digestive tract in favor of the skeletal muscles and brain. Regularly achieving a relaxed state (learning to calm the mind and body) is extremely important in relieving stress as well as improving digestion.

Indigestion

The term *indigestion* is often used by patients to describe heartburn and/or upper abdominal pain as well as a feeling of gassiness, swallowing, feelings of pressure or heaviness after eating, sensations of bloating after eating, stomach or abdominal pains or cramps, or fullness in the abdomen. The medical terms used to describe indigestion include *functional dyspepsia* (FD), *non-ulcer dyspepsia* (NUD), and *gastroesophageal reflux disorder* (GERD).

The dominant treatment of indigestion is the use of antacids and acid-blocker drugs. Acid-blocker drugs are divided into two general groups. One drug group is the older histamine-receptor antagonist drugs such as Zantac, Tagamet, and Pepcid AC. The other is the newer and more potent group of drugs called proton-pump inhibitors (PPIs), which includes Nexium, Prilosec, Protonix, Prevacid, and Aciphex. Use of antacid therapy, especially the newer drugs, is associated with an increased risk of osteoporosis, heart arrhythmias, intestinal infections, bacterial pneumonia, and multiple nutrient deficiencies. Most seriously, these drugs may increase the development of various gastrointestinal

cancers.[1] In regard to nutrient deficiencies, because the body uses gastric acid to release many nutrients from foods, people taking these acid-blocking drugs run the risk of multiple nutrient deficiencies. In particular, critical nutrients such as vitamin B_{12}, magnesium, and iron are generally low in patients on long-term use of proton-pump inhibitors.

The stomach's optimal pH range is 1.5 to 2.5, with hydrochloric acid being the primary stomach acid. The use of antacids and acid-blocker drugs will typically raise the pH above 3.5. This increase effectively inhibits the action of pepsin, an enzyme involved in protein digestion that can be irritating to the stomach. Although raising the pH can reduce symptoms, it must be pointed out that hydrochloric acid and pepsin are important factors in protein digestion. If their secretion is insufficient or their action inhibited, proper protein digestion and mineral disassociation will not occur. In addition, the change in pH can adversely affect the gut's microbial flora, including promoting overgrowth of *Helicobacter pylori*, which has been linked to several stomach disorders. Therefore, it is important to use antacids wisely and sparingly. In addition, many nutrition-oriented physicians believe that it is not too much acid but rather a lack of acid that is the problem. Typically, in addressing indigestion, naturopathic physicians use measures to enhance rather than inhibit digestion. Commonly used digestive aids include hydrochloric acid, pancreatic enzyme preparations, and enteric-coated peppermint oil products.

General Considerations

Gastroesophageal reflux disorder (GERD) is most often caused by the flow of gastric juices up the esophagus (reflux esophagitis), leading to a burning discomfort that radiates upward and is made worse by lying down. Reflux esophagitis is most often caused by overeating. Other common causes include obesity, cigarette smoking, chocolate, fried foods, carbonated beverages (soft drinks), alcohol, and coffee. These factors either increase intra-abdominal pressure, thereby causing the gastric contents to flow upward, or decrease the tone of the esophageal sphincter. The first step in treating reflux esophagitis is prevention. In most cases this step simply involves eliminating or reducing the causative factor.

For occasional heartburn, antacids may well be appropriate. However, they should not be abused. The best choices are antacid preparations that also include alginate, a type of soluble fiber. In a very detailed review of all published clinical trials, it was shown that compared with the placebo response in GERD, which ranged between 37% and 64%, the relative benefit increase beyond that was only 11% with antacids, 41% with histamine-2 receptor antagonists, and 60% with alginate/antacid combinations.[2] Be careful to avoid aluminum-containing antacids. Follow label instructions for any over-the-counter antacid preparation.

If heartburn is a chronic problem, it may be a sign of a hiatal hernia (outpouching of the stomach above the diaphragm). However, it is interesting to note that while 50% of people over the age of 50 have hiatal hernias, only 5% of patients with hiatal hernias actually experience reflux esophagitis.

Perhaps the most effective treatment of chronic reflux esophagitis and symptomatic hiatal hernias is to utilize gravity. The standard recommendation is to simply place 4-in. blocks under the bedposts at the head of the bed. This elevation of the head is very effective in many cases. Another recommendation is to use deglycyrrhizinated licorice (DGL, discussed below) to heal the esophagus,

A relatively new natural therapy for GERD is limonene, extracted from citrus fruit peel. Its mechanism of action is similar to enteric-coated peppermint oil in that it is thought to improve coordination of normal peristalsis. Surprisingly, taking 1,000 mg just once a week is helpful for many suffering from GERD.[3] The typical recommendation, however, is one 1000-mg capsule, every other day, for 20 days, or a total of 10 doses.

Hypochlorhydria

Although much is said about hyperacidity conditions, a more common cause of indigestion is a lack of gastric acid secretion. *Hypochlorhydria* refers to deficient gastric acid secretion, and *achlorhydria* refers to a complete absence of gastric acid secretion.

There are many symptoms and signs that suggest impaired gastric acid secretion, and a number of specific diseases have been found to be associated with insufficient gastric acid output.[4–12]

Common Signs and Symptoms of Low Gastric Acidity

Bloating, belching, burning sensation, and flatulence immediately after meals

Sense of excessive fullness after eating

Indigestion, diarrhea, or constipation

Multiple food allergies

Nausea after taking supplements

Itching around the rectum

Weak, peeling, and cracked fingernails

Dilated blood vessels in the cheeks and nose

Acne

Iron deficiency

Chronic intestinal parasites or abnormal flora

Undigested food in stool

Chronic candida infections

Upper digestive tract gassiness

Diseases Associated with Low Gastric Acidity

Addison's disease

Asthma

Autoimmune disorders

Celiac disease

Dermatitis herpetiformis

Diabetes

Eczema

Gallbladder disease

Graves' disease

Hepatitis

Hives (chronic)

Hyper- and hypothyroidism

Lupus erythematosus

Myasthenia gravis

Osteoporosis

Pernicious anemia

Psoriasis

Rheumatoid arthritis

Rosacea

Sjogren's syndrome

Thyrotoxicosis

Vitiligo

There is circumstantial evidence that the ability to secrete gastric acid decreases with age, but this association is now thought to be the result of increased overgrowth of the bacterium *H. pylori* in the stomach rather than any true effect of aging. Some older studies found low stomach acidity in over half of those over age 60.[13–15] The best method for

diagnosing a lack of gastric acid is a special procedure known as the Heidelberg gastric analysis.[16] This technique utilizes a electronic capsule attached to a string. The capsule is swallowed; once in the stomach, it measures the pH and sends a radio message to a receiver that records the pH level. After the test, the capsule is pulled up from the stomach by the string attached to it.

Not everyone can have detailed gastric acid analysis to determine the need for gastric acid supplementation. If you are experiencing any signs and symptoms of gastric acid insufficiency listed above, or have any of the diseases mentioned above:

- Begin by taking one tablet or capsule containing 500 to 600 mg hydrochloric acid at your next large meal. If this does not aggravate your symptoms, at every meal after that of the same size take one more tablet or capsule (two at the next meal, three at the meal after that, then four at the next meal).

- Continue to increase the dose until you reach seven tablets or when you feel warmth in your stomach, whichever occurs first. A feeling of warmth in the stomach means that you have taken too many tablets for that meal, and you need to take one less tablet for that meal size. It is a good idea to try the larger dose again at another meal to make sure that it was the HCl that caused the warmth and not something else.

- After you have found the largest dose that you can take at your large meals without feeling any warmth, maintain that dose at all of meals of similar size. You will need to take less at smaller meals.

- When you take multiple tablets or capsules, it is best to take them throughout the meal.

- As your stomach begins to regain the ability to produce the amount of HCl needed to properly digest your food, you will notice the warm feeling again and will have to cut down on the dose.

Helicobacter pylori Overgrowth

Overgrowth of the bacterium *Helicobacter pylori* in the stomach has been linked to GERD, achlorhydria, and hypochlorhydria, as well as peptic ulcer.[17,18] The presence of *H. pylori* is determined by measuring the level of antibodies to *H. pylori* in the blood or saliva, or by culturing material collected during an endoscopy as well as measuring the breath for urea.

Low gastric output is thought to predispose to *H. pylori* colonization, and *H. pylori* colonization increases gastric pH, thereby setting up a positive feedback scenario and increasing the likelihood that the stomach and duodenum will be colonized with other organisms.[19] This overgrowth chronically damages the lining of the stomach, resulting in progressive thinning and loss of the cells that secreted hydrochloric acid. Interestingly, it appears that habitual use of acid-blocking drugs may actually promote *H. pylori* overgrowth.[20]

If *H. pylori* gastritis leads to achlorhydria, the next obvious question is what factors lead to *H. pylori* gastritis. Consistent with its history, conventional medicine is obsessed with the infective agent rather than the host's defense factors. Proposed protective factors against *H. pylori*–induced intestinal damage are maintaining a low pH and adequate antioxidant defense mechanisms.[21–23] Low levels of vitamin C, vitamin E, and other antioxidant factors in the gastric juice appear to lead to the progression of *H. pylori* colonization. The fact that *H. pylori* damages the stomach and intestinal mucosa by oxidation also contributes to the microorganism's ulcer-causing potential.[24] Furthermore, antioxidant

status and gastric acid output appear to be the answer to the question why not everyone infected with *H. pylori* gets peptic ulcer disease or gastric cancer.

As for how to eradicate the organism as well as stimulate increased host defense factors, deglycyrrhizinated licorice (DGL) may prove useful. DGL has shown good results in healing both duodenal ulcers and gastric ulcers (discussed more fully in the chapter "Peptic Ulcer"). Rather than inhibit the release of acid, DGL stimulates the normal defense mechanisms that prevent ulcer formation. Specifically, DGL improves both the quality and the quantity of the protective substances that line the intestinal tract, increases the life span of the intestinal cell, and improves blood supply to the intestinal lining.

The active components of DGL are believed to be special flavonoid derivatives. These compounds have demonstrated impressive protection against chemically induced ulcer formation in animal studies. Several similar flavonoids have been shown to inhibit *H. pylori* in a clear-cut concentration-dependent manner.[25] In addition, unlike antibiotics, the flavonoids were also shown to augment natural defense factors that prevent ulcer formation. The activity of flavone, the most potent flavonoid in the study, was shown to be similar to that of bismuth subcitrate. Bismuth is a naturally occurring mineral that can act as an antacid as well as exert activity against *H. pylori*. The best-known and most widely used bismuth preparation is bismuth subsalicylate (Pepto-Bismol); however, bismuth subcitrate has produced the best results against *H. pylori* and in the treatment of non-ulcer-related indigestion as well as peptic ulcers.[26,27] In the United States, bismuth subcitrate preparations are available through compounding pharmacies [contact the International Academy of Compounding Pharmacists, www.iacprx.org, (800) 927-4227].

One of the advantages of bismuth preparations over standard antibiotic approaches to eradicating *H. pylori* is that while the bacterium may develop resistance to various antibiotics, it is very unlikely to develop resistance to bismuth. The usual dosage for bismuth subcitrate is 240 mg twice per day before meals. For bismuth subsalicylate the dosage is 500 mg (2 tablets or 30 ml standard-strength Pepto-Bismol) four times per day.

Bismuth preparations are extremely safe when taken at prescribed dosages and for periods of less than six weeks. Bismuth subcitrate may cause a temporary and harmless darkening of the tongue and/or stool. Bismuth subsalicylate should not be given to children recovering from the flu, chicken pox, or some other viral infection, as it may mask the nausea and vomiting associated with Reye's syndrome, a rare but serious illness.

Another useful natural product that helps relieve symptoms of GERD is enteric-coated peppermint oil capsules (ECPO), which are coated to prevent their breakdown in the stomach. The primary use of ECPO has been in improving gastrointestinal function in individuals suffering from irritable bowel syndrome (IBS) (see the heading "Irritable Bowel Syndrome" on page 142 and also the chapter "Irritable Bowel Syndrome"), but it can also be helpful for NUD, GERD, and *H. pylori*.

Several clinical studies in patients with IBS featured the combination of peppermint oil and caraway oil. The results of these trials indicate that this combination produces better results than peppermint oil alone against symptoms of IBS. Recent studies also indicate that the combination of peppermint and caraway oil is more helpful in improving non-ulcer dyspepsia (NUD).[28,29] In one double-blind study, 120 patients with NUD were given either the peppermint and caraway seed oil (ECPO) or the drug cisapride (Propulsid) for 4 weeks. The mean reduction of pain score was comparable in both groups (4.62 for ECPO, 4.6 for cisapride).[29] Other symptoms of NUD improved in a similar fashion. Positive results were also found in *H. pylori*–positive individuals.

While enteric-coated peppermint and caraway oil is extremely safe at recommended levels, cisapride (Propulsid) was pulled from the market in July 2000 after being linked to 341 reports of heart rhythm abnormalities.

The usual dosage of enteric-coated capsules containing peppermint and caraway seed oil is 1 or 2 capsules (200 mg/capsule) up to three times per day between meals. Side effects are rare but can include allergic reactions (skin rash), heartburn, and if the dosage is too high a burning sensation upon defecation. There are no known drug interactions.

Pancreatic Insufficiency

Both physical symptoms and laboratory tests can be used to assess pancreatic function. Common symptoms of pancreatic insufficiency include abdominal bloating and discomfort, gas, indigestion, and the passing of undigested food in the stool. For laboratory diagnosis, most nutrition-oriented physicians use the comprehensive stool and digestive analysis.

Pancreatic insufficiency is characterized by impaired digestion, malabsorption, nutrient deficiencies, and abdominal discomfort. The most severe level of pancreatic insufficiency is seen in cystic fibrosis. Although cystic fibrosis is quite rare, mild pancreatic insufficiency is thought to be a relatively common condition, especially in the elderly.

Pancreatic enzyme products are the most effective treatment for pancreatic insufficiency and are also quite popular digestive aids. Most commercial preparations include pancreatin prepared from fresh hog pancreas.

The dosage of pancreatic enzymes is based on the level of enzyme activity of the particular product. The United States Pharmacopeia (USP) has set a strict definition for level of activity. A 1X pancreatic enzyme (pancreatin) product has in each milligram not less than 25 USP units of amylase activity, not less than 2 USP units of lipase activity, and not less than 25 USP units of protease activity. Pancreatin of higher potency is given a whole-number multiple indicating its strength. For example, a full-strength undiluted pancreatic extract that is 10 times stronger than the USP standard would be referred to as 8-10X USP. Full-strength products are preferred to lower-potency products, which are often diluted with salt, lactose, or galactose to achieve the desired strength (e.g., 4X or 1X). The dosage recommendation for an 8-10X USP pancreatic enzyme product would be 350 to 1,000 mg three times a day immediately before meals when used as a digestive aid and 10 to 20 minutes before meals or on an empty stomach when anti-inflammatory effects are desired.

Enzyme products are often enteric-coated, that is, they are often coated to prevent digestion in the stomach, so that the enzymes will be liberated in the small intestine. However, numerous studies have shown that non-enteric-coated enzyme preparations actually outperform enteric-coated products.[30]

Alternatives to pancreatin include plant enzymes (e.g., bromelain, papain) and enzymes extracted from various microbes or yeast (e.g., *Aspergillus oryzae*). These enzymes are more resistant to digestive secretions and are active across a broader pH range. One double-blind, crossover trial involving 17 patients with severe pancreatic insufficiency compared the effects of a non-enteric-coated pancreatic enzyme preparation (360,000 lipase units/day), an enteric-coated pancreatic enzyme preparation (100,000 lipase units/day), and a fungal enzyme preparation (75,000 lipase units/day).[31] All three treatment preparations in both groups yielded significant reduction in total daily stool weight and total daily fecal fat excretion compared with controls. It is interesting to point out, however, that the fungal enzyme preparation produced similar benefit at three-fourths the dose of enteric-coated pancreatic enzyme and one-fifth the dose of non-enteric-coated pancreatic enzyme preparation.

Pancreatin and Food Allergies

Food allergies have been implicated as a causative factor in a wide range of conditions that affect many different parts of the body. The actual symptoms produced during an allergic response depend on the location of the immune system activation, the mediators of inflammation involved, and the sensitivity of the tissues to specific mediators. Since the gastrointestinal tract is a common site of immune system activation by a food allergy, it is not surprising that food allergies often produce gastrointestinal symptoms.

Both pancreatic insufficiency and hypochlorhydria play major roles in many cases of food allergies, particularly if a patient has multiple allergies. While starch and fat digestion can be carried out satisfactorily without the help of pancreatic enzymes, the proteases are critical to proper protein digestion. Incomplete digestion of proteins creates a number of problems for the body, including the development of food allergies. Typically individuals who do not secrete enough proteases will suffer from multiple food allergies.

In studies performed in the 1930s and 1940s, pancreatic enzymes were shown to be quite effective in preventing food allergies. The validity of this use has been verified in more recent studies.[32]

Small-Intestine Bacterial Overgrowth

The upper portion of the human small intestine is designed to be relatively free of bacteria. The reason is simple: when bacteria are present in significant concentrations in the duodenum and jejunum they compete with their host for nutrition. When bacteria (or yeast) get to the food first, problems can occur. The organism can ferment the carbohydrates and produce excessive gas, bloating, and abdominal distention. If this were not bad enough, the bacteria can also break down protein by the process of putrefaction to produce what are known as vasoactive amines. For example, bacteria and yeast contain enzymes (decarboxylases) that can convert the amino acid histidine to histamine and tyrosine to tyramine, in both cases causing inflammation and swelling. Even more dangerous-sounding (and smelly) are the compounds produced from the amino acids ornithine and lysine—namely, putrescine and cadaverine, respectively. All of these compounds are termed vasoactive amines to signify their ability to cause constriction and relaxation of blood vessels by acting on the smooth muscle that surrounds the vessels. In the intestinal tract, excessive vasoactive amine synthesis can lead to increased gut permeability ("leaky gut" syndrome), abdominal pain, altered gut motility, and pain. Vasoactive amines are also the primary cause of stool odor. The leaky gut syndrome results in the absorption of gut contents that normally do not enter the body and can lead to inflammation, joint pain, overwhelming of the immune and detoxification systems, and a variety of other symptoms.

Diagnosis of small-intestine overgrowth involves careful evaluation of the comprehensive digestive and stool analysis. There are also breath tests that measure hydrogen and methane after the administration of carbohydrates (lactulose and glucose). If there is small-intestine bacterial overgrowth, there will be higher than normal amounts of these gases.

Symptoms of small-intestine bacterial overgrowth are similar to those generally attributed to achlorhydria and pancreatic insufficiency—namely, indigestion and a sense of fullness (bloating)—but may also include symptoms generally associated with candida overgrowth (discussed below). More severe gastrointestinal symptoms may include nausea and diarrhea; arthritis may also be a result.[33]

The body has several protective measures that prevent bacterial overgrowth in the small intestine. The first is digestive secretions. In particular, hydrochloric acid, bile, and pancreatic enzymes play a critical role in preventing significant numbers of bacteria from migrating up the small intestine. Deficiencies in any of these may promote bacterial overgrowth. Normal peristalsis is another factor that prevents bacteria from overgrowing. Decreased motility in the small intestine due to a motility disorder (e.g., systemic sclerosis) or a meal high in refined sugar can contribute to small-intestine bacterial overgrowth. Under normal circumstances, secretory IgA, an antibody that protects and lines mucous membranes, is another safeguard. But low immune function, food allergies, stress, and other factors associated with a reduced level of secretory IgA can contribute to bacterial overgrowth in the small intestine. And finally, a weak ileocecal valve (the valve that separates the bacteria-rich colon contents from the ileum, the final segment of the small intestine) can lead to overpopulation of the small intestine with bacteria. A weak ileocecal valve is most often the consequence of long-term constipation or straining excessively at defecation; in both of these cases a low-fiber diet is most often responsible.

Factors Associated with Small-Intestine Bacterial Overgrowth

- Decreased digestive secretions due to:
  - Achlorhydria
  - Hypochlorhydria
  - Drugs that inhibit hydrochloric acid
  - Pancreatic insufficiency
  - Decreased bile output due to liver or gallbladder disease
- Decreased motility due to:
  - Scleroderma (progressive systemic sclerosis)
  - Systemic lupus erythematosus
  - Intestinal adhesions
  - Sugar-induced hypomotility
  - Radiation damage
- Low secretory IgA
- Weak ileocecal valve

Obviously, addressing the cause of the small-intestine bacterial overgrowth is the first step. The subject of decreased digestive secretions was discussed above. As for decreased motility, this most often is a result of a meal that is too high in sugar. The mechanism is simple: When blood sugar levels rise too rapidly, a signal is sent to the gastrointestinal tract to slow down. Since glucose is primarily absorbed in the duodenum and jejunum, the message most strongly affects this portion of the gastrointestinal tract. The result is that the duodenum and jejunum stop propelling chyme through the intestinal tract by peristalsis.

Restoring secretory IgA levels to normal involves eliminating food allergies (see the chapter "Food Allergy") and enhancing immune function. Stress is particularly detrimental to secretory IgA. This effect offers an additional explanation as to why stressful events tend to worsen gastrointestinal function and food allergies.

One possible natural medicine to use in cases of small-intestine bacterial overgrowth is berberine. In addition to exerting broad-spectrum antibiotic activity (including activity against the yeast *Candida albicans*), berberine has been shown to inhibit decarboxylase, the bacterial enzyme that converts amino acids into vasoactive amines.[34] Another natural medicine is pancreatic enzymes. As previously stated, the protein-digesting enzymes from the pancreas are largely responsible for keeping the small intestine free from bacteria and yeast as well as parasites such as protozoa and worms. A lack of proteases or other digestive secretions greatly increases an individual's risk of having intestinal infections, including chronic candida infections of the gastrointestinal tract.

An overgrowth in the gastrointestinal tract of the usually benign yeast *Candida albicans* is now becoming recognized as a complex medical syndrome, called yeast syndrome or chronic candidiasis (see the chapter "Candidiasis, Chronic"). The overgrowth of candida is believed to cause a wide variety of symptoms in virtually every system of the body, with the gastrointestinal, genitourinary, endocrine, nervous, and immune systems being the most susceptible.

Elimination and Colon Function

Just as important as digestion is the elimination of waste from the body. The health and function of the colon (the large intestine) are very important to proper elimination. The colon is really not involved in digestion to any significant extent. It does function in the absorption of water and electrolytes (salts). But its primary role is to provide temporary storage for waste products and a site for the formation of stool. The health of the colon is largely determined by the amount of dietary fiber a person consumes. Without enough dietary fiber, waste material tends to accumulate.

Constipation affects more than 4 million people in the United States on a regular basis. This high rate of constipation translates to over $500 million in annual sales of laxatives. There are a number of possible causes of constipation, but the most common is a low-fiber diet. For more information, see the chapter "Constipation."

Diverticular Disease

Diverticula are small sacs caused by the protrusion of the inner lining of the colon into areas of weakness in the colon wall. The term *diverticulosis* signifies the presence of diverticula in the colon. The incidence of diverticulosis increases with age, from less than 5% before age 40 to more than 65% by age 85. Most often the presence of diverticula causes no symptoms; however, if the diverticula become inflamed, perforated, or impacted, the condition is referred to as *diverticulitis*. Only about 20% of people with diverticulosis develop diverticulitis. Symptoms of diverticulitis include episodes of lower abdominal pain and cramping, changes in bowel habits (constipation or diarrhea), and a sense of fullness in the abdomen. In more severe cases, fever may be present along with tenderness and rigidity of the abdomen over the area of the intestine involved.

Treatment of diverticular disease involves a high-fiber diet. In severe cases of diverticulitis, an antibiotic may be warranted.

Irritable Bowel Syndrome

Irritable bowel syndrome (IBS) is a very common condition in which the large intestine, or colon, fails to function properly. Estimates suggest that approximately 15% of the population suffers from IBS (also known as nervous indigestion, spastic colitis, mucous colitis, and intestinal neurosis).

IBS has characteristic symptoms that can include a combination of any of the following: abdominal pain and distension, more frequent bowel movements with pain, or relief of pain with bowel movements; constipation; diarrhea; excessive production of mucus in the colon; symptoms of indigestion such as flatulence, nausea, or anorexia; and varying degrees of anxiety or depression.

Irritable bowel syndrome is usually caused by a lack of dietary fiber in the diet, by food allergies, or by stress. Simply increasing the intake of plant food in the diet is effective in most cases. Also, in several double-blind studies, enteric-coated peppermint oil has been shown to relieve all symptoms of IBS in approximately 70 to 85% of cases within a two- to four-week period. IBS is discussed in more detail in the chapter "Irritable Bowel Syndrome."

Dysbiosis

The human gastrointestinal tract is an incredibly complex ecosystem, with at least 500 different species of microflora normally found there. There are nine times as many bacteria in the gastrointestinal tract as there are cells in the human body. The type and number of gut bacteria play an important role in determining health and disease. A state of altered bacterial flora in the gut has become popularly known as *dysbiosis*. The term was first used by noted Russian scientist Élie Metchnikoff to reflect a state of living with intestinal flora that have harmful effects. He theorized that toxic compounds produced by the bacterial breakdown of food were the cause of degenerative disease. There is a growing body of research that supports and refines Metchnikoff's theory.

The major causes of dysbiosis are:

- Dietary disturbances
  - High protein intake
  - High sugar intake
  - High fat intake
  - Low fiber intake
- Food allergies
- Lack of digestive secretions
- Stress
- Antibiotics or other drug therapy
- Decreased immune function
- Malabsorption
- Intestinal infection
- Altered pH

Obviously, treatment of dysbiosis begins with addressing these major causes.

Probiotics

Probiotics, which literally means "for life," is a term used to refer to the health-promoting effects of "friendly" bacteria. The most important friendly bacteria are *Lactobacillus acidophilus* and *Bifidobacterium bifidum*. Because the intestinal flora play a major role in health, probiotic supplements can be used to promote overall good health. However, there are numerous specific uses for probiotics based upon clinical studies:

Benefits of Probiotic Supplementation Documented in Clinical Trials

- Promotion of proper intestinal environment

- Stimulation of gastrointestinal tract and systemic immunity
- Prevention and treatment of:
  - Antibiotic-induced diarrhea
  - Urinary tract infection
  - Vaginal yeast infections and bacterial vaginosis
  - Eczema
  - Food allergies
  - Cancer
  - Irritable bowel syndrome
  - Inflammatory bowel disease
  - Ulcerative colitis
  - Crohn's disease
  - Traveler's diarrhea
  - Lactose intolerance

Numerous analyses of commercially available probiotic supplements indicate there is a tremendous range of quality. The quality of probiotic supplements depends on the characteristics of the strains contained in the supplement and also on there being sufficient numbers of viable bacteria. Viability depends on a number of factors, such as proper manufacturing and the "hardiness" of the strain, as well as packaging and storage of the product at the correct temperature and humidity. Consumers should choose probiotics developed and manufactured by companies that have done the necessary research to ensure the viability of their products.

The dosage of probiotic supplements is based solely on the number of live organisms present in the product. Successful results are most often attained by taking between 5 billion and 20 billion viable bacteria per day.

Probiotics are very important in preventing the overgrowth of opportunistic organisms. For example, under normal circumstances the yeast *Candida albicans* lives in harmony with the host, but if the yeast overgrows and is out of balance with other gut microbes, it can result in problems.

In addition, probiotics help prevent parasitic infections. Most of the problems parasites cause involve interfering with digestion and/or damaging the intestinal lining, either of which can lead to diarrhea. Diarrheal diseases caused by parasites still constitute the greatest single worldwide cause of illness and death. The problem is magnified in underdeveloped countries with poor sanitation, but even in the United States diarrheal diseases are the third most frequent cause of sickness and death. Furthermore, the ease and frequency of worldwide travel and increased migration to the United States are resulting in growing numbers of parasitic infections in this country. These are discussed in greater detail in the chapter "Diarrhea."

While the most commonly reported symptoms of parasitic infection are diarrhea and abdominal pain, these symptoms do not occur in every case. In fact, there appears to be a growing number of individuals who have parasitic infections but are experiencing milder than usual gastrointestinal symptoms and/or symptoms not traditionally considered to be linked to parasitic infections. For example, many cases of irritable bowel syndrome, indigestion, and poor digestion may be the result of parasitic infection. In addition, parasitic infections are often an unsuspected cause of chronic illness and fatigue.

Signs and Symptoms of Parasitic Infections

Abdominal pain and cramps

Constipation

Depressed secretory IgA

Diarrhea

Fatigue

Fever

Flatulence

Food allergy

Foul-smelling stools

Gastritis

Headaches

Hives

Increased intestinal permeability

Indigestion

Irregular bowel movements

Irritable bowel syndrome

Loss of appetite

Low back pain

Malabsorption

Weight loss

Detection of parasites involves collecting multiple stool samples at intervals of two to four days. The stool samples are analyzed by microscopy, specialized staining techniques, and fluorescent antibodies (the antibodies attach to any parasites and can be seen when they fluoresce).

There are a number of natural compounds that can be useful in helping the body get rid of parasites. However, before selecting a natural alternative to an antibiotic for treatment of parasitic infections, try to discern what factors may have been responsible for setting up the internal terrain for a parasitic infection. For example, do you have achlorhydria or decreased pancreatic enzyme output? Proper treatment with either an antibiotic or a natural alternative requires monitoring by repeating multiple stool samples two weeks after therapy. For more information on dealing with parasites, see the chapter "Diarrhea."

Prebiotics

An important way to help the probiotics become well established is to take prebiotics—basically, soluble fiber compounds that help feed the healthful bacteria. Traditional dietary sources of prebiotics include soybeans, inulin sources (such as Jerusalem artichoke, jicama, and chicory root), oats, and whole grains; supplements are also available. The typical dose is 3 to 5 g per day.

Prevalence of Lactose Intolerance by Ethnic Group	
GROUP	PREVALENCE (%)
African blacks	97–100
Asians	90–100
North American blacks	70–75
Mexicans	70–80
People of Mediterranean descent	60–90
People of Jewish descent	60–80
North American whites	7–15
Northern Europeans	1–5

Lactose Intolerance

Lactose intolerance refers to the inability to properly digest lactose, the sugar found in milk and other dairy products. Most often lactose intolerance is due to a lack of lactase, an enzyme in the small intestine responsible for breaking the large molecule lactose into smaller, absorbable simple sugars. Lactose intolerance can lead to symptoms such as diarrhea, bloating, flatulence, and abdominal discomfort. Overall, lactose intolerance affects an estimated 25% of Americans and 75% of adults worldwide. However, the condition occurs more in some populations than in others. Many people with lactose intolerance are able to consume moderate amounts of lactose without symptoms, but in those with any symptoms avoidance of lactose or the use of lactose-reduced dairy products is a simple solution to lactose intolerance. Probiotic supplementation can often improve lactose tolerance.

QUICK REVIEW

- **Indigestion can be attributed to a great many causes, including not only increased secretion of stomach acid but also decreased secretion of stomach acid and other digestive factors and enzymes.**
- **GERD is most often caused by overeating (reflux esophagitis) and impaired digestion.**
- **The natural approach to chronic indigestion focuses on aiding digestion rather than on blocking the digestive process with antacids.**

- **Common symptoms of pancreatic insufficiency include abdominal bloating and discomfort, gas, indigestion, and the passing of undigested food in the stool.**
- **Just as important as digestion is the elimination of waste from the body.**
- **Achieving and maintaining good colon health are straightforward: eat a high-fiber diet, drink plenty of water, and maintain health-promoting microflora.**

Heart and Cardiovascular Health

Introduction

The cardiovascular system is composed of the heart and blood vessels. Its primary functions are to deliver oxygen and vital nutrition to cells throughout the body as well as aid in the removal of cellular waste products. In achieving this goal, the human heart beats 100,000 times each day, pumping 2,500 to 5,000 gallons of blood through the 60,000 miles of blood vessels within our bodies. In an average lifetime, the heart will beat 2.5 billion times and pump 100 billion gallons of blood.

Obviously, we need to support the heart in its tireless efforts. Unfortunately, as a nation we are doing a very poor job of keeping our hearts healthy. Heart disease and strokes are our nation's number one and number four killers, respectively. Together, these two conditions are responsible for at least 30% of all deaths in the United States. Both are referred to as "silent killers" because the first symptom or sign in many cases is a fatal event. The cause of both conditions is often atherosclerosis—hardening of the artery walls.

Atherosclerosis is the disease process underlying *cardiovascular disease (CVD)*, an umbrella term that encompasses atherosclerosis of the coronary arteries [called *coronary artery disease (CAD)* or *heart disease*], heart attack (the medical term is *myocardial infarction*), blockage of a main artery in the lung (called *pulmonary embolism*), and stroke (also called *cerebrovascular accident* or *CVA*) . The coronary arteries are blood vessels that supply the heart muscle with vital oxygen and nutrients. If the blood flow through these arteries is restricted or blocked, severe damage to or death of the heart muscle often occurs—a heart attack. In most cases, the artery blockage is due to a buildup of plaque, a combination of cholesterol, fatty material, and cellular debris. In the case of a stroke, it is an artery in the brain that is blocked.

Understanding Atherosclerosis

To fully understand the important ways that the various natural measures described in this chapter affect the health of the artery and the treatment of cardiovascular disease, it is necessary to examine closely the structure of an artery and the process of atherosclerosis.

Structure of an Artery

An artery is divided into three major layers:

1. The *intima* or *endothelium* is the internal lining of the artery. The intima consists

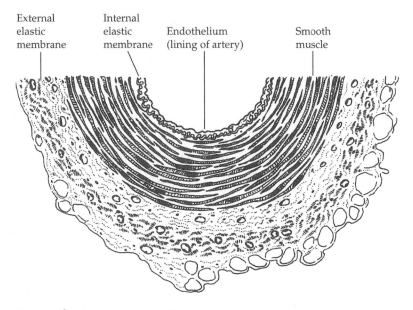

External elastic membrane

Internal elastic membrane

Endothelium (lining of artery)

Smooth muscle

Structure of an Artery

of a layer of cells known as endothelial cells. Molecules known as glycosaminoglycans (GAGs) line the exposed endothelial cells to protect them from damage as well as promote repair. Beneath the surface endothelial cells is an internal elastic membrane composed of a layer of GAGs and other ground substances that provide support to the endothelial cells and separate the intima from the smooth muscle layer.

2. The *media* or middle layer consists primarily of smooth muscle cells. Interposed among the cells are GAGs and other ground substances that provide support and elasticity to the artery.

3. The *adventitia* or external elastic membrane consists primarily of connective tissue, including GAGs, providing structural support and elasticity to the artery.

The Process of Atherosclerosis

No single theory of the development of atherosclerosis satisfies all investigators. However, the most widely accepted explanation theorizes that the lesions of atherosclerosis begin as a response to injury to the cells lining the inside of the artery, the intima. Details of the progression of atherosclerosis are illustrated below.

Causes of Atherosclerosis

Prevention of CVD involves reducing and, when possible, eliminating risk factors. Risk factors are divided into two primary categories: major risk factors and other risk factors. Keep in mind that some of the other risk factors have been shown to be more important than the so-called major risk factors. For example, a strong argument could be made that insulin resistance and elevations in high-sensitivity C-reactive protein (hsCRP), a marker for inflammation, are much more im-

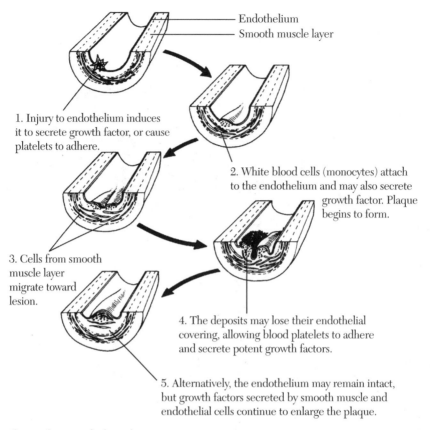

1. Injury to endothelium induces it to secrete growth factor, or cause platelets to adhere.

2. White blood cells (monocytes) attach to the endothelium and may also secrete growth factor. Plaque begins to form.

3. Cells from smooth muscle layer migrate toward lesion.

4. The deposits may lose their endothelial covering, allowing blood platelets to adhere and secrete potent growth factors.

5. Alternatively, the endothelium may remain intact, but growth factors secreted by smooth muscle and endothelial cells continue to enlarge the plaque.

Endothelium
Smooth muscle layer

The Development of Atherosclerosis

A. The initial step in the development of atherosclerosis is a weakening of the GAG layer that protects the endothelial cells. As a result, the endothelial cell is exposed to damage by free radicals and other injurious factors. Immune, physical, mechanical, viral, chemical, and drug factors have all been shown to induce damage to the endothelial cells and lead to plaque development.

B. Once the endothelial lining has been damaged, these sites of injury become more permeable to plasma constituents, especially lipoproteins (fat-carrying proteins). The binding of lipoproteins to glycosaminoglycans leads to a breakdown in the integrity of the ground substance matrix and causes an increased affinity for cholesterol. Once significant damage has occurred, monocytes (large white blood cells) and platelets adhere to the damaged area, where they release growth factors that stimulate smooth muscle cells to migrate from the media into the intima and replicate.

C. The local concentration of lipoproteins and platelets also leads to the migration of smooth muscle cells from the media into the intima, where they undergo proliferation. The smooth muscle cells dump cellular debris into the intima, leading to further development of plaque.

D. A fibrous cap (consisting of collagen, elastin, and glycosaminoglycans) forms over the intimal surface. Fat and cholesterol deposits accumulate.

E. Plaque continues to grow until eventually it either blocks the artery directly or ruptures to form a clot that travels throughout the general circulation until it occludes a blood vessel. Plaque instability is associated with a significantly greater risk for heart attack or stroke.[1] Thus, reducing inflammation and other factors that promote plaque instability is an important target.

portant than elevated cholesterol levels. It is also important to point out that the risk for a heart attack increases exponentially with the number of risk factors.

Risk Factors for Atherosclerosis

- Major risk factors
  - Smoking
  - Elevated blood cholesterol levels (especially oxidized LDL)
  - High blood pressure
  - Diabetes
  - Physical inactivity
- Other risk factors
  - Elevation in high-sensitivity C-reactive protein
  - Insulin resistance
  - Low thyroid function
  - Low antioxidant status
  - Low levels of essential fatty acids
  - Increased platelet aggregation
  - Increased fibrinogen formation
  - Low levels of magnesium and/or potassium
  - Elevated levels of homocysteine
  - Type A personality

Clinical Evaluation

Since CVD is such a major cause of death, we recommend consulting a physician in order to have a complete cardiovascular assessment that can include these tests:

Laboratory tests

- Total cholesterol (oxidized LDL is more predictive)
- Low-density-lipoprotein (LDL) cholesterol
- High-density-lipoprotein (HDL) cholesterol
- High-sensitivity C-reactive protein
- Lipoprotein(a), Lp(a)
- Fibrinogen
- Homocysteine
- Ferritin (an iron-binding protein)
- Lipid peroxides

Other procedures

- Exercise stress test
- Electrocardiography
- Echocardiography

Association of Major Risk Factors with the Incidence of Atherosclerosis	
MAJOR RISK FACTORS	**INCREASE IN INCIDENCE (%)**
Presence of one of the major risk factors	30
High cholesterol and high blood pressure	300
High cholesterol and a smoker	350
High blood pressure and a smoker	350
Smoker, high blood cholesterol, and high blood pressure	720

DETERMINING YOUR RISK

To help determine your overall risk for having a heart attack or stroke, we have developed the following risk-determinant scale. Although this risk assessment does not take into consideration several important factors such as your level of fibrinogen and your coping style, the score provides a good indication of your relative risk for a heart attack or stroke. Each of these risk factors is discussed below.

Risk Determination Scale for Heart Disease and Stroke					
	SCALE OF RISK				
	1	**2**	**3**	**4**	**5**
Blood pressure (systolic)	< 125	125–134	135–149	150–164	≥ 165
Blood pressure (diastolic)	< 90	90–94	95–104	105–114	≥ 115
Smoking (cigarettes per day)	None	1–9	10–19	20–29	≥ 30
Heredity I*	None	> 65	50–64	35–49	< 35
Heredity II†	0	1	2	4	≥ 4
Diabetes duration (years)	0	1–5	6–10	11–15	> 15
Total cholesterol (mg/dl)	< 200	200–224	225–249	250–274	≥ 275
HDL (high-density-lipoprotein) cholesterol (mg/dl)	≥ 75	65–74	55–64	35–54	< 35
Total cholesterol/HDL ratio‡	< 3	3–3.9	4–4.9	5–6.4	≥ 6.5
High-sensitivity CRP	< 1	1–2	2–3	3–4	> 4
Exercise (hours per week)	> 4	3–4	2–3	1–2	0–1
Supplemental EPA/DHA (mg) intake	> 600	400–599	200–399	100–199	< 100
Vitamin C, vitamin E, selenium, PCOs, lutein supplementation (number of items)	5	3	2	1	0
Average daily servings of fruits and vegetables	> 5	4–5	3	1–2	0
Age	< 35	36–45	46–55	56–65	> 65
Subtotals					

* Age of patient when he or she had a first heart attack or stroke.

† Number of immediate family members having had a heart attack before the age of 50.

‡ Total cholesterol divided by HDL.

Risk = sum of all five columns; 14–20 = very low risk; 21–30 = low risk; 31–40 = average risk; 41–50 = high risk; ≥ 51 = very high risk.

A Closer Look at Risk Factors

Smoking

Cigarette smoking is perhaps the most important risk factor for CVD, as statistical evidence reveals smokers have a 70% greater risk of death from CVD than nonsmokers.[2] The more cigarettes smoked and the longer a person has smoked, the greater the risk of dying from a heart attack or stroke. Overall, the average smoker dies seven to eight years sooner than the nonsmoker.

Tobacco smoke contains more than 4,000 chemicals, of which more than 50 substances have been identified as carcinogens. These chemicals are extremely damaging to the cardiovascular system. Specifically, these chemicals are carried in the bloodstream on low-density lipoprotein (LDL) cholesterol, where they either damage the lining of the arteries directly or damage the LDL molecule (creating oxidized LDL), which then damages the arteries. An elevated LDL level worsens the effect of smoking because more cigarette toxins travel through the cardiovascular system. Smoking contributes to elevated cholesterol presumably by damaging feedback mechanisms in the liver, which control how much cholesterol is being manufactured.[3] Smoking also promotes platelet aggregation and elevated fibrinogen levels, two other independent risk factors important for CVD because they tend to result in the formation of blood clots. In addition, it is a well-documented fact that cigarette smoking is a factor contributing to high blood pressure.[4]

Even passive exposure to cigarette smoke is damaging to cardiovascular health, as convincing evidence links environmental (secondhand or passive) smoke to CVD. Analysis of 10 population-based studies indicates a consistent dose-response effect related to exposure.[5] In other words, the more you are exposed to cigarette smoke, the greater your risk for CVD. Evidence indicates that nonsmokers appear to be more sensitive to smoke, including its deleterious effects on the cardiovascular system. Environmental tobacco smoke actually has a higher concentration of some toxic constituents. Data after short- and long-term exposure to environmental tobacco smoke show changes in the lining of the arteries and in platelet function as well as exercise capacity similar to those found in active smokers. In summary, passive smoking is a relevant risk factor for CVD. In the United States it is estimated that more than 37,000 heart disease deaths each year are attributable to environmental smoke.

The good news is that the magnitude of risk reduction achieved by smoking cessation in patients with CVD is quite significant. Results from a detailed meta-analysis showed a 36% reduction in relative risk of mortality for patients with coronary artery disease who quit compared with those who continued smoking.[6]

Various measures—including nicotine-containing skin patches or chewing gum, acupuncture, and hypnosis—have all been shown to provide some benefit in helping patients to quit smoking.[7] For more information on strategies to stop smoking, see the chapter "A Health-Promoting Lifestyle."

Elevated Blood Cholesterol Levels

The evidence overwhelmingly demonstrates that elevated cholesterol levels greatly increase the risk of death due to CVD, especially elevations in LDL cholesterol.[8] It is currently recommended that the total blood cholesterol level be less than 200 mg/dl. In addition, it is recommended that LDL be less than 130 mg/dl, HDL greater than

40 mg/dl in men and 50 mg/dl in women, and triglycerides less than 150 mg/dl.

Cholesterol is transported in the blood by lipoproteins. The major categories of lipoproteins are very-low-density lipoprotein (VLDL), LDL, and HDL. Because VLDL and LDL are responsible for transporting fats (primarily triglycerides and cholesterol) from the liver to body cells while HDL is responsible for returning fats to the liver, elevations of either VLDL or LDL are associated with an increased risk for developing atherosclerosis, the primary cause of a heart attack or stroke. In contrast, elevations of HDL are associated with a low risk of heart attacks.

The ratios of total cholesterol to HDL cholesterol and LDL to HDL are referred to as *cardiac risk factor ratios* because they reflect whether cholesterol is being deposited into tissues or broken down and excreted. The ratio of total cholesterol to HDL should be no higher than 4.2, and the ratio of LDL to HDL should be no higher than 2.5. The risk of heart disease can be reduced dramatically by lowering LDL while simultaneously raising HDL levels. For every 1% drop in the LDL level, the risk of a heart attack drops by 2%. Conversely, for every 1% increase in HDL level, the risk for a heart attack drops 3% to 4%.[8,9]

For more information on elevated blood cholesterol and lipoproteins, see the chapter "High Cholesterol and/or Triglycerides."

Diabetes

Atherosclerosis is one of the key underlying factors in the development of many chronic complications of diabetes. Individuals with diabetes have a two- to threefold higher risk of dying prematurely of heart disease or stroke than those who are not diabetic, and 55% of deaths in diabetic patients are caused by CVD. However, even mild insulin resistance and poor glucose control have

been shown to have a dramatic impact on the incidence and progression of CVD. For more information, see the chapter "Diabetes."

High Blood Pressure

Elevated blood pressure is often a sign of considerable atherosclerosis and a major risk factor for heart attack or stroke. In fact, the presence of hypertension is generally regarded as the most significant risk factor for stroke. For more information, see the chapter "High Blood Pressure."

Physical Inactivity/Lack of Exercise

A sedentary lifestyle is another major risk factor for CVD. Roughly 54% of adult Americans report little or no regular physical activity, and there is also a sharp decline in regular exercise among children and adolescents.[10] But not only does being active protect against the development of CVD, it also favorably modifies other CVD risk factors, including high blood pressure, blood lipid levels, insulin resistance, and obesity. Exercise is also important in the treatment and management of patients with CVD or increased risk, including those who have hypertension, stable angina, a prior heart attack, peripheral vascular disease, or heart failure, or who are recovering from a cardiovascular event. For more information, see the chapter "A Health-Promoting Lifestyle."

Other Risk Factors

In addition to the major risk factors for CVD (smoking, elevated cholesterol, high blood pressure, diabetes, physical inactivity, and obesity), a number of other factors have, on occasion, been shown to be more significant than the so-called major risk factors. In fact, more than 300 different risk factors have been identified. Although there is considerable evidence that all of these risk factors and more can play a significant role in the development of atherosclerosis, much of the current research has focused on the central roles of inflammatory processes and insulin resistance.[11]

Inflammatory mediators influence many stages in the development of atherosclerosis, from initial leukocyte recruitment to eventual rupture of the unstable atherosclerotic plaque. In particular, high-sensitivity C-reactive protein, a blood marker that reflects different degrees of inflammation, has been identified as an independent risk factor for CAD. The hsCRP level has been shown to be a stronger predictor of cardiovascular events than LDL level, but screening for both biological markers provides better prognostic information than screening for either alone.[12]

Elevations in hsCRP are closely linked to insulin resistance, a condition in which cells of the body become unresponsive to the hormone insulin (see the chapter "Diabetes" for more information).[13] Insulin resistance is a key underlying factor not only in type 2 diabetes but also in metabolic syndrome, defined as a combination of at least three of the following metabolic risk factors:

- A waist-to-hip ratio greater than 1 for men and greater than 0.8 for women

- Triglycerides greater than 150 mg/dl, and low HDL (below 40 mg/dl in men and below 50 mg/dl in women)

- High blood pressure (equal to or greater than 130/85 mm Hg)

- Insulin resistance or glucose intolerance (fasting blood sugar levels above 101 mg/dl)

- High blood levels of fibrinogen or plasminogen activator inhibitor

- Elevated high-sensitivity CRP

Metabolic syndrome has become increasingly common in the United States. It is now estimated that more than 60 million U.S. adults may have it.

Therapeutic Considerations

Prevention of a heart attack or stroke involves reducing risk factors. The major risk factors—smoking, obesity, physical inactivity, diabetes, and hypertension—are detailed in other chapters. The point we want to make here is that there is significant evidence that simply adopting a healthy diet and lifestyle dramatically reduces CVD-related mortality. In a prospective trial enrolling more than 20,000 men and women, it was found that the combination of four healthy behaviors (not smoking; being physically active; moderate alcohol intake; and consuming at least five servings of fruit and vegetables per day) reduced total mortality fourfold compared with the absence of all these behaviors.[14]

In addition to these healthful lifestyle behaviors, we will also discuss antioxidant status, elevated hsCRP, and fibrinogen levels.

Diet

The chapter "A Health-Promoting Diet" features a comprehensive dietary approach that will help both with the prevention and treatment of CVD and with the improvement of blood lipid profiles. In particular, it is important to reduce the intake of saturated fat and trans-fatty acids while increasing the consumption of vegetables, fruit, dietary fiber, monounsaturated fats, and omega-3 fatty acids. An important dietary goal is to improve the structure and composition of cell membranes by making available essential structural components like the monounsaturated and omega-3 fatty acids and by preventing oxidative and free radical damage to these structures by consuming a high level of antioxidants and phytochemicals.

One of the most widely studied dietary interventions in CVD is the traditional Mediterranean diet, which reflects food patterns typical of some Mediterranean regions in the early 1960s.[15] As we discussed in the chapter "A Health-Promoting Diet," the original Mediterranean diet had the following characteristics:

- Olive oil is the principal source of fat.
- The diet centers on an abundance of plant foods.
- Foods are minimally processed, and people focus on fresh, seasonal, locally grown foods.
- Fresh fruit is the typical everyday dessert, with sweets containing concentrated sugars or honey consumed only a few times a week at most.
- Dairy products (principally cheese and yogurt) are consumed in low to moderate amounts daily.
- Fish is consumed regularly.
- Poultry and eggs are consumed in moderate amounts (up to four times weekly) or not at all.
- Red meat is consumed in low amounts.
- Wine is consumed in low to moderate amounts, normally with meals.

In one study, the effect of the Mediterranean diet on the lining of blood vessels and hsCRP was examined in patients with metabolic syndrome.[16] Patients in the intervention group were instructed to follow the Mediterranean diet and received detailed advice on how to increase their consumption of whole grains, fruits, vegetables, nuts, and olive oil; patients in the control group followed the American Heart Association (AHA) diet. After two years, patients following the Mediterranean diet regularly ate more foods rich in monounsaturated fat, polyunsaturated fat, and fiber and had a lower ratio of omega-6 to omega-3 fatty acids. Compared with patients on the control diet, patients on the intervention diet had significantly reduced levels of hsCRP and other inflammatory mediators; improved blood vessel function; and greater weight loss.

Although several components of the Mediterranean diet deserve special mention, it is important to stress that the total benefits reflect an interplay among many beneficial compounds rather than any single factor.[17]

In addition, it is critical to follow a low-glycemic-load diet. A study of more than 48,000 participants following a low-glycemic diet for an average of eight years found that the consumption of foods with a high glycemic load increased the risk of CVD in women by 68%; women in the highest glycemic-load quartile had a relative risk of 2.2 for CHD compared with those in the lowest quartile.[18]

Olive Oil and Omega-3 Fatty Acids

One of the most important aspects of the Mediterranean diet may be the combination of olive oil and the intake of omega-3 fatty acids. Olive oil contains not only monounsaturated fatty acid (oleic acid) but also several antioxidant agents that may account for some of its health benefits. In addition to a mild effect in lowering LDL and triglycerides, olive oil increases HDL level and helps prevent LDL from being damaged by free radicals.[19]

In addition to olive oil, the benefits of the longer-chain omega-3 fatty acids EPA and DHA for cardiovascular health have been demonstrated in more than 300 clinical trials. These fatty acids exert considerable benefits in reducing the risk for CVD. Supplementation with EPA and DHA has little effect on cholesterol levels but does lower triglyceride levels significantly, as well as produce a myriad of additional beneficial effects, including reduced platelet aggregation, improved function of the lining of blood vessels and arterial flexibility, improved blood and oxygen supply to the heart, and a mild reduction in blood pressure.[20]

The levels of EPA and DHA within red blood cells have been shown to be highly significant predictors of heart disease. This laboratory value has been termed the omega-3 index. An omega-3 index of 8% was associated with the greatest protection, whereas an index of 4% was associated with the least. In one analysis, the omega-3 index was shown to be the most significant predictor of CVD compared with hsCRP, total cholesterol, LDL, HDL, and homocysteine. Researchers subsequently determined that a total of 1,000 mg EPA + DHA per day is required to achieve or surpass the 8% target of the omega-3 index.[21,22]

The findings about the omega-3 index are not surprising, as a wealth of information has documented a clear relationship between dietary intake of omega-3 fatty acids and the likelihood of developing CVD: the higher the omega-3 fatty acid intake, the lower the likelihood of CVD. It has been estimated that raising the levels of long-chain omega-3 fatty acids through diet or supplementation may reduce overall cardiovascular mortality by as much as 45%.[23,24]

In general, for preventive effects against CVD, the dosage recommendation is 1,000 mg EPA + DHA per day; for lowering triglycerides, the dosage is 3,000 mg per day. In a double-blind study, after eight weeks of supplementation, a daily dosage of 3.40 g EPA + DHA lowered triglycerides by 27%, while a lower dosage of 0.85 g had no effect. These results clearly indicate that lowering triglycerides requires dosages of 3 g EPA + DHA per day.[25]

Although the longer-chain omega-3 fatty acids exert more pronounced effects than alpha-linolenic acid, a shorter-chain omega-3 fatty acid (derived from vegetable sources such as flaxseed oil and walnuts), it is important to point out that the two populations with the lowest rates of heart attack have a relatively high intake of alpha-linolenic acid: the Japanese who inhabit Kohama Island and the inhabitants of Crete.[26,27] Typically, Cretans have a threefold higher serum concentration of alpha-linolenic acid than members of other European countries, owing to their frequent consumption of walnuts and the vegetable purslane.[26] Of course, another important dietary factor in both the Kohamans and the Cretans is their use of oleic-acid-containing oils. However, although the oleic acid content of the diet offers some degree of protection, the rates of heart attack among the Kohamans and Cretans are much lower than those in populations that consume only oleic acid sources and little alpha-linolenic acid. The intake of alpha-linolenic acid is viewed as a more significant protective factor than oleic acid.

Nuts and Seeds

Higher consumption of nuts and seeds has been shown to significantly reduce the risk of CVD in large population-based studies, including the Nurses Health Study, the Iowa Health Study, and the Physicians Health Study.[28] Researchers estimate that substituting nuts for an equivalent amount of carbohydrates in an average diet resulted in a 30% reduction in heart disease risk. Researchers calculated an even more impressive risk reduction, 45%, when fat from nuts was substituted for saturated fats (found primarily in meat and dairy products). Nuts have a cholesterol-lowering effect, which partly explains this benefit, but they are also a rich source of arginine. By increasing nitric oxide levels, arginine may help to improve blood flow, reduce blood clot formation, and improve blood fluidity (the blood becomes less viscous and therefore flows through blood vessels more easily).

Walnuts appear to be especially beneficial because they are also a rich source of both antioxidants and alpha-linolenic acid. In one study, men and women with high cholesterol were randomly assigned to a cholesterol-lowering Mediterranean diet or to a diet of similar energy and fat content in which walnuts replaced approximately 32% of the energy from monounsaturated fat (olive oil). Participants followed each diet for four weeks. Compared with the Mediterranean diet, the walnut diet improved endothelial cell function (it increased endothelium-dependent vasodilation and reduced levels of vascular cell adhesion molecule-1). The walnut diet also significantly reduced total cholesterol (–4.4%) and LDL (–6.4%).[29]

Vegetables, Fruits, and Red Wine

An important contributor to the benefits noted with the Mediterranean diet is the focus on carotenoid- and flavonoid-rich fruits, vegetables, and beverages (e.g., red wine). Numerous population studies have repeatedly demonstrated that a higher intake of dietary antioxidants significantly reduces the risk of heart disease and stroke. Higher blood levels of antioxidant nutrients are also associated with lower levels of hsCRP.[30] The importance of antioxidant intake in the prevention and treatment of CAD is discussed further below.

Two valuable sources of antioxidants in the Mediterranean diet are tomato products and red wine. Tomatoes are a rich source of the carotene lycopene. In large clinical studies evaluating the relationship between carotene status and heart attack, lycopene but not beta-carotene was shown to be protective.

Lycopene exerts greater antioxidant activity compared with beta-carotene in general but specifically against LDL oxidation.[31]

The cardiovascular protection offered by red wine is popularly referred to as the "French paradox." The French consume more saturated fat than people in the United States and the United Kingdom yet have a lower incidence of heart disease; red wine consumption has been suggested as the reason. Presumably this protection is the result of flavonoids and other polyphenols in red wine that protect against oxidative damage to LDL and help to reduce levels of inflammatory mediators.[16,32] However, moderate alcohol consumption alone has also been shown to be protective in some studies, exerting positive effects on ratios of HDL to LDL and CRP as well as levels of fibrinogen (although red wine typically has the most significant effects).[33] Importantly, the effects of alcohol on CVD risk, morbidity, and total mortality are counterbalanced by alcohol's addictive and psychological effects; excessive alcohol consumption results in depletion of glutathione and an increased risk of colon cancer.

The major benefits of red wine consumption in protecting against CVD may ultimately be the effects that the polyphenols have on improving the function of the cells that line the blood vessels.[34] The consumption of green tea and dark chocolate, like that of red wine, has also been shown in population studies to be associated with a reduced risk for CVD. As with red wine, much of the benefit from green tea and chocolate may be the result of several different mechanisms, including improving endothelial cell function.[35]

Other foods and beverages rich in antioxidant content have shown benefit in fighting atherosclerosis. Pomegranate (*Punica granatum*) juice appears to be particularly useful. It is remarkably rich in antioxidants, such as soluble polyphenols, tannins, and anthocyanins. Animal research has indicated that components of pomegranate juice can retard atherosclerosis, reduce plaque formation, and improve arterial health. Human clinical studies have supported the role of pomegranate juice (240 ml/day) in benefiting heart health.[36–38] An important caveat with pomegranate juice or any beneficial fruit juice (blueberry, cherry, grape, etc.) is that it can be a significant source of simple sugars, so consume in moderation. Keep the serving size no greater than 4 to 6 fl oz and drink it no more than twice per day.

Lowering Cholesterol Levels

Lowering total cholesterol as well as LDL and triglycerides is clearly associated with reducing CVD risk. For more information, see the chapter "High Cholesterol and/or Triglycerides."

Antioxidants

Dietary antioxidant nutrients such as lycopene, lutein, selenium, vitamin E, and vitamin C have been shown in population-based studies to offer significant protection against the development of CVD. Fats and cholesterol are particularly susceptible to free radical damage. When damaged, fats and cholesterol form lipid peroxides and oxidized cholesterol, which can then damage the artery walls and accelerate the progression of atherosclerosis. Antioxidants block the formation of these damaging compounds.

Although diets rich in antioxidant nutrients have consistently shown tremendous protection against CVD, clinical trials using antioxidant vitamins and minerals have produced inconsistent results.[39,40] This failure may be due to several factors, most impor-

tantly the fact that the human antioxidant system is a complex system of interacting components. It is unlikely that any single antioxidant would be proven to be effective, especially in the absence of a supporting cast. Most antioxidants require some sort of "partner" antioxidant, allowing them to work more efficiently. The most salient example of this is the partnership between the two primary antioxidants in the human body, vitamins C and E. Vitamin C is an aqueous-phase antioxidant, while vitamin E is a lipid-phase antioxidant. Although some studies have shown that supplementation with these nutrients reduces atherosclerotic lesions, more protection is probably required to ensure optimal effect.[41]

In addition to vitamin C, vitamin E also requires selenium and CoQ_{10} to work efficiently (as discussed in more detail later). Another shortcoming of many of the studies on antioxidant nutrients is the lack of consideration given to the importance of phytochemicals and plant-derived antioxidants, which, in addition to having benefits on their own, are well known to potentiate the activities of vitamin and mineral antioxidants. Phytochemicals such as carotenes (especially lycopene and lutein) and flavonoids are especially important in fighting free radical damage. Most scientific reviews on antioxidant supplements devote significant attention to studies of beta-carotene, because they have involved more than 70,000 subjects, but such studies fail to differentiate the facts that synthetic beta-carotene was used and that beta-carotene is of little importance in protecting against LDL oxidation. (Unlike lycopene and lutein, beta-carotene does not become incorporated into LDL effectively, although it may help protect the endothelium.)

Lutein may turn out to be the most significant carotene in the battle against atherosclerosis. On the basis of analysis of the different subtypes of LDL, lycopene, beta-carotene, and cryptoxanthin were mainly located in the larger, less dense LDL particles, whereas lutein and zeaxanthin tended to be found in the smaller, denser LDL particles. Because the smaller, denser LDL subtype is more easily oxidized, lutein and zeaxanthin are particularly important in protecting against damage to LDL.[42]

Other vitamins and minerals may also be important in supporting the effectiveness of antioxidants. Taking a multivitamin/multimineral supplement seems appropriate. In one double-blind study, CRP levels were significantly lower in the multivitamin group than in the placebo group, with the reduction in CRP levels most evident in patients who had elevated levels (equal to or greater than 1 mg/L) at baseline.[43] Researchers found that serum vitamin B_6 and vitamin C levels were inversely associated with CRP level.

Vitamin E

Although clinical studies have shown inconsistent effects, it is clear that vitamin E does play a role in the protection against oxidation of LDL because of its ability to be easily incorporated into the LDL molecule. Furthermore, there is a clear-cut dosage effect (i.e., the higher the dosage of vitamin E, the greater the degree of protection against oxidative damage to LDL). Although dosages as low as 25 mg were originally shown to offer some protection, it appears that doses greater than 400 IU are required to produce clinically significant effects.[44–46] However, what is probably of greatest importance is to use vitamin E within the context of a comprehensive dietary and supplementation strategy to boost antioxidant status.

Vitamin E supplementation may offer help in protecting against heart disease and strokes because of its ability to do the following:

- Reduce LDL oxidation and increase plasma LDL breakdown
- Inhibit excessive platelet aggregation
- Increase HDL levels
- Reduce CRP levels
- Improve endothelial cell function
- Improve insulin sensitivity

Two early large-scale studies with relatively low dosages of vitamin E supplementation demonstrated a significant reduction in the risk of heart attack or stroke. The Nurses Health Study of 87,245 female health care professionals concluded that those who took 100 IU of vitamin E daily for more than two years had a 41% lower risk of heart disease compared with nonusers of vitamin E supplements.[47] The Physicians Health Study of 39,910 male health care professionals found similar results: a 37% lower risk of heart disease with the intake of more than 30 IU of supplemental vitamin E daily.[48] Subsequent studies, however, have been inconsistent in showing any benefit at all. In fact, in some studies vitamin E supplementation was shown to be associated with an increased risk for CVD death.[49] Again, an important consideration is that vitamin E has a very narrow antioxidant effect and may not be effective unless paired with complementary antioxidants.

Some of the disappointing results may also have been due to the choice of synthetic vitamin E (D,L-alpha tocopherol) in one of the large studies vs. the more active natural form (D-alpha tocopherol). There is also the problem of the interference by statin drugs in vitamin E and CoQ_{10} metabolism; this interference increases the need for both compounds. Vitamin E and CoQ_{10} work synergistically, and each is required for the regeneration of the other. For example, CoQ_{10} is present in the blood in both oxidized (inactive) and reduced (active) form. During times of increased oxidative stress or low vitamin E levels, more CoQ_{10} will be converted to its oxidized form. Thus, by providing higher levels of vitamin E, the biological activity and function of CoQ_{10} are enhanced, and vice versa. Several studies in humans and animals have shown that the combination of vitamin E and CoQ_{10} works better than either alone. For example, in a study of baboons, where supplementation with vitamin E alone reduced CRP levels, co-supplementation with CoQ_{10} significantly enhanced this effect of vitamin E. Similar results have been seen in other animal studies of other factors associated with atherosclerosis, including LDL oxidation and lipid peroxide content within the aorta.[50–52]

In addition to CoQ_{10}, vitamin E also requires adequate selenium status for optimal antioxidant effects. Selenium functions primarily as a component of the antioxidant enzyme glutathione peroxidase. This enzyme works closely with vitamin E to prevent free radical damage to cell membranes. Studies looking only at vitamin E's ability to reduce cancer and heart disease are often faulty because they fail to factor in the critical partnership between selenium and vitamin E, not to mention the interrelationship between vitamin E and CoQ_{10}. Several studies have clearly demonstrated that low selenium status is significantly associated with coronary artery disease.[53,54] Failure to co-supplement with selenium as well as vitamin C and CoQ_{10} may be a major reason for the inconsistent results in intervention trials with vitamin E supplementation alone.

Finally, when you are taking vitamin E, it is important to take mixed tocopherols (that is, all the forms of vitamin E found in food) rather than simply d-alpha-tocopherol.

Vitamin C

Vitamin C works as an antioxidant in aqueous (watery) environments in the body, both outside and inside cells. It is the first line of antioxidant protection in the body. Its primary antioxidant partner is vitamin E, as this antioxidant is fat-soluble. Along with CoQ_{10}, vitamin C is also responsible for regenerating vitamin E after it has been oxidized in the body, thus potentiating the antioxidant benefits of vitamin E.[55] Vitamin C works along with antioxidant enzymes such as glutathione peroxidase, catalase, and superoxide dismutase as well. Vitamin C has been shown to be extremely effective in preventing LDL from being oxidized, even in smokers.[56] Vitamin C and E supplementation, 500 mg and 272 IU per day respectively for six years, has been shown to reduce the progression of carotid atherosclerosis by 53% in men and 14% in women.[57]

A high dietary intake of vitamin C has been shown to significantly reduce the risk of death from heart attacks and strokes, as well as all other causes, including cancer, in numerous population studies. One of the most detailed studies analyzed the vitamin C intake of 11,348 adults over five years and divided them into three groups: (1) less than 50 mg dietary intake per day, (2) more than 50 mg per day dietary intake with no vitamin C supplementation, and (3) more than 50 mg dietary intake plus vitamin C supplementation (estimated to be equal to or greater than 300 mg).[58] Analysis showed that the average death rate (for CVD and overall mortality) was up to 48% lower in the high-intake group than in the low-intake group. These differences correspond to an increase in longevity of five to seven years for men and one to three years for women.

Dozens of observational and clinical studies have shown that vitamin C levels correspond to total cholesterol and HDL.[59–61] In one of the best-designed studies, it was shown that the higher the vitamin C content of the blood, the lower the total cholesterol and triglycerides and the higher the HDL.[61] The benefits for HDL were particularly impressive. For each 0.5 mg/dl increase in vitamin C content of the blood, there was an increase in HDL of 14.9 mg/dl in women and 2.1 mg/dl in men. This study is significant in having demonstrated that the association of vitamin C and HDL levels persists even in well-nourished individuals with normal serum levels of vitamin C who supplement their diets with additional vitamin C.

In summary, vitamin C lowers the risk of CVD by doing the following:[62,63]

- Acting as an antioxidant
- Strengthening the collagen structures of the arteries
- Lowering total cholesterol, Lp(a), and blood pressure
- Raising HDL levels
- Inhibiting platelet aggregation
- Promoting the breakdown of fibrin (a component of blood clots and arterial plaque)
- Reducing markers of inflammation
- Regenerating vitamin E

Grape Seed and Pine Bark Extracts

One of the most beneficial groups of plant flavonoids is the procyanidolic oligomers (PCOs). Although PCOs exist in many plants as well as in red wine, commercially available sources of PCO include extracts from grape seeds and the bark of the maritime (Landes) pine. These extracts offer protection through several different mechanisms, including their antioxidant activity and effects on the endothelial cells that line blood vessels.[64,65]

Miscellaneous Risk Factors

Platelet Aggregation

Excessive platelet aggregation, or clumping, is another risk factor for heart disease and stroke. Once platelets aggregate, they release potent compounds that dramatically promote the formation of atherosclerotic plaque, or they can form a clot that can lodge in small arteries and produce a heart attack or stroke. The adhesiveness of platelets is determined largely by the type of fats in the diet and the level of antioxidants. While saturated fats and cholesterol increase platelet aggregation, omega-3 oils (both short-chain and long-chain) and monounsaturated fats have the opposite effect.[66–68]

In addition to the monounsaturated and omega-3 fatty acids, antioxidant nutrients, and flavonoids, vitamin B_6 also inhibits platelet aggregation and lowers blood pressure and homocysteine levels.[69,70] In one study, the effect of vitamin B_6 (pyridoxine HCl) supplementation on platelet aggregation, plasma lipids, and serum zinc levels was determined in 24 healthy male volunteers (19 to 24 years old) given either pyridoxine at a dosage of 5 mg/kg or a placebo for four weeks.[69] Results demonstrated that pyridoxine inhibited platelet aggregation by 41% to 48%, while there was no change in the control group. Pyridoxine prolonged both bleeding and coagulation time but not over physiologic limits. It had no effect on platelet count. Pyridoxine was also shown to lower total plasma lipids and cholesterol levels considerably from pretreatment levels. Total plasma lipids were reduced from 593 to 519 mg/dl, and total cholesterol was reduced from 156 to 116 mg/dl. HDL increased from 37.9 to 48.6 mg/dl. Serum zinc levels increased from 96 to 138 mg/dl.

In another study, a significant inverse graded relation was observed between the serum level of an active form of vitamin B_6—pyridoxal-5-phosphate (P5P)—and both CRP and fibrinogen.[70] Low P5P concentrations were associated with a calculated 89% increase in CVD. These results provide clear evidence of the possible role of vitamin B_6 supplementation in reducing the risk of atherosclerotic mortality.

Garlic preparations standardized for alliin content as well as garlic oil have also demonstrated inhibition of platelet aggregation. In one study, 120 patients with increased platelet aggregation were given either 900 mg per day of a dried garlic preparation containing 1.3% alliin or a placebo for four weeks.[71] In the garlic group, spontaneous platelet aggregation disappeared, the microcirculation of the skin increased by 47.6%, plasma viscosity decreased by 3.2%, diastolic blood pressure dropped from an average of 74 to 67 mm Hg, and fasting blood glucose concentration dropped from an average of 89.4 to 79 mg/dl.

Fibrinogen

Fibrinogen is a component of blood clots and atherosclerotic plaque. Elevated fibrinogen levels are another clear risk factor for CVD. Early clinical studies stimulated detailed population-based investigations into the possible link between fibrinogen and CVD. The first such study was the Northwick Park Heart Study in the United Kingdom. This large study involved 1,510 men 40 to 64 years of age who were randomly recruited and tested for a range of clotting factors including fibrinogen. At the four-year follow-up, there was a stronger association between cardiovascular deaths and fibrinogen levels than that for cholesterol. This association has now been confirmed in at least five other large population-based studies.[72]

Natural therapies designed to promote the breakdown of fibrin (fibrinolysis) include exercise, omega-3 oils, niacin, garlic, and nattokinase. Nattokinase is a protein-digesting enzyme isolated from a fermented soy product called natto. Nattokinase has potent fibrinolytic and thrombolytic (clot-busting) activity that has shown significant potential in improving CVD.[73] Typical dosage is 100 mg (2,000 FU) once or twice per day.

In addition, the Mediterranean diet alone significantly reduces fibrinogen and other markers of inflammation.[74] Adherence to the Mediterranean diet was shown to be associated with a 20% lower CRP level, 17% lower another marker of inflammation (interleukin-6 level), 15% lower homocysteine level, and 6% lower fibrinogen level.

Homocysteine

Homocysteine, an intermediate in the conversion of the amino acid methionine to cysteine, can damage the lining of arteries as well as the brain. If a person is functionally deficient in folic acid, vitamin B_6, or vitamin B_{12}, there will be an increase in homocysteine. Elevated homocysteine levels are an independent risk factor for heart attack, stroke, or peripheral vascular disease. Elevations in homocysteine are found in approximately 20 to 40% of patients with heart disease and are significantly associated with CVD.[75–78]

Although folic acid supplementation (400 mg per day) alone can reduce homocysteine levels in many subjects, given the importance of vitamins B_{12} and B_6 to proper homocysteine metabolism, all three should be used together. In one study the suboptimal levels of these nutrients in men with elevated homocysteine levels were 56.8%, 59.1%, and 25% for folic acid, vitamin B_{12}, and vitamin B_6, respectively, indicating that folic acid supplementation alone would not lower homocysteine levels in many cases.[79] In other words, folic acid supplementation will lower homocysteine levels only if there are adequate levels of vitamins B_{12} and B_6.

In 1998 the FDA mandated the fortification of food products with folic acid. Although homocysteine levels have decreased modestly since then, the effect on mortality has been minor at best.[80] This indicates the importance of more aggressive supplementary measures to reduce homocysteine-associated cardiovascular risk and the need to address all three nutrients, not just one.

Type A Personality

Type A behavior is characterized by an extreme sense of time urgency, competitiveness, impatience, and aggressiveness. This behavior carries with it a twofold increase in CHD compared with non-type-A behavior.[81–83] Particularly damaging to the cardiovascular system is the regular expression of anger. In one study, the relationship between habitual anger as a coping style, especially anger expression, and serum lipid concentrations was examined in 86 healthy subjects.[82] Habitual anger expression was measured on four scales: aggression, controlled affect, guilt, and social inhibition. A positive correlation between serum cholesterol level and aggression was found. The higher the aggression score, the higher the cholesterol level. A negative correlation was found between the ratio of LDL to HDL and controlled affect score—the greater the ability to control anger, the lower this ratio. In other words, those who learn to control anger experience a significant reduction in the risk for heart disease, while an unfavorable lipid profile is linked with a predominantly aggressive (hostile) anger coping style.

Anger expression also plays a role in CRP levels. In one study, greater anger and severity of depressive symptoms, separately and in combination with hostility, were significantly associated with elevations in CRP in apparently healthy men and women.[83] Other mechanisms explaining the link between the emotions, personality, and CVD include increased cortisol secretion, endothelial dysfunction, hypertension, and increased platelet aggregation and fibrinogen levels.[84]

Ten Tips to Help You Improve Your Coping Strategies

1. Do not starve your emotional life. Foster meaningful relationships. Provide time to give and receive love in your life.

2. Learn to be a good listener. Allow the people in your life to really share their feelings and thoughts uninterruptedly. Empathize with them; put yourself in their shoes.

3. Do not try to talk over somebody. If you find yourself being interrupted, relax; do not try to outtalk the other person. If you are courteous and allow someone else to speak, eventually (unless the person is extremely rude) he or she will respond likewise. If not, explain that he or she is interrupting the communication process. You can do this only if you have been a good listener.

4. Avoid aggressive or passive behavior. Be assertive, but express your thoughts and feelings in a kind way to help improve relationships at work and at home.

5. Avoid excessive stress in your life as best you can by avoiding excessive work hours, poor nutrition, and inadequate rest. Get as much sleep as you can.

6. Avoid stimulants such as caffeine and nicotine. Stimulants promote the fight-or-flight response and tend to make people more irritable in the process.

7. Take time to build long-term health and success by performing stress-reduction techniques and deep breathing exercises.

8. Accept gracefully those things over which you have no control. Save your energy for those things that you can do something about.

9. Accept yourself. Remember that you are human and will make mistakes from which you can learn along the way.

10. Be more patient and tolerant of other people. Follow the golden rule.

Magnesium and Potassium Deficiency

Magnesium and potassium are absolutely essential to the proper functioning of the entire cardiovascular system. Their critical roles in preventing heart disease and strokes are now widely accepted. In addition, there is a substantial body of knowledge demonstrating that supplementation of magnesium, potassium, or both is effective in treating a wide range of cardiovascular disease, including angina, arrhythmias, congestive heart failure, and high blood pressure. In many of these applications, magnesium or potassium supplementation has been used for more than 50 years.

The average intake of magnesium by healthy adults in the United States ranges from 143 to 266 mg per day. This level is well below even the recommended daily intake (RDI) of 350 mg for men and 300 mg for women. Food choices are the main reason. Because magnesium occurs abundantly in whole foods, many nutritionists and dietitians assume that most Americans get enough magnesium in their diets. But most Americans are not eating whole, natural foods. They are consuming large quantities of processed foods. Because food processing removes a large portion of a food's magnesium,

most Americans are not getting the RDI for magnesium.

The best dietary sources of magnesium are tofu, legumes, seeds, nuts, whole grains, and green leafy vegetables. Fish, meat, milk, and most commonly eaten fruits are quite low in magnesium. Most Americans consume a low-magnesium diet because their diet is high in low-magnesium foods such as processed foods, meat, and dairy products.

People dying of heart attacks have been shown to have lower heart magnesium levels than people of the same age dying of other causes.[85] Low magnesium levels contribute to atherosclerosis and CVD via many mechanisms including disruption of the protective factors within the lining of the arteries.[86]

Intravenous magnesium therapy has now emerged as a valued treatment measure in acute heart attack.[87–89] The major obstacle to its becoming the preferred method for saving a person's life may be a financial interest. Magnesium is cheap compared with new high-tech, high-priced, genetically engineered drugs currently being promoted by drug companies. The treatment of heart attacks is big business in the United States: each year more than 1.5 million U.S. citizens experience one. Although many other parts of the world are now using magnesium therapy for heart attack because of its effectiveness, low cost, safety, and ease of administration, it plays second fiddle to the high-tech drugs in the United States.

During the past decade, eight well-designed studies involving more than 4,000 patients have demonstrated that intravenous magnesium supplementation during the first hour of admission to a hospital for acute heart attack reduces immediate and long-term complications as well as death rates. The beneficial effects of magnesium in heart attack relate to its ability to do the following:

- Improve energy production within the heart
- Dilate the coronary arteries, resulting in improved delivery of oxygen to the heart
- Reduce peripheral vascular resistance, resulting in reduced demand on the heart
- Inhibit platelets from aggregating and forming blood clots
- Reduce the size of the blockage
- Improve heart rate and arrhythmias

Vitamin D Deficiency

Data from a detailed study involving more than 8,000 subjects indicate that individuals with vitamin D levels below 30 ng/ml had at higher risk for CVD.[90] Another study of more than 3,000 men and women found that those in the lowest quartile of vitamin D blood levels had a more than a twofold increase in CVD mortality.[91]

Preventing a Second Heart Attack

People who have experienced a heart attack or stroke and live through it are extremely likely to experience another. To prevent future cardiovascular events, the primary focus is, of course, still on controlling the major cardiac risk factors (e.g., high cholesterol levels, hypertension, cigarette smoking, diabetes, physical inactivity). But many physicians recommend low-dose aspirin (e.g., usually 325 mg per every other day or 81 mg—one "baby" aspirin—per day) to reduce the risk of a subsequent heart attack. However, there may be more effective alternatives, especially for those who cannot tolerate aspirin therapy. Furthermore, although it is becoming increasing popular to recommend dosages of aspirin lower than 325 mg every other day

there are few (if any) data to support these lower dosage recommendations.

Aspirin Therapy

Let's first take a look at studies with aspirin. It has been shown to decrease the risk of CVD events (heart attack or stroke) in people who have never had a heart attack as well as in those with a history of a heart attack. In the Physicians Health Study, there was a 44% reduction in the risk of a first heart attack with the use of 325 mg aspirin every other day. Since this study, three additional randomized trials including both men and women have shown aspirin to be effective in the prevention of a first heart attack. Among the 55,580 subjects, aspirin use was associated with a statistically significant 32% reduction in the risk of a first heart attack and a significant 15% reduction in the risk of all other important vascular events, but it had no significant effects on nonfatal stroke or death due to a heart attack or stroke. Evaluation of the data from the Physicians Health Study indicated that those with the highest CRP had the greatest decrease in risk, 55.7%, vs. 13.9% in those with the lowest CRP. It seems reasonable to reserve the use of aspirin as a primary prevention strategy for individuals with high CRP values.[92]

As of 2012 there have been seven prospective randomized placebo-controlled trials involving almost 15,000 survivors of heart attack that have examined the use of aspirin to reduce the incidence of recurrent heart attack and death due to a heart attack. These trials have used several doses of aspirin ranging from 325 to 1,500 mg per day, and enrolled patients at various intervals after the heart attack, ranging from four weeks to five years. None of the studies demonstrated a statistically significant reduction in mortality with aspirin use. However, when all the results from these studies were pooled, aspirin was shown to reduce the mortality rate from all causes as well as cardiovascular deaths. The mortality rate for all causes in the aspirin group was 5.8%, compared with 8.3% in the placebo group, indicating a reduction in mortality by 30% with aspirin.[93,94]

Aspirin and other nonsteroidal anti-inflammatory drugs (NSAIDs) are associated with a significant risk of peptic ulcer. However, most studies documenting the relative frequency of peptic ulcers as a consequence of NSAIDs have focused on the drugs' use in the treatment of arthritis and headaches. The risk of gastrointestinal bleeding due to peptic ulcers has been evaluated for aspirin at daily dosages of 300, 150, and 75 mg. Essentially there is an increased risk of gastrointestinal bleeding due to peptic ulcers at all dosage levels. However, the dosage of 75 mg per day was associated with a lower risk, a 2.3-fold increased risk of ulcers compared with 3.9-fold increased risk at 300 mg per day and 3.2-fold risk at 150 mg per day.[95]

Because it is unknown whether 75 mg per day of aspirin is helpful in preventing a second heart attack or stroke, most physicians recommend at least 300 mg. To prevent death due to a stroke, the dosage necessary appears to be 900 mg. However, these dosage recommendations carry with them a significant risk for developing a peptic ulcer but may be appropriate for high-risk patients unwilling to adopt the natural approach.

Dietary Alternatives to Aspirin

The best approach to preventing subsequent heart attacks may not be low-dose aspirin, especially in aspirin-sensitive patients. The first alternative to aspirin to be examined here is one too often overlooked by many physicians—diet. Several studies have shown that dietary modifications not only are more

effective in preventing recurrent heart attack than aspirin but also can reverse the blockage of clogged arteries. In addition to the studies with the Mediterranean diet, three famous studies deserve special mention. The first was the Lifestyle Heart Trial, conducted by Dean Ornish.[96] In this study, subjects with heart disease were divided into a control group and an experimental group. The control group received regular medical care, while the experimental group members were asked to eat a low-fat vegetarian diet for at least one year. The diet included fruits, vegetables, grains, legumes, and soybean products. Subjects were allowed to consume as many calories as they wished. No animal products were allowed except egg whites and 1 cup of nonfat milk or yogurt per day. The diet contained approximately 10% fat, 15% to 20% protein, and 70% to 75% carbohydrates (predominantly complex carbohydrates from whole grains, legumes, and vegetables).

The experimental group members were also asked to perform stress reduction techniques such as breathing exercises, stretching exercises, meditation, imagery, and other relaxation techniques for an hour each day and to exercise for at least three hours each week. At the end of the year, the subjects in the experimental group showed significant overall regression of atherosclerosis of the coronary blood vessels. In contrast, subjects in the control group who were being treated with regular medical care and following the standard AHA diet actually showed progression of their disease. Ornish stated: "This finding suggests that conventional recommendations for patients with CHD (such as a 30% fat diet) are not sufficient to bring about regression in many patients."

Two other famous studies showing that diet can prevent further heart attacks in patients suffering a first heart attack highlight the importance of omega-3 fatty acids and again show the ineffectiveness of the AHA's dietary recommendations. As stated previously, numerous population studies have demonstrated that people who consume a diet rich in omega-3 oils from either fish or vegetable sources have a significantly reduced risk of developing heart disease. Two famous intervention trials upheld this protective effect. In the Dietary and Reinfarction Trial (DART), it was only when the intake of omega-3 fatty acids (from fish) was increased that future heart attacks were reduced.[97] In another study, the Lyon Diet Heart Study, increasing the intake of omega-3 fatty acids from plant sources (alpha-linolenic acid) was found to offer the same degree of protection as increased fish intake.[98]

Finally, we can't emphasize enough that there are no side effects of a healthy diet comparable to the increased risk of ulcers and other problems from taking aspirin.

Other Considerations

Angiography, Coronary Artery Bypass Surgery, or Angioplasty?

A significant challenge for patients is weighing the benefits against the risks when they are referred for angiography, coronary artery bypass surgery, or angioplasty. As is fully discussed in the chapter "Angina," these procedures are used far more frequently than is justified by objective evaluation of their appropriateness and efficacy. That chapter also gives advice for patient care when angiography, coronary artery bypass surgery, or angioplasty is unavoidable.

In one study, angiography performed on 205 consecutive patients showed an 82% accuracy in predicting heart disease, with a false-positive rate of 12% and a false-negative rate of 18%.

Earlobe Crease

The presence of a diagonal earlobe crease has been recognized as a sign of CVD since 1973. More than 30 studies have been reported in the medical literature. The earlobe is richly vascularized, and a decrease in blood flow over an extended period of time is believed to result in collapse of the vascular bed. This leads to a diagonal crease.[99,100]

In a study of 112 consecutive patients, the earlobe crease was highly correlated with demonstrable heart disease and less strongly with previous heart attack.[99]

The crease is seen more commonly with advancing age, until the age of 80, when the incidence drops dramatically. However, the association with heart disease is independent of age. Although the presence of an earlobe crease does not prove heart disease, it strongly suggests it, and examination of the earlobe is an easy screening procedure. The correlation does not hold with Asians, Native Americans, or children with Beckwith's syndrome.[100]

· ·

QUICK REVIEW

- **Atherosclerosis—hardening of the artery walls—is the underlying disease process in cardiovascular disease (CVD).**

- **Prevention of CVD involves reducing and, when possible, eliminating various risk factors.**
- **Cigarette smoking is perhaps the most**

important risk factor for CVD, as statistical evidence reveals smokers have a 70% greater risk of death from CVD than nonsmokers.

- The evidence overwhelmingly demonstrates that elevated cholesterol levels, especially elevations in LDL cholesterol, greatly increase the risk of death due to CVD.

- Physical activity and regular exercise protect against the development of CVD and also favorably modify other CVD risk factors including high blood pressure, blood lipid levels, insulin resistance, and obesity.

- High-sensitivity C-reactive protein, a blood marker that reflects different degrees of inflammation, has been identified as an independent risk factor for coronary artery disease.

- One of the most important aspects of the Mediterranean diet may be the combination of olive oil (a source of monounsaturated fats and antioxidants) and the intake of omega-3 fatty acids.

- Higher consumption of nuts and seeds has been shown to significantly reduce the risk of CVD in large population-based studies including the Nurses Health Study, the Iowa Health Study, and the Physicians Health Study.

- Dietary antioxidant nutrients such as lycopene, lutein, selenium, vitamin E, and vitamin C have been shown in population-based studies to offer significant protection against the development of CVD.

- Several studies have shown that dietary modifications not only are more effective in preventing recurrent heart attack than aspirin but also can reverse the blockage of clogged arteries.

- The presence of a diagonal earlobe crease has been recognized as a sign of CVD since 1973.

. . . .

TREATMENT SUMMARY

There is little doubt that in most cases atherosclerosis is directly related to diet and lifestyle. Treatment and prevention include reducing all known risk factors. In particular, it is important to work with your physician in identifying risk factors via laboratory evaluation of such factors as cholesterol, triglyceride, and CRP levels.

Lifestyle

- Do not smoke.
- Achieve and maintain ideal body weight.
- Exercise on a regular basis.

Diet

- Follow the dietary guidelines given in the chapter "A Health-Promoting Diet."

Specifically, it is important to do the following:

○ Eat less saturated fat and cholesterol by reducing or eliminating the amounts of animal products in the diet.

○ Increase consumption of fiber-rich plant foods (fruits, vegetables, grains, legumes, nuts, and seeds).

○ Increase consumption of monounsaturated fats (e.g., nuts, seeds, and olive oil) and omega-3 fatty acids.

○ Follow a low-glycemic diet.

Nutritional Supplements

• Take a high-potency multivitamin and mineral formula according to the guidelines given in the chapter "Supplementary Measures."

• Key individual nutrients:

○ Vitamin C: 250 to 500 mg one to three times per day

○ Vitamin E (mixed tocopherols): 100 to 200 IU per day

○ Vitamin D: 2,000 to 4,000 IU per day (ideally, measure blood levels and adjust dosage accordingly)

○ Vitamin B_6: 25 to 50 mg per day

○ Folic acid: 800 mcg per day

○ Vitamin B_{12}: 800 mcg per day

○ Magnesium: 250 to 400 mg per day

○ Fish oils: minimum 1,000 mg EPA + DHA per day

○ One of the following:

– Grape seed extract (> 95% procyanidolic oligomers): 100 to 300 mg per day

– Pine bark extract (> 95% procyanidolic oligomers): 100 to 300 mg per day

– Some other flavonoid-rich extract with a similar flavonoid content, super greens formula, or other plant-based antioxidant that can provide an oxygen radical absorption capacity (ORAC) of 3,000 to 6,000 units or higher per day

○ Consider:

– Nattokinase: 100 mg (2,000 FU) per day

Immune System Support

Introduction

The immune system is one of the most complex and fascinating systems of the human body. Its primary function is to protect the body against infection and the development of cancer. Too often conventional medicine overlooks the importance of susceptibility to infection or disease. Support and enhancement of the immune system are perhaps the most important and vital steps in reducing susceptibility to colds, flu, and cancer.

Determining Immune Function

The criteria that we use to determine whether the immune system is going to be an area of focus is an answer of yes to any of the following questions:

- Do you catch colds or flu easily?
- Do you get colds or flu more than three times a year?
- Are you suffering from chronic infection?
- Do you get frequent cold sores or fungal nail infections, or do you have genital herpes?
- Are your lymph glands sore and swollen at times?
- Do you have now or have you ever had cancer?

Recurrent or chronic infections, even very mild colds, happen only when the immune system is weakened. What makes it difficult for susceptible people to overcome their tendency for infection is a repetitive cycle: a weakened immune system leads to infection, and chronic infection leads to depletion of the immune system, further weakening resistance. Enhancing the immune system by following the guidelines in this chapter may provide the means of breaking the cycle.

Components of the Immune System

The immune system is composed of the lymphatic vessels and organs (thymus, spleen, tonsils, and lymph nodes), white blood cells (lymphocytes, neutrophils, basophils, eosinophils, monocytes, etc.), specialized cells residing in various tissue (macrophages, mast cells, etc.), and specialized serum factors.

The Thymus

The thymus is the major gland of our immune system. It is composed of two soft pinkish gray lobes lying like a bib just below the thyroid gland and above the heart. To a very large extent, the health of the thymus determines the health of the immune system. Individuals who get frequent infections or suffer from chronic infections typically have impaired thymus activity. Also, people affected with hay fever, allergies, migraine headaches, or rheumatoid arthritis usually have altered thymus function.

The thymus is responsible for many immune system functions, including the production of T lymphocytes, a type of white blood cell responsible for cell-mediated immunity (immune mechanisms not controlled or mediated by antibodies). Cell-mediated immunity is extremely important in the resistance to infection by mold-like bacteria, yeast (including *Candida albicans*), fungi, parasites, and viruses (including herpes simplex, Epstein-Barr, and viruses that cause hepatitis). If an individual is suffering from an infection from these organisms, it is a good indication that his or her cell-mediated immunity is not functioning up to par. Cell-mediated immunity is also critical in protecting against the development of cancer, autoimmune disorders such as rheumatoid arthritis, and allergies.

The thymus gland releases several hormones, such as thymosin, thymopoeitin, and serum thymic factor, which regulate many immune functions. Low levels of these hormones in the blood are associated with depressed immunity and an increased susceptibility to infection. Typically, thymic hormone levels will be very low in the elderly (thymus function decreases with age), individuals prone to infection, cancer and AIDS patients, and individuals exposed to undue stress.

Lymph, Lymphatic Vessels, and Lymph Nodes

Approximately one-sixth of the entire body is the space between cells. Collectively this space is referred to as the interstitium and the fluid contained within the space is referred to as the interstitial fluid. This fluid flows into the lymphatic vessels and becomes the lymph.

Lymphatic vessels usually run parallel to arteries and veins. The vessels serve to drain waste products from tissues. The lymphatic vessels transport the lymph to lymph nodes, which filter the lymph. The cells responsible for filtering the lymph are macrophages. These large cells engulf and destroy foreign particles, including bacteria and cellular debris.

The lymph nodes also contain B lymphocytes, white blood cells capable of initiating antibody production in response to the presence of viruses, bacteria, yeast, and other organisms.

The Spleen

The spleen is the largest mass of lymphatic tissue in the body. Weighing about 7 oz, the spleen is a fist-sized, spongy, dark purple organ that lies in the upper left abdomen behind the lower ribs. The spleen's functions include producing white blood cells; engulfing and destroying bacteria and cellular debris, and destroying worn-out red blood cells and platelets. The spleen also serves as a blood reservoir. During times of demand, such as hemorrhage, the spleen can release its stored blood and prevent shock.

Like the thymus, the spleen also releases many potent immune-system-enhancing compounds. For example, tuftsin and splenopentin, two small proteins secreted by the spleen, have been shown to exert profound immune-enhancing activity.

White Blood Cells

There are several types of white blood cells, including neutrophils, eosinophils, basophils, lymphocytes, and monocytes.

Neutrophils
These cells actively phagocytize—engulf and destroy—bacteria, tumor cells, and dead particulate matter. Neutrophils are especially important in preventing bacterial infection.

Eosinophils and Basophils

These cells are involved in allergic conditions. They secrete histamine and other compounds designed to break down antigen-antibody complexes, but they also promote allergic mechanisms.

Lymphocytes

There are several types of lymphocytes, including T cells, B cells, and natural killer cells.

T cells are thymus-derived lymphocytes. These cells orchestrate many immune functions and are the major components of cell-mediated immunity (discussed above). There are different types of T cells, including helper T cells, which help other white blood cells to function; suppressor T cells, which inhibit white blood cell functions; and cytotoxic T cells, which attack and destroy foreign tissue, cancer cells, and virus-infected cells.

The ratio of helper T cells to suppressor T cells is a useful determinant of immune function. If the ratio is low, immunodeficiency is present. For example, AIDS is characterized by a very low ratio of helper T cells to suppressor T cells. If the ratio of helper T cells to suppressor T cells is high, most often allergies or autoimmune disorders such as rheumatoid arthritis or lupus are present. Both high and low T cell ratios have been found in chronic fatigue syndrome.

B cells are responsible for producing antibodies, which are large protein molecules which bind to foreign molecules (antigens) on bacteria, viruses, other organisms, and tumor cells. After the antibody binds to the antigen it sets up a sequence of events that ultimately destroys the infectious organism or tumor cell.

Natural killer cells or NK cells received their name because of their ability to destroy cells that have become cancerous or infected with viruses. They are the body's first line of defense against cancer development. The level of activity of natural killer cells in chronic fatigue syndrome, cancer, and chronic viral infections is usually low.

Monocytes

Monocytes are the garbage collectors of the body. These large white blood cells are responsible for cleaning up cellular debris after an infection. Monocytes are also responsible for triggering many immune responses.

Special Tissue Cells

Macrophages

As stated earlier, the lymph is filtered by specialized cells known as macrophages. Macrophages are actually monocytes that have taken up residence in specific tissues such as the liver, spleen, and lymph nodes. These large cells phagocytize or engulf foreign particles including bacteria and cellular debris. Macrophages are essential in protecting against invasion by microorganisms as well as against damage to the lymphatic system.

Mast Cells

Mast cells are basophils that have taken up residence primarily along blood vessels. The mast cell, like the basophil, is responsible for releasing histamine and other compounds involved in allergic reactions.

Special Chemical Factors

There are a number of special chemical factors that enhance the immune system (interferon, interleukins, complement, etc.). These compounds are produced by various white blood cells—for example, interferon is produced primarily by T cells, interleukins are produced by macrophages and T cells, and complement fractions are manufactured in the liver and spleen. These special chemical factors are extremely important in activating the white blood cells to destroy cancer cells and viruses.

Supporting the Immune System

There really isn't any single magic bullet that can immediately restore immune function. The immune system is a complex integration of parts that are continuously protecting the body from microbial and cancerous attack. The immune system is truly holistic, as evidenced by the close association of psychological, neurological, nutritional, environmental, and hormonal factors with immune function. Supporting the immune system is critical to good health. Conversely, good health is critical to supporting the immune system. The best approach to supporting immune function is a comprehensive plan involving lifestyle, stress management, exercise, diet, nutritional supplementation, avoidance of toxins, and the use of botanical medicines.

Emotional State and Immune Function

The first step in supporting immune function is employing the healing power of the mind and attitude. *Psychoneuroimmunology* (PNI) is the term used to describe the interactions between emotional state, nervous system function, and the immune system.[1] Investigations into these interactions have documented that the mind and attitude play a significant role in the functioning of the immune system. However, a complete and detailed account of the many facets of PNI, or behavioral immunology, is beyond the scope of this chapter, so we will focus on the basics.

Our mood and attitude have a tremendous bearing on the function of our immune system. When we are happy and up, our immune system functions much better. Conversely, when we are depressed, our immune system tends to be impaired. Employing measures outlined in the chapter "A Positive Mental Attitude" can be quite useful in improving the immune system.

It was easily accepted by conventional medical authorities that negative emotional states adversely affect the immune system, but for some reason the medical community initially scoffed at the notion that positive emotional states can actually enhance immune function.

Although a stressor does not have to be a major life event to cause depressed immune function, it is safe to say that the more significant the stressor, the greater the impact on the immune system. The loss of a spouse, perhaps the most stressful life event, was strongly associated with increased sickness and death well before a link between the mind and immune function was documented. In fact, it was not until 1977 that a study of 26 bereaved spouses documented that grief led to a significant depression in immune function (natural killer cell activity was significantly reduced).[2] Subsequent studies have further demonstrated that bereavement, depression, and stress significantly diminish important immune functions.[1,3]

Positive Emotional State and Immune Function

By the end of the 1970s, several studies had shown that negative emotions suppress immune function. But in 1979, Norman Cousins' popular book *Anatomy of an Illness* caused a significant stir in the medical community. Cousins's book provided an autobiographical anecdotal account that positive emotional states can cure the body of even a quite serious disease.[4] Cousins watched *Candid Camera* and Marx Brothers films and read humorous books.

Originally physicians and researchers scoffed at Cousins's account. But they soon demonstrated in numerous studies that laughter and other positive emotional states can in fact enhance the immune system.[5,6] In addition, guided imagery, hypnosis, and other meditative states have been shown to enhance immune system function.[1,7]

If you want to have a healthy immune system, you need to laugh often, view life with a positive eye, and put yourself in a relaxed state of mind on a regular basis.

Stress

Many clinical and experimental studies have clearly demonstrated that stress, personality, attitude, and emotion are etiologic or contributory in suppressing the immune system as well as leading to the development of many and diverse diseases.[1] Reaction to stressful stimuli is entirely individual, reinforcing the fact that people differ significantly in their perceptions of and responses to various life events. The variations in response help account for the wide diversity of stress-induced illnesses. Stress causes increases in blood levels of the adrenal hormones adrenaline and cortisol, leading to an immune-suppressed state and leaving the host susceptible to infectious and carcinogenic illnesses. This immune suppression is proportional to the level of stress, and although the effects are numerous, they appear to involve a common mechanism: increases in cortisol, pro-inflammatory compounds known as cytokines, and adrenaline, resulting in significant decrease in white blood cell function, thymic function, and the formation of new white blood cells. More than 150 clinical studies have now shown that stress can alter immune function and contribute to the development of significant disease and poor health.[1,3] Stress not only disrupts the immune system's ability to fight infection but also can lead to the

development of allergies and/or autoimmune disease.[8–10]

Studies have documented the relationship between psychosocial stress and the development of infectious illness. Research studies often use the response to a vaccine to simulate the response to an infectious organism as a measure of immune system function. For example, the chronic stress associated with caring for a spouse with Alzheimer's disease or, for younger people, experiencing stressful life events was associated with a poorer antibody response to an influenza virus vaccine than was the case in well-matched control subjects.[11,12] The premise is that the production of a delayed, weaker, and shorter-lived immune response to a vaccine is the same as an impaired immune responses to disease-causing organisms in the real world. Consistent with this concept, subjects who show poorer responses to vaccines also experience higher rates of clinical illness as well as longer-lasting infectious episodes.

Fortunately, the effects of stress on the immune system can be attenuated or even overcome with positive mood, effective stress reduction techniques, humor, laughter, and guided imagery.[1,13] For more information on dealing with stress, see the chapter "Stress Management."

Lifestyle

A healthful lifestyle, as detailed in the chapter "A Health-Promoting Lifestyle," goes a long way in establishing a healthy immune system. This benefit is perhaps most obvious when one looks at the effects of lifestyle on natural killer cell activity.[14–16] Below is a list of the lifestyle practices associated with higher natural killer cell activity. One particular lifestyle factor that is absolutely critical to healthy immune function is adequate sleep. In healthy humans, sleep deprivation has consistently been demonstrated to impair different components of immune function and mood. Interestingly, the deterioration of immune function precedes the plummeting of subjective well-being and psychosocial performance in sleep-deprived subjects.[17]

Lifestyle Practices Associated with Higher Natural Killer Cell Activity

Not smoking

Increased intake of green vegetables

Regular meals

Maintaining proper body weight

Getting more than seven hours of sleep per night

Exercising regularly

A vegetarian diet

Diet

The health of the immune system gland is greatly affected by a person's nutritional status. Dietary factors that depress immune function include nutrient deficiency, excessive consumption of sugar, consumption of allergenic foods, and high cholesterol levels in the blood. Dietary factors that enhance immune function include all essential nutrients, antioxidants, carotenes, and flavonoids. Consistent with good health, optimal immune function requires a healthy diet that:

- Is rich in whole, natural foods, such as fruits, vegetables, grains, beans, seeds, and nuts

- Is low in fats and refined sugars

- Contains adequate but not excessive amounts of protein

In addition, individuals are encouraged to drink five or six 8-fl.-oz glasses of water per day. These dietary recommendations, along with a positive mental attitude, a good high-potency multivitamin and mineral supplement, a regular exercise program, daily deep breathing and relaxation exercises (meditation, prayer, etc.), and at least seven hours of sleep per day, will go a long way in helping the immune system function at an optimal level.

Nutrient Deficiency. Nutrient deficiency is the most common cause of a depressed immune system. Although research relating nutritional status to immune function has historically concerned itself with severe malnutrition states (i.e., kwashiorkor and marasmus), attention is now shifting toward marginal deficiencies of single or multiple nutrients and the effects of too many calories. The large body of clinical and experimental data has made inevitable the conclusion that a single nutrient deficiency can profoundly impair the immune system.

Given the widespread problem of multiple marginal (subclinical) nutrient deficiencies in Americans, it can be concluded that many people are suffering from impaired immunity that would be amenable to nutritional supplementation. This statement is particularly true of the elderly. Numerous studies have shown that almost all elderly Americans are deficient in at least one nutrient, and most are deficient in many. Likewise, numerous studies show that taking a multivitamin and mineral supplement enhances immune function in elderly subjects (whether they suffer from overt nutritional deficiency or not).[18–20] These findings have considerable fundamental, clinical, and public health significance.

Sugar. The oral administration of 100 g portions of carbohydrate as glucose, fructose, sucrose, honey, or orange juice significantly reduces neutrophil phagocytosis, while starch has no effect. As can be seen in the figure below, effects start within half an hour and last for more than five hours, and typically

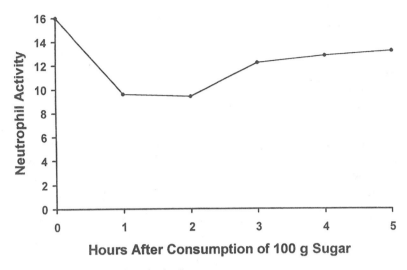

The Effects of Sugar on White Blood Cell Function

there is a 50% reduction in phagocytic activity at the peak of inhibition (usually two hours after ingestion).[21,22] Because neutrophils constitute 60 to 70% of the total white blood cell (WBC) count and are a major portion of the defense mechanism, impairment of phagocytic activity leads to an immune-compromised state. Oral administration of increasing amounts of glucose progressively lowers neutrophil phagocytosis, with maximal inhibition corresponding to maximal blood glucose levels.

In addition, oral ingestion of 75 g glucose has been shown to depress lymphocyte response; lymphocytes are the primary white blood cells that fight viruses.[23] Other parameters of immune function are also undoubtedly affected by sugar consumption.

It has been hypothesized that the ill effects of high glucose levels are a result of elevation of insulin values and competition with vitamin C for membrane transport sites.[24,25] This hypothesis is based on evidence that vitamin C and glucose appear to compete for absorption into white blood cells, which requires insulin to happen. Once inside the white blood cell, glucose and vitamin C appear to have opposite effects on immune function.

Considering that the average American consumes 125 g sucrose plus 50 g other refined simple sugars each day, the conclusion that most Americans have chronically depressed immune systems is inescapable. It is clear, particularly during an infection, that the consumption of simple sugars, even in the form of fruit juice, is harmful to the host's immune status.

Fasting during the first phase of an infection might be helpful because it results in a significant increase (up to 50%) in the phagocytic index.[21] The fast should not be continued beyond the first 24 hours, however, because eventually the white blood cells' energy sources will become depleted.

Obesity

Obesity is associated with decreased immune status, as evidenced by the reduced ability of the white blood cells of obese individuals to destroy bacteria. Obesity is also associated with higher infection rates as well as an increase in risk for certain cancers.[26] Obesity also increases the risk of asthma and autoimmune diseases by inducing decreased immunological tolerance, a consequence of immunological changes brought about by hormones known as adipokines and cytokines, secreted by fat cells.[27] In addition, cholesterol and lipid values are usually elevated in obese individuals; this may explain their impaired immune function. Increased blood levels of cholesterol, free fatty acids, triglycerides, and bile acids inhibit various immune functions, including:[28,29]

- Formation of new white blood cells
- Response to infectious agents
- Antibody response
- Movement of white blood cells to areas of infection
- Phagocytosis

Optimal immune function therefore depends on control of these serum components. Interestingly, carnitine, even at minimal concentrations, has been shown to neutralize lipid-induced immunosuppression.[30] This effect is probably due to carnitine's role as a rate-limiting factor in the removal of fatty substances from the blood. Individuals with elevations in blood lipids experiencing frequent infections may want to supplement with carnitine (900–1,500 mg per day).

Alcohol

Alcohol consumption increases the susceptibility to experimental infections in animals, and alcoholics are known to be more susceptible to infections, especially pneumonia. Studies of immune function in alcoholics show a profound depression in most indicators of immunity.[31]

Vitamins and Minerals

Vitamin A and Carotenes

Vitamin A plays an essential role in maintaining the integrity of the skin and linings of the respiratory and gastrointestinal tract as well as their secretions. These tissues constitute a primary nonspecific host defense mechanism. Vitamin A has also been shown to stimulate and/or enhance numerous immune processes. Also, vitamin A deficiency may predispose an individual to an infection, and during the course of an infection vitamin A stores typically plummet. Vitamin A may be helpful in boosting immune function beyond reversal of vitamin A deficiency, because many immune functions are further enhanced by the administration of (supposedly) excessive levels of vitamin A.[20,32] In addition, vitamin A prevents and reverses stress-induced thymus gland shrinkage (involution), and additional vitamin A can actually promote thymus growth.[33]

Carotenes have also demonstrated a number of immune-enhancing effects. In addition to being converted into vitamin A, carotenes function as antioxidants. Because the thymus gland is so susceptible to damage by free radicals, beta-carotene has advantages in enhancing the immune system that are different from vitamin A (retinol) through its ability to protect the thymus. However, taking sufficient vitamin A is still important, as about 25% of the population does not effectively convert beta-carotene to vitamin A.

Vitamin C

Vitamin C (ascorbic acid) plays an important role in the natural approach to immune enhancement. Although vitamin C has been shown to be antiviral and antibacterial, its main effect is improvement of host resistance. Many different immunostimulatory effects have been demonstrated, including enhancing lymphoproliferative response to mitogens and lymphotrophic activity and increasing interferon levels, antibody responses, immunoglobulin levels, secretion of thymic hormones, and integrity of ground substance.[20,34] Vitamin C also has direct biochemical effects similar to those of interferon.[35]

Numerous clinical studies support the use of vitamin C in the treatment of infectious conditions and possibly even cancer at very high intravenous dosages. In addition to its effects on the common cold, vitamin C has also been shown to be useful in other infectious conditions.[36] Vitamin C levels are quickly depleted during the stress of an infection as well as in chronic disease.[37]

It is useful to supplement vitamin C concurrently with flavonoids, which raise the concentration of vitamin C in some tissues and potentiate its effects as well as exert their own effects.[38]

Vitamin D

The importance of vitamin D to the regulation of cells of the immune system has gained increased appreciation over the past decade with the discovery of the vitamin D receptor on white cells and key vitamin D metabolizing enzymes expressed by cells of the immune system. Vitamin D has been shown to produce a wide range of immune-enhancing effects, including:[39–43]

- Upregulation of antimicrobial peptides, to enhance clearance of bacteria at various barrier sites and in immune cells

- Modulation of the immune system by direct effects on T cell activation

- Protection against the development of autoimmune diseases (e.g., Crohn's disease, type 1 diabetes, multiple sclerosis, asthma, and rheumatoid arthritis)

- Reduction of the frequency of viral upper respiratory infections

Vitamin D appears to be especially important in protection against viral or bacterial upper respiratory infection.[44]

Vitamin E

Vitamin E enhances both antibody production and cell-mediated immunity. A vitamin E deficiency results in atrophy of lymphoid tissue and decreases white blood cell response and function. Vitamin E supplementation (30–150 IU) has been shown to:[45]

- Increase white blood cell response
- Prevent free-radical-induced thymus atrophy
- Enhance helper T cell activity
- Increase antibody response and phagocytosis

Elderly subjects may benefit from even higher dosages of vitamin E. One study sought to determine the effect of vitamin E supplementation at different dosages on immune function in 88 patients older than 65 years.[20,46] The researchers measured T cell function by a number of assessments. Vitamin E was given at 60, 200, or 800 IU for 235 days. Although the placebo group experienced only an 8% increase in T cell function, the 60 IU group had a 20% increase, the 200 IU group a 58% increase, and the 800 IU group a 65% increase. With regard to antibody production, the best results were observed in the patients receiving 200 IU per day. No effect on autoimmune antibodies was noticed. No adverse effects were observed at any of the three dosage schedules of vitamin E.

In another double-blind study of 451 elderly participants in a nursing home, vitamin E supplementation (200 IU per day) demonstrated a protective effect against upper respiratory tract infections, particularly the common cold.[47]

Vitamin B$_6$

Vitamin B$_6$ deficiency results in depressed cellular and humoral immunity; the thymus, spleen, and lymph nodes shrink; the number of white blood cells plummets; there is a tremendous reduction in the quantity and quality of antibodies produced; and there is decreased activity of thymus hormones. Factors predisposing to vitamin B$_6$ deficiency are low dietary intake, excess protein intake, high consumption of yellow (hydralazine) food dyes, alcohol consumption, and use of oral contraceptives.

Folic Acid and Vitamin B$_{12}$

A deficiency of vitamin B$_{12}$ and/or folate results in significantly reduced production of white blood cells and abnormal white blood cell responses. Folic acid deficiency (the most common vitamin deficiency in the United States) has been shown to result in shrinkage of the thymus and lymph nodes and impaired white blood cell function. A B$_{12}$ deficiency produces identical findings and is especially harmful to the ability of white blood cells to engulf and destroy infecting organisms.

Other B Vitamins

Thiamine, riboflavin, and pantothenic acid deficiencies lead to reduced antibody response, decreased white blood cell response, and atrophy of the thymus and lymph tissue.

Iron

Iron deficiency is a common nutritional deficiency state that causes immune dysfunction in large numbers of people, in particular menstruating women, elderly individuals taking aspirin and other drugs that can cause gastrointestinal bleeding due to ulcer formation,

and children. Marginal iron deficiency, even at levels that do not lower blood values, can influence the immune system. Thymus and lymph node atrophy, decreased white blood cell response and function, and decreased ratio of T cells to B cells are common findings.

Iron is an important nutrient to bacteria as well as humans. During infection, one of the body's nonspecific defense mechanisms to limit bacterial growth is to reduce plasma iron, and in vitro studies have shown that the natural protectors in the blood against bacterial infection are eliminated by the addition of iron to the serum.[48] As body temperature rises, plasma iron levels drop, and when temperature is raised to fever levels the growth of bacteria is inhibited, though not at high iron concentrations.

These observations lead us to the conclusion that iron supplementation is probably contraindicated during acute infection, especially in patients with low transferrin levels. However, in patients with impaired immune function, chronic infections, and subnormal iron levels, adequate supplementation is essential.

Zinc

The hereditary zinc deficiency disease acrodermatitis enteropathica (AE) offers an excellent model for understanding the role of zinc in immunity. In AE, the number of T cells is reduced, white blood cell function is significantly impaired, and thymic hormone levels are lower. All of these effects are reversible upon adequate zinc administration and absorption.

Some studies have shown that zinc serves a vital role in many immune system reactions. For example, it promotes the destruction of foreign particles and microorganisms, acts as a protectant against free radical damage, acts synergistically with vitamin A, is required for proper white blood cell function, and is a necessary cofactor in activating serum thymic factor.[49,50]

Zinc also directly inhibits the growth of several viruses, including common cold viruses and the herpes simplex virus.[51,52] Throat lozenges containing zinc have become popular in the treatment of the common cold for good reason—they work (as discussed further in the chapter "Common Cold").

Selenium

With the vital role it plays in the antioxidant enzyme glutathione peroxidase, selenium affects all components of the immune system, including the development and expression of all white blood cells. Selenium deficiency results in depressed immune function, whereas selenium supplementation results in augmentation and/or restoration of immune functions. Selenium deficiency has been shown to inhibit resistance to infection as a result of impaired white blood cell and thymus function, while selenium supplementation (200 mcg per day) has been shown to stimulate white blood cell and thymus function.[53–56]

The ability of selenium supplementation to enhance immune function goes well beyond simply restoring selenium levels in selenium-deficient individuals. For example, in one study selenium supplementation (200 mcg per day) to individuals with normal selenium concentrations in their blood resulted in a 118% increase in the ability of lymphocytes to kill tumor cells and an 82.3% increase in the activity of natural killer cells.[56] These effects were apparently related to the ability of selenium to support the expression of the immune-enhancing compound interleukin-2 and, consequently, the rate of white blood cell proliferation and differentiation into forms capable of killing tumor cells and microorganisms. The supplementation regimen did not produce significant changes in the blood selenium levels of the participants. The results indicated that the immune-enhancing effects of selenium in humans require supplementation above the normal dietary intake.

Enhancing Thymus Function

Perhaps the most effective method of reestablishing a healthy immune system is employing measures to improve thymus function. Promoting optimal thymus gland activity involves the following:

- Prevention of thymic involution or shrinkage by ensuring adequate dietary intake of antioxidant nutrients
- Use of nutrients that are required in the manufacture or action of thymic hormones

Antioxidants

The thymus gland shows maximum development immediately after birth. During the aging process, the thymus gland undergoes a process of shrinkage, or involution. The reason for this involution is that the thymus gland is extremely susceptible to free radical and oxidative damage caused by stress, radiation, infection, and chronic illness.

Many patients with impaired immune function as well as conditions associated with impaired immunity (e.g., chronic fatigue syndrome, cancer, AIDS) suffer from a state of oxidative imbalance characterized by a greater number of pro-oxidants than antioxidants in their system. This situation is quite detrimental to thymus function. One of the primary ways in which antioxidants affect the immune system, particularly cell-mediated immunity, may be by protecting the thymus gland from damage. The antioxidant nutrients most important for protecting the thymus include the carotenes, vitamin C, vitamin E, zinc, and selenium.

Nutrients

Many nutrients function as important co-factors in the manufacture, secretion, and function of thymic hormones. A deficiency of any one of these results in decreased thymic hormone action and impaired immune function. Zinc, vitamin B_6, and vitamin C are among the most important. Supplementation with these nutrients has been shown to improve thymic hormone function and cell-mediated immunity.

Zinc is perhaps the critical mineral involved in thymus gland function and thymus hormone action, taking part in virtually every aspect of immunity. When zinc levels are low, the number of T cells is reduced, thymic hormone levels are lower, and many white blood cell functions critical to the immune response are severely lacking. All of these effects are reversible with adequate administration and absorption of zinc.[57,58]

Adequate zinc levels are particularly important in the elderly, and zinc supplementation in elderly subjects results in increased numbers of T cells and enhanced cell-mediated immune responses.[58]

Botanical Medicine

Many herbs have been shown to have antibacterial, antiviral, and immunostimulatory effects. A complete discussion is outside the scope of this chapter, though several immune-enhancing botanicals, such as *Echinacea* species, goldenseal (*Hydrastis canadensis*), and umka (*Pelargonium sidoides*), are discussed in the chapters on upper respiratory tract infections (common cold, bronchitis, sinusitis, and sore throat), as that context reflects their primary use. One herb that will be described in this chapter is the root of *Astragalus membranaceus*, a traditional Chinese medicine used for infections. Clinical studies in China have shown it to be effective when used as a preventive measure against the common cold.[59] It has also been shown to reduce the duration and severity of symptoms in acute treatment of the common cold as well as to raise WBC counts in people with chronic low levels of WBCs.

Research on animals has shown that astragalus apparently works by stimulating several factors of the immune system, including enhancing the phagocytic activity of monocytes and macrophages, increasing interferon production and natural killer cell activity, improving T cell activity, and potentiating other antiviral mechanisms.[59–61] Astragalus appears particularly useful in cases in which the immune system has been damaged by chemicals or radiation. In immunodepressed mice, astragalus has been found to reverse the T cell abnormalities caused by an immune-suppressing drug (cyclophosphamide), radiation, and aging.[62]

In terms of supporting immune function, extracts and preparations of baker's yeast and medicinal mushrooms such as maitake (*Grifola frondosa*), shiitake (*Lentinus edodes*), reishi (*Ganoderma lucidum*), and *Cordyceps sinensis* exert significant immune-enhancing effects. Much of this activity is due to the presence of molecules known as beta-glucans. Numerous experimental and clinical studies have shown that yeast and mushroom beta-glucans activate white blood cells by binding to receptors on the outer membranes of neutrophils, macrophages, natural killer (NK) cells, and cytotoxic T cells. Just like a key in a lock, the binding of the beta-glucan to cellular receptors flips white blood cells on and triggers a chain reaction leading to increased immune activity. In addition to increasing the ability of the neutrophils and macrophages to engulf and destroy microbes, cancer cells, and other foreign cells, the binding stimulates the production of important signaling proteins of the immune system, such as interleukin-1, interleukin-2, and lymphokines. These immune activators ramp up defenses by activating immune cells.[63,64]

One of the best-researched beta-glucan sources is Wellmune WGP—a whole glucan particle composed of 1,3/1,6-beta-glucan derived from the cell walls of a highly purified, proprietary baker's yeast (*Saccharomyces cerevisiae*). Once absorbed, Wellmune is taken up by macrophages, digested into smaller fragments, and slowly released over a number of days. The fragments bind to neutrophils via complement receptor 3 (CR3), enhancing their activity. As of 2011, six double-blind clinical studies have been conducted with Wellmune WGP demonstrating positive results in reducing the signs, symptoms, frequency, and duration of upper respiratory infections. In a study of marathon runners (who experience increased infections after long runs like marathons), Wellmune WGP significantly reduced symptoms of upper respiratory tract infection (sore throat, stuffy nose, etc.) in the test subjects. Furthermore, the Wellmune group reported 22% higher scores in vigor, 48% reduction in fatigue, 38% reduction in tension, and 38% reduction in confusion compared with the control groups.[65]

In a double-blind study during the cold and flu season, the Wellmune WGP group reported (1) no incidence of fever, compared with an incidence of 3.5 in the control group over a 90-day period; (2) no need to take a sick day from work or school, compared with 1.38 days of work or school missed for the placebo group; and (3) an increase in general health, including physical energy and emotional well-being.[66]

In the latest study of 122 healthy volunteers, participants taking 250 mg Wellmune WGP per day for 12 weeks reported a 58% reduction in upper respiratory tract infection symptoms, compared with individuals taking a placebo. These subjects also experienced improvement in energy levels compared with the placebo group.[67]

QUICK REVIEW

- **The immune system protects the body against infection and the development of cancer.**
- **Recurrent or chronic infections, even very mild colds and flu, are signs that the immune system is weakened.**
- **Supporting immune function involves a comprehensive approach.**
- **The mind and emotions have a tremendous impact on immune function.**
- **Stress depresses immune function.**
- **Too much sugar in the diet leads to lowered white blood cell activity.**
- **Nutrient deficiency is the most common cause of low immune function.**

- **Key nutrients for supplementation to support the immune system are vitamin A, vitamin C, vitamin E, B vitamins, zinc, and selenium.**
- **Supporting the thymus, the major gland of the immune system, is one of the primary goals of therapy.**
- **The herb astragalus exerts broad-spectrum effects on immune function.**
- **One of the best-researched beta-glucan sources is Wellmune WGP, a whole glucan particle derived from the cell walls of baker's yeast.**

TREATMENT SUMMARY

The regimen given here is meant as a general approach to supporting immune function during an active infection. It is designed to be supportive but is not intended to be a replacement for proper medical care. Though most common infections, such as the common cold, are self-limiting conditions, others can be life-threatening. Proper medical care should be sought when there is any sign or symptom associated with a more serious infection: fever, redness, excessive swelling, severe fatigue, pus formation, etc.

General Recommendations

- Rest (bed rest is best).
- Drink large amount of fluids (preferably diluted vegetable juices, soups, and herb teas—no fruit juice).
- Limit your simple sugar consumption (including fruit sugars) to less than 50 g per day.

Nutritional Supplements

- High-potency multivitamin and mineral formula as described in the chapter "Supplementary Measures"
- Vitamin C: 500 mg every two hours
- One of the following:
  - Bioflavonoids (mixed): 1,000 mg per day
  - Grape seed or pine bark extract, 50 to 100 mg per day
- One of the following:
  - Vitamin A: 2,500 IU per day
  - Beta-carotene 25,000 IU per day
- Vitamin D: 2,000 to 4,000 IU per day (ideally, measure blood levels and adjust dosage accordingly)
- Zinc: 20 to 30 mg per day

Botanical Medicines

- *Astragalus membranaceus:*
  - Dried root (or as decoction): 1 to 2 g three times per day
  - Tincture (1:5): 2 to 4 ml three times per day
  - Fluid extract (1:1): 2 to 4 ml three times per day
  - Solid (dry powdered) extract (0.5% 4-hydroxy-3-methoxy isoflavone): 100 to 150 mg three times per day
- Beta-glucan sources:
  - Wellmune WGP: 250 to 500 mg per day.
  - Maitake: dosage is based upon body weight and beta-glucan content stated as MD- or D-fraction (typically 0.5 mg to 1.0 mg/kg per day).
  - Shiitake or reishi: equivalent of 6 to 9 g dried mushrooms per day.

Longevity and Life Extension

. . . .

Introduction

Life extension has been a goal of humans since long before Ponce de León's search for the mythical fountain of youth. Since the early 1980s, a number of books advocating the use of vitamins, minerals, hormones, drugs, and other compounds to extend life have made the best-seller lists. Many—though not all—of the recommendations to slow down the aging process do make sense and appear to be scientifically sound. This chapter will focus on such recommendations.

First, some definitions: *life expectancy* refers to the average number of years of life a person in a given population is expected to live, while *life span* refers to the maximal age obtainable by a member of a species. *Health span* refers to the number of years of healthy life—our true goal. After all, why live longer if you are debilitated, live in a nursing home, and don't recognize your children?

On the surface it appears that in the United States, impressive gains in extending life have been made since the beginning of the 20th century. In 1900 the average life expectancy was 45 years. Now it is 75.6 years for men and 80.8 years for women.[1] However, if we examine what was really responsible for this increase in life expectancy, it is almost entirely due to decreased infant mortality. If infant mortality is taken out of the calcula-

tions, life expectancy really improved only a maximum of six years during this time. In adults reaching 50 years of age, life expectancy has increased a few years at best.

The primary strategy for increasing life expectancy involves reducing causes of premature death. Obesity, smoking, and alcohol abuse contribute greatly to premature death and in many cases are the underlying contributors to the majority of the top 10 causes of death. As detrimental as smoking is, obesity has become equal to or greater than smoking as the most important risk factor for premature death as well as shortened health span.[2]

Top 10 Causes of Death in 2009[1]	
CONDITION	**NUMBER OF DEATHS**
1. Heart disease	598,607
2. Cancer	568,668
3. Chronic lung disease	137,082
4. Stroke	128,603
5. Accidents	117,176
6. Alzheimer's disease	78,889
7. Diabetes	68,504
8. Influenza and pneumonia	53,582
9. Kidney failure	48,714
10. Suicide	36,547

Longevity: Myths and Reality

Myths still circulate about certain groups of people (the Hunzas of Pakistan, Georgians in the Caucasus region of Europe, and inhabitants of Andean villages in Ecuador, for example) who are reported to live to an extremely old age, between 125 and 150 years. However, detailed scientific reports have refuted these claims.[3-5]

For example, one group of investigators studying the people of Vilcabamba, Ecuador, to determine whether the degree of bone loss that occurred during aging was different in that population compared with the U.S. population, made a revealing discovery.[3] They did an initial survey and went back for a follow-up five years later, at which time a number of individuals reported being 10 years older than they had been during the first survey. From studying existing birth records it became obvious that there was considerable exaggeration of age. In this society as well as in the other societies associated with longevity, social standing increases with increasing age.

In the country of Georgia, in the Caucasus region of Europe, it has been demonstrated that the majority of reported centenarians (people older than 100 years) are actually in their 70s and 80s; they just look as if they are 140 years old as a result of their arduous existence.[4]

The current official world record of longevity is 122 years, reached by a Frenchwoman, Jeanne Louise Calment. Born on February 21, 1875, she lived through France's Third and Fourth Republics, and into its Fifth. She was 14 when the Eiffel Tower was completed in 1889. She died on August 28, 1997. In her later years, she lived mostly off the income from her apartment, which she sold cheaply in 1966 to a lawyer, André-François Raffray. He had agreed to make monthly payments on the apartment in exchange for taking possession when she died, but he never got to move in. He died at the age of 77, a year before Jeanne Calment; his family was required to keep making the payments.

RANK	NAME	SEX	REPORTED BIRTH DATE	DEATH DATE	REPORTED AGE	PLACE OF DEATH
1	Jeanne Calment	F	2/21/1875	8/4/1997	122 years, 164 days	France
2	Sarah Knauss	F	9/24/1880	12/30/1999	119 years, 97 days	United States
3	Lucy Hannah	F	7/16/1875	3/21/1993	117 years, 248 days	United States
4	Marie-Louise Meilleur	F	8/29/1880	4/16/1998	117 years, 230 days	Canada
5	María Capovilla	F	9/14/1889	8/27/2006	116 years, 347 days	Ecuador
6	Tane Ikai	F	1/18/1879	7/12/1995	116 years, 175 days	Japan
7	Elizabeth Bolden	F	8/15/1890	12/11/2006	116 years, 118 days	United States
8	Carrie C. White	F	11/18/1874	2/14/1991	116 years, 88 days	United States
9	Kamato Hongo	F	9/16/1887	10/31/2003	116 years, 45 days	Japan
10	Maggie Barnes	F	3/6/1882	1/19/1998	115 years, 319 days	United States

The 10 Oldest Living People at Their Time of Death, Based on Confirmed Records

What Causes Aging?

Answers to the question "What causes aging?" are coming rapidly as a result of research in gerontology, the science of aging. There are many interesting theories of aging; however, only the most significant will be briefly discussed below. There are basically two types of aging theories: programmed theories and damage theories. Programmed theories believe there is some sort of genetic clock ticking away that determines when old age sets in, while damage theories believe aging is a result of cumulative damage to cells and genetic materials. Our opinion is that both are valid. Arguments like this seem to repeat themselves in science—a case in point is the nature of light, which functions as both a particle and a wave. Well, human aging is the result of both programmed cell life and cellular damage.

The Hayflick Limit

In 1912 in a laboratory at the Rockefeller Institute, Dr. Alexis Carrel, one of the foremost biologists of his time, began an experiment that would last for more than 34 years. Dr. Carrel set out to find out how long he could keep chicken fibroblasts dividing. Fibroblasts are connective tissue cells that manufacture collagen. Fed with a special broth containing an extract of chick embryo, the chicken fibroblasts grew quite well in flasks. They would divide and form new cells, with the excess cells being periodically discarded by the researchers. The tissue culture system kept dividing for 34 years, until two years after the death of Dr. Carrel, when his coworkers finally discarded the culture. Dr. Carrel's work prompted the idea that cells are inherently immortal if given an ideal environment.[6]

This idea was not discarded until the early 1960s, when Dr. Leonard Hayflick observed that human fibroblasts in tissue culture wouldn't divide more than about 50 times.[7] Why the discrepancy? It appears Dr. Carrel had inadvertently added new "fresh" fibroblasts contained in the embryo broth used as nutrition for the tissue culture. New cells had repeatedly been added to the tissue cultures.

Hayflick found that if he froze cells in culture after 20 divisions, they would "remember" that they had 30 doublings left when they were thawed and refed. Fifty cell divisions or doublings are called the *Hayflick limit*. As fibroblasts approach 50 divisions, they begin looking old. They become larger and accumulate an increased amount of lipofuscin, the yellow-brown pigment responsible for age spots—those brownish spots that appear on the skin as the result of cellular debris and lipofuscin clumping together.

The Telomere-Shortening Theory

Based on the Hayflick limit, experts on aging theorized there is a genetic clock ticking away within each cell that determines when old age sets in. The latest, and most likely, programmed theory of aging is the telomere shortening theory. Telomeres are the end-cap segments of DNA (our genetic material). The concept that shortening of the telomere with each cellular replication leads to aging was first proposed by a Russian scientist, Alexaie Olovnikov, in 1971, and also by James Watson (the codiscoverer of the structure of DNA) in 1972. But it wasn't until 1990 that the telomere theory of aging really began to be accepted.[8] New evidence supports the notion that telomeres are, in fact, the "clocks of aging."

Each time a cell replicates, a small piece

of DNA is taken off the end of each chromosome. At conception, telomeres are about 10,000 base pairs long. By birth they will have already been shortened by 5,000 base pairs. Compared with the rest of the chromosome, the telomere is small. An average chromosome is 130 million base pairs long, or about 25,000 times as long as the telomere at birth. Every time a body cell replicates, the telomere gets shorter. The shorter the telomere gets, the more it affects gene expression. The result is cellular aging.

In addition to serving as a clock for aging, the telomere is also involved in protecting the end of the chromosome from damage, allowing for complete replication of the chromosome, controlling gene expression, and aiding in the organization of the chromosome. The telomere determines not only the aging of the cell but our risk for cancer, Alzheimer's disease, and other degenerative diseases.[9]

Perhaps the greatest support for the telomere theory of aging is Hutchinson-Gilford syndrome. You most likely have never heard of this condition, but you are likely to have heard of its common name, progeria. This syndrome was first described in 1886. Children with progeria are extraordinarily rare, 1 in 8 million births, but if you have ever seen one, you will never forget it. The child typically shows symptoms of aging during the first year of life and generally dies of "old age" by the age of 13. Another rare syndrome known as Werner's syndrome is less severe—typically symptoms begin to manifest themselves in the early 20s and death usually occurs by age 50.

Much has been learned from children with progeria. If progeria is a reflection of accelerated aging—and few would argue that it isn't—it may hold the key to understanding how to truly extend life expectancy and even life span. Researchers have been working intensively to find the mechanism responsible

for the accelerated aging of progeria. The answer appears to be telomere shortening. Compared with normal children, at birth children with progeria have telomeres like those of a 90-year-old. In Werner's syndrome, telomeres are of normal length at birth but appear to shorten faster than normal.

The key to extending maximal human life span will ultimately involve preserving or restoring telomere length (as well as decreasing chromosomal damage, cellular oxidation, and many other factors). Several measures have already been shown to achieve this goal. Simply adopting a comprehensive dietary and lifestyle change consistent with good health has been shown to preserve telomere length.[10] Physical exercise has been shown to be associated with preserving telomere length.[11] And meditation has also been shown to preserve telomere length by reducing the negative effects of stress.[12] Higher vitamin D levels are associated with longer telomeres (as discussed in more detail below).[13] Last, strategies that reduce inflammation are very important in reducing the rate pf telomere shortening.[14] Levels of inflammatory markers in the blood correlate with telomere shortening. For more information on natural ways to reduce these inflammatory markers, see the chapter "Silent Inflammation."

The Free Radical Theory

The best damage theory is the free radical theory of aging. This theory contends that damage caused by free radicals contributes to aging and age-associated disease.[15,16] Free radicals are defined as highly reactive molecules that can bind to and destroy cellular compounds. Free radicals may be derived from our environment (sunlight, X-rays, radiation, chemicals) or from ingested foods or drinks, or they may be produced within our bodies during chemical reactions. The majority of free radicals present within the body are actually produced within the body. However, exposure to environmental and dietary free radicals greatly increases the free radical load of the body. In addition to aging, free radicals have been linked to virtually every disease associated with aging, including atherosclerosis, cancer, Alzheimer's disease, cataracts, osteoarthritis, and immune deficiency.

Telomeres appear to be especially susceptible to oxidative damage, so telomere shortening may actually fit very nicely as the underlying result of cumulative free radical damage.

Cigarette smoking is a good example of how to increase free radical load. Many of the deleterious health effects of smoking are related to the inhalation of extremely high levels of free radicals. Other external sources of free radicals include radiation; air pollutants; pesticides; anesthetics; aromatic hydrocarbons (petroleum-based products); fried, barbecued, and charbroiled foods; alcohol; coffee; and solvents such as formaldehyde, toluene, and benzene, found in cleaning fluids, paints, gasoline and furniture polish. Obviously, reduced exposure to these sources of free radicals is recommended in a life extension program.

Most free radicals in the body are toxic oxygen-containing molecules. It is ironic that the oxygen molecule is the major source of free radical damage in our bodies. Oxygen sustains our lives in one sense, yet in another it is responsible for much of the destruction and aging of the cells of our bodies. Similar to the way oxygen reacts with iron to form rust, oxygen, in its toxic state, is able to oxidize molecules in our bodies. As you probably already know, compounds that prevent this type of damage are referred to as antioxidants.

In addition to damaging cell membranes and proteins, free radical damage extends to our DNA. The genetic material is responsible for transmitting the characteristics of one generation of cells to another. Damage to the DNA structure results in mutations (expression of different genetic material), or the cells simply die or are destroyed. DNA is constantly bombarded by free radicals and other compounds that can cause damage. Fortunately, the body has enzymes that (mostly) repair damaged DNA. The differences in life spans among mammals are largely a result of an animal's or human's ability to repair damaged DNA. For example, the maximal life span of a human (about 120 years) is more than twice as long as that of a chimpanzee (about 50 years) because our DNA repair is much more effective.[17]

Research has shown that old cells are not able to repair DNA as rapidly as young cells. It appears that nature has set the rate of DNA repair at less than the rate of damage, so that animals can accumulate mutations and evolve. If repair were perfect, there would be no evolutionary processes.

Glycosylation and Aging

Another damage theory that deserves mentioning is the glycosylation theory. In a nutshell, this theory involves the continued attachment of blood sugar (glucose) molecules to cellular proteins until finally the protein ceases to function properly. For example, cholesterol-carrying proteins that have been glycosylated do not bind to receptors on liver cells that halt the manufacture of cholesterol. As a result, too much cholesterol is manufactured. Excessive glycosylation and the formation of what are referred to as advanced glycation end products (AGEs) have many adverse effects: inactivation of enzymes, damaging structural and regulatory proteins, impaired immune function, and increased likelihood of autoimmune diseases. Like free radical damage, AGEs are associated with many chronic degenerative diseases.[18] Diets that promote glycosylation and poor glucose control are also linked to telomere shortening.

Obviously we want to avoid excessive glycosylation. This can be done by keeping blood sugar levels under control by consuming a low-glycemic diet (and, if needed, using special nutritional factors such as PolyGlycopleX, alpha-lipoic acid, and others). For more information, see the chapter "Diabetes."

Extending Life Span

Can life span be increased and the aging process slowed? The answer is definitely yes. However, we want to discourage readers from seeking a single "magic bullet" to halt the aging process. Instead we want you to realize that the best steps that can be taken to slow down the aging process and reduce your risk of the major causes of premature death is to adopt the guidelines described in Section II, "The Four Cornerstones of Good Health":

- A positive mental attitude
- A health-promoting lifestyle
- A health-promoting diet
- Supplementary measures

Caloric Restriction

Severe restriction of calories is a consistent and reproducible way of dramatically increasing life span in laboratory rats, mice, and primates.[19] However, it is not known if caloric restriction has the same value for humans. From population data accumulated by insurance companies and others, the following

conclusion can be made: individuals who are either overweight or severely underweight (the latter condition is typically due to severe disease, such as end-stage cancer) have the shortest life span, while those individuals whose weight is just below the average weight for height have the longest life span.

Exercise

As stated in the chapter "The Healing Power Within," the better shape you are in physically, the greater your odds of enjoying a healthier and longer life. Most studies have showed that individuals who are not physically fit have an eightfold greater risk of having a heart attack or stroke than do physically fit individuals. Researchers have estimated that for every hour of exercise, there is a two-hour increase in longevity. That is quite a return on an investment.

Maintaining muscle mass must be a major goal in any life extension plan. Muscle mass increases in childhood and peaks during the late teens through the mid- to late 20s. After that there starts a decline in muscle mass that is rather slow but unfortunately very consistent. From 25 to 50 the decline in muscle mass is roughly 10%. In our 50s the rate of decline accelerates slightly, but the real decline usually begins at 60. By the time people reach the age of 80 their muscle mass is a little more than half of what it was in their 20s.

Sarcopenia is the term for degenerative loss of skeletal muscle mass and strength as we age. Sarcopenia is to our muscle mass what osteoporosis is to our bones. The degree of sarcopenia as we age is a predictor of mortality and disability.[20] It is linked not just to a significantly shorter life expectancy but also to decreased vitality, poor balance, slower gait speed, more falls, and increased fractures. In the prevention of osteoporosis, we want to build bone while we are young to help us preserve it longer through the aging process; the same is true for muscle tissue. And just as it is important to engage in dietary, lifestyle, and exercise strategies to fight osteoporosis in our later years, we must do the same to fight sarcopenia. You must build muscle to maintain your health.[21]

Interestingly, the same dietary factors linked to accelerated aging are linked to sarcopenia, while the dietary practices associated with good health are associated with protection against sarcopenia. While diet is unquestionably critical, for most people perhaps the most important step to preventing sarcopenia is to engage in a regular strength training program—that is, to lift weights or perform resistance exercises.[22] The benefits of strength training are vast, particularly for women and for people over 50. In addition to helping burn more fat, a larger muscle mass is associated with a healthier heart, improved joint function, relief from arthritis pain, better antioxidant protection, better blood sugar control, and higher self-esteem. While many women do not strength-train because they fear gaining weight, just the opposite occurs: building muscle mass actually helps to more effectively burn calories.

Dietary protein is also essential in supporting muscle growth and fighting sarcopenia, especially when combined with exercise.[22] The best choice for protein supplementation is whey. Whey protein has the highest biological value of all proteins. Biological value is used to rate protein based on how much of the protein consumed is actually absorbed, retained, and used in the body. One of the reasons the biological value of whey protein is so high is that it has the highest concentrations of glutamine and branched-chain amino acids found in nature. These amino acids are critical to cellular health, muscle growth, and protein synthesis. Whey protein is also high in cysteine, which promotes the synthesis of glutathione—which, as we discuss in the chapter "Detoxification and Internal Cleansing," plays a major role in helping us get rid of toxins.

Although the most popular use of whey protein is by bodybuilders and athletes looking to increase their protein intake, whey protein is also used to support recovery from surgery, to prevent the wasting syndrome seen with AIDS, and to offset some of the negative effects of radiation therapy and chemotherapy. This increased efficiency of protein use is particularly important in battling sarcopenia. Whey protein supplementation has also been demonstrated in clinical trials to produce greater strength and muscle mass gains in elderly subjects involved in a weight training program, compared with a placebo as well as other types of protein.[23]

The typical recommendation to boost protein levels is 25 to 50 g per day, though for severe sarcopenia the dosage recommendation is 1 g/kg.

A Comprehensive Nutritional Approach to Preventing Sarcopenia

- Reduce the amount of saturated fat, trans-fatty acids, cholesterol, and total fat in the diet by eating only lean sources of protein and more plant foods.

- Increase intake of omega-3 oils by eating flaxseed oil, walnuts, and cold-water fish such as salmon. Eat at least two, but no more than three, servings of fish per week.

- Increase the intake of monounsaturated fats and the amino acid arginine by eating regular but moderate amounts of nuts and seeds, such as almonds, Brazil nuts, coconut, hazelnuts, macadamia nuts, pecans, pine nuts, pistachios, and sesame and sunflower seeds, and by using a monounsaturated oil, such as olive, macadamia, or canola oil, for cooking purposes.

- Eat five or more servings per day of a combination of vegetables and fruits, especially green, orange, and yellow vegetables, dark-colored berries, and citrus fruits.

- Limit the intake of refined carbohydrates. Sugar and other refined carbohydrates lead to the development of insulin resistance, which in turn is associated with increased silent inflammation, a major contributor to sarcopenia.

- Utilize the benefits of whey protein by taking 25 to 50 g whey protein per day.

Glutathione- and Sulfur-Containing Amino Acids

Whey protein is also a rich source of the sulfur-containing amino acids methionine and cysteine, which are important components of a life extension plan. Typically, as people age the content of these amino acids in the body decreases.[24] Since research has shown that supplementing the diets of mice and guinea pigs with cysteine increases life span considerably, it has been suggested that maintaining optimal levels of methionine and cysteine may promote longevity in humans.

The mechanism may be because methionine and cysteine levels are a major determinant in the concentration of sulfur-containing compounds, such as glutathione, within cells. Glutathione assumes a critical role in the body's defense against a variety of injurious compounds, combining directly with these toxic substances to aid in their elimination. When increased levels of toxic compounds or free radicals are present, the body needs higher levels of glutathione, and hence methionine and cysteine. Good dietary sources are whey protein, fish, eggs, brewer's yeast, garlic, onions, and nuts.

Antioxidants

The free radical theory of aging really lends itself to nutritional intervention by antioxidant compounds, which act as free radical "scavengers." The body has several enzymes that prevent the damage induced by specific types of free radicals. For example, superoxide dismutase prevents the damage caused by the toxic oxygen molecule known as superoxide. Catalase and glutathione peroxidase are two other antioxidant enzymes found in the human body.

The level of antioxidant enzymes and the level of dietary antioxidants determine the life span of mammals. Human beings live longer than chimpanzees, cats, dogs, and many other mammals because we have a greater quantity of antioxidants within our cells.[25,26] Some strains of mice live longer than other strains because they have higher levels of antioxidant enzymes. Presumably, the reason some people outlive others is that they have higher levels of antioxidants in their cells. This line of thinking is largely why many cutting-edge physicians recommend increasing the level of antioxidant mechanisms within cells.

A significant number of studies have clearly demonstrated that diets rich in antioxidants can definitely increase life expectancy. In addition, diets rich in antioxidants reduce the risk for cancer, heart disease, and many other diseases linked to premature death.

Dietary antioxidants of extreme significance in life extension include vitamins C and E, selenium, beta-carotene, flavonoids, and sulfur-containing amino acids. Not surprisingly, these same nutrients are also of great significance in cancer prevention, as aging and cancer share many mechanisms.

Carotenes

An important class of dietary antioxidants for longevity is the carotenes, the most wide-spread group of naturally occurring plant pigments. For many people (physicians included) the term *carotene* is synonymous with provitamin A, but only 30 to 50 of the more than 400 carotenoids that have been identified are believed to have vitamin A activity.

Considerable evidence now demonstrates that carotenes do much more than just serve as a precursor to vitamin A. For example, carotenes have potent antioxidant effects. Although research has primarily focused on beta-carotene, other carotenes such as lycopene, lutein, and astaxanthin are more potent in their antioxidant activity and are deposited in tissues to a greater degree. It should also be kept in mind that while research tends to focus on beta-carotene intake, eating a diet rich in beta-carotene means that you are also getting many other carotenes.

It appears that tissue carotenoid content is one of the most significant factors in determining life span in mammals, including humans.[26] Since tissue carotenoids appear to be the most significant factor in determining a species' maximal life span potential, it only seems logical that individuals with the optimal level of carotenoids in their tissues would be the ones that would live the longest.

Consumption of foods rich in carotenes (green leafy vegetables, pumpkin, sweet potatoes, carrots, etc.) and supplementation with palm oil carotene complex, carotene complexes from algae (as opposed to isolated, synthetic beta-carotene), lycopene, lutein, or astaxanthin are the best methods of increas-

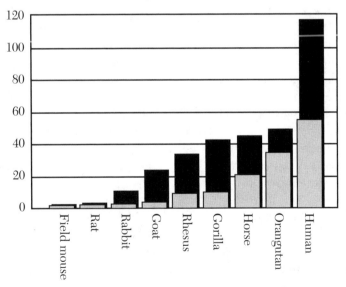

Concentration of Carotenoids and Maximum Life-span Potential

Concentration of carotenoids, in mcg/dl
Maximum life-span potential, in years

The Influence of Carotene Content on Life Span Potential

ing tissue carotenoid levels. High carotene intake may also offer significant benefit to the immune system—the thymus gland is largely composed of epithelial cells, and carotenes concentrated in those cells are able to significantly reduce the shrinkage the thymus gland undergoes during normal aging and stress. In addition, studies have shown that thymus-gland-mediated immune functions could be improved with carotene supplementation (see the chapter "Immune System Support").

Flavonoids

Another group of plant pigments with remarkable protection against free radical damage is the flavonoids. These compounds are largely responsible for the colors of fruits and flowers. However, these compounds serve other functions in plant metabolism besides contributing to the plants' aesthetic quality. In plants, flavonoids serve as protectors against environmental stress. In humans, flavonoids appear to function as biological response modifiers. That is, they modify the body's reaction to other compounds, such as allergens, viruses, and carcinogens, as evidenced by flavonoids' anti-inflammatory, anti-allergenic, antiviral, and anticancer properties. Flavonoid molecules are also quite unusual in their antioxidant and free radical scavenging activity, in that they are active against a wide variety of oxidants and free radicals.

The best way to ensure an adequate intake of flavonoids is to eat a varied diet rich in colorful fruits and vegetables. The richest dietary sources of flavonoids include citrus fruits, berries, onions, parsley, legumes, green tea, and red wine. As far as flavonoid supplements go, the best choices are flavonoid-rich extracts, particularly procyanidolic oligomers (PCOs) such as grape seed and pine bark.[27,28] Green tea and Ginkgo

biloba extracts also offer significant benefits in promoting longevity.

While there is significant overlap among these flavonoid-rich extracts, Ginkgo biloba deserves some special mention. In herbal medicine, for centuries it was believed that plants were signed by the Creator with some visible or other clue that would indicate their therapeutic use. This concept is commonly referred to as the "doctrine of signatures." Ginkgo's signature is its long life and resistance to the environment. Ginkgo biloba is the world's oldest living tree species. The sole surviving species of the family Ginkgoaceae, the ginkgo tree can be traced back more than 200 million years to the fossils of the Permian period and for this reason is often referred to as a "living fossil."

Once common in North America and Europe, the ginkgo was almost destroyed during the Ice Age in all regions of the world except China, where it is has long been cultivated as a sacred tree. The ginkgo tree was brought to America in 1784 to the garden of William Hamilton near Philadelphia. The ginkgo is now planted throughout much of the United States as an ornamental tree, as it will grow where other trees quickly die. Ginkgo is the tree most resistant to insects, disease, and pollution. As a result, it is frequently planted along streets in cities.

Although the notion of a doctrine of signatures is fanciful, the bottom line is that Ginkgo biloba extract can be very useful in increasing the quality of life in the elderly. Many symptoms common in the elderly are a result of insufficient blood and oxygen supply. Ginkgo biloba extract has demonstrated beneficial effects in improving blood and oxygen supply to the brain and as a result may help improve a number of common symptoms of aging, including short-term memory loss, dizziness, headache, ringing in the ears, hearing loss, and depression.[29,30]

Resveratrol

Resveratrol is a plant compound similar to flavonoids. It is found in low levels in the skin of red grapes, red wine, cocoa powder, baking chocolate, dark chocolate, peanuts, and the skin of mulberries. Red wine is perhaps the most widely recognized source of resveratrol; however, red wine contains only 1 mg per glass. Most resveratrol supplements use Japanese knotweed (*Polygonum cuspidatum*) as the source. Resveratrol occurs naturally in two forms: cis-resveratrol and trans-resveratrol. Trans-resveratrol is much more bioactive and clinically beneficial than cis-resveratrol.

Resveratrol has received a lot of attention as a longevity aid, but the scientific basis for this relies on test tube and animal studies—there are only a few published human studies at this time, and many questions remain to be answered.[31,32] We do know that resveratrol activates an enzyme, sirtuin 1, that plays an important role in the regulation of cellular life span; it also promotes improved insulin sensitivity. The effects of resveratrol in animal studies are very similar to the benefits noted with calorie restriction, but are obtained without actually reducing calorie intake. Its longevity-promoting effects have been demonstrated in yeast, fish, and mice but have not yet been properly assessed in humans. At this time we prefer to recommend less expensive and more substantiated measures, such as ensuring optimal vitamin D levels (discussed below).

Vitamin D

The list of the benefits of vitamin D supplementation is growing at a rapid pace. Perhaps the greatest benefit may be in extending life. An analysis of studies of vitamin D supplementation showed that participants who took vitamin D supplements had a 7% lower risk of death compared with those who did not.[33] Of course, this result is not surprising. It is now known that virtually every cell in our body has receptors for vitamin D. It has been shown to protect against certain cancers (particularly breast and prostate), autoimmune diseases such as multiple sclerosis and type 1 diabetes, and heart disease.[34]

A 2007 study added another major benefit for vitamin D and also provides an explanation for its longevity-promoting effects: vitamin D may slow aging by increasing the length of telomeres.[35] In the study, scientists examined the effects of vitamin D on the length of telomeres in white blood cells of 2,160 women ages 18 to 79. The higher the vitamin D levels, the longer the telomere length. In terms of the effect on aging, there was a five-year difference in telomere length in those with the highest levels of vitamin D compared with those with the lowest levels. Obesity, smoking, and lack of physical activity can shorten the telomere length, but the researchers found that increasing vitamin D levels overcame these effects. What this five-year difference means is that a 70-year-old woman with higher vitamin D levels would have a biological age of 65.

DHEA

The primary role of the adrenal hormone dehydroepiandrosterone (DHEA) is as a precursor for all other steroid hormones in the human body, including sex hormones and corticosteroids. Because DHEA levels tend to decline with aging, it has been postulated that raising DHEA through supplementation may offer some protection against the effects of aging. In fact, the benefits of DHEA supplementation may extend well beyond an antiaging effect. Over the last decade a number of studies have demonstrated that declining levels of DHEA are linked to such conditions as diabetes, obesity, elevated cholesterol levels, heart disease, arthritis, and autoimmune diseases. In addition, DHEA shows promise in enhancing memory and improving mental function in the elderly as well as increasing muscle strength and lean body mass, improving immune function, and enhancing quality of life in aging men and women.[36–38] It also has been shown to improve insulin sensitivity. In a two-year study, 57 men and 68 women ages 65 to 75 were randomly assigned to take 50 mg DHEA or a placebo once per day. Year one was a randomized, double-blind trial. Year two was an open-label continuation. DHEA replacement improved insulin sensitivity, reduced plasma triglycerides, and lowered inflammatory markers (cytokines IL6 and TNFα).[39]

Although DHEA may prove useful in maintaining vim and vigor, we think it is not likely to significantly increase a person's life span. While some strains of rats live longer when taking DHEA, others do not. But probably the biggest argument against DHEA as something that will dramatically extend a healthy person's life is the observation that DHEA levels are normal in children with progeria. Surely if DHEA were a significant factor in aging, levels would be low in such children.

Nonetheless, although DHEA probably will not extend a person's life span, it will often improve the health span. Our opinion is that DHEA offers significant benefits when used appropriately. One of the concerns that we have with DHEA is that it is not like vitamin C or many other nutrients that have virtually no toxicity. DHEA is a hormone, and there is relatively little information on its long-term safety. It is safe if used appropriately, but it is a big gamble if abused.

For men ages 40 to 50, we recommend DHEA for reduced libido, fatigue, diabetes,

and extended high levels of stress. We suggest basing the dosage on blood levels of DHEA and testosterone; typically, the dosage will range from 15 to 25 mg per day. For women who have not yet passed through menopause, we do not recommend DHEA unless there is confirmation that their DHEA levels are in fact low. The reason is that as many women approach menopause there is actually a rise in DHEA levels. Taking extra DHEA may lead to acne and increased facial hair. After menopause we recommend using DHEA with caution and in low dosages ranging from 5 to 15 mg unless the woman has an autoimmune disease or diabetes. For men over 50, again we recommend using blood or saliva measurements to determine the dosage. For men desiring to increase their libido, improve their sense of well-being, and feel younger, our goal has been to raise their testosterone and DHEA levels to those of men in their early 20s. Typically, we have found the dosage required to achieve this goal is between 25 and 50 mg. As men and women reach their 70s, they may require higher levels, but until more is known about DHEA we would rather err on the side of being conservative.

Melatonin

Melatonin (not to be confused with melanin, the compound responsible for producing skin pigment) is a hormone manufactured from serotonin and secreted by the pineal gland. The pineal gland, a small pea-sized gland at the base of the brain, has been a source of curiosity since antiquity. The ancient Greeks considered the pineal gland the seat of the soul, a concept that was extended by the philosopher Descartes. In the 17th and 18th centuries physicians associated "madness" with the pineal gland. Physicians in the early 1900s believed the pineal gland was somehow involved with the endocrine system. The identification of melatonin in 1958 provided the first solid scientific evidence of an essential role for the pineal gland. It is now thought that the sole function of the pineal gland is to manufacture and secrete melatonin.

Melatonin is critically involved in the synchronization of hormone secretion. The natural biorhythm of hormone secretion is referred to as the circadian rhythm. The human body is governed by an internal clock that signals the secretion of various hormones at different times to regulate body functions. Melatonin plays a key role as the biological timekeeper of hormone secretion. Melatonin also helps control periods of sleepiness and wakefulness. Release of melatonin is stimulated by darkness and suppressed by light.

In addition to its role in synchronizing hormone secretion, melatonin has shown antioxidant and longevity-promoting effects in animal studies.[40] For example, studies of rats showed that melatonin supplementation led to longer lives (31 months vs. 25 months). However, the clinical significance of melatonin's antioxidant effects has not been fully determined in humans. What is known is that melatonin is very important in initiating a good night's sleep, and this alone may have profound effects on life expectancy.[40]

Inadequate or poor-quality sleep accelerates the aging process, especially in the brain.[41] With age, the percentage of deep slow-wave sleep has been shown to decrease, and interrupted sleep is extremely common. Poor sleep quality at any age triggers the stress response and leads to an increase in inflammation, but it is especially a problem as we get older. A number of lifestyle interventions, such as taking short daytime naps, maintaining a routine, and using bright light therapy in the morning, as well as supplemental interventions, have been found to increase deep slow-wave sleep, improve sleep quality, and prolong overall sleep time.[42,43] For more information, see the chapter "Insomnia."

QUICK REVIEW

- **If infant mortality is taken out of the calculations, life expectancy really improved a maximum of only six years during the past century, while the burden of degenerative disease has skyrocketed out of proportion to the increase in longevity.**

- **Based on confirmed records, the oldest person lived to an age of 122 years 164 days.**

- **Increasing life expectancy involves reducing causes of premature death.**

- **The real goal is improving health span, not just life span.**

- **The latest, and most likely, programmed theory of aging is the telomere shortening theory.**

- **Telomeres, the end cap of our DNA molecules, are the "clocks of aging."**

- **Free radical damage causes, and antioxidant nutrients prevent, cellular aging.**

- **Individuals who are either overweight or severely underweight have the shortest life span, while those individuals** whose weight is just below the average weight for height have the longest life span.

- Researchers have estimated that for every hour of exercise, there is a two-hour increase in longevity.
- Maintaining muscle mass must be a major goal in any life extension plan.
- The level of antioxidant enzymes and the level of dietary antioxidants determine the life span of mammals.
- Ginkgo biloba extract has demonstrated beneficial effects in improving many symptoms associated with aging.
- Resveratrol has received a lot of attention as a longevity aid, but its scientific basis relies on test tube and animal studies—there are only a few published human studies at this time, and many questions remain to be answered.
- Vitamin D may slow aging by increasing the length of telomeres.
- Obesity, smoking, and lack of physical activity can shorten telomere length, but researchers have found that increasing vitamin D levels overcame these effects.
- Because DHEA levels tend to decline with aging, it has been postulated that raising DHEA through supplementation may offer some protection against the effects of aging
- Melatonin is not likely to extend life in humans based solely on its antioxidant effects; its benefits may be related to improved sleep quality.

TREATMENT SUMMARY

The best way to ensure a long, healthy, high-quality life is to adopt the guidelines described in Section II, "The Four Cornerstones of Good Health," and address any issue associated with premature death (smoking, obesity, alcohol abuse, etc.) as well as any health conditions that could prove fatal, such as atherosclerosis, diabetes, and cancer.

Specific recommendations and dosages of supplements for slowing the aging process are given below. While trying to lengthen your life span is important, we want to encourage you to focus on improving the quality of your life as well.

Diet

Follow the dietary guidelines in the chapter "A Health-Promoting Diet." In particular, a high intake of colorful vegetables and fruits is essential to a life extension program because of the vitamins, minerals, carotenes, flavonoids, and dietary fiber found in these foods. It is also especially important to follow the dietary recommendations for reducing the risk of heart disease (atherosclerosis), such as increasing the intake of dietary fiber (especially soluble fiber, found in legumes, flaxseed, oat bran, pectin, etc.), olive oil, and fish, while reducing the consumption of saturated fats, cholesterol, sugar, and animal proteins.

Nutritional Supplements

- A high-potency multiple vitamin and mineral formula as described in the chapter "Supplementary Measures"
  - Key individual nutrients:
  - Vitamin C: 500 to 1,000 mg per day
  - Selenium: 100 to 200 mcg per day
  - Vitamin E (mixed tocopherols): 100 to 200 IU per day
  - Vitamin D$_3$: 2,000 to 4,000 IU per day (ideally, measure blood levels and adjust dosage accordingly)
  - Fish oil: 1,000 mg EPA + DHA per day
- One of the following:
  - Grape seed extract (> 95% procyanidolic oligomers): 150 to 300 mg per day
  - Pine bark extract (> 95% procyanidolic oligomers): 150 to 300 mg per day
  - Green tea extract (> 80% polyphenol content): 300 to 500 mg per day
  - Ginkgo biloba extract (24% ginkgo flavonglycosides): 240 to 320 mg per day
  - Some other flavonoid-rich extract with a similar flavonoid content, super greens formula, or other plant-based antioxidant that can provide an oxygen radical absorption capacity (ORAC) of 3,000 to 6,000 units or higher per day
- Consider:
  - DHEA: as above on page 193
  - Melatonin: 3 mg at bedtime

Silent Inflammation

. . . .

Introduction

Inflammation is a reaction designed to protect us after an injury or infection. The term owes its origin to the Latin word *inflammare*, which means "to set on fire." In the classic response to injury or infection, the injured area becomes red, swollen, hot, and painful. But there is another type of inflammation that is not so obvious. This silent inflammation reflects an underlying low-grade stimulation of the inflammatory process with no outward signs of inflammation. The only time that it becomes apparent is when the blood is tested for markers of inflammation such as C-reactive protein (discussed in detail below). Silent inflammation is a major factor in the development of virtually every major chronic degenerative disease, including cardiovascular disease, allergies, type 2 diabetes, cancer, and Alzheimer's disease.

There are many factors that trigger silent inflammation, including insulin resistance, obesity, emotional stress, environmental toxins, low antioxidant intake, increased exposure to free radicals (from, e.g., radiation or smoking), chronic infections, imbalances of dietary fats, and increased intestinal permeability.

Markers of Inflammation

The most common test to measure silent inflammation is a blood test for C-reactive

protein (CRP).[1,2] Technically, CRP is classified as an acute-phase protein. Its physiological role is to bind to the surface of dead or dying cells (and some types of bacteria) in order to activate the complement system, a system of other blood proteins that go on to help destroy the cell, bacteria, or other particulate matter.

In an acute infection or injury, levels of CRP rapidly increase within 2 hours and reach a peak at 48 hours. When the acute inflammation is dealt with effectively, the CRP declines rapidly. Because there are a large number of conditions that can increase CRP production, an elevated CRP level does not diagnose a specific disease. But it does tell us how much inflammation is occurring in the body. Rapid elevations in CRP as high as 50,000 times the normal value of 1 mg/l can occur with inflammation, infection, trauma, tissue necrosis, malignancies, and autoimmune disorders such as rheumatoid arthritis.[3]

Interest in measuring CRP is the result of significant research showing it to be a very sensitive marker for the prediction for cardiovascular disease.[1,2] Indeed, of all the current inflammatory markers used in clinical practice, CRP provides the most conclusive information with regard to cardiovascular risk. Results are typically divided into three different risk categories: low risk (<1 mg/l), average risk (1–3 mg/l), and high risk (>3 mg/l).

Patients with high CRP concentrations are more likely to have a stroke or heart attack or to develop severe peripheral vascular disease. Research also indicates that elevations of CRP are linked to diabetes, some forms of cancer, Alzheimer's disease, and many other chronic degenerative diseases. Though other candidates for measuring silent inflammation may emerge, there is no question that measuring CRP is the most well-recognized assessment. The best determination is referred to as high-sensitivity CRP (hsCRP), as this test gives results in 25 minutes with a sensitivity down to 0.04 mg/l.

Therapeutic Considerations

There is little doubt that diet is a major contributor to silent inflammation. First, diet is the major contributor to the development of insulin resistance. Decreased responsiveness of body tissues to insulin leads to elevations in blood sugar and increased oxidative (free radical) stress. CRP levels generally parallel insulin resistance. Insulin resistance is largely the result of increased abdominal obesity and excessive consumption of calories, particularly carbohydrates. In fact, abdominal obesity is the strongest independent predictor of silent inflammation and CRP levels.[4,5] Therefore, the guidelines given in the chapter "Obesity and Weight Management" should be regarded as the first step in reducing silent inflammation in overweight or obese individuals.

In addition to weight loss, a diet low in refined carbohydrates and starchy foods that can raise blood sugar levels (i.e., a low-glycemic-load diet) is critical in reducing silent inflammation. In a study of more than 200 apparently healthy women, glycemic load was found to be significantly and positively associated with CRP levels.[6]

In addition to a low-glycemic diet, the Mediterranean diet has also been found to be of great benefit in lowering CRP levels.[7] A diet rich in plant pigments, especially flavonoids, found in soy, apples, berries, and other fruits and vegetables, is associated with lower CRP levels as well.[8,9]

Omega-3 to Omega-6 Ratio

The ratio of omega-3 to omega-6 fatty acids is also a major factor in determining the degree of silent inflammation and CRP levels. The typical Western diet promotes inflammation because it is particularly high in sources of the omega-6 fatty acid linoleic acid and low in sources of both short-chain (alpha-linolenic acid) and long-chain omega-3 fatty acids (EPA and DHA).[10] The last 150 years have seen a dramatic increase in foods high in omega-6 fatty acids along with a dramatic decrease of foods rich in omega-3 fatty acids. As a result, the ratio of omega-6 to omega-3 in the Western diet ranges between 15:1 and 20:1—far different from the nearly 1:1 ratio that humans evolved with.

Both omega-6 and omega-3 fatty acids are utilized by the body as building blocks for mediators of inflammation. It is simplistic, but still fairly accurate, to say that most mediators formed from omega-3 fatty acids are anti-inflammatory, while those derived from omega-6 are pro-inflammatory.[11] Particularly pro-inflammatory is the omega-6 fatty acid arachidonic acid, which is found in animal foods but also can be formed from linoleic acid. So in fighting inflammation it is a good idea to eliminate common sources of linoleic acid such as soy, safflower, sunflower, and corn oil. The bottom line is that to reduce inflammation there must be a reduced intake of omega-6 fatty acids combined with an increase in omega-3 fatty acids. Ultimately, the goal is to improve the composition and function of the cell membrane. To accomplish this goal, observe the following dietary guidelines:

- Be aware of the fat content of foods. Limit total dietary fat intake to no more than 30% of calories consumed (400–600 calories a day from fat, based on a standard 2,000-calorie-a-day diet). Reduce the amount of saturated fats and total fat in the diet. In general, animal products are high in fat, while most plant foods are very low in fat. While most nuts and seeds are relatively high in fat, the calories they supply come mostly from monounsaturated fats.

- Reduce the intake of meat and dairy products from corn-fed animals while increasing the intake of fish. Particularly beneficial are cold-water fish such as wild salmon, mackerel, herring, and halibut because of their high levels of omega-3 fats.

- Cook with olive, canola, or macadamia nut oil. Use flaxseed oil or olive oil as your base in salad dressings.

- Eliminate margarine and other foods containing trans-fatty acids and partially hydrogenated oils.

- Take a high-quality fish oil supplement providing at least 1,000 mg EPA + DHA daily.

Exercise and Physical Activity

Physical activity is tightly linked to inflammation in a very complex manner. It does not appear to affect CRP, but rather affects other markers of silent inflammation such as interleukins. Regular, moderate exercise reduces the level of silent inflammation, while high-intensity training for a prolonged period increases silent inflammation.[12–14]

Gastrointestinal Permeability

Increased permeability of the intestinal lining can be the result of food allergies, microbial toxins, food and environmental toxins, some drugs such as aspirin, or the consequence of diseases that affect this tissue, such as inflammatory bowel disease (Crohn's disease and ulcerative colitis) and celiac disease (sensitivity to gluten). The latter diseases have been used as models of how impaired intestinal permeability initiates a chronic inflammatory process. To reduce silent inflammation, it is important to rule out food allergies (See the chapter "Food Allergy"), avoid drugs that damage the intestines, and maintain a healthy and intact intestinal lining. If you have inflammatory bowel disease, psoriasis, or celiac disease, consult the chapters that deal with these issues and follow the recommendations given.

Nutritional Supplements

The general supplementation guidelines given in the chapter "Supplementary Measures" collectively will ensure some anti-inflammatory effects. In particular, supplementation with EPA + DHA in the form of fish oils as well as with various flavonoid-rich extracts has shown anti-inflammatory effects, including an ability to lower CRP. Pine bark and grape seed extract appear very useful, as they exert a number of anti-inflammatory effects that in clinical trials have been shown to lower CRP.[15,16] In a double-blind study in patients with osteoarthritis of the knee those who took 100 mg pine bark extract (Pycnogenol) per day saw their CRP levels decrease from baseline 3.9 mg/l to 1.1 mg/l, whereas the control group had no significant change. Other markers of inflammation also declined with pine bark extract.

Botanical Medicines

Specific botanical medicines to reduce silent inflammation are usually not necessary, as the recommendations for diet are far more important. Nonetheless, there may be some specific situations where CRP is stubbornly resistant to falling. In these situations, curcumin, the yellow pigment of turmeric (*Curcuma longa*), may be helpful because of its variety of anti-inflammatory effects.[17]

One concern regarding curcumin has been absorption, but there now exist a number of methods and products that enhance the absorption of curcumin. One of those products, Meriva, complexes the curcumin with soy phospholipids. Absorption studies in animals indicate that peak plasma levels of curcumin after administration of Meriva were five times higher than those after administration of regular curcumin.[18] Studies with another advanced form of curcumin, Theracurmin, show even greater absorption (27 times greater than regular curcumin).[19] In a study in patients with osteoarthritis a dosage of 1,000 mg Meriva (providing 200 mg curcumin) for three months decreased the level of CRP from 168 to 11.3 mg/L.[20]

Turmeric can also be consumed liberally in the diet, but since curcumin is so poorly absorbed, Meriva at a dosage of 1,000–1,200 mg per day or Theracurmin at a dosage of 300 mg per day can be used.

WHAT IS THE DIFFERENCE BETWEEN AN HERB AND A SPICE?

Technically, an herb is a plant that does not have a woody stem. If a plant has a woody stem, it is referred to as a shrub, bush, or tree. The term *herb* is also used to describe a plant or plant part that is used for medicinal purposes. A spice, on the other hand, is technically a plant product that has aromatic properties and is used to season or flavor foods. Most spices are derived from bark (e.g., cinnamon), fruit (e.g., red and black pepper), seeds (e.g., nutmeg), or other parts of an herb, tree, or shrub, while herbs for cooking typically use the leaves and stem. This makes for an easy way of distinguishing an herb from a spice. But can herbs be spices and can spices be herbs? Yes, of course. Many herbs are used to flavor foods, thus meeting the definition of a spice, and most spices can be used for medicinal purposes, thus meeting the second definition of an herb. To reduce silent information, make liberal use of spices in particular—turmeric, ginger, cayenne pepper, cinnamon, and other spices all exert significant anti-inflammatory effects, ideal for reducing silent inflammation.

QUICK REVIEW

- **Silent inflammation is a major factor in the development of virtually every major chronic degenerative disease, including cardiovascular disease, allergies, type 2 diabetes, cancer, and Alzheimer's disease.**

- **The most common test to measure silent inflammation is blood determination of C-reactive protein (CRP).**

- **Abdominal obesity is the strongest predictor of silent inflammation and CRP levels.**

- The higher the diet is in foods that raise blood sugar levels, the higher the CRP level will be.
- The Mediterranean diet and a diet rich in flavonoids (found in soy, apples, berries, and other fruits and vegetables) are also associated with lower CRP levels.
- The ratio of omega-3 to omega-6 fatty acids is a major factor in determining the degree of silent inflammation and CRP levels.

- Regular, moderate exercise reduces the level of silent inflammation.
- Pine bark and grape seed extract appear very useful, as they exert a number of anti-inflammatory effects that lower CRP.
- Curcumin may help lower CRP in cases not responsive to diet and general supplementation guidelines.

TREATMENT SUMMARY

Research has left little room for doubt that diet is a major factor in silent inflammation. Diet is the major contributor to the development of insulin resistance. Decreased sensitivity of body tissues to insulin results in elevations in blood sugar and increased oxidative stress. Insulin resistance is largely the result of abdominal obesity and excessive consumption of calories, particularly carbohydrates. In fact, abdominal obesity is the strongest independent predictor of silent inflammation and CRP levels.[4,5] Therefore, the guidelines given in the chapter "Obesity and Weight Management" should be regarded as the first step in reducing silent inflammation in overweight or obese individuals. CRP levels generally correspond to insulin sensitivity. In other words, when insulin sensitivity is good, CRP levels are much lower than when insulin sensitivity is poor. Not surprisingly, diabetics' CRP levels are generally high.

Lifestyle

- Do not smoke.
- Achieve and maintain ideal body weight.
- Exercise on a regular basis.

Diet

Follow the dietary guidelines in the chapter "A Health-Promoting Diet." Specifically, it is important to do the following:

- Follow a low-glycemic, Mediterranean-style diet and increase consumption of fiber-rich plant foods (fruits, vegetables, grains, and legumes).
- Consume less saturated fat and cholesterol by reducing or eliminating the amounts of animal products in the diet.
- Increase consumption of monounsaturated fats (e.g., nuts, seeds, and olive oil) and omega-3 fatty acids.

Nutritional Supplements

- A high-potency multivitamin and mineral formula according to the guidelines given in the chapter "Supplementary Measures."
- Key individual nutrients:
  - Vitamin C: 250 to 500 mg one to three times per day
  - Vitamin D: 2,000 to 4,000 IU per day (ideally, measure blood levels and adjust dosage accordingly)
- Fish oil: minimum 1,000 mg EPA + DHA per day
- One of the following:
  - Grape seed extract (>95% procyanidolic oligomers): 100 to 300 mg per day
  - Pine bark extract (>95% procyanidolic oligomers): 100 to 300 mg per day
  - Some other flavonoid-rich extract with a similar flavonoid content, super greens formula, or another plant-based antioxidant that can provide an oxygen radical absorption capacity (ORAC) of 3,000 to 6,000 units or higher per day

Botanical Medicines

If the high-sensitivity C-reactive protein test shows that CRP is not responding to the above recommendations after a three-month trial, add one of the following curcumin products:

- Meriva: 500 to 1,000 mg twice daily
- BCM95 Complex: 750 to 1,500 mg twice daily
- Theracurmin: 300 mg one to three times daily

Stress Management

· ·

Introduction

Stress is defined as any disturbance—for example, heat or cold, chemical toxin, microorganism, physical trauma, strong emotional reaction—that can trigger the "stress response." How an individual handles stress plays a major role in determining his or her level of health. Comprehensive stress management involves a truly holistic approach designed to counteract the everyday stresses of life. Most often the stress response is so mild it goes entirely unnoticed. However, if stress is extreme, unusual, or long-lasting, the stress response can be overwhelming and becomes quite harmful to virtually every body system.

Before we discuss methods for helping to deal effectively with stress, it is important to understand the stress response. Ultimately, the success of any stress management program depends on its ability to improve an individual's immediate and long-term responses to stress.

The General Adaptation Syndrome

The stress response is actually part of a larger response known as the *general adaptation syndrome*, a term coined by the pioneering stress researcher Hans Selye. The syndrome is composed of three phases: alarm, resistance, and exhaustion.[1] These phases are

largely controlled and regulated by the adrenal glands.

The initial response to stress is the alarm reaction, which is often referred to as the *fight-or-flight response*. The fight-or-flight response is triggered by activation of the sympathetic nervous system and ultimately the hypothalamic-pituitary-adrenal axis, which causes the adrenals to secrete adrenaline and other stress-related hormones.

The fight-or-flight response is designed to counteract danger by mobilizing the body's resources for immediate physical activity. As a result, the heart rate and force of contraction increase to provide blood to areas necessary for response to the stressful situation. Blood is shunted away from the skin and internal organs, except the heart and lung, while the amount of blood supplying required oxygen and glucose to the muscles and brain is increased. The rate of breathing rises to supply necessary oxygen to the heart, brain, and working muscle. Sweat production increases to eliminate toxic compounds produced by the body and to lower body temperature. Production of digestive secretions is severely reduced because digestive activity is not critical for counteracting stress. Blood sugar levels rise dramatically as the liver converts stored glycogen into glucose for release into the bloodstream.

Although the alarm phase is usually short-lived, the next phase—the resistance reaction—allows the body to continue fighting a stressor long after the effects of the fight-or-flight response have worn off. Other hormones, such as cortisol and other corticosteroids secreted by the adrenal cortex, are largely responsible for the resistance reaction. For example, these hormones stimulate the conversion of protein to energy, so that the body has a large supply of energy long after glucose stores are depleted; the hormones also promote the retention of sodium to keep blood pressure elevated.

As well as providing the necessary energy and circulatory changes required to deal effectively with stress, the resistance reaction provides the changes required to handle an emotional crisis, perform strenuous tasks, and fight infection. The effects of adrenal cortex hormones are quite necessary when the body is faced with danger, but prolongation of the resistance reaction or continued stress increases the risk of significant disease (including diabetes, high blood pressure, and cancer) and results in the final stage of the general adaptation syndrome, exhaustion.

Exhaustion may be manifested as a partial or total collapse of a body function or specific organ. Two of the major causes of exhaustion are loss of potassium ions and depletion of adrenal glucocorticoid hormones like cortisone. Loss of potassium results in cellular dysfunction and, if severe, cell death. Adrenal glucocorticoid depletion diminishes glucose control, leading to hypoglycemia.

Another cause of exhaustion is weakening of the organs. Prolonged stress places a tremendous load not just on the adrenals but also on many other organ systems, especially the heart, blood vessels, and immune system, and is associated with many common diseases.

Diseases Strongly Linked to Stress

Angina

Asthma

Autoimmune disease

Cancer

Cardiovascular disease

Common cold

Depression

Diabetes (type 2)

Headaches

Hypertension

Immune suppression

Irritable bowel syndrome

Menstrual irregularities

Premenstrual tension syndrome

Rheumatoid arthritis

Ulcerative colitis

Ulcers

Stress: A Healthy View

The father of modern stress research was Hans Selye. Having spent many years studying this subject, Selye developed valuable insights into the role of stress in disease. According to Selye, stress in itself should not be viewed in a negative context. It is not the stressor that determines the response; instead it is the individual's internal reaction, which then triggers the response. This internal reaction is highly individualized. What one person may experience as stress, the next person may view entirely differently. Selye perhaps summarized his view best in the following passage from his book *The Stress of Life*:[2]

No one can live without experiencing some degree of stress all the time. You may think that only serious disease or intensive physical or mental injury can cause stress. This is false. Crossing a busy intersection, exposure to a draft, or even sheer joy are enough to activate the body's stress mechanisms to some extent. Stress is not even necessarily bad for you; it is also the spice of life, for any emotion, any activity causes stress. But, of course, your system must be prepared to take it. The same stress which makes one person sick can be an invigorating experience for another.

The key statement Selye made may be "your system must be prepared to take it." A significant body of knowledge has now accumulated on strategies to develop healthful, rather than disease-facilitating, responses to both short-term and long-term stress.

The Stress Scale

Evaluating the impact of stress on a person's health status requires a complete clinical assessment (review of systems, medical history, physical exam, sleep history, etc.). Many people who are stressed out may not be able to identify exactly what is causing them to feel stressed. Typical presenting symptoms are insomnia, depression, fatigue, headache,

upset stomach, digestive disturbances, and irritability.

One useful tool to assess the role that stress may play is the social readjustment rating scale developed by Holmes and Rahe (see below).[3] The scale was originally designed to predict the risk of a serious disease due to stress. Various life-changing events are rated according to their potential to cause disease. Notice that even events commonly viewed as positive, such as an outstanding personal achievement, carry stress.

If a person is under a great deal of immediate stress or has endured a fair amount of stress for a few months or longer, it is appropriate to assess adrenal dysfunction more accurately with laboratory methods.

The standard interpretation of the social readjustment rating scale is that a total of 200 or more units in one year is considered to be predictive of a high likelihood of experiencing a serious disease. However, rather than using the scale solely to predict the likelihood of serious disease, anyone can use it to determine his or her level of stressor exposure, because everyone reacts differently to stressful events.

The Social Readjustment Rating Scale		
RANK	**LIFE EVENT**	**MEAN VALUE**
1	Death of spouse	100
2	Divorce	73
3	Marital separation	65
4	Jail term	63
5	Death of a close family member	63
6	Personal injury or illness	53
7	Marriage	50
8	Fired at work	47
9	Marital reconciliation	45
10	Retirement	45

The Social Readjustment Rating Scale		
RANK	**LIFE EVENT**	**MEAN VALUE**
11	Change in health of family member	44
12	Pregnancy	40
13	Sex difficulties	39
14	Gain of a new family member	39
15	Business adjustment	39
16	Change in financial state	38
17	Death of a close friend	37
18	Change to different line of work	36
19	Change in number of arguments with spouse	35
20	Large mortgage	31
21	Foreclosure of mortgage or loan	30
22	Change in responsibilities at work	29
23	Son or daughter leaving home	29
24	Trouble with in-laws	29
25	Outstanding personal achievement	28
26	Spouse begins or stops work	26
27	Beginning or end of school	26
28	Change in living conditions	25
29	Revision of personal habits	24
30	Trouble with boss	23
31	Change in work hours or conditions	20
32	Change in residence	20
33	Change in schools	20
34	Change in recreation	19
35	Change in church activities	19
36	Change in social activities	18
37	Small mortgage	17
38	Change in sleeping habits	16
39	Change in number of family get-togethers	15
40	Change in eating habits	15
41	Vacation	13
42	Christmas	12
43	Minor violations of the law	11

Salivary Cortisol Levels

A popular assessment of the impact of stress is based on salivary levels of the stress hormone cortisol. Salivary cortisol levels are reproducible, comparable to plasma levels, and easy to assess.[4,5] Salivary cortisol levels generally show a sharp rise when a person wakes up and during the first hour afterward. Generally, an initially overactive acute stress response results in elevated cortisol levels, but chronic stress, insomnia, or depression may blunt this effect.[6,7]

Another popular test is measuring salivary cortisol levels at awakening and in the evening, usually along with DHEA. The classic pattern associated with chronic stress is elevated cortisol combined with reduced DHEA, indicating a shift toward stress hormone production and away from sex hormone steroid production. This pattern is often associated with anxiety and depression. Adrenal exhaustion is characterized by low cortisol and low DHEA. Adrenal exhaustion is a common side effect of continual high stress as well as of steroid drugs such as prednisone, used in the treatment of allergic or inflammatory diseases.

Therapeutic Considerations

Whether you are aware of it or not, you have developed a pattern for coping with stress. Unfortunately, most people have found patterns and methods that ultimately do not support good health. Negative coping patterns must be identified and replaced with positive ways of coping. Try to identify any negative or destructive coping patterns listed below and replace those patterns with more positive measures for dealing with stress.

Stress management can be substantially improved by focusing on the following six equally important areas:

- Techniques to calm the mind, promote parasympathetic tone, and promote a positive mental attitude
- Lifestyle factors
- Exercise
- A healthful diet designed to nourish the body and support physiological processes
- Dietary and botanical supplements designed to support the body as a whole, but especially the adrenal glands
- Supervised stress management program

Negative Coping Patterns

Dependence on chemicals: legal and illicit drugs, alcohol, smoking

Overeating

Too much television

Emotional outbursts

Feelings of helplessness

Overspending

Excessive behavior

Calming the Mind and Body

Learning to calm the mind and body is extremely important in relieving stress. Among the easiest methods for the patient to learn are relaxation exercises. The goal of relaxation techniques is to produce a physiological response known as a *relaxation response*—a response that is exactly opposite to the stress response that reflects activation of the parasympathetic nervous system. Although an individual may relax by simply sleeping, watching television, or reading a book, relaxation techniques are designed specifically to produce the relaxation response.

The term *relaxation response* was coined

STRESS RESPONSE	RELAXATION RESPONSE
The heart rate and force of contraction of the heart increase to provide blood to areas necessary for response to the stressful situation.	The heart rate is reduced and the heart beats more effectively. Blood pressure is reduced.
Blood is shunted away from the skin and internal organs, except the heart and lung, while the amount of blood supplying required oxygen and glucose to the muscles and brain is increased.	Blood is shunted toward internal organs, especially those organs involved in digestion.
The rate of breathing rises to supply necessary oxygen to the heart, brain, and exercising muscle.	The rate of breathing decreases as oxygen demand is reduced during periods of rest.
Sweat production increases to eliminate toxic compounds produced by the body and to lower body temperature.	Sweat production diminishes, because a person who is calm and relaxed does not experience nervous perspiration.
Production of digestive secretions is severely reduced because digestive activity is not critical to counteracting stress.	Production of digestive secretions is increased, greatly improving digestion.
Blood sugar levels rise dramatically as the liver dumps stored glucose into the bloodstream.	Blood sugar levels are maintained in the normal physiological range.

by Harvard professor and cardiologist Herbert Benson in the early 1970s to describe a physiological response that he found in people who meditate.[1] The relaxation response is just the opposite of the stress response. With the stress response, the sympathetic nervous system dominates. With the relaxation response, the parasympathetic nervous system dominates. The parasympathetic nervous system controls bodily functions such as digestion, breathing, and heart rate during periods of rest, relaxation, visualization, meditation, and sleep. Although the sympathetic nervous system is designed to protect against immediate danger, the parasympathetic system is designed for repair, maintenance, and restoration of the body.

The relaxation response can be achieved through a variety of techniques. It doesn't matter which technique you choose, because all have the same physiological effect—a state of deep relaxation. The most popular techniques are meditation, prayer, progressive relaxation, self-hypnosis, and biofeed-

back. To produce the desired long-term health benefits, use the relaxation technique for at least 5 to 10 minutes each day.

Breathing

Producing deep relaxation with any technique requires learning how to breathe properly. One of the most powerful methods of producing less stress and more energy in the body is by breathing with the diaphragm. Diaphragmatic breathing activates the relaxation centers in the brain and the parasympathetic nervous system. Following is a technique for teaching diaphragmatic breathing.

Instructions for Diaphragmatic Breathing

1. Find a comfortable and quiet place to lie down or sit.

2. Place your feet slightly apart. Place one hand on your abdomen near your navel. Place the other hand on your chest.

3. You will be inhaling through your nose and exhaling through your mouth.

4. Concentrate on your breathing. Note which hand is rising and falling with each breath.

5. Gently exhale most of the air in your lungs.

6. Inhale while slowly counting to four. As you inhale, slightly extend your abdomen, causing it to rise about one inch. Make sure that you are not moving your chest or shoulders.

7. As you breathe in, imagine the warmed air flowing in. Imagine this warmth flowing to all parts of your body.

8. Pause for one second, then slowly exhale to a count of four. As you exhale, your abdomen should move inward.

9. As the air flows out, imagine all your tension and stress leaving your body.

10. Repeat the process until a sense of deep relaxation is achieved.

Progressive Relaxation

One of the most popular techniques for producing the relaxation response is progressive relaxation. The technique is based on a very simple procedure of comparing tension with relaxation. Many people are not aware of the sensation of relaxation. In progressive relaxation, an individual is taught what it feels like to relax by comparing relaxation with muscle tension.

The basic technique is to contract a muscle forcefully for a period of one to two seconds and then give way to a feeling of relaxation in that muscle. The procedure systematically goes through all the muscles of the body, progressively producing a deep state of relaxation. The procedure begins with contracting the muscles of the face and neck, then the upper arms and chest, followed by the lower

arms and hands. The process is repeated progressively down the body, from the abdomen through the buttocks, the thighs, and the calves to the feet. This whole process is repeated two or three times. This technique is often used in the treatment of anxiety and insomnia.

Progressive relaxation, deep breathing, or some other stress reduction technique is an important component of a comprehensive stress management program.

Lifestyle

A person's lifestyle is a major determinant of his or her stress levels. In addition to those factors described in the chapter "A Health-Promoting Lifestyle," two areas of concern are time management and relationship issues.

One of the biggest stressors for most people is time. They simply do not feel they have enough of it. Here are some tips on time management.

Tips for Improved Time Management

- **Set priorities.** Realize that you can accomplish only so much in a day. Decide what is important, and limit your efforts to that goal.

- **Organize your day.** There are always interruptions and unplanned demands on your time, but create a definite plan for the day on the basis of your priorities. Avoid the pitfall of always letting the immediate demands control your life.

- **Delegate authority.** Delegate as much authority and work as you can. You can't do everything yourself. Learn to train and depend on others.

- **Tackle tough jobs first.** Handle the most important tasks first, while your energy levels are high. Leave the busywork or running around for later in the day.

- **Minimize meeting time.** Schedule meetings to bump up against the lunch hour or quitting time; that way they can't last forever.

- **Avoid putting things off.** Work done under pressure of an unreasonable deadline often has to be redone. That creates more stress than if it had been done right the first time. Plan ahead.

- **Don't be a perfectionist.** You can never really achieve perfection anyway. Do your best in a reasonable amount of time, then move on to other important tasks. If you find time, you can always come back later and polish the task some more. The old adage "The perfect is the enemy of the good" contains much wisdom.

Another major cause of stress for many people is interpersonal relationships. Interpersonal relationships can be divided into three major categories: marital, family, and job-related. The quality of any relationship ultimately comes down to the quality of the communication. Learning to communicate effectively goes a very long way toward reducing the stress and conflicts of interpersonal relationships. Here are seven tips for effective communication, regardless of the type of interpersonal relationship.

Keys to Improving Communication

- **Learn to be a good listener.** Allow the person you are communicating with to really share his or her feelings and thoughts uninterrupted. Empathize; put yourself in the other person's shoes. If you first seek to understand, you will find yourself being better understood.

- **Be an active listener.** This means that you must be truly interested in what the other person is communicating. Listen to what he or she is saying instead of thinking about your response. Ask questions to gain more information or clarify what the other person is telling you. Good questions open lines of communication.

- **Be a reflective listener.** Restate or reflect back to the other person your interpretation of what he or she is telling you. This simple technique shows the other person that you are both listening to and understanding what he or she is saying. Restating what you think is being said may cause some short-term conflict in some situations, but it is certainly worth the risk.

- **Wait to speak until the person you want to communicate with is listening.** If the person is not ready to listen, your message will not be heard no matter how well you communicate it.

- **Don't try to talk over somebody.** If you find yourself being interrupted, relax; don't try to outtalk the other person. If you are courteous and allow the other person to speak, chances are he or she will eventually respond likewise. If that doesn't happen, point out that the other person is interrupting the communication process. You can do this only if you have been a good listener. Double standards in relationships seldom work.

- **Help the other person become an active listener.** This can be done by asking whether the other person has understood what you were communicating. Ask him or her to tell you what he or she heard. If the other person doesn't seem to understand what you are saying, keep trying.

- **Don't be afraid of long silences.** Human communication involves much more than human words. A great deal can be communicated during silences; unfortunately, in many situations silence can make us feel uncomfortable. Relax. Some people need silence to collect their thoughts and feel safe in communicating. The important thing to remember during silences is that you must remain an active listener.

Exercise

The immediate effect of exercise is stress on the body. However, with a regular exercise program the body adapts, and exercise becomes an effective stress reduction technique. With regular exercise, the body becomes stronger, functions more efficiently, and has greater endurance. Exercise is a vital component of a comprehensive stress management program and overall good health.

People who exercise regularly are much less likely to suffer from fatigue and depression. Tension, depression, feelings of inadequacy, and worries diminish greatly with regular exercise.

Exercise alone has been demonstrated to have a tremendous effect in terms of improving mood and the ability to handle stressful life situations. This effect is seen in adolescents as well as adults. In one study, 2,223 boys and 2,838 girls (mean age 16.3 years) from 10 teams and 25 different individual sports were studied for the relationship between emotional well-being and psychological well-being. Engagement in sports and in vigorous recreational activity was positively associated with emotional well-being independent of other variables.[8]

Diet

An individual suffering from stress or anxiety must support the biochemistry of the body by following some important dietary guidelines:

- Eliminate or restrict the intake of caffeine.
- Eliminate or restrict the intake of alcohol.
- Eliminate refined carbohydrates from the diet.
- Eat a diverse range of colorful, whole foods.
- Increase the potassium-to-sodium ratio.
- Eat regular planned meals in a relaxed environment.
- Control food allergies.

According to Selye, whether or not stress is harmful is based on the strength of the system.[2] From a purely physiological perspective, it can be strongly argued that delivery of high-quality nutrition to the cells of the body is the critical factor in determining the strength of the system.

When the eating habits of Americans are examined as a whole, it is little wonder that so many people are suffering from stress, anxiety, and fatigue. Most Americans are not providing their bodies with the high-quality nutrition they need. Instead of eating foods rich in vital nutrients, most Americans focus on refined foods high in calories, sugar, fat, and cholesterol.

Caffeine

The average American consumes 150 to 225 mg caffeine per day, or roughly the amount of caffeine in two cups of coffee. Although some people can handle this amount, others are more sensitive to the effects of caffeine. Even small amounts of caffeine can affect sensitive people, whereas those with normal sensitivity respond to large amounts. Excessive caffeine consumption can produce "caffeinism," which is characterized by symptoms of depression, nervousness, irritability, recurrent headache, heart palpitations, and insomnia. People prone to feeling stress and anxiety tend to be especially sensitive to caffeine.[9] One way to determine if you are suffering caffeinism is to stop drinking coffee and all other sources of caffeine (chocolate, tea, medications with caffeine, etc.). Developing headaches is a sure sign you are consuming too much.

Alcohol

Alcohol produces chemical stress on the body and increases oxidative stress, resulting in the depletion of the critical intracellular antioxidant glutathione. It also increases adrenal hormone output and interferes with both normal brain chemistry and normal sleep cycles. Although many people believe that alcohol has a calming effect, a study of 90 healthy male volunteers given either a placebo or alcohol demonstrated significant increases in anxiety scores after consumption of alcohol.[10]

Refined Carbohydrates and Glycemic Volatility

One of the consequences of the stress response is abdominal fat cell growth and loss of muscle mass, a scenario that obviously leads to insulin resistance and obesity. A complex set of events orchestrated by cortisol, released as a result of the stress response, is ultimately responsible for the fact that stress promotes weight gain. Cortisol is also a factor contributing to rapidly fluctuating blood sugar levels, which are generally related to some degree of insulin resistance and made worse by overconsumption of foods with a high glycemic impact. Refined carbohydrates (e.g., sugar and white flour) are known to contribute to problems with blood sugar control, especially hypoglycemia as well as glycemic volatility. The association between hypoglycemia and impaired mental function is well known. Numerous studies have shown that hypoglycemia frequently develops in depressed patients.[11,12] As depression is one of the most common causes of anxiety, this finding provides a link between hypoglycemia and feelings of stress. Simply eliminating refined carbohydrate from the diet may be all that is needed for patients who have depression or anxiety due to hypoglycemia.

Potassium-to-Sodium Ratio

One of the key dietary recommendations to support the adrenal glands is to ensure adequate potassium levels within the body. This can best be done by consuming foods rich in potassium and avoiding foods high in sodium. Most Americans have a dietary potassium-to-sodium (K:Na) ratio of less than 1:2. In contrast, most researchers recommend a dietary K:Na ratio higher than 5:1. However, even this recommendation may not be optimal. A natural diet rich in fruits and vegetables can produce a K:Na ratio higher than 50:1, as most fruits and vegetables have a K:Na ratio of more than 100:1.

Meal Planning

Mealtimes should be spent in a relaxed environment. As noted previously, digestion is a process largely controlled by the parasympathetic nervous system. Eating in a rushed manner or in a noisy or hurried environment is not conducive to good digestion or good health.

Food Allergies

People with symptoms of anxiety or chronic fatigue must be concerned about food allergies. As far back as 1930, pioneering allergist Albert Rowe began noticing that anxiety and fatigue were key features of food allergies.[13] Originally Rowe described a syndrome known as "allergic toxemia," which included symptoms such as anxiety, fatigue, muscle and joint aches, drowsiness, difficulty of concentration, and depression. Around the 1950s, this syndrome began to be referred to as the "allergic tension-fatigue syndrome." With the current focus on chronic fatigue syndrome, many physicians and other people are forgetting that food allergies can lead to anxiety as well as chronic fatigue.

Nutritional Supplements and Botanical Medicines

Nutritional and botanical support for the individual experiencing signs and symptoms of stress largely involves supporting the adrenal glands. Long-term stress and corticosteroids cause the adrenal glands to shrink and become dysfunctional, aggravating anxiety, depression, and chronic fatigue.

An abnormal adrenal response, either deficient or excessive hormone release, significantly alters an individual's response to stress. Often the adrenals become "exhausted" as a result of constant demands put on them. An individual with adrenal exhaustion usually suffers from chronic fatigue and may complain of feeling "stressed out" or chronically anxious. He or she typically has a reduced resistance to allergies and infection.

Nutritional Supplements

The nutrients especially important for supporting adrenal function are vitamin C, vitamin B_6 (pyridoxine), zinc, magnesium, and pantothenic acid (vitamin B_5). All of these nutrients play a critical role in the health of the adrenal gland as well as the manufacture of adrenal hormones. During stress, the levels of these nutrients in the adrenals decrease substantially.

For example, during chemical, emotional, psychological, or physiological stress, the urinary excretion of vitamin C is increased. Examples of chemical stressors are cigarette smoke, pollutants, and allergens. Extra vitamin C in the form of supplementation and a higher intake of vitamin C–rich foods is often recommended to keep the immune system working properly during times of stress.

Equally important during high periods of stress or in individuals needing adrenal support is pantothenic acid. Pantothenic acid deficiency results in adrenal atrophy, characterized by fatigue, headache, sleep disturbances, nausea, and abdominal discomfort. Pantothenic acid is found in whole grains, legumes, cauliflower, broccoli, salmon, liver, sweet potatoes, and tomatoes. In patients who suffer from chronic stress or have a history of corticosteroid (prednisone) use, the typical level of supplementation is 100 to 500 mg per day.

Gamma-Aminobutyric Acid (GABA)

Gamma-aminobutyric acid (GABA) is a major neurotransmitter that is abundantly and widely distributed throughout the central nervous system. A low level of GABA or decreased GABA function in the brain is associated with several psychiatric and neurological disorders, but primarily anxiety, depression, insomnia, and epilepsy. Currently, many popular antianxiety drugs—the sedative-hypnotics—interact primarily with GABA receptors. These drugs include the benzodiazepine drugs such as alprazolam (Xanax) and diazepam (Valium), as well as drugs such as flurazepam (Dalmane), quazepam (Doral), temazepam (Restoril), triazolam (Halcion), zolpidem (Ambien), and baclofen (Kemstro and Lioresal).

Clinical studies with a product called PharmaGABA, naturally manufactured by a fermentation process that utilizes *Lactobacillus hilgardii*, have shown it to produce significant antistress effects.[14] Specifically, PharmaGABA has been shown to produce relaxation, as evidenced by changes in brain wave patterns, diameter of the pupil, and heart rate, as well as reduce markers of stress, including salivary cortisol levels. These effects are thought to be the result of activation of the parasympathetic nervous system rather than the PharmaGABA crossing the blood-brain barrier. The typical dosage is 100 to

200 mg up to three times per day. The general guideline is to take no more than 1,000 mg within a 4-hour period and no more than 3,000 mg within a 24-hour period.

Botanical Medicines

Several botanical medicines support adrenal function. Most notable are Chinese ginseng (*Panax ginseng*) and Siberian ginseng (*Eleutherococcus senticosus*), rhodiola (*Rhodiola rosea*), and ashwagandha (*Withania somnifera*). All of these plants exert beneficial effects on adrenal function and enhance resistance to stress and are often referred to as "adaptogens." These plants have historically been used to:

- Restore vitality in debilitated and feeble individuals
- Increase feelings of energy
- Improve mental and physical performance
- Prevent the negative effects of stress and enhance the body's response to stress

Both Siberian and Chinese ginseng have been shown to enhance the ability to cope with various stressors, both physical and mental.[15,16] Presumably this antistress action is mediated by mechanisms that control the adrenal glands. Ginseng delays the onset of the alarm phase of the general adaptation syndrome and reduces its severity.

People taking either of the ginsengs typically report an increased sense of well-being. Clinical studies have confirmed that both Siberian and Chinese ginsengs significantly reduce feelings of stress and anxiety. For example, in one double-blind clinical study, nurses who had switched from day to night duty rated themselves for competence, mood, and general well-being and were given a test for mental and physical performance along with blood cell counts and blood chemistry evaluation.[17] The group who were given Chinese ginseng demonstrated higher scores in competence, mood, and mental and physical performance compared with those receiving placebos. The nurses taking the ginseng felt more alert, yet more tranquil, and were able to perform better than the nurses who were not taking the ginseng.

In addition to these human studies, several animal studies have shown the ginsengs to exert significant antianxiety effects. In several of these studies, the stress-relieving effects were comparable to those of Valium; however, while Valium causes behavior changes, sedative effects, and impaired motor activity, ginseng has none of these negative effects.[15,16]

On the basis of the clinical and animal studies, ginseng appears to offer significant benefit to people suffering from stress and anxiety. Chinese ginseng (*P. ginseng*) is generally regarded as being more potent than Siberian ginseng. *P. ginseng* is probably better for the person who has experienced a great deal of stress, who is recovering from a long illness, or who has taken corticosteroids such as prednisone for a long time. For the person who is under mild to moderate stress and is experiencing less obvious impairment of adrenal function, Siberian ginseng may be the better choice. Dosages are as follows:

Panax ginseng (Chinese or Korean ginseng)

- High-quality crude ginseng root: 1.5 to 2 g one to three times per day
- Fluid extract (containing a minimum of 10.5 mg/ml ginsenosides with Rg1:Rb1 greater than or equal to 0.5 by HPLC): 2 to 4 ml (½ to 1 tsp) one to three times per day
- Dried powdered extract standardized to contain 5% ginsenosides with an Rb1/Rg1 ratio of 2:1: 250 to 500 mg one to three times per day

Siberian ginseng (*Eleutherococcus senticosus*):

- ○ Dried root: 2 to 4 g one to three times per day

- ○ Fluid extract (1:1): 2 to 4 ml (½ to 1 tsp) 2 to 4 g one to three times per day

- ○ Solid (dry powdered) extract (20:1 or standardized to contain more than 1% eleutheroside E): 100 to 200 mg 2 to 4 g one to three times per day

Another useful botanical medicine to support stress management is *Rhodiola rosea* (Arctic root), a popular plant in traditional medical systems in Eastern Europe and Asia, where it has traditionally been recommended to help combat fatigue and restore energy. Modern research has confirmed these effects and its qualities as an adaptogen. However, the adaptogenic actions of rhodiola are different from those of Chinese and Siberian ginsengs, which act primarily on the hypothalamus-pituitary-adrenal axis. Rhodiola seems to exert its adaptogenic effects by working on neurotransmitters and endorphins. Rhodiola appears to offer an advantage over other adaptogens in circumstances of acute stress because it produces a greater feeling of relaxation and antianxiety effects. A single dose of rhodiola extract prior to acute stressful events has been shown to prevent stress-induced disruptions in function and performance, but like the ginsengs, *R. rosea* has also shown positive results with long-term use.[18–21] In one randomized, placebo-controlled trial of 60 patients with stress-related fatigue, rhodiola was found to have an antifatigue effect that increased mental performance, particularly the ability to concentrate; it also decreased the cortisol response to the stress of awakening from sleep.[21]

On the basis of results of clinical trials with a standardized *R. rosea* extract, the therapeutic dose varies according to the rosavin content. For a dosage target of 3.6 to 7.2 mg rosavin, the daily dose would be 360 to 600 mg for an extract standardized for 1% rosavin, 180 to 300 mg for 2% rosavin, and 100 to 200 mg for 3.6% rosavin. When rhodiola is used as an adaptogen, long-term administration is normally begun several weeks before a period of expected increased physiological, chemical, or biological strain and continued throughout the duration of the challenging event or activity. When rhodiola is used as a single dose for acute stress (e.g., for an examination or athletic competition), the suggested dose is three times the dose used for long-term supplementation. No side effects have been reported in the clinical trials, but at higher dosages some individuals might experience greater irritability and insomnia.

Clinical studies with Sensoril, a patented proprietary extract of roots and leaves from ashwagandha (*Withania somnifera*), have shown considerable antistress and adaptogenic effects. In one double-blind study, chronically stressed subjects taking Sensoril had significant reductions in anxiety, serum cortisol, C-reactive protein, pulse rate, and blood pressure compared with the placebo group, as well as significant increases of serum DHEA and hemoglobin. In addition, there were dose-dependent responses in lowering fasting blood glucose and improving blood cholesterol levels. Dosage is 125 to 250 mg per day.[22]

Additional Therapies

DHEA (Dehydroepiandrosterone)

With prolonged stress, levels of DHEA tend to be reduced. One of the key indicators of too much stress or a poor stress response is a reduction in salivary DHEA and an increase in salivary cortisol. DHEA supplementation is being recognized for its important health-supporting effects, including an ability to lower cortisol levels.[23] For men age 40 to 50, we recommend DHEA if they are complaining of reduced libido or fatigue, if they have diabetes, or if they have been subject to high levels of stress for a long period of time. We recommend basing the dosage on blood levels of DHEA and testosterone; typically the dosage ranges from 15 to 25 mg per day. For men over 50, typically, the dosage we recommend is between 25 and 50 mg. For women who have not yet passed through menopause, we do not recommend DHEA unless there is confirmation that DHEA levels are in fact low. The reason is that as many women approach menopause there is actually an increase in DHEA levels. Taking extra DHEA may lead to acne and increased facial hair. After menopause, DHEA may be used with caution and in low dosages ranging from 5 to 15 mg unless the woman has an autoimmune disease or diabetes.

Stress Management Programs

Supervised stress management programs are thought to offer greater compliance and better results than unsupervised, patient-directed programs. In one study, stress management experts evaluated six widely used occupational stress management interventions (relaxation, physical fitness, cognitive restructuring, meditation, assertiveness training, and stress inoculation) on the basis of 10 practicality criteria and 7 effectiveness objectives. They found that relaxation was the most practical intervention, and that meditation and stress inoculation were the least practical. Physical fitness was rated as the most effective intervention, and both meditation and assertiveness training were rated overall as the least effective. These results imply that although relaxation training may be the most practical intervention, physical exercise was the most effective intervention.[24]

Although in this evaluation meditation was shown to be the least practical and least effective method, when it is part of supervised program it can be very effective. In one trial of 103 adults, 59% and 61% of the meditation and control groups, respectively, completed the study.[25] The intervention program consisted of an eight-week group stress reduction program in which subjects learned, practiced, and applied mindfulness meditation to daily life situations. Those in the control group received educational materials and were encouraged to use community resources for stress management. Compared with the control group, intervention subjects reported significant decreases in the effect of daily hassles (24%), psychological distress (44%), and medical symptoms (46%); these were maintained at the three-month follow-up.

· ·

QUICK REVIEW

- **How an individual handles stress plays a major role in determining his or her level of health.**

- **Stress management can be substantially improved by focusing on the following six equally important areas:**

○ Techniques to calm the mind, promote parasympathetic tone, and promote a positive mental attitude

○ Lifestyle factors

○ Exercise

○ A healthful diet designed to nourish the body and support physiological processes

○ Dietary and botanical supplements designed to support the body as a whole, but especially the adrenal glands

○ Supervised stress management program

• One of the most powerful methods of producing less stress and more energy in the body is breathing with the diaphragm.

• Learning to manage time and communicate effectively goes a very long way in reducing stress.

• Exercise is a vital component of a comprehensive stress management program and contributes to overall good health.

• Excessive caffeine consumption can produce "caffeinism," characterized by symptoms of depression, nervousness, irritability, recurrent headache, heart palpitations, and insomnia.

• One of the consequences of the stress response is abdominal fat cell growth and loss of muscle mass, a scenario that leads to insulin resistance and obesity.

• One of the key dietary recommendations to support the adrenal glands is to ensure adequate potassium levels within the body.

• The nutrients especially important for supporting adrenal function are vitamin C, vitamin B$_6$, zinc, magnesium, and pantothenic acid.

• Clinical studies with PharmaGABA have shown it to produce significant antistress effects.

• Chinese ginseng (*Panax ginseng*) and Siberian ginseng (*Eleutherococcus senticosus*), rhodiola (*Rhodiola rosea*), and ashwagandha (*Withania somnifera*) exert beneficial effects on adrenal function and enhance resistance to stress.

• DHEA supplementation can help lower cortisol levels.

• Formal stress management programs produce measurable benefits.

· ·

TREATMENT SUMMARY

A comprehensive approach to a healthier, calmer life is an absolute must in modern life. Below are guidelines based upon an individual's need for support.

Level 1 Support

In addition to the general lifestyle and dietary guidelines discussed above and the regular utilization of techniques to calm the mind and body, Level 1 support simply involves the four cornerstones of good health presented in Section II:

- A positive mental attitude
- A health-promoting lifestyle
- A health-promoting diet
- Supplementary measures

Level 2 Support

Level 2 support encompasses Level 1 support plus the use of PharmaGABA (100 to 200 mg up to six times per day) to deal with situational stress and nervousness.

Level 3 Support

In the more anxious individual, Level 3 support encompasses Level 2 support plus the use of an herbal adaptogen (dosages given above).

Level 4 Support

For people who are experiencing significant signs of adrenal fatigue, generalized exhaustion, and/or anxiety, Level 4 support encompasses Level 3 support plus the recommendations in the chapter "Anxiety," and/or those in the chapter "Insomnia." In particular, improving sleep quality is essential to restoring adrenal function, a positive mood, physical and mental energy, and healing.

Obesity and
Weight Management

Introduction

Each year obesity-related conditions cost over $100 billion and cause an estimated 300,000 premature deaths in the United States, making a very strong case that the obesity epidemic is the most significant threat to the future of this country as well as other nations. In 1962, 13% of Americans were obese. By 1980 the proportion had risen to 15% and by 1994 it was up to 23%, and by the year 2004 obesity in America had reached a rate of one out of three, or 33%. Approximately 65 million adult Americans are now obese—more than the population of Britain, France, or Italy. As alarming as these statistics are, it must be pointed out that there is no end in sight. In particular, the percentage of children who are obese is also rising at an alarming rate. It is now estimated that 16.9% of children and adolescents from 2 to 19 years old are obese. Given the health challenges associated with obesity, the significance of these increases is staggering.[1-5]

Obesity and Health

Can you be both fat and healthy? No. According to detailed studies, obesity is more damaging to health than smoking, high levels of alcohol consumption, or poverty.[4,5] Obe-sity affects all major bodily systems—heart, lung, muscles, and bones. The health effects associated with obesity include, but are not limited to, the following:

- **High blood pressure.** Additional fat tissue in the body needs oxygen and nutrients in order to live, and therefore the blood vessels must circulate more blood to the fat tissue. This increases the workload of the heart because it must pump more blood through additional blood vessels. More circulating blood also means more pressure on the artery walls. Higher pressure on the artery walls increases blood pressure. In addition, extra weight can raise the heart rate and reduce the body's ability to transport blood through the vessels.

- **Diabetes.** Obesity, particularly abdominal obesity, is the major cause of type 2 diabetes. Obesity can cause resistance to insulin, the hormone that regulates blood sugar. When obesity causes insulin resistance, the body's blood sugar levels becomes elevated. Even moderate obesity dramatically increases the risk of diabetes.

- **Heart disease.** Atherosclerosis (hardening of the arteries) is present 10 times more often in obese people compared with those who are not obese. Coronary artery disease is also more prevalent because fatty deposits build up in arteries that supply the heart. Narrowed arteries and reduced blood flow to the heart can cause chest pain (angina) or a heart attack. Blood clots can also form in narrowed arteries and cause a stroke.

- **Cancer.** In women, being overweight contributes to an increased risk for a variety of cancers, including those of the breast, colon, gallbladder, and uterus. Men who are overweight have a higher risk of colon and prostate cancers.

- **Joint problems, including osteoarthritis.** Obesity can affect the knees and hips because of the stress placed on the joints by extra weight. Joint replacement surgery, while commonly performed on damaged joints, may not be advisable for an obese person because the artificial joint has a higher risk of loosening and causing further damage.

- **Sleep apnea and respiratory problems.** Sleep apnea, which causes people to stop breathing for brief periods, interrupts sleep throughout the night; the result is sleepiness during the day. It also causes heavy snoring. Respiratory problems associated with obesity occur when the added weight of the chest wall squeezes the lungs and causes restricted breathing. Sleep apnea is also associated with high blood pressure.

- **Psychosocial effects.** In a culture where often the ideal of physical attractiveness is to be overly thin, people who are overweight or obese frequently suffer disadvantages. Overweight and obese individuals are often blamed for their condition and may be considered lazy or weak-willed. It is not uncommon for overweight or obese people to have lower incomes or fewer or no romantic relationships. Disapproval of overweight people expressed by some individuals may progress to bias, discrimination, and even torment.

Obese individuals have a life expectancy that is on average five to seven years shorter compared with normal-weight individuals, with greater obesity associated with a greater relative risk for early mortality.[4,5] Most of the increased risk for early mortality is due to cardiovascular disease, as obesity carries with it a tremendous risk for type 2 diabetes, elevated cholesterol levels, high blood pressure, and other factors contributing to atherosclerosis. In 2009 annual medical spending due to overweight and obesity was estimated to be $147 billion.[6]

Health Problems Resulting from Obesity

- Cardiovascular problems
  - Angina
  - Atherosclerosis
  - Congestive heart failure
  - Deep vein thrombosis
  - Heart attack
  - High blood pressure
  - High cholesterol levels
  - Pulmonary embolism
  - Stroke
- Skin problems
  - Cellulitis
  - Hirsutism
  - Intertrigo
  - Lymphedema
  - Stretch marks
- Endocrine and reproductive problems
  - Complications during pregnancy
  - Diabetes
  - Infertility
  - Menstrual disorders

- o Intrauterine fetal death
- o Polycystic ovarian syndrome
- Gastrointestinal problems
  - o Gastroesophageal reflux disease
  - o Gallstones
  - o Fatty liver disease
- Neurological problems
  - o Carpal tunnel syndrome
  - o Dementia
  - o Idiopathic intracranial hypertension
  - o Migraine headaches
  - o Multiple sclerosis
- Cancer
- Mental health issues
  - o Depression
  - o Social stigmatization
- Respiratory problems
  - o Asthma
  - o Obstructive sleep apnea
- Rheumatological and orthopedic problems
  - o Chronic low back pain
  - o Gout
  - o Osteoarthritis
- Genital and urinary problems
  - o Chronic renal failure
  - o Erectile dysfunction
  - o Hypogonadism
  - o Urinary incontinence

Obesity Defined

The basic definition of obesity is an excessive amount of body fat. A simple measure known as the body mass index (BMI) is now the accepted standard for classifying individuals with regard to their body composition, and generally correlates well with a person's total body fat. (This may not be true for some very muscular athletes, whose body weight may place them in the category of overweight even though they have a low percentage of body fat.) BMI is calculated by dividing a person's weight in kilograms by height in meters squared. On the opposite page is a simple table to use to determine your BMI. To use the table, find your height in the left-hand column. Move across the row to your weight. The number at the top of the column is the BMI for that height and weight.

A BMI of 25 to 29.9 is a marker for being overweight, while someone who has a BMI of 30 or greater is considered obese. To put the BMI into perspective, a 5-foot-4-inch woman with a BMI of 30 is about 30 pounds above her ideal body weight. So obesity is not a matter of simply being a few pounds overweight. It reflects a significant amount of excess fat.

There is one more calculation that is important—your waist size. The combination of your BMI and your waist circumference is very good indicator of your risk for all of the diseases associated with obesity, especially the major killers: heart disease, stroke, cancer, and diabetes.

Abdominal Obesity

Abdominal obesity is highly associated with metabolic syndrome, insulin resistance, elevated inflammatory markers, high cholesterol and/or triglycerides, and high blood pressure. It is much more strongly linked to these issues than body mass index. So it appears that it is not how much you weigh but rather where you store your fat that determines your risk for cardiovascular disease.

Abdominal fat tissue was previously regarded as an inert storage depot; however, the emerging concept describes adipose tissue as a complex and highly active meta-

Body Mass Index Chart

BMI (KG/M²)	19	20	21	22	23	24	25	26	27	28	29	30	35	40
Height (inches)	Weight (pounds)													
58	91	96	100	105	110	115	119	124	129	134	138	143	167	191
59	94	99	104	109	114	119	124	128	133	138	143	148	173	198
60	97	102	107	112	118	123	128	133	138	143	148	153	179	204
61	100	106	111	116	122	127	132	137	143	148	153	158	185	211
62	104	109	115	120	126	131	136	142	147	153	158	164	191	218
63	107	113	118	124	130	135	141	146	152	158	163	169	197	225
64	110	116	122	128	134	140	145	151	157	163	169	174	204	232
65	114	120	126	132	138	144	150	156	162	168	174	180	210	240
66	118	124	130	136	142	148	155	161	167	173	179	186	216	247
67	121	127	134	140	146	153	159	166	172	178	185	191	223	255
68	125	131	138	144	151	158	164	171	177	184	190	197	230	262
69	128	135	142	149	155	162	169	176	182	189	196	203	236	270
70	132	139	146	153	160	167	174	181	188	195	202	207	243	278
71	136	143	150	157	165	172	179	186	193	200	208	215	250	286
72	140	147	154	162	169	177	184	191	199	206	213	221	258	294
73	144	151	159	166	174	182	189	197	204	212	219	227	265	302
74	148	155	163	171	179	186	194	202	210	218	225	233	272	311
75	152	160	168	176	184	192	200	208	216	224	232	240	279	319
76	156	164	172	180	189	197	205	213	221	230	238	246	287	328

Risk of Disease According to BMI and Waist Size

BMI	WAIST SIZE LESS THAN OR EQUAL TO 40 INCHES (MEN) OR 35 INCHES (WOMEN)	WAIST SIZE GREATER THAN 40 INCHES (MEN) OR 35 INCHES (WOMEN)
18.5 or less (underweight)	No increased risk of disease	No increased risk of disease
18.5–24.9 (normal weight)	No increased risk of disease	No increased risk of disease
25.0–29.9 (overweight)	Increased risk of disease	High risk of disease
30.0–34.9 (obese)	High risk of disease	Very high risk of disease
35.0–39.9 (obese)	Very high risk of disease	Very high risk of disease
40 or greater (extremely obese)	Extremely high risk of disease	Extremely high risk of disease

bolic and endocrine organ. Fat cells secrete hormone-like compounds known as adipokines that control insulin sensitivity and appetite. As abdominal fat accumulates, it leads to alterations in adipokines that ultimately promote insulin resistance and increased appetite, thereby adding more abdominal fat. Fortunately, reduction of abdominal fat through diet and increased physical activity can reestablish insulin sensitivity and reduce appetite.

To determine your waist circumference, place a measuring tape around the abdomen just above the upper hip bone, ensuring that the tape measure is horizontal. The tape measure should be snug but not tight. If you are a man and your waist circumference is greater than 40 inches, or if you are a woman and your waist circumference is greater than 35 inches, there is no need to do any further calculation, as this measurement alone has been shown to be a major risk factor for both cardiovascular disease and type 2 diabetes. If your waist circumference is less than these values, you need to determine your waist/hip ratio. To do this, measure the circumference of your hips at the widest part. Divide the waist circumference by the hip circumference. A waist/hip ratio above 1.0 for men and above 0.8 for women increases the risk of developing cardiovascular disease, type 2 diabetes, high blood pressure, and gout.

1. Measure the circumference of your waist: _____

2. Measure the circumference of your hips: _____

3. Divide the waist measurement by the hip measurement: _____ (this is your waist/hip ratio)

Body Fat vs. Body Weight

The number on the scale represents your total weight, not body composition (proportion of fat to muscle). It is increased body fat that is associated with poor health outcomes, not increased body weight. For example, people with a normal BMI can develop type 2 diabetes if they have an increased body fat percentage, especially if that excess fat is collecting around the waist. To more accurately determine body composition, we recommend using a scale that utilizes a safe, very low-level amount of electricity to measure body fat percentage by bioelectrical impedance. Since fat does not conduct much bioelectricity, a higher degree of impedance of the electrical charge is associated with a higher percentage of body fat. The most popular scales of this sort are manufactured by Tanita (www.tanita.com) and range in cost from $55 to $200 depending upon features. Ideally, women should strive to keep their body fat below 25% and men below 20%.

Causes of Obesity

Although there may or may not be a specific "obesity gene," the tendency to be overweight is definitely inherited. Nonetheless, even high-risk individuals can avoid obesity, and this indicates that dietary and lifestyle factors (primarily little or no physical activity) are chiefly responsible for obesity. In looking at possible causes beyond diet and lifestyle, researchers have focused on both psychological factors and physiological factors.

Psychological Factors

In the past, psychological factors were thought to be largely responsible for obesity. An early popular theory proposed that over-

Body Fat Rating Chart for Use with a Body Fat Measuring Scale					
MALES					
Age	**Risky**	**Excellent**	**Good**	**Fair**	**Poor**
19–24	<6%	10.8%	14.9%	19.0%	23.3%
25–29	<6%	12.8%	16.5%	20.3%	24.4%
30–34	<6%	14.5%	18.0%	21.5%	25.2%
35–39	<6%	16.1%	19.4%	22.6%	26.1%
40–44	<6%	17.5%	20.5%	23.6%	26.9%
45–49	<6%	18.6%	21.5%	24.5%	27.6%
50–54	<6%	19.8%	22.7%	25.6%	28.7%
55–59	<6%	20.2%	23.2%	26.2%	29.3%
60+	<6%	20.3%	23.5%	26.7%	29.8%
FEMALES					
Age	**Risky**	**Excellent**	**Good**	**Fair**	**Poor**
19–24	<9%	18.9%	22.1%	25.0%	29.6%
25–29	<9%	18.9%	22.0%	25.4%	29.8%
30–34	<9%	19.7%	22.7%	26.4%	30.5%
35–39	<9%	21.0%	24.0%	27.7%	31.5%
40–44	<9%	22.6%	25.6%	29.3%	32.8%
45–49	<9%	24.3%	27.3%	30.9%	34.1%
50–54	<9%	26.6%	29.7%	33.1%	36.2%
55–59	<9%	27.4%	30.7%	34.0%	37.3%
60+	<9%	27.6%	31.0%	34.4%	38.0%

weight individuals were insensitive to internal signals for hunger and satiety while simultaneously being extremely sensitive to external stimuli (sight, smell, and taste) that can increase the appetite. One source of external stimuli that has clearly been shown to be associated with obesity is watching television.

Watching TV has been demonstrated to be linked to the onset of obesity, and there is a dose-related effect. Increased TV viewing and decreased physical activity are thought to be primary causes of the growing number of obese children in the United States. TV viewing in childhood and adolescence is associated not only with being overweight but also with poor fitness and with obesity, smoking, and raised cholesterol levels in adulthood, indicating that excessive viewing has long-lasting adverse effects on health.[7]

TV viewing also contributes to being overweight in adults. In one study 50,277 women who had a BMI less than 30 completed questions on physical activity. During six years of follow-up, 3,757 (7.5%) became obese (BMI ≥30) and 1,515 new cases of type 2 diabetes occurred. Time spent watching TV was positively associated with risk of obesity and type 2 diabetes. Each two-hour-per-day increment in TV watching was associated with a 23% increase in obesity and a 14%

increase in risk of diabetes. In contrast, each two-hour-per-day increment in sitting at work was associated with a 5% increase in obesity and a 7% increase in diabetes.[8]

Although watching TV fits nicely with the psychological theory (increased sensitivity to external cues), several physiological effects of watching television promote obesity, such as reducing physical activity and the lowering of basal metabolic rate to a level similar to that experienced during trancelike states. These factors clearly support the physiological view.

Physiological Factors

Although the psychological theories primarily propose that obese individuals have a decreased sensitivity to internal cues of hunger and satiation, an emerging theory of obesity states almost the opposite: that obese individuals appear to be extremely sensitive to specific internal cues.[4] Unfortunately, these cues lead to dysfunctional appetite control, thanks to a combination of genetic, dietary, and lifestyle factors. At the center of this dysfunction in many cases is resistance to the hormone insulin, a conditioned response to a high-glycemic diet. The development, progression, and maintenance of obesity form a vicious circle of positive feedback consisting of insulin resistance, abdominal obesity, alterations in the fat cell hormones known as adipokines, loss of appetite control, impaired diet-induced thermogenesis, and low brain serotonin levels. All of these factors are interrelated and support the theory that obesity is primarily an adaptive response that is out of control. Failure to address these underlying areas and provide proper psychological support results in only temporary weight loss at best.

The Set Point

Body weight is closely tied to what is referred to as the "set point"—the weight that a body tries to maintain by regulating the amount of food and calories consumed. Research with animals and humans has found that each person has a programmed set point weight. It has been postulated that individual fat cells control this set point: when the enlarged fat cells in obese individuals become smaller, they either send powerful messages to the brain to eat or block the action of appetite-suppressing compounds.

The existence of this set point helps to explain why most diets do not work. Although the obese individual can fight off the impulse to eat for a time, eventually the signals become too strong to ignore. The result is rebound overeating, with individuals often exceeding their previous weight. In addition, their set point is now set at a higher level, making it even more difficult to lose weight. This has been termed the "ratchet effect" and "yo-yo dieting."

The key to overcoming the fat cells' set point appears to be increasing the sensitivity of the fat cells to insulin. This sensitivity apparently can be improved, and the set point lowered, by exercise, a specially designed diet, and several nutritional supplements (discussed later). The set point theory suggests that a diet that does not improve insulin sensitivity will most likely fail to provide long-term results.

When fat cells, particularly those around the abdomen, become full of fat, they secrete a number of biological products (e.g., resistin, leptin, tumor necrosis factor, and free fatty acids) that dampen the effect of insulin, impair glucose utilization in skeletal muscle, and promote glucose production by the liver. Also important is that as the number and size of fat cells increase, they lead to a reduction in the secretion of compounds that promote insulin action, including adiponectin, a protein produced by fat cells. Not only is adiponectin associated with improved insulin sensitivity, but it also has anti-inflammatory activity, lowers triglycerides, and blocks the development of atherosclerosis. The net effect of all these actions by fat cells is that they severely stress blood sugar control mechanisms, as well as lead to the development of the major complication of diabetes—atherosclerosis. Because of all these newly discovered hormones secreted by fat cells, many experts now consider adipose tissue a member of the endocrine system.[9,10]

Adipokine and Gut-Derived Hormone Alterations

It could be argued that obese individuals are more sensitive to internal signals to eat. Appetite reflects a complex system that has evolved to help humans deal with food shortages. As a result, it is extremely biased toward weight gain. It makes sense that people who survived famines were those who were more adept at storing fat than burning it. So humans have a built-in tendency to overeat, even though in developed countries food is readily available.

To combat the tendency to eat more than is required, it is important to accentuate the normal physiological processes that curb the appetite. An elaborate system exists that is supposed to tell the hypothalamus when the body requires more food, as well as when enough food has been consumed. Many of these strong signals of appetite control actually originate from the gastrointestinal tract. In addition to nerve signals feeding back to the central nervous system, researchers have identified a growing list of gut-derived hormones and peptides that affect appetite, such as PYY, ghrelin, and cholecystokinin.[11,12] While some of these compounds promote feelings of satiety, others cause increased appetite. For example, the stomach-derived hormone ghrelin increases appetite. Ghrelin levels are highest when the stomach is empty and during calorie restriction. Obese individuals tend to have elevated ghrelin levels, and when they try to lose weight, ghrelin levels increase even more. Part of the reason gastric bypass surgery is successful in producing permanent weight loss is thought to be that it significantly reduces ghrelin levels.[13]

Although using various appetite regulators as therapeutic agents in human obesity is possible, preliminary studies seem to indicate that in humans compensatory actions may negate the effect. The perfect drug or natural product to affect appetite must possess an ability to increase insulin sensitivity and produce a targeted effect of reducing factors that increase appetite while simultaneously increasing factors that decrease appetite. Highly viscous dietary fiber seems ideal for this (a good example, PolyGlycopleX, is discussed below).

Diet-Induced Thermogenesis

Another physiological difference between obese and thin people is how much of the food consumed is converted immediately to heat. This process is known as diet-induced thermogenesis. Researchers have found that in lean individuals a meal may stimulate up to a 40% increase in diet-induced thermogenesis. In contrast, overweight individuals often display an increase of only 10% or less.[14] In overweight individuals the food energy is stored instead of being converted to heat as it is in lean individuals.

A major factor for the decreased thermogenesis in overweight people is, once again, insulin insensitivity.[15] Therefore enhancing insulin sensitivity may go a long way toward reestablishing normal thermogenesis, as well as resetting the set point in overweight individuals.

Researchers have also shown that even after weight loss has been achieved, individuals predisposed to obesity still have decreased diet-induced thermogenesis compared with lean individuals.[16] Therefore it is important to continue to support insulin sensitivity and proper metabolism indefinitely if weight loss is to be maintained.

In addition to insulin insensitivity and reduced sympathetic nervous system activity, another factor determines diet-induced thermogenesis—the amount of brown fat. Most fat in the body is white fat: an energy reserve that contains triglycerides stored in a single compartment. Tissue composed of white fat looks white or pale yellow. Brown fat cells contain multiple fat storage compartments. The triglycerides are localized in smaller droplets surrounding numerous mitochondria. An extensive blood vessel network and the density of the mitochondria give the tissue its brown appearance, as well as its increased capacity to metabolize fatty acids.[17]

Brown fat does not metabolize fatty acids to chemical energy as efficiently as other tissues of the body, including white fat. This inefficiency results in increased heat production. Brown fat plays a major role in diet-induced thermogenesis.

Some theories suggest that lean people have a higher ratio of brown fat to white fat than overweight individuals. Evidence supports this theory. The amount of brown fat in modern humans is extremely small (estimates are 0.5 to 5% of total body weight), but because of its profound effect on diet-induced thermogenesis, as little as 1 oz brown fat (0.1% of body weight) could make the difference between maintaining body weight and putting on an extra 10 lb/year.[17]

Lean individuals also tend to respond to excess calories differently from overweight individuals. In one experiment, lean individuals were overfed to increase their weight. In order to maintain the excess weight, they had to increase their caloric intake by 50% over their previous intake.[18] The opposite appears

to be the case in overweight and formerly overweight individuals. They require fewer calories to gain and maintain their weight; in addition, studies have shown that in order to maintain a reduced weight, formerly obese persons must restrict their food intake to approximately 25% less than a lean person of similar weight and body size.[19]

Individuals predisposed to obesity because of decreased diet-induced thermogenesis have been shown to be extremely susceptible to significant weight gain when consuming a high-fat diet, compared with lean individuals.[20] Not only are these individuals more sensitive to the weight-gain-promoting effects of a high-fat diet, but they tend to consume much more dietary fat than lean individuals and exercise less.

The Low Serotonin Theory

A considerable body of evidence demonstrates that levels of serotonin in the brain play a major role in influencing eating behavior. Initial studies showed that when animals and humans are fed diets deficient in tryptophan, appetite is significantly increased, resulting in binge eating of carbohydrates.[21,22] A diet low in tryptophan leads to low brain serotonin levels, a condition the brain interprets as starvation, resulting in the stimulation of the appetite control centers. This stimulation results in a preference for carbohydrates. Feeding animals or humans a carbohydrate meal leads to increased tryptophan delivery to the brain, resulting in the elevated manufacture of serotonin. This scenario has led to the idea that low serotonin levels contribute to carbohydrate cravings and play a major role in the development of obesity.

Furthermore, it has been demonstrated that concentrations of tryptophan in the bloodstream and subsequent brain serotonin levels plummet with dieting.[23] In response to severe drops in serotonin levels, the brain simply puts out such a strong message to eat that it cannot be ignored. This explains why most diets do not work.

Cravings for carbohydrates due to low serotonin levels can be mild or quite severe. They may range in severity from the desire to nibble on a piece of bread or a cookie to uncontrollable binging. At the upper end of the spectrum of carbohydrate addiction is bulimia, a potentially serious eating disorder characterized by binge eating and purging of the food through forced vomiting or the use of laxatives. The medical consequences of bulimia can be quite severe (e.g., rupture of the stomach, erosion of the dental enamel, and heart disturbances due to loss of potassium).

Therapeutic Considerations

Long-term control of obesity is one of the greatest clinical challenges. Few people want to be overweight, and most overweight people express a strong desire to lose weight, yet only 5% of obese individuals can attain and maintain normal body weight for a year or more, while 66% of those just a few pounds or so overweight are able to do the same.

The successful program for obesity is consistent with the basic foundations of good health—a positive mental attitude, a healthful lifestyle (especially important is regular exercise), a health-promoting diet, and supplementary measures. All of these components are interrelated, creating a situation in which no single component is more important than the others. Improvement in one facet may be enough to result in some positive changes, but incorporating all components yields the greatest results.

Literally hundreds of diets and diet programs claim to be the answer to the problem of obesity. Dieters are constantly bombarded with new reports of yet another "wonder" diet. However, the basic calculation for losing weight never changes. In order for an individual to lose weight, energy intake must be less than energy expenditure. This goal can be achieved by decreasing caloric intake or by increasing the rate at which calories are metabolized; the best results are achieved by doing both.

To lose 1 pound, a person must consume 3,500 fewer calories than he or she expends. The loss of 1 lb each week requires a negative caloric balance of 500 calories a day. This can be achieved by decreasing the amount of calories ingested or by increasing exercise. Reducing a person's caloric intake by 500 calories is often difficult, as is increasing metabolism by an additional 500 calories a day through exercise (accomplished by a 45-minute jog, playing tennis for an hour, or a brisk walk for 1.25 hours). The most sensible approach to weight loss is to both decrease caloric intake and increase energy expenditure through exercise.

Most individuals begin to lose weight if they decrease their caloric intake below 1,500 calories a day and exercise for 15 to 20 minutes three to four times per week. Starvation and crash diets usually result in rapid weight loss (largely of muscle and water) but cause rebound weight gain. The most successful approach to long-term, sustainable weight loss is gradual weight reduction (0.5 to 1 lb per week) through adopting long-term dietary and lifestyle habits that promote health and the attainment and maintenance of ideal body weight. Exercise is critical to maintaining muscle mass and bone mineral density and to preventing the accumulation of abdominal fat, both during active weight loss and after weight loss has been achieved.[24,25]

Although many obese individuals may need to lose considerable weight to achieve their long-term goals, it is important to stress that even modest reductions in body weight can produce significant health benefits. For example, a 5 to 10% reduction in weight is accompanied by clinically meaningful improvements in cholesterol, blood pressure, and blood glucose levels.

Behavioral Therapy

Although clinical studies indicate that behavioral approaches to the management of obesity are often successful in achieving clinically significant weight loss, the lost weight is generally regained. The great majority of patients return to their pretreatment weight within three years. In order to provide the best insights on effective interventions, it is important to examine the psychological characteristics of people who have lost significant amounts of weight and experienced only minimal weight regain.[26] Six main behavioral characteristics have been identified in individuals who avoid significant weight regain:

- Maintaining high levels of physical activity (approximately one hour a day)
- Eating a low-calorie, low-fat, low-glycemic diet
- Eating breakfast regularly
- Self-monitoring weight
- Maintaining a consistent eating pattern across weekdays and weekends
- Avoiding depression

These characteristics are intertwined within a whole host of additional factors that provide necessary leverage for successful weight loss. For example, most obese patients who see a doctor about weight loss want to lose 20 to 30% of their body weight. Because most people lose only modest amounts of weight, many quickly lose the motivation and determination to keep the weight off.

However, if people feel a significant boost to self-esteem and self-confidence, as well as have the experience of improving their appearance, feeling more attractive, and being able to wear more fashionable clothing, it can provide tremendous impetus for continued weight loss until goals are achieved.

Remember that the majority of people want to lose weight for the changes in their physical appearance, not the health benefits. Although there is widespread awareness that being overweight is associated with increased health risks, relatively few patients give this as their reason for seeking treatment. Identifying patients' primary goals for losing weight is a key step in helping them achieve success.

Diet

The dietary strategy that we recommend for obesity is the one given in the chapter "A Health-Promoting Diet." The principles and goals detailed there reinforce some of the key goals in achieving weight loss and maintaining ideal body weight. It is important to stress the importance of adequate protein consumption. We recommend 2 g protein daily per kg of body weight unless a person is showing signs of kidney failure.

The importance of higher protein consumption was demonstrated in the Diogenes Study (*Diogenes* is an acronym for "Diet, Obesity, and Genes"). The five-year program involved 29 world-class centers in diet and health studies, epidemiology, dietary genomics, and food technology across Europe. More than 700 overweight adults from eight European countries who had lost at least 8% of their initial body weight with an 800-calorie diet (mean initial weight loss was 24.2 lb) were randomly assigned to one of five diets to prevent weight regain: a low-protein and low-glycemic diet, a low-protein and high-glycemic diet, a high-protein and low-glycemic diet, a high-protein and high-glycemic diet, or a control diet. The participants were to stay on the diet for 26 weeks, and the amount they could eat was not controlled. Fewer participants dropped out in the high-protein/high glycemic and high-protein/low-glycemic groups than in the low-protein/high-glycemic group (26.4% and 25.6%, respectively, vs. 37.4%). Among participants who completed the study, only the low-protein/high-glycemic diet was associated with subsequent significant weight regain (3.7 lbs). The weight regain was 2.0 lb less in the groups assigned to a high-protein diet than in those assigned to a low-protein diet and 2.1 lb less in the groups assigned to a low-glycemic-index diet than in those assigned to a high-glycemic-index diet. The groups did not differ significantly with respect to diet-related adverse events.[27]

Water Consumption

It is well established that water consumption can acutely reduce the amount of calories eaten during a meal, especially among middle-aged and older adults. In the most recent study, 48 adults ages 55 to 75 with a BMI of 25 to 40 were assigned to one of two groups: (1) a low-calorie diet plus 500 ml water prior to each meal (water group), or (2) a low-calorie diet alone (non-water group). Weight loss was about 4.4 lb greater in the water group than in the non-water group, and the water group showed a 44% greater decline in weight over the 12 weeks than the non-water group.[28]

The Atkins Diet

Although hundreds of fad diets have been promoted over the years, we would be remiss if we did not mention the most famous weight loss diet of all time, the Atkins Diet. This high-protein, high-fat, low-carbohydrate diet was developed by Robert Atkins, M.D., dur-ing the 1960s. In the early 1990s Dr. Atkins brought his diet back into the nutrition spotlight with the publication of his best-selling book *Dr. Atkins' New Diet Revolution.* An estimated 50 million people worldwide have tried the Atkins Diet, which emphasizes the consumption of protein and fat. Individuals following the Atkins Diet are permitted to eat unlimited amounts of all meats, poultry, fish, and eggs, plus most cheeses.

The Atkins Diet is divided into four phases: induction, ongoing weight loss, pre-maintenance, and maintenance. During the induction phase (the first 14 days of the diet), carbohydrate intake is limited to no more than 20 g per day. No fruit, bread, grains, starchy vegetables, or dairy products except cheese, cream, and butter are allowed during this phase. During the ongoing weight loss phase, dieters experiment with various levels of carbohydrate consumption until they determine the most liberal level of carbohydrate intake that allows them to continue to lose weight. Dieters are encouraged to maintain this level of carbohydrate intake until their weight loss goals are met. Then, during the pre-maintenance and maintenance phases, dieters determine the level of carbohydrate consumption that allows them to maintain their weight. To prevent regaining weight, dieters must stick to this level of carbohydrate consumption, perhaps for the rest of their lives.

Although we agree with the underlying principle of the Atkins Diet, that diets high in sugar and refined carbohydrates cause weight gain and ultimately lead to obesity, we disagree with several aspects of the solution. One of the big reasons why the Atkins Diet is so attractive to dieters who have tried unsuccessfully to lose weight on low-fat, low-calorie diets is that while on the Atkins Diet, they can eat as many calories as desired from protein and fat, as long as carbohydrate consumption is restricted. As a result, many Atkins dieters are spared the feelings of hunger and deprivation that accompany other weight loss regimens. However, we simply do not agree that such a diet is conducive to long-term health.

Despite its enormous popularity, the Atkins program was not evaluated in a proper clinical trial until 2003. In this initial study, although people following the Atkins Diet did experience initial weight loss (probably as a result of water loss rather than true fat loss), in the long run they gained it all back plus more. In the study, 63 obese men and women were randomly assigned to the Atkins Diet or a low-calorie, high-carbohydrate, low-fat diet. Professional contact was minimal to replicate the approach used by most dieters. Although at 6 months subjects on the Atkins Diet had lost more weight than subjects on the conventional diet, the difference at 12 months was not significant. Adherence was poor, and attrition was high in both groups.[29]

Since this initial clinical evaluation, other studies have shown similar results. For example, in one study of 34 adults with impaired glucose tolerance, 12 weeks of a low-fat (18% of total calories), high-complex-carbohydrate (62% of total calories) diet alone (high-CHO) or paired with an aerobic exercise training program (high-CHO-ex) was compared with the effects of an Atkins-style diet (41% fat, 14% protein, 45% carbohydrate). Fiber intake averaged 58 to 61 g per day in the two high-carbohydrate groups vs. 18.5 g per day in the control group. Participants engaged in aerobic exercise for 45 minutes per day, four days per week, at 80% of peak oxygen consumption in the high-CHO-ex group. All participants were instructed not to limit their food intake. Although caloric intake was similar in all three groups, both high-CHO groups (with and without exercise) lost more weight (mean loss was 10.5 lb with exercise

and 7 lb without exercise) than the control group (mean loss was a fraction of 1 lb). Similarly, a higher percentage of body fat was lost by the high-CHO-ex group (3.5%) and the high-CHO without exercise group (2.2%) than by controls (0.2% increase in body fat). Thigh fat area also decreased significantly in both high-CHO groups but not in the control group. Resting metabolic rate and rate of fat oxidation were not decreased in the high-CHO (or control) groups.[30]

In another study, 132 obese adults (BMI >35), of whom 83% had type 2 diabetes or metabolic syndrome, were counseled to consume either an Atkins-like diet limited to less than 30 g carbohydrates per day or a diet restricted by 500 calories per day with less than 30% of calories from fat. Although the Atkins Diet did promote weight loss during the first 6-month period, this effect began to disappear during the second 6-month period. At 12 months, the difference in average weight loss in the groups was no longer statistically significant (11 lb in the Atkins group vs. 7 lb in the low-fat group), though changes in triglyceride levels favored the Atkins Diet (−57 mg/dl vs. −4 mg/dl), as did HgA1c reductions (−0.7 vs. −0.1%) in the patients with type 2 diabetes.[31]

Another study worth commenting on was funded by the Atkins Foundation. In this study, 120 overweight but otherwise healthy adult subjects with elevated lipid levels followed either the Atkins Diet or a diet containing fewer than 30% calories from fat, 10% or fewer calories from saturated fat, less than 300 mg cholesterol, and a deficit of 500 to 1,000 calories. At 24 weeks, the Atkins group had lost a mean of 26 lb. vs. a mean loss of 14 lb. in the reduced-fat group. Triglyceride levels fell more in the Atkins group (−74 mg/dl) than in the restricted-fat group (−28 mg/dl) as well, and HDL levels increased in the Atkins group (5.5 mg/dl) while they decreased in the low-fat group (–1.6 mg/dl). The main criticism of this dietary study was that the so-called low-fat group received almost 30% of its caloric intake from fat, and the dieticians administering the dietary recommendations made no clear attempt to significantly restrict sugar and refined carbohydrate sources. Thus, the control diet with which the Atkins Diet was compared was significantly less than ideal.[32]

The findings from these clinical trials indicate that while adhering strictly to the Atkins Diet (dramatically reducing carbohydrate intake while allowing free access to high-fat and high-protein foods) can lead to more weight loss in the first six months, eating the diet described in the chapter "A Health-Promoting Diet" is associated with greater efficacy in the long run and is considerably better for health. Although the low-carbohydrate diet was associated with a greater improvement in some risk factors, on the basis of the current evidence we do not recommend the Atkins Diet. Furthermore, since the high protein content of the Atkins Diet stresses the liver and kidneys, we do not recommend it for anyone with impaired liver or kidney function. Our final concern is that on the Atkins Diet there is not much differentiation between high-quality proteins and fats and those of lower quality. For example, a person eating an Atkins-type diet can consume excessive amounts of carcinogens from meats and omega-6 fatty acids from corn-fed animals that can result in silent inflammation (see the chapter "Silent Inflammation" for a more complete discussion).

Natural Weight Loss Aids

Several natural weight loss aids can help to either reduce appetite or enhance metabolism. In decreasing order of efficacy, we rate these items as follows:

- Fiber supplements
- Meal replacement formulas
- Chromium
- 5-hydroxytryptophan (5-HTP)
- Hydroxycitrate
- Medium-chain triglycerides

Fiber Supplements

A tremendous amount of clinical evidence indicates that increasing the amount of dietary fiber promotes weight loss. The best supplemental fiber for weight loss is PolyGlycopleX, or PGX (discussed below), followed by glucomannan, gum karaya, psyllium, chitin, guar gum, and pectin, because they are highly viscous, soluble fibers. When taken with water before meals, these fiber sources bind to the water in the stomach to form a gelatinous mass that induces a sense of satiety. As a result, individuals are less likely to overeat.

The benefits of fiber go well beyond this mechanical effect, however. Fiber supplements have been shown to enhance blood sugar control, decrease insulin levels, and reduce the number of calories absorbed by the body. In some of the clinical studies demonstrating weight loss, fiber supplements were shown to reduce the number of calories absorbed by 30 to 180 per day. Although modest, this reduction in calories would, over the course of a year, result in a 3- to 18-lb weight loss.[33,34]

When choosing a fiber supplement, avoid products that contain a lot of sugar or other sweeteners to camouflage the taste. Be sure to drink adequate amounts of water when taking any fiber supplement, especially if it is in pill form.

Several studies have used guar gum, a soluble fiber obtained from the Indian cluster bean *(Cyamopsis tetragonoloba)*, glucomannan from konjac root *(Amorphophallus konjac)*, and pectin, with good results.[35–40] In one study, nine women weighing between 160 and 242 lb were given 10 g guar gum immediately before lunch and dinner. They were told not to consciously alter their eating habits. After two months, the women reported an average weight loss of 9.4 lb. Reductions were also noted for cholesterol and triglyceride levels.[35]

An important consideration is that the effectiveness of fiber in reducing appetite, blood sugar, and cholesterol is directly proportional to the amount of water the fiber is able to absorb (water holding capacity) and the degree of thickness or viscosity it imparts when in the stomach and intestine. For instance, this ability to bind water and form a viscous mass is why oat bran lowers cholesterol and controls blood sugar better gram for gram than wheat bran.

Although there are many varieties of soluble fiber, PolyGlycopleX (PGX) is a completely novel matrix produced from natural soluble fibers (xantham gum, alginate, and glucomannan). PGX produces a higher level of viscosity, gel-forming properties, and expansion with water than the same quantity of any other fiber alone.[41,42] PGX is able to bind roughly six hundred times its weight in water, resulting in volume and viscosity three to five times greater than those of other highly soluble fibers such as psyllium or oat beta-glucan. To put this in perspective, a 5 g serving of PGX in a meal replacement formula or on its own produces volume and viscosity that would be equal to as much as those produced by four bowls of oat bran. In this way, small quantities of PGX can be added to foods or taken as a drink before meals to have an impact on appetite and blood sugar control equivalent to eating enormous and impractical quantities of any other form of fiber.

Detailed clinical studies published in major medical journals and presented at the world's major diabetes conferences have shown PGX to exert the following benefits:[43-47]

- Reduces appetite and promotes effective weight loss, even in the morbidly obese

- Increases the level of compounds that block the appetite and promote satiety

- Decreases the level of compounds that stimulate overeating

- Reduces postprandial (after-meal) blood glucose levels when added to or taken with foods

- Reduces the glycemic index of any food or beverage

- Increases insulin sensitivity and decreases blood insulin

- Improves diabetes control and dramatically reduces the need for medications or insulin

- Stabilizes blood sugar control in the overweight and obese

- Lowers blood cholesterol and triglycerides

Groundbreaking research by Michael R. Lyon, M.D., has shown that people who are overweight spend much of their day on a virtual "blood sugar roller coaster." Specifically, by using new techniques in two-hour blood sugar monitoring, it has been shown that excessive appetite and food cravings in overweight subjects are directly correlated with rapid fluctuations in blood glucose throughout the day and night. Furthermore, by utilizing PGX these same subjects can dramatically restore their body's ability to tightly control blood sugar levels and that this accomplishment is powerfully linked to remarkable improvements in insulin sensitivity and reductions in calories consumed.

To gain the benefits of PGX it is important to ingest 1.5 to 5 g PGX at major meals, perhaps double that for those with an appetite more difficult to tame. PGX is available in a

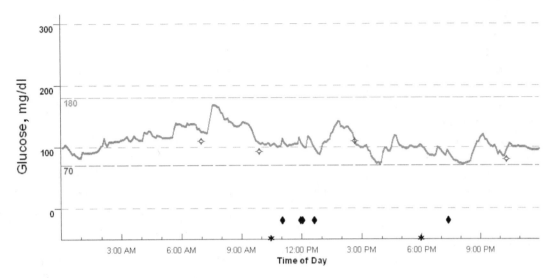

CGMS Graph 1

Uncontrolled and erratic blood sugar levels of an overweight woman over 24 hours with a poor diet and no physical activity.

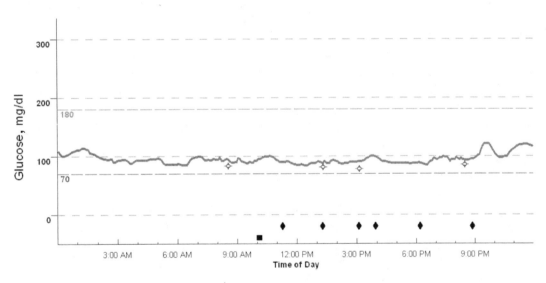

CGMS Graph 2

Controlled and balanced blood sugar levels of the same woman after consuming PGX for six weeks and experiencing a healthy weight loss of 2 lbs. per week.

variety of forms: soft gelatin capsules, a zero-calorie drink mix, granules to be added into food and beverages, and a meal replacement drink mix. The key to effective use of PGX is to take it before every meal with a glass of water. Detailed studies in both humans and animals have shown that PGX is very safe and well tolerated. There are no specific drug interactions, but it is best to take any medication either an hour before or an hour after taking PGX. For more information, see www.PGX.com.

Meal Replacement Formulas

Meal replacement formulas are a popular weight-loss strategy. Their effectiveness has been confirmed in several clinical trials.[48–54] In these studies, dietary compliance and convenience were viewed more favorably by participants who consumed meal replacement (MR) formulas than by those in a conventional weight-loss program. Ideally MR formulations should be of high nutritional quality: high in protein, low in glycemic load, and high in soluble fiber. A protein target of 2.2 g per kg of body weight per day is recommended.

Medifast is a popular physician-supervised weight loss program that relies heavily on MR formulas. In one 40-week randomized, controlled clinical trial that included 90 obese adults with a BMI between 30 and 50, subjects were randomly assigned to one of two weight loss programs for 16 weeks and then followed for a 24-week period of weight maintenance. The dietary intervention was either a meal replacement program (Medifast) or a self-selected food-based meal plan (FB) with an amount of calories equal to the Medifast plan. The Medifast plan included five meal replacement drinks (90–110 calories each), 5–7 oz lean protein, 1½ cups nonstarchy vegetables, and up to two fat servings per day, providing a total of 800–1,000 calories. The meal replacements used in this study were low-fat, low-glycemic, and low-sugar; provided a balanced ratio of carbohydrates to proteins; and were based on either soy and/or whey protein. The food-based plan included 3 oz grains, 1 cup vegetables, 1 cup fruit, 16 fl oz milk, 5–7 oz lean protein, and 3 tsp fat per day, providing a total of about 1,000 calories per day. The FB group was also instructed to take a multivitamin and additional calcium to ensure that micronutrient needs were met while following a low-calorie meal plan. Weight loss at 16 weeks was significantly better in the Medifast group vs. the food-based group: 12.3% of starting weight vs. 6.9%, respectively. Significantly more of the Medifast participants had lost 5% or more of their initial weight at week 16 (93% vs. 55%) and week 40 (62% vs. 30%). Significant improvements in body composition were also observed in Medifast participants compared with FB at week 16 and week 40. At week 40, mean body fat had dropped among the subjects in the Medifast group by 2.9%, whereas the FB group decreased by 1.8%; lean muscle mass as a percentage of total weight was significantly increased by 4.5% from baseline to week 40 in the Medifast group, whereas the FB group did not experience any significant change. Blood pressure also dropped: at week 40, the Medifast group saw a reduction in systolic blood pressure of 6.0 mm Hg (4.5%), and the FB group experienced a drop of 8.3 mm Hg (6.5%). Diastolic blood pressure decreased by 5.5 mm Hg (6.20%) for the Medifast group, compared with 0.9 mm Hg (0.45%) in the FB group.[53]

Chromium

One of the goals for enhancing weight loss is to increase the sensitivity of the cells throughout the body to insulin. Chromium has recently gained a great deal of attention as an aid to weight loss, as it plays a key role in cellular sensitivity to insulin. The importance of this trace mineral in human nutrition was not discovered until 1957, when it was shown that it was essential to proper blood sugar control. Although there is no recommended dietary intake (RDI) for chromium, good health requires a dietary intake of at least 200 mcg per day. Chromium levels can be depleted by refined sugars, white flour products, and lack of exercise.[54]

In some clinical studies of type 2 diabetics, supplementing the diet with chromium has been shown to decrease fasting glucose levels, improve glucose tolerance, lower insulin levels, and decrease total cholesterol and triglyceride levels, while increasing HDL cholesterol levels.[55] Obviously chromium is a critical nutrient in diabetes, but it is also important in hypoglycemia. In one study, eight female patients with hypoglycemia given 200 mg per day for three months demonstrated alleviation of their symptoms.[56] In addition, glucose tolerance test results were improved and the number of insulin receptors on red blood cells was increased.

Chromium supplementation has been demonstrated to lower body weight yet increase lean body mass, presumably as a result of increased insulin sensitivity.[57] In one study, patients were given either a placebo or chromium picolinate in one of two doses (200 mcg or 400 mcg) per day for 2.5 months.[58] Patients taking the 200 and 400 mcg doses of chromium lost an average of 4.2 lb of fat. The group taking the placebo lost only 0.4 lb. Even more impressive was the fact that the chromium groups gained more muscle (1.4 vs. 0.2 lb) than those taking a placebo. The results were most striking in elderly subjects and in men. The men taking chromium picolinate lost more than seven times as much body fat as those taking the placebo (7.7 vs. 1 lb). The 400-mcg dose was more effective than the 200-mcg dose.

The results of these preliminary studies with chromium are encouraging. Particularly interesting is the fact that in these initial studies, chromium picolinate promoted an increase in lean body weight percentage, as it led to fat loss but also to muscle gain.[59] Greater muscle mass means greater fat-burning potential. However, two clinical trials with women involved in an exercise program did not find any significant changes in body composition.[60,61]

All of the effects of chromium appear to be due to increased insulin sensitivity. Several forms of chromium are on the market. Chromium picolinate, chromium polynicotinate, chromium chloride, and chromium-enriched yeast are each touted by their respective suppliers as providing the greatest benefit. No firm evidence indicates that one is a significantly better choice than another.

5-Hydroxytryptophan (5-HTP)

5-HTP is the direct precursor to the brain chemical serotonin. More than three decades ago, researchers demonstrated that administering 5-HTP to rats that were genetically bred to overeat and be obese resulted in a significant reduction in food intake. Further research revealed that these rats have decreased activity of the enzyme tryptophan hydroxylase, which converts tryptophan to 5-HTP, itself subsequently converted to serotonin. In other words, these rats are fat as a result of a genetically determined low level of activity of the enzyme that starts the manufacture of serotonin from tryptophan. These rats don't get the message to stop eating until they have consumed far greater amounts of food than normal rats. Circumstantial evidence indicates that many humans are genetically predisposed to obesity. This predisposition may involve the same mechanism as that in these genetically predisposed rats (i.e., decreased conversion of tryptophan to 5-HTP and, as a result, decreased serotonin levels). When preformed 5-HTP is provided, this genetic defect is bypassed and more serotonin is manufactured.

The early animal studies with 5-HTP as a weight loss aid have been followed by a series of three human clinical studies of overweight women.[62-64] The first study showed that 5-HTP was able to reduce calorie intake and promote weight loss despite the fact that the women made no conscious effort to lose weight.[62] The average amount of weight loss during the 5-week period of 5-HTP supplementation was a little more than 3 lb.

The second study sought to determine if 5-HTP helped overweight individuals adhere to dietary recommendations.[63] The 12-week study was divided into two 6-week periods. For the first 6 weeks there were no dietary recommendations, and for the second 6 weeks the women were placed on a 1,200-calorie diet. The women taking the placebo lost 2.28 lb, while the women taking the 5-HTP lost 10.34 lb.

As in the previous study, 5-HTP appeared to promote weight loss by promoting satiety, leading to consumption of fewer calories at meals. All women taking 5-HTP reported early satiety.

A third study with 5-HTP was similar to the second study: for the first 6 weeks there were no dietary restrictions, and for the second 6 weeks the women were placed on a diet of 1,200 calories per day.[64] The group receiving the 5-HTP lost an average of 4.39 lb after the first 6 weeks and an average of 11.63 lb after 12 weeks. In comparison, the placebo group lost an average of only 0.62 lb after the first 6 weeks and 1.87 lb after 12 weeks. The lack of weight loss during the second 6-week period in the placebo group obviously reflects the fact that the women had difficulty adhering to the diet.

Early satiety was reported by 100% of the subjects taking 5-HTP during the first 6-week period. During the second 6-week period, even with severe caloric restriction, 90% of the women taking 5-HTP reported early satiety. Many of the women receiving the 5-HTP (300 mg three times per day) reported mild nausea during the first 6 weeks of therapy. However, the symptom was never severe enough for any of the women to drop out of the study. No other side effects were reported.

Hydroxycitrate

Hydroxycitrate (HCA) is a natural substance isolated from the fruit of the Malabar tamarind (*Garcinia cambogia*), a yellowish fruit that is about the size of an orange, with a thin skin and deep furrows similar to an acorn squash. It is native to southern India, where it is dried and used extensively in curries. The dried fruit contains about 30% hydroxycitric acid.

HCA has been shown to be a powerful inhibitor of fat formation in animals.[65,66] Whether it demonstrates this effect in humans has not yet been determined. The weight-loss-promoting effects in animals are perhaps best exemplified in a study that shows HCA producing a "significant reduction in food intake, and body weight gain," in rats.[67] Not only may HCA be a powerful inhibitor of fat production; it may also suppress appetite. It is critical in using an HCA formula that a low-fat diet be maintained, as it inhibits only the conversion of carbohydrates into fat.

By itself, HCA may offer a safe, natural aid for weight loss when taken at a dosage of 1,500 mg three times per day. In two clinical trials, a total of 90 moderately obese subjects (ages 21 to 50, BMI greater than 26) were randomly divided into three groups. Group A was administered HCA 4,667 mg; group B was administered a combination of HCA 4,667 mg, niacin-bound chromium 4 mg, and *Gymnema sylvestre* extract 400 mg; and group C was given a placebo. All subjects were provided a 2,000-calorie-per-day diet and participated in a supervised walking program for 30 minutes a day, five days a week. Eighty-two subjects completed the study. At the end of eight weeks, in group A, both body weight and BMI decreased by 5.4%, LDL cholesterol and triglycerides levels were reduced by 12.9% and 6.9% respectively, HDL cholesterol levels increased by 8.9%, and urinary excretion of fat metabolites increased between 32 and 109%. Group B demonstrated similar beneficial changes, but generally to a greater extent. Specifically, group B reduced body weight and BMI by 7.8% and 7.9%, respectively; food intake was reduced by 14.1%; total cholesterol, LDL, and triglyceride levels were reduced by 9.1, 17.9, and 18.1%, respectively, while HDL levels increased by 20.7%; and the excretion of urinary fat metabolites increased between 146 and 281%. No significant adverse effects were observed in either trial.[68]

Medium-Chain Triglycerides
Medium-chain triglycerides (MCTs) are saturated fats (extracted from coconut oil) that range in length from 6 to 12 carbon chains. MCTs are used by the body differently from the long-chain triglycerides (LCTs), which are the most abundant fats found in nature. LCTs, which range in length from 18 to 24 carbon chains, are the storage fats for both humans and plants. This difference in length makes a substantial difference in how MCTs and LCTs are metabolized. Unlike regular fats, MCTs appear to promote weight loss rather than weight gain.

MCTs may promote weight loss by increasing thermogenesis and energy expenditure.[69–73] In contrast, the LCTs are usually stored in the fat deposits, and because their energy is conserved, a high-fat diet tends to decrease the metabolic rate. In one study the thermogenic effect of a high-calorie diet containing 40% fat as MCTs was compared with one containing 40% fat as LCTs. The thermogenic effect (calories wasted six hours after a meal) of the MCTs was almost twice as high as that of the LCTs, 120 calories vs. 66 calories. The researchers concluded that the excess energy provided by fats in the

QUICK REVIEW

- **A successful program for weight loss must be consistent with the four cornerstones of good health—proper diet, adequate exercise, a positive mental attitude, and the right support for the body through natural measures.**

- **Atherosclerosis (hardening of the arteries) is present 10 times more often in obese people compared with those who are not obese.**

- **Obese individuals have a life expectancy that is on average five to seven years shorter than that of normal-weight individuals, with a greater rela-** tive risk for early mortality associated with a greater degree of obesity.

- **As abdominal fat accumulates it leads to alterations in adipokines that ultimately promote insulin resistance and an increased appetite, thereby adding more abdominal fat.**

- **The reason why most Americans are overweight is that they eat too much fat and sugar and do not get enough physical activity.**

- **Television watching has been demonstrated to be linked to the onset of obesity, and there is a dose-related effect:**

- the more TV watched, the greater the degree of obesity.
- Physiological theories of obesity are tied to brain serotonin levels, diet-induced thermogenesis, activity of the sympathetic nervous system, metabolism of fat cells, and sensitivity to the hormone insulin.
- Fiber supplements, especially PGX, have been shown to enhance blood sugar control and insulin effects, as well as reduce the number of calories absorbed by the body.
- 5-hydroxytryptophan reduces the number of calories consumed and promotes weight loss.

- One of the key goals for enhancing weight loss is to increase the sensitivity of cells throughout the body to the hormone insulin.
- Chromium supplementation has been demonstrated to lower body weight yet increase lean body mass, presumably as a result of increased insulin sensitivity.
- Medium-chain triglycerides (MCTs) may promote weight loss by increasing thermogenesis.
- Hydroxycitrate has been shown to be a powerful inhibitor of fat formation in animals.

TREATMENT SUMMARY

A successful program for weight loss must be consistent with the four cornerstones of good health detailed in these chapters:

- "A Positive Mental Attitude"
- "A Health-Promoting Lifestyle"
- "A Health-Promoting Diet"
- "Supplementary Measures"

All of these components are essential and interrelated.

Nutritional Supplements

- Foundational supplements as described in the chapter "Supplementary Measures":
  - PGX: 1.5 to 5 g before meals
  - Chromium: 200 to 400 mcg per day
  - Medium-chain triglycerides (optional): up to 1 to 2 tbsp per day
  - 5-HTP: for the first two weeks, 50 to 100 mg 20 minutes before meals; after two weeks, if weight loss has been less than 1 lb per week, double the dosage, to a maximum of 300 mg (high dosages can cause nausea, but this symptom disappears after six weeks of use)

Botanical Medicines

- Hydroxycitrate (from *G. cambogia*): 1,500 mg three times per day form of medium-chain triglycerides would not be efficiently stored as fat, but rather would be wasted as heat. A follow-up study demonstrated that MCT oil given over a six-day period can increase diet-induced thermogenesis by 50%.[74]

In another study, researchers compared single meals of 400 calories composed entirely of MCTs or LCTs.[75] The thermic effect of MCTs over six hours was three times greater than that of LCTs. In addition, while the LCTs elevated blood fat levels by 68%, MCTs had no effect on the blood fat level. Researchers concluded that substituting MCTs for LCTs would produce weight loss as long as the calorie level remained the same.

In order to gain the benefit from MCTs, a diet must remain low in LCTs. MCTs (or coconut oil) can be used as an oil for salad dressing or as a bread spread, or simply taken as a supplement. A good dosage recommendation for MCTs is 1 to 2 tbsp a day.

SPECIFIC HEALTH PROBLEMS

Acne

- Blackheads: dilated skin follicles with central dark, horny plugs

- Whiteheads: red, swollen follicles with or without white pustules

- Nodules: tender collections of pus deep in the skin that discharge to the surface of the skin

- Cysts: deep nodules that fail to discharge contents to surface

- Large deep pustules: cysts that contain inflammatory compounds that break down adjacent skin tissue, leading to scar formation

Acne is the most common of all skin problems. There are two major forms: acne vulgaris and acne conglobata. *Acne vulgaris* is characterized as a superficial disease that affects the hair follicles and oil-secreting glands of the skin; it is manifested as blackheads, whiteheads, and inflammation (redness). Acne vulgaris is the least severe form of acne. On the other hand, *acne conglobata* is a more severe form, with cyst formation and subsequent scarring. *Rosacea* is a chronic acne-like eruption on the face of middle-aged and older adults, associated with facial flushing (see the chapter "Rosacea"). In both superficial (acne vulgaris) and cystic (acne conglobata) acne, the lesions occur predominantly on the face and, to a lesser extent, on the back, chest, and shoulders.

Causes

Acne has its origin in the skin pore or, to use a more accurate term, the *pilosebaceous unit.* Such units usually consist of a hair follicle and the associated sebaceous glands, which are connected to the skin by the follicular canal through which the hair shaft passes. The *sebaceous glands* produce *sebum,* a mixture of oils and waxes that lubricates the skin and prevents the loss of water. Sebaceous glands are concentrated most highly on the face and to a lesser extent on the back, chest, and shoulders.

Acne is more common among males, and onset is typically at puberty (somewhat later for the cystic form). This occurs because male sex hormones, such as testosterone, stimulate the cells that line the follicular canal to produce *keratin,* a fibrous protein that is the main component of the outermost layer of skin as well as of hair and nails. Overproduction of keratin can block skin pores. In addition, testosterone causes the sebaceous glands to enlarge and produce more sebum. So higher testosterone levels increase the likelihood that pores will become blocked by either excessive keratin or too much sebum. While boys are at greater risk, there is an increase in testosterone level in girls during puberty, making them susceptible as well.

While the onset of acne usually reflects an increase in testosterone level, the severity and progression of acne are determined by a complex interaction among hormonal factors, keratin-producing cells, sebum, and bacteria. Here is the basic scenario: Pimples begin forming near the surface of the skin pore when the cells that line the canal start producing an excess of keratin; this eventually leads to blockage of the canal, resulting in ballooning and thinning. Eventually a whitehead or blackhead is formed. A blackhead will form if the blockage is incomplete, allowing the sebum to make its way to the surface, thereby avoiding the inflammation of a whitehead (discussed below), and a whitehead will form if the blockage is complete.

With the blockage of the canal, a bacterium known as *Propionibacterium acnes* (*Corynebacterium acnes*) can overgrow and release enzymes that break down sebum and promote inflammation. The redness of pimples is a result of this inflammation. If the bacterium grows out of control or if the inflammation is severe, the condition can result in the rupture of the wall of the hair canal and damage to surrounding tissue. If this happens at the skin surface, it simply causes superficial redness and pustules. However, if it occurs deeper within the skin, a nodule or cyst can form, leading to more significant damage and possibly scar formation.

As noted above, male hormones control sebaceous gland secretion and exacerbate the development of abnormal growth of the hair-follicle cells. But excessive secretion of male hormones is not necessarily the cause, since there is only a poor correlation between blood levels of these hormones and the severity of the disease.[1–3] What may be more important is that the skin of patients with acne shows greater activity of an enzyme called 5-alpha-reductase, which converts testosterone to a more potent form known as dihydrotestosterone (DHT).[4,5]

One key factor in acne is genetics. It is inherited in an autosomal dominant pattern. What this means is that if both parents had

acne, three of four children will have acne. If one parent had acne, then one of four children will have acne.[6]

Dietary factors also play a major role in acne, from both a preventive perspective and a therapeutic one, and are discussed below. Another contributor to acne that is seldom recognized is intestinal toxemia. One study showed that 50% of patients with severe acne had increased blood levels of toxins absorbed from the intestines.[7] This situation has not yet been fully evaluated, but it is an interesting finding given that naturopathic physicians in the early 1900s viewed acne as largely a condition reflecting poor colon health.

In 1948, Dr. M. B. Sulzberger stated, "There is no single disease which causes more psychic trauma and more maladjustment between parents and children, more general insecurity and feelings of inferiority and greater sums of psychic assessment than does acne vulgaris." Acne has always been associated with emotional stress and depression, but it is possible that the emotional stress also plays a role in the disease progression. In the 1940s dermatologists John H. Stokes and Donald M. Pillsbury first proposed a gastrointestinal mechanism for the overlap between depression, anxiety, and skin conditions such as acne. These doctors hypothesized that emotional states might alter the normal intestinal microflora, increase intestinal permeability, and contribute to systemic inflammation and increased sebum production. They also noted that as many as 40% of those with acne have hypochlorhydria, and they hypothesized that inadequate stomach acid would set the stage for migration of bacteria from the colon toward the distal portions of the small intestine, as well as an alteration of normal intestinal microflora. The remedies these authors discussed as a means to cut off the stress-induced cycle included administration of *Lactobacillus aci-*

dophilus cultures (long before they were known as probiotics) and also cod liver oil. Many aspects of this gut-brain-skin unifying theory proposed by Stokes and Pillsbury have recently been validated. The ability of the gut microflora and oral probiotics to influence systemic inflammation, oxidative stress, glycemic control, tissue lipid content, and even mood itself, may have important implications in acne.[8] In addition, probiotic supplementation is often indicated, given that a common treatment for acne is antibiotics, which kill off the important healthful bacteria in the intestines.

If a person appears to have acne, it is important to make sure that it truly is acne. Exposure to a variety of compounds can produce the characteristic lesions of acne.

Agents That Cause Acne-like Lesions

Drugs: steroids, diphenylhydantoin, lithium carbonate

Industrial pollutants: machine oils, coal tar derivatives, chlorinated hydrocarbons

Local actions: use of cosmetics or pomades, excessive washing, repetitive rubbing

Therapeutic Considerations

Acne requires an integrated therapeutic approach. Also, because many individuals have undergone long-term treatment with broad-spectrum antibiotics, they often develop in-

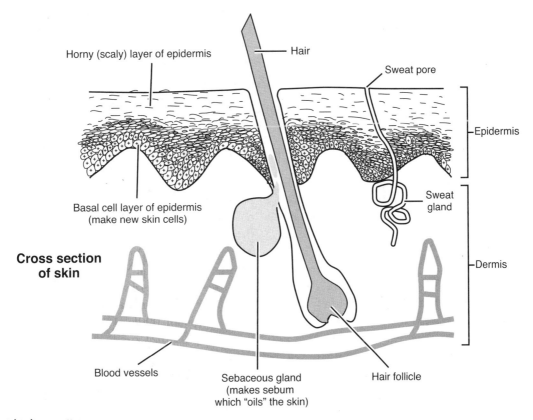

Cross section of skin

Horny (scaly) layer of epidermis

Hair

Sweat pore

Epidermis

Basal cell layer of epidermis (make new skin cells)

Sweat gland

Dermis

Blood vessels

Sebaceous gland (makes sebum which "oils" the skin)

Hair follicle

Pilosebaceous Unit

testinal overgrowth of the yeast *Candida albicans*. This chronic yeast infection may actually make acne worse and must be treated when present. (See the chapter "Candidiasis, Chronic.")

Conventional Therapies

In addition to orally administered antibiotics, another acne treatment is oral isotretinoin (Accutane), a derivative of vitamin A. It is approved only for severe acne and recalcitrant nodular acne. This drug has received a lot of attention regarding its safety. Specifically, reports of intracranial hypertension, depression, and suicidal ideation have prompted an examination of Accutane's life-threatening potential. It is also not to be taken by pregnant women. A warning was added to its product label with regard to signs of depression and suicidal ideation, and a U.S. Food and Drug Administration–mandated registry is now in place for all individuals prescribing, dispensing, or taking isotretinoin, to help decrease the risks associated with isotretinoin therapy.

Another popular treatment for acne is the use of over-the-counter preparations containing benzoyl peroxide (e.g., Oxy 5/Oxy 10, Clearasil, Benoxyl). Benzoyl peroxide acts as a skin antiseptic to keep the growth of bacteria down. It is most effective for superficial pimples that are inflamed. In order to be effective, benzoyl peroxide preparations must be applied on a daily basis. The primary side effect of benzoyl peroxide preparations is a tendency to dry out the skin and/or cause redness and peeling. The prescription topical medicine most often used is tretinoin (Retin-A). Side effects are more common with Retin-A than with benzoyl peroxide. The peeling and drying can be quite severe, as Retin-A improves acne by chemically burning the skin.

Diet

Although there is some controversy about diet in the etiology of acne, there is clear evidence of an association. In westernized societies, acne vulgaris is a nearly universal skin disease, afflicting 79 to 95% of the adolescent population. In men and women older than 25 years, 40 to 54% have some degree of facial acne, and clinical facial acne persists into middle age in 12% of women and 3% of men. In contrast, epidemiological evidence shows that acne incidence rates are considerably lower in non-westernized societies.[9]

A number of dietary factors have been identified. Milk is a significant problem for many acne sufferers. In addition to trans-fatty acids, milk contains hormones, including precursors to DHT, and it promotes an increase in insulin-like growth factor 1 (IGF-1). Receptors for IGF-1 are present on the sebaceous gland. When IGF-1 binds to these receptors it stimulates sebum production. Elimination of all milk and dairy products and high-sugar foods is recommended.[10–13]

For those who are iodine sensitive, foods high in iodine should be eliminated (including foods with a high salt content, as most salt is iodized). Also, foods containing trans-fatty acids (milk and milk products; margarine, shortening, and other synthetically hydrogenated vegetable oils) or oxidized fatty acids (fried food) should be avoided, as these may aggravate acne by increasing inflammation in sebaceous glands.

A diet high in refined carbohydrates is associated with acne. In the early 1940s dermatologists reported that insulin is effective in the treatment of acne, suggesting impaired skin glucose tolerance, insulin insensitivity, or both.[14,15] The insulin was either given systemically (5 to 10 units two to three times a week) or injected directly into the lesion. Interestingly, one study comparing the results of oral glucose tolerance tests in acne patients showed no differences from controls in blood glucose measurements. However, repetitive skin biopsies revealed that the acne patients' skin glucose tolerance was significantly disturbed.[11] One researcher even coined the term *skin diabetes* to describe acne.[16] Acne sufferers generally have a diet higher in glycemic load than that of even the typical American.[17] This is problematic for several reasons, including the influence dietary ratios of carbohydrates, protein, and fat have on the metabolism of testosterone in the skin. Basically, a high-carbohydrate diet increases the conversion of testosterone to the more potent DHT in the skin, which in turn increases sebum production and worsens acne. In contrast, a diet in the range of 45% protein, 35% carbohydrate, and 20% fat produces substantially less DHT formation and enhances the elimination of estrogen, both therapeutic goals.[18]

High-chromium yeast is known to improve glucose tolerance and enhance insulin sensitivity;[19] it has been reported in an uncontrolled study to induce rapid improvement in patients with acne.[20] Other forms of chromium may offer similar benefits.

Nutritional Supplements

Vitamin A (Retinol)

Many studies have demonstrated that oral vitamin A in the retinol form can reduce sebum production and the overproduction of keratin. Retinol has been shown to be effective in treating acne when used at high—and potentially toxic—dosages (i.e., 300,000 to 400,000 IU per day for five to six months).[21] Although dosages of vitamin A below 300,000 IU per day for a few months rarely cause toxic symptoms, we do not recommend this therapy unless it is conducted under the direct supervision of a physician. In fact, we do not recommend dosages

greater than 150,000 even under a physician's supervision. And high dosages of vitamin A should never be ingested by anyone with significant liver disease.

The first significant toxic symptom is usually headache followed by fatigue, emotional volatility, and muscle and joint pain. Laboratory tests appear unreliable for monitoring toxicity, since serum vitamin A levels correlate poorly with toxicity, and liver enzymes are elevated only in symptomatic patients. Of far greater concern is the risk of birth defects caused by high dosages of vitamin A. Women of childbearing age must have at least two negative pregnancy test results prior to the initiation of vitamin A therapy, and they should use effective birth control during treatment and for at least one month after discontinuation. Women who are pregnant or may become pregnant need to limit their daily intake of vitamin A to 3,000 IU, as higher dosages increase the risk for birth defects. The baseline laboratory examination should also include cholesterol and triglyceride assessment, liver enzymes, and a CBC (complete blood count). These tests should be repeated monthly during treatment. Again, we recommend that this therapy be used only under strict physician supervision.

Zinc

Zinc is an important nutrient in the treatment of acne. It is involved in local hormone activation, retinol-binding protein formation, wound healing, immune system activity, and tissue regeneration.

Zinc supplementation in the treatment of acne has been the subject of much controversy and many double-blind studies. Inconsistent results may be due to the differing absorbability of the various zinc salts used. For example, studies using effervescent zinc sulfate show efficacy similar to that of the antibiotic tetracycline, with fewer side effects from chronic use,[22] while those using plain zinc sulfate have shown less beneficial results.[23] The majority of patients required 12 weeks of supplementation before good results were demonstrated, although some patients experienced dramatic improvement immediately.

In another study, 66 patients with inflammatory acne were given zinc gluconate (30 mg elemental zinc) or a placebo for two months.[24] On the basis of the number and severity of lesions, an "inflammatory score" was given to each patient. In the placebo group the inflammatory score dropped from 58 to 47, while in the treatment group the score dropped from 49 to 27. Physicians rated 24 of 32 patients in the zinc group as responders, compared with only 8 of 34 in the placebo group. At least two other double-blind studies with zinc gluconate provide additional support.[25,26] Unfortunately, there have been no studies to date using better-absorbed forms of zinc, such as zinc picolinate, citrate, acetate, or monomethionine.

The importance of zinc to normal skin function is well recognized, especially in light of the zinc deficiency syndrome called acrodermatitis enteropathica. As noted above, zinc is essential for retinol-binding protein and thus for serum retinol levels.[27] Although low levels of zinc increase the formation of DHT, high concentrations significantly inhibit its formation.[28] Interestingly, serum zinc levels are lower in 13- and 14-year-old males than in any other age group.[29]

Vitamin E and Selenium
Serum vitamin A levels in rats on a vitamin-E-deficient diet remain low regardless of the amount of oral or intravenous vitamin A supplementation. Serum levels return to normal after vitamin E is restored to the diet. Vitamin E has been shown to regulate retinol levels in humans.

Male acne patients have significantly decreased levels of the antioxidant enzyme glutathione peroxidase, which normalize with vitamin E and selenium treatment. The acne of both men and women improves with this treatment.[30] This improvement is probably due to inhibition of lipid peroxide formation and suggests that the use of other antioxidants may be valuable.

Topical Treatments

Various topical gels, ointments, and creams containing natural products are available to treat acne. Like benzoyl peroxide, these preparations aim to reduce both the bacteria level and inflammation. Although there are many choices, the most popular natural formulas are those with tea tree oil and azelaic acid.

Tea Tree Oil
Melaleuca alternifolia, or tea tree, is a small tree native to only one area of the world: the northeast coastal region of New South Wales, Australia. The leaves, the portion of the plant that is used medicinally, are the source of tea tree oil.

Tea tree oil possesses significant antiseptic properties and is regarded by many as an ideal skin disinfectant. This claim is supported by its efficacy against a wide range of organisms (including 27 of 32 strains of *P. acnes*),[31] its good penetration, and the fact that usually it does not irritate the skin. The therapeutic uses of tea tree oil are based largely on its antiseptic and antifungal properties.

In a study conducted at the Royal Prince Hospital in New South Wales, a 5% tea tree oil solution demonstrated beneficial effects similar to those of 5% benzoyl peroxide, but with substantially fewer side effects.[32] However, this 5% tea tree oil solution is probably not strong enough for moderate to severe acne. Stronger solutions (up to 15%) should provide even better results. Numerous studies have shown that tea tree oil is extremely safe for use as a topical antiseptic, but it can occasionally produce contact dermatitis.

Azelaic Acid

This naturally occurring nine-carbon dicarboxylic acid, extracted from grains such as wheat and barley, has demonstrated much pharmacological activity, including antibiotic activity against *P. acnes*. Clinical studies with 20% azelaic acid cream have shown it to produce results equal to those achieved with benzoyl peroxide, tretinoin, and oral tetracycline.[33] It has been shown to be effective in all of the different forms of acne. In order to achieve benefits, azelaic acid must be applied to affected areas twice per day for a period of at least four weeks. Treatment usually must be continued for at least six months to maintain the benefits produced after the first month.

One review article found a topical cream containing 20% azelaic acid to be as effective as 5% benzoyl peroxide, 4% hydroquinone cream, 0.05% tretinoin, 2% erythromycin, and 0.5 to 1 g per day oral tetracycline in improving acne vulgaris but less effective than oral isotretinoin at a daily dose of 0.5 to 1 mg/kg in reducing acne conglobata. The authors suggested that the few side effects of topical azelaic acid and lack of overt systemic toxicity offer a clear advantage over conventional drugs.[34]

. . . .

QUICK REVIEW

- **Acne is the most common skin problem.**
- **Acne is dependent upon male hormones, especially testosterone, that stimulate the manufacture of sebum.**
- **Acne is most common among males during puberty, due to hormonal changes.**
- **Long-term use of antibiotics may result in an overgrowth of the yeast *Candida albicans* in the intestines.**
- **The key dietary recommendation is to avoid sugar, trans-fatty acids, milk, fried foods, and iodine.**
- **Nutrients to aid in the treatment of acne include chromium, vitamin A, vitamin E, selenium, and zinc.**
- **Topical treatment with tea tree oil or azelaic acid has produced results equal to benzoyl peroxide without the side effects.**

. . . .

TREATMENT SUMMARY

Acne is a multifactorial disease requiring an integrated therapeutic approach in order to avoid supplement toxicity while attaining the desired clinical results. Patients should be checked for treatable causes and underlying hormonal abnormalities before specific therapies are initiated.

Diet

The recommendations given in the chapter "A Health-Promoting Diet" should be the foundation of treatment. In addition, eliminate all refined and concentrated carbohydrates and limit consumption of high-fat and high-carbohydrate foods. Avoid fried foods, iodine, and foods containing trans-fatty acids. Keep the intake of milk and other dairy products low.

Nutritional Supplements

- A high-potency multiple vitamin and mineral formula as described in the chapter "Supplementary Measures"
- Key individual nutrients:
  - Vitamin A: 150,000 IU per day for three months under a physician's supervision (women who are pregnant or who may become pregnant should not take more than 3,000 IU per day)
  - Vitamin C: 1,000 mg per day
  - Zinc: 50 mg per day (picolinate is best)
  - Selenium: 200 mcg per day
  - Chromium: 200 to 400 mcg per day
  - Vitamin D_3: 2,000 to 4,000 IU per day (ideally, measure blood levels and adjust dosage accordingly)
- Fish oils: 3,000 mg EPA + DHA per day
- One of the following:
  - Grape seed extract (>95% procyanidolic oligomers): 100 to 300 mg per day
  - Pine bark extract (>95% procyanidolic oligomers): 100 to 300 mg per day
  - Some other flavonoid-rich extract with a similar flavonoid content, super greens formula, or another plant-based antioxidant that can provide an oxygen radical absorption capacity (ORAC) of 3,000 to 6,000 units or higher per day
- Probiotic (active lactobacillus and bifidobacteria cultures): a minimum of 5 billion to 10 billion colony-forming units per day

Physical Medicine

- Exposure to sun or ultraviolet lamp
- Fruit acid peels
- Light therapy (blue and red light), intense pulsed light, laser, photodynamic therapy, fractionated light (for acne scars)

Topical Treatments

- Thorough daily cleansing
- Application of one of the following:
  - Tea tree oil, 5% to 15% preparation
  - Azelaic acid, 20% preparation

Acquired Immunodeficiency Syndrome (AIDS) and HIV Infection

- Positive test for the human immunodeficiency virus (HIV)

- Primary risk factors: sexual contact with an HIV-infected person, intravenous drug user sharing needles, being born to a mother who has HIV

- Onset may vary:
  - May present with sudden onset (duration of up to 14 days) of fevers, sweats, malaise, fatigue, joint and muscle pain, headaches, sore throat, diarrhea, generalized swelling of lymph glands, rash on the trunk
  - May present insidiously, as unexplained progressive fatigue, weight loss, fever, diarrhea, and generalized swelling of the lymph glands
  - May present first as an opportunistic infection such as thrush (oral candidiasis) or *Pneumocystis carinii* pneumonia

- Advanced stages will show neurological changes including dementia and loss of nerve function (partial paralysis, vertigo, visual disturbances, etc.)

Acquired immunodeficiency syndrome (AIDS) is characterized by a profound defect in immune functions. The primary cause of AIDS is infection with the human immunodeficiency virus (HIV). The spectrum of HIV infection ranges from a person with a positive test for HIV without any signs of immune deficiency to the person with full-blown AIDS characterized by all of the now classic components of the disease. The HIV virus does not kill; what it does is cripple the immune system to such an extent that a person dies from severe infection or cancer. AIDS is now viewed as a late stage of HIV infection.

HIV is diagnosed when an individual has a positive blood test for HIV antigen and antibodies. AIDS is diagnosed when certain criteria are met, such as the presence of one of the 23 opportunistic infections (infections caused by normally non-infectious organisms) and cancers linked to AIDS, or a positive HIV test plus a CD4 count (a count of important white blood cells, also called T helper cells) of less than $200/\mu l$ or a ratio of T helper cells to total lymphocytes (CD4/CD8 count) of less than 14%. The current average time from becoming infected with HIV to the development of AIDS is 10 years.[1]

Estimates today are that more than 1 million Americans are infected with HIV and a little under 200,000 meet the requirements to be diagnosed as having AIDS. In the

253

United States, African-Americans make up 10% of the population but about half of the HIV/AIDS cases nationwide. There are also geographic disparities in AIDS prevalence in the United States: it is most common in rural areas and in the southern states, particularly in the Appalachian and Mississippi Delta regions and along the border with Mexico. HIV infection is more prevalent in these populations due to a lack of information about AIDS and to people's perception that they are not vulnerable, as well as to limited access to health care resources and a higher likelihood of sexual contact with at-risk male sexual partners.[1]

Globally, more than 30 million people are infected with HIV. Sub-Saharan Africa remains by far the worst affected region. In 2007 it accounted for an estimated 68% of all people living with AIDS and 76% of all AIDS deaths, with 1.7 million new infections bringing the number of people there living with HIV to 22.5 million; there are also 11.4 million AIDS orphans living in the region. Adult prevalence in 2007 was an estimated 5.0%, and AIDS continued to be the single largest cause of mortality in this region.[1]

AVOID CONTRACTING HIV

While this chapter focuses on treatment for HIV infection and AIDS, those who are not HIV-positive should take the following steps in order to avoid contracting the virus:

- Do not have sexual intercourse with people who are known to have or are suspected of having HIV or who use intravenous drugs.
- Practice safe sex.
- Do not share a toothbrush, a razor, or any other implement that could become contaminated with blood from someone with an HIV infection.
- Do not share needles with others.

HIV

The human immunodeficiency virus (HIV) is now regarded as the primary causative agent in AIDS by virtually every expert in the field. Our perspective is that nutritional status, lifestyle, and mental/emotional state play significant roles in the progression of HIV to AIDS, as does the susceptibility to infection in the first place.

Classified as a retrovirus, HIV has the ability to insert its RNA into human DNA through the activity of an enzyme called reverse transcriptase. When the cell is activated, the inserted DNA produces new viruses. The cells most affected by this process are the T4 inducer/helper subset of lymphocytes. HIV is highly selective for and easily isolated from these white blood cells, but it is also found in other white blood cells. It actively replicates in these cells, especially when they are activated to mount a response to an infection. This infection-replication process renders the T cells nonfunctional, eventually destroying them and dramatically reducing their number, thus contributing to the profound disruption of the immune system.

Therapeutic Considerations

Conventional medical management of HIV/AIDS is continually changing but basically revolves around two treatment principles: (1) inactivate or slow the replication of HIV, and (2) provide antibiotics to patients with abnormally low CD4 counts. Progress was made in the treatment of AIDS in 1996 with the use of highly active anti-retroviral therapy (HAART). The five main classes of HAART that are currently being used in the care of HIV-positive patients in various combinations are:

1. Nucleoside and nucleotide reverse transcriptase inhibitors (NRTIs, or "nukes")

2. Non–nucleoside reverse transcriptase inhibitors (NNRTIs, or "non-nukes")

3. Protease inhibitors (PIs)

4. Entry inhibitors (including fusion inhibitors and CCR5 inhibitors)

5. Integrase inhibitors

The use of these drugs appears to be very much appropriate in HIV-positive patients with CD4 counts less than 500. More controversial is the use of these drugs in HIV-positive patients showing no signs of immune deficiency. Our current recommendation for HIV-positive individuals is to monitor immune function by having CD4 counts every six months as long as levels stay above 500 and every three months if levels drop below 500. There are also specialized tests to measure viral load and activity (such as p24 antigen levels, PCR-based HIV-RNA levels) that can be used as monitors.

In short, at this time we recommend conventional therapies for all individuals with CD4 counts below 500. That isn't to say that natural measures should be abandoned at this point. Quite the contrary—with HIV infection, it is absolutely vital to employ aggressive natural measures that promote good health and immune function from the very start, and certainly when AIDS develops. It is important to remember that the HIV virus does not kill. It is the opportunistic infections allowed by a suppressed immune system that set into motion an accelerating downward spiral that ultimately results in death.

The basic therapeutic goals from a natural perspective are to optimize nutrition and enhance immune function. Studies indicate that more than 70% of HIV-positive persons are using some form of complementary or alternative medicine in their treatment, resulting in improvement in quality of life and better outcomes. Our goal is to provide some guidance in navigating the best course.

Nutrition and HIV/AIDS

The immune system requires a constant supply of nutrients to function properly. Unfortunately, in this regard the AIDS patient has many obstacles to overcome, chief among them gastrointestinal tract infection and the wasting (muscle breakdown) promoted by the progressing infection. It is easier to institute nutritional therapies early on instead of after AIDS has developed.

There is a very strong association between nutritional status, immune function, and the progression from HIV to AIDS.[2–4] It is

Relationship of CD4 Count to Development of Opportunistic Infection			
600	**400 TO 600**	**100 TO 400**	**LESS THAN 100**
No opportunistic infections	Bacterial infections	Pneumocytosis	Cytomegalovirus retinitis
	Tuberculosis	Toxoplasmosis	Brain lymphoma
	Herpes simplex	Cryptococcosis	Severe infection of any body tissue is possible
	Herpes zoster	Histoplasmosis	
	Vaginal candidiasis	Cryposporidiosis	
	Hairy leukoplakia		
	Kaposi's sarcoma		

vitally important to supply optimal levels of all nutrients. There is considerable debate over what is optimal for the general population, but there is a growing consensus that HIV/AIDS patients require higher levels of virtually all known nutrients. While recommendations here are in line with those in the chapter "Supplementary Measures," aggressive supplementation is necessary. Supplementation with multiple vitamin and mineral formulas has shown significant value in improving immune status and delaying progression to AIDS in HIV-positive patients.[5–8]

The HIV-positive individual should consume a diet that promotes health, as defined in the chapter "A Health-Promoting Diet." The diet should be rich in whole, natural foods, such as fruits, vegetables, grains, beans, seeds, and nuts, and should be low in fats and refined sugars; it is important to consume adequate but not excessive amounts of protein. On top of this, individuals are encouraged to drink five or six 8-fl-oz glasses of water per day. These dietary recommendations, along with a positive mental attitude, a good high-potency multivitamin-mineral supplement, a regular exercise program, daily deep breathing and relaxation exercises (meditation, prayer, etc.), and at least seven to eight hours of sleep per day will go a long way in helping the immune system function at an optimal level—a critical goal in HIV/AIDS.[9–12]

HIV-positive patients commonly require digestive support and may require the use of digestive enzymes to combat the adverse effects of HIV, HAART, and prophylactic antibiotics on the GI system.[13,14] For information on the use of digestive enzymes, see the chapter "Digestion and Elimination." HIV-positive patients should avoid high-sodium foods, high-fructose corn syrup in processed foods, alcohol, caffeine, and fried foods as well as raw eggs, unpasteurized milk, un-

dercooked meat or fish, and any potentially contaminated food.

Diarrhea is a common complaint and an issue that can greatly affect quality of life. There are many reasons an HIV-positive person might develop diarrhea, and the specific cause guides the choice of treatment. Since there is an increased incidence of gluten intolerance in HIV-positive individuals, all sources of gluten should be eliminated in any HIV-positive patient with diarrhea (see the chapter "Celiac Disease" for more information).[15] Lactose intolerance often develops in cases of chronic diarrhea, and so all milk and dairy products containing lactose should also be eliminated. The recommendations given in the chapter "Diarrhea" are appropriate in most cases, especially the use of probiotics.[16,17]

In addition to these basic recommendations, the person with HIV/AIDS has higher protein requirements. While the typical person does quite well with 0.8 g protein per kg of body weight, the individual with HIV/AIDS requires at least 1.5 g per kg.[18] Supplementing the diet with whey protein, which is high in the amino acid glutamine, appears particularly useful in AIDS because of its possible ability to address the wasting syndrome of AIDS as well as its ability to heal the gastrointestinal tract and increase the level of the important antioxidant glutathione within body cells.[19,20]

Wasting syndrome (severe breakdown of body tissues) is a common complication of HIV infection and is marked by progressive weight loss and weakness, often associated with fever and diarrhea. The mechanisms responsible for this syndrome are not well defined, but it is clear that this is a multifactorial process. Contributors to wasting syndrome include inadequate dietary protein intake, malabsorption, increased metabolism, and increased levels of inflammatory com-

PROTEIN FOR AIDS PATIENTS

In order to assess the quality of a protein, scientists measure the proportion of the amino acids that are absorbed, retained, and used in the body. These determine the protein's *biological value*. The protein with the highest biological value is found in whey, a natural by-product of the cheese-making process. Cow's milk has about 6.25% protein. Of that protein, 80% is casein (another type of protein), and the remaining 20% is whey protein. Cheese making uses the casein molecules, leaving whey. Whey protein is collected by filtering off the other components of whey, such as lactose, fats, and minerals.

Whey protein is a complete protein, in that it contains all essential and nonessential amino acids. One of the reasons the biological value of whey protein is so high is that it has the highest concentrations of glutamine and branched-chain amino acids found in nature; these substances are critical to cellular health, muscle growth, and protein synthesis.

Although the most popular use of whey protein is by bodybuilders and athletes looking to increase their protein intake, whey protein can also be used to support recovery from surgery, to offset some of the negative effects of radiation therapy and chemotherapy, and to help prevent wasting syndrome seen in both cancer and AIDS.

The protein found in eggs is a close second to whey protein.

Biological Value of Selected Protein Sources	
PROTEIN SOURCE	**BIOLOGICAL VALUE**
Whey (ion exchange, microfiltered)	100
Whole egg	93.7
Milk	84.5
Fish	76.0
Beef	74.3
Soybeans	72.8

pounds, known as cytokines, secreted by the immune system (e.g., tumor necrosis factor, interleukins, and alpha-interferon). These cytokines stimulate the breakdown of fat and muscle.

Nutritional Supplements

While general broad-spectrum nutritional support is required, including a high-potency multiple vitamin and mineral formula, there are several nutrients that deserve special attention.

- Vitamin A (15,000–30,000 IU taken with food) slows progression to AIDS and decreases mortality, improves growth in infants and decreases stunting associated with chronic diarrhea, and prevents GI deterioration in mothers and infants.[21,22]

- Beta-carotene (60–120 mg [150,000 IU] taken with food) increased CD4+ count, CD4/CD8 ratios, and total lymphocyte count; it also decreased mortality.[23] Deficiency found in all HIV+ patients is likely to be due to poor digestion, decreased free radical elimination, and high lipid peroxidation.[24]

- Folic acid (400 mcg) is important to offset the toxicity of the drug AZT on red blood cell formation.[25,26]

- Thiamine (vitamin B_1, 50 mg) supplementation is associated with increased survival in HIV+ patients and decreased progression to AIDS.[27–29]

- Vitamin B_6 (50 mg) is essential in nucleic acid and protein metabolism and cellular and humeral immune responses.[30,31] B_6 supplementation both alone and in conjunction with CoQ_{10} increased circulating IgG, CD4+ cells, and CD4/CD8 ratios.[32]

- Vitamin B_{12} (1,000 mcg per day) can improve lymphocyte counts, CD4/CD8 ratios, and NK cell activity.[33] Supplementation has also been found to reverse AIDS dementia complex when that condition is associated with low levels of the vitamin.[34] Deficiency has been associated with increased risk of progression to AIDS.[35–37]

- Vitamin C (500 to 1,000 mg three times per day) has been shown in test tube studies to exert some beneficial effects against HIV replication. Other studies have shown that HIV-positive people with the highest levels of vitamin C intake had the slowest progression to AIDS.[4,38]

- Vitamin E (400 to 800 IU per day as mixed tocopherols) also slows down the progression of HIV to AIDS.[39–42] Men with the highest levels of vitamin E in their blood showed a 34% decrease in risk of progression to AIDS compared with those with the lowest levels. Deficiency is found in most HIV+ patients, with wasting, and in progression to AIDS.[43]

- Vitamin D deficiency is commonly found in urban HIV-infected men with suppressed viral load and a CD4 count over 200; tobacco use was correlated with severe deficiency.[44] Undetectable levels of vitamin D in HIV-positive patients correlated with more advanced HIV infection, lower CD4 count, and higher levels of inflammation.[45] Recommended dosage is 5,000 IU.

- Copper (2 mg) can inhibit HIV protease and viral replication.[46] Deficiencies of copper are associated with AZT therapy and AIDS.[47,48]

- Magnesium deficiency is found in AIDS patients.[49,50] Recommended dosage is 300 mg.

- Selenium (400 mcg) suppresses the progression of HIV, reduces viral burden, and provides indirect improvement of CD4 count.[51] Selenium supplementation has been shown to decrease HIV-associated mortality, reduce the number of hospitalizations, and lower the costs of caring for HIV-positive patients.[52–54] Deficiency in patients progressing to AIDS may be due to decreased caloric and protein intake, malabsorption, and various infections.[55]

- Zinc (15–30 mg) has been found to decrease frequency of infections.[56,57] Zinc deficiency is very common in HIV+ patients progressing to AIDS.[58]

Antioxidants

Numerous studies have shown that individuals infected with HIV have a compromised antioxidant defense system.[59] Furthermore, HAART is associated with oxidative damage to cellular components, including mitochondria.[60] Blood levels of antioxidants are decreased in HIV-positive patients, and peroxidation products of lipids (fats) and proteins are increased. This blood profile may contribute to the progression of AIDS, because antioxidants such as glutathione prevent viral replication, while reactive oxidants tend to stimulate the virus. Consequently, it has been suggested that HIV-infected patients may benefit from antioxidant supplementation therapy. Antioxidant therapy, especially vitamin E and selenium, does in fact appear to slow down the progression from HIV to AIDS as well as offset the free radical damage caused by HAART.[39–42,51,61]

One of the more controversial antioxidants in HIV infection is N-acetylcysteine (NAC). It was proposed that NAC may act as an effective antioxidant and raise tissue glutathione levels in AIDS patients at dosages of 2 to 8 g per day.[62–64] However, supplementation at a dosage of 1.8 g NAC failed to increase glutathione in white blood cells in patients with AIDS.[65] Nonetheless, NAC inhibits HIV replication. Better options to raise glutathione levels may be vitamin E, beta-carotene, vitamin C, selenium, and alpha-lipoic acid.

Alpha-lipoic acid (also known as thioctic acid) is a sulfur-containing vitamin-like substance that plays an important role as the necessary cofactor in two vital energy-producing reactions involved in the production of cellular energy. Alpha-lipoic acid is not considered a vitamin because it is thought that either the body can usually manufacture sufficient levels or the nutrient can be acquired in sufficient quantities from food. However, as with many of the other compounds described in this section, a relative deficiency can occur in certain situations, and alpha-lipoic acid supplementation provides benefits beyond its role in normal metabolism. Alpha-lipoic acid is an effective antioxidant, unique in that it is effective against both water-soluble and fat-soluble free radicals.

Based on alpha-lipoic acid's antioxidant effects as well as its ability to significantly inhibit the replication of HIV by reducing the activity of reverse transcriptase, it was suggested that it might be of value in HIV-positive patients.[66,67] To test this hypothesis, a small pilot study was designed to determine the short-term effect of alpha-lipoic acid supplementation (150 mg three times per day) in HIV-positive patients.[68] Alpha-lipoic acid supplementation increased plasma ascorbate in 9 of 10 patients, total glutathione in 7 of 7 patients, total plasma sulfur groups in 8 of 9 patients, and T helper lymphocytes and T helper/suppressor cell ratio in 6 of 10 patients, while the lipid peroxidation product malondialdehyde decreased in 8 of 9 patients. The results of this pilot study indicated that alpha-lipoic acid supplementation led to significant beneficial changes in the blood of HIV-infected patients. Perhaps the most significant of these effects was the increase in the glutathione content, since the level of glutathione is directly linked to preventing the progression to AIDS. Alpha-lipoic acid (600 mg) protected the liver, inhibited viral replication, increased intracellular glutathione, and increased CD4/CD8 ratios; it has the potential to decrease peripheral neuropathy pain because of its antioxidant effect on nervous tissue.

Coenzyme Q_{10} also seems to be an important consideration. CoQ_{10} levels are often deficient in HIV-positive patients, leading to impaired energy production. Supplementation with CoQ_{10} increases circulating antibodies, helper T cells, and CD4/CD8 ratios in normal subjects and may produce similar effects in HIV-positive patients.[69,70]

Carnitine

Several reports indicate that systemic carnitine deficiency may be a problem in patients with AIDS. Reduced levels of carnitine are often found in the blood and blood cells in AIDS patients. Increasing the carnitine content of the white blood cells has been shown to strongly improve their function, a finding that highlights the importance of carnitine to the immune system.[71]

Carnitine has also been shown to prevent the toxicity of the drug AZT on muscle cells. AZT poisons the mitochondria of the muscle, leading to abnormal energy production within the muscle, which manifests itself clinically as muscle fatigue and pain. Because L-carnitine is able to prevent this negative effect of AZT and similar drugs, it is critically important in these patients.[72–74]

Clinical studies indicate that carnitine supplementation can improve immune function. When AIDS patients being treated with AZT were given 6 g L-carnitine per day, it led to significant increased white blood cell proliferation and reduced circulating tumor necrosis factor—a known trigger of HIV replication.[75] Supplementation has also been shown to be effective for the painful peripheral nerve pain common to HIV-positive patients.[76]

Botanical Medicines

There are many different herbs and herbal components that are showing great promise as antiviral agents active against HIV. In our opinion, the three that are presented here offer the most promise.

Milk Thistle

Milk thistle (*Silybum marianum*) extract (silymarin) is strongly indicated for all patients on HAART to improve liver function, decrease liver damage, and increase antioxidant activity of blood cells. Even HIV-positive individuals not on HAART may benefit from the liver support provided by milk thistle. For more information see the chapter "Hepatitis."

Curcumin from Turmeric

HIV infection and progression to AIDS are associated with activation of a latent virus. This activation is governed by the long terminal repeat (LTR) sequence in the viral DNA. The virus remains in an inactive form until the LTR tells it to replicate. Whether or not LTR signals the latent provirus to become active is determined by a complex interaction of positive and negative regulators that bind to specific sites within the LTR. It is thought that if the stimuli that activate LTR can be reduced while, simultaneously, compounds that block activation of LTR are used, the progression of HIV infection or AIDS could be halted or at least delayed.

In March 1993, researchers at Harvard Medical School published results of a study showing that curcumin inhibits the replica-

tion of HIV by blocking LTR expression.[77] Curcumin is the yellow pigment and active ingredient of the spice turmeric (*Curcuma longa*), an important ingredient in curry. The research may have been performed as a follow-up to a population study in Trinidad. About 40% of Trinidad's population is of Indian descent and these Trinidadians use curry extensively in their diet. Another 40% of the population is of African descent; these people rarely use curry. Population studies in Trinidad indicated that people of African descent were more than 10 times as likely to have HIV as people of Indian descent. Whether this was due to dietary factors or culturally determined sexual behaviors remains to be shown; however, given the recent antiviral studies with curcumin, a strong case could be made for the former.

In another study, curcumin was shown to inhibit HIV integrase, the enzyme that integrates a double-stranded DNA copy of the RNA genome, synthesized by reverse transcriptase, into a host chromosome.[78,79] Curcumin has also been shown to inhibit other factors that stimulate HIV to replicate, such as tumor necrosis factor (TNF) and NF-kappa B.[80-82] TNF, a chemical mediator of inflammation, is part of the immune system's inflammatory response, which, when working properly, is used to kill disease-causing organisms. TNF production, however, triggers the production of NF-kappa B, a chemical messenger that plays a critical role in initiating HIV replication.

In addition, curcumin is a powerful antioxidant showing activity as much as 300 times greater than that of vitamin E. Preliminary studies of its effect on HIV/AIDS are encouraging. For example, in a controlled clinical study, a group of 18 HIV-positive patients with CD4 counts ranging from 5 to 615 took an average of 2,000 mg curcumin per day.[83] This regimen resulted in an increase in CD4 counts compared with control treatment. Unfortunately, with the development of HAART, the interest in curcumin as an anti-HIV agent has waned. The only other clinical study of curcumin evaluated its effect in eight patients with HIV-associated diarrhea, who were given an average daily dose of 2,000 mg curcumin and followed for an average of 41 weeks.[84] All had resolution of diarrhea and normalization of stool quality, usually within two weeks. The average number of bowel movements per day dropped from 7 to 1.7. Seven of eight patients also had considerable weight gain on curcumin (10.8 lb). Five of six patients had resolution of bloating and abdominal pain. Patients on anti-retroviral therapy experienced no discernible drug interactions, changes in CD4 count, or changes in HIV viral load while taking curcumin.

The curcumin content of turmeric is about 1%. To reach an effective dosage (1.2 to 2 g per day) of curcumin, a person would need to consume 100 to 200 g (roughly 3 to 6 oz) of turmeric. For this reason, pure curcumin preparations are preferred to turmeric when medicinal effects are desired. Although the benefit of curcumin in HIV and AIDS remains to be proved, given the safety of curcumin along with its possible benefit, supplemental curcumin makes sense.

One concern regarding curcumin has been absorption, but there now exist a number of methods and products that enhance the absorption of curcumin. One of those methods is complexing the curcumin with soy phospholipids, as in the product Meriva. Absorption studies in animals indicate that peak plasma levels of curcumin after administration of Meriva were five times higher than those after administration of regular curcumin.[85] Studies with another advanced form of curcumin, Theracurmin, show even greater absorption.[86]

Turmeric can be consumed liberally in the diet, but since curcumin is so poorly absorbed, Meriva at a dosage of 1,000–1,200 mg per day or Theracurmin at a dosage of 300 mg per day may produce significantly better clinical results.

Licorice

The primary active components of licorice (*Glycyrrhiza glabra*) root are glycyrrhizin and its backbone structure glycyrrhetinic acid (glycyrrhizin minus a small sugar molecule). These are showing promise in the treatment of AIDS as well as chronic hepatitis (see the chapter "Hepatitis"). Although much of the research has featured intravenous administration, this route of administration may not be necessary, as glycyrrhizin and glycyrrhetinic acid are easily absorbed orally and well tolerated.

The benefit of oral administration is most evident in a recent double-blind study on the clinical effectiveness of glycyrrhizin by long-term oral administration to 16 hemophiliac patients who were HIV-positive.[87] The patients received daily doses of 150 to 225 mg glycyrrhizin for three to seven years. Helper T cell and total T cell numbers, other immune system indicators, and glycyrrhizin and glycyrrhetinic acid levels in the blood were monitored. The results indicated that orally administered glycyrrhizin was converted into glycyrrhetinic acid without producing any side effects. None of the patients given the glycyrrhizin suffered progression to AIDS or deterioration of immune function. In contrast, in the group not receiving glycyrrhetinic acid showed decreases in helper and total T cell counts and antibody levels. Two of the 16 patients in the control group developed AIDS.

Glycyrrhizin in HIV-positive and AIDS patients produces almost immediate improvement in immune function. In one study, nine symptom-free HIV-positive patients received

200 to 800 mg glycyrrhizin intravenously per day. After eight weeks, the groups had increased CD4 count, improved CD4/CD8 ratio, and improved liver function. In another study, six AIDS patients received 400 to 1,600 mg glycyrrhizin intravenously per day. After 30 days, five of the six showed a reduction or disappearance of the P24 antigen (an indicator of viral load and severity of active disease).[88]

In a more recent study, high-dose glycyrrhizin (Stronger Neo-Minophagen C, SNMC) was shown to prevent the liver damage produced by HAART in four hemophiliacs infected with both HIV and hepatitis C. Two of the patients had previously had to discontinue HAART because of the liver damage. After SNMC administration, these patients were able to resume HAART.[89]

The results of these studies and others with HIV-positive and AIDS patients are encouraging. The big concern is that licorice root at a dosage of more than 3 g per day or glycyrrhizin at more than 100 mg per day for more than six weeks may cause sodium and water retention, leading to high blood pressure. Monitoring of blood pressure and increasing dietary potassium intake are suggested.

Exercise

Regular exercise has been demonstrated to provide benefit to individuals with immunodeficiency diseases, particularly through stress alleviation and mood enhancement. HIV-positive individuals had increases in CD4, CD8, and natural killer (NK) cells immediately following aerobic exercise, and long-term exercise has demonstrated increases in other immune indicators.[90,91] HIV-positive individuals practicing tai chi demonstrated greater overall perception of health and significant improvements in several measures of physical function when compared with controls.[92] Other patients practicing yoga reported increased self-confidence and quicker return to athletic activities after medical interventions.[93]

. . . .

QUICK REVIEW

- **Acquired immunodeficiency syndrome (AIDS) is characterized by a profound defect in cell-mediated immunity.**
- **The HIV virus does not kill; what it does is cripple the immune system to such an extent that a person dies from severe infection or cancer.**
- **Nutritional status, lifestyle, and mental/emotional state play significant roles in the progression of HIV to AIDS.**
- **At this time we recommend that conventional therapies be used for all individuals with CD4 counts below 500.**

- **There is a very strong association between nutritional status, immune function, and the progression from HIV to AIDS.**
- **Optimal levels of all nutrients are vitally important in patients with HIV/AIDS.**
- **Supplementation with multiple vitamin and mineral formulas has shown significant value in improving immune status and delaying progression to AIDS in HIV-positive patients.**
- **Supplementing the diet with whey protein appears particularly useful in AIDS**

because of its possible ability to address the wasting syndrome of AIDS as well as its ability to heal the gastrointestinal tract and increase the level of the important antioxidant glutathione within body cells.

- Numerous studies have shown that individuals infected with HIV have a compromised antioxidant defense system.

- Antioxidant therapy, especially vitamin E and selenium, does in fact appear to slow down the progression from HIV to AIDS as well as offset the free radical damage caused by HAART.

- Alpha-lipoic acid is demonstrating extremely encouraging results in HIV patients.

- Clinical studies indicate that carnitine supplementation can improve immune function and reduce the level of HIV-induced immune suppression.

- Milk thistle extract (silymarin) is strongly indicated for all patients on HAART to improve liver function, decrease liver damage, and increase antioxidant activity of blood cells.

- Curcumin exhibits potent anti-HIV activity and is showing promise in clinical trials.

- Licorice components have shown tremendous benefits in clinical studies.

- HIV-positive individuals had increases in CD4, CD8, and natural killer cells immediately following aerobic exercise, and long-term exercise has demonstrated increases in other immune indicators.

· ·

TREATMENT SUMMARY

The goal of treatment for HIV-positive individuals is to slow down the progression of HIV to AIDS. That goal is accomplished by optimizing nutritional status, following a health-promoting lifestyle, and employing measures to enhance immune function. In the treatment of AIDS the goal shifts to supporting the conventional therapies available at this time. It is particularly important to maintain high nutritional and antioxidant status.

Lifestyle

- Perform a relaxation exercise (deep breathing, meditation, prayer, visualization, etc.) for 10 to 15 minutes each day.

- Get regular exercise (non-strenuous walking, tai chi, stretching, etc.).

Diet

- Follow the dietary recommendations in the chapter "A Health-Promoting Diet."

- Consume adequate amounts of protein; consider supplementation with a high-quality whey protein at a dosage of 1 g/kg.

- Eliminate alcohol, caffeine, and sugar.
- Drink at least 48 fl oz water per day.

Nutritional Supplements

- A high-potency multiple vitamin and mineral formula as described in the chapter "Supplementary Measures"
- Key individual nutrients:
  - Vitamin C: 500 to 1,00 mg three times per day
  - Vitamin E: 400 to 800 IU per day
  - Vitamin D: 5,000 IU per day (ideally, measure blood levels and adjust dosage accordingly)
  - Carotene complex: 50,000 to 100,000 IU per day
  - Methylcobalamin (active form of vitamin B_{12}): 1,000 mcg per day
- Flaxseed oil: 1 tbsp per day
- Fish oils: 3,000 mg EPA + DHA per day
- One of the following:
  - Grape seed extract (>95% procyanidolic oligomers): 100 to 300 mg per day
  - Pine bark extract (>95% procyanidolic oligomers): 100 to 300 mg per day
  - Some other flavonoid-rich extract with a similar flavonoid content, super greens formula, or another plant-based antioxidant that can provide an oxygen radical absorption capacity (ORAC) of 3,000 to 6,000 units or higher per day
- Probiotic (active lactobacillus and bifidobacteria cultures): a minimum of 5 billion to 10 billion colony-forming units per day

- Specialty nutrients:
  - Alpha-lipoic acid: 150 mg three times per day.
  - Carnitine: 2,000 mg one to three times per day

Botanical Medicines

- Milk thistle (*Silybum marianum*):
  - The standard dose of milk thistle is based on its silymarin content. For this reason, standardized extracts are preferred. The best results are achieved at higher dosages, i.e., 140 mg to 210 mg silymarin three times per day. The dosage for silymarin phytosome is 120 mg two to three times per day between meals.
- Curcumin, one of the following:
  - Curcumin: 600–800 mg three times per day with meals
  - Meriva: 1,000 to 1,200 mg per day
  - Theracurmin: 300 mg per day
- Licorice root (*Glycyrrhiza glabra*), one of the following:
  - Powdered root: 1 to 2 g three times per day
  - Fluid extract (1:1): 2 to 4 ml three times per day
  - Solid (dry powdered) extract (10% glycyrrhetinic acid content): 250 to 500 mg three times per day
  - *Note:* If licorice is to be used over a long period of time, increase the intake of potassium-rich foods.

Alcohol Dependence

- Psychological/social signs of excessive alcohol consumption: depression, loss of friends, arrest for driving while intoxicated, drinking before breakfast, frequent accidents, unexplained work absences
- Alcohol dependence as manifested when alcohol is withdrawn: delirium tremens, convulsions, hallucinations
- Alcoholic binges, benders (48 hours or more of continuous drinking associated with failure to meet usual obligations), or blackouts
- Physical signs of excessive alcohol consumption: alcohol odor on breath, flushed face, tremor, unexplained bruises

Alcohol dependence—or, as it was formerly known, alcoholism or alcohol-use disorder—is a disabling addictive disorder characterized by alcohol consumption that exceeds acceptable cultural limits or injures health or social relationships. Estimates are that in the United States, 12.5% of the population will have a problem with alcohol dependence at some point during their lifetime, while 3.8% have had a problem with alcohol dependence in the last twelve months.[1]

Alcohol dependence is significantly more prevalent among men, whites, Native Americans, younger adults, unmarried adults, and those with lower incomes. Alcohol dependence is one of the most serious health problems facing society today.[1] The total number of Americans affected, either directly or indirectly, is much greater when one consid-ers disruption of family life, automobile accidents, crime, decreased productivity, and mental and physical illness. With more than 100,000 deaths annually attributed to alcohol misuse, alcohol-related problems are a considerable cause of mortality.[2]

Consequences of Alcoholism
Increased mortality

- 10-year decrease in life expectancy
- Double the usual death rate in men, triple in women
- Six times greater suicide rate
- Major factor in the four leading causes of death in men between the ages of 25 and 44: accidents, homicides, suicides, cirrhosis

Health effects

- Metabolic damage to every cell
- Intoxication
- Abstinence and withdrawal syndromes
- Nutritional diseases
- Brain degeneration
- Psychiatric disorders
- Esophagitis, gastritis, ulcer
- Increased cancer of mouth, pharynx, larynx, esophagus
- Pancreatitis
- Liver fatty degeneration and cirrhosis
- Heart disease

265

- Hypertension
- Angina
- Hypoglycemia
- Decreased protein synthesis
- Increased serum and liver triglycerides
- Decreased serum testosterone
- Muscle wasting
- Osteoporosis
- Acne rosacea
- Psoriasis
- Fetal alcohol syndrome

Causes

The cause of alcohol dependence remains obscure. It represents a multifactorial condition with genetic, physiological, psychological, and social factors, all of which seem to be equally important. Serious drinking often starts in younger people: approximately 35% of alcoholics develop their first symptoms between 15 and 19 years of age, and more than 80% develop their first symptoms before age 30.[3]

Although alcohol dependence is most common in men, the incidence has been increasing in women: the female-to-male ratio for alcohol dependence has tapered to 1:2.[1,2] Women generally seem to develop disease at a lower quantity of intake than men do. This may be partially due to women's lower body weight and may also be related to increased gut permeability to endotoxins.[4]

Research indicates that genetic factors may be most important.[5] The finding of a genetic marker for alcohol dependence could result in the diagnosis of the disease in its initial and most reversible stage. Some case-control studies suggest that non-gender-based gene polymorphisms encoding cytokines and other immune modulators may play a role in the predisposition to alcohol dependence. The gene patterns associated with risk reveal that antibody-mediated mechanisms could play a role in disease pathogenesis.[4] The genetic basis of alcohol dependence has also been supported by the following:

- Genealogical studies show that alcohol dependence is a family condition.
- The biological children of alcoholics who have been raised by adoptive parents demonstrate a continued higher risk of alcohol dependence.
- Twin studies show differences in alcohol dependence rates between identical and fraternal twins.
- Alcohol dependence has an association with genetic markers for color vision, non-secretor ABH, HLA-B13, and low platelet monoamine oxidase (MAO).
- Biochemical studies show the importance of alcohol dehydrogenase polymorphism in racial susceptibility to alcohol dependence.[5]

Although a biological marker would be useful, it may not be ultimately necessary, as an individual's family history can suggest when it may be helpful to implement a relatively innocuous primary prevention program.

Signs of Alcohol Intoxication

The signs of alcoholic intoxication are typical of a central nervous system depressant: drowsiness, errors of commission, disinhibition, and disturbed body movements. In cases of alcohol dependence, withdrawal symptoms usually occur one to three days after the last drink. They typically range from anxiety and tremors to mental confusion, increased sensitivy to sensory stimulation, visual hallucinations, excessive sweating, dehydration, electrolyte disturbances, seizures, and cardiovascular abnormalities.

Metabolic Effects of Alcohol and Alcohol Dependence

Alcohol Metabolism

The primary metabolic processes that regulate the rate of alcohol breakdown in normal individuals are:[6]

- The rate of alcohol absorption from the intestines

- The concentration and activity of the liver enzymes alcohol dehydrogenase (ADH) and aldehyde dehydrogenase (ALDH)

- The ratio of active niacin to inactive niacin within liver cells.

It is generally accepted that the availability and regeneration of active niacin are the dominant factors affecting the rate at which alcohol is broken down.[7] Alcohol is converted to acetaldehyde by the liver enzyme ADH, with active niacin as a necessary cofactor. Acetaldehyde is believed to be responsible both for many of the harmful effects of alcohol consumption and for the addictive process itself. Normally acetaldehyde is converted by another liver enzyme (ALDH) to either energy or long-chain fatty acids.[6] But higher than normal blood aldehyde levels have been found in alcoholics and their relatives after alcohol consumption, suggesting either increased ADH activity or depressed ALDH activity in people susceptible to alcohol dependence.[7]

Fatty Liver

All active alcoholics display fatty infiltration of the liver, with the severity roughly proportional to the duration and degree of alcohol abuse. Even moderate doses of alcohol may produce both acute and chronic fatty liver infiltrates. The development of fatty liver is due to the following:[6,8]

- Increased fatty acid manufacture stimulated by alcohol

- Diminished triglyceride utilization

- Impaired ability to carry fatty acids away from the liver

- Direct damage to cell structures by free radicals produced by alcohol metabolism

- The high-fat diet of the alcoholic (as is typical of the average American diet)

Leptin is a peptide hormone involved in the regulation of appetite and energy metabolism. It is most likely directly related to liver pathology in alcoholics. High levels of leptin are known to contribute to fatty infiltration of the liver and other types of liver damage.[9] Research has demonstrated increased circulating leptin levels in a dose-dependent manner in chronic alcohol dependence, regardless of nutritional status.[10]

Hypoglycemia

Alcohol consumption often results in reactive hypoglycemia, in which a rapid increase in blood glucose levels is followed by a subsequent drop. The drop in blood glucose produces a craving for food, particularly foods that quickly elevate blood glucose, such as sugar and more alcohol. Increased sugar consumption aggravates the reactive hypoglycemia, particularly in the presence of alcohol. Hypoglycemia aggravates the mental and emotional problems of the alcoholic, producing such symptoms as sweating, tremor, anxiety, hunger, dizziness, headache, visual disturbance, decreased mental acuity, confusion, and depression.

Therapeutic Considerations

Nutrition is a primary focus in alcohol dependence. Although many of the nutritional problems of alcoholics relate directly to the effects of alcohol, a major contributing factor is that alcoholics tend not to eat, instead substituting alcohol for food. As a result, the alcoholic has to deal not only with nutritional deficiencies caused by excessive alcohol consumption but also with deficiencies due to inadequate intake.

Zinc

One of the key nutrients involved in the metabolic detoxification of alcohol is zinc, as both ADH and ALDH are zinc-dependent enzymes, with the latter being more sensitive to deficiency.[11] Both acute and chronic alcohol consumption result in zinc deficiency.[11,12] Several factors contribute to the development of zinc deficiency in alcoholics:

• Decreased dietary intake
• Decreased absorption
• Increased urinary excretion

Low serum zinc levels are associated with impaired alcohol metabolism, a predisposition to cirrhosis, impaired testicular function, and other complications of alcohol abuse.[11,13] Zinc supplementation, particularly when combined with ascorbic acid, greatly increases alcohol detoxification and survival in rats.[14]

Vitamin A

Vitamin A deficiency is also common in alcoholics and appears to work synergistically with zinc deficiency to produce the major complications of alcohol dependence.[8,13] The mechanism has been hypothesized as follows: reduced intestinal absorption of zinc and vitamin A (alcohol damages the intestines), in conjunction with impaired liver function (reduced extraction of zinc, mobilization of retinol binding protein [RBP], and storage of vitamin A), results in reduced blood levels of zinc, vitamin A, RBP, and transport proteins, as well as a shift to nonprotein ligands. These conditions cause the tissues to have reduced concentrations of zinc and vitamin A, abnormal enzyme activities and glycoprotein synthesis, and impaired DNA/RNA metabolism; they also cause the kidneys to increasingly lose zinc. These metabolic abnormalities then lead to the common disorders of alcohol dependence:

• Night blindness
• Skin disorders
• Cirrhosis of the liver
• Slow skin healing
• Decreased testicular function
• Impaired immune function

Vitamin A supplementation inhibits alcohol consumption in female rats (though this effect is inhibited by testosterone administration and removal of the ovaries).[15,16]

Vitamin A supplementation in the alcoholic has improved night blindness and sexual function.[8] However, great care must be employed in recommending vitamin A supplementation, as a liver damaged by excessive alcohol consumption significantly loses its ability to store vitamin A. As a result, the alcoholic is at great risk for developing vitamin A toxicity when the vitamin is supplemented at dosages above 5,000 IU per day.

Antioxidants

Alcohol consumption increases the formation of damaged fats (lipid peroxides) in both the liver and the blood. Matters are made even worse by the fact that alcoholics are typically deficient in key antioxidant nutrients, particularly vitamin E, selenium, and vitamin C, that protect against lipid peroxide formation.[17,18] There is a significant link between serum lipid peroxide levels and liver damage, as shown by an elevation of the liver enzyme serum glutamate oxaloacetate transaminase (SGOT) in the blood.[19] Antioxidant administration, either before or simultaneously with alcohol intake, inhibits lipoperoxide formation and prevents fatty infiltration of the liver.[20] Effective antioxidants include vitamins C and E, zinc, selenium, and cysteine (in the form of N-acetylcysteine or whey protein powder).

Carnitine

The usual nutritional compounds that support liver function, such as choline, niacin, and cysteine, appear to have little value in improving liver function in the alcoholic.[21,22] In contrast, carnitine significantly inhibits alcohol-induced fatty liver disease. It has been suggested that chronic alcohol consumption results in either a reduced manufacture of carnitine or an increased need.[23,24] Carnitine is normally manufactured in sufficient quantities by the body. It serves a critical role in the transport of fatty acids into the mitochondria, the energy-producing structures of the cells. Supplemental carnitine improves liver function in alcoholics; it also reduces serum triglycerides and SGOT levels while elevating HDL cholesterol.[24]

Amino Acids

Blood levels of the various amino acids (building blocks of protein molecules) are imbalanced in alcoholics.[25-27] Since the liver is the primary site for amino acid metabolism, it is not surprising that alcoholics develop abnormal amino acid patterns. Correction of this disturbance greatly aids the alcoholic, especially when there are signs or symptoms of cirrhosis or depression.[28] Although there are some characteristic amino acid abnormalities in alcoholics, an individual approach is indicated to address differences in nutritional status, biochemistry, and the amount of liver damage. Correction of the imbalances probably requires seeing a nutritionally oriented physician for proper analysis and treatment. That said, the branched-chain amino acids—valine, isoleucine, and leucine—can be of significant benefit for an alcoholic with cirrhosis.[28]

One of the typical findings in alcoholics is a very low level of tryptophan, the amino acid that is converted to serotonin. Low serotonin levels are a hallmark feature of depression. The recommendations in the chapter "Depression" are definitely appropriate to aid in recovery, especially using 5-hydroxytryptophan (5-HTP) to raise brain serotonin levels.

When there is severe alcohol-induced liver damage, the liver will be unable to convert the amino acid methionine to S-adenosylmethionine (SAM-e), a valuable compound in normal physiology. Supplementation with SAM-e is required.[29]

For the alcoholic with severe liver damage, it may be necessary to lighten the load on the liver by temporarily eating a low-protein diet and supplementing the diet with free-form amino acids according to the recommendations of a physician.

Vitamin C

Vitamin C deficiency is common in alcohol-related disease—in one study, a deficiency of vitamin C was found in 91% of patients.[30] Supplemental vitamin C helped ameliorate the effects of acute and chronic alcohol toxicity in experimental studies involving humans and guinea pigs, two species unable to synthesize their own vitamin C.[14,31] There is a direct correlation between levels of vitamin C in leukocytes (a good index of the body's actual vitamin C status), the rate of alcohol clearance from the blood, and the activity of the liver enzymes responsible for clearing alcohol.[13] In other words, the higher the vitamin C, the better able the liver is able to clear alcohol.

Selenium

Blood selenium levels are lower in patients with alcohol dependence.[18] Low selenium status contributes to depressed mood, whereas high dietary or supplementary selenium has been shown to improve mood.[32] Research has consistently reported that low selenium status is associated with a significantly increased incidence of depression, anxiety, confusion, and hostility.[18] Furthermore, when alcohol dependence and depression occur together in an individual, there is an increased risk for suicide.[33] Given the frequency of low selenium status in alcoholics and the relationship between selenium levels and depression, selenium supplementation is warranted.

B Vitamins

Alcoholics are classically deficient in most of the B vitamins.[1,8,30] These deficiencies result from various mechanisms:

- Low dietary intake
- Deactivation of the active form

- Impaired conversion to the active form
- Impaired absorption
- Decreased storage capacity

Alcohol diminishes thiamine (vitamin B_1) absorption in the intestine and reduces liver thiamine storage. It also decreases the formation of thiamine into its most active form, and this effect may also contribute to the development of functional thiamine deficiency.[34] A thiamine deficiency is both the most common (55% in one study)[30] and the most serious of the B vitamin deficiencies, since a deficiency causes the clinical conditions beriberi and Wernicke-Korsakoff syndrome. In addition, evidence indicates that a thiamine deficiency results in greater intake of alcohol, suggesting that thiamine deficiency is a predisposing factor for alcohol dependence.[35] It should be noted that once present, Wernicke-Korsakoff syndrome is unresponsive to oral doses of thiamine, so rapid replacement of depleted brain thiamine levels by repeated intravenous therapy is required.[36]

A functional vitamin B_6 (pyridoxine) deficiency is also common in alcoholics, due not so much to inadequate intake as to impaired conversion to its active form, pyridoxal-5-phosphate, and enhanced degradation.[37] In addition to inhibiting conversion to more active forms, alcohol decreases the absorption and utilization by the liver and increases the urinary excretion of many B vitamins, especially folic acid.[38]

Magnesium

Magnesium deficiency is very common in alcoholics. In fact, one study found deficiency in as many as 60% of alcoholics and a strong link to delirium tremens (a state of confusion and trembling during alcohol withdrawal).[39] It is thought to be the major reason for the increased cardiovascular disease noted in alcoholics. This deficiency is due primarily to a reduced magnesium intake coupled with alcohol-induced excessive excretion of magnesium by the kidneys, which continues during withdrawal despite low serum magnesium levels. Alcoholic cardiomyopathy, often associated with thiamine deficiency, may instead be due to a magnesium deficiency.

Essential Fatty Acids

Alcohol has been shown to interfere with essential fatty acid (EFA) metabolism and may produce symptoms of essential fatty acid deficiency if consumed in excess.[40] In a five-year study, alcohol-consuming rhesus monkeys developed alcoholic amblyopia, a rare neurological disorder characterized by blurred vision, diminished retinal function, and a significant reduction in visual acuity; biopsies showed that the omega-3 fatty acid DHA level in the monkeys' brains and retinas had decreased significantly compared with that in controls.[41] Given the importance of long-chain fatty acids to brain function, it may be useful to supplement EPA + DHA in alcoholics.

Glutamine

Supplementation of the amino acid glutamine (1 g per day) has been shown to reduce voluntary alcohol consumption in uncontrolled human studies and experimental animal studies.[42-44] Although this research occurred more than 50 years ago, there has never been any follow-up to these preliminary studies. This is unfortunate, as the results were promising and showed the supplement to be safe and relatively inexpensive.

Psychosocial Aspects

Psychological and social measures are critical in the treatment of alcohol dependence, as it can be a chronic, progressive, and potentially fatal disease.[1] Social support for both the alcoholic and his or her family is important, and treatment success is often proportional to the involvement of Alcoholics Anonymous (AA), counselors, and other social agencies. Because most physicians have not had adequate training or experience in handling the psychosocial aspects of this problem, it is important to establish a close working relationship with an experienced counselor and AA. Al-Anon and Ala-Teen are useful resources for family members. Successful initiation of treatment requires the following:

- The alcoholic's agreement that he or she has an alcohol problem
- Education about the physical and psychosocial effects of alcohol dependence
- Immediate involvement in a treatment program

Successful programs (such as AA) usually include strict control of drinking, strongly supported by family, friends, and peers. Although strict abstinence may not be absolutely necessary, at this time it appears the safest and most effective choice.[1]

Depression

Depression is common in alcoholics and is known to lead to their high suicide rate. In some cases depressed individuals become alcoholic (primary depressives), while others become alcoholic first and later develop a depressive condition in the context of their alcohol dependence (secondary depressives). Alterations in the metabolism of brain chemicals such as serotonin and the availability of its precursor, tryptophan, have been implicated in some forms of depression, while other forms have been linked to alterations in catecholamine metabolism and tyrosine availability.

As mentioned above, alcoholics have severely depleted levels of tryptophan, which may explain both the depression and the sleep disturbances common in alcohol dependence, since brain serotonin levels depend on circulating tryptophan levels.[45] Alcohol impairs tryptophan transport into the brain and increases the enzyme that breaks down tryptophan.[25] In one study, five of six chronic alcoholics had no detectable plasma tryptophan on withdrawal.[26] The tryptophan levels returned to normal after six days of treatment and abstinence.

Another factor influencing tryptophan uptake into the brain is competition from amino acids that share the same transport mechanism, especially tyrosine and phenylalanine, which are elevated in malnourished alcoholics. Alcoholics have significantly depressed ratios of tryptophan to these amino acids when compared with normal controls, with depressed alcoholics having the lowest ratios.[26,46]

Following the recommendations in the chapter "Depression" is definitely appropriate to aid in recovery, especially using 5-hydroxytryptophan (5-HTP) to raise brain serotonin levels.

Intestinal Flora

The intestinal microflora is severely deranged in alcoholics.[47] Colonization of the small intestine by bacteria that produce endotoxins may lead to malabsorption of fats, carbohydrates, protein, folic acid, and vitamin B_{12}. This mechanism is probably the cause of the abnormalities of the small intestine commonly found in alcoholics. Alcohol ingestion also increases intestinal permeability to endotoxins and large particles that can activate the immune system adversely.[48]

Exercise

The involvement of the alcoholic patient in an individually tailored fitness program has been shown to improve the likelihood of maintaining abstinence.[49] Research has shown that regular exercise is effective in alleviating anxiety and depression and enables individuals to respond better to stress. Improved fitness may allow more effective responses to emotional upset, thereby reducing the likelihood of resorting to alcohol when the patient is involved in conflict.

Botanical Medicines

Kudzu

Kudzu (*Pueraria lobata*) was one of the earliest medicinal plants used in traditional Chinese medicine. It has many profound pharmacological actions, including helping prevent alcohol abuse.[50] Two of its isoflavones, daidzin and daidzein, account for this effect.[51] These compounds are also found in soy foods. Rodent studies have been impressive, but in human studies the results have been mixed. In one study, kudzu treatment resulted in significant reduction in the number of beers consumed: the time to consume each beer increased, with the number of sips increasing and the volume of each sip decreasing.[52] However, in a double-blind trial, kudzu root extract (1.2 g twice per day) produced no statistically significance difference in craving and sobriety scores compared with the placebo group.[53] It may be that kudzu reduces alcohol intake without significantly affecting cravings.

Milk Thistle

The flavonoid complex of milk thistle (*Silybum marianum*, or silymarin) appears to be useful for the alcoholic, especially when there is considerable liver involvement or cirrhosis. Silymarin has been shown to be effective in the treatment of the full spectrum of alcohol-related liver disease, from relatively mild to serious cirrhosis. Perhaps the most significant benefit is extending the life span of these patients. In one study 87 cirrhotics (46 with alcoholic cirrhosis) received silymarin, while 83 cirrhotics (45 with alcoholic cirrhosis) received a placebo.[54] The average observation period was 41 months. In the silymarin group, there were 24 deaths with 18 related to liver disease, while in the control group there were 37 deaths with 31 related to liver disease. The four-year survival rate was 58% in the silymarin group, compared with 39% in the controls.

Silymarin can also improve immune function in patients with cirrhosis.[55] Whether this effect is involved in the liver protective action or a result of improved liver function has yet to be determined.

QUICK REVIEW

- **Genetic factors play a big role in the development of alcohol dependence.**
- **All active alcoholics display signs of injury to the liver.**
- **Hypoglycemia aggravates the mental and emotional problems of the alcoholic.**
- **Zinc is one of the key nutrients involved in the breakdown of alcohol.**
- **Vitamin A deficiency is also common in alcoholics and appears to work together with zinc deficiency to produce the major complications of alcohol dependence.**
- **Antioxidants taken either prior to or along with alcohol inhibit free radical damage and the development of a fatty liver.**
- **Carnitine inhibits alcohol-induced fatty liver.**
- **There is a direct link between the level of vitamin C in white blood cells and the rate of clearance of alcohol from the blood.**
- **Thiamine (vitamin B_1) deficiency is both the most common and the most serious of the B vitamin deficiencies in the alcoholic.**
- **Low magnesium levels are present in as many as 60% of alcoholics and are linked to delirium tremens.**
- **Glutamine supplementation (1 g per day) has been shown to reduce voluntary alcohol consumption in uncontrolled human studies.**
- **Kudzu, an ancient Chinese herbal medicine, has shown good results in reducing alcohol consumption in human studies.**

TREATMENT SUMMARY

Alcohol dependence is a difficult condition to treat. Although many therapeutic regimens have been attempted, there has been little documented long-term success,

except for Alcoholics Anonymous (and even the overall success of this program is highly controversial). All alcoholics, at whatever stage, benefit the most from simultaneous counseling, lifestyle, and nutrition-oriented approaches.

Lifestyle

Follow the recommendations given in the chapter "A Health-Promoting Lifestyle," as well as those in the chapter "Stress Management." It is especially important to:

- Identify stressors
- Eliminate or reduce sources of stress
- Identify negative coping patterns and replace them with positive patterns
- Perform a relaxation/breathing exercise for a minimum of five minutes twice per day
- Manage time effectively
- Enhance your relationships through better communication
- Get regular exercise

Diet

Stabilization of blood sugar levels is critical to successful treatment. The recommendations given in the chapter "A Health-Promoting Diet" should serve as the foundation for the dietary treatment of alcohol dependence. Key dietary recommendations include elimination of all simple sugars (foods containing added sucrose, fructose, or glucose; fruit juice; dried fruit; and low-fiber fruits such as grapes and citrus fruits); limitation of processed carbohydrates (white flour, instant potatoes, white rice); and an increase in complex carbohydrates (whole grains, vegetables, beans).

Nutritional Supplements

- A high-potency multiple vitamin and mineral formula as described in the chapter "Supplementary Measures"
- Key individual nutrients:
  - Vitamin A: 2,500 to 5,000 IU per day (use beta-carotene if suffering from liver impairment)
  - Vitamin B complex: 20 times the RDI
  - Vitamin C: 1 g two times per day
  - Vitamin E: 100 to 200 IU per day
  - Magnesium (citrate or aspartate): 250 mg two times per day
  - Selenium: 200 mcg per day
  - Zinc: 30 mg per day
- Fish oils: 3,000 mg EPA + DHA per day
- One of the following:
  - Grape seed extract (>95% procyanidolic oligomers): 100 to 300 mg per day
  - Pine bark extract (>95% procyanidolic oligomers): 100 to 300 mg per day
  - Some other flavonoid-rich extract with a similar flavonoid content, super greens formula, or another plant-based antioxidant that can provide an oxygen radical absorption capacity (ORAC) of 3,000 to 6,000 units or higher per day
- Specialty supplements:
  - Probiotic (active lactobacillus and bifidobacteria cultures): a minimum of 5 billion to 10 billion colony-forming units per day

- ○ Carnitine: 500 mg two times per day (L-carnitine)
- ○ Glutamine: 1 g per day
- ○ If depression is an issue, 5-hydroxy-tryptophan: 50 to 100 mg three times per day

Botanical Medicines

- Kudzu (*Pueraria lobata*) root extract: 1.2 g twice per day
- Milk thistle extract (70 to 80% silymarin): 70 to 210 mg three times per day, with higher dosages if there is significant liver involvement; dosage for silymarin phytosome is 120 mg two to three times per day between meals

Other Considerations

- Establish a good working relationship with Alcoholics Anonymous or an experienced counselor who has particular expertise in working with alcoholics.
- It is important to establish a strong network of caring family, friends, and peers for support. Get involved and busy with intense, people-oriented activities. Develop better strategies to deal with stress and the challenges of life.

Alzheimer's Disease

- Progressive mental deterioration, loss of memory and cognitive function, inability to carry out activities of daily life
- Characteristic symmetrical, usually diffuse brainwave pattern seen on EEG
- Diagnosis usually made by exclusion; imaging techniques can help rule out other causes of dementia
- At this time, definitive diagnosis can be made only by brain biopsy after death.

Alzheimer's disease (AD) is a degenerative brain disorder associated with progressive dementia—a deterioration of memory and cognition. In the United States, Alzheimer's disease is now estimated to affect 1.6% of the population younger than 74, with the rate increasing to 19% in those between 75 and 84 and to 42% in those older than 84. These numbers are striking when compared with data from the 1960s indicating an incidence of only 2% in people over the age of 85. The tremendous increase in AD in people over 85 is often referred to as the "Alzheimer's epidemic."[1]

Causes

AD is the result of damage to many aspects of brain structure and function. One characteristic feature of AD is the development of distinctive brain lesions called plaques and tangles.[1] Plaques are hard deposits of a protein, beta-amyloid, that are found be-

tween neurons. *Amyloid* is a general term for protein fragments that the body produces normally, and beta-amyloid is a fragment snipped from an amyloid precursor protein (APP). In a healthy brain, these fragments are broken down and eliminated, but in Alzheimer's disease they accumulate to form plaques. Another type of lesion, neurofibrillary tangles, occurs within brain cells. In the healthy brain cell, a protein called tau forms structures called microtubules. In Alzheimer's disease, however, the tau protein is abnormal and the microtubules collapse into a twisted mass. It is thought that the buildup of beta-amyloid triggers the changes in the tau protein. Both types of lesions disrupt message transmittal within the brain and eventually cause cell death.

Genetic factors play a major role and are estimated to account for up to 70% of cases of AD. The key appears to be genetically linked alterations in the ability of the immune system to regulate inflammation in the brain. Although the immune cells in the brain normally remove beta-amyloid, research is beginning to characterize a chronic and excessive inflammatory reaction to amyloid proteins in the brain that can promote AD in susceptible individuals.[2] Therapies designed to affect these immune cells in the brain are being investigated. Chief among these strategies is to immunize AD patients with beta-amyloid peptides so they will generate antibodies that bind to beta-amyloid and enhance its clearance.[3] Although preclinical studies were successful, the initial human clinical trial of an active beta-amyloid vaccine was halted owing to the development of severe inflammation in the brain in approximately 6% of the vaccinated AD patients.

Although genes have a big part in determining susceptibility to AD, lifestyle and environmental factors also play a significant role, as they do in most chronic degenerative disease. Emerging research reveals that dietary factors are especially important. Poor-quality diets with excessive amounts of saturated or trans-fatty acids may predispose neurons to environmental toxicities.[4,5] Some studies suggest that abnormal sleep-wake cycles and decreased morning light exposure may play a role in the expression of AD (see the section on melatonin later in this chapter). Traumatic injury to the head; chronic exposure to aluminum, silicon (most often due to occupational exposures in the construction, sandblasting, and mining industry), or both; exposure to neurotoxins such as mercury from environmental sources; and free radical damage have all been implicated as causative factors as well. As with other chronic degenerative diseases, there is considerable evidence that increased oxidative damage plays a central role. Therapies designed to support antioxidant mechanisms (discussed later) may be quite helpful in the prevention of AD.[6]

The tremendous increase in AD parallels the rise in type 2 diabetes and insulin resistance, suggesting a possible connection. It is well established that type 2 diabetics have a 1.5- to 4-fold increased risk for AD as well as for non-Alzheimer's dementia caused by damage to the blood vessels of the brain. Impaired insulin signaling, insulin resistance in the brain, and a decrease in cerebral insulin receptors associated with aging may be other important factors in the development of AD.

Measures to improve blood sugar control and improve insulin sensitivity appear to be important steps in the prevention of AD.[7,8]

Diagnostic Considerations

Comprehensive Evaluation

A comprehensive diagnostic workup is critical, as there are many conditions that can cause dementia. For example, depression is frequently seen in the elderly and can mimic dementia, and the most common reversible cause of dementia is drug toxicity. Other important causes are metabolic and nutritional disorders such as hypoglycemia, thyroid disturbances, and deficiency in vitamin B_{12}, folate, or thiamine. A comprehensive evaluation should include the following:[9]

- A detailed history
- Neurological and physical examination
- Psychological evaluation with particular attention to depression
- A general medical evaluation with emphasis on the detection of subtle metabolic, toxic, or cardiopulmonary disorders that can precipitate confusion, especially in the elderly
- A series of standardized neurophysiology tests such as the mini–mental state examination (MMSE) or Folstein test to document the type and severity of cognitive impairment
- Appropriate laboratory assessment (see below for recommended tests)
- An electroencephalogram (EEG)
- Imaging techniques such as computed tomography (CT), magnetic resonance imaging (MRI), positron emission tomography (PET), or others

Recommended Laboratory Tests for Dementia	
TEST	**RATIONALE**
CBC	Anemia, infection
Electrolytes	Metabolic dysfunction
Liver function tests	Hepatic dysfunction
BUN	Renal dysfunction
TSH, T4, T3, T3U	Thyroid dysfunction
Serum B_{12} and RBC folate	Deficiency
Urinalysis	Kidney/liver dysfunction
Hair mineral analysis	Heavy metal intoxication
ECG	Heart function
EEG	Focal vs. diffuse brain lesions
CT scan	Atrophy, intracranial mass

Fingerprint Patterns

Abnormal fingerprint patterns are associated with both AD and Down syndrome.[10] Compared with the normal population, Alzheimer and Down patients show an increased number of ulnar loops on the fingertips, with a decrease in whorls, radial loops, and arches. Ulnar loops (pointing toward the ulnar bone, away from the thumb) are frequently found on all 10 fingertips. Radial loops (pointing toward the thumb), when they do appear, tend to be shifted away from the index and middle fingers—where they most commonly occur—to the ring and little fingers. In patients with this fingerprint pattern, it is recommended that an aggressive, preventive approach be instituted immediately.

Therapeutic Considerations

The primary areas of intervention from a natural medicine perspective are prevention (addressing suspected causative factors) and treatment with natural measures (to improve mental function in the early stages of the disease). In the advanced stages of AD, natural measures will usually provide little benefit.

Diet

Dietary factors are clearly important in the development of AD. Food choices consistent with the standard American diet are associated with significant risk for the development of AD. A diet high in saturated fat and transfatty acids and low in dietary antioxidants may lead to increased serum and brain concentrations of aluminum and transition metal ions, which are implicated in oxidative stress. In addition, a poor-quality diet may cause inflammation in the brain.[4,5,11]

Many dietary risk factors are the same for both AD and atherosclerosis. Likewise, recent studies have provided clear evidence that following a Mediterranean-type diet does not just reduce the risk of heart disease but also is definitely associated with slower cognitive decline, lower risk for both pre-dementia syndromes and AD, and decreased mortality from all causes in AD patients.[11,12]

The key dietary factors that reduce

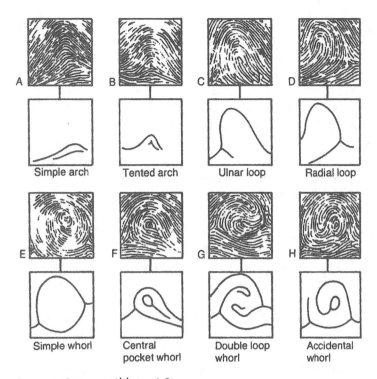

| Simple arch | Tented arch | Ulnar loop | Radial loop |

| Simple whorl | Central pocket whorl | Double loop whorl | Accidental whorl |

Fingerprint Patterns in Alzheimer's Disease

AD risk are higher fish consumption (and omega-3 fatty acids), monounsaturated fatty acids (primarily from olive oil), light to moderate alcohol use (primarily red wine), and increased consumption of nonstarchy vegetables and fruits. It is likely that it is the combination of all of these factors that provides the highest degree of protection, rather than any single dietary factor.[11,12]

One study in particular produced some very interesting findings. Given the ability of the Mediterranean diet to reduce inflammation and improve insulin sensitivity, many people assume that this plays a significant role in its ability to reduce AD. However, in a four-year prospective study, the lower risk of AD with the Mediterranean diet did not seem to be due to reducing atherosclerosis.[13] It is therefore thought that other aspects of the diet or specific foods are probably re-

sponsible, possibly working directly on reducing beta-amyloid formation or deposition.[14–21] For example, polyphenols found in grapes, grape seed extract, and red wine have been shown to prevent beta-amyloid formation and promote disassembly of the neurofibrillary tangles.[19–21] Animal studies using grape polyphenols marked with radioactive particles show absorption into the brain after oral administration.[22]

Even something as simple as eating celery (*Apium graveolens*) may offer significant protection against AD. Celery and celery seed extracts contain a unique compound, 3-n-butylphthalide (3nB), that is responsible for both the characteristic odor of celery and its health benefits. In an animal model of AD, 3nB treatment significantly improved learning deficits as well as long-term spatial memory, significantly reduced total cerebral beta-amyloid plaque deposition, and lowered brain beta-amyloid levels. It was also shown that 3nB markedly directed amyloid precursor protein processing toward a pathway that precludes beta-amyloid formation. The researchers concluded that "3nB shows promising preclinical potential as a multitarget drug for the prevention and/or treatment of Alzheimer's disease."[23]

The research on grape polyphenols and 3nB raises a powerful question: how many other foods contain unique compounds that address the pathophysiology of Alzheimer's disease? From preliminary investigations it looks as if there may be a great many. Especially promising are sources of phenols, polyphenols, and flavonoids.

Estrogen

Estrogen has been touted as offering protective and possibly therapeutic benefits in AD. However, the evidence to support the potential benefits of estrogen is contradictory. Yes, 16 population-based studies indicated that women on hormone replacement therapy (HRT) had a lower rate of AD.[24] But the problem with these studies was that women taking HRT were much healthier before taking the hormones compared with the control group, who were more likely to have hypertension, diabetes, and a history of stroke.[25] Data from the only large randomized controlled trial published to date, the Women's Health Initiative Memory Study, did not confirm these observations and have even suggested an increase in dementia risk for women using HRT (and especially those given HRT after menopause) compared with controls.[26] Clinical trials involving women with AD have concluded that estrogen therapy does not improve dementia symptoms in women with AD.[27–29] Given the cloud of uncertainty about the benefits of HRT, at this

point it seems most reasonable to consider the risks of estrogen therapy as outweighing any possible benefit in the prevention of AD.

Aluminum

Considerable attention has been focused on aluminum concentrations in neurofibrillary tangles. Whether the aluminum accumulates in the tangles in response to the formation of lesions or whether it actually initiates the lesions has not yet been determined, but significant evidence shows that it contributes, possibly significantly, to the disease.[30] There is a great deal of circumstantial evidence linking chronic aluminum exposure to AD. Increasing aluminum concentrations in the brain could explain why the frequency of AD rises with increasing age. And those with AD have significantly higher aluminum levels than both normal people and patients with other types of dementia, such as those from alcohol, atherosclerosis, and stroke.[31] The aluminum appears to come from the water supply, food, antacids, and antiperspirants. The most significant source is probably drinking water, as the aluminum in water is in a more bioavailable and thus potentially toxic form. Researchers measuring the absorption of aluminum from tap water added a small amount of soluble aluminum in a radioactive form to the stomachs of animals. They discovered that the trace amounts of aluminum from this single exposure immediately entered the animals' brain tissue. The frightening news is that aluminum in water not only occurs naturally but also is added (in the form of alum) to treat some water supplies.[32]

Avoiding all known sources of aluminum—aluminum-containing antacids, aluminum-containing antiperspirants, cooking in aluminum pots and pans, wrapping food with aluminum foil, nondairy creamers containing the food additive sodium aluminosilicate, and some types of baking powder and table salt—certainly seems appropriate. In addition, citric acid and calcium citrate supplements appear to increase the efficiency of absorption of aluminum (but not lead) from water and food.[33] Aluminum absorption can be decreased by magnesium, because magnesium competes with aluminum for absorption not only in the intestines but also at the blood-brain barrier.[34] Focus on unprocessed foods, avoid milk and dairy products, and increase consumption of vegetables, whole grains, nuts, and seeds—all good sources of magnesium.

Nutritional Considerations

Nutritional status is directly related to mental function in the elderly.[35] Given the frequency of nutrient deficiency in the elderly population, it is likely that many cases of impaired mental function may have a nutritional basis.

As pointed out above, diet is critically important in the prevention and arrest of AD, with various components working together in a synergistic fashion to address many of the underlying features of AD.

Antioxidants

As noted previously, considerable evidence indicates that oxidative damage plays a major role in the development and progression of AD.[6,36,37] Population-based evidence suggests that antioxidant nutrients offer significant protection against AD.[4,38] Prospective and clinical studies have primarily focused on vitamin C, vitamin E, and beta-carotene, with somewhat favorable results (see the table below).[36,39–42] As with other chronic degenerative diseases, better results may be achieved with a broader range of supplemental nutrients. For example, in a French study of middle-aged adults, 13 years of

Prospective Studies of Antioxidants and Risk of AD		
STUDY	**FOLLOW-UP**	**FINDINGS**
Rotterdam Study	6 years	Dietary vitamin E effective (more among current smokers)
Canadian Study of Health and Aging	5 years	Combination of vitamin E and vitamin C supplements and/or multivitamin consumption effective
Chicago Health Aging Study	3.9 years	Dietary vitamin E was effective only among a subset of individuals lacking a genetic risk factor (non-apoE4 carriers)
Washington Heights–Inwood Columbia Aging Project	4 years	No effect of vitamin E (diet or supplement)
Cache County Study	3 years	Vitamin E alone was not effective, but combined with vitamin C it was effective
Honolulu-Asia Aging Study	30 years	Dietary vitamin E was not effective
Duke Established Populations for Epidemiologic Studies of the Elderly	10 years	No effect of vitamin C and/or vitamin E
Group Health Cooperative	5.5 years	No effect of supplemental vitamin E and vitamin C alone or in combination

daily supplementation with 120 mg vitamin C, 30 mg vitamin E, 6 mg beta-carotene, 100 mcg selenium, and 20 mg zinc compared with a placebo were significantly associated with better verbal memory, which is a cognitive domain that is particularly vulnerable to AD. These results appear to be significantly better than those achieved with vitamin C, vitamin E, and beta-carotene either alone or in combination without the minerals.

It is entirely possible (and very likely) that vitamin E, vitamin C, and beta-carotene may simply be markers of increased phytochemical antioxidant intake and do not play a significant role on their own. Fruit and vegetables contain an array of antioxidant compounds beyond these three, and some of the other compounds may have considerable benefit in AD. Often researchers make the mistake of thinking that the antioxidant activity of a particular fruit or vegetable is due solely to its vitamin C, vitamin E, or beta-carotene content. However, these nutrient antioxidants often account for a very small fraction of a food's antioxidant effect—for example, only about 0.5% of the total antioxidant activity of an apple. The overwhelming antioxidant activity of fruit and vegetables comes from phytochemicals such as flavonoids, phenols, polyphenols, and other carotenoids.[16] In particular, as detailed above, phytochemicals are showing tremendous promise in protecting against AD beyond their antioxidant effects by interfering with beta-amyloid formation and deposition.

Thiamine (Vitamin B$_1$)

Although severe thiamine deficiency is relatively uncommon (except in alcoholics), many Americans, and especially the elderly, do not consume even the RDI of 1.5 mg. In an attempt to gauge the prevalence of thiamine deficiency in the geriatric population, 30 people visiting a university outpatient clinic in Tampa, Florida, were tested for thiamine levels. Depending on the thiamine measurement (plasma or red blood cell thiamine), low levels were found in 57% and 33%, respectively, of the people studied.[43]

In addition to its role as a nutrient, thiamine demonstrates some pharmacological effects on the brain. Specifically, it both potentiates and mimics acetylcholine, an important neurotransmitter involved in memory.[44] This effect explains the positive clinical results that have been noted for thiamine (3 to 8 g per day) in improving mental function in people with AD or age-related impaired mental function.[45,46] High-dosage thiamine supplementation has no side effects.

These results highlight the growing body of evidence that a significant percentage of the geriatric population is deficient in one or more of the B vitamins. Given the essential role of thiamine and other B vitamins in normal human physiology, especially cardiovascular and brain function, routine B vitamin supplementation appears to be worthwhile in this age group. AD may simply be the result of chronic low intake of essential nutrients—key among which are the B vitamins.

Vitamin B$_{12}$

Another B vitamin linked to AD is vitamin B$_{12}$. Vitamin B$_{12}$ deficiency results in impaired nerve function, which can cause numbness, tingling sensations, or a burning feeling in the feet, as well as impaired mental function, which in the elderly can mimic AD.[47,48] Vitamin B$_{12}$ deficiency also is a major cause of depression in this age group.

Several investigators have found that the level of vitamin B$_{12}$ declines with age (probably due to gastric atrophy) and that vitamin B$_{12}$ deficiency is found in 3% to 42% of people 65 and older. One way to determine whether there is a deficiency is by measuring the level of cobalamin in the blood. In one study of 100 geriatric outpatients who were seen in office-based settings for various acute and chronic medical illnesses, 11 had serum cobalamin levels of 148 pmol/l or below, 30 had levels between 148 and 295 pmol/l, and 59 patients had levels above 296 pmol/l.[49] After the initial cobalamin determination, the subjects were followed for up to three years. The patients with cobalamin levels below 148 pmol/l were treated and not included in the analysis of declining cobalamin levels. The average annual decline in serum cobalamin level was 18 pmol/l for patients who had higher initial serum cobalamin levels (224 to 292 pmol/l). For patients with lower initial cobalamin levels, the average annual decline was much higher, 28 pmol/l. These results indicate that screening for vitamin B_{12} deficiency appears to be indicated in the elderly given the positive cost-benefit ratio.[50–52] Other ways of screening for B_{12} deficiency involve measuring the level of methylmalonic acid in the urine or measuring the level of plasma homocysteine (which also serves to determine the status of folate). Having a high homocysteine level (>14 mmol/l) nearly doubles the risk of AD.[53]

The importance of detailed examination in elderly patients with mental symptoms is highlighted by results from a study that analyzed the plasma homocysteine, serum cobalamin, and blood folate in 296 patients referred to a geriatric psychiatric ward in Sweden for diagnosis of mental disease.[54] Patients who were deficient in vitamin B_{12} or folic acid or who had elevated levels of homocysteine were given vitamin B_{12} (dosage not specified), folic acid (10 mg per day), or both. When individuals with low cobalamin levels were supplemented with vitamin B_{12}, significant clinical improvements were noted.

In other studies, supplementation has shown tremendous benefit in reversing impaired mental function when there are low levels of vitamin B_{12}.[47] In one large study, a complete recovery was observed in 61% of cases of mental impairment due to low levels of vitamin B_{12}.[55] The fact that 39% did not respond is probably a result of long-term low levels of vitamin B_{12} causing irreversible damage. Several studies have shown that the best clinical responders are those who have been showing signs of impaired mental function for less than six months.[16] In one study, 18 subjects with low serum cobalamin levels and evidence of mental impairment were given vitamin B_{12}. Only those patients who had had symptoms for less than one year showed improvement.[56] The importance of diagnosing and correcting low vitamin B_{12} levels in the elderly cannot be overstated.

Serum vitamin B_{12} levels are significantly low in AD patients.[47,57,58] It has recently been demonstrated that an oral dose as low as 50 mcg per day can significantly increase serum vitamin B_{12} levels in vitamin B_{12}–deficient elderly people.[59] Supplementation of B_{12}, folic acid, or both may result in complete reversal in some patients, but generally there is little improvement in mental function in patients who have had Alzheimer's symptoms for more than six months.[60]

Vitamin B_{12} is available in several forms. The most common form is cyanocobalamin; however, vitamin B_{12} is active in the human body in only two forms, methylcobalamin and adenosylcobalamin. Although methylcobalamin and adenosylcobalamin are active immediately upon absorption, cyanocobalamin must be converted to either methylcobalamin or adenosylcobalamin. The body's ability to make this conversion may decline with aging and may be another factor responsible for the vitamin B_{12} disturbances noted in the elderly population.

Finally, the damaging effects of low vitamin B_{12} levels are aggravated by high levels of folic acid that mask a vitamin B_{12} deficiency. While the addition of folic acid to the food supply in 1998 helped decrease neural tube defects in infants, it may also have worsened the problems caused by low vitamin B_{12}.

Zinc

Zinc deficiency is one of the most common nutrient deficiencies in the elderly and has been suggested as a major factor in the development of AD, as most enzymes involved in DNA replication, repair, and transcription contain zinc.[61] It has been suggested that dementia may represent the long-term cascading effects of error-prone or ineffective DNA-handling enzymes in nerve cells, possibly because of a long-term zinc deficiency.[62] In addition, zinc is required by many antioxidant enzymes, including superoxide dismutase. With insufficient zinc, the end result could be the destruction of nerve cells and the formation of neurofibrillary tangles and plaques. Levels of zinc in the brain and cerebrospinal fluid in patients with AD are markedly decreased, and there is a strong inverse correlation between serum zinc levels and plaque count.[63]

Zinc supplementation has demonstrated good benefits in AD. In one study, 10 patients with AD were given 27 mg per day of zinc (as zinc aspartate). Only two patients failed to show improvement in memory, understanding, communication, and social contact. In one 79-year-old patient, the response was labeled "unbelievable" by both the medical staff and the family.[64] Unfortunately, there does not seem to be much interest in the scientific community in following up these impressive results with zinc therapy.

There is ambivalence in recent medical literature about zinc because in vitro, zinc accelerates the formation of insoluble beta-amyloid peptide.[65,66] Although zinc is neurotoxic at high concentrations and accumulates at sites of degeneration, total tissue zinc is markedly reduced in the brains of Alzheimer patients. Other research has shown a much higher concentration of copper-zinc superoxide dismutase in and around the damaged brain tissue of AD patients.[67] This suggests that the increased concentration of zinc in the damaged areas is due to the body's efforts to neutralize free radicals through the increased local production of dismutases. A possible explanation is that the higher localized levels of zinc result in increased amyloid formation when the free-radical-scavenging mechanisms have been inadequate.

Phosphatidylcholine and Other Sources of Choline

Because dietary phosphatidylcholine can increase acetylcholine levels in the brain in normal patients and AD is characterized by a decrease in acetylcholine function, it seems reasonable to assume that phosphatidylcholine supplementation would benefit Alzheimer's patients by providing more choline. However, the basic defect in many patients with AD relates to impaired activity of the enzyme acetylcholine transferase. This enzyme combines choline (as provided by phosphatidylcholine) with an acetyl molecule to form acetylcholine, the neurotransmitter. Providing more choline does not necessarily increase the activity of this key enzyme, so phosphatidylcholine supplementation is not beneficial in the majority of patients with AD. In addition, choline levels are elevated in the cerebrospinal fluid in AD. When researchers measured the levels of the water-soluble metabolites of phosphatidylcholine (glycerophosphocholine [GPC], phosphocholine, and choline) in normal patients and age-matched AD patients, they found increased levels in the AD patients. GPC was increased by 76%, phosphocholine by 52%, and free choline by 39%. What these data demonstrate is that AD is associated not only with reduced acetylcholine manufacture but also with increased breakdown of phosphatidylcholine, which is a component of brain cell membranes.[68]

Not surprisingly, clinical trials using phosphatidylcholine have largely been disappointing. Studies have shown inconsistent improvements in memory from choline supplementation in both normal and Alzheimer patients.[69–72] The studies have been criticized for small sample size, low dosage of phosphatidylcholine, poor design, and poor choice of choline form.[73] Clinical studies with glycerophosphocholine (GPC) and citicoline (also known as cytidine diphosphate-choline or CDP-choline) have shown benefit in improving age-related memory decline; however, studies investigating the use of these agents in AD have usually shown only very slight benefits.[73] In one double-blind study patients affected by mild to moderate AD were treated with GPC or a placebo for 180 days.[74] Scores on standard assessments (e.g., the Alzheimer's Disease Assessment Scale and the Global Improvement Scale) after 90 and 180 days showed improvement in the GPC group, whereas in the placebo group they remained unchanged or worsened. Study results with citicoline in AD have been inconsistent.[75,76]

Despite the questionable benefit specifically related to AD, in cases of mild to moderate dementia we recommend a 90-day trial of either GPC or CDP at dosages of 1,200 mg and 1,000 mg per day, respectively. Given the difficulty with diagnosing AD, it is possible that many cases of dementia are related to other factors that may respond to choline supplementation. If there is no noticeable improvement within the 90-day time frame, supplementation should be discontinued.

Phosphatidylserine

Phosphatidylserine (PS) is the major phospholipid in the brain, where it plays a significant role in determining the integrity and fluidity of cell membranes. Normally the brain can manufacture sufficient levels of phosphatidylserine, but a deficiency of methyl donors (such as S-adenosyl-methionine [SAM-e], folic acid, and vitamin B_{12}) or essential fatty acids may inhibit production of sufficient PS. Low levels of phosphatidylserine in the brain are associated with impaired mental function and depression in the elderly. To date, 11 published double-blind studies have all reported the successful use of PS in the treatment of age-related cognitive decline, AD, or depression.[77–86] In the largest study a total of 494 patients between 65 and 93 years old with moderate to severe dementia were given either phosphatidylserine (100 mg three times per day) or a placebo for six months.[72] The patients were assessed for mental performance, behavior, and mood at the beginning and end of the study. Statistically significant improvements were noted in mental function, mood, and behavior for the phosphatidylserine group.

L-Acetylcarnitine

A great deal of research has been conducted with L-acetylcarnitine (LAC; also called acetyl-L-carnitine) in the treatment of AD, senile depression, and age-related memory defects. LAC is composed of acetic acid and L-carnitine bound together. This reaction occurs naturally in the human brain. Therefore it is not exactly known how much greater an effect is achieved with LAC vs. L-carnitine. However, LAC is thought to be substantially more active than other forms of carnitine in conditions involving the brain.[87,88]

The close structural similarity between

LAC and acetylcholine led to an interest in using LAC in AD. Research has shown that LAC both enhances and mimics acetylcholine and is of benefit not only in patients with early-stage AD but also in elderly patients who are depressed or who have impaired memory.[88] It has been shown to act as a powerful antioxidant within the brain cell, stabilize cell membranes, and improve energy production within the brain cell as well.[89]

In an analysis of studies of LAC in mild cognitive impairment and mild (early) AD, patients taking doses ranging from 1.5 to 3 g a day were assessed at 3, 6, 9, and 12 months. This analysis showed a significant advantage for LAC compared with a placebo. The advantage for LAC was seen by the time of the first assessment at three months and increased over time. Additionally, LAC was well tolerated in all studies.[90]

Further studies also show its efficacy in situations where AD patients were unresponsive to standard drug therapy (acetylcholinesterase inhibitors). One study showed LAC at 2 g per day increased the effectiveness of drugs such as donepezil and rivastigmine.[91]

Memory impairment need not be as severe as it usually is in AD in order for LAC to demonstrate a benefit.[92–94] In one double-blind study of 236 elderly subjects with mild mental deterioration, as evidenced by detailed clinical assessment, the group receiving 1,500 mg per day of LAC demonstrated significant improvement in mental function, particularly in memory and constructional thinking.[94]

Dehydroepiandrosterone (DHEA)

DHEA is the most abundant hormone in the bloodstream and is found in extremely high concentrations in the brain. Because DHEA levels decline dramatically with aging, low levels of DHEA in the blood and brain are thought to contribute to many symptoms associated with aging, including impaired mental function. In some studies DHEA supplementation has shown promise in enhancing memory and improving cognitive function.[95] However, no effect was noted in the largest study as well as others.[96,97] The only double-blind study in actual AD was a small pilot study (58 subjects) in which 50 mg DHEA was given twice a day. Although some benefit was reported at three months, DHEA did not significantly improve cognitive performance or overall change in severity.[98]

We feel that the failure of DHEA to provide benefits may have been due to not properly qualifying the patients. Measuring DHEA levels in the blood or saliva can help determine if DHEA may be of benefit. It is not likely to be of benefit in those with satisfactory levels for their age and sex. The dose of DHEA necessary to improve brainpower in men older than 50 appears to be 25 to 50 mg per day. For women, a dosage of 15 to 25 mg appears to be sufficient in most cases. As men and women reach their 70s, they may require higher levels (e.g., 50 to 100 mg). Excessive dosages of DHEA can cause acne and, in younger women, menstrual irregularities.

Melatonin and Bright Light Therapy

Test tube studies have shown that melatonin protects brain cells from heavy metal damage. For example, melatonin treatment prevented oxidative damage and beta-amyloid release caused by cobalt. Since cobalt is another toxic metal found in high levels in AD patients, melatonin may prove an important preventive treatment in AD.[99]

One double-blind study of AD patients involved subjects who got 3 mg melatonin or a placebo at 8:30 p.m. every day for a month. Based on standard dementia and AD assessment scales, the melatonin group had significantly increased sleeping time and decreased nighttime activity, with improved levels of mental function.[100]

Melatonin may also be helping by improving the disturbance in circadian (daily) rhythm common in AD. Circadian rhythm affects body functions such as sleep cycles, temperature, alertness, and hormone production. Impaired sleep and nocturnal restlessness place great burdens on both those who suffer from AD and their caregivers. Clinical research has shown that exposure to full-spectrum light throughout the day and darkness at night can help improve some aspects of AD, reducing agitation, increasing sleep efficiency (percentage of time in bed spent asleep), decreasing nighttime wakefulness, and decreasing nighttime activity. If natural sunlight exposure is not possible for at least an hour in the morning, light boxes are available that can simulate sunlight. Full-spectrum lightbulbs are available that can replace conventional bulbs as well.[101–103]

Although bright light therapy during the day is often effective on its own, combining it with melatonin produces the best results.[104]

Botanical Medicines

Ginkgo Biloba Extract

Ginkgo biloba extract (GBE) has been extensively investigated in cases of dementia, including Alzheimer's disease. In addition to GBE's ability to increase functional brain capacity, it has been shown to normalize acetylcholine receptors in the brains of aged animals, increase cholinergic transmission, inhibit beta-amyloid deposition, and address many of the other major elements of AD.[105] However, while preliminary studies with established AD patients were quite promising, it now appears that at best GBE can help to reverse or delay mental deterioration only in the early stages of AD. Even this may be in doubt, as in several double-blind studies no benefit over a placebo was observed in halting cognitive decline.[106–108] In other double-blind studies, though, the benefits of GBE in early-stage AD were quite evident, as they were in a meta-analysis of studies of more than six months' duration.[109] In one study, 216 patients with AD or multi-infarct dementia were given either 240 mg per day of GBE or a placebo for 24 weeks.[110] Improvements were noted in several clinical areas, including the Clinical Global Impressions scale (described below). Similar results were seen in another double-blind study where the 240 mg dose was administered once per day.[111]

One study worth special mention was the first U.S. clinical study on GBE published in the *Journal of the American Medical Association*.[112] The study was conducted at six research centers. Harvard Medical School and the New York Institute for Medical Research approved the design of the study, in which 202 patients with AD were given either a modest dose of GBE (120 mg per day) or a placebo for one year. GBE not only stabilized AD but also led to significant improvements in mental function in 64% of the patients. There were no side effects with GBE.

Ginkgo has been used extensively as a

Clinical Global Impression Ratings: Ginkgo Biloba Extract (GBE) vs. Placebo		
STATUS	**GBE (%)**	**PLACEBO (%)**
Very much improved	3	1
Much improved	29	16
Slightly improved	41	38
Unchanged	28	30
Moderately worse	0	14
Much worse	0	1

medicinal agent worldwide for centuries. It is the most frequently prescribed medicinal herb in Europe, with hundreds of studies reporting positive effects from taking ginkgo for both prevention and treatment of various health complaints. The most dramatic benefits are reported in improving circulation in the elderly. This can enhance memory, possibly delaying the onset of Alzheimer's disease, reducing other forms of dementia, and improving tinnitus and vertigo. Ginkgo's memory-enhancing effects are reported in younger populations as well.

In the most recent study, 410 patients with mild to moderate dementia were randomly assigned to receive either 240 mg GBE or a placebo per day for 24 weeks. The results revealed that treatment with the ginkgo biloba extract led to significant improvements in the symptoms of apathy/indifference, sleep/nighttime behavior, irritability/lability, depression/dysphoria, and aberrant motor behavior. These results indicate that even if GBE does not improve cognitive function, it may produce significant improvements in mood and behavior.[112] This would at the very least help enable patients to maintain a normal life and avoid being institutionalized.

It is important to point out that studies directly comparing gingko with standard drug regimens indicate that they offer similar efficacy in AD, but ginkgo has fewer side effects. A comparative analysis of studies of at least six months' duration demonstrated that GBE and second-generation cholinesterase inhibitors (tacrine, donepezil, rivastigmine, metrifonate) were equally effective in treating mild to moderate AD.[113] In a meta-analysis of 50 studies that examined the effect of ginkgo on objective measures of cognitive function in patients with AD using standardized measures of cognition, it was concluded that GBE produced benefits comparable to those of standard drug therapy.[114]

In addition to possibly being beneficial in early-stage AD, if the mental deficit is due to vascular insufficiency or depression and not AD, GBE is usually effective in reversing the deficit. GBE should be taken consistently for at least 12 weeks in order to determine its effectiveness. Although in some people with AD benefits are reported within two or three weeks, most will need to take GBE for a longer period.

Huperzine A

Huperzine A, an alkaloid isolated from the moss *Huperzia serrata*, has been shown to potentiate the effects of acetylcholine in the brain by inhibiting the enzyme acetylcholinesterase, which breaks down acetylcholine. It is significantly more selective and substantially less toxic than the acetylcholine esterase inhibitors currently used in conventional medicine (physostigmine, tacrine, and donepezil). In contrast, huperzine A has been used as a prescription drug in China since the early 1990s and has reportedly been used by more than 100,000 people with no serious adverse effects.[115]

In one of the first double-blind clinical studies, huperzine A at a dose of 200 mcg twice per day produced measurable improvements in memory, cognitive function, and behavioral factors in 58% of AD patients.[116] In contrast, in the placebo group only 36% showed improvement.

In a more recent double-blind study, 210 individuals with AD were randomly assigned to receive a placebo or huperzine A (200 mcg or 400 mcg twice per day) for at least 16 weeks. The 200-mcg dose did not produce any change in cognitive assessment score, but patients taking the 400-mcg dose showed a 2.27-point improvement in this score after 11 weeks compared with a 0.29-point decline in the placebo group, and a 1.92-point improvement after 16 weeks compared with a 0.34-point improvement in the placebo group.[117]

Adverse reactions have been noted with huperzine A, including hyperactivity, nasal obstruction, nausea, vomiting, diarrhea, insomnia, anxiety, dizziness, thirst, and constipation. One trial reported abnormalities in electrocardiogram patterns (cardiac ischemia and arrhythmia).

Curcumin

There is considerable experimental evidence that curcumin protects against age-related brain damage and in particular Alzheimer's disease. Researchers began exploring this effect after noting that elderly residents of rural India who eat large amounts of turmeric have been shown to have the lowest incidence of Alzheimer's disease in the world: 4.4 times lower than that of Americans. In test tube and animal studies curcumin has been shown to inhibit beta-amyloid and have other effects beneficial in AD. Unfortunately, the two clinical trials conducted to date failed to show any benefit.[118] However, the failure to produce positive results may have been due to the poor absorption profile of the curcumin used in the trials. There now exist a number of methods and products that enhance the absorption of curcumin. In one product, Meriva, the curcumin is complexed with soy phospholipids. Absorption studies in animals indicate that peak plasma levels of curcumin after administration of Meriva were five times higher than those after administration of regular curcumin.[119] Studies with another advanced form of curcumin, Theracurmin, show even greater absorption (27 times greater than regular curcumin).[120]

....

QUICK REVIEW

- **AD is the result of damage to the brain that affects the activity of the neurotransmitter acetylcholine.**
- **Research is beginning to identify a chronic and excessive inflammatory reaction to amyloid proteins in the brain in individuals susceptible to AD.**
- **Although genes play a big part in determining susceptibility to AD, lifestyle and environmental factors also have a significant role.**
- **Traumatic injury to the head; chronic exposure to aluminum, silicon, or both; exposure to neurotoxins from environmental sources; and free radical damage have all been implicated as causative factors.**

- **Measures to improve blood sugar control and improve insulin sensitivity appear to be important steps in the prevention of AD. Abnormal fingerprint patterns are associated with both Alzheimer's disease and Down syndrome.**
- **From the perspective of natural medicine, the primary goals of intervention are prevention and using natural measures to improve mental function in the early stages of the disease.**
- **In the advanced stages of AD, natural measures will usually provide little benefit.**
- **There is evidence to suggest that antioxidants offer significant protection**

against Alzheimer's disease as well as therapeutic benefits.

- Aluminum absorption can be decreased by magnesium, as magnesium competes with aluminum for absorption pathways.

- Polyphenols found in grapes, grape seed extract, and red wine have been shown to prevent beta-amyloid formation and promote disassembly of neurofibrillary tangles.

- A significant percentage of the geriatric population is affected by B vitamin deficiencies linked to Alzheimer's disease.

- Zinc supplementation is demonstrating good results in the treatment of Alzheimer's disease.

- The results of using L-acetylcarnitine to delay the progression of Alzheimer's disease have been outstanding.

- DHEA shows promise in enhancing memory and improving mental function in the elderly.

- It appears that ginkgo biloba helps reverse or delay mental deterioration only during the early stages of Alzheimer's disease.

- Huperzine A is more selective and substantially less toxic than the acetylcholine esterase inhibitors currently used in conventional medicine.

- There is considerable experimental evidence that curcumin protects against age-related brain damage and, in particular, Alzheimer's disease.

TREATMENT SUMMARY

The primary therapeutic goal is prevention; follow the recommendations below under "Lifestyle," "Diet," and "Nutritional Supplements." When symptoms begin to appear, it is important to increase nutritional support, as described under "Therapeutic Supplements"; we also offer suggestions under "Botanical Medicines." Keep in mind that in advanced AD, treatment is less likely to be of benefit. In general, we recommend a trial for a minimum of 90 days in attempting to improve AD with natural measures. If no benefit is seen during this time, further therapy is unlikely to provide benefit.

Lifestyle

- Follow the recommendations given in the chapter "A Health-Promoting Lifestyle."

- Avoid aluminum (often found in antiperspirants, antacids, and cookware).

Diet

Follow the recommendations given in the chapter "A Health-Promoting Diet." In particular, apply the principles of the Mediterranean diet; increase whole food products, including fish, cereals, vegetables, and monounsaturated fats; avoid high-glycemic foods and unhealthy fats;

achieve ideal body weight; and take measures to improve insulin sensitivity.

Nutritional Supplements

- A high-potency multiple vitamin and mineral formula as described in the chapter "Supplementary Measures"
- Vitamin C: 500 to 1,000 mg per day
- Vitamin E: 100 to 200 IU per day
- Fish oils: 1,000 mg EPA + DHA per day
- Grape seed or pine bark extract (>95% procyanidolic content): 150 to 300 mg per day
- In high-risk individuals, choose one of the following forms of bioavailable curcumin:
  ○ Meriva: 1,000–1,200 mg per day
  ○ Theracurmin: 300 mg per day

Therapeutic Supplements

The following are in addition to all of the supplements listed under "Nutritional Supplements" above:

- Thiamine: 3 to 8 g per day
- One of the following:
  ○ Glycerophosphocholine: 1,200 mg per day
  ○ Citicoline: 1,000 mg per day
- Phosphatidylserine: 100 mg three times per day
- L-acetylcarnitine: 1,500 mg per day
- Methylcobalamin: 1,000 mcg upon arising each day
- Melatonin: 3 mg in the evening at least a half hour before bedtime

Botanical Medicines

- Ginkgo biloba (24% ginkgo flavonglycosides): 240 to 320 mg per day
- Huperzine A: 200 to 400 mcg per day
- Curcumin, one of the following:
  ○ Meriva: 500 to 1,000 mg twice daily
  ○ BCM95 Complex: 750 to 1,500 mg twice daily
  ○ Theracurmin: 300 mg one to three times daily

Anemia

· ·

- Pallor, weakness, and a tendency to become fatigued easily
- Low volume of blood, low level of total red blood cells, or abnormal size or shape of red blood cells

Anemia is a condition in which the blood is deficient in red blood cells or the hemoglobin (iron-containing) portion of red blood cells. The primary function of the red blood cell (RBC) is to transport oxygen from the lungs to the tissues of the body and then bring carbon dioxide from the tissues to the lungs, where it is exhaled. The symptoms of anemia, such as extreme fatigue, reflect a lack of oxygen being delivered to tissues and a buildup of carbon dioxide.

There are three major classifications of anemia.

1. Anemia due to excessive blood loss
2. Anemia due to excessive red blood cell destruction
3. Anemia due to deficient red blood cell or hemoglobin production

Anemia Due to Excessive Blood Loss

Anemia can be produced during acute (rapid) or chronic (slow but constant) blood loss. Acute blood loss can be fatal if more than one-third of total blood volume is lost (roughly 1.5 l). Since acute blood loss is usu-

ally quite apparent, there is little difficulty in diagnosis. Often blood transfusion is required.

Chronic blood loss from a slow-bleeding peptic ulcer, hemorrhoids, or menstruation can also produce anemia. This highlights the importance of identifying the cause through a complete diagnostic workup by a qualified health care professional.

Anemia Due to Excessive Red Blood Cell Destruction

Old red blood cells, as well as abnormal RBCs, are removed from the circulation primarily by the spleen. If destruction of old or abnormal RBCs exceeds the body's ability to manufacture new RBCs, anemia can result. The most common cause of excessive destruction of RBCs is abnormal RBC shape.

A number of things can lead to abnormal RBC shape, including synthesis of defective hemoglobin, as seen in hereditary conditions such as sickle-cell anemia; mechanical injury due to trauma or turbulence within arteries; hereditary RBC enzyme defects; and vitamin or mineral deficiency.

Anemia Due to Deficient Red Blood Cell or Hemoglobin Production

Insufficient production of RBCs or hemoglobin is the most common category of anemia, and by far the most common cause is nutritional deficiency. Although a deficiency of any of several vitamins and minerals can produce anemia, only the most common—iron, vitamin B_{12}, and folic acid—will be discussed here. Iron deficiency anemia is characterized as *microcytic anemia* because the RBCs become very small, while folic acid and B_{12} deficiency anemias are classified as *macrocytic anemias* because the RBCs become quite large.

Iron Deficiency Anemia

Iron is critical to human life. It plays the central role in the hemoglobin molecule of our red blood cells, where it transports oxygen from the lungs to the body's tissues and carbon dioxide from the tissues to the lungs. Iron also functions in several key enzymes in energy production and metabolism including DNA synthesis.

Iron deficiency is the most common nutrient deficiency in the United States and the most common cause of anemia. The groups at highest risk for iron deficiency are infants under two years of age, teenage girls, pregnant women, and the elderly. Studies have found evidence of iron deficiency in as many as 30 to 50% of people in these groups. For example, some degree of iron deficiency occurs in 35 to 58% of young, healthy women. During pregnancy, the number is even higher. However, it must be pointed out that anemia is the last stage of iron deficiency. Iron-dependent enzymes involved in energy production and metabolism are the first to be affected by low iron levels. Serum ferritin is the best laboratory test for determining body iron stores.[1]

Iron deficiency may be caused by an increased iron requirement, decreased dietary intake, diminished iron absorption or utilization, blood loss, or a combination of factors. Increased requirements for iron occur during the growth spurts of infancy and adolescence and during pregnancy and lactation. Currently, the vast majority of pregnant women are routinely given iron supplements during their pregnancy, as the dramatically increased need for iron during pregnancy cannot usually be met through diet alone. Inadequate intake of iron is common in many parts of the world, especially areas where people consume a primarily vegetarian diet.

Typical infant diets in developed countries are high in milk and cereals and thus are also low in iron. The adolescent who eats a lot of junk food is at high risk for iron deficiency. However, those at greatest risk for a diet deficient in iron are the low-income elderly. This situation is complicated by the fact that decreased absorption of iron is very frequently found in the elderly. Decreased absorption of iron is often caused by a lack of hydrochloric acid secretion in the stomach, an extremely common condition in the elderly.

Other causes of decreased absorption include chronic diarrhea or malabsorption, the surgical removal of the stomach, and use of antacids or acid-blocking drugs. Blood loss is the most common cause of iron deficiency in women of childbearing age. This blood loss is most often due to excessive menstrual bleeding. Interestingly enough, iron deficiency is a common cause of excessive menstrual blood loss.[2,3] Other frequently seen causes of blood loss include bleeding from peptic ulcers, bleeding from hemorrhoids, and donating blood.

The negative effects of iron deficiency are

due largely to the impaired delivery of oxygen to the tissues and the impaired activity of iron-containing enzymes in various tissues. Iron deficiency can lead to anemia, excessive menstrual blood loss, learning disabilities, impaired immune function, and decreased energy levels and physical performance.[1]

It has been clearly demonstrated that even a slight iron deficiency leads to a reduction in physical work capacity and productivity. The iron-dependent enzymes involved in energy production and metabolism will be impaired long before anemia occurs.[1] Supplementation with iron has produced rapid improvements in work capacity among iron-deficient individuals.

Vitamin B$_{12}$ Deficiency Anemia

Vitamin B$_{12}$ deficiency is most often due to a defect in absorption, not a dietary lack. In order for vitamin B$_{12}$ to be absorbed from food, it must be liberated from food by hydrochloric acid and bound to a substance known as intrinsic factor within the small intestine. Intrinsic factor is secreted by the parietal cells of the stomach. These same cells are responsible for the secretion of hydrochloric acid. Hence the secretion of intrinsic factor parallels that of hydrochloric acid. The B$_{12}$–intrinsic factor complex is absorbed in the small intestine with the aid of the pancreatic enzyme trypsin.

In order for vitamin B$_{12}$ to be absorbed, an individual must secrete enough hydrochloric acid, intrinsic factor, and pancreatic enzymes, including trypsin, and have a healthy and intact ileum (the end portion of the small intestine, where the vitamin B$_{12}$–intrinsic factor complex is absorbed).

Lack of intrinsic factor results in a condition known as pernicious anemia. The defect is rare before the age of 35, and it is more common in individuals of Scandinavian, English, and Irish descent. It is much less common in southern Europeans, Asians, and blacks. Pernicious anemia is frequently associated with iron deficiency as well.

A dietary lack of vitamin B$_{12}$ is most often associated with a vegan diet (a vegetarian diet that includes no milk products or eggs). Unlike other water-soluble nutrients, vitamin B$_{12}$ is stored in the liver, kidney, and other body tissues. As a result, signs and symptoms of vitamin B$_{12}$ deficiency may not show themselves until after five to six years of poor dietary intake or inadequate secretion of intrinsic factor. The classic symptom of vitamin B$_{12}$ deficiency is pernicious anemia. However, it appears that a deficiency of vitamin B$_{12}$ will affect the brain and nervous system before anemia develops.

The diagnosis of vitamin B$_{12}$ deficiency is best made by measuring the vitamin B$_{12}$ level in the blood. Most physicians, however, simply rely on the presence of large red blood cells and characteristic symptoms. Symptoms of severe B$_{12}$ deficiency can include paleness; easy fatigability; shortness of breath; a sore, beefy red, and swollen tongue; diarrhea; and heart and nervous system disturbances.

The nervous system disturbances of a vitamin B$_{12}$ deficiency can be quite serious. Common symptoms include numbness and tingling of the arms or legs, depression, mental confusion, loss of the ability to sense vibration, and loss of deep tendon reflexes. In the elderly, a vitamin B$_{12}$ deficiency can mimic Alzheimer's disease.

Folic Acid Deficiency

Folic acid deficiency is the most common vitamin deficiency in the world. The body does not store a large surplus of folic acid (unlike vitamin B$_{12}$); it stores only enough to sustain itself for one to two months. Folic acid deficiency will result in the same type of anemia as that caused by a vitamin B_{12} deficiency: an anemia characterized by enlarged RBCs (macrocytic anemia). Other symptoms of folic acid deficiency include diarrhea, depression, and a swollen, red tongue.

Folic acid deficiency is extremely common among alcoholics, as alcohol consumption impairs absorption of folic acid, disrupts its metabolism, and causes the body to excrete it.

Folic acid deficiency is also common among pregnant women because of the developing fetus's high demands. Folic acid is vital to cell reproduction within the fetus. If the fetus does not have a constant source of folic acid, birth defects such as neural tube defects may result. If alcohol is consumed during pregnancy, the alcohol may lower folic acid levels, leading to fetal alcohol syndrome or neural tube defects.

In addition to alcohol, there are a number of drugs that can induce folic acid deficiency, including anticancer drugs, drugs for epilepsy, and oral contraceptives.

Folic acid deficiency is quite common among patients who have chronic diarrhea or malabsorption states such as celiac disease, Crohn's disease, or tropical sprue. Since a deficiency of folic acid will result in diarrhea and malabsorption, often a vicious circle ensues. The administration of folic acid as a preventive measure is warranted for anyone experiencing chronic diarrhea. Often this has a therapeutic effect as well.

NOTE: It is always necessary to supplement vitamin B_{12} with folic acid to prevent the folic acid supplement from masking a vitamin B_{12} deficiency. Supplementing with folic acid will correct the anemia of a vitamin B_{12} deficiency, but it cannot overcome the problems that vitamin B_{12} deficiency causes in the brain. Also, a high level of folic acid will actually aggravate the problems caused by vitamin B_{12} deficiency.

The most sensitive test to assess folic acid deficiency is determining the folic acid content of the serum and RBC.

Therapeutic Considerations

The treatment of anemia is dependent on proper clinical evaluation by a physician. It is imperative that a comprehensive laboratory analysis of the blood be performed. Do not be satisfied with the diagnosis of "anemia." It is critical that the underlying cause of the anemia be uncovered so that the correct therapy can be employed.

General Nutritional Support for All Types of Anemia

Perhaps the best food for an individual with any kind of anemia is calf liver. It is rich not only in iron but also in all B vitamins. Green leafy vegetables are also of great benefit to individuals with any kind of anemia. These vegetables contain natural fat-soluble chlorophyll (a molecule similar to the hemoglobin molecule) as well as other important nutrients, including iron and folic acid. Only fat-soluble chlorophyll can be absorbed from the gastrointestinal tract; the water-soluble form cannot and so has no use in the treatment of anemia.

Since a large percentage of individuals with anemia do not secrete enough hydrochloric acid, it is often important to take hydrochloric acid supplements with meals. See the chapter "Digestion and Elimination" for more information and dosage instructions.

Support for Iron Deficiency Anemia

Again, treatment of any type of anemia should focus on underlying causes. For iron deficiency anemia, this typically involves finding a reason for chronic blood loss or for why an individual is not absorbing sufficient amounts of dietary iron. Lack of hydrochloric acid is a common reason for impaired iron absorption, especially among the elderly.

Increasing iron intake through food may partially or completely overcome poor iron absorption. There are two forms of dietary iron: heme iron and non-heme iron. Heme iron, found only in animal foods such as meat, poultry, and fish, is bound to the oxygen-binding proteins hemoglobin and myoglobin. It is the most efficiently absorbed form of iron. The absorption rate of non-heme iron, which is the kind found in plant food and in supplements such as ferrous sulfate and ferrous fumarate, is 2.9% on an empty stomach and 0.9% with food, much less than the absorption rate of heme iron, which is as high as 35%. In addition, heme iron is without the side effects associated with non-heme sources of iron, such as nausea, flatulence, constipation, and diarrhea.[4]

Despite the superiority of heme iron, non-heme iron salts are the most popular iron supplements. One reason is that even though heme iron is better absorbed, it is easy to take higher quantities of non-heme iron salts, so the net amount of iron absorbed is about equal. In other words, if you take 3 mg heme iron and 50 mg non-heme iron, the net absorption for each will be about the same.

Ferrous sulfate is the most popular iron supplement, but it is certainly less than ideal, as it often causes constipation or other gastrointestinal disturbances. The best forms of non-heme iron are ferrous succinate, glycinate, fumarate, and pyrophosphate. Of these, we prefer ferrous pyrophosphate that is micronized (made into a very small particle size) and then microencapsulated. The advantages of this form include that it is extremely stable, has no taste or flavor, is free from gastrointes-

tinal side effects, and provides a sustained-release form of iron (up to 12 hours) with a high relative bioavailability, especially if it is taken on an empty stomach.[5]

For iron deficiency, the usual recommendation for any non-heme source is generally up to 60 mg per day in divided doses. High intakes of other minerals, particularly calcium, magnesium, and zinc, can interfere with iron absorption, so in treating iron deficiency it is recommended to take iron away from other mineral supplements. In contrast, vitamin C enhances iron absorption.

The best dietary sources of iron are red meat, especially liver. Good nonmeat sources of iron include fish, beans, molasses, dried fruits, whole grain and enriched breads, and green leafy vegetables.

The table below provides the iron content per serving of some of the better sources of iron. The table does not factor in absorption. For example, the absorption rate for the iron in calf liver is nearly 30%, while the absorption rate for the iron in vegetable sources is approximately 5%.

Several foods and beverages contain sub-

Dietary Sources of Iron		
FOOD	**AVERAGE SERVING SIZE (G)**	**IRON PER SERVING (MG)**
Calf or lamb liver	60	9.6
Beef or chicken liver	60	5.2
Beef	90	2.7
Beans, cooked	100	2.3
Prunes	100	1.8
Bread (3 slices)	70	1.7
Chicken or turkey	90	1.6
Greens, cooked	75	1.5
Peas	75	1.5
Eggs	50	1.1

Recommended Dietary Intakes (RDI) for Iron	
GROUP	**DAILY DOSE (MG)**
Infants (7 months) up to age 10	10
Males 11–18 years old	12
Males 19 years and older	8
Females 11 years and older	18
Pregnant women	27

CAUTIONS AND WARNINGS: Keep all iron supplements out of the reach of children. Acute iron poisoning in infants can result in serious consequences: damage to the intestinal lining, liver failure, nausea and vomiting, and shock.

---

stances that inhibit iron absorption, including tea, coffee, wheat bran, and egg yolk. Antacids and overuse of calcium supplements also decrease iron absorption. These items should be restricted by individuals who have iron deficiency.[1]

Support for Vitamin B_{12} Deficiency Anemia

In 1926, it was shown that injectable liver extracts were effective in the treatment of pernicious anemia. Soon after, active concentrates of liver became available for intramuscular as well as oral administration. Today, the use of liver and liver extracts has fallen out of favor in mainstream medicine. For pernicious anemia, standard medical treatment involves injecting vitamin B_{12} at a dose of 1,000 mcg per day for one week, but oral therapy has shown equal effectiveness (discussed in the section "Oral Versus Injectable B_{12}," below).

Vitamin B_{12} is found in significant quantities only in animal foods. The richest sources are liver and kidney, followed by eggs, fish, cheese, and meat. Vegans are often told that fermented foods such as tempeh and miso are excellent sources of vitamin B_{12}. However, in addition to tremendous variation of B_{12} content in fermented foods, there is some evidence that the form of B_{12} in these foods is not the form that meets the human body's requirements and is therefore useless. The same holds true for certain cooked sea vegetables. Although the vitamin B_{12} content of these foods is in the same range as beef, it is not known how well this form is utilized. Therefore, at this time we recommend that vegetarians, and particularly vegans, supplement their diets with vitamin B_{12}.

Vitamin B_{12} is available in several forms. The most common form is cyanocobalamin. However, vitamin B_{12} is active in only two forms: methylcobalamin and adenosylcobalamin. Methylcobalamin is the only active form of vitamin B_{12} that is available commercially in tablet form in the United States. While methylcobalamin is active immediately upon absorption, cyanocobalamin must be converted by the body to either methylcobalamin or adenosylcobalamin. Cyanocobalamin is not active in many experimental models, while both methylcobalamin and adenosylcobalamin demonstrate exceptional activity.

Oral vs. Injectable B_{12}

Although it is popular to inject vitamin B_{12}, injection is not necessary; the oral administration of an appropriate dosage, even in the absence of intrinsic factor, can result in effective elevations of vitamin B_{12} levels in the blood. This fact has gone relatively ignored among most physicians. In the United States, oral vitamin B_{12} therapy is rarely used despite the fact that it has been shown to be fully (100%) effective in the long-term treatment of pernicious anemia.[6]

Almost as soon as vitamin B_{12} was isolated in 1948, it was introduced in an injectable form, and researchers busily sought an oral alternative. Oral preparations containing intrinsic factor were tried, but some patients developed antibodies against intrinsic factor and therefore would not respond. Studies in the 1950s and 1960s soon documented that a small but constant proportion of an oral dose of cyanocobalamin was absorbed even without intrinsic factor through the process of diffusion, so by sufficiently increasing the dose, adequate absorption could be attained. A study in 1978 described 64 Swedish patients with pernicious anemia and other vitamin B_{12} deficiency states who were treated with 1,000 mcg of oral cyanocobalamin per day.[7] Complete normalization of serum levels and liver stores for vitamin B_{12}, as well as full clinical remission, was observed in all patients studied over a three-year period. Since that time numerous other studies have all confirmed the effectiveness of oral therapy with vitamin B_{12} for pernicious anemia.[6]

Despite the research, oral vitamin B_{12} therapy is still not used in the United States. Why? The short answer is education and bias. Physicians have erroneously been educated by medical texts that state that oral vitamin B_{12} therapy for pernicious anemia is "unpredictable," has poor patient compliance, and is more costly. These same texts then state that oral cobalamin is effective and can be used when injection therapy is problematic, but the bias against oral treatment has already been established. In a survey of internists, 91% erroneously believed that vitamin B_{12} could not be absorbed in sufficient quantities without intrinsic factor. Interestingly, 88% of these doctors also stated that an effective oral vitamin B_{12} therapy would be useful in their practice and further added that it would be their preferred method of delivery if it was effective. Let's reassure these doctors by answering the concerns regarding oral therapy.

- *Is oral vitamin B_{12} therapy unpredictable?* No, not at an effective dosage. Some of the early studies with oral B_{12} therapy used only 100 to 250 mcg per day. These reports led the U.S. Pharmacopoeia Anti-Anemia Preparations Advisory Board in 1959 to caution against oral therapy for pernicious anemia as being, "at best, unpredictably effective." However, based on what is now known about oral vitamin B_{12} absorption, the response to these low doses must now be considered predictable. It has been established that the average absorption rate of oral cyanocobalamin by patients with pernicious anemia is 1.2% across a wide range of dosages. Thus an oral dosage of 100 to 250 mcg per day results in a average absorption of 1.2 to 3 mcg, respectively—a dosage that is sufficient for many, but not all, patients. The bottom line is that higher dosages are necessary in order for most patients to benefit from oral therapy.

- *How high must the dosage be to produce predictable improvements?* The first month the dosage should be 2,000 mcg per day. After that a dosage of 1,000 mcg per day is recommended.

- *Does oral vitamin B_{12} lead to poor patient compliance?* No. The concern about patient compliance cited by the medical texts is irrational. Why is vitamin B_{12} singled out from all other oral therapies? It simply does not make any sense, especially since studies with oral cobalamin have shown excellent compliance. In many cases, the compliance is higher with an oral preparation, since many patients prefer taking a pill over getting a shot.

- *Does oral vitamin B_{12} cost more than injectable?* No way! The facts are that the two forms—injectable and oral—do not differ much in price for the vitamin B_{12} itself. The difference is in the cost charged to administer the vitamin B_{12} injection— anywhere from $20 in a private practice to $100 in a nursing home. As a result, the injectable form is considerably more expensive.

It should be obvious that there is no basis for the dogmatic belief that vitamin B_{12} must be administered by injection in order to produce clinical benefit. In the treatment of pernicious anemia, the usual dosage recommended by most medical texts is 1,000 mcg weekly for eight weeks, then once a month for life. For oral vitamin B_{12}, the recommended dosage is 2,000 mcg per day (14,000 mcg weekly) for at least one month, followed by a daily intake of 1,000 mcg. Methylcobalamin, the active form of B_{12}, is preferred over cyanocobalamin.

Support for Folic Acid Deficiency Anemia

The diet should focus on foods high in folic acid: liver, asparagus, dried beans, brewer's yeast, dark green leafy vegetables, and whole grains. Since folic acid is destroyed by heat and light, fruits and vegetables should be eaten fresh or with very little cooking. Poor sources of folic acid include most meats, milk, eggs, and root vegetables.

To replenish folic acid stores, 800–1,000 mcg of folic acid should be taken every day for up to one month. Folic acid is available as folic acid (folate) and folinic acid (5-methyltetrahydrofolate). In order to utilize folic acid, the body must first convert it to tetrahydrofolate and then add a methyl group to form 5-methyltetrahydrofolate (folinic acid). Therefore, supplying the body with 5-methyltetrahydrofolate bypasses these steps and is needed for those with a genetic inability to make the conversion. Folinic acid is the most active form of folic acid and has been shown to be more efficient at raising body stores than folic acid.[8]

. . . .

QUICK REVIEW

- **Identifying the cause of anemia through a complete diagnostic workup by a qualified health care professional is essential.**

- **Anemia caused by deficient red blood cell (RBC) production is almost always due to nutrient deficiency. The three most common forms are due to deficiencies of either iron, vitamin B_{12}, or folic acid.**

- **Iron deficiency is the most common cause of anemia.**

- **Perhaps the best food for an individual with any kind of anemia is calf liver.**

- **Although it is popular to inject vitamin B_{12} in the treatment of vitamin B_{12} deficiency, injection is not necessary, as oral administration of an appropriate dosage has been shown to produce excellent results.**

TREATMENT SUMMARY

Effective therapy for anemia is dependent on proper diagnosis of its cause. The following recommendations are given with this in mind. Blood tests should be performed monthly to determine effective treatment.

Diet

The ingestion of 4 to 6 oz calf liver three to five times per week is recommended until the anemia is resolved, along with the liberal consumption of green leafy vegetables. Otherwise, follow the recommendations given in the chapter "A Health-Promoting Diet."

Nutritional Supplements

In addition to the recommendations given in the chapter "Supplementary Measures," here are specific recommendations for each type of anemia.

- For iron deficiency anemia:
  - Iron: 30 mg, bound to either pyrophosphate, succinate, glycinate, or fumarate, twice per day between meals (if this recommendation results in abdominal discomfort, take 30 mg with meals three times per day)
  - Vitamin C: 1 g three times per day with meals
- For vitamin B_{12} deficiency anemia:
  - Oral vitamin B_{12}: 2,000 mcg per day for at least one month, followed by 1,000 mcg per day (methylcobalamin, the active form of vitamin B_{12}, supplied in sublingual tablets, is preferable to cyanocobalamin)
  - Folic acid: 800 to 1,200 mcg three times per day
- For folic acid deficiency anemia:
  - Folic acid: 800 to 1,200 mcg three times per day
  - Vitamin B_{12}: 1,000 mcg per day (it is always necessary to supplement vitamin B_{12} with folic acid to prevent the folic acid supplement from masking a vitamin B_{12} deficiency)

Angina

· ·

- Squeezing or pressure-like pain in the chest occurring immediately after exertion (other precipitating factors include emotional tension, cold weather, or large meals), possibly radiating to the left shoulder blade, left arm, or jaw, and typically lasting for only 1 to 20 minutes

- Stress, anxiety, and high blood pressure typically present

- An abnormal ECG reading (transient ST segment depression) in response to light exercise (stress test)

Angina pectoris is caused by an insufficient supply of oxygen to the heart muscle, which produces a squeezing or pressure-like pain in the chest. Angina usually precedes a heart attack. Since physical exertion and stress increase the heart's need for oxygen, they are often the triggering factors. The pain may radiate to the left shoulder blade, left arm, or jaw. The pain typically lasts for only 1 to 20 minutes.

Angina is almost always due to *atherosclerosis*, the buildup of cholesterol-containing plaque that progressively narrows and ultimately blocks the blood vessels supplying the heart (the coronary arteries). This blockage results in a decreased supply of blood and oxygen to the heart tissue. When the flow of

---

WARNING: An acute angina attack can be a medical emergency. If you are suffering from an acute attack, consult your physician or an emergency room immediately.

---

oxygen to the heart muscle is substantially reduced, or when there is an increased need by the heart, it results in angina. Hypoglycemia (low blood sugar) can also cause angina.[1]

There is another type of angina that is not related to a buildup of plaque in the coronary arteries. It is known as *Prinzmetal's variant angina* and is caused by spasm of a coronary artery. This form of angina is more apt to occur at rest, may occur at odd times during the day or night, and is more common in women under age 50. It usually responds to magnesium supplementation.

Therapeutic Considerations

Angina is a serious condition that requires careful treatment and monitoring. Prescription medications may be necessary in severe cases, as well as in the initial stages of mild to moderate angina. Eventually it should be possible to control the condition with the help of natural measures. If there is significant blockage of the coronary artery, angioplasty, coronary artery bypass, or intravenous EDTA chelation therapy (discussed below) may be appropriate.

Coronary Angiogram, Angioplasty, and Artery Bypass Surgery

An *angiogram* (cardiac catheterization) is an X-ray procedure in which dye is injected

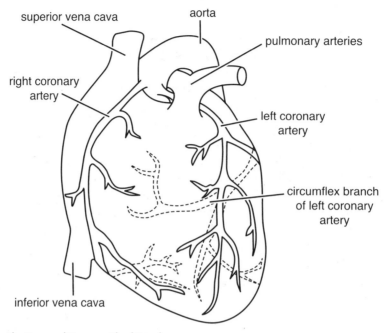

The Heart and Coronary Blood Vessels

into the coronary arteries to locate blockages. These blockages are then most often opened with *balloon angioplasty* (a surgical procedure in which the diameter of the blocked artery is increased with the aid of a very small balloon attached to a flexible tube), the placement of a stent (a tiny wire mesh tube that acts as a scaffolding to maintain and support the opening of an artery), and/or coronary artery bypass surgery (a procedure in which the coronary artery is bypassed by constructing an alternative route using a portion of a vein from the patient's leg). All of these procedures are often agreed to by patients without careful consideration of the risks and benefits.

Angiograms, angioplasty, and bypass surgery are big business. More than 1 million heart angiograms are performed each year, for a total annual cost of over $10 billion. But based upon extensive analysis, it appears that most of this money is wasted.

Several studies have challenged the widespread recommendation of angiograms made by most cardiologists.[2] One study evaluated 168 patients who were told they needed to have an angiogram to determine the degree of blockage, followed by bypass surgery or angioplasty. Using noninvasive tests, such as the exercise stress test, the echocardiogram (an ultrasound exam that measures the size and functional status of the heart), and the Holter heart monitor (a portable heart monitor that is worn for 24 hours and measures the pulse and characterizes beats as normal or abnormal), the researchers determined that 134, or 80%, did not need the catheterization. Over a five-year period, this group of 168 patients had only a 1.1% rate of fatal heart attacks annually. This rate is much lower than the mortality rates associated with either coronary artery bypass surgery (5 to 10%) or angioplasty (1 to 2%). The researchers concluded that "in a large fraction of medically stable patients with coronary disease who are urged to undergo coronary angiography (heart catheterization), the procedure can be safely deferred." Noninvasive testing to determine the functional state of the heart is far more important than the dangerous search for blocked arteries in determining the type of therapy that is needed. If the heart is not functioning well, *then* an angiogram may be needed to see if surgery should be done.

Furthermore, blockages found by an angiogram are usually not relevant to the patient's risk of heart attack. For instance, in the most sophisticated study to date of bypass surgery, the Coronary Artery Surgery Study (CASS), it was demonstrated that heart patients with healthy hearts but with one, two, or all three of the major heart vessels blocked did surprisingly well without surgery.[3–5] Regardless of the number or severity of the blockages, each group had the same low death rate of 1% per year.

That same year, the average death rate from bypass surgery was 10.1%, or about 1 death per 10 operations. In other words, the operation being recommended supposedly to save lives was 5 to 10 times more deadly than the disease. The best that can be said about bypass surgery and balloon angioplasty is that they are irrelevant to the course of the disease in all but the most serious cases. Patients who elect not to have the surgery live just as long as or longer than those who have the surgery.[6]

The severity of blockage does not necessarily correlate with reduction in blood flow in the artery. In one study, Iowa researchers measured blood flow in 44 blockages demonstrated by angiogram.[7] Much to their surprise, they found no correlation between blood flow and the severity of the heart artery blockage. In other words, the angiogram did not provide clinically relevant information. The researchers found in one case that a cor-

onary artery with a 96 percent blockage had a better blood flow than an artery with only a 40 percent blockage. The authors concluded that the blockages found by the heart catheterization simply do not correlate with blood flow restriction, and noted that these results were "profoundly disturbing . . . Information cannot be determined accurately by conventional angiographic approaches."

The bottom line is this: when patients are advised to have a coronary angiogram, chances are 8 out of 10 that they do not need it. The critical factor in whether a patient needs coronary artery bypass surgery or angioplasty is how well the left ventricular pump is working, not the degree of blockage or the number of arteries affected. The left ventricle (chamber) of the heart is responsible for pumping oxygenated blood through the aorta (the large artery emanating from the heart) to the rest of the body. Bypass surgery is helpful only when the *ejection fraction*, the amount of blood pumped by the left ventricle, is less than 40% of capacity.[8] Up to 90% of all bypass procedures are done when the ejection fraction is greater than 50%, which is adequate for circulatory needs. In other words, as many as 90% of all bypass procedures may be unnecessary.

Coronary artery bypass has largely been replaced by angioplasty—or, as it is known in research circles, percutaneous coronary intervention (PCI). The results from large studies with these procedures, including the use of stents that release drugs to prevent blockage (drug-eluting stents), show the same lack of benefit as bypass operations. For example, the Clinical Outcomes Utilizing Revascularization and Aggressive Drug Evaluation (COURAGE) trial revealed that PCI showed no significant differences over medical therapy alone in the primary end point of all-cause mortality or nonfatal heart attacks, or major secondary end points (composites of death, heart attack, and stroke; hospitalization for angina or heart attack) over a 4.6-year follow-up in 2,287 patients with stable coronary artery disease.[8]

When coronary artery bypass surgery or angioplasty is necessary, based on these accepted criteria, it definitely increases long-term survival and gives relief of symptoms for 85% of patients. However, the surgery is not without risk. Complications arising from coronary bypass operations are common, as this surgery represents one of the most technically difficult procedures in modern medicine. Considering the cost of the procedure, the lack of long-term survival benefit, and the high level of complications, it appears that electing to have this surgery is unwise for the majority of patients.

This is particularly true in light of the availability of effective natural alternatives to coronary bypass surgery. Numerous studies have shown that dietary and lifestyle changes can significantly reduce the risk of heart attack and other causes of death due to atherosclerosis (see the chapter "Heart and Cardiovascular Health"). Simple dietary changes—decreasing the amount of saturated fat and cholesterol in the diet; increasing the consumption of dietary fiber, complex carbohydrates, fish oils, and magnesium; eliminating alcohol consumption and cigarette smoking; and reducing high blood pressure—would greatly reduce the number of coronary bypass operations performed in westernized countries. In addition, clinical studies have shown that several nutritional supplements and botanical medicines improve heart function in even the most severe angina cases. Another important alternative is intravenous EDTA chelation therapy (discussed later in this chapter). Although this therapy is controversial, considerable clinical research has proved its efficacy.

When an Angiogram Is Unavoidable

When an angiogram or angioplasty is deemed necessary, the goal is then to prevent the damaging effects produced by this procedure. This can be accomplished with a high-potency multiple vitamin and mineral formula, along with additional vitamin C (minimum 500 mg three times per day) and CoQ_{10} (300 mg per day two weeks prior to surgery and for three months afterward). *Note:* It is generally recommended that garlic supplementation and high dosages of vitamin E (greater than 200 IU) be avoided prior to any surgery because of their ability to possibly promote excessive bleeding by inhibiting platelet aggregation, a key aspect of blood clot formation.

Vitamin C supplementation is rarely employed in hospitals, despite the fact that it may provide significant benefits; low vitamin C status is quite common in hospitalized patients. In a study analyzing the vitamin C status of patients undergoing coronary artery bypass, the plasma concentration of vitamin C was shown to plummet by 70% in the 24 hours after coronary artery bypass surgery; this level persisted in most patients for up to two weeks after surgery.[9] In contrast, vitamin E and carotene levels did not change to any significant degree, presumably because these nutrients are fat-soluble and are therefore retained in the body for longer periods of time. Given the importance of vitamin C, this serious depletion may deteriorate defense mechanisms against free radicals, infection, and wound repair in these patients. Supplementation appears to be essential in patients recovering from heart surgery, or any surgery, for that matter.

Return of blood flow (*reperfusion*) after coronary artery bypass surgery results in oxidative damage to the vascular endothelium and myocardium and thus greatly increases the risk of subsequent coronary artery disease. Coenzyme Q_{10} is recommended in an attempt to prevent such oxidative damage after bypass surgery or angioplasty. In one study, 40 patients undergoing elective surgery either served in the control group or received 150 mg CoQ_{10} each day for seven days before the surgery.[10] The concentrations of lipid peroxides and the enzyme creatine kinase, which indicate myocardial damage, were significantly lower in patients who received CoQ_{10} than in the control group. The treatment group also showed a statistically significant lower incidence of ventricular arrhythmias during the recovery period. These results clearly demonstrate that pretreatment with CoQ_{10} can play a protective role during routine bypass surgery by reducing oxidative damage.

Therapeutic Considerations

Nutritional Supplements

From a natural perspective, there are two primary therapeutic goals in the treatment of angina: improving energy metabolism within the heart and improving blood supply to the heart. These goals are interrelated, as an increased blood flow means improved energy metabolism and vice versa. The heart uses fats as its major metabolic fuel. It converts free fatty acids to energy in much the same way as an automobile uses gasoline. Defects in the utilization of fats by the heart greatly increase the risk of atherosclerosis, heart attack, and angina pain. Specifically, impaired utilization of fatty acids by the heart results in accumulation of high concentrations of fatty acids within the heart muscle. This

makes the heart extremely susceptible to cellular damage, which ultimately leads to a heart attack.

Carnitine, pantethine, and coenzyme Q_{10} are essential compounds in normal fat and energy metabolism and are of extreme benefit to sufferers of angina. These nutrients prevent the accumulation of fatty acids within the heart muscle by improving the conversion of fatty acids and other compounds into energy.

Antioxidants

Using antioxidant supplementation is important for patients with angina. In an analysis of normal controls and patients with either stable or unstable angina, the plasma level of antioxidants has been shown to be a more sensitive predictor of unstable angina than the severity of atherosclerosis.[11,12] One group of researchers concluded: "These data are consistent with the hypothesis that the beneficial effects of antioxidants in coronary artery disease may result, in part, by an influence on lesion activity rather than a reduction in the overall extent of fixed disease."[11]

Antioxidant nutrients are also important for patients on oral nitroglycerin therapy. Oral nitroglycerin is widely used in the conventional treatment of angina, but its continuous use can result in the development of tolerance (loss of effectiveness). Experimental findings indicate that tolerance is associated with increased vascular production of superoxide, a free radical form of oxygen. The superoxide molecules generated quickly degrade the nitric oxide formed from the administration of nitroglycerin and result in lower levels of intracellular regulators that promote relaxation of the coronary arteries. Because vitamin C is the main aqueous (water) phase antioxidant and free radical scavenger of superoxide and vitamin E is the main lipid (fat) phase antioxidant, their importance is obvious. Clinical trials have upheld this connection, showing that high-dose vitamin C and E supplementation can prevent the development of tolerance.[13,14]

Carnitine

Carnitine, a vitamin-like compound, stimulates the breakdown of long-chain fatty acids by the mitochondria, the energy-producing units in cells. Carnitine is essential in the transport of fatty acids into the mitochondria. A deficiency in carnitine results in a decrease in fatty acid concentrations in the mitochondria and reduced energy production.

Normal heart function is critically dependent on adequate concentrations of carnitine. Although the normal heart stores more carnitine than it needs, if the heart does not have a good supply of oxygen, carnitine levels become depleted. This leads to decreased energy production in the heart and increased risk for angina and heart disease. Since angina patients have a decreased supply of oxygen, carnitine supplementation makes good sense.

Several clinical trials have demonstrated that carnitine improves angina and heart disease.[15–19] Supplementation with carnitine normalizes heart carnitine levels and allows the heart muscle to use its limited oxygen supply more efficiently. This translates to an improvement in cases of angina. Improvements have been noted in exercise tolerance and heart function. The results indicate that carnitine is an effective alternative to drugs in cases of angina.

In one study of patients with stable angina, oral administration of 900 mg carnitine increased average exercise time and the time necessary for abnormalities to occur on a stress test (6.4 minutes in the placebo group compared with 8.8 minutes in the carnitine-treated group).[19]

These results indicate that carnitine may be an effective alternative to other anti-angina agents such as beta-blockers, calcium channel blockers, and nitrates, especially in patients with chronic stable angina pectoris.

Carnitine, by improving fatty acid utilization and energy production in the heart muscle, may also prevent the production of toxic fatty acid metabolites. These compounds are extremely damaging, as they activate various inflammatory enzymes and disrupt cellular membrane structures. The changes in the properties of cardiac cell membranes induced by fatty acid metabolites are thought to contribute to impaired heart muscle contractility, increased susceptibility to irregular beats, and eventual death of heart tissue. Supplemental carnitine increases heart carnitine levels and prevents the production of toxic fatty acid metabolites. This has been demonstrated clinically: the early administration of carnitine (40 mg/kg per day) in patients having heart attacks was found to considerably reduce heart damage.[20]

Pantethine

Pantethine is the stable form of pantetheine, the active form of pantothenic acid, which is the fundamental component of coenzyme A (CoA). CoA is involved in the transport of fatty acids to and from cells, as well as to the mitochondria. The synthetic pathway from pantethine to CoA is much shorter than that of pantothenic acid, making pantetheine the preferred therapeutic substance. In addition, pantetheine has significant lipid-lowering activity, while pantothenic acid has very little (if any) effect in lowering cholesterol and triglyceride levels.

The standard dose for pantethine is 900 mg per day. Like carnitine, pantethine has been shown in clinical trials to significantly reduce serum triglyceride and cholesterol levels while increasing HDL cholesterol levels.[21-23] Its lipid-lowering effects are most impressive when its toxicity (virtually none) is compared with that of conventional lipid-lowering drugs. Its mechanism of action is due to inhibiting cholesterol synthesis and accelerating fatty acid breakdown in the mitochondria.

Pantethine is well indicated in angina. Like carnitine levels, heart pantethine levels decrease during times of reduced oxygen supply. Demonstrated effects in animals indicate that pantethine would greatly benefit individuals with angina.[24]

Coenzyme Q_{10} (CoQ_{10})

CoQ$_{10}$ is another essential component of the mitochondria, where it plays a major role in energy production. Like carnitine and pantethine, CoQ$_{10}$ can be synthesized within the body. Nonetheless, deficiency states have been reported. Deficiency can be a result of impaired CoQ$_{10}$ synthesis due to nutritional deficiencies, a genetic or acquired defect in CoQ$_{10}$ synthesis (e.g., statin drugs block CoQ$_{10}$ formation), or increased tissue needs.[25]

Cardiovascular diseases including angina, hypertension, mitral valve prolapse, and congestive heart failure are examples of diseases that require increased tissue levels of CoQ$_{10}$.[25] In addition, many of the elderly may have increased CoQ$_{10}$ requirements: the decline of CoQ$_{10}$ levels that occurs with age may be partly responsible for the age-related deterioration of the immune system.

CoQ$_{10}$ deficiency is common in individuals with heart disease. Heart tissue biopsies in patients with various heart diseases show a CoQ$_{10}$ deficiency in 50 to 75% of cases.[25] One of the most metabolically active tissues in the body, the heart may be unusually susceptible to the effects of CoQ$_{10}$ deficiency. Accordingly, CoQ$_{10}$ has shown great promise in the treatment of angina. In one study 12 patients with stable angina pectoris were treated with CoQ$_{10}$ (150 mg per day for four weeks) in a double-blind crossover trial.[26] Compared with placebo, CoQ$_{10}$ reduced the frequency of angina attacks by 53%. In addition, there was a significant increase in treadmill exercise tolerance (time to onset of chest pain and time to development of ECG abnormalities) during CoQ$_{10}$ treatment. The results of this study and others suggest that CoQ$_{10}$ is a safe and effective treatment for angina pectoris.

Magnesium

Magnesium deficiency may play a major role in angina, including Prinzmetal's variant. A magnesium deficiency has been shown to produce spasms of the coronary arteries and is thought to be a cause of nonocclusive heart attacks.[27] Furthermore, it has been observed that men who die suddenly of heart attacks have significantly lower levels of heart magnesium, as well as potassium, than matched controls.[28]

Making magnesium the treatment of choice for angina due to coronary artery spasm has been suggested by some researchers.[28-30] Magnesium administration has also been found to be helpful in the management of arrhythmias and in angina due to atherosclerosis. Its benefit in these situations is presumably via the same mechanisms responsible for its effects in an acute heart attack.

Since the mid-1980s, eight well-designed studies involving more than 4,000 patients have demonstrated that intravenous magnesium supplementation during the first hour of admission to a hospital for an acute heart attack reduces immediate and long-term complications as well as death rates.[31-33]

The beneficial effects of magnesium in an acute heart attack relate to its ability to do the following:

- Improve energy production within the heart

- Dilate the coronary arteries, improving delivery of oxygen to the heart
- Reduce peripheral vascular resistance, reducing demand on the heart
- Inhibit platelets from aggregating and from forming blood clots
- Reduce the size of the blockage
- Improve heart rate and arrhythmias

Arginine

Arginine supplementation has been shown to be beneficial in a number of cardiovascular diseases, including angina pectoris. Its benefit is thought to occur because it increases nitric oxide levels, thereby improving blood flow and reducing blood clot formation (thrombosis). The degree of improvement offered by arginine supplementation in angina and other cardiovascular diseases can be quite significant. In double-blind studies it has been shown to be especially effective in increasing exercise tolerance. The typical dosage is 6 g per day in divided doses.[34–36] In a short-term study, involving 3 g per day for 15 days, arginine supplementation resulted in increased activity of free-radical-scavenging enzyme superoxide dismutase (SOD) and other antioxidant protective mechanisms.[37] One caution is provided by a study in which heart attack survivors who supplemented with arginine (9 g per day for six months) had an increase in mortality compared with the placebo group (8.6% vs. 0%).[38] This effect may have been an aberration or due to higher dosages of arginine being used.

Botanical Medicines

Hawthorn

Hawthorn (*Crataegus* species) berry and flowering top extracts are widely used in Europe for their cardiovascular activity. They exhibit a combination of effects that are of great value to patients with angina and other heart problems. Studies have demonstrated that hawthorn extracts are effective in reducing angina attacks, as well as in lowering blood pressure and serum cholesterol levels and improving heart function.[39–41]

The beneficial effects in the treatment of angina are due to improvement in the blood and oxygen supply of the heart resulting from dilation of the coronary vessels, as well as improvement of the metabolic processes in the heart.[39–41]

Hawthorn's ability to dilate coronary blood vessels has been repeatedly demonstrated in experimental studies. In addition, hawthorn extracts have been shown to improve cardiac energy metabolism in human and experimental studies. This combined effect is extremely important in the treatment of angina, as it results in improved myocardial function with more efficient use of oxygen. The improvement results not only from increased blood and oxygen supply to the heart muscle but also from hawthorn flavonoids interacting with key enzymes to enhance the heart's ability to contract properly.

Khella

Khella (*Ammi visnaga*) is an ancient medicinal plant native to the Mediterranean region, where it has been used in the treatment of angina and other heart ailments for thousands of years. Several of its components have demonstrated effects in dilating the coronary arteries. Its mechanism of action appears to be similar to that of the calcium-channel-blocking drugs.

Since the late 1940s, there have been numerous scientific studies on the clinical effect of khella extracts in the treatment of angina. More specifically, khellin, a derivative of the plant, was shown to be extremely effective in relieving angina symptoms, improving exercise tolerance, and normalizing ECG tests. The concluding statement in a 1952 study reads: "The high proportion of favorable results, together with the striking degree of improvement frequently observed, has led us to the conclusion that khellin, properly used, is a safe and effective drug for the treatment of angina pectoris."[42]

At higher doses (120 to 150 mg per day), pure khellin was associated with mild side effects such as loss of appetite, nausea, and dizziness. Although most clinical studies used high dosages, several studies show that as little as 30 mg khellin per day appears to offer equally good results with fewer side effects.[43,44]

Rather than the isolated compound khellin, khella extracts standardized for khellin content (typically 12%) are the preferred form. Dose of such an extract would be 250 to 300 mg per day. Khella appears to work well with hawthorn extracts.

Other Therapies

Acupuncture

Several studies have shown acupuncture to be of benefit in improving angina, specifically in reducing nitroglycerin use, decreasing the number of angina attacks, and improving exercise tolerance and ECG readings.[45–48]

Relaxation and Breathing Exercises

Relaxation and breathing exercises may be helpful in improving angina symptoms, especially when anxiety is a significant contributor.[49] In one study in patients with cardiac syndrome X, a form of angina in people with otherwise normal coronary arteries, transcendental meditation (20 minutes twice per day of silently chanting a mantra with eyes closed) was found to reduce angina-like chest pain and to normalize ECGs.[50]

Intravenous Ethylenediaminetetraacetic Acid Chelation (EDTA) Therapy

EDTA chelation therapy is promoted as an alternative to coronary artery bypass surgery and angioplasty. EDTA is an amino-acid-like molecule that, when slowly infused into the bloodstream, binds with minerals such as calcium, iron, copper, and lead and carries them to the kidneys, where they are excreted. EDTA chelation has been commonly used for lead poisoning, but in the late 1950s and early 1960s it was found to help patients with atherosclerosis.

The discovery of EDTA chelation therapy in the treatment of angina and other conditions associated with atherosclerosis happened accidentally. In 1956 a battery worker whom Dr. Norman Clarke was treating with EDTA for lead poisoning noticed that his symptoms of angina disappeared. Clarke and others began using EDTA chelation therapy in patients with angina, cerebral vascular insufficiency, and occlusive peripheral vascular disease.

In a series of 283 patients treated by Clarke and his colleagues from 1956 to 1960, 87% showed improvements in their symptoms. Heart patients improved, and patients with blocked arteries in the legs, particularly those with diabetes, avoided amputation.[51,52]

It was originally thought that EDTA opened blocked arteries by chelating out the calcium deposits in the cholesterol plaque. However, it now seems more related to chelating out excess iron and copper, minerals that, in the presence of oxygen, stimulate free radicals. Free radicals damage the cells in the artery and are a primary reason for atherosclerosis. In a review of the progression and regression of atherosclerosis, the authors write that the process of atherosclerosis is "dependent on the presence of some metals (copper and iron) and can be completely inhibited by chelating agents such as EDTA."[53]

Despite obvious benefits to heart patients, EDTA fell out of favor in the mid-1960s. Advocates believe this occurred for two reasons: (1) the lucrative surgical approach to heart and vessel disease was on the rise and (2) the patent on EDTA that was held by Abbott Laboratories expired, so there was no financial interest for drug companies to fund any research.

Fortunately, in 1972 a small group of practicing physicians using EDTA chelation therapy founded an organization now called the American College for the Advancement of Medicine to continue education and research in this important area.

In the early days of EDTA chelation therapy, several serious problems were discovered. Giving too much EDTA or giving it too fast was soon noted to be dangerous. In fact, several deaths attributed to kidney failure were caused by toxicity in reaction to EDTA. Fortunately, additional research resulted in more appropriate protocols, and EDTA chelation therapy as used now is safe. No deaths or significant adverse reactions have occurred in more than 500,000 patients who have undergone EDTA chelation therapy. Because EDTA chelation improves blood flow throughout the body, the "side

- -

QUICK REVIEW

- **Angina is a serious condition that requires careful treatment and monitoring.**
- **As many as 90% of all bypass procedures may be unnecessary.**
- **The critical factor in whether a patient needs coronary artery bypass surgery or angioplasty is how well the left ventricular pump is working, not the degree of blockage or the number of arteries affected.**
- **Bypass surgery is helpful only when the ejection fraction (the amount of blood pumped by the left ventricle) is less than 40% of capacity.**
- **The two primary therapeutic goals in the natural treatment of angina are:**
  - ○ **Improving energy metabolism within the heart**
  - ○ **Improving the blood supply to the heart**
- **Carnitine and coenzyme Q_{10} (CoQ_{10}) have been shown to improve angina in well-designed double-blind clinical trials.**
- **Magnesium deficiency plays a major role in angina.**
- **Hawthorn extracts improve the supply of blood and oxygen to the heart.**
- **Since the late 1940s, there have been numerous scientific studies that demonstrate the clinical effectiveness of khella extracts in the treatment of angina.**
- **EDTA chelation therapy is an alternative to coronary artery bypass surgery and angioplasty; it may prove to be more effective, and it is definitely safer and less expensive.**

effects" are usually beneficial and only a few adverse effects are noticed.

A substantial body of scientific evidence exists on the use of EDTA chelation therapy in the treatment of angina, peripheral vascular disease, and cerebral vascular disease.[54–58] Nonetheless, there is a lack of well-designed, placebo-controlled studies to definitively assess the efficacy of this approach. This shortcoming is unfortunate considering the early successes. The conclusion from a Cochrane review summarizes the situation well: "At present, there is insufficient evidence to decide on the effectiveness or ineffectiveness of chelation therapy in improving clinical outcomes of patients with atherosclerotic cardiovascular disease."[59]

For more information, contact the American College of Advancement in Medicine (ACAM), 8001 Irvine Center DriveSte 825, Irvine, CA 92618, Phone 949-309-3520; www.acam.org.

TREATMENT SUMMARY

The primary therapy for angina is prevention because angina is usually secondary to atherosclerosis. Once angina has developed, restoring proper blood supply to the heart and enhancing energy production within the heart are necessary. Particularly important nutrients for accomplishing these results are vitamins C and E, carnitine, pantethine, CoQ$_{10}$, magnesium, and arginine. Magnesium is of additional benefit because of its ability to relax spastic coronary arteries and improve heart function.

Hawthorn berries or extracts offer a number of benefits to individuals with angina, including coronary artery dilation and improved heart muscle metabolism.

Individuals with unstable angina pectoris (characterized by a progressive increase in the frequency and severity of pain, increased sensitivity to precipitating factors, progression of symptoms over several days, and prolonged coronary pain) require immediate medical attention.

Diet

The dietary guidelines given in the chapter "A Health-Promoting Diet," as well as in the chapter "Heart and Cardiovascular Health," are appropriate here. In particular, an increase of soluble dietary fiber is recommended (e.g., flaxseed, oat bran, pectin). Onions and garlic (both raw and cooked), vegetables, and fish should also be increased, while the consumption of saturated fats, cholesterol, sugar, and animal proteins should be reduced. All fried foods and food allergens should be avoided. Patients with reactive hypoglycemia should eat regular meals and carefully avoid simple carbohydrates of all forms (e.g., sugar, honey, dried fruit, fruit juice). A Mediterranean-type diet is recommended.

Lifestyle

The individual with angina should not smoke or drink alcohol or coffee. Stress should be decreased by the use of stress

management techniques such as progressive relaxation, meditation, and guided imagery. A carefully graded, progressive aerobic exercise program (30 minutes three times per week) is a necessity. Walking is a good exercise to start with.

Nutritional Supplements

- A high-potency multiple vitamin and mineral formula as described in the chapter "Supplementary Measures"
- Key individual nutrients:
  - Vitamin C: 500 to 1,000 mg per day
  - Vitamin E (mixed tocopherols): 200 to 400 IU per day
  - Magnesium, preferably bound to aspartate, citrate, glycinate or malate: 200 to 400 mg three times per day
- Fish oils: 3,000 mg EPA + DHA per day
- One of the following:
  - Grape seed extract (>95% procyanidolic oligomers): 100 to 300 mg per day
  - Pine bark extract (>95% procyanidolic oligomers): 100 to 300 mg per day
  - Some other flavonoid-rich extract with a similar flavonoid content, super greens formula, or another plant-based antioxidant that can provide an oxygen radical absorption capacity (ORAC) of 3,000 to 6,000 units or higher per day
- Carnitine: 500 mg three times per day
- Pantethine: 300 mg three times per day
- Coenzyme Q_{10}: 100 mg two to three times per day
- Arginine: 1,000 to 2,000 mg three times per day

Botanical Medicines

- Hawthorn (*Crataegus oxyacantha*):
  - Berries or flowers (dried): 3 to 5 g or as a tea three times per day
  - Fluid extract (1:1): 1 to 2 ml (¼ to ½ tsp) three times per day
  - Solid extract (10% proanthocyanidins or 1.8% vitexin-4'-rhamnoside): 150 to 250 mg three times per day
- Khella (*Ammi visnaga*):
  - Dried powdered extract (12% khellin content): 100 mg three times per day

Anxiety

· ·

- Nervousness, anxiety, or inappropriate sense of fear
- Shortness of breath, heart palpitations, and tingling sensations in the extremities

More than 20 million Americans suffer from anxiety, an unpleasant emotional state that can range from mild unease to intense fear. Anxiety differs from fear in that while fear is a rational response to a real danger, anxiety usually lacks a clear or realistic cause. Though some anxiety is normal and even healthy, higher levels of anxiety not only are uncomfortable but also can lead to significant problems.

Anxiety is often accompanied by a variety of symptoms. The most common symptoms relate to the chest, such as heart palpitations (awareness of a more forceful or faster heart beat), throbbing or stabbing pains, a feeling of tightness or inability to take in enough air, and a tendency to sigh or hyperventilate. Tension in the muscles of the back and neck often leads to headaches, back pains, and muscle spasms. Other symptoms can include excessive sweating, dryness of the mouth, dizziness, digestive disturbances, and the constant need to urinate or defecate.

Anxious individuals usually have a constant feeling that something bad is going to happen. They may fear that they have a chronic or dangerous illness—a belief that is reinforced by the symptoms of anxiety. Inability to relax may lead to difficulty in getting to sleep and constant waking in the night.

Panic Attacks

Severe anxiety will often produce what are known as "panic attacks"—intense feelings of fear. Panic attacks may occur independently of anxiety but are most often associated with generalized anxiety or agoraphobia. *Agoraphobia* is an intense fear of being in public places. As a result, most people with agoraphobia become housebound.

Panic attacks are very common; about 15% of the U.S. population will experience a panic attack in their lifetime. Among adults ages 25 to 54, about 1.5 to 3% experience frequent panic attacks.

Causes

Clinical anxiety, including panic attacks, can be produced by psychological problems as well as by biochemical factors such as caffeine, certain other drugs, and the infusion of lactate into the blood. The fact that these compounds can produce anxiety and panic attacks can be put to good use in understanding the underlying biochemical features of anxiety.

Perhaps the most significant biochemical disturbance noted in people with anxiety and panic attacks is an elevated blood lactic acid level and an increased ratio of lactic acid to pyruvic acid. Lactate (the soluble form of lactic acid) is the final product in the breakdown of blood sugar (glucose) when there is a lack of oxygen.

To illustrate how lactic acid is produced, let's take the classic example of the exercising muscle. Muscles prefer to use fat as their energy source, but when you exercise vigorously there isn't enough oxygen, so the muscle must burn glucose. Without oxygen, there is a buildup of lactic acid within the muscle; this is what causes muscle fatigue and soreness after exercise. Let's look more closely at this process.

The first few steps of normal glucose breakdown can occur without oxygen, until pyruvic acid is produced. The next steps require oxygen and end in the complete breakdown of pyruvic acid to carbon dioxide and water. But what happens if there is not enough oxygen? Because the exercising muscle needs energy, the muscle cells continue to convert glucose to pyruvic acid in a process referred to as *anaerobic metabolism*. The pyruvic acid is then converted into a temporary waste product, lactic acid. With good circulation, the lactic acid is removed from the muscle and transported to the liver,

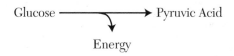

Glucose Breakdown to Pyruvic Acid

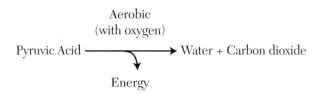

Breakdown of Pyruvic Acid to CO2 and H2O

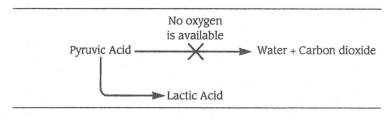

Pyruvic Acid Conversion to Lactic Acid

Lactic Acid Conversion to Pyruvic Acid or Glucose

where it can be turned back into pyruvic acid or even glucose if needed.

All of this biochemistry plays a role in anxiety, because individuals with anxiety have elevated blood levels of lactate and a higher ratio of lactic acid to pyruvic acid when compared with normal controls. Furthermore, if people who get panic attacks are injected with lactate, severe panic attacks are produced. In normal individuals nothing happens. So it appears that individuals with anxiety may be sensitive to lactate. In other words, lactate may be causing their anxiety. Reducing the level of lactate is a critical goal in the treatment of anxiety and panic attacks.

Therapeutic Considerations

The natural approach to anxiety builds upon the recommendations given for stress in the chapter "Stress Management." After all, anxiety is usually a symptom of severe stress. If you suffer from mild anxiety, follow all of the recommendations given in that chapter for diet, exercise, nutritional supplementation, calming the mind and body, and taking an adrenal adaptogen. If you suffer from moderate to severe anxiety, follow all of the recommendations in that chapter as well as those discussed below; substitute kava for the adrenal adaptogen.

Lactate Levels

As pointed out previously, increased lactic acid levels may be an underlying factor in panic attacks and anxiety. The goal is to prevent the conversion of pyruvic acid to lactic acid and to improve the conversion of lactic acid back to pyruvic acid. Nutrition appears to play a key role in achieving this goal. There

are at least six nutritional factors that may be responsible for elevated lactate levels or ratios of lactic acid to pyruvic acid:[1]

1. Alcohol
2. Caffeine
3. Sugar
4. Deficiency of the B vitamins niacin, pyridoxine, and thiamine
5. Deficiency of calcium or magnesium
6. Food allergens

By avoiding alcohol, caffeine, sugar, and food allergens, people with anxiety can go a long way toward relieving their symptoms. Simply eliminating coffee can result in complete relief from symptoms. This recommendation may seem too simple to be valid, but substantial clinical evidence indicates that in many cases it is all that is necessary. For example, one study dealt with four men and two women who had generalized anxiety or panic disorder. Their caffeine consumption ranged from 1½ to 3½ cups of coffee per day. Avoiding caffeine for one week brought about significant relief of symptoms.[2] The degree of improvement was so noticeable that all patients volunteered to continue abstaining from caffeine. Previously, these patients had been only minimally helped by drug therapy. Follow-up exams 6 to 18 months afterward indicated that five out of the six patients were completely without symptoms; the sixth patient became asymptomatic with a very low dose of Valium.

By following the guidelines in the chapter "A Health-Promoting Diet," as well as the recommendations for nutritional supplementation given in the chapter "Supplementary Measures," you will provide your body with the kind of nutritional support it needs to counteract the biochemical derangements found in patients with anxiety and panic attacks.

Nutritional Supplements

Omega-3 Fatty Acids

Anxiety and depression appear to be linked to lower levels of omega-3 fatty acids.[3] The mechanism appears to be that both depression and anxiety can enhance the production of pro-inflammatory compounds known as cytokines. A high intake of omega-6 fatty acids (found in corn-fed animal products, dairy products, and common vegetable oils such as corn, soy, safflower, and sunflower) and a low intake of omega-3 fatty acids (found in fish, fish oils, and flaxseed oil) can lead to an amplification in the production of these cytokines. Cytokines not only promote inflammation but also appear to affect the way we feel. So increasing the intake of omega-3 fatty acids and lowering the intake of omega-6 fatty acids may help to reduce anxiety and depression. The positive results seen with fish oil supplements in clinical depression are well documented. In regard to anxiety, one clinical study showed that fish oil supplementation decreased feelings of anger and anxiety in substance abusers.[4] In a detailed study involving medical students, 2.5 g long-chain omega-3 fatty acids (2,085 mg EPA and 348 mg DHA) from fish oils per day produced a 14% decrease in cytokine production and a 20% reduction in anxiety symptoms.[5]

Flaxseed oil, a source of the short-chain omega-3 fatty acid alpha-linolenic acid, has also shown antianxiety effects. In one study, three out of four patients with a history of agoraphobia for 10 or more years improved within two to three months after taking flaxseed oil at a dosage of 2 to 6 tbsp per day, in divided doses depending upon response.[6] All patients had signs of essential fatty acid deficiency, such as dry skin, dandruff, brittle fingernails that grow slowly, and nerve disorders.

Kava

The area of Oceania—the island communities of the Pacific, including Micronesia, Melanesia, and Polynesia—is one of the few geographic areas in the world that did not have alcoholic beverages before European contact in the 18th century. However, these islanders did possess a magical drink that was used in ceremonies and celebrations because of its calming effect and ability to promote sociability. The drink, called kava, is still used today in this region, where the people are often referred to as the happiest and friendliest in the world. Preparations of kava root *(Piper methysticum)* gained popularity in Europe and the United States up until 2001, when safety concerns (discussed below) derailed their popularity.

Several clinical trials utilized a special kava extract standardized to contain 70% kavalactones. However, this high percentage of kavalactones may be sacrificing some of the other constituents that may contribute to the pharmacology of kava. Therefore, preparations around 30% may prove to be the most effective. More important than the actual percentage of kavalactones is the total dosage of the kavalactones and the assurance that the full range of kavalactones is present.

In one of the first double-blind studies, a 70% kavalactone extract was shown to exhibit significant therapeutic benefit in patients suffering from anxiety.[7] Twenty-nine patients were assigned to receive 100 mg kava extract three times per day, while another 29 patients received a placebo. Therapeutic effectiveness was evaluated using several standard psychological assessments, including the Hamilton Anxiety Scale. The results of this four-week study indicated that individuals who took kava extract had a statistically significant reduction in symptoms of anxiety, including feelings of nervousness and somatic complaints such as heart palpitations, chest pains, headache, dizziness, and feelings of gastric irritation. No side effects were reported with the kava extract.

Studies have also compared the effects of a kava extract with antianxiety drugs such as buspirone and opipramol. In one double-blind study, 129 patients with generalized anxiety disorder were given either 400 mg kava (30% kavalactones), 10 mg buspirone, or 100 mg opipramol per day for eight weeks. Detailed analysis showed that no significant differences could be observed in terms of efficacy and safety. About 75% of patients were classified as responders (at least a 50% reduction of the anxiety score) in each treatment group, and about 60% achieved full remission.[8]

Kava has also been shown to be particularly effective in relieving anxiety in perimenopausal and postmenopausal women.[9–11] In one double-blind study, two groups of 20 women with menopause-related symptoms were treated with 70% kavalactone extract (100 mg three times per day) or a placebo.[11] The measured variable was once again the Hamilton Anxiety Scale. The group receiving the kava extract demonstrated significant improvement at the end of the very first week of treatment. Scores continued to improve over the course of the eight-week study. In addition to symptoms of stress and anxiety, a number of other symptoms also improved. Most notably there was an overall improvement in subjective well-being, mood, and general symptoms of menopause, including hot flashes. As with previous studies, no side effects were noted.

Additional studies have shown that unlike benzodiazepines (Valium-like drugs), alcohol, and other drugs, kava extract is not associated with depressed mental function or impairment in driving or the operation of heavy equipment.[12,13] In one of these studies, 12 healthy volunteers were tested in a double-blind crossover manner to assess the effects of oxazepam, 70% kavalactone extract (200 mg three times per day for five days), and a placebo.[13] The subjects' task was to identify within a list of visually presented words those that were shown for the first time and those that were being repeated. Like other benzodiazepines, oxazepam inhibited the recognition of both new and old words. In contrast, kava allowed a slightly greater recognition rate and a larger difference between old and new words. The results of this study once again demonstrate the unusual effects of kava. In this case, it relieves anxiety, but unlike standard antianxiety drugs, kava actually improves mental function and, at the recommended levels, does not promote sedation.

In 2009, the first documented human clinical trial assessing the antianxiety and antidepressant efficacy of a water-based extract of kava was published.[14] The Kava Anxiety Depression Spectrum Study was a three-week placebo-controlled, double-blind crossover trial that recruited 60 adult participants with one month or more of elevated generalized anxiety. The kava preparation produced significant antianxiety and antidepressant activity and raised no liver toxicity or safety concerns at the dose and duration studied. Specifically, kava reduced participants' Hamilton Anxiety Scale score in the first controlled phase by –9.9 vs. –0.8 for the placebo and in the second controlled phase by –10.3 vs. +3.3. Pooled analyses also revealed highly significant relative reductions in other anxiety and depression scale scores.

The dosage of kava preparations is based on their level of kavalactones. As a result of clinical studies, the recommendation for anxiety-relieving effects is 45 to 70 mg kavalactones three times per day. For sedative effects, the same daily quantity (135 to 210 mg) can be taken as a single dose one hour before retiring.

To put the therapeutic dosage in perspective, it is important to point out that a standard bowl of traditionally prepared kava drink contains approximately 250 mg kavalactones, and several bowls may be consumed at one sitting.

Kava can have significant side effects. In November 2001, German health authorities announced that 24 cases of liver disease (including hepatitis, liver failure, and cirrhosis) associated with the use of kava had been reported; of the affected individuals, one died and three required a liver transplant. As a result, in December 2001 the U.S. Food and Drug Administration began advising consumers of the potential risk of severe liver injury associated with the use of kava-containing dietary supplements. Kava was subsequently withdrawn form the market in the European Union, the United Kingdom, and Canada. In 2007, Germany reevaluated the data and allowed kava back on the market.

In the initial report the true nature of kava-induced liver damage was clouded by the fact that in 18 of these cases, conventional prescription or over-the-counter pharmaceutical drugs with known or potential liver toxicity were also being used. Proponents of kava quickly argued that it was entirely possible that the use of kava by these individuals was a coincidence rather than the cause of the liver problem. As of 2007 of the approximately 100 cases of liver toxicity that had been reported worldwide, only in 14 cases was causality deemed to be "probable."[15] Two drug monitoring studies, including a total of 7,078 patients taking 120 to 150 mg kava extract per day, had not found a single case of kava-induced liver toxicity. Nonetheless, as of 2011, the liver toxicity of kava cannot be ruled out.

The existing data are complex, but it looks as if the major factor in any kava-induced liver toxicity was the use of non-root parts such as stems and leaves as well as stem peelings.[16] It turns out that there wasn't enough kava root to meet skyrocketing demand. Suppliers then knowingly or unknowingly bought the leaves and peelings of kava. Up until that development, the only parts of the kava plant

QUICK REVIEW

- Perhaps the most significant biochemical disturbance noted in people with anxiety and panic attacks is an elevated blood lactate level.
- There are at least six nutritional factors that may be responsible for an elevated ratio of lactic acid to pyruvic acid:
  - Alcohol
  - Caffeine
  - Sugar
  - Deficiency of the B-vitamins niacin, pyridoxine, and thiamine
  - Deficiency of calcium or magnesium
  - Food allergens
- Kava extract has produced relief from anxiety comparable to that from drugs such as Valium, but it must be used with caution and is contraindicated for those with liver disease.

that were traditionally used throughout its 3,000-year history were the roots, never the peelings or the leaves. According to a WHO report, German pharmaceutical industries preferred to buy kava stem peelings to extract kavalactones to make kava drugs; kava stem peelings were sold at almost one-tenth of the price of kava roots.[17] In addition, dosage may also have been a factor in some of the cases of liver toxicity. A survey of 400 German medical practices showed that 78% of the kava prescriptions that were written prior to 2001 significantly exceeded the recommended intake.[18] Nonetheless, there have been reports of hepatitis in patients using kava at dosages equal to or only slightly higher than recommended levels, indicating other factors beyond dosage.[19] Flavokawain B, a chalcone from kava root, has been identified as a potent liver toxin.

Measures suggested to address the liver toxicity issue include (1) use of a noble kava cultivar that is at least five years old at time of harvest, (2) use of peeled and dried rhizomes and roots, (3) dosage recommendation of ≤250 mg kavalactones per day (for medicinal use), and (4) manufacturer quality control systems enforced by strict policing.[16] Another important step may be determination of flavokawain B. It should be mentioned that while it has been suggested that traditional aqueous extracts should be used instead of alcoholic or acetonic extracts, the toxicity is linked to the kava plant itself, possibly with a low-quality plant or wrong plant part, rather than the method of extraction or solvent.[20]

At this time, kava is not recommended for use by anyone who has any liver problems or who is a regular consumer of alcohol. Use of kava for more than four weeks requires close monitoring of liver enzymes once every four to six weeks. Patients should be instructed to discontinue use of kava if symptoms of jaundice (e.g., dark urine, yellowing of the eyes) occur. Nonspecific symptoms of liver disease include nausea, vomiting, light-colored stools, unusual tiredness, weakness, stomach or abdominal pain, and loss of appetite. Kava is not recommended for use by pregnant or breastfeeding women.

Kava has the potential to interact with a wide range of medications and may also potentiate the effects of benzodiazepines, barbiturates, and prescription sedative drugs (sleeping pills).[21] There is also evidence that kava interferes with dopamine or other drugs used in the treatment of Parkinson's disease; therefore, until this issue is resolved, kava extract should not be used by patients with Parkinson's disease.[22]

. . . .

TREATMENT SUMMARY

Effective treatment for anxiety must address psychological as well as physiological factors. In that regard, it is important to follow these recommendations:

- **Reduce or eliminate the use of stimulants.**
- **Follow the dietary, lifestyle, and supplement recommendations in the chapter "Stress Management," as well as those given below.**

Note: **If you are currently taking a sedative-hypnotic or antidepressant drug, you will need to work with a physician to get off the drug. Stopping the drug on** your own can be dangerous; you absolutely must have proper medical supervision.

Diet

Follow the guidelines in the chapter "A Health-Promoting Diet." It is especially important to:

- Eliminate or restrict caffeine
- Eliminate or restrict alcohol
- Eliminate refined carbohydrates
- Increase the potassium-to-sodium ratio of the diet
- Eat regular planned meals in a relaxed environment
- Control food allergies

Lifestyle

Follow the recommendations in the chapter "A Health-Promoting Lifestyle" and the chapter "Stress Management." It is especially important to:

- Identify stressors
- Eliminate or reduce sources of stress
- Identify negative coping patterns and replace them with positive ones
- Perform a relaxation/breathing exercise for a minimum of five minutes twice a day
- Manage time effectively
- Enhance relationships through better communication
- Get regular exercise

Nutritional Supplements

- A high-potency multiple vitamin and mineral formula as described in the chapter "Supplementary Measures"
- Key individual nutrients:
  - Calcium: 1,000 mg per day
  - Magnesium: 350 to 500 mg per day.
  - Vitamin D_3: 2,000 to 4,000 IU per day (ideally, measure blood levels and adjust dosage accordingly)
  - Vitamin B_6: 25 to 50 mg per day
  - Folic acid: 800 mcg per day
  - Vitamin B_{12}: 800 mcg per day
  - Vitamin K_2 (MK-7): 100 mcg per day
- Fish oils: 1,000 to 3,000 mg EPA + DHA per day
- Flaxseed oil: 1 tbsp per day
- One of the following:
  - Grape seed extract (>95% procyanidolic oligomers): 100 to 300 mg per day
  - Pine bark extract (>95% procyanidolic oligomers): 100 to 300 mg per day
  - Or some other flavonoid-rich extract with a similar flavonoid content, "super greens formula," or another plant-based antioxidant that can provide an oxygen radical absorption capacity (ORAC) of 3,000 to 6,000 units or more per day

Botanical Medicines

- One of the following:
  - *Panax ginseng* (Chinese or Korean ginseng):
    - High-quality crude ginseng root: 1.5 to 2 g one to three times per day

- Fluid extract (containing a minimum of 10.5 mg/ml ginsenosides with an Rb1/Rg1 ratio of 2:1): 2 to 4 ml (½ to 1 tsp) one to three times per day
- Solid (dry powdered) extract (standardized to contain 5% ginsenosides with an Rb1/Rg1 ratio of 2:1): 250 to 500 mg one to three times per day
○ Siberian ginseng (*Eleutherococcus senticosus*):
- Dried root: 2 to 4 g one to three times per day
- Fluid extract (1:1): 2 to 4 ml (½ to 1 tsp) or 2 to 4 g one to three times per day

- Solid (dry powdered) extract (20:1, or standardized to contain more than 1% eleutheroside E): 100 to 200 mg or 2 to 4 g one to three times per day
○ *Rhodiola rosea* (Arctic root): For a dosage target of 3.6 to 7.2 mg rosavin, the daily dose would be 360 to 600 mg for an extract standardized for 1% rosavin, 180 to 300 mg for 2% rosavin, and 100 to 200 mg for 3.6% rosavin.
○ *Withania somnifera* (ashwagandha), equivalent to Sensoril: 125 to 250 mg per day[22]
○ Kava (*Piper methysticum*): dosage equivalent to 45 to 70 mg kavalactones three times per day

Asthma

- Recurrent attacks of shortness of breath, cough, and coughing up thick mucus
- Prolonged expiration phase with generalized wheezing and abnormal breath sounds
- Laboratory signs of allergy (increased levels of eosinophils in blood, increased serum IgE levels, positive food and/or inhalant allergy tests)

Asthma is a breathing disorder characterized by spasm and swelling of the bronchial airways along with excessive excretion of a viscous mucus that can also make breathing difficult. Asthma affects approximately 7% of the population of the United States and causes 4,210 deaths per year. Although it occurs at all ages, it is most common in children younger than 10. There is a 2:1 male-to-female ratio among affected children, which equalizes by the age of 30.[1]

The incidence of asthma is rising rapidly in the United States, especially in children. Reasons often given to explain the rise in asthma include the following:

- Increased stress on the immune system due to factors such as greater chemical pollution in the air, water, insect allergens (mostly from dust mites), and food
- Earlier weaning and earlier introduction of solid foods to infants
- Food additives
- Higher incidence of obesity[2]

- Genetic manipulation of plants, resulting in food components with greater allergenic tendencies

In addition, certain genetic variables may make certain individuals more susceptible to asthma.[3–6]

Major Categories

Asthma has typically been divided into two categories: extrinsic and intrinsic. *Extrinsic* or *atopic asthma* is generally considered an allergic condition with a characteristic increase in IgE—the antibody produced by white blood cells that can bind to specialized white blood cells, known as mast cells, and cause the release of mediators such as histamine. *Intrinsic asthma* is associated with a bronchial reaction that is due not to an allergy but rather to such factors as chemicals, cold air, exercise, infection, and emotional upset.

Asthma is often clinically classified according to the frequency of symptoms, forced expiratory volume in 1 second (FEV_1), and peak flow rate.

WARNING: An acute asthma attack can be a medical emergency. If you are suffering from an acute attack, consult your physician immediately or go to an emergency room.

Clinical Classification of Asthma Severity				
SEVERITY IN PATIENTS 12 AND OLDER	**SYMPTOM FREQUENCY**	**NIGHTTIME SYMPTOMS**	**FEV_1, % OF PREDICTED**	**FEV_1 VARIABILITY**
Intermittent	Less than 2 times week	1 or 2 times a month	≥80%	<20%
Mild persistent	2 or more times a week but not every day	3 or 4 times a month	≥80%	20–30%
Moderate persistent	Every day	More than 1 time a week but not nightly	60–80%	>30%
Severe persistent	Throughout the day	Frequent (often 7 times a week)	<60%	>30%

Diagnostic Considerations

The U.S. National Asthma Education and Prevention Program (NAEPP) guidelines for the diagnosis and management of asthma state that a diagnosis of asthma begins by determining if any of the following indicators are present:

- Wheezing (high-pitched whistling sounds during breathing out), especially in children. (Lack of wheezing and a normal chest examination do not exclude asthma.)

- History of any of the following:
  - Cough, worse particularly at night
  - Recurrent wheezing
  - Recurrent difficulty breathing
  - Recurrent chest tightness

- Symptoms occur or worsen in the presence of:
  - Exercise
  - Viral infection
  - Animals with fur or hair
  - Dust mites (in mattresses, pillows, upholstered furniture, carpets)
  - Mold
  - Smoke (from tobacco or wood)
  - Pollen
  - Changes in weather
  - Strong emotional expression (laughing or crying hard)
  - Airborne chemicals or dusts
  - Onset of menstruation

- Symptoms occur or worsen at night, awakening the patient

Determining respiratory function with the use of a spirometer plays a central role in the management of asthma and should be performed at the time of initial diagnosis, after treatment is initiated and symptoms are stabilized, whenever control of symptoms deteriorates, and every one or two years on a regular basis.

Causes

Asthma is caused by a complex interaction of environmental and genetic factors. The strongest risk factor for developing asthma is a history of allergies such as eczema (atopic dermatitis) and hay fever. The presence of atopic dermatitis increases the risk of asthma three- to fourfold. Allergies and the response of the immune system are obviously involved in asthma. The specific imbalance is an increase in the number or function of specialized white blood cells known as Th2 helper T cells. These cells ultimately lead to an increase in the release of compounds that heighten the allergic response.[2-4]

Both extrinsic and intrinsic factors trigger the release from mast cells of chemicals that mediate (produce or control) inflammation. The inflammatory mediators are responsible for the signs and symptoms of asthma. They are either preformed in little packets (granules) within mast cells or generated from fatty acids that reside in cell membranes.

The preformed mediators include histamine and compounds known as leukotrienes. These compounds are responsible for producing much of the allergic reaction seen in asthma. Some leukotrienes are 1,000 times more potent than histamine as stimulators of bronchial constriction and allergy. It has been observed that asthmatics have a tendency to form higher levels of leukotrienes.[5] This abnormality is further aggravated in patients with aspirin-induced asthma. Aspirin and other nonsteroidal anti-inflammatory drugs (NSAIDs, such as indomethacin and ibuprofen) result in the production of excessive levels of leukotrienes in sensitive individuals.[6,7] Tartrazine (yellow dye #5) produces similar effects on leukotriene levels and is often a cause of asthma, particularly in children. Tartrazine is added to most processed foods and can even be found in vitamin preparations and anti-asthma prescription drugs. Tartrazine may also indirectly support the asthmatic process via its role as an antimetabolite of vitamin B_6 (see the discussion in "Tryptophan Metabolism and Pyridoxine Supplementation," later in this chapter).

The Autonomic Nervous System and Adrenal Glands

The autonomic nervous system and adrenal glands are also involved in asthma.[8] Some of the inflammatory mediators block the beta-2 receptors for the neurotransmitter epinephrine (adrenaline), secreted by the adrenal gland. This ultimately results in constriction of the smooth muscle of the airway, as well as the release of histamine and other allergic compounds from mast cells and basophils. Also, if the adrenal gland is not producing sufficient levels of cortisol and epinephrine, it can set the stage for bronchial constriction.

Pertussis Vaccine

An evaluation of 448 children and adolescents in Britain who had received only breast milk for the first six months of life, and in particular on the first day after birth, produced some interesting findings. All of the children were weaned after one year of age and were older than four years at the time the parents responded. The mean age was 7.87 years. In response to the question "Has your child ever been diagnosed as asthmatic?" there were 30 positive answers (6.72%). The surprise came when the researchers classified the respondents according to whether or not they had received the pertussis (whooping cough) vaccine.[9]

Among the 243 immunized children, 26 were diagnosed as having asthma (10.69%). In contrast, of the 203 children who had not been immunized, only 4 had asthma (1.97%). The relative risk of developing asthma from the pertussis vaccine was 5.43 in this study.

Even though all of the children who received the pertussis vaccine received other vaccinations, the researchers suspected that the statistical evidence focused on pertussis. Among the children who did not receive the pertussis vaccine, most had received some other vaccination. Of the 91 subjects of the study who received no vaccines, only one had asthma, compared with 3 of the 112 who had other vaccinations. Therefore the relative risk of developing asthma is about 1% in children receiving no immunizations, 3% in those receiving vaccinations other than pertussis, and 11% for those receiving the pertussis vaccine. Another finding to weigh is that in the group not immunized against pertussis, 16 developed the disease, compared with only 1 in the immunized group.

Influenza Vaccine

One evaluation of more than 9,600 children was employed to determine the safety of intranasal influenza virus vaccine in children. Although this relatively new vaccination was deemed safe for children and adolescents, there was a four times greater risk in children 18 to 35 months old of asthma and associated reactive airway disease.[10]

Antibiotics, Probiotics, and Mucosal IgA

In a combined analysis of seven studies involving more than 12,000 youngsters, researchers at the University of British Columbia found that those prescribed antibiotics before their first birthday were more than twice as likely as untreated children to develop asthma.[11] If they had had multiple courses of antibiotics, that bumped up the risk even higher—16% for every course of the drugs taken before age one. There are a couple of explanations for this association between antibiotic use and asthma. One is that antibiotics contribute to a state of "excess hygiene," leading to reduced exposure to microbes, which in turn creates an oversensitive immune system that mounts an over-the-top allergic reaction to pollen and dust mites, ultimately leading to asthma. The second explanation is that antibiotics have a negative effect on the normal flora of the gastrointestinal and respiratory passages. Some studies have shown that giving probiotics (active lactobacillus and bifidobacteria cultures) lowers the risk of atopic allergic disease such as asthma and eczema. Some of this protective effect may be mediated by mucosal IgA, an antibody that participates in antigen elimination. In a group of 237 allergy-prone infants given either a combination of four probiotic strains or a placebo, researchers found that the probiotic supplementation increased fecal IgA while reducing inflammatory markers.[12] In infants with high fecal IgA concentration at the age of six months, the risk of having any allergic disease or any IgE-associated (atopic) disease before the age of two years was cut by nearly 50%. High intestinal IgA in early life is associated with minimal intestinal inflammation and indicates reduced risk for IgE-associated allergic diseases.

Therapeutic Considerations

The first step in the natural approach to asthma is to reduce allergic tendencies. Allergens can be viewed as straws on a camel's back. Adding enough straws to the camel's back will ultimately cause the camel's back to break. Similarly, increasing the exposure to allergens will ultimately cause symptoms. By reducing allergic tendencies, as well as the offending allergens in many cases, the allergic process can be prevented. There are two primary ways to increase the allergic threshold: reduce exposure to airborne allergens and reduce intake of food allergens.

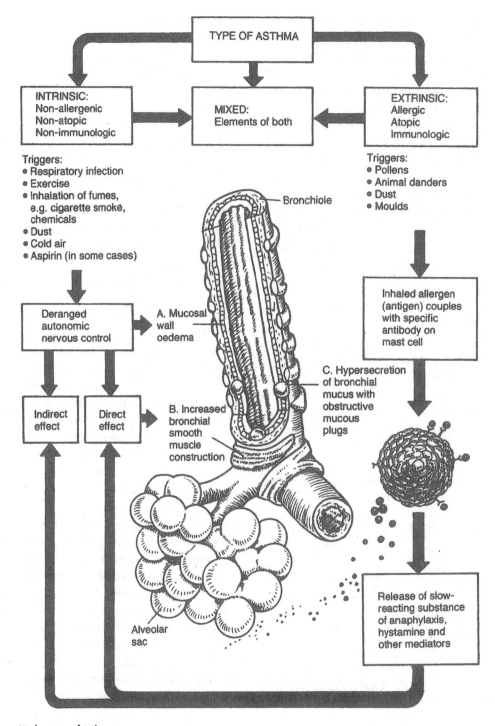

TYPE OF ASTHMA

INTRINSIC:
Non-allergenic
Non-atopic
Non-immunologic

MIXED:
Elements of both

EXTRINSIC:
Allergic
Atopic
Immunologic

Triggers:
• Respiratory infection
• Exercise
• Inhalation of fumes,
  e.g. cigarette smoke,
  chemicals
• Dust
• Cold air
• Aspirin (in some cases)

Triggers:
• Pollens
• Animal danders
• Dust
• Moulds

Bronchiole

Deranged
autonomic
nervous control

A. Mucosal
wall
oedema

Inhaled allergen
(antigen) couples
with specific
antibody on
mast cell

Indirect
effect

Direct
effect

B. Increased
bronchial
smooth
muscle
construction

C. Hypersecretion
of bronchial
mucus with
obstructive
mucous
plugs

Alveolar
sac

Release of slow-
reacting substance
of anaphylaxis,
hystamine and
other mediators

Mechanisms of Asthma

Airborne Allergens

Airborne allergens, such as pollen, dander, and dust mites, are often difficult to avoid entirely, but measures can be taken to reduce exposure. Removing dogs and cats as well as surfaces where allergens can collect (carpets, rugs, upholstered furniture) is a great first step. If this can't be done entirely, make sure that the bedroom is as allergy-proof as possible. Encase the mattress in an allergen-proof plastic; wash sheets, blankets, pillowcases, and mattress pads every week in hot water with additive- and fragrance-free detergent; consider using bedding material made from Ventflex, a special hypoallergenic synthetic material; and install an air purifier. The best mechanical air purifiers are HEPA (high-efficiency particulate air) filters, which can be put into rooms or attached to central heating and air-conditioning systems.

For high-risk children, breastfeeding can produce significant benefits. First, there is substantial evidence that breastfeeding alone has some effect in the prevention of asthma.[13,14] But when breastfeeding is combined with allergy avoidance, even better results are seen. For example, the Canadian Asthma Primary Prevention study collected two years of data in which researchers chose 545 infants who were considered at high risk of asthma on the basis of family history.[15] These children were broken down into control and intervention groups. The interventions included (1) house dust control measures; (2) recommendations for avoidance of pets, environmental tobacco smoke, and day care during the first year; and (3) only breastfeeding or use of partially hydrolyzed whey formula until at least the age of four months. At one year of age, asthma was significantly reduced by 34% in the intervention group. At two years of age, the intervention group had 60% fewer children with persistent asthma

and a 90% reduction in recurrent wheezing. Studies such as this one are quite useful in order to show the effectiveness of a combined approach vs. a single intervention.

Food Allergies

Many studies have indicated that food allergies can play an important role in asthma.[16–20] Adverse reactions to food may be immediate or delayed. Double-blind food challenges in children have shown that immediate-onset sensitivities are usually due to (in decreasing order of frequency) eggs, fish, shellfish, nuts, and peanuts, while foods most commonly associated with delayed onset include (in decreasing order of frequency) milk, chocolate, wheat, citrus, and food colorings. Elimination diets have been successful in identifying allergens and treating asthma and are a particularly valuable diagnostic and therapeutic tool in infants.[17] Elimination of common allergens during a child's first two years has been shown to reduce allergic tendencies in high-risk children (e.g., those with a strong family history).[13]

The presence of food allergies greatly lowers the threshold for asthma. In other words, it sets the stage for overreactivity of the airways to airborne allergens. Something as simple as lack of stomach acid production may be responsible for food allergies in asthmatics. Gastric analyses in 200 asthmatic children in 1931 showed that 80% of them had gastric acid secretions below normal levels.[21] This high occurrence suggests that decreased gastric acid output may predispose these children to food allergies, have a major impact on the success of rotation or elimination diets, and if not corrected lead to the development of additional food allergies.

Food allergies are thought to be responsible for "leaky gut" syndrome in asthmatics.[22] Another important consideration is an overgrowth of the common yeast *Candida albicans*.[23] As a result of increased gut permeability due to either a leaky gut or candida, there is a greater antigen load on the immune system. This subsequently overwhelms the immune system and the ability of the Kupfer cells in the liver to clear immune complexes and incompletely digested proteins from the intestines, increasing the likelihood of developing additional allergies as well as increasing the amount of bronchoconstrictive compounds in circulation. It is essential to identify offending foods as soon as possible to avoid the development of further allergies. For more information, see the chapter "Food Allergy."

Food Additives

Vitally important in the control of asthma is the elimination of food additives.[24] Artificial dyes and preservatives are widely used in foods, beverages, and drugs. In particular, the dye tartrazine and the preservatives benzoate, sulfur dioxide, and sulfite have been reported to cause asthma attacks in susceptible individuals.[24,25] It is estimated that 2 to 3 mg sulfites are consumed each day by the average U.S. citizen, while an additional 5 to 10 mg are ingested by wine and beer drinkers.

It has been postulated that a deficiency of the trace mineral molybdenum may be responsible for sulfite sensitivity.[26] Sulfite oxidase, the enzyme responsible for neutralizing sulfites, is molybdenum dependent.

Salt

Strong evidence indicates that an increased intake of salt raises bronchial reactivity and mortality from asthma.[27,28] The degree of bronchial reactivity to histamine is positively correlated with two-hour urinary sodium excretion and rises with increased dietary sodium. Because the severity of asthma correlates with the degree of bronchial reactivity, the severity of asthma can clearly be influenced by alterations in dietary sodium consumption.

Beneficial Foods

A number of research studies corroborate the notion that people who have a diet rich in fruit and vegetables have a lower risk of poor respiratory health.[29–31] This effect is most likely due to the increased levels of antioxidants. One study found that among children, consumption of fresh fruit, particularly fruit high in vitamin C, has been related to a lower prevalence of asthma symptoms and higher lung function.[32] The effect was observed even at low levels of fruit consumption (one or two servings per week, compared with less than one serving per week); this suggests that even a small increase in fruit intake could be beneficial. This same review discussed consumption of fish as also being related to lower airway hyperreactivity among children and higher lung function in adults.

A study of Scottish adults also found a dose-response relationship between fruit consumption and pulmonary function, whereby increased fruit consumption led to decreases in phlegm and better pulmonary function.[33] Another study of 607 asthma patients and 864 controls highlighted apples and moderate amounts of red wine (preferably low in sulfites) as sources of antioxidants that decreased asthma severity.[34]

Dietary intake of soy foods may be helpful, as the soy isoflavone genistein is associated with reduced severity of asthma and improved lung function.[35] While this effect may be due to some antioxidant action, studies have also shown that genistein is able to block the manufacture of allergic mediators, including leukotrienes, in asthma patients.[36,37] However, when increasing soy consumption, be sure to check for an allergic reaction.

Vegan Diet

A long-term trial of a vegan diet (elimination of all animal products) provided significant improvement in 92% of the 25 treated patients who completed the study (nine dropped out).[38] Improvement was determined by a number of clinical variables, including lung capacity, FEV_1, and physical working capacity. The researchers also found a reduction in susceptibility to infectious disease. Note, however, that although 71% of the patients responded within four months, one year of therapy was required before the 92% level was reached.

The diet excluded all meat, fish, eggs, and dairy products. Drinking water was limited to spring water (chlorinated tap water was specifically prohibited); and coffee, ordinary tea, chocolate, sugar, and salt were excluded. Herbs were allowed for seasoning, and water and herbal teas were allowed up to 1.5 l a day. Vegetables used freely were lettuce, carrots, beets, onions, celery, cabbage, cauliflower, broccoli, nettles, cucumber, radishes, Jerusalem artichokes, and all beans except soybeans and green peas. Potatoes were allowed in restricted amounts. A number of fruits were also used freely: blueberries, cloudberries, raspberries, strawberries, black currants, gooseberries, plums, and pears. Apples and citrus fruits were not allowed, and grains were either restricted or eliminated.

The beneficial effects of this dietary regimen are probably related to three factors:

- Elimination of food allergens
- Altered prostaglandin metabolism
- Increased intake of antioxidant nutrients and magnesium

The importance of avoiding food allergies was discussed earlier. The avoidance of dietary sources of arachidonic acid (derived from animal products) appears to be quite significant, as well, as the prostaglandins and leukotrienes derived from arachidonic acid contribute significantly to the allergic reaction in asthma. The benefits of altering prostaglandin metabolism are further discussed later, as is the role of increased dietary antioxidants in preventing asthma.

Perhaps the most significant effects noted in the trial of the vegan diet, besides the patients' improvement in health, were the great reduction in health care costs (the patients had been receiving corticosteroids and other drugs and therapies for an average of 12 years) and, according to the authors, patients' changed attitude toward increased responsibility for their own health.

Omega-3 Fatty Acids

Population-based studies have shown that children who eat fish more than once a week have one-third the asthma risk of children who do not eat fish regularly.[39] Several clinical studies have shown that increasing the intake of omega-3 fatty acids through supplementation with fish oils (which contain EPA and DHA) offers significant benefits in asthma, as demonstrated by improvements in airway responsiveness to allergens, as well as improvements in respiratory function.[40,41] These benefits are related to increasing the ratio of omega-3 to omega-6 fatty acids in cell membranes, thereby reducing the availability of arachidonic acid, which can lead to the production of inflammatory leukotrienes. Omega-3 fatty acid ingestion leads to a significant shift in leukotriene synthesis, from the extremely inflammatory 4-series to the less inflammatory 5-series leukotrienes. This shift is directly related to improvements in asthma symptoms.[42] It may take as long as one year before benefits are apparent, as it appears to take time to produce new cellular membranes that include the omega-3 fatty acids.

Tryptophan Metabolism and Pyridoxine Supplementation

Children with asthma have been shown to have a metabolic defect in tryptophan metabolism and reduced platelet transport for serotonin.[43,44] These defects may be related to low vitamin B_6 (pyridoxine) levels. In one study, plasma and red blood cell vitamin B_6 levels were significantly lower in 15 adult patients with asthma than in 16 controls.[45] Oral supplementation with 50 mg pyridoxine twice per day given to seven of the patients failed to produce a substantial elevation of these low levels. However, all patients reported a dramatic decrease in frequency and severity of wheezing and asthmatic attacks while taking the supplements. In a study of 76 asthmatic children, pyridoxine at a dosage of 200 mg per day produced significant reductions in symptoms and in the dosages of bronchodilators and corticosteroids required. However, a double-blind study failed to demonstrate any significant improvement with B_6 supplementation in patients who depended on steroids for control of symptoms.[46]

Although vitamin B_6 supplementation may not help patients on steroids, it is definitely indicated for asthmatics being treated with the drug theophylline. Theophylline significantly depresses pyridoxal-5-phosphate levels.[47] In addition, another study has shown that vitamin B_6 supplementation can significantly reduce the typical side effects of theophylline (e.g., headaches, nausea, irritability, sleep disorders).[48]

Nutritional Supplements

Antioxidants

The substantial increase in the prevalence of asthma over the past 20 years can be partially explained by the reduced dietary intake of antioxidant nutrients such as beta-carotene and vitamins A, C, and E, as well as the mineral cofactors essential for antioxidant defense mechanisms, such as zinc, selenium, and copper.[49] Patients in acute asthmatic distress are known to have lowered serum total antioxidants.[50] Genetic influences may also play a role in the need for antioxidants.

One study of 158 children with moderate to severe asthma revealed that supplementation with 50 mg per day of vitamin E and 250 mg per day of vitamin C produced significant protection against reduction in pulmonary function caused by an ozone challenge.[51] Antioxidants are thought to provide important defense mechanisms against the oxidizing agents that can both stimulate bronchoconstriction and increase hyperreactivity to other agents.[52] Acetaminophen, which is known to deplete antioxidant levels such as glutathione in animals, should be used with caution in asthmatic patients.

Vitamin C. Vitamin C is very important to the health of the lungs, as it is the major antioxidant substance present in the extracellular fluid lining the airway surfaces. Vitamin C intake in the general population appears to inversely correlate with asthma: low vitamin C (in the diet and the blood) is an independent risk factor for asthma. In a survey of 771 people with current asthma, 352 people with former asthma, and 15,418 people without asthma, lower vitamin C concentrations were observed among those with current or former asthma than among people who had never had asthma.[53] Additional support is offered by the fact that children of smokers have a higher rate of asthma (cigarette smoke is known to deplete respiratory vitamin C and E levels), and symptoms of ongoing asthma in adults appear to be increased by exposure to environmental oxidizing agents and decreased by vitamin C supplementation.[57]

Both treated and untreated asthmatic patients have been shown to have significantly lower levels of ascorbic acid in serum and leukocytes.[53] From a clinical perspective, it appears that asthmatics have a higher need for vitamin C. From 1973 to 1994 there were 11 clinical studies of vitamin C supplementation in asthma.[54] Seven of these studies showed significant improvements in respiratory measures and asthma symptoms as a result of supplementing the diet with 1 to 2 g vitamin C per day. This dosage recommendation appears extremely wise based on the increasing exposure to inhaled oxidants today, along with the growing appreciation of the antioxidant function of vitamin C in the respiratory system.

High-dose vitamin C therapy may also help asthma by lowering histamine levels.[55] The importance of vitamin C as a natural antihistamine has emerged in the context of concern over the safety of antihistamine medications and the recently recognized immune-suppressing effects of histamine. In the initial stages of an immune response, histamine amplifies the immune response by increasing capillary permeability and smooth muscle contraction, thus enhancing the flow of immune factors to the site of infection. Subsequently, histamine exerts a suppressive effect on the accumulated white blood cells in an attempt to contain the inflammatory response.

Vitamin C acts in a number of ways against histamine. Specifically, it prevents the secretion of histamine by white blood cells and increases the detoxification of histamine. One study examined the antihistamine effect of short- and long-term vitamin C administration and its effect on neutrophil function in healthy men and women. In the long-term part of the study, 10 subjects ingested a placebo during weeks one, two, five, and six and 2 g per day of vitamin C during weeks three and four. Fasting blood samples were collected at the end of weeks two, four, and six. Blood vitamin C levels rose significantly following vitamin C administration, while blood histamine levels fell by 38% during the weeks vitamin C was given. The ability of white blood cells to respond to an infection (chemotaxis) increased by 19% during vitamin C administration and fell 30% after vitamin C withdrawal. Interestingly, these changes were linked to histamine concentrations. Chemotaxis was greatest when histamine levels were the lowest. In the part of the study looking at the short-term effects of vitamin C, blood histamine concentrations and chemotaxis did not change four hours after a single dose of vitamin C. This result suggests that vitamin C will lower blood histamine only if taken over a period of time. Individuals prone to allergy or inflammation are encouraged to increase their consumption of vitamin C through supplementation.[55]

In a small study, asthmatic subjects with documented exercise-induced bronchoconstriction participated in a randomized, placebo-controlled double-blind crossover trial.[56] Subjects entered the study on their usual diet and were placed on either two weeks of vitamin C supplementation (1,500 mg per day) or a placebo, followed by a one-week washout period, before crossing over to the alternative treatment. The vitamin C group significantly reduced the maximum fall in postexercise FEV_1 (–6.4 %) compared with the usual diet (–14.3%) and the placebo (–12.9%). Asthma symptom scores significantly improved with vitamin C supplementation compared with the placebo and the usual diet. Postexercise inflammatory mediators were also significantly lower with ascorbic acid supplementation.

Flavonoids. Flavonoids appear to be key antioxidants in the treatment of asthma. Various flavonoids, chief among them being quercetin, have been shown to have beneficial effects in preventing the formation and release of allergic mediators.[57–60] In addition, flavonoids have both a vitamin-C-sparing effect and a direct stabilizing effect on membranes, including those of mast cells.

Quercetin or more bioavailable forms of quercetin can be used (e.g., enzymatically modified isoquercitrin, or EMIQ). However, flavonoid-rich extracts such as those from grape seed, pine bark, green tea, or ginkgo biloba may prove even more helpful in the treatment of asthma. In particular, the proanthocyanidins, from grape seed or pine bark extracts, appear to have an affinity for the lungs. In a randomized, placebo-controlled, double-blind study involving 60 subjects between 6 and 18 years old, a proprietary pine bark extract (Pycnogenol) significantly improved pulmonary function and asthma symptoms compared with a placebo. Specifically, the subjects in the Pycnogenol group were able to reduce or discontinue their use of rescue inhalers more often than the placebo group. There was also a significant reduction of urinary leukotrienes in the Pycnogenol group.[61]

In another study, a flavonoid preparation derived from purple passion fruit peel (PFP) was studied in a four-week randomized, placebo-controlled, double-blind trial in asthma patients. The dosage of the PFP extract was 150 mg per day. The prevalence of wheezing, coughing, and shortness of breath was reduced significantly in the group treated with PFP extract, whereas the placebo caused no significant improvement.

Supplementation with PFP extract also resulted in a marked increase in the ability to breathe while the placebo showed no effect.[62]

Carotenes. Carotenes are powerful antioxidants that may increase the integrity of the epithelial lining of the respiratory tract and decrease inflammatory leukotriene formation.[63] Some studies have shown that asthmatics have reduced plasma antioxidant potential due to low whole-blood levels of carotenoids (beta-carotene, alpha-carotene, beta-cryptoxanthin, lutein, and zeaxanthin)[64] and in particular low lycopene levels,[65] and thus are more susceptible to the damaging effects of oxidative stress. This highlights the potential role for carotenoid supplementation in these subjects. Lycopene may emerge as the most useful supplemental carotenoid. In animal models of asthma, lycopene supplementation suppresses allergic responses in the bronchioles, lung tissue, and blood and also reduces the number of mucus-secreting cells in the airways.[66]

In a proof-of-concept human study, 32 asthmatic adults consumed a low-antioxidant diet for 10 days, then commenced a randomized crossover trial involving three 7-day treatment arms: placebo, tomato extract (45 mg lycopene a day), and tomato juice (45 mg lycopene a day).[67] With consumption of a low-antioxidant diet, plasma carotenoid concentrations decreased, the asthma control score worsened, lung function (as measured by FEV_1) decreased, and sputum white blood cells (neutrophils) increased. Treatment with both tomato juice and extract reduced airway neutrophil influx. Treatment with tomato extract also reduced sputum neutrophil elastase activity. This short-term study indicates that antioxidant status, particularly carotenoids, modifies some signs and symptoms of asthma.

There have been two double-blind studies of lycopene supplementation (30 mg per day) in exercise-induced asthma. One study failed to show any benefit,[68] while another showed that in some patients it prevents airway constriction and reduced breathing capacity.[69]

Selenium. Reduced selenium levels have been demonstrated in asthma patients.[70–72] Glutathione peroxidase, a selenium-dependent enzyme, is important for reducing leukotriene formation. Reduced levels of glutathione peroxidase have also been reported for asthmatics. Supplemental selenium appears warranted to address any deficiency of glutathione peroxidase.

Vitamin B$_{12}$

Noted physician Jonathan Wright believes that "B$_{12}$ therapy is the mainstay treatment for childhood asthma."[73] In one clinical trial, weekly 1,000 mcg intramuscular injections produced definite improvement in asthmatic patients.[74] Of 20 patients, 18 showed less shortness of breath on exertion, as well as improved appetite, sleep, and general condition. Vitamin B$_{12}$ appears to be especially effective in sulfite-sensitive individuals.

Magnesium

In 1912 P. Trendelenburg demonstrated that magnesium relaxed bovine bronchial smooth muscle in test tube studies.[75] Later, uncontrolled clinical studies revealed magnesium's beneficial effect in the treatment of patients with acute attacks of bronchial asthma.[76] Now, intravenous magnesium (2 g magnesium sulfate infused every hour, up to a total of 24.6 g) is a well-proved and clinically accepted measure to halt an acute asthma attack as well as acute exacerbations of chronic obstructive pulmonary disease (COPD).[77–81]

Although these initial studies used injectable magnesium, it has been demonstrated that oral magnesium is just as effective at restoring magnesium status (except in the case of an emergency situation such as an acute heart attack or acute asthma attack), although it will usually take six weeks to achieve significant elevations in tissue magnesium concentrations.[82] Oral supplementation appears to be warranted because low levels of plasma magnesium have been found in asthmatic patients[83] and dietary magnesium intake is independently related to lung function and asthma severity.[84] Several double-blind studies of oral magnesium supplementation in adults and children with asthma have demonstrated an improvement in respiratory function, antioxidant status (i.e., increased glutathione concentrations), reduced reactivity to chemical challenge with methacholine, and measures of asthma control and quality of life.[85–87] Dosages ranged from 300 mg a day in children to 340 mg a day in adults, usually in divided dosages.

Nebulized magnesium has also proved useful as an adjunct to standard bronchodilation therapies in severe asthmatics, with a greater response in those with life-threatening asthma.[88]

Vitamin D

Vitamin D deficiency is linked to increased airway reactivity, reduced lung function, and worse asthma control.[89] One study of more than 1,000 children with asthma showed that 35% had insufficient levels of vitamin D (30 ng/ml or less 25-hydroxyvitamin D).[90] After adjusting for age, sex, body mass index, income, and treatment group, insufficient vitamin D status was associated with higher odds of any hospitalization or emergency department visit. In addition to correcting a vitamin D insufficiency, vitamin D supplementation may improve asthma control by blocking the cascade of inflammation-causing proteins in the lung. Preliminary clinical evidence is encouraging, especially in childhood asthma prevention at a dosage of 1,200 IU per day of vitamin D$_3$.[91] This study, done in Japan, looked at the efficacy of supplemental vitamin D for preventing influenza infection. The researchers were surprised to find that the vitamin D not only decreased flu by 42% but also decreased asthma attacks by a remarkable 83%.

Botanical Medicines

Asthma patients commonly employ botanical self-treatments. A cross-sectional analysis of 601 adults with asthma found that 14% of asthma sufferers use either herbal products, coffee, or black tea in order to treat their condition. Unfortunately, this study illustrated that those who used these methods had a higher incidence of hospitalization.[92] Because of the possibility of improper use of botanicals and the inability of the users to recognize the need for acute conventional interventions, we recommend that before using natural therapies, patients with asthma consult a naturopathic physician or another qualified practitioner who understands the proper use of botanicals and can assess the asthmatic patient's risk severity.

The most popular historical herbal treatment of asthma involved the use of *Ephedra sinensis* (ma huang) in combination with herbal expectorants. This approach appeared to have considerable merit, as ephedra and its alkaloids have proved effective as bronchodilators in treating mild to moderate asthma and hay fever.[93] However, ephedra preparation are no longer sold in the United States owing to safety concerns when excessive dosages were used as a weight loss aid.

Ivy (*Hedera helix*)

In Europe, herbal preparations containing extracts from the leaves of ivy (*Hedera helix*) enjoy great popularity for the relief of coughing as well as asthma. In 2007, more than 80% of herbal expectorants prescribed in Germany included ivy extract, amounting to nearly 2 million prescriptions nationwide. Ivy leaf contains saponins (alpha-hederin and hederacoside C) that show expectorant, mucolytic, spasmolytic, bronchodilatory, and antibacterial effects.[94] A 2003 meta-analysis of three double-blind studies in children showed that the ivy preparations used were significantly superior to a placebo.[95] One study compared ivy leaf extract cough drops with a placebo, one compared suppositories with drops, and one tested syrup against drops. The reviewers concluded that ivy leaf extract preparations improve a variety of respiratory functions in children with chronic bronchial asthma, but noted the data were meager. In the only placebo-controlled, double-blind study reviewed, 24 children with asthma between the ages of 4 and 12 were given a dry ivy leaf extract (35 mg) in cough drops or a placebo for three days with a washout of three to five days before crossing over to the other treatment. Superiority of the ivy leaf extract over the placebo was noted by small improvements in airway resistance, residual volume, and breathing capacity when the baseline measurements were compared with the third day at three hours after the morning dose.

Licorice

Licorice (*Glycyrrhiza glabra*) root has a long history of use as an anti-inflammatory and antiallergic agent, and there is considerable documentation in the scientific literature. The primary active component of licorice root in this application is glycyrrhetinic acid, a compound that has shown cortisol-like activity. In particular, glycyrrhetinic acid has been shown to inhibit phospholipase A$_2$, the enzyme responsible for cleaving arachidonic acid from the phospholipid membrane pool and initiating the formation of inflammatory prostaglandins and leukotrienes.[96] Licorice is also an expectorant, which is useful to treat asthma.

Capsaicin from Cayenne Pepper

Experimental evidence has shown that capsaicin, the major active component of cayenne pepper (*Capsicum frutescens*), desensitizes airway mucosa to various mechanical and chemical irritants.[97] This effect is probably due to capsaicin-induced depletion of substance P (which normally increases vascular permeability and flow) in the respiratory tract nerves.[98] The respiratory and gastrointestinal tracts have large numbers of neurons that contain substance P. Because of the location of substance P and its physiological action, it is believed to play an important role in atopic conditions such as asthma and atopic dermatitis. Therefore, depletion of substance P may be desirable in these conditions.

Jujube Plum

The jujube plum (*Zizyphi fructus*) has been used extensively in Chinese medicine for the treatment of asthma and allergic rhinitis.[99] It contains cyclic AMP—a compound that promotes bronchial relaxation—at a level of 100 to 500 nmol/g of dry weight, a concentration 10 times greater than that of any other plant or animal tissue thus far reported in the literature.[100] These experimental findings, in conjunction with the jujube plum's long historical use, strongly support its clinical use.

Tylophora

The leaves of tylophora (*Tylophora asthmatica*) have been used extensively in ayurvedic medicine for asthma and other respiratory tract disorders. Tylophora's mode of action is unknown but is thought to be due to its alkaloids, especially tylophorine, which have been reported to possess antihistamine and antispasmodic activity, as well as inhibition of mast cell degranulation.[101,102] However, a more central mechanism may be responsible for the clinical effects in asthma.

Several double-blind clinical studies have shown tylophora to produce good results.[103,106] In one study of 135 patients, those given 200 mg tylophora leaves twice per day for six days demonstrated improvements in symptoms and respiratory function during the treatment period and for up to two weeks after treatment.[103] Side effects such as nausea and vomiting occurred in 9.8% of subjects in the tylophora group and 14% in the placebo group.

In another double-blind study of 103 patients, those receiving 40 mg of the dry alcoholic extract of *Tylophora indica* per day for only six days demonstrated significant improvement in symptoms of asthma compared with a placebo group.[105] At the end of the first week, 56% had complete to moderate improvement, as compared with 31.6% of the 92 patients receiving the placebo. At the end of 4 weeks, the respective figures were 32% and 23.8%; at 8 weeks, 23.8% and 8.4%; and at 12 weeks, 14.8% and 7.2%. The incidence of side effects such as nausea, partial diminution of taste for salt, and slight mouth soreness was 16.3% in the tylophora group and 6.6% in the placebo group. These results, as well as the results from an additional study, indicate that the benefits of tylophora are short-lived.[106]

Ginkgo Biloba Extract (GBE)

Ginkgo biloba contains several unique terpene molecules, known collectively as *ginkgolides*, that antagonize platelet-activating factor (PAF), a key chemical mediator in asthma, inflammation, and allergies. Ginkgolides compete with PAF for binding sites and inhibit the various events induced by PAF. The antiasthmatic effects of orally administered or inhaled ginkgolides have been shown to produce improvements in respiratory function and reduce bronchial reactivity in several double-blind studies.[107,108] Treatment consisted of 120 mg of the pure ginkgolides per day—a dosage that is currently expensive to achieve using GBE with 24% ginkgo flavonglycosides and 6% total terpenoids.

Aloe Vera

Administration of aloe vera preparations may be effective for patients who are not dependent on corticosteroids. In one study, the oral administration of an aloe vera extract for six months was shown to produce good results in the treatment of asthma in some individuals of various ages.[109] The extract was produced from fresh leaves stored in the dark at 4°C for seven days. Subjecting the leaves to dark and cold results in an increase in the polysaccharide fraction—1 g of crude extract obtained from leaves stored in cold and dark produced 400 mg neutral polysaccharide compared with only 30 mg produced from leaves not subjected to cold or dark. The dosage was 5 ml of a 20% solution of the aloe vera extract in saline twice per day for 24 weeks; 11 of 27 patients (40%) without corticosteroid dependence felt much better at the study's conclusion. The mechanism of action is thought to be restoration of protective mechanisms, plus augmentation of the immune system.

Coleus

Coleus forskohlii extract may be particularly useful in asthma, as its active component, forskolin, has been shown to have remarkable effects in relaxing constricted bronchial muscles in asthmatics.[110–111] However, these studies used inhaled doses of pure forskolin. Whether orally administered forskolin in the form of *C. forskohlii* extract would produce similar bronchodilator effects has yet to be determined. However, on the basis of the plant's historical use and additional mechanisms of action, it appears likely.

Boswellia

The Indian ayurvedic botanical *Boswellia serrata* exerts anti-inflammatory and anti-allergy effects. In one double-blind, placebo-controlled study, bronchial asthma was reduced in 70% of 40 patients treated with boswellia gum resin at 300 mg three times per day for six weeks, whereas only 27% of the control group improved. Improvement was seen in physical symptoms and signs such as shortness of breath, the number of attacks, breathing capacity, and eosinophil counts.[112]

Acupuncture and Acupressure

In traditional Chinese medicine (TCM), chronic asthmatic symptomology is usually characterized as a lung or spleen deficiency. This model considers that acute symptoms may be caused by invasion from cold wind (environmental factors) or by an internal condition stemming from a lung heat condition (increased inflammation and eosinophilia). Chronic asthma is considered more of a weakness in the lung itself or a weakness of the spleen, which is responsible for nourishing the lung chi. In TCM, the emotion of grief is also known to weaken lung chi.

In one study, 41 patients with chronic obstructive asthma were randomly assigned to receive acupuncture plus standard care, acupressure plus standard care, or standard care alone. For each subject, 20 acupuncture treatments were given, and self-administered acupressure was performed daily for eight weeks. According to a standard respiratory questionnaire, the acupuncture subjects showed an average 18.5-fold improvement, whereas the improvement for the acupressure-only subjects was 6.57-fold. Additionally, for patients who received acupressure, the irritability domain score exhibited an 11.8-fold improvement.[113] Another study involved 44 patients receiving bona fide or sham acupressure.

Each received five 16-minute treatments per week for four weeks. On the basis of breathing function and shortness of breath scores, 6-minute walking distance measurements, and state anxiety scale scores, the acupressure group had significant improvements in breathing and less anxiety compared with the sham group.[114]

. . . .

QUICK REVIEW

- **Cases of asthma are growing in number and severity.**
- **The first step in the natural approach to asthma is to reduce the allergic threshold by avoiding airborne and food allergens.**
- **Elimination diets have been successful in identifying allergens and treating asthma.**
- **A vegan diet can be very effective in reducing asthma symptoms.**
- **Omega-3 fatty acids can relieve asthma.**
- **Food additives can trigger allergic reactions and asthma.**

- **Vitamin B_6 supplementation is recommended for the treatment of asthma, especially if the asthmatic has to take the drug theophylline.**
- **Antioxidants, especially high doses of vitamin C and flavonoid-rich extracts such as grape seed or pine bark, are highly recommended for the treatment of asthma.**
- **Magnesium can help open the airways.**
- **Asthmatics should avoid salt.**
- **Ivy extract has shown benefits in improving lung function in asthmatics.**

. . . .

TREATMENT SUMMARY

The effective treatment of asthma requires the consideration of many environmental, dietary, and supplement factors. We recommend consulting a naturopathic physician or another medical practitioner who can help coordinate all of these different factors.

Environment

Airborne allergens such as pollen, dander, and dust mites are often difficult to avoid entirely, but measures described above must be taken to reduce exposure.

Diet

All food allergens and food additives should be eliminated. The patient who has many food allergies may need to use a four-day rotation diet. Garlic and onions should be liberally used unless the patient reacts to them. If the patient is willing, or if his or her asthma is unresponsive to recommended therapy, a vegan diet (with the possible inclusion of cold-water fish) should be tried for a minimum of four months to one year. Moderate fruit consumption, especially apples, should also be encouraged, along with the liberal use of green tea. For dietary guidelines, see the chapter "A Health-Promoting Diet."

Nutritional Supplements

- A high-potency multiple vitamin and mineral formula as described in the chapter "Supplementary Measures"
- Key individual nutrients:
  - Vitamin B$_6$: 25 to 50 mg two times per day
  - Vitamin B$_{12}$: 800 to 1,000 mcg per day
  - Vitamin C: 10 to 30 mg/kg in divided doses
  - Vitamin E (mixed tocopherols): 100 to 200 IU per day
  - Magnesium (citrate, malate, aspartate, or glycinate): 200 to 400 mg three times per day
  - Selenium: 200 mcg per day
  - Vitamin D$_3$: 2,000 to 4,000 IU per day (ideally, measure blood levels and adjust dosage accordingly)
- Fish oils: 1,000 to 3,000 mg EPA + DHA per day
- One of the following:
  - Grape seed extract (>95% procyanidolic oligomers): 100 to 300 mg per day
  - Pine bark extract (>95% procyanidolic oligomers): 100 to 300 mg per day
  - Some other flavonoid-rich extract with a similar flavonoid content, super greens formula, or another plant-based antioxidant that can provide an oxygen radical absorption capacity (ORAC) of 3,000 to 6,000 units or more per day
- Quercetin: 400 mg 20 minutes before meals, or enzymatically modified isoquercitrin (EMIQ) 100 mg per day.
- Lycopene: 15 to 30 mg per day

Botanical Medicines

- Take one or more of the following:
  - Ivy leaf (*Hedera helix*), available as tincture, fluid extract, and dry powdered extract in capsules and tablets; typical dosage for adults and children over 12 years of age for a 4:1 dry powdered extract is 100 mg per day (the equivalent of 420 mg dried herbal substance); for children 1–5 years old, dosage is the equivalent of 150 mg dried herbal substance; for children 6–12 years old, the equivalent of 210 mg dried herbal substance
  - *Glycyrrhiza glabra:*
    - Powdered root: 1 to 2 g three times per day
    - Fluid extract (1:1): 2 to 4 ml three times per day
    - Solid (dry powdered) extract (4:1): 250 to 500 mg three times per day
  - *Tylophora asthmatica:* 200 mg tylophora leaves or 40 mg dry alcoholic extract twice per day
  - *Coleus forskohlii:* 50 mg of an extract standardized to contain 18% forskolin two to three times per day

Counseling

For patients who respond to emotional stress with asthmatic attacks, counseling is important. Counseling is also important for children with moderate to severe asthma, who may develop behavioral problems.

Acupuncture and Acupressure

Regular acupuncture and home acupressure treatments should be used.

Attention-Deficit/
Hyperactivity Disorder

- A brain and behavioral disorder that begins in early childhood and persists into adolescence and adulthood

- Typified by one or more symptoms of disabling inattentiveness, hyperactivity, and impulsivity

- Commonly accompanied by mood disorders or learning disabilities

The term attention-deficit/hyperactivity disorder (ADHD) encompasses three separate ADHD forms: predominantly inattentive (often referred to as simply attention deficit disorder, or ADD), predominantly hyperactive, and combined type. Depending on the region and the investigator, ADHD has been found in 5 to 15% of school-age children, or about 10 million children in the United States. Clinical observation and epidemiological surveys typically report a greater incidence in boys than girls (approximately 2:1). More than 5.5 million children in the United States take amphetamine-type drugs for ADHD each day. Onset is usually by the age of three, although the diagnosis is often not made until later, when the child is in school.[1]

The characteristics of ADHD in order of frequency are: (1) hyperactivity, (2) emotional instability (mood swings, outbursts, etc.), (3) clumsiness, (4) disorders of attention (short attention span, distractibility, failure to finish things off, not listening, poor concentration), (5) impulsiveness (action before thought, abrupt shifts in activity, poor organizing, jumping up in class), (6) disorders of memory and thinking, (7) specific learning disabilities, (8) disorders of speech and hearing, and (9) various neurological signs and brainwave pattern irregularities.

These characteristics are frequently associated with difficulties in school, both in learning and in behavior. If not intensively managed, a child with ADHD will be likely to experience academic impairment, increased risk of injuries, and problems with self-esteem and socialization. Later in adolescence and adulthood, those with ADHD have a high risk of experiencing depression or anxiety, substance abuse and addictions, traffic accidents, financial problems, vocational underachievement, and social problems. Nevertheless, ADHD is a condition that can be transcended—many people with ADHD have achieved a high level of personal success.

Causes

There are many factors linked to ADHD, with the leading factor being diminished function of certain circuits in the executive centers of the brain responsible for impulse control and the ability to maintain sustained attention. Evidence from studies using sophisticated brain imagery techniques such as MRI, PET scanning, CT imaging, and EEGs indicates that the brains of those with ADHD exhibit differences in both structure and function compared with normal controls, particularly with regard to the executive centers.

Research into what causes these changes has focused on genetic, environmental, and nutritional factors. There is little doubt that genetics is a predisposing factor.[2] However, as with most health conditions, environmental and dietary factors appear to play a significant role in whether and how these genetic factors are manifested.

Therapeutic Considerations

The role of nutritional and environmental factors in ADHD is becoming increasingly widely recognized. Despite significant advances in the use of nutritional therapies for ADHD, however, the prevailing conventional approach to the treatment of ADHD relies almost entirely on amphetamine drugs for purely symptomatic relief. These drugs, such as Ritalin and Concerta (methylphenidate), Adderall (amphetamine), and Vyvanse (lisdexamfetamine) improve ADHD symptoms primarily by potentiating the neurotransmitter dopamine within all brain regions, including those most affected in ADHD. These medications reportedly improve behavior and cognitive functioning in approximately 75% of children in formal placebo-controlled trials. However, the success of treatment when studied in actual clinical practice may be significantly lower. Furthermore, follow-up studies have failed to demonstrate long-term benefits with these stimulant medications. Additionally, these drugs are associated with a high prevalence of adverse effects such as

decreased appetite, sleep problems, anxiety, and irritability. Some of the long-term effects of these drugs could be extremely detrimental to both brain function and behavior.[3–5]

Nonstimulant drugs such as atomoxetine (Strattera) have been promoted as a safe alternative. However, atomoxetine has its own set of problems, including the fact that children and teenagers with ADHD who take atomoxetine are more likely to have suicidal thoughts.[6]

The bottom line is that every effort should be made to treat ADHD without the long-term reliance of medications.

Environmental Factors

Environmental factors that contribute to the development of ADHD may begin at or even before conception. Maternal-to-fetal transport of various neurotoxins can occur readily during pregnancy. A woman who has an ongoing exposure to or a significant body burden of neurotoxic substances (e.g., heavy metals such as lead and mercury, solvents, pesticides, PCBs, alcohol, and other drugs of abuse) may herself exhibit features consistent with ADHD and give birth to a child who manifests symptoms of ADHD. In such cases it might be assumed that ADHD is inherited when it is actually acquired. Children remain susceptible to neurotoxins following birth, and some of these agents have been shown to be common among children in North America.[7,8]

Maternal tobacco and drug use has been associated with a higher risk of ADHD.[9–11] One study suggested that up to 25% of all behavioral disorders in children can be attributed to exposure to cigarette smoking during pregnancy.[9] In addition, there is an alarmingly high incidence of chronic, low-level lead intoxication in North American children.[8,12] The Centers for Disease Control and Prevention estimated that about 2% of American children younger than age six currently meet the criteria for lead toxicity at a level that has been associated with cognitive deficits and behavioral disturbances (>10 mg/dl whole blood lead).[12] Low-level lead intoxication has also been associated with addictive behaviors and impulsivity, suggesting neurological changes.[13] Pilot studies have demonstrated improvement in ADHD behaviors in some children with moderate elevations in blood lead levels who have been treated with intravenous EDTA chelation.[14]

In addition to lead, other heavy metals such as mercury, cadmium, and aluminum, as well as pesticides and PCBs, are nearly ubiquitous contaminants arising from dental amalgam fillings, food, air, and drinking water, and these agents may act synergistically to impair neurological function and development in susceptible children. Consumers Union recently conducted the largest study to date looking at the level of human exposure to a wide range of pesticides in the U.S. food supply, demonstrating that human exposure to pesticides is far greater than ever previously estimated and that children are at particularly high risk for neurotoxic effects from regular inadvertent pesticide exposure from common foodstuffs.[15]

A recent study has shown a direct correlation between the levels of organophosphates in a child's urine and the incidence of ADHD.[16] Children eating conventionally grown foods have a level of organophosphates nine times as high as those eating organically grown foods.[17] This level results in a 50% increase in ADHD—not surprisingly, as these pesticides are neurotoxins.

Food Additives, Sugar, and the Feingold Hypothesis

The hypothesis that food additives can cause ADHD in children was popularized by the research of Benjamin Feingold, M.D., and is now commonly referred to as the "Feingold hypothesis." According to Feingold, many hyperactive children, perhaps 40 to 50%, are sensitive to artificial food colors, flavors, and preservatives.[18]

Feingold's claims were based on his experience with more than 1,200 cases in which food additives were linked to learning and behavior disorders. Since Feingold's presentation on this subject to the American Medical Association in 1973, the role of food additives as a contributing cause of hyperactivity has been hotly debated in the scientific literature. In actuality, however, researchers have focused on only 10 food dyes, though Feingold was concerned with 3,000 food additives.

At first glance, it appears that the majority of the double-blind studies designed to test the hypothesis have shown essentially negative results. However, upon closer examination of these studies and further investigation into the literature, it becomes evident that food additives do, in fact, play a major role in hyperactivity. In several of the studies, overwhelming evidence was produced.[19,20]

In a recent study, 153 three-year-old and 144 eight- and nine-year-old children from the general population (in other words, the study was not focused on children with a specific diagnosis of ADHD) were given either a drink that contained sodium benzoate and an artificial food coloring mix or a placebo mix. The main outcome measure was a global hyperactivity aggregate (GHA), based on observed behaviors and ratings by teachers and parents, plus, for the older children, a computerized test of attention. The results showed that the children given the artificial food coloring agents had a statistically significant adverse increase in hyperactivity.[21]

It is interesting to note that while U.S. studies have been largely negative, reports from the United Kingdom, Australia, and Canada have been more supportive. Feingold contended that there is a conflict of interest on the part of the Nutrition Foundation, an organization supported by major U.S. food manufacturers—Coca-Cola, Nabisco, General Foods, and others. It seems significant that the Nutrition Foundation has financed most of the negative studies. The conflict of interest arises because these companies would suffer economically if food additives were found to be harmful. Other countries have significantly restricted the use of artificial food additives because of possible harmful effects.

Virtually every study (either negative or positive) that looked at the role of food additives in ADHD demonstrated that some hyperactive children consistently react with behavioral problems when challenged by specific food additives. Critics of the hypothesis ignore the significance of these clear, reproducible individual results. The bottom line is that some children react strongly enough to food additives to warrant eliminating these compounds in the diet for at least 10 days to judge their significance in a particular child.

Sugar consumption also appears to be a factor. One study demonstrated that destructive-aggressive and restless behavior significantly correlated with the amount of sugar consumed.[22] The higher the sugar intake, the worse the behavior. In another study, researchers performed five-hour oral glucose tolerance tests on 261 hyperactive children; 74% displayed abnormal glucose tolerance or hypoglycemia.[23]

Essential Fatty Acids

Numerous studies have now shown that children with ADHD have a measurable reduction in tissue levels of the omega-3 fatty acids eicosapentaenoic acid (EPA) and docosahexaenoic acid (DHA) when compared with age-matched controls. This should not be surprising: omega-3 fatty acids are critical in the structure and function of brain cells. Omega-3 (EPA + DHA) supplementation in ADHD has now been studied extensively and is considered a sensible intervention even by many mainstream physicians. Omega-3 fatty acid supplementation improves many symptoms of ADHD, including impulsive-oppositional behavior, a symptom not typically helped by the pharmaceutical treatment of ADHD.[24] DHA deficiency has also been shown in animal studies to result in increased permeability of the blood-brain barrier, which plays a critical role in protecting the brain from an influx of neurotoxic compounds such as pesticides and mercury.[25,26]

Human breast milk is rich in DHA, and several studies have shown that children who are fed formula are at twice as high a risk of developing ADHD as those who are breastfed.[27] The role of DHA in brain development, intelligence, and possible protection against ADHD finally led to its inclusion in many infant formulas and other foods.

Individual Nutrients and ADHD

Besides fatty acids, inadequate provision of other nutrients during fetal development and early childhood may also play a significant role in the development of ADHD.[28,29] In addition, children with ADHD often show multiple nutrient deficiencies, highlighting the importance of broad-spectrum nutritional support. In particular, the following minerals are critical supplements in the management of ADHD:

- **Magnesium.** Magnesium levels in serum, red blood cells, and hair have all been shown to be low in the majority of children with ADHD.[30] These children also demonstrated improved behavior when administered magnesium supplements.[31]

- **Zinc.** Low levels of zinc in hair and serum have both been shown to frequently accompany ADHD.[32] Children with low serum zinc were also more frequently found to have lower free fatty acid levels, suggesting that abnormalities in fatty acid metabolism may result, at least in part, from zinc deficiency.[33] It has also been shown that lower hair zinc levels correlate with a poorer response to treatment with amphetamines. Several clinical trials have now demonstrated positive effects of zinc supplementation in hyperactive children.[34,35]

- **Iron.** Anemia from iron deficiency is estimated to affect approximately 20% of infants, and many more are thought to suffer milder iron deficiencies without anemia, leaving them at risk for impairment of brain development.[36] Iron deficiency has been found to be even more common in children with ADHD. One study demonstrated that iron supplementation in nonanemic children with ADHD resulted in diminished ADHD symptoms within 30 days.[37] A more recent study demonstrated improvement in ADHD symptoms in children with ADHD and low iron stores.[38]

Food Allergies

There is a very strong relationship between allergies, including food allergies, and ADHD.[39–43] In one study demonstrable brainwave changes occurred immediately following ingestion of a previously identified food allergy.[43] Food allergies and other allergic disorders have also been associated with a higher incidence of recurrent ear infections (otitis media).[44] In turn, recurrent otitis media has been associated with an increased risk of ADHD.[45] Both food allergy and ADHD have been associated with sleep disturbances, which may, in turn, contribute to a worsening of ADHD symptoms. Heavy snoring and sleep apnea are particularly prevalent in allergic children and may significantly contribute to ADHD symptoms.[46–48] Studies have demonstrated improved sleep in children with ADHD who are on a low-allergy-potential (oligoantigenic) diet. In fact, food allergy elimination or desensitization can be as effective as drug therapy in reducing ADHD symptoms.[49–52]

Probiotic supplementation with active bifidobacteria and lactobacillus cultures may be helpful in the treatment of ADHD. These organisms function as part of the first line of defense in gut immunity and have been shown to counteract altered gut permeability due to food allergies.[53,54]

Nutritional Supplements

Grape Seed or Pine Bark Extract

Extracts of grape seed and the bark of the maritime pine (Pycnogenol) are rich sources of proanthocyanidins are one of the most beneficial groups of plant flavonoids. These extracts may prove useful in the treatment of ADHD due to their broad-spectrum antioxidant effects alone, as increased oxidative damage is believed to be a central factor in ADHD.

To date, four studies have been conducted on the use of Pycnogenol in children with ADHD. In two of the studies, children supplemented with Pycnogenol (1 mg/kg per day) showed improved antioxidant status.[55,56] A third study not only confirmed this antioxidant effect but also demonstrated that Pycnogenol produced improvements in hyperactivity.[57] In the most detailed study, which involved 61 children with ADHD supplemented with 1 mg/kg Pycnogenol or a placebo daily over a period of four weeks, the children taking Pycnogenol showed a significant reduction of hyperactivity, along with improved attention, visual-motor coordination, and concentration.[58] These results point to an option to use grape seed or pine bark extract as a nutritional adjunct in ADHD.

Ginkgo Biloba Extract (GBE)

Two pilot studies, one of children (testing GBE in combination with American ginseng) and the other of adults, showed some beneficial effects attributed to supplementation with GBE.[59,60] Specifically these studies showed improvements in inattentiveness, hyperactivity, and socialization.

L-theanine

L-theanine, an amino acid found in green tea, shows promise in improving sleep quality in children with ADHD. This amino acid is also known to reduce anxiety and increase concentration. A recently completed double-blind trial of L-theanine in ADHD showed significant improvements in sleep quality with supplementation.[61] L-theanine was given at a dosage of 200 mg twice daily. These results are extremely promising, as disturbances in sleep quality are a very common occurrence in ADHD.

Biofeedback

In biofeedback training treatment, individuals are provided with real-time feedback about their brainwave activity through electronic instrumentation. This feedback allows the subject to learn self-regulation of brainwave intensity and frequency. Biofeedback treatment is designed to train individuals with ADHD to reduce or eliminate abnormal brain wave activity (cortical slowing) and thus reduce or eliminate many symptoms associated with ADHD. Evidence supporting the use of biofeedback as an effective treatment in ADHD is accumulating; some studies show that children using biofeedback may be able to stop taking Ritalin.[62–65]

QUICK REVIEW

- **More than 5.5 million children in the United States take amphetamine-type drugs for ADHD each day.**
- **There are many factors linked to ADHD, with the leading one being diminished function of certain circuits in the executive centers of the brain responsible for impulse control and for the ability to maintain sustained attention.**
- **The role of nutritional and environmental factors as the underlying cause of ADHD is increasingly being recognized.**
- **According to the Feingold hypothesis, many ADHD children, perhaps 40 to 50%, are sensitive to artificial food additives.**
- **There is growing research showing an association between the amount of organophosphate pesticides consumed and the incidence of ADHD.**
- **Numerous studies have now shown that**

children with ADHD have a measurable reduction in tissue levels of the omega-3 fatty acids EPA and DHA.

- Omega-3 fatty acid supplementation improves many symptoms of ADHD including impulsive-oppositional behavior, a symptom not typically helped by the pharmaceutical treatment of ADHD.
- Children with ADHD often show multiple nutrient deficiencies, highlighting the importance of broad-spectrum nutritional support.
- Supplementation with magnesium, zinc, or iron has shown benefit in ADHD, particularly in those subjects with confirmed deficiency.

- There is a very strong relationship between allergies, including food allergies, and ADHD.
- Food allergy elimination or desensitization can be as effective as drug therapy in reducing ADHD symptoms.
- Pycnogenol caused a significant reduction of hyperactivity while improving attention, visual-motor coordination, and concentration in children with ADHD.
- Evidence is accumulating to support the use of biofeedback as an effective treatment in ADHD.

TREATMENT SUMMARY

The treatment plan for ADHD involves the detection and elimination of any heavy metal or environmental toxicity; establishment of optimal nutrition, including the use of a high-potency multiple vitamin and mineral formula and fish oil supplement; elimination of food additives and sugar from the diet; and elimination of food allergens.

Diet

An allergy elimination (oligoantigenic) diet for a period of four weeks, followed by reintroduction of (challenge with) suspected foods (full servings at least once a day, one food introduced every three to four days), is the most sensible and economical approach for identifying food allergies; for more information see the chapter "Food Allergy." Where possible, eat only organically grown foods.

Nutritional Supplements

- High-potency multiple vitamin and mineral formula as described in the chapter "Supplementary Measures"
- Key individual nutrients:
  - Vitamin B_6: 25 to 50 mg per day
  - Folic acid: 400 to 800 mcg per day
  - Vitamin B_{12}: 400 to 800 mcg per day
  - Zinc: 20 to 30 mg per day
  - Vitamin C: 500 to 1,000 mg per day
  - Vitamin E (mixed tocopherols): 100 to 200 IU per day

- ○ Vitamin D$_3$: 2,000 to 4,000 IU per day (ideally, measure blood levels and adjust dosage accordingly)
- ○ Magnesium: 5 mg/kg per day in divided doses
- ○ Iron: 30 mg per day, bound to either pyrophosphate, succinate, glycinate, or fumarate between meals (if this recommendation results in abdominal discomfort, take 30 mg with meals two times per day or use iron pyrophosphate)
- Fish oils: 1,000 to 3,000 mg EPA + DHA per day

- One of the following:
  - ○ Grape seed extract (>95% procyanidolic oligomers): 150 to 300 mg per day
  - ○ Pine bark extract (>95% procyanidolic oligomers): 150 to 300 mg per day
  - ○ Ginkgo biloba extract (24% ginkgo flavonglycosides): 120 to 320 mg per day
- Consider:
  - ○ L-theanine: 100 to 200 mg up to three times per day
  - ○ Melatonin: 1 to 3 mg at bedtime

Autism Spectrum Disorder

- Characterized by difficulties with social interaction, problems with verbal and non-verbal communication, and repetitive behaviors or narrow, obsessive interests that usually become apparent before a child is three years old.
- Males are four times more likely than females to have an autism spectrum disorder.
- Autism spectrum disorders (ASDs) have three primary forms:
  - Classic autism
  - Asperger syndrome
  - Pervasive developmental disorder, not otherwise specified (PDD-NOS)

The use of the word *spectrum* signifies the broad range of autistic-type disorders, including severe autism, high-functioning autism, mild Asperger syndrome, and minor PDD-NOS. Asperger syndrome differs from autism in that it does not involve delays in mental development and language. PDD-NOS is the term used when not all the criteria for autism or Asperger syndrome are met. There have been proposals to eliminate all of these classifications of ASD as separate disorders and simply merge them under a single ASD diagnosis; physicians would then rate the severity of clinical presentation of ASD as severe, moderate, or mild.

Parents of infants with ASD often notice early on that their child is unresponsive to people or focuses intently on one item for long periods of time. In many cases the child appears to be developing normally but then suddenly becomes silent, withdrawn, self-abusive, or indifferent to social overtures.

The appearance of any of the warning signs of ASD is reason to have a child evaluated by a professional specializing in these disorders. Diagnosis is now possible in many cases at 18 months and in some cases as early as 12 months. Early intervention greatly improves outcomes. Early behavioral or cognitive intervention can help autistic children gain self-care, social, and communication skills. For many children, autism symptoms improve with treatment and with age. Some children with autism grow up to lead normal or near-normal lives.

The number of reported cases of autism increased dramatically in the 1990s and early 2000s. With the new diagnostic practices and classifications, the rate of ASD in the United States is now estimated at 9 cases per 1,000 compared with 1 to 2 per 1,000 worldwide.

Early and Later Signs of ASD
Early indicators

- No babbling or pointing by age 1
- No single words by 16 months or two-word phrases by age 2
- No response to name
- Loss of language or social skills
- Poor eye contact
- Excessive lining up of toys or objects
- No smiling or social responsiveness

Later indicators

- Impaired ability to make friends with peers
- Impaired ability to initiate or sustain a conversation with others
- Absence or impairment of imaginative and social play
- Repetitive or unusual use of language
- Restricted patterns of interest that are abnormal in intensity or focus
- Preoccupation with certain objects or subjects
- Inflexible adherence to specific routines or rituals

Cause

The cause of autism is extremely controversial. It does have a strong genetic component, but as with most health conditions, dietary and environmental factors play a huge role in whether and how the genetic predisposition is manifested. Perhaps more important than a specific genetic marker are the factors that determine how genes are expressed, such as environmental and nutritional factors. Although controversies surround the various proposed environmental causes, such as heavy metals, pesticides, or childhood vaccines, there is little doubt that genetic factors on their own are insufficient to lead to autism.

Therapeutic Considerations

Children with ASD require a combination of specialized and supportive educational programming, communication training (such as speech/language therapy), social skills support, and behavioral intervention. In general, the earlier these interventions are initiated the better the prognosis. Fortunately, the resources available to support children with ASD and their parents have grown considerably as the prevalence has increased.

The Individuals with Disabilities Education Act (IDEA) is a federally mandated program that ensures a free and appropriate public education for children with diagnosed learning deficits. Usually children are placed in public schools and the school district pays for all necessary services. These include, as needed, services by a speech therapist, occupational therapist, school psychologist, social worker, school nurse, or aide. By law, the public schools must prepare and carry out a set of instruction goals, or specific skills, for every child in a special education program. The list of skills is known as the child's Individualized Education Program (IEP). The IEP is an agreement between the school and the family on the child's goals.

Diet

Common dietary approaches to ADHD (see the chapter "Attention-Deficit/Hyperactivity Disorder") are also appropriate to ASD, as they aim to enhance brain function. Such dietary recommendations are not a cure, but some children experience significant improvements when food allergies are identified and food additives eliminated. Specifically, sensitivity to gluten and milk (casein protein in particular) seems to be a significant factor in some children with ASD.[1,2] Results of a gluten- and casein-free diet are entirely individualized but sometimes can be dramatic. In one study, 19 children with ASD were treated with either a gluten-free and milk-reduced diet or a milk-free and gluten-reduced diet.[3] After the diet was followed for one year, social contact had increased, self-mutilating behaviors such as head banging had ceased, and "dreamy state" periods had decreased. These improvements were accompanied by a significant decrease in urinary peptide excretion. The possible mechanism is that children with autism suffer from one or more peptidase defects that fail to break down certain peptides found in milk and wheat.[4,5] These peptides then gain entry into the brain, where they significantly disrupt brain chemistry. At the very least, a trial of a gluten- and casein-free diet for at least three months seems to be worth the effort.

The presence of other food allergies may also contribute to some of the symptoms of ASD. In fact, determining food allergies may be very important in dealing with the increased intestinal permeability noted in these patients.[5] For more information, see the chapter "Food Allergy."

Nutritional Supplements

Omega-3 Fatty Acids

Omega-3 fatty acids (such as in fish oils providing EPA + DHA) are thought to be an important nutritional supplement in ASD.[6] Despite the potential benefit, there are only a few, very small clinical studies evaluating omega-3 fatty acids in ASD. In the first double-blind study, 13 children ages 5 to 17 with ASD accompanied by severe tantrums, aggression, or self-injurious behavior were given 1.5 g EPA + DHA a day for six weeks.[7] Children taking the EPA + DHA showed improvements in hyperactivity and repetitive or ritualistic movement compared with children taking a placebo. In another controlled trial, 27 children ages 3 to 8 with ASD were given 1.3 g EPA + DHA a day for 12 weeks.[8] The children showed improvements primarily in hyperactivity. Results may be more significant in younger children than in adults: an open-label study of young adults failed to

show the same positive results as the studies of children.[9]

Vitamin B$_6$ and Magnesium

Abnormalities in serotonin and other neurotransmitters have been reported in ASD. To address these issues, vitamin B$_6$ supplementation in autistic children has been investigated in several double-blind clinical studies.[10–13] The results indicate that there is a small subgroup that improves with B$_6$ supplementation. On the average, only about 20% of patients will show moderate improvement in symptom scores, while about 10% will demonstrate dramatic clinical improvement. It has also been observed that B$_6$ supplementation had a greater effect when used in combination with magnesium.[11–13]

In a 1985 study of 60 autistic children, the children were divided into two groups and given various combinations of vitamin B$_6$, magnesium, and a placebo. Therapeutic effects were measured using behavioral rating scales and urinary excretion of homovanillic acid (HVA). The combination of B$_6$ and magnesium resulted in significant improvement in behavior that was closely associated with decreases in HVA. However, magnesium and vitamin B$_6$ were not significantly effective when used alone.[13] More recent studies have shown the same synergistic effect between B$_6$ and magnesium.[14]

Folic Acid, Vitamin B$_{12}$, and Vitamin C

The abnormalities in serotonin and other neurotransmitters reported in ASD may be due to a decrease in activity of the enzyme tryptophan hydroxylase. This enzyme is dependent on a molecule known as tetrahydrobiopterin (BH4) that has been shown to be low in people with ASD. Since the mid-1980s, several clinical trials have suggested that treatment with BH4 improves ASD in some individuals. Children with ASD who had low BH4 metabolites in the cerebrospinal fluid or urine were treated with a daily dose of 20 mg/kg BH4. The majority of children (63%) responded positively to treatment. Further research is under way, but it is believed that BH4 therapy will gain wider use if these studies show similar results.[15] Unfortunately, BH4 is not readily available, but folic acid, vitamin B_{12}, and vitamin C supplementation may improve the brain's ability to manufacture its own BH4.

Melatonin

Sleep disturbances are very common in ASD. Clinical studies have demonstrated abnormalities in the production of melatonin or its release in individuals with ASD. Several clinical studies have also shown that melatonin produces significant benefit in improving sleep quality in ASD at dosages ranging from 0.75 mg to 6 mg prior to bedtime. In fact, several meta-analyses of existing data have concluded that melatonin administration in ASD is associated with improved sleep, better daytime behavior, and minimal side effects.[16,17] The studies reviewed included three double-blind studies. All three of these studies showed a significantly shorter time to fall asleep and longer sleep duration with melatonin (2–5 mg dosage) compared with a placebo.[18–20]

In an open trial, 86% of parents of autistic children reported that melatonin produced either complete elimination or significant improvement of sleep disturbance. Of the 107 children treated with melatonin, only three had mild side effects (morning sleepiness).[21]

L-carnosine

L-carnosine is a small protein that was demonstrated in one double-blind placebo-controlled trial involving 31 children with autism to improve expressive and receptive vocabulary; there was also subjective improvement on an autism rating scale over an eight-week trial at a dosage of 800 mg per day.[22]

. . . .

QUICK REVIEW

- **Although there is a strong genetic component to ASD, there is little doubt that diet and environmental factors play a role in the expression of a genetic tendency.**
- **Children with ASD require a combination of specialized and supportive educational programming, communication training (such as speech/language therapy), social skills support, and behavioral intervention.**
- **Sensitivity to gluten and milk seems to be a significant factor in some children with ASD.**

- **Omega-3 fatty acid supplementation has been showed to reduce hyperactivity and repetitive or ritualistic movement.**
- **There is a small subgroup of ASD patients who respond to magnesium and vitamin B_6 supplementation.**
- **Several clinical trials have suggested that treatment with tetrahydrobiopterin (BH4) improves ASD in some individuals.**
- **Melatonin produces significant benefit in improving sleep quality in ASD.**
- **At this time there is no credible evidence that secretin is effective for treatment of ASD.**

Secretin

Secretin is a gastrointestinal hormone that has been extensively studied in autism. It came to light as a potential treatment after a television show highlighted a report of three children showing improvement in symptoms of autism after administration of secretin during endoscopy to examine pancreatic secretions.[23] Since then, more than a dozen well-designed studies have failed to demonstrate efficacy of secretin for symptoms of autism.[24,25] At this time there is no credible evidence that single or multiple dose intravenous secretin is effective for treatment of ASD.

· ·

TREATMENT SUMMARY

ASD requires a comprehensive approach to help facilitate the best possible outcomes. Every aspect of supporting a child with ASD should be maximized including appropriate social, speech, nutritional, and medical care. In particular, it is critical to try to address the underlying issues associated with ASD as described above.

Diet

Eliminate those dietary factors that play a role in aggravating brain dysfunction including gluten and casein sensitivity, food allergies, nutrient deficiency, and low omega-3 fatty acid levels. Otherwise, follow the general recommendations given in the chapter "A Health-Promoting Diet."

Nutritional Supplements

- **A high-potency multiple vitamin and mineral formula as described in the chapter "Supplementary Measures"**
- **Key individual nutrients:**
  - Vitamin B_6: 25 mg two to three times per day
  - Folic acid: 400 to 800 mcg per day
  - Vitamin B_{12}: 400 to 800 mcg per day
  - Vitamin D_3: 1,000 to 2,000 IU per day
  - Magnesium: 250 to 400 mg per day
- **Fish oils: 1,500 to 3,000 mg EPA + DHA per day**
- **L-carnosine: 800 mg per day**
- **One of the following:**
  - Grape seed extract (>95% procyanidolic oligomers): 150 to 300 mg per day
  - Pine bark extract (>95% procyanidolic oligomers): 150 to 300 mg per day
  - Ginkgo biloba extract (24% ginkgo flavonglycosides): 120 to 320 mg per day
- **Also consider the following (see the chapter "Attention-Deficit/Hyperactivity Disorder"):**
  - L-theanine: 100 to 200 mg up to three times per day
  - Melatonin: 1 to 3 mg at bedtime
  - Carnosine: 800 mg per day

Boils

· ·

- Painful inflammatory swelling of a hair follicle that forms an abscess; typically appears as a small rounded or conical nodule surrounded by redness, progressing to a localized pus pocket with a white center.
- There is tenderness and pain and, if the condition is severe, mild fever.
- *Staphylococcus aureus* can be cultured from the abscess.

A boil (furuncle) is a deep-seated infection (abscess) involving the entire hair follicle and adjacent tissue. The most commonly involved sites are hairy parts of the body that are exposed to friction, pressure, or moisture, such as the neck, armpits, and buttocks. Using petroleum-based skin lotions or creams can plug the hair follicles and increase the risk of boil formation. Since the infection can spread, several boils are often found at one location. When several furuncles join together, they are called a carbuncle.

Causes

There is no particular cause of boils, although occasionally they may indicate an underlying disease that is associated with poor immune function, such as diabetes, AIDS, or cancer. Most lesions will resolve within one to two weeks. Recurrent boils can indicate a highly infective form of bacteria, poor hygiene, industrial exposure to chemicals, or depression of the immune system.

Therapeutic Considerations

Recurrent attacks of boils can also indicate a depressed immune system, which may be caused by nutritional deficiencies, food allergies, and/or excessive consumption of sugar and other concentrated refined carbohydrates (see the chapter "Immune System Support," for further discussion). The treatment goals are to address any underlying immune disorder, achieve higher skin levels of vitamin A and zinc, and disinfect the area with topical application of herbal antiseptics. However, in severe cases consult a physician immediately.

Botanical Medicines

The best herbal treatment for boils is the topical application of tea tree oil. The tea tree (*Melaleuca alternifolia*) is a small tree native to only one area of the world: the northeast coastal region of New South Wales, Australia. Tea tree oil possesses significant antiseptic properties and is regarded by many as the ideal skin disinfectant. It is effective against a wide range of organisms, penetrates the skin well, and does not cause irritation.[1] Organisms inhibited by tea tree oil include:

- *Candida albicans*
- *Propionibacterium acnes*
- *Pseudomonas aeruginosa*

- *Staphylococcus aureus*
- *Streptococcus pyrogenes*
- *Trichomonas vaginalis*
- *Trichophyton mentagrophytes*

A clinical trial involving patients with boils demonstrated that tea tree oil encouraged more rapid healing without scarring, compared with matched controls.[2] Presumably the positive clinical effects were due to the oil's antibiotic activity against *Staphylococcus aureus*. The method of application included cleaning the site, followed by painting the surface of the boil freely with tea tree oil two or three times a day.

For boils and most skin infections, the most effective treatment appears to be direct application of full-strength, undiluted oil at the site of infection. If irritation occurs, try diluting the oil.

Poultices

Various herbal poultices are commonly used in the treatment of abscesses. Folk healers have used burdock root, castor oil, chervil, licorice root, and others. Poultices, although quite simple, appear to be highly effective. Historically, naturopathic physicians commonly used a poultice made from a paste of goldenseal root powder. Its efficacy is probably due to berberine, the most active alkaloid in goldenseal. Berberine is well documented as an antimicrobial agent.[3] It is toxic to the bacteria commonly associated with boils, particularly *Staphylococcus aureus*.[4] It has also been found to stimulate immune system function and decrease inflammatory processes. An advantage of goldenseal poultices, as compared with hot packs and other types of poultices, is that they usually will not cause the boil to rupture.

QUICK REVIEW

- **Recurrent attacks of boils can indicate a depressed immune system.**
- **Tea tree oil is an effective topical treatment for boils.**
- **If the boil is severe or does not resolve within two to three days, consult a physician.**

TREATMENT SUMMARY

Eliminate from the diet any foods that may suppress immune function (sugar, refined simple carbohydrates, and food allergens). If the boil is severe or does not resolve within two to three days, consult a physician, since the infection can spread under the skin, causing cellulitis (inflammation of the connective tissue), or into the bloodstream, causing bacteremia (bacteria in the blood). Cleanliness should be rigorously maintained. The infected area should be immobilized and not handled, except when necessary to change the poultice. If tea tree oil or goldenseal poultices are not available, a pack of hot Epsom salts (mix 2 tbsp Epsom salts in a cup of hot water, soak a washcloth in the solution, and apply to the boil) will bring an abscess to a head.

Nutritional Supplements

- In addition to the general recommendations given in the chapter "Supplementary Measures," take:
  - ○ Vitamin C: 500 to 1,000 mg three times per day
  - ○ Vitamin A: 5,000 IU per day (do not use more than 3,000 IU per day of vitamin A if you are pregnant or may become pregnant)
  - ○ Zinc: 30 to 45 mg per day for up to one month, then 20 to 30 mg per day

Botanical Medicines

- Tea tree oil (*Melaleuca alternifolia*): Apply undiluted oil to the affected area two to three times per day
- Goldenseal (*Hydrastis canadensis*) poultice: Mix 1 tbsp root powder with water to form a paste, then apply to abscess and cover with an absorbent bandage; use twice per day

Breast Cancer (Prevention)

- Breast cancer is most often discovered when a woman feels a lump in her breast.
  - A mammogram can detect early breast cancer.
  - Other than a lump, changes in breast size or shape such as skin dimpling, nipple inversion, or spontaneous single-nipple discharge may signal breast cancer.

Breast cancer is a cancer originating from breast tissue, most commonly from the inner lining of milk ducts or the lobules that supply the ducts with milk. Cancers originating from ducts are known as ductal carcinomas; those originating from lobules are known as lobular carcinomas.

Although breast cancer can occur in men, it is over 100 times more common in women. It is currently estimated that one out of eight women in the United States will develop breast cancer in her lifetime. It is the second most common cancer (after skin cancer) and the most common cause of cancer death in women. Breast cancer causes more than 40,000 deaths in the United States each year.

Causes

Genetics is an important risk factor, but in most cases a genetic predisposition is strongly affected by dietary, lifestyle, and environmental factors. In other words, breast cancer risk is largely a result of diet and lifestyle. The rate of breast cancer is typically five times higher for women in the United States compared with women in many other parts of the world. It is interesting to note that in Japan the rate of breast cancer is about one-fifth the rate in the United States, but in second- or third-generation Japanese women living in America and eating the typical American diet, the rate of breast cancer is identical to that of other women living in the United States.

There are many risk factors associated with breast cancer. Here is a brief overview:

- **Age.** The risk of breast cancer increases as a woman gets older. Breast cancer is uncommon in women under age 35. Most breast cancers occur in women over the age of 50, and the risk is especially high for women over 60.

- **Genetics.** The presence of certain genes (BRCA1, BRCA2, and others) increases the risk of breast cancer, although this is mainly true if many women in your family have actually developed breast or ovarian cancer. A woman's risk for developing breast cancer increases if her mother, sister, or daughter has had breast cancer, especially at a young age. Women of Ashkenazi (Central and Eastern European) Jewish ancestry also tend to have a higher than average rate of breast cancer.

- **Race.** Breast cancer occurs more often in white women than among black, Hispanic, or Asian women.

- **Estrogen.** The female hormone estrogen stimulates breast cells. The longer a woman is exposed to estrogen in any form (made by the body, taken as a drug, or delivered by a patch), the more likely she is to develop breast cancer. For example, risk is higher among women who began menstruation at an early age (before age 12), experienced menopause late (after age 55), never had children, or took hormone replacement therapy for long periods of time.

- **Later childbearing.** Women who have their first child after about age 30 have a greater chance of developing breast cancer than women who have a child at a younger age. The most protection comes from childbirth followed by breastfeeding.

- **Breast density.** Breast cancers nearly always develop in dense tissue (lobes and ducts), not in fatty tissue. That's why cancer is more likely to occur in women who have dense breast tissue than in those with fattier breast tissue. Complicating the picture is that abnormal areas in dense breasts are harder to detect on a mammogram.

- **Environmental factors.** Among the factors that have been linked to breast cancer in varying degrees are exposure to xenoestrogens (synthetic compounds that mimic estrogen), secondhand smoke, pesticides, herbicides, power lines, electric blankets, and radiation, and lack of exposure to sunlight.

- **Exercise.** Taking into account other established risk factors for breast cancer, women who exercise regularly have up to a 60% reduction in the risk of breast cancer compared with women with low levels of activity.

- **Alcohol consumption.** Women who have one drink a day have a 10% greater risk;

those who drink two drinks have a 20% increased risk, and so on.

- **Smoking.** Like most other cancers, cigarette smoking increases the risk of developing breast cancer.

- **Dietary factors.** Important dietary factors include body weight (the more overweight you are, the greater the risk); increased intake of saturated fat; and decreased intakes of antioxidants, dietary fiber, omega-3 fatty acids (particularly alpha-linolenic acid), and dietary phytoestrogens (estrogen-like compounds found in foods such as legumes, nuts, and seeds).

Detecting Breast Cancer

Conventional wisdom dictates that early detection of breast cancer improves the chances of survival. Monthly breast self-exams have been stressed as important steps toward this goal. Mammography (a special type of breast X-ray) can detect breast cancer long before it can be felt. The National Cancer institute recommends that women age 40 and older have mammograms every one to two years.

Recently, however, this practice of routine mammography has come under fire. An increasing number of studies suggest that for women under 50 who have not yet gone through menopause, screening mammograms may not be a good idea. According to many experts in the field, screening mammograms don't work very well for these women because:

- They have a high rate of false negatives (results that show no cancer when in fact cancer is present). The dense, healthy breast tissue of younger women can resemble or obscure tumors. Routine mammograms miss approximately 40% of the breast cancers that develop among women ages 40 to 49.

- Mammograms expose women to radiation that may cause breast cancer. With modern mammography equipment the risk is small (no more than 1 in 2,700). On the downside, the risk is cumulative, meaning that the chances increase with each subsequent mammogram.

- Screening mammography has not always been shown to increase the chances that premenopausal women will survive breast cancer.

- In women over the age of 50 it appears that mammography is best used to evaluate suspicious lumps, rather than screen for cancer (that is, to look for cancers when there is no sign the woman might have the disease).

- Results from a major study, the Canadian National Breast Screening Study 2, involving nearly 40,000 women, showed that yearly mammograms in women 50 to 59 did not lower breast cancer mortality compared with yearly physical examination alone. The authors of the study concluded that for women older than 50, thorough annual physical breast examinations, plus teaching of breast self-examination, may be a valid alternative to yearly mammography.[1]

- A Cochrane review in 2009 concluded that mammograms reduce mortality from breast cancer by 15% but also result in unnecessary surgery and anxiety.[2]

All of this information may be a bit confusing. There is no easy answers, as there are a lot of conflicting studies. Our recommendation is to get a baseline mammography after the age of 40, perform regular breast self-exam, get a yearly physical that includes a breast exam, and discuss the appropriateness

of regular mammography with your physician.

Alternatives to a mammogram include thermography (computerized regulation thermography or thermal imaging thermography), which can help identify inflammation of the breast tissue and/or the existence of any breast tumors, but these techniques are still considered less reliable than a mammogram.

Therapeutic Considerations

The therapeutic goal is to reduce as many risk factors as possible while simultaneously maximizing dietary and lifestyle factors associated with breast cancer prevention. Most of the lifestyle factors linked to causing or preventing cancer in general, such as avoiding cigarette smoke and excessive intake of alcohol, also apply to breast cancer. The same is true for dietary factors. Therefore, we recommend strengthening the four cornerstones of good health detailed in Section II of this book. Focusing on these key foundations provides the strongest general protection against cancer:

- A positive mental attitude
- A health-promoting lifestyle
- A health-promoting diet
- Supplementary measures

Breastfeeding

One of the most interesting protective factors appears to be breastfeeding. Numerous scientific studies show that the longer a woman breastfeeds her child, the greater the degree of protection. The minimum amount of time required to see beneficial effects is three months. Breastfeeding may be protective because it will extend the period before a woman begins to ovulate again, thus reducing her overall total lifetime burden of estrogen exposure. The total number of ovulatory cycles experienced by women was much lower in preindustrial societies than in today's society, in which women begin to have periods sooner, have children later, and have fewer children.

Preliminary evidence suggests that breastfeeding an infant girl may also help protect her from developing breast cancer as an adult. This protection may be due to the hormones and immune factors present in breast milk. Of course, there are many other important health benefits associated with breastfeeding, for both mother and baby. Babies who are breastfed have a lower incidence or severity of several childhood illnesses, including diarrhea, lower respiratory infections, ear infections, and bacterial meningitis. Other possible protective effects have been reported against sudden death infant syndrome, allergic diseases, and chronic digestive diseases.[3,4]

Exercise

Many studies have shown that exercise reduces the risk of breast cancer. Taking into account other established risk factors for breast cancer, women who regularly engage in exercise have up to a 60% lower risk of developing breast cancer compared with women with low levels of activity.[5] Exercise is even helpful in women with breast cancer, both during and after conventional treatments such as surgery, chemotherapy, and radiation.[6–8] In particular, women with breast cancer who exercised reported having higher self-esteem, improved body image, less nausea during chemotherapy treatment, and less fatigue, depression, and insomnia. Women who exercised also had improvements in physical performance and a higher quality of life. For example, in one study, women who walked at their own pace for 20 to 30 minutes four to five times per week reported feeling less fatigued and less emotionally distressed and had an improved level of physical performance.[8] Also, weight gain is a troublesome and potentially serious problem for breast cancer patients undergoing chemotherapy. In one study, the patients who gained more weight during treatment were more likely to relapse and more likely to die of their breast cancer than patients who gained less weight.[9] Breast cancer patients who exercise while undergoing treatment may gain less weight compared with patients who do not exercise.

Diet

Diet appears to be one of the most critical aspects in the prevention of breast cancer. Obesity is perhaps the most significant factor, as it carries with it at least a 30% increased risk for developing breast cancer. Just as with heart disease and other chronic degenerative disease, eating a traditional Mediterranean diet is associated with lower risk. This diet features a high intake of vegetables, fiber, fruit, and fish and unsaturated oils, particularly omega-3 fatty acids, while a typical Western diet features a high intake of total and saturated fat, refined carbohydrates, and processed and red meat, plus a low fiber intake.[10]

Research on specific dietary factors is a bit muddy because investigators often look only at dietary factors in the United States. For example, let's take a look at the research on saturated fats and breast cancer. It is difficult to determine true risk in looking at women in the United States because what is considered a low intake of saturated fat in the United States often translates to a high intake in other countries. To gauge all dietary risk factors in breast cancer, it is extremely important to examine data from a global perspective. When these sorts of analyses have been done, the results provide some sound evidence as to which dietary factors appear to promote breast cancer and which appear to be preventive.[11]

Nutritional Factors in Breast Cancer

Factors that may increase risk

Meats

High total fat intake

Saturated fats

Dairy

Refined sugar

Excess intake of total calories

Alcohol

Factors that may lower risk

Fish

Whole grains

Soy and other legumes

Cabbage

Other vegetables

Nuts

Fruits

It may not be simply that meat intake is associated with breast cancer; what may eventually be shown is that cooking method determines whether it is carcinogenic. Perhaps the most important foods to avoid are meats grilled or broiled at high temperatures, because this preparation produces many potent carcinogens, including lipid peroxides and heterocyclic amines.

Researchers from the University of South Carolina gave questionnaires to 273 women who were diagnosed with breast cancer between 1992 and 1994 as well as 657 women who were cancer-free. They found that women who routinely ate three meats—very well done hamburger and beefsteak, and bacon—had a 462% greater chance of developing breast cancer. Women who regularly consumed these meats individually had lower increases in risk for breast cancer compared with those that ate all three, but they still had an increase in breast cancer risk. The risk for very well done vs. rare or medium was 50 to 70% greater for hamburger and bacon, and 220% greater for beefsteak. These results, coupled with other evidence, suggest that avoiding well-done meats can dramatically reduce breast cancer risk.[12]

One of the most interesting aspects of the population study was the tremendous protective effect of fish consumption. Fish, particularly cold-water fish such as salmon, mackerel, halibut, and herring, are rich sources of omega-3 fatty acids. These fats have shown tremendous anticancer effects and are especially important in fighting breast cancer.[13–15] In contrast, the omega-6 fatty acids found in most animal products as well as common vegetable oils such as corn, safflower, and soy are associated with promoting breast cancer.

To evaluate the hypothesis that omega-3 fatty acids protect against breast cancer and omega-6 fatty acids promote breast cancer, the fatty acid composition of breast fatty tissue (adipose tissue) was examined from 241 patients with breast cancer and compared with that of 88 patients with benign breast disease. Women with higher levels of omega-3 fatty acids (alpha-linolenic acid, DHA) had a risk for breast cancer that was 61 to 69% less than women with lower levels. And women with the highest ratio of the long-chain omega-3 fatty acids EPA + DHA to omega-6 fatty acids had a 67% reduced risk of breast cancer.[16]

Flaxseed

In addition to a diet that features fish and fish oil supplementation, supplementing the diet with flaxseed oil and ground flaxseed appears to offer significant protection against breast cancer, for at least two reasons.

Flaxseed oil provides the short-chain omega-3 fatty acid alpha-linolenic acid. In addition to the study looking at alpha-linolenic acid (ALA) in breast fatty tissue described above, other studies have shown lower levels of ALA in breast cancer patients.[17] And in another study, of 121 women with initially localized breast cancer, a low level of ALA was associated with the spread of the cancer into the lymph nodes of the armpit as well as tumor invasiveness.[18] Since the main cause of death in breast cancer patients is the development of cancer in other tissues, this finding is extremely important. We recommend supplementing with 1 tbsp flaxseed oil (approximately 58% ALA) per day.

Flaxseed oil can be used as a salad dressing, mixed with yogurt or cottage cheese, or used as a dip for bread. Because its fats can be damaged by high heat, never cook with flaxseed oil—use olive or canola oil instead. Flaxseed oil should be bought in small, opaque bottles and kept refrigerated at all times. Some manufacturers also add antioxidants such as vitamin E or rosemary to the oil to further protect it. If a bottle of flaxseed oil is not used up within three months, throw it out and replace it with a fresh bottle, Also dispose of any flaxseed oil that has a bitter or rancid taste.

Flaxseed is also the best source of lignans, one of a group of substances called phytoestrogens that are capable of binding to estrogen receptors and interfering with the cancer-promoting effects of estrogen on breast tissue. Other foods that contain phytoestrogens include soy and whole grains. In addition to competing with estrogen for binding sites on breast cells, lignans and other phytoestrogens increase the production of a compound known as sex hormone binding globulin, which regulates estrogen levels by escorting excess estrogen from the body. Population studies, as well as experimental studies involving humans and animals, have demonstrated that lignans exert significant anticancer effects, especially against breast cancer.[19,20] For example, in one study researchers followed 28 postmenopausal nuns for a year and tracked blood levels of two cancer-related estrogens: estrone sulfate and estradiol. In addition to their normal diets, the nuns were assigned to receive supplements of either 5 or 10 g ground flaxseed per day or to a control group. Estrogen levels fell significantly among the women taking the ground flaxseed but remained stable in the control group.[21]

In another study, 50 women who had recently been diagnosed with breast cancer were divided into two groups. One group received a muffin containing 25 g ground flaxseed (about 2 tbsp) each day. The others were given ordinary muffins. When their tumors were removed a month later, the researchers examined them for signs of how fast the cancer cells had been growing. The women who had received the flaxseed muffins had slower-growing tumors than the others.[22]

Ground flaxseed provides more digestible nutritional benefits than whole seed. That's because flaxseed is very hard, making it difficult to crack, even with careful chewing. Flaxseed is easily ground with a coffee grinder, food processor, or blender. We recommend 1 or 2 tbsp per day added to foods such as hot cereals, salads, or smoothies.

Soy Products

Since the 1970s, there has been a marked increase in the consumption of both traditional soy foods (such as tofu, tempeh, and miso) and "second-generation" soy foods that simulate traditional meat and dairy products (such as soy milk, soy hot dogs, soy sausage, soy cheese, and soy frozen desserts). One of the big reasons for the increase in soy consumption is that there is now considerable evidence from test tube, animal, and population studies that soy may have an anticancer effect, particularly in hormone-sensitive cancers such as breast and prostate cancer.

Much of the latest research on soy has focused on the soy isoflavone compounds daidzein and genistein. These substances are often classified as phytoestrogens, which bind to estrogen receptor sites. However, other factors beyond isoflavones appear to contribute to soy's anticancer properties. Researchers at the University of Illinois tested the effects of purified isoflavones against soy protein mixes with and without isoflavones in female rats. Although all the compounds studied reduced the incidence of mammary gland tumors, the soy protein mix without isoflavones was the most effective in decreasing the number of tumors.

Anticancer Effects of Soy Isoflavonoids

- They act as antioxidants.
- They reduce estrogen levels, particularly free estrogen. Lower levels of estrogen have been associated with a decreased risk of breast cancer.
- They have anti-angiogenesis effects (that is, they prevent the formation of new blood vessels). This prevents tumors from obtaining the increased blood supply necessary for their continued growth.
- They prevent tumor cells from dividing and growing by inhibiting certain enzymes required during cellular replication.
- They replace animal-based protein in the diet, thus reducing intake of saturated fats, which are a known risk factor.

Population studies have offered clear evidence that soy offers some protection against breast cancer. Women in Asian countries, such as China and Japan, who traditionally consume more soy products than most women in Western countries, have a lower risk of breast cancer. There are also a growing number of clinical and experimental studies offering support for the contention that soy consumption reduces the risk for breast cancer. When healthy women add soy products to their diets, the change leads to lower levels of estrogen and other hormones in their bodies.[23–25]

The most protective benefit of soy consumption may occur before and during adolescence. Animal studies appear to show that intake of soy before adulthood enhances the maturation (differentiation) of breast cells. These more mature cells are less susceptible to carcinogens. Population-based studies seem to support the importance of intake during adolescence. Soy eaten after adolescence appears to have a more significant protective effect against premenopausal breast cancer compared with postmenopausal breast cancer.[24]

The amount and frequency of soy intake are also important. The amount necessary to protect against the development of breast cancer is thought to be 25–100 mg of isoflavones per day. We strongly recommend getting this amount from food rather than taking a dietary supplement containing purified isoflavones. Labels on any soy foods now state the level of isoflavones per serving. As the table below shows, you do not need to consume huge amounts of soy foods to get the recommended levels.

Vegetables in the Brassica Family

Vegetables in the brassica family, such as broccoli, cauliflower, cabbage, and kale, contain anticancer phytochemicals known as

Soy Foods and Their Isoflavone Content		
PRODUCT	**SERVING SIZE**	**APPROXIMATE ISOFLAVONE CONTENT (MG)**
Cooked soybeans	½ cup	40
Roasted soybeans (soy nuts)	½ cup	40
Tempeh	4 oz	40
Tofu	4 oz	40
Soy protein	½ cup	35
Soy milk	1 cup	40

glucosinolates. The chief glucosinolate is indole-3-carbinol (I3C), a compound formed whenever cruciferous vegetables are crushed, chewed, or cut. (Crushing, chewing, or cutting the cells in cruciferous vegetables activates the enzyme that makes the I3C.) I3C and other glucosinolates are antioxidants and potent stimulators of natural detoxifying enzymes in the body. I3C is converted in the stomach to several other compounds, including diindolylmethane (DIM). Both IC3 and DIM are especially protective against breast and cervical cancer (see the chapter "Cervical Dysplasia") because of a number of actions, including an ability to accelerate the breakdown of estrogen. Studies have shown that increasing the intake of brassica vegetables or taking I3C or DIM as a dietary supplement significantly increased the conversion of estrogen from cancer-producing forms to nontoxic breakdown products.[26–29]

Specifically, the body can break down estrogen into either 16-alpha-hydroxyestrone, a compound that promotes the growth of breast tumors; or 2-hydroxyestrone, which does not stimulate breast cancer cells. Adding 500 g per day of broccoli to the diet or taking IC3 (400 mg per day) or DIM (a daily dose of 2 mg/kg) improves the ratio of good to bad estrogen breakdown products, as determined by measuring these compounds in the urine. In high-risk women, we

WARNING: For women with estrogen-receptor-positive breast cancer, we recommend no more than one serving of soy per day, providing no more than 40 mg isoflavones. In test tube and animal studies, genistein has been shown to inhibit breast cancer cells that do not have estrogen receptors, but in certain situations it may actually encourage growth of breast cancer cells with estrogen receptors. Exactly how all of this research in test tubes relates to human consumption is not clear, but given the potential for harm, we recommend that until this issue is clarified, women with a history of estrogen-receptor-positive breast cancer should restrict soy intake and definitely avoid soy isoflavone supplements.

Soy consumption is also contraindicated for women who are taking the anticancer drug tamoxifen. Genistein and tamoxifen have a similar affinity for estrogen receptors. In test tube studies, when isolated human breast cells are exposed to both genistein and tamoxifen at the same time, genistein can stimulate cell growth and override the growth-inhibition effect of tamoxifen. Until researchers show us what happens when tamoxifen, genistein, and naturally occurring estrogen are all together at the same time in the human body, it is prudent to restrict soy intake while on tamoxifen.

recommend either making sure to eat large amounts of vegetables in the brassica family or supplementing the diet with IC3 or DIM. Broccoli sprouts have been reported to have the highest levels of these compounds, with 1 lb of broccoli sprouts being equivalent to 40 lbs of fresh broccoli.

Glucuronidase

One of the key ways in which the body gets rid of estrogen is by attaching glucuronic acid to estrogen in the liver and then excreting this complex in the bile. Glucuronidase is a bacterial enzyme that breaks the bond between estrogen and glucuronic acid, leading to less excretion of estrogen. Thus it is not surprising that excessive glucuronidase activity is associated with an increased cancer risk, particularly for estrogen-dependent breast cancer. The activity of this enzyme is increased when the diet is high in fat and low in fiber. The level of glucuronidase activity may be one of the factors explaining why certain dietary factors cause breast cancer and why other dietary factors are preventive.

The activity of glucuronidase can be reduced by making sure you have a good balance of health-promoting intestinal bacteria.

QUICK REVIEW

- **The rate of breast cancer is typically five times higher for women in the United States than for women in many other parts of the world.**
- **Genetics is an important risk factor, but in most cases a genetic predisposition is secondary to dietary, lifestyle, and environmental factors.**
- **Early detection of breast cancer improves the likelihood of survival.**
- **The therapeutic goal is to reduce as many risk factors as possible while simultaneously incorporating dietary and lifestyle factors associated with breast cancer prevention.**
- **Women who exercise regularly have a statistically significant lower risk of developing breast cancer.**
- **Obesity is perhaps the most significant dietary factor, as it carries with it at least a 30% increased risk for developing breast cancer.**
- **Women with the highest ratio of omega-3 fatty acids to omega-6 fatty acids have a 67% reduced risk of breast cancer.**
- **Flaxseed and flaxseed oil provide the omega-3 fatty acid alpha-linolenic acid and anticancer compounds known as lignans.**
- **There is a growing amount of evidence that soy consumption reduces the risk for breast cancer.**
- **Increasing the intake of vegetables in the brassica family or taking I3C or DIM as a dietary supplement significantly increases the conversion of estrogen from cancer-producing forms to nontoxic breakdown products.**
- **Women working the graveyard shift have an increased risk of developing breast cancer.**
- **Studies suggest that green tea offers a protective effect against breast cancer.**

Eat a diet high in plant foods and supplement it with the "friendly" bacteria *Lactobacillus acidophilus* and *Bifidobacterium bifidum*. Another dietary factor that can dramatically reduce the activity of this enzyme is the consumption of onion, garlic, and foods high in glucaric acid such as apples, brussels sprouts, broccoli, cabbage, and lettuce.

Calcium D-glucarate is a dietary supplement used to inhibit glucuronidase. Researchers at M. D. Anderson Cancer Center, Memorial Sloan-Kettering Cancer Center, and other major cancer centers have conducted preliminary research with calcium D-glucarate in the prevention and treatment of breast cancer, and the results have been quite encouraging. The recommended daily dosage for prevention is 200 to 400 mg. Higher dosages (i.e., 400 to 1,200 mg) may be necessary for individuals with existing cancer. There are no known side effects or drug interactions.[30,31]

The Night Shift—Melatonin—Breast Cancer Connection

Several studies have shown quite dramatically that women working the so-called graveyard shift have an increased risk of developing breast cancer.[32–34] In fact, in one study graveyard shift work was associated with a 60% increased breast cancer risk.[33]

The risk seems to rise with the amount of time spent working this shift.

The explanation given for this link is that exposure to artificial light at night appears to suppress the normal nighttime production of melatonin, a hormone secreted by the pineal gland (a small pea-sized gland at the base of the brain). Melatonin is critically involved in regulating the natural biorhythm of hormone secretion, and it has significant anticancer effects, especially against breast cancer. To offset the increased risk of breast cancer that comes with night shift work, we recommend taking 3 mg melatonin at bedtime for night shift workers (regardless of when that bedtime might be).

Green Tea

Population studies have shown that increasing green tea (*Camellia sinensis*) consumption reduces the risk of breast cancer. For example, studies have suggested that breast cancer rates are lower in Japan in part because, per day, people there typically drink about three cups of green tea, which provide roughly 240 to 320 mg polyphenols, substances that have an anticancer effect. To achieve the same degree of protection from supplements containing green tea extract, standardized for 80% total polyphenol content, takes 300 to 400 mg per day.[35]

- -

TREATMENT SUMMARY

Focus on reducing risk factors and incorporating dietary and lifestyle factors associated with breast cancer prevention.

Lifestyle

- **Follow the recommendations in the chapter "A Health-Promoting Lifestyle."**

Diet

- **Follow the dietary guidelines in the chapter "A Health-Promoting Diet." In particular, apply the principles of the Mediterranean-style diet: increase consumption of whole food products, including fish, cereals, vegetables, and** monounsaturated fats; eat soy foods and vegetables in the brassica family on a regular basis; avoid high-glycemic foods and unhealthy fats; and achieve and maintain ideal body weight. Take 1 or 2 tbsp ground flaxseed per day.

Nutritional Supplements

- A high-potency multiple vitamin and mineral formula as described in the chapter "Supplementary Measures"
- Key individual nutrients:
  - Vitamin D: 2,000 to 4,000 IU per day
  - Selenium: 200 mcg per day
- Fish oils: 1,000 to 3,000 mg EPA + DHA per day
- Flaxseed oil: 1 tbsp per day (in addition to the 1 tbsp of ground flaxseeds)
- One of the following:
  - Grape seed extract (>95% procyanidolic oligomers): 100 to 300 mg per day
  - Pine bark extract (>95% procyanidolic oligomers): 100 to 300 mg per day
  - Some other flavonoid-rich extract with a similar flavonoid content, super greens formula, or another plant-based antioxidant that can provide an oxygen radical absorption capacity (ORAC) of 3,000 to 6,000 units or higher per day
- Probiotic supplement (active lactobacillus and bifidobacteria cultures): a minimum of 5 billion to 10 billion colony-forming units per day
- For night shift workers: melatonin, 3 mg at bedtime
- In high-risk cases, one of the following:
  - I3C: 200 to 400 mg per day
  - DIM: 150 to 200 mg per day
  - Calcium-D-glucarate: 200 to 400 mg per day

Botanical Medicines

- Green tea extract (>80% total polyphenol content): 300 to 400 mg per day

Bronchitis and Pneumonia

....

- Cough with or without the production of mucus (sputum)
- Usually proceeded by upper respiratory tract infection or irritation of the airways
- Pneumonia shows classic signs of lung involvement (shallow breathing, cough, abnormal breath sounds, etc.)
- In pneumonia: X-ray shows infiltration of fluid and lymph in lungs

Bronchitis is inflammation of the mucous membranes of the bronchi, the passages that carry air from the trachea into the lungs. Pneumonia is inflammation of the lungs. Both acute bronchitis and pneumonia are characterized by the development of a cough with or without the production of mucus. Acute bronchitis often occurs during the course of an acute viral illness such as the common cold or influenza. Viruses cause about 90% of cases of acute bronchitis.

Although pneumonia may occur in healthy individuals, it is usually seen in those who are immune-compromised, particularly drug and alcohol abusers, individuals with chronic lung diseases, and those on chemotherapy and other drugs that suppress the immune system. Hospital-acquired pneumonia is also a serious problem and carries with it a high mortality rate. Acute pneumonia is still the seventh-leading cause of death in the United States.[1] It is particularly dangerous in the elderly.

In individuals who are not taking drugs to suppress their immune system or who are suffering from diseases associated with impaired immunity, pneumonia most often follows a viral infection (especially influenza) or an insult to the host defense mechanisms: cigarette smoke and other noxious fumes, impairment of consciousness (which depresses the gag reflex, allowing aspiration), cancer, or hospitalization (being hospitalized for any purpose increases the risk of developing pneumonia). Cigarette smoking is the strongest independent risk factor for severe pneumonia.[2]

Differentiating Between Bronchitis and Pneumonia

Since both acute bronchitis and pneumonia are characterized by a cough, it is sometimes difficult to know which is which. A chest X-ray clears up the diagnosis, but an X-ray should not be done every time someone has a cough. In patients with an acute cough, the following findings suggest the need for a chest X-ray: (1) heart rate greater than 100 beats per minute, (2) respiratory rate greater than 24 breaths per minute, (3) body temperature above 100.4°F (measured orally), and (4) characteristic chest sounds in a chest examination by a physician. Typically when a person has pneumonia there are characteristic chest sounds:

- Rales (a bubbling or crackling sound) heard on one side of the chest or while the patient is lying down

- Rhonchi (abnormal rumblings indicating the presence of thick fluid).
- On percussion, instead of a healthy hollow-drum-like sound, a dull thud that suggests consolidation (a condition in which the lung becomes firm and inelastic) and pleural effusion (fluid buildup in the space between the lungs and the lining around it)

Special Considerations with Pneumonia

The three most common forms of pneumonia are the viral, mycoplasmal, and pneumococcal types.

Viral Pneumonia

Viral pneumonia is most often caused by adenovirus, influenza virus, parainfluenza virus, or respiratory syncytial virus. Viral pneumonia is responsible for about 30% of cases of pneumonia and will often develop as a complication of an upper respiratory infection caused by one of the viruses. People who are at risk for more serious viral pneumonia include those with impaired immune function (e.g., cancer patients undergoing chemotherapy, and elderly patients with multiple nutrient deficiencies). Antibiotics are of no value in viral pneumonia.

Clinical Summary for Viral Pneumonia

- People who are at risk for more serious viral pneumonia are often immunocompromised.
- Antibiotics are of no value in viral pneumonia.
- Symptoms of viral pneumonia often begin slowly and may not be severe at first.

- The most common symptoms of viral pneumonia are
  - Cough (with some pneumonias patients may cough up mucus or even bloody mucus)
  - Fever, which may be mild or high
  - Shaking chills
  - Shortness of breath (may occur only upon mild exertion, such as climbing stairs)

Mycoplasmal Pneumonia

Mycoplasmal pneumonia is caused by *Mycoplasma pneumoniae*. *Mycoplasma* is a genus of bacteria that lack cell walls. Various studies suggest that *M. pneumoniae* is responsible for 15 to 50% of all cases of pneumonia in adults and even more than that in school-age children. It is often referred to as "walking pneumonia." Antibiotics are usually not necessary but may speed recovery. Effective classes of antibiotics that may be effective against *M. pneumoniae* include macrolides, quinolones, and tetracyclines.

Clinical Summary for Mycoplasmal Pneumonia

- Most commonly occurs in children or young adults.
- Onset is insidious, over several days.
- Nonproductive cough, minimal physical findings, temperature generally less than 102°F.
- Headache and malaise are common early symptoms.
- White blood cell count is normal or slightly elevated.
- X-ray pattern is patchy.

Pneumococcal Pneumonia

Pneumococcal pneumonia (due to *Strepto-coccus pneumoniae*) is the most common bacterial pneumonia and the most common cause of pneumonia requiring hospitalization. Antibiotics are almost always indicated in pneumococcal pneumonia. Unfortunately, antibiotics are becoming less effective, as there has been an increase in resistant strains of bacteria.[3–5] In two multinational studies, the worldwide prevalence of penicillin- and macrolide-resistant *S. pneumoniae* ranged from 18 to 22% and from 24 to 31%, respectively.[6,7] This is why it is important to consider natural treatments in cases resistant to antibiotics or as an adjunct to antibiotics.

Clinical Summary for Pneumococcal Pneumonia

- Pneumonia is usually preceded by upper respiratory tract infection.
- There is a sudden onset of shaking, chills, fever, and chest pain.
- Sputum is pinkish or blood-specked at first, then becomes rusty at the height of the infection, and finally becomes yellow and green during resolution.
- A rapid urine test (BinaxNOW) for *S. pneumoniae* antigens is positive.
- Initially breath sounds are suppressed and fine inspiratory rales are heard.
- Later, classic signs of consolidation appear (deeper rales, dullness).
- X-ray shows lung consolidation.

Therapeutic Considerations

The natural approach to bronchitis and pneumonia involves three primary goals:

(1) stimulation of normal processes that promote the expectoration (removal) of mucus; (2) thinning the mucus to aid expectoration; and (3) enhancement of immune function.

Bacterial pneumonia can be quite serious, and any individual with symptoms suggestive of pneumonia should consult a physician immediately, as antibiotics may be required. However, antibiotics offer no benefit in viral pneumonia. Nor are they useful in bronchitis, as demonstrated in more than a dozen double-blind studies over the past 30 years. According to the guidelines of the American College of Chest Physicians, "The widespread use of antibiotics for the treatment of acute bronchitis is not justified, and vigorous efforts to curtail their use should be encouraged."[8] Nonetheless, roughly 70% of doctors regularly prescribe an antibiotic for acute bronchitis even though it provides no benefit and significant risk. The risks include overgrowth of *Candida albicans*, disruption of normal gut microflora, and the possibility of developing antibiotic-resistant strains of bacteria.

Many doctors persist in prescribing antibiotics for acute bronchitis, despite the scientific facts, because of their own misconceptions—such as that a fever is a sign antibiotics are required, or that antibiotics are required to prevent progression to pneumonia. They may also prescribe antibiotics because of pressure from patients who mistakenly believe antibiotics are necessary.[9]

Expectorants

Botanical expectorants act to increase the quantity of mucus produced by the respiratory tract, decrease its viscosity, and promote its expulsion. Botanical expectorants have a long history of use in bronchitis and pneumonia. Because impaired cough reflexes have been thought to play a role in recurrent bronchitis and pneumonia, it seems reasonable that these botanicals would be useful in helping to relieve this condition and prevent recurrences.[10] Many also have antibacterial and antiviral activity. Some expectorants are also cough suppressants; however, *Lobelia inflata,* a commonly used expectorant, actually helps promote the cough reflex.[11] Therefore *Lobelia* may be more effective at clearing the lungs than other expectorants when the cough is productive. Other commonly used expectorants include *Glycyrrhiza glabra* (licorice), *Pelargonium sidoides* (South African geranium), *Hedera helix* (ivy), and wild cherry bark.

South African Geranium (*Pelargonium sidoides*)

Pelargonium sidoides is a medicinal plant in the geranium family that is native to South Africa. Its common name, *umckaloaba,* is a close approximation of a Zulu word that means "severe cough" and is a testimony to its effect in bronchitis. Extracts from the underground parts of the plant (rhizomes and tubers) have been shown to have a number of effects beneficial in upper respiratory tract infections, particularly bronchitis. Almost all of the research has been conducted using an extract known as EPs 7630 (also marketed as Umcka), and it is an approved drug for the treatment of acute bronchitis in Germany. The primary active ingredients include highly oxygenated coumarins (e.g., umckalin) and polyphenolic compounds.[12]

Research with EPs 7630 shows that it provides a three-pronged approach in acute bronchitis: (1) it enhances immune function; (2) it has some antimicrobial effects, including antimycobacterial[13] and antiviral activity,[14] and it appears to inhibit the attachment of bacteria, viruses, and perhaps other organisms to mucous membranes of the respiratory tract;[12] and (3) it acts as an expectorant.[12] In

regard to its antiviral effects, EPs 7630 has been shown to interfere with the replication of seasonal influenza A virus strains (H1N1, H3N2), respiratory syncytial virus, human coronavirus, parainfluenza virus, and coxsackievirus, but did not affect replication of avian influenza A virus (H5N1), adenovirus, or rhinovirus.[14]

A 2008 meta-analysis of four randomized clinical trials of EPs 7630 comprising 1,647 patients with acute bronchitis support its safety and efficacy.[15] On average, participants who received EPs 7630 were able to return to work two days earlier than those given a placebo. In another study, 742 children with acute bronchitis showed a drop of at least 80% in the severity of symptoms within two weeks of therapy, and over 88% of the treating physicians rated the treatment as "successful."

Since the 2008 meta-analysis there have been additional studies that offer additional evidence of the safety and efficacy of EPs 7630 in acute bronchitis as well as further insight on dosage. In the most recent of these, 406 patients with acute bronchitis were randomly assigned to one of four parallel treatment groups—10-mg EPs 7630 tablets three times a day (30 mg group), 20-mg EPs 7630 tablets three times a day (60 mg group), 30-mg EPs 7630 tablets three times a day (90 mg group), or a placebo three times a day (control group)—for seven days.[16] Effects were measured by change in the total bronchial symptom score (BSS). Between day 0 and day 7, the mean BSS score decreased by 2.7 (control group), 4.3 (30-mg group), 6.1 (60-mg group), and 6.3 (90-mg group). These results indicated that the 20-mg tablets of EPs 7630 taken three times per day constitute the optimal dose. Similar results were seen in a study of 400 children with acute bronchitis using the same dosage assessment.[17]

Ivy (*Hedera helix*)

In Europe, herbal preparations containing extracts from the leaves of ivy (*Hedera helix*) enjoy great popularity for the relief of cough as well as asthma. In 2007, more than 80% of herbal expectorants prescribed in Germany, totaling nearly 2 million prescriptions, included ivy extract. Ivy leaf contains saponins that show expectorant, mucolytic, spasmolytic, bronchodilatory, and antibacterial effects. The mucolytic and expectorant action of ivy is due to the saponins alpha-hederin and hederacoside C, the latter of which is metabolized to alpha-hederin when ingested.[18]

Ivy is often used as a sole therapy in both acute and chronic bronchitis and has very good safety, compliance, and efficacy ratings.[19,20] One double-blind study used a combination of ivy and thyme (*Thymus vulgaris*) in 361 patients with acute bronchitis suffering from 10 or more coughing fits during the day, bronchial mucus production with impaired ability to cough up the mucus, and a BSS score of 5 or more. Patients were randomly assigned to an 11-day treatment with either thyme-ivy combination syrup (5.4 ml three times per day) or placebo syrup. The average reduction in coughing fits on days seven to nine was 68.7% with the thyme-ivy combination compared with 47.6% with the placebo. In the thyme-ivy combination group, a 50% reduction in coughing fits was reached two days earlier compared with the placebo group. Symptoms as assessed by BSS score improved rapidly in both groups, but regression of symptoms was faster and responder rates were higher at the second visit (83.0% vs. 53.9%) and third visit (96.2% vs. 74.7%) with the thyme-ivy combination. Treatment was well tolerated, with no difference in the frequency or severity of side effects between the thyme-ivy combination and placebo groups.[21]

Mucolytics

A mucolytic agent should be used to thin the mucous secretions so as to promote expectoration. Guaifenesin (also known as glycerol guiacolate) is a derivative of a compound originally isolated from beech wood. Guaifenesin is an approved over-the-counter expectorant and mucolytic. It is available in many over-the-counter preparations. Alternatives include N-acetylcysteine and bromelain.

N-Acetylcysteine

N-acetylcysteine (NAC) has an extensive history of use as a mucolytic in the treatment of acute and chronic lung conditions. It directly splits the sulfur linkages of mucoproteins, thereby reducing the viscosity of bronchial and lung secretions. As a result, it improves bronchial and lung function, reduces cough, and improves oxygen saturation in the blood.

NAC is helpful in all lung and respiratory tract disorders, especially chronic bronchitis and chronic obstructive pulmonary disease. Detailed analyses of 39 trials suggest that oral NAC reduces the risk of exacerbation (severe worsening) and improves symptoms in patients with chronic bronchitis, compared with a placebo.[22]

In addition to its effects as a mucolytic, NAC can increase the manufacture of glutathione, a major antioxidant for the entire respiratory tract. The typical dosage for NAC is 200 mg three times per day.

Bromelain

Bromelain is a useful adjunctive therapy for bronchitis and pneumonia owing to its fibrinolytic, anti-inflammatory, and mucolytic actions and enhancement of antibiotic absorption.[23] Bromelain's mucolytic activity is responsible for its particular effectiveness in respiratory tract diseases, including pneumonia, bronchitis, and sinusitis.[24]

Nutritional Supplements

Vitamin C

In the early part of the 20th century, before the advent of effective antibiotics, many controlled and uncontrolled studies demonstrated the efficacy of large doses of vitamin C in bronchitis and pneumonia, but only when they were started on the first or second day of infection.[25] If administered later, vitamin C tended only to lessen the severity of the disease. Researchers also demonstrated that in pneumonia, white blood cells take up large amounts of vitamin C.

The value of vitamin C supplementation in elderly patients with pneumonia was demonstrated clearly in a double-blind study of 57 elderly patients hospitalized for severe acute bronchitis and pneumonia.[26] The patients were given either 200 mg per day of vitamin C or a placebo. Patients were assessed by clinical and laboratory methods (vitamin C levels in the plasma, white blood cells, and platelets; sedimentation rates; and white blood cell counts and differential). Patients receiving this modest dosage of vitamin C demonstrated substantially increased vitamin C levels in all tissues even in the presence of an acute respiratory infection. Using a clinical scoring system based on major symptoms of respiratory infections, patients receiving the vitamin C fared significantly better than those on the placebo. The benefit of vitamin C was most obvious in patients with the most severe illness, many of whom had low plasma and white blood cell levels of vitamin C on admission.

Vitamin A

Vitamin A supplementation appears to be of value, especially in children with measles, which has pneumonia as one of its complications. This may be because of the increased rate of excretion of vitamin A found during severe infections such as pneumonia. One study evaluated 29 patients with pneumonia and sepsis and found that their mean excretion rate of vitamin A was significantly greater than normal. A remarkable 34% of the patients excreted more than 1.75 mmol a day of vitamin A (retinol), which is equivalent to 50% of the U.S. recommended dietary intake.[27] This may be particularly important for children. A randomized, double-blind trial of 189 children with measles (average age 10 months) in South Africa evaluated the efficacy of vitamin A in reducing complications. Providing 400,000 international units (120 mg retinyl palmitate), half on admission and half on the day after admission, reduced the death rate by more than 50% and the duration of pneumonia, diarrhea, and hospital stay by 33%.[28] However, another study did not show any benefit from vitamin A supplementation. The difference may be due to the lower dose (100,000 IU) used in the second study or to the fact that it was not limited to children with pneumonia as a complication of measles.[29]

Evidence also indicates there are positive results from the use of vitamin A and concomitant zinc supplementation. One study of 2,482 children from six months to three years old revealed that those children given initial high doses of vitamin A followed by four months of elemental zinc (10 mg per day for infants and 20 mg per day for children older than one year) brought about a reduced incidence of pneumonia, which was not seen in the group given only vitamin A.[30]

In the United States, we do not think it is necessary to give such extreme dosages of vitamin A, but we do feel that in children especially, reasonable dosages of vitamin A (e.g., 10,000 IU per day for one week) may provide benefit and that it should be accompanied by zinc at the levels given above. (Note that women of childbearing age should not take more than 3,000 IU of vitamin A per day.)

Bottle Blowing and Salt Pipes

A Swedish study carried out with 145 adults hospitalized for pneumonia showed that the patients who were instructed to sit up and blow bubbles in a bottle containing 10 ml water through a plastic tube 20 times on 10 occasions per day had shorter hospital stays.[31] Another study found this also helped decrease impairment of pulmonary function and an increase in total lung capacity in patients who had undergone coronary artery bypass surgery.[32] Bottle blowing or another similar activity, such as a playing a wind instrument, may well prove useful as a means of decreasing the frequency and duration of respiratory events in patients who are vulnerable to respiratory infections such as pneumonia.

An alternative to bubble blowing is the use of a salt pipe. These pipes are inhaler-type devices containing tiny salt particles said to ease breathing. The practice originated in central Europe, where individuals with respiratory complaints would spend time in salt caves or mines to help relieve their breathing problems.

Postural Draining

One of the main treatment goals in bronchitis, sinusitis, and pneumonia is to help the lungs and air passages get rid of the excessive mucus. We recommend applying a heating pad, hot water bottle, or mustard poultice to the chest for up to 20 minutes twice per day. A mustard poultice is made by mixing 1 part dry mustard with three parts flour and adding enough water to make a paste (the strength of mustard powder varies greatly, so test a small amount on the skin first to be sure it is not too strong, as indicated by excessive redness). The paste is spread on thin cotton (an old pillowcase works very well) or cheesecloth, and the folded cloth is placed on

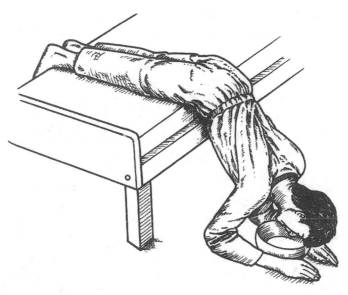

Postural Drainage Position

the chest. Check often, as mustard can cause blisters if left on too long. After the hot pack or mustard poultice, perform postural drainage by lying with the top half of the body off the bed, using the forearms as support, for a 5- to 15-minute period while trying to cough and expectorate into a basin or newspaper on the floor.

QUICK REVIEW

- **Most cases of bronchitis and/or pneumonia do not require antibiotics.**
- **The natural approach to bronchitis and pneumonia involves three primary goals: (1) stimulate normal processes that promote the expectoration (removal) of mucus; (2) thin the mucus to aid expectoration; and (3) enhance immune function.**
- **Despite sufficient data showing no clinical benefit for antibiotics in acute bronchitis, many doctors prescribe these drugs for patients with acute bronchitis.**
- **Botanical expectorants act to increase the quantity, decrease the viscosity, and promote expulsion of the secretions of the respiratory mucous membranes.**
- **A 2008 meta-analysis of randomized clinical trials of EPs 7630 (Umcka) supports its safety and efficacy**
- **N-acetylcysteine has shown good results in the treatment of bronchitis.**
- **Vitamin C supplementation is warranted in all elderly patients with acute respiratory infection, especially those who are severely ill.**
- **The application of local heat followed by postural drainage can help get rid of excessive mucus.**

TREATMENT SUMMARY

As stated above, the basic approach is to use expectorants, mucolytics, and immune-supportive nutrients to help resolve the condition. Some general physical measures may also be helpful, including the use of a mustard poultice or hot pack along with postural drainage and the use of a salt pipe or bottle blowing. In addition, it is important to:

- **Get plenty of rest.**
- **Drink enough liquids.**
- **Use a humidifier.**

Expectorants

- **One or more of the following:**
  - *Lobelia inflata:*
    - **Dried herb: 0.2 to 0.6 g three times per day**
    - **Tincture: 15 to 30 drops three times per day**
    - **Fluid extract: 8 to 10 drops three times per day**
  - **Licorice root (*Glycyrrhiza glabra*):**
    - **Powdered root: 1 to 2 g**
    - **Fluid extract (1:1): 2 to 4 ml**

- Solid (dry powdered) extract (4:1): 250 to 500 mg
○ *Pelargonium sidoides* (EPs 7630 or equivalent):
  - Adults: 1.5 ml three times per day or 20 mg tablets three times per day for up to 14 days
  - Children: ages 7 to 12, 20 drops (1 ml) three times per day; 6 years or less, 10 drops (0.5 ml) three times per day
○ Ivy (*Hedera helix*), available as tincture, fluid extract, and dry powdered extract in capsules and tablets; typical dosage for adults and children over 12 years of age for a 4:1 dry powdered extract is 100 mg per day (the equivalent of 420 mg dried herbal substance); for children 1–5 years old, dosage is the equivalent of 150 mg dried herbal substance; for children 6–12 years old, the equivalent of 210 mg dried herbal substance

Mucolytics

- One or more of the following:
  ○ Guaifenesin
    - Adults and children 12 years of age and older: 200 to 400 mg every four hours (do not take more than 2,400 mg in a 24-hour period)
    - Children 6 to 11 years old: 100 to 200 mg every 4 hours (do not take more than 1,200 mg in a 24-hour period)

- Children 2 to 5 years old: 50 to 100 mg every four hours (do not take more than 600 mg in 24 hours)
- Children under 2 years of age: not recommended
○ N-acetylcysteine: 200 mg three times per day
○ Bromelain (1,200 to 1,800 MCU or GDU): 500 to 750 mg three times per day between meals

Nutritional Supplements

- A high-potency multiple vitamin and mineral formula as described in the chapter "Supplementary Measures"
- Key individual nutrients:
  ○ Vitamin A: 10,000 international units per day for 1 week (women who are pregnant or who may become pregnant should not take more than 3,000 IU per day)
  ○ Vitamin C: 500–1,000 mg every two hours
  ○ Zinc: 20–30 mg per day
- One of the following:
  ○ Bioflavonoids (mixed citrus): 1,000 mg per day
  ○ Grape seed extract (>95% procyanidolic oligomers): 150 to 300 mg per day
  ○ Pine bark extract (>95% procyanidolic oligomers): 150 to 300 mg per day.

Candidiasis, Chronic

- Positive demonstration of yeast overgrowth on stool culture
- Higher than normal levels of candida antibodies or antigens in the blood

In the past 30 years, overgrowth in the gastrointestinal (GI) tract of the usually benign yeast *Candida albicans* has become increasingly recognized as a complex medical syndrome known as *chronic candidiasis* or *yeast syndrome*.[1,2] Specifically, the overgrowth of candida is believed to cause a wide variety of symptoms in virtually every system of the body, with the GI, genitourinary, endocrine, nervous, and immune systems being most susceptible.[3]

Although chronic candidiasis has been clinically defined for a long time, it was not until Orion Truss published *The Missing Diagnosis* and William Crook published *The Yeast Connection* that the public and many physicians became aware of the magnitude of the problem.[1,2]

Normally, *C. albicans* lives harmoniously in the inner warm creases and crevices of the digestive tract (and in the vaginal tract in women). However, when this yeast overgrows, when immune system mechanisms are depleted, or when the normal lining of the intestinal tract is damaged, the body can absorb yeast cells, particles of yeast cells, and various toxins.[3] As a result, there may be significant disruption of body processes, resulting in the development of yeast syndrome.

Patients who have chronic candidiasis generally say they "feel sick all over." Fatigue, allergies, immune system malfunction, depression, chemical sensitivities, and digestive disturbances are just some of the symptoms patients with yeast syndrome may experience.[3]

The typical patient with yeast is female, as women are eight times more likely to experience yeast syndrome compared with men owing to the effects of estrogen, birth control pills, and the higher number of prescriptions for antibiotics (see box).[4]

TYPICAL CHRONIC CANDIDIASIS PATIENT PROFILE

Sex: Female

Age: 15–50 years

General symptoms:
- Chronic fatigue
- Loss of energy
- General malaise
- Decreased libido

Gastrointestinal symptoms:
- Thrush
- Bloating, gas
- Intestinal cramps
- Rectal itching
- Altered bowel function

Genitourinary system complaints
- Vaginal yeast infection
- Frequent bladder infections

Endocrine system complaints:
- Primarily menstrual complaints

Nervous system complaints:
- Depression
- Irritability
- Inability to concentrate

Immune system complaints:
- Allergies
- Chemical sensitivities
- Low immune function

Past history:
- Chronic vaginal yeast infections
- Chronic antibiotic use for infections or acne
- Oral birth control usage
- Oral steroid hormone usage

Associated conditions:
- Premenstrual syndrome
- Sensitivity to foods, chemicals, and other allergens
- Endocrine disturbances
- Eczema
- Psoriasis
- Irritable bowel syndrome

Other:
- Craving for foods rich in carbohydrates or yeast

Causes

Chronic candidiasis is a classic example of a multifactorial condition, as shown in the list below. Therefore, the most effective treatment involves addressing and correcting the factors that predispose to *C. albicans* overgrowth. It involves much more than killing the yeast with antifungal agents, whether synthetic or natural.

Predisposing Factors in *Candida albicans* Overgrowth

Decreased digestive secretions

Dietary factors

Impaired immunity

Nutrient deficiency

Drugs

Prolonged antibiotic use

Impaired liver function

Underlying disease states

Altered bowel flora

Prolonged antibiotic use is believed to be the most important factor in the development of chronic candidiasis in most cases. By suppressing normal intestinal bacteria that prevent yeast overgrowth and suppression of the immune system, antibiotics strongly promote the overgrowth of candida.

There is little argument that, when used appropriately, antibiotics save lives. However, there is also little argument that antibiotics are seriously overused, both clinically and in animals raised for food. Although the appropriate use of antibiotics makes good medical sense, what does not make sense is reliance on them for such conditions as acne, recurrent bladder infections, chronic ear infections, chronic sinusitis, chronic bronchitis, and nonbacterial sore throats. Relying on antibiotics in the treatment of these conditions does not make sense, as either the antibiotics rarely provide benefit or these conditions are effectively treated with natural measures. Equally problematic is the heavy use of antibiotics in animals raised for food. According to the FDA, 80% of antibiotics in the United States are used in animals. This contributes to antibiotic resistance as well as human exposure to antibiotics.

CANDIDIASIS QUESTIONNAIRE

History | Score

1. Have you taken broad-spectrum or other antibiotics for acne for one month or longer? — 25

2. Have you ever taken broad-spectrum antibiotics for respiratory, urinary, or other infections for two months or longer, or in short courses four or more times in a one-year period? — 20

3. Have you ever taken any broad-spectrum antibiotic, even a single course? — 6

4. Have you ever been bothered by persistent prostatitis, vaginitis, or other problems affecting your reproductive organs? — 25

5. Have you been pregnant . . .
   One time? — 3
   Two or more times? — 5

6. Have you taken birth control pills . . .
   For six months to two years? — 8
   For more than two years? — 15

7. Have you taken prednisone or other cortisone-type drugs . . .
   For two weeks or less? — 6
   For more than two weeks? — 15

8. Does exposure to perfumes, insecticides, fabric shop odors, and other chemicals provoke . . .
   Mild symptoms? — 5
   Moderate to severe symptoms? — 20

9. Are your symptoms worse on damp, muggy days or in moldy places? — 20

10. If you have ever had athlete's foot, ringworm, jock itch, or other chronic infections of the skin or nails, have the infections been . . .
    Mild to moderate? — 10
    Severe or persistent? — 20

11. Do you crave sugar? — 10
12. Do you crave breads? — 10
13. Do you crave alcoholic beverages? — 10
14. Does tobacco smoke *really* bother you? — 10

Total score for this section _____

Major Symptoms

For each of your symptoms, enter the appropriate figure in the Score column.

> If a symptom is occasional or mild — score 3 points
> If a symptom is frequent and/or moderately severe — score 6 points
> If a symptom is severe and/or disabling — score 9 points

1. Fatigue or lethargy ____
2. Feeling of being "drained" ____
3. Poor memory ____
4. Feeling "spacey" or "unreal" ____
5. Depression ____
6. Numbness, burning, or tingling ____
7. Muscle aches ____
8. Muscle weakness or paralysis ____
9. Pain and/or swelling in joints ____
10. Abdominal pain ____
11. Constipation ____
12. Diarrhea ____
13. Bloating ____
14. Persistent vaginal itch ____
15. Persistent vaginal burning ____
16. Prostatitis ____
17. Impotence ____
18. Loss of sexual desire ____
19. Endometriosis ____

20. Cramps and/or other menstrual irregularities ____

21. Premenstrual tension ____

22. Spots in front of eyes ____

23. Erratic vision ____

Total score for this section _____

Other Symptoms

For each of your symptoms, enter the appropriate figure in the Score column.

If a symptom is occasional or mild	score 1 point
If a symptom is frequent and/or moderately severe	score 2 points
If a symptom is severe and/or disabling	score 3 points

1. Drowsiness ____

2. Irritability ____

3. Lack of coordination ____

4. Inability to concentrate ____

5. Frequent mood swings ____

6. Headache ____

7. Dizziness/loss of balance ____

8. Pressure above ears, feeling of head swelling and tingling ____

9. Itching ____

10. Other rashes ____

11. Heartburn ____

12. Indigestion ____

13. Belching and intestinal gas ____

14. Mucus in stools ____

15. Hemorrhoids ____

16. Dry mouth ____

17. Rash or blisters in mouth ____

18. Bad breath ____

19. Joint swelling or arthritis ____

20. Nasal congestion or discharge ____

21. Postnasal drip ____

22. Nasal itching ____

23. Sore or dry throat ____

24. Cough ____

25. Pain or tightness in chest ____

26. Wheezing or shortness of breath ____

27. Urinary urgency or frequency ____

28. Burning on urination ____

29. Failing vision ____

30. Burning or tearing of eyes ____

31. Recurrent infections or fluid in ears ____

32. Ear pain or deafness ____

Total score for this section _____

Total score for all three sections _____

Interpretation

If your score is:

Women	Men	
>180	>140	Yeast-connected health problems are almost certainly present
120–180	90–140	Yeast-connected health problems are probably present
60–119	40–89	Yeast-connected health problems are possibly present
<60	<40	Yeast-connected health problems are less likely to be present

Diagnostic Considerations

Although the candida questionnaire can help, the best method for diagnosing chronic candidiasis is clinical evaluation by a physician knowledgeable about yeast-related illness. It is more than likely that the doctor will take a detailed medical history and ask you to fill out a patient questionnaire. He or she may also employ laboratory techniques such as stool cultures for *C. albicans* and measurement of levels of antibodies to *C. albicans* or *C. albicans* antigens in the blood. Although these laboratory examinations are useful diagnostic aids, they should be used to confirm the diagnosis. In other words, the diagnosis is best made by evaluation of a patient's history and clinical picture.

Comprehensive Stool and Digestive Analysis

Compared with simply culturing a stool sample for the presence of *C. albicans*, the comprehensive digestive stool analysis (CDSA) is more clinically useful. This battery of integrated diagnostic laboratory tests evaluates digestion, intestinal function, intestinal environment, and absorption by carefully examining the stool. It is a useful tool in determining the digestive disturbance that is likely to be the underlying factor responsible for *C. albicans* overgrowth. In addition, the CDSA may determine that the symptoms are related not to *C. albicans* overgrowth but rather to a condition such as small-intestine bacterial overgrowth or leaky gut syndrome.

Antibody and Antigen Levels

Another laboratory method to confirm the presence of *C. albicans* overgrowth involves measuring the level of antibodies to candida or the level of antigens in the blood.[5]

However, our feeling is that these tests are rarely necessary, as the results typically only confirm what the patient history, physical examination, and CDSA reveal. Hence the test does not change the course of action. Nonetheless, some patients and physicians may desire confirmation that *C. albicans* is a significant factor in the patient's health. In this situation, blood studies can be helpful and can also be used as a way of monitoring therapy.

Therapeutic Considerations

A comprehensive approach is more effective in treating chronic candidiasis than simply trying to kill the *C. albicans* with a drug such as nystatin, ketoconazole, or fluconazole, or with a natural antifungal agent. These rarely produce significant long-term results because they fail to address the underlying factors that promote *C. albicans* overgrowth. It's a bit like trying to weed a garden by simply cutting the weeds, instead of pulling them out by the roots. Nonetheless, in many cases it is useful to try to eradicate *C. albicans* from the system, preferably with the help of natural antiyeast therapies described below. A follow-up stool culture and *C. albicans* antigen determination will confirm if the candida has been eliminated. If it has and symptoms are still apparent, it is likely that the symptoms are unrelated to an overgrowth of *C. albicans*. Symptoms similar to those attributed to chronic candidiasis can be caused by small-intestine bacterial overgrowth, for example. In such a case, pancreatic enzymes and berberine-containing plants such as goldenseal can be helpful.

In addition to using natural agents to eradicate *C. albicans*, it is important to address predisposing factors, go on a diet that helps control candida, and support various body systems according to your individual needs.

Diet

A number of dietary factors appear to promote the overgrowth of *C. albicans*. The most important factors are a high intake of sugar; milk and other dairy products; foods containing a high content of yeast or mold; and food allergies.

Sugar

Sugar is the chief nutrient for *C. albicans*. It is well accepted that restriction of sugar intake is an absolute necessity in the treatment of chronic candidiasis. Most patients do well by simply avoiding refined sugar and large amounts of honey, maple syrup, and fruit juice.[1–4]

Milk and Other Dairy Products

There are several reasons to restrict or eliminate the intake of milk in patients with chronic candidiasis:

- High lactose content promotes the overgrowth of candida.
- Milk is one of the most frequent food allergens.
- Milk may contain trace levels of antibiotics, which can further disrupt the GI bacterial flora and promote candida overgrowth.

Mold- and Yeast-Containing Foods

Many experts generally recommend that individuals with chronic candidiasis avoid foods with a high content of yeast or mold, including alcoholic beverages, cheeses, dried fruits, and peanuts. Even though many patients with chronic candidiasis may be able to tolerate these foods, we think it is still a good idea to avoid them until the situation is under control.

Food Allergies

Food allergies are another common finding in patients with yeast syndrome.[3] ELISA tests, which can identify both IgE- and IgG-mediated food allergies, are often helpful.

Hypochlorhydria

An important step in treating chronic candidiasis in many cases is improving digestive secretions. Gastric hydrochloric acid, pancreatic enzymes, and bile all inhibit the overgrowth of *C. albicans* and prevent its penetration into the absorptive surfaces of the small intestine. Decreased secretion of any of these important digestive components can lead to overgrowth of yeast in the GI tract. For example, people on acid-blocking drugs, including over-the-counter varieties, can develop yeast overgrowth in the stomach.[6] And pancreatic enzymes are largely responsible for keeping the small intestine free from parasites (including bacteria, yeast, protozoa, and intestinal worms).[7,8] Therefore, restoration of normal digestive secretions through the use of supplemental hydrochloric acid, digestive enzymes, and substances that promote bile flow is critical in the treatment of chronic candidiasis. The comprehensive digestive stool analysis can provide valuable information to help identify which factor is most important. See the chapter "Digestion and Elimination" for more information.

Enhancing Immunity

Recurrent or chronic infections, including chronic candidiasis, are signs of a depressed immune system. What makes it difficult for people to overcome chronic candidiasis is a repetitive cycle—a compromised immune system leads to infection, and infection leads to damage to the immune system, further weakening resistance.

The importance of a healthy immune system in protecting against *C. albicans* overgrowth is well known by any physician who has seen a patient suffering from AIDS or taking drugs that suppress the immune system. In either case, severe yeast overgrowth is a hallmark feature. The occurrence of candida overgrowth in these conditions provides considerable evidence that improving the functioning of the immune system is absolutely essential in the patient with chronic candidiasis.

In addition, patients with chronic candidiasis often suffer from other chronic infections, presumably due to a depressed immune system. Typically, this depression of immune function is related to decreased thymus function and is manifested primarily as depressed cell-mediated immunity. Although expensive laboratory tests can document this depression, it is better to rely on the history of repeated viral infections (including the common cold), outbreaks of cold sores or genital herpes, and prostatic (in men) or vaginal (in women) infections.

Causes of Depressed Immune Function in Candidiasis

As we've noted, the person with chronic candidiasis is typically stuck in a vicious circle. A triggering event such as antibiotic use or nutrient deficiency can lead to immune suppression, allowing *C. albicans* to overgrow and become more firmly entrenched in the lining of the GI tract. Once the organism attaches itself to the intestinal cells, it competes with the cell and ultimately the entire body for nutrition, potentially robbing the body of vital nutrients. In addition, this kind of yeast secretes a large number of mycotoxins and antigens.[9,10] Candida is referred to as a *polyantigenic* organism because more than 79 distinct antigens have been identified. Because of this tremendous number of antigens, an overgrowth of *C. albicans* greatly taxes the immune system.

Triggers to Impaired Immunity in Candidiasis

Antibiotic use

Corticosteroid use

Other drugs that suppress the immune system

Nutrient deficiency

Food allergies

High-sugar diet

Stress

Restoring Proper Immune Function

Restoring proper immune function is one of the key goals in the treatment of chronic candidiasis. No single magic bullet exists to immediately bring the immune system back to an optimal state. Instead, we recommend a comprehensive approach involving lifestyle, stress management, exercise, diet, nutritional supplementation, and the use of plant-based medicines. For more information, see the chapter "Immune System Support."

Perhaps the most effective intervention in reestablishing a healthy immune system is measures designed to improve thymus gland function.[11,12] Promoting optimal thymus activity primarily involves prevention of thymus gland atrophy (shrinkage) by ensuring adequate dietary intake of antioxidant nutrients such as carotenes, vitamin C, vitamin E, zinc, and selenium.

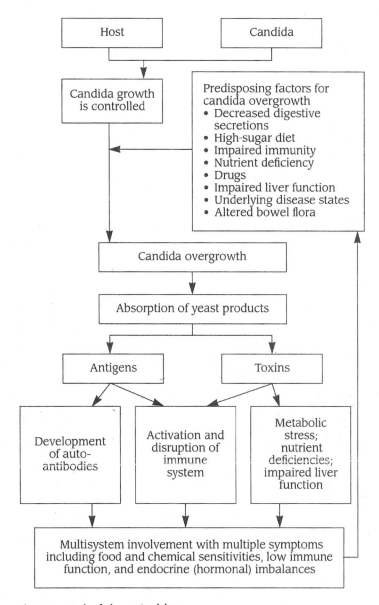

The Vicious Circle of Chronic Candidiasis

Promoting Detoxification

People with chronic candidiasis usually exhibit multiple chemical sensitivities and allergies, an indication that the body's detoxification reactions are stressed. Supporting liver function will help promote detoxification and may be one of the most critical factors in the successful treatment of candidiasis.

Damage to the liver is often an underlying factor in chronic yeast overgrowth, as well as in chronic fatigue (see the chapter "Chronic

Fatigue Syndrome"). When the liver is even slightly damaged by chemical toxins, immune function is severely compromised.

The immune-system-suppressing effect of nonviral liver damage has been repeatedly demonstrated in experimental animal studies and human studies. For example, when the liver of a rat is damaged by a chemical toxin, immune function is severely hindered.[13] Liver injury is also linked to *C. albicans* overgrowth, as evident in studies with mice.[14]

A rational approach to aiding the body's detoxification involves the following:

- A diet focused on fresh fruits and vegetables, whole grains, legumes, nuts, and seeds
- A healthful lifestyle, including exercising regularly and avoiding alcohol
- A high-potency multiple vitamin and mineral supplement
- Lipotropic formulas and silymarin to protect the liver and enhance liver function
- A three-to-seven-day nutritional cleansing program or fast at the change of each season

Indications of the Need for Detoxification

More than 20 lb overweight

Diabetes

Gallstones

History of heavy alcohol use

Psoriasis

Natural and synthetic steroid hormone use

- ○ Anabolic steroids
- ○ Estrogens
- ○ Oral contraceptives

High exposure to certain chemicals or drugs

- ○ Cleaning solvents
- ○ Pesticides
- ○ Antibiotics
- ○ Diuretics
- ○ Nonsteroidal anti-inflammatory drugs
- ○ Thyroid hormone

History of viral hepatitis

Lipotropic Factors

The nutrients choline, betaine, and methionine are often beneficial in enhancing liver function and detoxification reactions in patients with chronic candidiasis. These compounds, referred to as *lipotropic agents*, promote the flow of fat and bile to and from the liver. In essence, they produce a "decongesting" effect on the liver and help improve liver function and fat metabolism. Nutrition-oriented physicians have used lipotropic formulas for a wide variety of conditions, including liver disorders such as hepatitis, cirrhosis, and chemical-induced liver disease. The daily dosage should be 1,000 mg choline and 1,000 mg methionine or cysteine (or both).

Lipotropic formulas appear to increase levels of two important liver substances: SAM-e (S-adenosyl-methionine), the major lipotropic compound in the liver; and glutathione, one of the major detoxifying compounds in the liver.[15,16] Alternatively, SAM-e can be taken at a dosage of 200 mg three times per day.

Promoting Elimination

In addition to directly supporting liver function, proper detoxification involves proper elimination. A diet that focuses on high-fiber plant foods should be sufficient to promote proper elimination. If additional support is needed, fiber formulas can be prescribed. These formulas may include natural plant fibers derived from psyllium seed, kelp, agar, pectin, and plant gums such as karaya and guar. Alternatively, they may include purified semisynthetic polysaccharides such as methylcellulose and carboxymethyl cellulose. During treatment of candidiasis, take 3 to 5 g soluble fiber at bedtime, to ensure that dead yeast cells are excreted and not absorbed.

Probiotics

Intestinal flora plays a major role in the health of the host, especially in the battle against GI tract infection.[17,18] The kind of bacteria found in the intestinal tract is intimately involved in the body's nutritional status and affects immune system function, cholesterol metabolism, carcinogenesis, and aging. Probiotic supplements can be used both to support overall good health and during treatment for chronic candidiasis.

The dosage of a commercial probiotic supplement containing lactobacillus or bifidobacteria cultures is based on the number of live organisms. A dosage of 5 billion to 10 billion viable cells per day is sufficient for most people. Amounts exceeding these may induce mild GI disturbances, while smaller amounts may not be able to colonize the GI tract.

Natural Antiyeast Agents

A number of natural agents have proven activity against *C. albicans*. As we have noted, however, rather than relying on these agents as a primary therapy, it is important to address the underlying factors that predispose to chronic candidiasis.

The four approaches we feel most comfortable in recommending as natural agents against *C. albicans* are:

- Berberine-containing plants
- Garlic
- Enteric-coated volatile oil preparations like oregano
- Propolis

Most but not all patients can achieve benefits from the natural agents described here.

Use of any effective antiyeast therapy alone, without the other supportive measures we recommend, may result in a Herxheimer reaction (die-off). When an antiyeast agent rapidly kills off the candida, the body must deal with large quantities of yeast toxins, cell particles, and antigens, and symptoms may worsen. The Herxheimer reaction can be minimized by the following measures:

- Following the dietary recommendations for a minimum of two weeks before taking an antiyeast agent
- Supporting the liver by following the recommendations made earlier
- Starting any of the previously described antiyeast medications in low doses and gradually increasing the dose over the course of one month to achieve full therapeutic value

Berberine-Containing Plants

Berberine-containing plants include goldenseal (*Hydrastis canadensis*), barberry (*Berberis vulgaris*), Oregon grape (*Berberis aquifolium*), and goldthread (*Coptis chinensis*). Berberine, an alkaloid, has been extensively studied in both experimental and clinical settings for its antibiotic activity. Berberine exhibits a broad spectrum of antibiotic activity, having shown activity against bacteria, protozoa, and fungi, including *C. albicans*.[19-25]

Berberine's antibiotic action against some of these pathogens is actually stronger than that of some commonly used pharmaceutical antibiotics. And because berberine inhibits *C. albicans* as well as pathogenic bacteria, it can help prevent the overgrowth of yeast that is a common side effect of antibiotic use.

Berberine has shown remarkable antidiarrheal activity in even the most severe cases, including cholera, amebiasis, giardiasis, and other causes of acute GI infection. It may also relieve the diarrhea seen in patients with chronic candidiasis.[26–32]

The dosage of any berberine-containing plant should be based on berberine content. The recommended dosage of berberine is 25 to 50 mg three times per day. (For children, a dosage based on body weight is appropriate: a total of 5 to 10 mg/kg berberine per day.) With goldenseal, for example, standardized extracts are preferred, as there is a wide range of quality in goldenseal preparations. For goldenseal, the dosage would be:

- Dried root or as infusion (tea), 2 to 4 g three times a day

- Tincture (1:5), 6 to 12 ml (1.5 to 3 tsp) three times a day

- Fluid extract (1:1), 2 to 4 ml (0.5 to 1 tsp) three times a day

- Solid (powdered dry) extract (4:1 or 8% to 12% alkaloid content), 250 to 500 mg three times a day

Berberine and berberine-containing plants are generally nontoxic at the recommended dosages; however, berberine-containing plants are not recommended for use during pregnancy, and higher dosages may interfere with B vitamin metabolism.[33]

Garlic

Garlic has demonstrated significant antifungal activity. In fact, its inhibition of *C. albicans* in both animal and test tube studies has shown it to be more potent than nystatin, gentian violet, and six other reputed antifungal agents.[34–36] The active component is allicin, which is also responsible for garlic's pungent odor. Modern clinical use of garlic features the use of commercial enteric-coated preparations designed to offer the benefits of garlic without the odor (the allicin is released in the small and large intestine).

The treatment of chronic candidiasis requires a daily dose of at least 10 mg allicin or a total allicin potential of 4,000 mg. This amount is equal to approximately one clove (4 g) of fresh garlic. Going beyond this dosage, even with these odorless preparations, usually results in a detectable odor of garlic.

Enteric-Coated Volatile Oils

Volatile oils from oregano, thyme, peppermint, and rosemary are all effective antifungal agents. One study with oregano oil showed the minimum inhibitory concentration was less than 0.1 mg/ml.[37] These results indicate that the anti–*C. albicans* activity of oregano oil is more than 100 times as potent as caprylic acid—a popular natural product to fight candida. Because volatile oils are quickly absorbed and may induce heartburn, an enteric coating is recommended to ensure delivery to the small and large intestine. An effective dosage for an enteric-coated volatile oil preparation is 0.2 to 0.4 ml twice per day between meals—the same dosage used in the treatment of irritable bowel syndrome (see the chapter "Irritable Bowel Syndrome").

Nutritional Supplements

Tea Tree Oil

Tea tree (*Melaleuca alternifolia*) oil is another option, especially in the topical treatment of candida infections such as thrush or vaginal yeast infection. In one open study, 27 patients with AIDS and oral candidiasis that did not respond to fluconazole were randomly assigned to receive either an alcohol-based or an alcohol-free *Melaleuca alternifolia* oral solution four times per day for two to four weeks. Overall, 60% of patients demonstrated a clinical response to this oral solution (seven patients cured and eight patients clinically improved).[38]

Propolis

Propolis is the resinous substance collected by bees from the leaf buds and barks of trees, especially poplar and conifer trees. The bees use the propolis, along with beeswax, to construct the hive. Propolis has antimicrobial activities that help the hive block out viruses, bacteria, and other organisms.

The primary use of propolis has been in immune system enhancement and infections. Propolis has shown considerable in vitro antimicrobial activity against *C. albicans*, as well as an ability to enhance the effectiveness of conventional antifungal drugs.[39–42] Its cytotoxic activity against *C. albicans*, along with its immune-enhancing effects, makes propolis a strong candidate for treatment of chronic candidiasis. The typical dosage is 100 to 500 mg three times per day.

QUICK REVIEW

- **Prolonged antibiotic use is believed to be the most important factor in the development of chronic candidiasis.**
- **A physician knowledgeable about yeast-related illness can help in diagnosing, treating, and monitoring chronic candidiasis.**
- **A comprehensive approach is more effective in treating chronic candidiasis than simply trying to kill the candida with a drug or natural antiyeast agent.**
- **Recurrent or chronic infections, including chronic candidiasis, are characterized by a depressed immune system.**

- **Restoring proper immune function is one of the key goals in the treatment of chronic candidiasis.**
- **Enteric-coated volatile oil preparations may be effective natural anti-candida compounds.**
- **Propolis has shown considerable in vitro antimicrobial activity against *C. albicans*, as well as an ability to enhance the effectiveness of conventional antifungal drugs.**

TREATMENT SUMMARY

The following is a comprehensive step-by-step approach to the successful elimination of chronic candidiasis.

1. Identify and address predisposing factors:

o Eliminate the use of antibiotics, steroids, immune-suppressing drugs, and birth control pills unless there is an absolute medical necessity.

o Follow a health care professional's specific recommendations if the identifiable predisposing factor is diet, impaired immunity, impaired liver function, or an underlying disease state.

2. Follow the *C. albicans* control diet:
   - Eliminate refined and simple sugars.
   - Eliminate milk and other dairy products.
   - Eliminate foods with a high content of yeast or mold, including alcoholic beverages, cheeses, dried fruits, melons, and peanuts.
   - Eliminate all known or suspected food allergies.

3. Get nutritional support by taking a high-potency multiple vitamin and mineral formula.

4. Support the immune system:
   - Develop a positive mental attitude.
   - Use positive techniques for coping with stress.
   - Avoid alcohol, sugar, smoking, and elevated cholesterol levels, which can impair immune system function.
   - Get plenty of rest, and make sure that sleep is of good quality.
   - To support thymus gland function, take 750 mg crude polypeptide fractions per day.

5. Promote detoxification and elimination:
   - Consume 3 to 5 g water-soluble fiber from sources such as guar gum, psyllium seed, or pectin at night.
   - If necessary, take lipotropic factors and silymarin to enhance liver function.

6. Take probiotics: 5 to 10 billion viable lactobacillus and bifidobacteria cells per day.

7. Use appropriate antiyeast therapy:
   - Ideally, take the recommended nutritional or herbal supplements, or both, to help control yeast overgrowth and promote healthful bacterial flora.
   - If necessary, take prescription antiyeast drugs appropriately.

These steps should take care of chronic candidiasis in most cases. If a patient follows these guidelines and fails to achieve significant improvement or complete resolution, further evaluation is necessary to determine if chronic candidiasis is in fact the issue. Repeat stool cultures and antigen levels are often helpful here. If the organism has not been eradicated, stronger prescription antibiotics can be used, along with the other general recommendations.

Canker Sores

....

- Single or clustered shallow, painful ulcers found anywhere in the oral cavity
- Ulcerations usually resolve in 7 to 21 days but are recurrent in many people

Canker sores (the medical term is *aphthous stomatitis*) are quite common, but in 20% of the U.S. population they tend to recur often (in which case they are called *recurrent aphthous ulcers*, or RAU). Although the lesions generally heal on their own, some individuals seem to have canker sores all the time.

Causes

Local chemical or physical trauma often initiates ulcers in susceptible individuals. Stress is frequently a precipitating factor in RAU, suggesting a breakdown in normal host protective factors.[1] Allergies, gluten sensitivity, and nutrient deficiency are also common causes. One controlled study has shown a statistically significant increase in RAU in subjects taking nonsteroidal anti-inflammatory drugs (NSAIDs) such as aspirin and ibuprofen.[2]

Allergies

Allergies, particularly food allergies to milk and gluten, are a common cause. The oral cavity is obviously the first site of contact for ingested allergens and many inhaled ones. The lesions and the association of RAU with increased serum antibodies to food antigens strongly suggest that an allergic reaction

is involved.[3] Furthermore, the presence of higher levels of allergic antibodies (IgE) and white blood cells associated with allergies (mast cells and basophils) are characteristic of RAU.[4,5] Mast cells and basophils contain granules of histamine and other allergic mediators that are released in response to allergens. The sensitivity is not necessarily to a food; it can also be to a food additive or contact metal. Frequent nonfood allergens inducing RAU include:[6]

Benzoic acid

Cinnamaldehyde

Nickel

Parabens

Dichromate

Sorbic acid

Gluten Sensitivity

Considerable evidence indicates that sensitivity to gluten is associated with RAU. The incidence of RAU is increased in patients with celiac disease (see the chapter "Celiac Disease").[7-11] Withdrawing gluten from the diet results in complete remission of RAU in patients with celiac disease and some improvement in others.[7-11]

Nutrient Deficiency

The oral cavity is often the first place that nutritional deficiency becomes visible because of the high turnover rate of the cells that line it (the mucosal epithelium). Although a number of nutrient deficiencies can lead to canker sores, thiamine deficiency appears to be the most significant. In one study seeking to examine whether thiamine deficiency is associated with RAU, levels of transketolase (a thiamine-dependent enzyme) were determined in 70 patients with RAU and 50 patients from a control group.[12] Low levels of transketolase were found in 49 of 70 patients with RAU, compared with only 2 of 50 among the controls.

Several other studies show that nutrient deficiencies are much more common in RAU sufferers than others. For example, a study of 330 patients with RAU found that 47 (14.2%) were deficient in iron, folate, vitamin B_{12}, or a combination of these nutrients.[13] In another study of 60 patients, 28.2% were deficient in thiamine, riboflavin, or pyridoxine.[14]

Low nutrient status may explain why patients with RAU have an impaired antioxidant defense system, leading to higher levels of free radicals and damaged fats in the blood.[15]

Therapeutic Considerations

For RAU, the most effective treatments involve identifying the cause. Food allergies, gluten sensitivity, and nutrient deficiency should all be addressed and corrected. Correction of the cause will stop the cycle of RAU. For example, an allergy elimination diet has been shown to have good therapeutic results;[16,17] elimination of gluten is curative in those with gluten sensitivity; and when nutrient deficiencies are corrected, most RAU patients have a complete remission.[18] Even taking extra vitamin B_{12} (1,000 mcg per day) alone has shown benefit regardless of whether deficiency exists or not.[19]

Zinc supplementation has also been shown to be helpful. In one double-blind study, 40 patients with RAU were given either zinc sulfate (220 mg, providing 50 mg elemental zinc) or a placebo once per day for one month.[20] Results showed that the levels of serum zinc before treatment were below normal in 42.5% of the patients with RAU. After one month of zinc therapy, the sores were reduced and did not reappear for three months.

A small study of adolescents showed a reduction in the incidence of RAU and associated pain from 2,000 mg per day of vitamin C.[21]

Deglycyrrhizinated licorice (DGL) may be effective in promoting the healing of RAU. In one study, 20 patients were instructed to use a solution of DGL as a mouthwash (200 mg powdered DGL dissolved in 200 ml of warm water) four times per day.[22] Of the 20 patients, 15 (75%) experienced 50 to 75%

QUICK REVIEW

- **Recurrent canker sores can be caused by trauma, food sensitivities (especially milk and gluten sensitivities), stress, and/or nutrient deficiency.**
- **Eliminating food allergens, sources of**

gluten, and nutritional deficiencies results in a complete cure in most cases.
- **Deglycyrrhizinated licorice (DGL) may be effective in promoting the healing of RAU.**

improvement within one day, followed by complete healing of the ulcers by the third day. DGL in tablet form may be more convenient and effective. For more information on DGL, see the chapter "Peptic Ulcer."

• •

TREATMENT SUMMARY

Food allergies, gluten sensitivity, and nutrient deficiency should all be addressed and corrected. Considerable evidence suggests that gluten sensitivity may be a contributing factor in some patients.

Diet

The diet should be free of known allergens and, if gluten sensitivity is present, all gluten sources. Otherwise, the guidelines in the chapter "A Health-Promoting Diet" are appropriate.

Nutritional Supplements

- **A high-potency multiple vitamin and mineral formula as described in the chapter "Supplementary Measures"**
- **Key individual nutrients:**
  - ○ **Thiamine (vitamin B$_1$): 50 to 100 mg per day**
  - ○ **Vitamin B$_6$: 25 to 50 mg per day**
  - ○ **Folic acid: 400 to 800 mcg per day**
  - ○ **Vitamin B$_{12}$ (methylcobalamin): 1,000 mcg per day**
  - ○ **Vitamin C: 500 to 1,000 mg twice per day**
  - ○ **Zinc: 20 to 30 mg per day**
- **Fish oils: 1,000 mg EPA + DHA per day**
- **One of the following:**
  - ○ **Grape seed extract (>95% procyanidolic oligomers): 100 to 300 mg per day**
  - ○ **Pine bark extract (>95% procyanidolic oligomers): 100 to 300 mg per day**
  - ○ **Some other flavonoid-rich extract with a similar flavonoid content, super greens formula, or another plant-based antioxidant that can provide an oxygen radical absorption capacity (ORAC) of 3,000 to 6,000 units or higher per day**

Botanical Medicines

- **DGL: one to two 380-mg chewable tablets 20 minutes before meals**

Carpal Tunnel Syndrome

- Numbness, tingling, and/or burning pain in the first three fingers of the hand, particularly at night
- Appearance or worsening of symptoms caused by flexing of the wrist for 60 seconds and relieved by extending the wrist

Carpal tunnel syndrome (CTS) is a common, painful disorder caused by compression of the median nerve, which passes between the bones and ligaments of the wrist. Compression of this nerve causes weakness; pain in gripping; and burning, tingling, or aching that may radiate to the forearm and shoulder. Symptoms may be occasional or constant and usually occur most at night. CTS is more prevalent among women and occurs frequently between the ages of 40 and 60. It occurs most often in pregnant women, women taking oral contraceptives, menopausal women, or patients on hemodialysis due to kidney failure.[1] These groups tend to have a greater need for vitamin B_6.

CTS also occurs in people who perform repetitive strenuous work with their hands (e.g., carpenters), and it may occur in people who do repetitive lighter work (e.g., typists and keyboard operators). It may also follow injuries of the wrist. More frequently, however, there is no history of significant trauma.

Causes

Any factor that causes the carpal tunnel to get smaller or its contents to swell can lead to carpal tunnel syndrome. Common causes include:[2]

- Increased volume of canal contents/edema (inflammation of the carpal tunnel tendons, obesity, pregnancy, oral contraceptives)
- Trauma (fracture, repetitive wrist flexion)
- Abnormal anatomy (cysts, fatty tumors, bone spurs)
- Metabolic conditions (diabetes, hypothyroidism)
- Inflammatory conditions (rheumatoid arthritis, gout, connective tissue disease)

Therapeutic Considerations

Many cases of CTS respond on their own in a month or two. Surgery for CTS should definitely not be considered before more conservative treatment has been tried for six months, and should be reserved for cases that are persistent (not resolving after one year) or deteriorating (worsening clinically, along with nerve conduction studies showing deterioration). To prevent permanent nerve damage, however, surgery should not be delayed be-

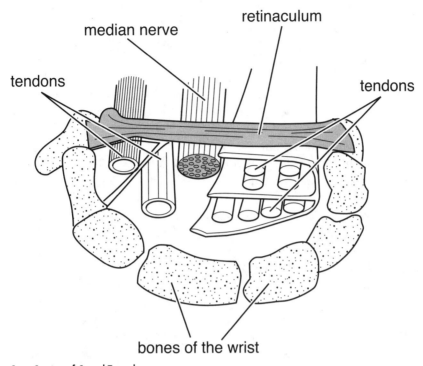

median nerve

retinaculum

tendons

tendons

bones of the wrist

Cross Section of Carpal Tunnel

yond three years after first onset of symptoms. Open carpal tunnel release surgery is one of the most commonly performed outpatient surgeries and is less expensive than the newer endoscopic procedures. A detailed review reported no difference in long-term results between the procedures, but pain is reduced the first two weeks following the endoscopic surgery compared with open procedures.[3] Surgery with early mobilization allowing movement of the hand and wrist versus immobilization,[4] surgery with oral homeopathic arnica and topical arnica ointment,[5] and surgery with controlled cold therapy all showed benefits over surgery alone.[6]

The most recommended initial treatment is four weeks in a neutral wrist splint worn full-time. Splinting is most effective when started within three months of onset of CTS. Specialized splints have not been proven more effective than a good-quality, well-fitted over-the-counter splint.[7,8]

Alternating Hot and Cold Water Treatment

Inflammation and swelling are present in many cases of CTS. Alternating hot and cold water treatment (contrast hydrotherapy) provides a simple, efficient way to increase circulation to the area and reduce swelling. Immersion of the hand past the wrist in hot water for three minutes, followed by immersion in cold water for 30 seconds, repeated three to five times, will increase local circulation, thereby increasing local inflow of nutrients, increasing elimination of waste products, and decreasing pain.

Nutritional Supplements

The increased incidence of CTS since its initial description in 1950 parallels the increased presence of dietary compounds, drugs, and environmental toxins that block the action of vitamin B_6 (hydrazine dyes such as yellow dye #5; drugs such as isoniazid, hydralazine, dopamine, penicillamine, and oral contraceptives; and excessive protein). Several clinical studies demonstrated the efficacy of vitamin B_6 supplementation for CTS; the initial dose was 50 mg initially, increased to 200 to 300 mg.[9–11] Even greater effect was seen when B_6 and B_2 (riboflavin) were given together,[11] possibly owing to riboflavin-dependent enzymes that convert pyridoxine to its active form, pyridoxal-5-phosphate (P5P). While two studies failed to show that B_6 was better than a placebo,[12,13] given the safety profile and possible effectiveness of B_{12} it is definitely worth trying in the treatment of CTS. We recommend dosages no greater than 100 mg per day, however. If B_6 does not produce results within a few weeks, P5P should be tried at 10 mg per day.

Celadrin

Celadrin is a proprietary mixture of cetylated fatty acids that has been shown to affect several key factors that contribute to inflammation. Studies have assessed both the oral and the topical use of Celadrin in the treatment of osteoarthritis (see the chapter "Osteoarthritis"). Although there are no studies of Celadrin in CTS, we feel that the topical application of Celadrin cream may help when CTS is associated with inflammation. Apply to the affected area twice per day.

Acupuncture

A randomized controlled study comparing an oral steroid (prednisolone 20 mg for two weeks, then 10 mg for two weeks) vs. eight sessions of acupuncture over four weeks showed acupuncture to be as effective as the steroid in CTS symptom control. In addition, acupuncture improved muscle function but prednisolone did not.[14] Another acupuncture study demonstrated a positive response in 35 of 36 patients (14 of whom were previously treated unsuccessfully with surgery).[15]

. . . .

QUICK SUMMARY

- **Any factor that causes the carpal tunnel to get smaller or its contents to swell can lead to carpal tunnel syndrome.**
- **Surgery for CTS should definitely not be considered before six months of more conservative treatment.**
- **The most recommended initial treatment is four weeks in a neutral wrist splint worn full-time.**
- **Alternating hot and cold water treatment (contrast hydrotherapy) provides a simple, efficient way to increase circulation to the area and reduce swelling.**
- **Several clinical studies demonstrated the efficacy of vitamin B_6 supplementation for CTS.**

TREATMENT SUMMARY

Physical Medicine

- Identify and reduce causes of strain and vibration, and prevent repeated trauma.
- Full-time splinting in a neutral position as a first step.
- Acupuncture can be helpful.
- Contrast hydrotherapy: immerse hand past the wrist for three minutes in hot water; this is followed by a 30-second immersion in cold water. Repeat three to five times per day.

Diet

Follow the general recommendations given in the chapter "A Health-Promoting Diet."

Nutritional Supplements

- A high-potency multiple vitamin and mineral formula as described in the chapter "Supplementary Measures"
- Vitamin B_6 (pyridoxine): 50 to 100 mg per day; if no response, try 10 mg P5P per day
- Fish oils: 3,000 mg EPA + DHA per day
- One of the following:
  - Grape seed extract (>95% procyanidolic oligomers): 100 to 300 mg per day
  - Pine bark extract (>95% procyanidolic oligomers): 100 to 300 mg per day
  - Some other flavonoid-rich extract with a similar flavonoid content, super greens formula, or another plant-based antioxidant that can provide an oxygen radical absorption capacity (ORAC) of 3,000 to 6,000 units or more per day

Topical Treatment

- Celadrin: Apply a cream containing Celadrin to the affected areas twice per day.

Cataracts

· ·

- Clouding or opacity in the crystalline lens of the eye
- Gradual loss of vision

Cataracts are white, opaque blemishes on the normally transparent lens of the eye. They occur as a result of damage to the protein structure of the lens, similar to the damage that occurs to the protein of eggs when they are boiled or fried. Cataracts are the leading cause of impaired vision and blindness in the United States. Approximately 6 million Americans have some degree of vision-impairing cataract, and among Medicare recipients, cataract surgery is the most common major surgical procedure, with nearly 1 million procedures each year.

Cataracts can be classified by location and appearance of the lens opacities, by cause or significant contributing factor, and by age of onset. Many factors may cause or contribute to the progression of lens opacity, including ocular disease, injury, or surgery; systemic diseases (e.g., diabetes); exposure to toxins, radiation, or ultraviolet and near-ultraviolet light; and hereditary disease. Aging-related cataracts (senile cataracts) are discussed in this chapter, and diabetic and galactose-induced cataracts (sugar cataracts) are discussed in the chapter "Diabetes."

The lens of the eye is, obviously, a vital component of the visual system, owing to its ability to focus light (by changes in shape) while maintaining optical transparency. Unfortunately, this transparency diminishes with age. The majority of the geriatric population displays some degree of cataract formation. Even with normal aging there is a progressive increase in size, weight, and density of the lens.

Causes

In cataract formation, the normal protective mechanisms are unable to prevent free radical damage to the cells of the lens. The lens, like many other tissues of the body, depends on adequate levels and activities of antioxidant enzymes such as superoxide dismutase (SOD), catalase, and glutathione peroxidase, and adequate levels of the accessory antioxidants such as lutein, vitamins E and C, and selenium, to aid in prevention of damage by free radicals.[1–6]

Therapeutic Considerations

Nutritional Supplements

Individuals with higher dietary intakes of vitamin C and E, selenium, and carotenes (especially lutein) have a much lower risk for development of cataracts.[7] Several studies have shown that various nutritional supplements—multiple vitamin formulas, vitamins C and E, B vitamins (especially B_{12} and folic acid), and vitamin A—also offer significant protection against cataracts.[8–11] Studies conducted by the Age-Related Eye Disease Study (AREDS) Research Group and others indicate that a combination of these nutrients will be likely to produce better results in the prevention of age-related macular degeneration and cataracts than any single nutrient alone, or even limited combinations of three or fewer nutrients (see the chapter "Macular Degeneration" for more information).

Lutein

Lutein, a yellow-orange carotene that offers significant protection against macular degeneration, also helps protect against cataract formation.[12] Like the macula, the human lens concentrates lutein. In 1992 a study showed that consumption of spinach (high in lutein) was inversely related to the risk of cataracts severe enough to require extraction.[13] This initial investigation was followed by three studies that were more detailed showing that intake of lutein was inversely associated with cataract surgery (20 to 50% risk reduction).[14–16] In a double-blind intervention trial, 17 patients clinically diagnosed with age-related cataracts were randomly assigned to receive dietary supplementation with either lutein (15 mg), vitamin E (100 mg), or a placebo three times a week for up to two years.[17] Visual performance (visual acuity and glare sensitivity) actually improved in the lutein group, whereas there was trend toward the maintenance of visual acuity with vitamin E and a decrease with the placebo.

Vitamin C

A high dietary intake of vitamin C from either dietary sources or supplements has been shown to protect against cataract formation.[8–11] In addition to preventing cataracts, antioxidant nutrients such as vitamin C may offer some therapeutic effects. Several

clinical studies have demonstrated that vitamin C supplementation can halt cataract progression and, in some cases, significantly improve vision. For example, in one study conducted in 1939, 450 patients with cataracts were started on a nutritional program that included 1 g per day of vitamin C, which resulted in a significant reduction in cataract development.[1] Similar patients had previously required surgery within four years, but in this study only a small handful of the patients treated with vitamin C needed surgery, and in most there was no evidence that the cataracts had progressed over the 11-year study period.

It appears that the dosage of vitamin C necessary to increase the vitamin C content of the lens is 1,000 mg.[2] The lens of the eye and active tissues of the body require higher concentrations of vitamin C. The average level of vitamin C in the blood is about 0.5 mg/dl; in the liver, spleen, and lens of the eye, the vitamin C level is increased by at least a factor of 20. In order for these concentrations to be maintained in these tissues, the body has to generate enormous amounts of energy to pull vitamin C out of blood against this tremendous gradient. Keeping blood vitamin C concentrations elevated helps the body concentrate vitamin C into active tissue by reducing the gradient. That is probably why such high dosages are required to raise the vitamin C content of the lens.

In another study, 450 patients with incipient cataracts were started on a nutritional program that included 1,000 mg per day of vitamin C, which led to a significant reduction in cataract development.[3]

In a large double-blind trial, 11,545 apparently healthy U.S. male physicians 50 years or older without a diagnosis of cataracts were randomly assigned to receive 400 IU of vitamin E or a placebo on alternate days and 500 mg vitamin C or a placebo per day.[18]

After eight years of treatment and follow-up, there was no significant difference in cataract formation in the groups. This study may have failed to show benefit because it was below the threshold of 1,000 mg per day of vitamin C.

Glutathione

Glutathione (GSH) is a key antioxidant found at very high concentrations in the lens. GSH plays a vital role in maintaining a healthy lens and has been postulated as a key protective factor against cataract formation. GSH functions as an antioxidant and acts as a vital coenzyme of various enzyme systems within the lens.[4] Low GSH levels predispose the lens to cataract formation.

Selenium and Vitamin E

Selenium and vitamin E are antioxidants known to function synergistically. Maintaining proper selenium levels appears to be especially important because the lens antioxidant enzyme glutathione peroxidase requires selenium. Low selenium levels greatly promotes cataract formation; early studies have shown that selenium content in the human lens with a cataract is only 15% of normal levels.[5]

A more recent study was conducted to better examine the role of selenium in cataract formation.[6] Selenium levels in the serum, lens, and fluid of the eye (aqueous humor) were determined in 48 patients with cataracts and compared with levels in matched controls. Selenium levels in the serum and aqueous humor were found to be significantly lower in the patients with cataracts (serum, 0.28 mcg/ml; aqueous humor, 0.19 mcg/ml) than in normal controls (serum, 0.32 mcg/ml; aqueous humor, 0.31 mcg/ml). However, selenium levels in the lens itself did not significantly differ between the patients with cataracts and the controls.

The most important finding of the study was the decreased level of selenium in the aqueous humor in patients with cataracts. Excessive hydrogen peroxide levels, up to 25 times normal, are found in the aqueous humor in patients with cataracts and are a key underlying factor in cataract formation. Because selenium-dependent glutathione peroxidase is responsible for the breakdown of hydrogen peroxide, it is quite obvious why low selenium levels appear to be a major factor in the development of cataracts.

As previously described, vitamin E supplementation alone does not slow the progression of cataract formation.[17] A double-blind study in which vitamin E was given at a dose of 500 IU per day also found that supplementation did not slow cataract formation.[19] In a seven-year trial, supplemental vitamin E (400 IU) combined with vitamin C (500 mg) and beta-carotene (15 mg) had no effect on the development or progression of cataracts.[20] In order for vitamin E to function in protecting the lens against free radical damage, it requires selenium, and vice versa.

Superoxide Dismutase

The activity of the important antioxidant enzyme SOD is lower in the human lens than in other tissues as a result of the greater ascorbate and glutathione levels in the lens. Nonetheless, SOD is a very important protector against free radical damage in the lens, and as SOD levels decline, cataracts progress. Oral supplementation is probably of little value, because it does not affect tissue SOD activity.[21] Of greater value is supplementation with the trace mineral components of SOD, such as zinc, copper, and manganese. Levels of these necessary cofactors are greatly reduced in lenses with cataracts; copper and zinc levels are reduced by more than 90%, and manganese by 50%.[5]

Tetrahydrobiopterin

Tetrahydrobiopterin is a molecule similar to folic acid and is believed to play a protective role against cataract formation by preventing oxidation and damage from ultraviolet light. This action prevents the formation of high-molecular-weight proteins in the lens. Studies of human senile cataracts have demonstrated decreased levels of tetrahydrobiopterin and pteridine-synthesizing enzymes.[22] Supplemental folic acid may help compensate for this deficiency by increasing the ability to manufacture pteridines.

Riboflavin

In order to maintain GSH in its active form, the lens requires riboflavin (vitamin B_2).[23,24] Deficiency of riboflavin is believed to enhance cataract formation. However, no more than 10 mg per day of riboflavin should be taken by people with cataracts, because it is a photosensitizing substance—that is, riboflavin reacts with the light to form superoxide free radicals. In animal studies, riboflavin supplementation and light have been used experimentally to induce cataracts. The evidence appears to suggest that excess riboflavin does more harm than good in patients with cataracts.

Cysteine

Cysteine, one of the key amino acids of GSH, has been shown to be of some aid in cataract treatment.[25] N-acetylcysteine is the preferred supplemental form of cysteine.

Zinc, Vitamin A, and Beta-Carotene

Zinc, vitamin A, and beta-carotene are known antioxidant nutrients vital to the health of the eye. In particular, beta-carotene may act as a filter, protecting against light-induced damage to the fiber portion of the lens.[26] However, beta-carotene supplementation on its own (50 mg on alternate days) has no impact on cataract prevention in long-term studies in either women or men.[27,28]

Flavonoid-Rich Extracts

The occurrence of cataracts in rats can be slowed down by changing their diet from a commercial laboratory chow to a diet that includes flavonoids.[29] Of the flavonoid-rich extracts, bilberry anthocyanosides may offer the greatest protection. In one human study, bilberry extract plus vitamin E stopped progression of cataract formation in 97% of 50 patients with senile cortical cataracts.[30] Grape seed and pine bark extracts are also excellent choices in cataract prevention.

· ·

QUICK REVIEW

- **In cataract formation, the normal protective mechanisms are unable to prevent free radical damage.**
- **Individuals with higher dietary intakes of antioxidants have a much lower risk for developing cataracts.**
- **Several clinical studies have demonstrated that vitamin C supplementation can halt cataract progression and, in some cases, significantly improve vision.**
- **Bilberry extract plus vitamin E stopped progression of cataract formation in 48 of 50 patients.**

Heavy Metals

A number of heavy metals have been shown to have higher concentrations in both the aging lens and those with cataracts.[5] The cadmium concentration is two to three times higher in cataract lenses than in lenses of age-matched controls without cataracts. Because cadmium displaces zinc from binding as a coenzyme in enzymes, it may contribute to deactivation of free radical quenching and other protective/repair mechanisms.

Other elements of unknown significance are bromine, cobalt, iridium, and nickel.[5]

TREATMENT SUMMARY

In cases of marked vision impairment, cataract removal and lens implant may be the only alternative. As with most diseases, prevention or treatment at an early stage is most effective. Free radical damage appears to be the primary factor in the induction of senile cataracts, so avoidance of oxidizing agents and greatly increased intake of antioxidants are critical to successful treatment. Because the elderly population is especially susceptible to nutrient deficiencies, every effort should be made to ensure optimal nutrition. Wear sunglasses when outdoors. Progression of the disease process can be stopped and early lesions can be reversed. However, significant reversal of well-developed cataracts does not appear possible at this time.

Diet

Follow the guidelines given in the chapter "A Health-Promoting Diet." Avoid fried foods, overly well-done or charbroiled meat, and other dietary sources of free radicals while increasing the consumption of antioxidant-rich foods such as legumes (high in sulfur-containing amino acids), yellow vegetables (carotenes), berries and citrus (flavonoids), and foods rich in vitamins C.

Nutritional Supplements

- A high-potency multiple vitamin and mineral formula as described in the chapter "Supplementary Measures"
- Key individual nutrients:
  - Vitamin B_6: 25 to 50 mg per day
  - Folic acid: 800 mcg per day
  - Vitamin B_{12}: 800 mcg per day
  - Vitamin C: 500 to 1,000 mg twice per day
  - Vitamin E (mixed tocopherols): 100 to 200 IU per day
  - Copper: 0.5 to 1 mg per day
  - Selenium: 100 to 200 mcg per day
  - Zinc: 20 to 30 mg per day
  - Vitamin D_3: 2,000 to 4,000 IU per day (ideally measure blood levels and adjust dosage accordingly)
- Fish oils: 1,000 mg EPA + DHA per day
- Specialty supplements:
  - Lutein: 5 to 15 mg per day
  - N-acetylcysteine: 200–400 mg per day

Botanical Medicines

- **One or more of the following:**
  - Bilberry (*Vaccinium myrtillus*) extract (25% anthocyanidin content): 160 to 240 mg day
  - Grape seed extract (>95% procyanidolic oligomers): 100 to 300 mg per day
  - Pine bark extract (>95% procyanidolic oligomers): 100 to 300 mg per day
  - Some other flavonoid-rich extract with a similar flavonoid content, super greens formula, or another plant-based antioxidant that can provide an oxygen radical absorption capacity (ORAC) of 3,000 to 6,000 units or more per day

Celiac Disease

....

- A chronic intestinal malabsorption disorder caused by an intolerance to gluten
- Bulky, pale, frothy, foul-smelling, greasy stools with increased fecal fat
- Weight loss and signs of multiple vitamin and mineral deficiencies
- Increased blood levels of endomysial, anti-tissue transglutaminase, and anti-gliadin antibodies

Celiac disease, also known as nontropical sprue, gluten-sensitive enteropathy, or celiac sprue, is characterized by symptoms of varying severity, from very mild gastrointestinal discomfort to serious malabsorption (e.g., diarrhea, malodorous flatulence, abdominal bloating, and increased amounts of fat and undigested food particles in the stool). It is also characterized by abnormalities in small intestine structure that revert to normal with removal of gluten and more specifically its smaller derivative, gliadin, found primarily in wheat, barley, and rye grains. Symptoms most commonly appear during the first three years of life, after gluten-containing foods are introduced into the diet. However, a second peak incidence occurs during early adulthood. While celiac disease is often thought of as a disease diagnosed early in life, more diagnoses are made in adulthood than childhood.[1]

The prevalence of celiac disease has increased dramatically, and this is not simply due to increased detection. Until a few decades ago celiac disease was believed to be relatively rare (estimated before as 1 case in 5,000 in the United States), but celiac disease is now thought to affect as many as 1% of all Americans, though it remains largely undiagnosed.[1–3] Undetected celiac disease carries with it an increased risk of morbidity (disease) and early mortality (death), so widespread screening may be economically justified.

In the past, the definitive diagnosis of celiac disease involved taking a biopsy of the small intestine. Now there are blood tests that measure specific antibodies to gluten components. These tests include endomysial antibodies, anti-tissue transglutaminase antibodies, and anti-gliadin antibodies. In patients with celiac disease, anti-gliadin antibody is an antibody produced against gliadin in the diet, and endomysial and anti-tissue transglutaminase antibodies are antibodies produced against the body's own tissues as an unfortunate side effect of the immune system's reaction to gliadin.

Causes

Celiac disease appears to have a strong genetic component. There is an increased frequency of celiac disease in people with some specific genetic markers known as HLA-B8 and DRw3 that appear on the surface of cells, similar to the genetic markers of blood type.[3,4] For example, the HLA-B8 marker has been found in 85 to 90% of celiac patients, as compared with 20 to 25% of normal subjects. There is a low frequency of HLA-B8 within long-standing agrarian (farming) populations, as in Asia, while the frequency in northern and central Europe and the northwest part of the Indian subcontinent is much higher.[3] Wheat cultivation in these high HLA-B8 areas is a relatively recent development (1000 B.C.). The prevalence of celiac disease is much higher in these areas than in other parts of the world. In the United States, with its diverse genetic background, the frequency rate is now roughly 1 in 100. The early introduction of cow's milk is also believed to be a major causative factor.[1–4] Research in the past few years has clearly indicated that breastfeeding and delayed administration of cow's milk and cereal grains are the primary preventive steps that can greatly reduce the risk of developing celiac disease.[5–7]

Mortality and Morbidity Risks

A landmark study that looked at almost 30,000 patients from 1969 to 2008 found a higher than normal risk of early death associated with sensitivity to gluten.[8] Those with full-blown celiac disease had a 39% increased risk of early death compared with controls; those with inflammation of the intestine but not full-blown celiac disease had a 72% increased risk; and those with gluten sensitivity (elevated gluten antibodies) but negative intestinal biopsy had a 35% increased risk.

A review article listed 55 health conditions linked to celiac disease and gluten sensitivity, including irritable bowel disease, inflammatory bowel disease, anemia, migraines, epilepsy, fatigue, canker sores, osteoporosis, rheumatoid arthritis, lupus, multiple sclerosis, and almost all other autoimmune diseases.[9] Thyroid abnormalities, insulin-dependent diabetes, psychiatric disturbances (including schizophrenia), dermatitis herpetiformis, and urticaria have also been linked to gluten intolerance.[1] A more ominous association is the increased risk for malignant cancers seen in celiac patients, especially for non-Hodgkin lymphoma.[10]

There is also evidence from population-based, clinical, and experimental studies that gluten is a contributing factor in some cases of schizophrenia.[11–13] Digested particles of wheat gluten have demonstrated activity similar to opiates (morphine-like compounds).[14] This opiate activity is believed to be the factor responsible for the association between wheat consumption and schizophrenia.

Gluten sensitivity has also been weakly linked to lower mood scores, impairment of mental function, and autism.[15–17]

Therapeutic Considerations

Celiac disease often leads to the development of multiple food allergies, lactose intolerance, and increased intestinal permeability.[18] Improving nutritional status appears to produce significant improvement in quality of life in patients with celiac disease. Even something as simple as taking a B-complex supplement produces considerable benefits. In one double-blind study, 65 celiac patients on a strict gluten-free diet for several years were randomly assigned to either a daily dose of 800 mcg folic acid, 500 mcg vitamin B_{12} (cyanocobalamin), and 3 mg vitamin B_6 (pyridoxine) or a placebo for six months.[19] Following vitamin supplementation, the levels of homocysteine, a factor implicated in cardiovascular disease and some cancers, dropped an average of 34%, and this decrease led to significant improvement in feelings of well-being, reduced anxiety, and improved mood.

Diet

Once the diagnosis has been established, a gluten-free diet is indicated. This diet does not contain any wheat, rye, barley, triticale, or oats. Buckwheat and millet are often excluded as well; although buckwheat is not in the grass family and millet appears to be more closely related to rice and corn, buckwheat and millet contain compounds known as prolamins with antigenic activity similar to that of gliadin.

Many gluten-free products are available in natural foods stores and online catalogs, but it's important to read labels carefully, because some "wheat-free" products add gluten—the source of gliadin—to improve the quality of baked goods. Grains that can be used to replace gluten-containing grains include amaranth, quinoa, and various types of rice (brown, red, black, and wild). In addition, recent evidence suggests that complete elimination of gluten-related compounds (e.g., secalins, hordeins, and avenins) may not be necessary for many patients. This statement is particularly true of oats. In a five-year study in which one group followed a gluten- and oat-free diet and another followed a gluten-free diet while consuming oats, no differences were seen with respect to duodenal villous architecture, inflammatory cell infiltration of the duodenal mucosa, or antibody titers.[20]

Detailed studies of celiac disease patients who eat oats have shown no evidence of immune activation.[21-24] For example, in one study, 116 children with newly diagnosed celiac disease were randomly assigned to one of two groups: one group was given a standard gluten-free diet (GFD-std) and one group was given a GFD with additional wheat-free oat products (GFD-oats). After one year, the GFD-oats and GFD-std groups did not differ significantly regarding blood markers for

Gluten and Gliadin Content of Selected Foods					
FOOD	TOTAL PROTEIN	PROLAMINES[a] (% OF TOTAL PROTEIN)	GLIADIN (MG/100 G)	GLUTELINS[b] (% OF TOTAL PROTEIN)	CROSS-REACTIVITY WITH GLIADIN
Wheat	10–15	40–50	6,900	30–40	++++ —
Rye	9–14	30–50	580	30–50	+++ —
Oats	8–14	10–15	100	5	++ —
Corn (maize)	7–13	50–55	0	30–45	+ —
Rice	8–10	1–5	0	85–90	—
Sorghum	9–13	>60	NA	NA	NA
Millet	7–16	57	0	30	NA
Buckwheat	13–15	NA	4	High	—

NA = No data available; + to +++ = degree of reactivity; — = no reactivity

[a] Primarily gliadin.

[b] Primarily gluten.

Data from Baker PG, *Lancet* 1975;ii:1307; Friis SU, *Clin Chim Acta* 1988;178:261–270; Chartrand LJ, Russo PA, Duhaime AG, et al. *J Am Diet Assoc* 1997;97:612–618.

celiac disease or small bowel mucosal architecture, including numbers of lymphocytes within intestinal cells.[21]

One point, however, is that while oat ingestion may not activate the disease, it may increase gastrointestinal symptoms. In one study, 39 celiac disease patients were randomly assigned to take either 50 g oats-containing gluten-free products per day or to continue without oats for one year.[24] Patients taking oats suffered significantly more often from diarrhea, but there was a simultaneous trend toward a more severe average constipation symptom score. The lining of the intestine was not disturbed, but more signs of inflammation and allergy were evident in the oats group. It appears that oats provide an alternative in the gluten-free diet, but celiac patients should be aware of the possible increase in intestinal symptoms. If symptoms appear or become exacerbated, oats can be excluded. Ultimately, it depends on the sensitivity of each person. While many with celiac can eat rice and oats, some cannot.

In addition, other foods should be rotated, and milk and milk products should be eliminated until the patient redevelops an intestinal structure and function returns to normal.

Usually with gluten elimination, clinical improvement will be obvious within a few days or weeks (30% respond within three days, another 50% within a month, and 10% within another month). However, 10% of patients respond only after 24 to 36 months of gluten avoidance.[1] If a patient does not appear to respond, either the diagnosis is not correct or there may be some obstacle to a cure, such as zinc deficiency (celiac disease symptoms will not respond to gluten elimination if an underlying zinc deficiency is present).[25] The importance of a multivitamin and mineral supplement in celiac disease cannot be emphasized enough. In addition to treating any underlying deficiency, supplementation provides the necessary cofactors for growth and repair.

Nutritional Supplements

Pancreatic Enzymes

The effect of pancreatic enzyme therapy in the two months following the initial diagnosis of celiac disease was investigated in one double-blind study.[26] The study sought to clarify the benefit of pancreatic enzyme therapy because previous studies had shown

QUICK REVIEW

- **Celiac disease is characterized by varying symptoms of severity, from very mild gastrointestinal discomfort to malabsorption (e.g., diarrhea, malodorous flatulence, abdominal bloating, increased amounts of fat and undigested food particles in the stool).**

- **Celiac disease is caused by the immune system's response to a protein known as gluten.**

- **A gluten-free diet is curative.**

- **Pancreatic enzyme supplementation enhances the benefit of a gluten-free diet during the first 30 days after the initial diagnosis.**

- **Preparations containing DPP-IV are often recommended in order to safeguard against any hidden sources of gluten.**

pancreatic insufficiency in 8% to 30% of celiac patients. In this study patients followed a gluten-free diet, the standard treatment for celiac disease, and received with each meal either two capsules of pancreatic enzymes (each capsule containing 5,000 IU lipase, 2,900 IU amylase, and 330 IU protease) or two placebo capsules. Results indicated that pancreatic enzyme supplementation enhanced the clinical benefit of a gluten-free diet during the first 30 days but did not provide any greater benefit than the placebo after 60 days. These results support the use of pancreatic enzyme preparations in the first 30 days after diagnosis of celiac disease.

Alternatively, a better choice than pancreatic enzymes may be enzyme preparations containing dipeptidyl peptidase IV (DPP-IV) from fungal sources. This enzyme targets both gliadin and casein (milk protein) and is resistant to breakdown by other digestive enzymes. DPP-IV is thought to be one of the key enzymes responsible for the digestion of these proteins and is known to be found in lower amounts in the intestinal mucosa of individuals with celiac disease and also to have an inverse correlation with the level of mucosal damage among those with celiac disease as well as those without the disease. In other words, the lower the DPP-IV the more significant the damage to the intestinal lining. Use of preparations containing DPP-IV is often recommended in order to safeguard against any hidden sources of gluten.

. . . .

TREATMENT SUMMARY

The therapeutic approach is quite straightforward: eliminate all sources of gluten (see the table earlier in this chapter), eliminate dairy products initially, correct underlying nutritional deficiencies, treat any associated conditions, and determine and eliminate all food allergens.

Diet

Maintenance of a strict gluten-free diet is quite difficult in the United States because of the ubiquitous presence of gliadin and other activators of celiac disease in processed foods. People with celiac disease must read labels carefully in order to avoid hidden sources of gliadin, such as some brands of soy sauce, modified food starch, **ice cream, soup, beer, wine, vodka, whiskey, and malt. We also recommend consulting the following resources.**

Gluten Intolerance Group
15110 10 Ave. SW, Suite A
Seattle, WA 98166-1820
www.gluten.net

Celiac Sprue Association
P.O. Box 31700
Omaha, NE 68131-0700
www.csaceliacs.org

Celiac Disease Foundation
13251 Ventura Blvd., Suite 1
Studio City, CA 91604
http://celiac.org

Nutritional Supplements

- A high-potency multiple vitamin and mineral formula as described in the chapter "Supplementary Measures"
- Vitamin D_3: 2,000 to 4,000 IU per day (ideally, measure blood levels and adjust dosage accordingly)
- Fish oils: 1,000 mg EPA + DHA per day
- One of the following:
  - Grape seed extract (>95% procyanidolic oligomers): 100 to 300 mg per day
  - Pine bark extract (>95% procyanidolic oligomers): 100 to 300 mg per day
  - Some other flavonoid-rich extract with a similar flavonoid content, super greens formula, or another plant-based antioxidant that can provide an oxygen radical absorption capacity (ORAC) of 3,000 to 6,000 units or more per day
- Specialty supplements:
  - Probiotic (active lactobacillus and bifidobacteria cultures): a minimum of 5 billion to 10 billion colony-forming units per day
  - Enzyme preparations containing dipeptidyl peptidase IV (DPP-IV)

Cerebral Vascular Insufficiency

....

- Indicated by the presence of one or more of the following symptoms:
  - Short-term memory loss
  - Dizziness (vertigo)
  - Headache
  - Ringing in the ears
  - Depression
  - Blurred vision
  - Reduced blood flow to the brain based on ultrasound exam

Cerebral vascular insufficiency (CVI)— decreased blood supply to the brain—is extremely common among the elderly in developed countries owing to the high prevalence of atherosclerosis (hardening of the arteries). The artery affected in most cases is the carotid artery. A pair of carotid arteries— one on each side of the neck running parallel to the jugular vein—are the main arteries that supply blood to the brain.

Typically, the problem develops at the carotid bifurcation—the splitting of the carotid artery into the internal branch (supplying the brain) and the external branch (supplying the face and scalp). This bifurcation is similar to a stream splitting into two branches. At the bifurcation, just as at the splitting of the stream, debris and sediment accumulate. Significant symptoms begin to appear in most cases only when the blockage of the artery

has reached 90%. This situation is similar to what occurs in angina (see the chapter "Angina").

Symptoms of cerebral vascular insufficiency are caused by reduced blood flow and oxygen supply to the brain. Severe disruption of blood and oxygen supply results in a stroke. The official definition of a stroke is loss of nerve function for at least 24 hours due to lack of oxygen. Some strokes are quite mild; others can leave a person paralyzed, in a coma, or unable to talk, depending on which part of the brain is affected. Smaller "mini-strokes," or transient ischemic attacks (TIAs), may result in loss of nerve function for an hour or more, but less than 24 hours. TIAs may produce transient symptoms of CVI: dizziness, ringing in the ears, blurred vision, confusion, and so on. Repeated TIAs are serious, as over time they can result in substantial, progressive damage to brain function. What makes this so insidious is that the lack of a sudden event can mask the problem, so it is not recognized until too late.

Diagnostic Considerations

Anyone who experiences signs and symptoms of CVI should consult a physician immediately for proper evaluation. In the past, evaluation of blood flow to the brain involved invasive techniques such as cerebral angiography. This procedure was similar to a cardiac (heart) angiogram (see the chapter "Angina") and carried a relatively high side-effect rate: it caused a stroke in roughly 4% of the subjects. The modern evaluation of blood flow to the brain primarily involves the use of ultrasound techniques. These techniques determine the rate of blood flow and the degree of blockage by using sound waves.

Therapeutic Considerations

The considerations and recommendations in the chapter "Heart and Cardiovascular Health" are appropriate here, since the primary goal is to improve blood flow by making the arteries healthier. Diet is particularly important, as stroke patients, especially those with significant blockage of the carotid arteries, tend to have an unfavorable dietary pattern (high intake of saturated fatty acids; low intake of fruits, vegetables, and omega-3 fatty acids) that may have been a key factor leading to their stroke.[1] It is also important to address any other underlying factors, such as high cholesterol levels or high blood pressure. Beyond these general recommendations, we will offer a discussion of two natural medicines with proven benefits in CVI: fish oils and ginkgo biloba extract.

Before we discuss these natural approaches, it is important to take a look at a surgical procedures that is often recommended for patients with CVI: *carotid endarterectomy*. The internal, common, and external carotid arteries are clamped, the lining of the internal carotid artery is opened, and the atherosclerotic plaque is removed. This surgery is risky: approximately 6 to 10% of patients will either die or suffer severe neurological damage as a result of a stroke

during the surgery, and about 7 to 11% of the patients will die during or soon (less than one month) after having a carotid endarterectomy. Newer, less invasive procedures include angioplasty done by threading catheters through the femoral artery in the leg and up through the aorta to the carotid, then inflating a balloon to dilate the artery. Often a wire-mesh stent (tube) is placed in the artery. However, it remains controversial whether angioplasty is actually safer or produces better outcomes. What is known is that carotid endarterectomies or angioplasties are of no value to patients with less than 70% blockage (as determined by an angiograph).[2–6]

If you have symptoms of severe CVI, including frequent TIAs or a past stroke, along with severe (greater than 70%) blockage of the carotid artery, then carotid endarterectomy or angioplasty may be appropriate. However, we recommend that you consult a qualified EDTA chelation specialist before electing to go ahead with these procedures. For a discussion of EDTA and referrals, see the chapter "Angina."

Nutritional Supplements

The importance of fish oils for the patient with CVI cannot be overstated. Just as the long-chain omega-3 fatty acids eicosapentaenoic acid (EPA) and docosahexaenoic acid (DHA) protect against heart disease, they are also protective against a stroke. Low levels of EPA and DHA are found in the atherosclerotic plaque in the carotid arteries of patients with significant carotid blockage, while supplementation with EPA + DHA is associated with reducing inflammation within the atherosclerotic plaque, thereby reducing the likelihood that the plaque will rupture and lead to blood clots that may cause a stroke.[7,8] The recommended dosage for prevention is 1,000 mg EPA + DHA.

Botanical Medicines

Ginkgo biloba extract (GBE) has been the subject of more than 40 double-blind studies on the treatment of cerebral vascular insufficiency. In well-designed studies, GBE has produced statistically significant improvement in the major symptoms of CVI as well as in impaired mental performance. These symptoms included short-term memory loss, vertigo, headache, ringing in the ears, lack of vigilance, and depression. These results suggest that vascular insufficiency, not a true degenerative process, may be the major cause of these so-called age-related cerebral disorders.[9]

There has been some concern that GBE may increase bleeding risk when used with warfarin (Coumadin), aspirin, and antiplatelet therapies. However, a study evaluating the use of GBE and warfarin concurrently revealed no change in the international normalized ratio (INR), which is the blood test used to monitor a patient's possible bleeding risk in response to anticoagulation therapy.[10] Results from controlled studies consistently indicate that ginkgo does not significantly affect bleeding time or platelet aggregation, nor does it adversely affect the safety of aspirin or warfarin.[11]

. . . .

QUICK REVIEW

- **Symptoms of cerebral vascular insufficiency are associated with reduced blood flow and oxygen supply to the brain.**
- **Anyone who experiences signs and symptoms of cerebral vascular insufficiency should consult a physician immediately.**
- **The modern evaluation of blood flow to the brain involves the use of ultrasound techniques.**
- **Carotid endarterectomy and angioplasty are highly controversial surgical procedures because approximately 6 to 10% of patients will either die or suffer severe neurological damage as a result of a stroke during the procedure.**
- **Fish oils are especially helpful for reducing the inflammation associated with strokes.**
- **In well-designed studies, ginkgo biloba extract has produced a statistically significant regression of the major symptoms of cerebral vascular insufficiency and impaired mental performance.**

. . . .

TREATMENT SUMMARY

In most cases, CVI is a consequence of atherosclerosis. Appropriate treatment involves following the recommendations in the chapter "Heart and Cardiovascular

Health." It may also be appropriate to consult the chapters "High Cholesterol and/or Triglycerides" and "High Blood Pressure." The primary therapeutic goal in the treatment of CVI is to enhance the blood and oxygen supply to the brain. Ginkgo biloba extract has shown excellent results in this regard. The recommended dosage of GBE (24% ginkgo flavonglycosides) is 240 to 320 mg per day.

Cervical Dysplasia

• A Pap smear of the cervix showing abnormal (but not cancerous) cells

The cervix is a small, cylindrical organ that comprises the lower part and neck of the uterus. The cervix contains a central canal (the endocervical canal) for passage of sperm and menstrual blood, and for childbirth. Both the canal and the outer surface of the cervix are lined with two types of cells: mucus-producing (glandular) cells and protective (squamous) cells.

The term *dysplasia* refers to abnormal cells that are not cancerous but have the potential to become cancer. So cervical dysplasia is a precancerous lesion of the cervix. Cervical dysplasia is diagnosed by a Pap smear—a sampling of cells from the surface of the cervix. Before any cancer appears, abnormal changes occur in cells on the surface of the cervix. Cancer of the cervix is one of the most common cancers affecting women. Fortunately, cervical cancer is one of the few cancers with well-defined precancerous stages, so when detected early it usually can be treated quite successfully. Women routinely receive Pap smears on a yearly basis.

Understanding a Pap Smear

A Pap smear examines the cells that cover the cervix. Most laboratories in the United States use a standard set of terms, called the Bethesda System, to report Pap test results. The Bethesda System considers abnormalities of squamous cells (the thin, flat cells that form the surface of the cervix) and glandular cells (mucus-producing cells found in the endocervical canal or in the lining of the uterus) separately. Glandular cell abnormalities are much less common than squamous cell abnormalities. Samples with cell abnormalities are divided into the following categories, ranging from the mildest to the most severe.

Squamous Cell Abnormalities

• **ASC** (atypical squamous cells). This is the most common abnormal finding in Pap tests. The Bethesda System divides this category into two groups:
  ○ **ASC-US** (atypical squamous cells of undetermined significance).
  ○ **ASC-H** (atypical squamous cells, cannot exclude a high-grade squamous intraepithelial lesion). The cells do not appear normal, but doctors are uncertain about what the cell changes mean. ASC-H lesions may be at higher risk of being precancerous compared with ASC-US lesions.

• **LSIL** (low-grade squamous intraepithelial lesion). *Low-grade* means that there are early changes in the size and shape of cells. *Intraepithelial* refers to the layer of cells that forms the surface of the cervix. LSILs are considered mild abnormalities caused by human papillomavirus (HPV) infection. LSILs are sometimes referred to as mild dysplasia. They may also be referred to as cervical intraepithelial neoplasia (CIN 1). *Neoplasia* means an abnormal growth of cells, and the number describes how much of the thickness of the lining of the cervix contains abnormal cells—only the top layer, in this case.

- **HSIL** (high-grade squamous intraepithelial lesion). *High-grade* means that there are more evident changes in the size and shape of the abnormal (precancerous) cells and that the cells look very different from normal cells. HSILs are more severe abnormalities that have a higher likelihood of progressing to cancer. HSILs include lesions with moderate or severe dysplasia or carcinoma in situ. (With carcinoma in situ, abnormal cells are present only on the surface of the cervix. Although they are not cancer, these abnormal cells may become cancer and spread into nearby healthy tissue.) HSIL lesions are sometimes referred to as CIN 2, CIN 3, or CIN 2/3, indicating that the abnormal cells occupy most of the layers of the lining of the cervix.

- **Squamous cell carcinoma.** Cervical cancer occurs when abnormal cervical squamous cells invade deeper into the cervix or to other tissues or organs. In a well-screened population, such as that in the United States, a finding of cancer on a Pap test is extremely rare.

Glandular Cell Abnormalities

- **AGC** (atypical glandular cells). The glandular cells do not appear normal, but doctors are uncertain about what the cell changes mean.

- **AIS** (endocervical adenocarcinoma in situ). Precancerous cells are found in the glandular tissue.

Causes

Since cervical dysplasia is a precancerous lesion, the risk factors for cervical dysplasia are identical to those for cervical cancer. These risk factors include exposure to human papillomavirus (HPV), early age of first intercourse, multiple sexual partners, low income, smoking, oral contraceptive use, and many nutritional factors.[1]

Of these factors, the most significant is HPV, as it is implicated in virtually all (99.8%) of the 320,000 cases of cervical cancer that occur annually in women throughout the world. In addition, HPV is detected in

Terms Used to Describe Pap Smear and Biopsy Results		
BETHESDA SYSTEM	**DYSPLASIA**	**CIN**
Negative	Benign	Benign
ASC-US	Benign with inflammation	Benign with inflammation
Low-grade SIL	Mild dysplasia	CIN 1
High-grade SIL	Moderate dysplasia	CIN 2
High-grade SIL	Severe dysplasia	CIN 3
High-grade SIL	Carcinoma in situ	CIN 3
Carcinoma	Carcinoma	Invasive cancer

CIN = cervical intraepithelial neoplasia; SIL = squamous epithelial lesion; carcinoma = squamous cell carcinoma.

approximately 50 to 80% of vaginal, 50% of vulvar, and nearly all penile and anal cancers.

HPV, which is easily transmitted by genital-to-genital contact, can cause genital warts. The time from exposure to the appearance of a genital wart or an abnormal Pap smear can range from a few weeks to decades. The number of medical visits for HPV disease has increased more than 500% in the past 30 years, and HPV infection is often considered epidemic. At least 60% of young women have evidence of HPV in their cervix; however, less than 10% develop any signs of an infection or cervical change. This suggests that the immune system is able to defend against the development of clinical infection, cervical dysplasia, and cancer.

A complex interaction of defense mechanisms, including immunity, viral load, viral type, and host susceptibility, determines the natural course of the disease. One of three things can happen following infection with HPV: (1) the infection remains permanently latent (silent) or produces only temporary cellular changes in the cervix; (2) women develop low-grade HPV-associated cervical dysplasia or cellular changes; and (3) women develop the more serious high-grade squamous intraepithelial lesion (HSIL). The other risk factors given above are largely what determines which of these possibilities will occur. For example, smoking is a significant risk factor for cervical cancer and cervical dysplasia: smokers have an approximately threefold increased incidence compared with nonsmokers, with one study showing the increase to be as high as 17-fold in women ages 20 to 29.[2–6] Possible explanations offered for this association are:

- Smoking may depress immune function, allowing a sexually transmitted agent to promote abnormal cellular development.

- Smoking induces vitamin C deficiency, since vitamin C levels are significantly depressed in smokers.

- Cervical cells may be especially sensitive to the harmful free radicals from cigarette smoke.

- There may be unrecognized associations between smoking and sexual behavior.

Therapeutic Considerations

A follow-up Pap test is always indicated to determine what course of action is needed. Many cases of mild cervical dysplasia (LSIL) will go away. The median time required for progression from cervical dysplasia to carcinoma in situ ranges from 86 months for LSIL to 12 months for HSIL. In LSIL, there is time to try the natural approaches provided in this chapter, with a follow-up Pap smear and colposcopy at three months. A colposcopy is a procedure in which a colposcope—an instrument much like a microscope—is used to examine the vagina and the cervix. During a colposcopy, the doctor inserts a speculum to widen the vagina and may apply a dilute vinegar solution to the cervix; this solution causes abnormal areas to turn white. The doctor then uses the colposcope (which remains outside the body) to observe the cervix. If colposcopy finds abnormal tissue, the doctor may perform endocervical curettage—a type of biopsy that involves scraping cells from inside the endocervical canal with a small spoon-shaped tool called a curette.

If testing shows carcinoma in situ or HSIL, conventional medical treatment is recommended. Current treatment options include the following:

- LEEP (loop electrosurgical excision procedure) uses an electrical current that is passed through a thin wire loop to act like a knife to remove tissue.

- Cryotherapy destroys abnormal tissue by freezing it.

- Laser therapy uses a narrow beam of intense light to destroy or remove abnormal cells.

- Conization removes a cone-shaped piece of tissue using a knife, a laser, or the LEEP technique.

In the event that these methods are not indicated for or desired by the patient who has HSIL, the natural approach can be tried, with the same follow-up recommended above—Pap smear and colposcopy at three-month intervals. However, the patient who has CIN 3 should definitely be treated with one of the conventional options above if there is no regression after three months.

Diet

Numerous nutritional factors have been implicated as cofactors for cervical dysplasia. A large proportion (67%) of patients with cervical cancer are deficient in at least one nutrient (particularly beta-carotene and vitamin A, folic acid, vitamin B[6], and vitamin C), while 38% show more than one deficiency.[7] In addition, many patients have a marginal nutritional status, on the lower end of normal.[8]

General dietary factors are important as well. A high fat intake has been associated with an increased risk for cervical cancer, while a diet rich in fruits and vegetables is believed to offer significant protection against carcinogenesis, probably owing to the higher intake of fiber, beta-carotene, and vitamin C.[5] Increasing concentrations of serum lycopene and higher dietary intakes of dark green and deep yellow vegetables and fruits decrease the risk of cervical dysplasia and cervical cancer.[9] Significant reductions (approximately 40% to 60%) in risk of cervical cancer were observed for women who had the highest intakes of dietary fiber, vitamin C, vitamin E, vitamin A, alpha-carotene, beta-carotene, lutein, and folate.[10]

Nutritional Supplements

Several key individual supplements are discussed below, but a combination of products may work best. One study showed that multiple vitamin and mineral formulas, vitamins A and E, and calcium were significantly associated with a lower risk of cervical cancer and a lower HPV load.[11]

Vitamin A and Beta-Carotene

There is a strong inverse relationship between dietary beta-carotene intake and the risk of cervical cancer or dysplasia.[8,12–16] Unfortunately, the response to intervention with supplemental beta-carotene has been inconsistent. In a double-blind, randomized, placebo-controlled trial with more than 100 women who used either 30 mg per day of beta-carotene or a placebo, beta-carotene did not appear to promote the regression of carcinoma in situ, especially in HPV-positive subjects.[17] Although one study found higher regression rates of mild to severe dysplasia with 30 mg per day beta-carotene vs. a placebo,[18] for the most part other studies failed to show much, if any, benefit:

- No difference in regression of mild dysplasia after 12 months with 30 mg beta-carotene per day vs. placebo[19]

- No regression of cervical dysplasia with 10 mg per day of beta-carotene vs. placebo[20]

- Slightly increased progression of mild dysplasia with 30 mg per day of beta-carotene vs. no treatment[21]

One of the shortcomings of these studies may be the use of isolated, synthetic beta-carotene. Mixed natural carotenoids are preferred by naturopathic physicians.

Several studies have shown that topical vitamin A therapy produces rather impressive results. In one study, 301 women received either four consecutive two-hour applications (using a collagen sponge in a cervical cap) of vitamin A or a placebo followed by two more applications at three and six months. Vitamin A (retinoic acid) increased the complete regression rate of moderate dysplasia from 27% in the placebo group to 43% in the treatment group. However, the women with severe dysplasia did not improve.[22] In another study, vitamin A was delivered to 20 women via a cervical cap. In 10 of 20 women, cervical dysplasia completely disappeared. Of the 10 patients with a complete response, 5 had had mild dysplasia and 5 had had moderate dysplasia.[23] There were too few patients with severe dysplasia to be evaluated.

Vitamin C

A significant decrease in vitamin C intake and plasma levels occurs in patients with cervical dysplasia, and it has been documented that inadequate vitamin C intake is an independent risk factor for the development of cervical dysplasia and carcinoma in situ.[24,25] Vitamin C is known to do the following:

- Act as an antioxidant
- Strengthen and maintain normal epithelial integrity
- Improve wound healing
- Enhance immune function

Selenium

Selenium levels in the diet and blood have been reported to be significantly lower in patients with cervical dysplasia. In one study,

significantly lower selenium and zinc levels were found in both HSIL and cervical cancer patients compared with controls. The activity of the selenium-containing antioxidant enzyme glutathione peroxidase was significantly lower in patients with HSIL or cancer as well, and total antioxidant ability decreased from controls to CIN to cancer. Increased glutathione peroxidase activity resulting from increased selenium intake is believed to be the factor responsible for selenium's anticarcinogenic effect, although other factors may be of equal significance.[26]

Folic Acid

Low folic acid levels have been implicated in many cases of cervical dysplasia, though this may change now that there is widespread folic acid fortification of the food supply. When cells lack folic acid, they display abnormal shapes or size. For example, folic acid deficiency in red blood cells causes the cells to become macrocytic, or larger than normal. Interestingly, abnormal cell structure due to folic acid insufficiency is visible in the cervix before it is visible in the red blood cells.[27,28] Prior to fortification of the food supply with folic acid it was the most common vitamin deficiency in the world and was especially common in women who were pregnant or taking oral contraceptives.[28,29] It is probable that many abnormal Pap smears in the past reflected folate deficiency rather than true dysplasia.[28,30,31]

Even with food fortification, folic acid is still a factor in many cases of cervical dysplasia. This observation is particularly applicable to patients taking oral contraceptives. It has been hypothesized that the hormones induce a localized interference with folate metabolism, so although serum levels may be increased, tissue levels at end-organ targets such as the cervix may be inadequate.[30,31] This is consistent with the observation that tissue status (as measured by erythrocyte folate) is typically decreased, especially in those with cervical dysplasia, while serum levels may be normal or even increased.[32] In controlled clinical studies of women with cervical dysplasia taking oral contraceptives, a very high dosage of folic acid (10 mg per day) resulted in the improvement or normalization of Pap smears.[30,33,34] Regression rates for patients with untreated cervical dysplasia are typically 1.3% for mild dysplasia and 0% for moderate dysplasia. When patients were treated with folic acid, the regression-to-normal rate, as determined by colposcopy/biopsy examination, was observed to be 20% in one study,[34] 63.7% in another,[33] and 100% in yet another.[30] Furthermore, the progression rate of cervical dysplasia in untreated patients is typically 16% at four months, a figure matched in the placebo group in one study, while the folate-supplemented group had a 0% progression rate.[31] These figures were achieved despite the fact that the women remained on oral contraceptives.

Lower folic acid status has been shown to enhance the effect of other risk factors for cervical dysplasia. For example, low red blood cell folate appears to be a major risk factor for HPV infection of the cervix.[33–35] In particular, higher circulating concentrations of folate are independently associated with a lower likelihood of becoming positive for high-risk human papillomaviruses (HR-HPVs) and of having a persistent HR-HPV infection and a greater risk for HSIL.

Vitamin B_{12} supplementation should always accompany folate supplementation to rule out the possibility that the latter may be masking an underlying vitamin B_{12} deficiency. In addition, women with higher concentrations of plasma folate who also had sufficient plasma vitamin B_{12} had a 70% lower risk of being diagnosed with cervical dysplasia.[36]

Indole-3-Carbinol/Diindolylmethane

Indole-3-carbinol (I3C) is a phytochemical found in vegetables in the brassica (cabbage) family. It is converted in the stomach to several compounds including diindolylmethane (DIM). I3C and DIM are antioxidants and potent stimulators of natural detoxifying enzymes in the liver. Studies have shown that increasing the intake of brassica vegetables or taking I3C or DIM as a dietary supplement significantly increases the conversion of estrogen from cancer-producing forms to nontoxic breakdown products.[37,38] The body breaks down estrogen in several ways. It can be converted into a substance called 16-alpha-hydroxyestrone, a compound that promotes estrogen-dependent cancer. Another method of breakdown produces 2-hydroxyestrone, which does not stimulate cancer cells. Women with HSIL have altered estrogen metabolism with a higher level of 16-alpha hydroxyestrone and fewer 2-hydroxyestrogen metabolites than normal.[39]

Given the ability of I3C or DIM to improve estrogen metabolism and possibly exert anti-HPV activity, these agents would seem to be very good candidates for the treatment of cervical dysplasia.[37,38] Preliminary studies are very encouraging. In one double-blind, placebo-controlled study of 30 women with HSIL (biopsy-proven CIN 2 or 3), the women were given either 200 or 400 mg I3C or a placebo for 12 weeks.[39] In 4 of 8 patients in the group who took 200 mg per day of I3C and 4 of 9 in the 400-mg group there was complete regression of their severe dysplasia, compared with none of the placebo group. HPV was detected in 7 of 10 placebo patients, in 7 of 8 in the 200-mg group, and in 8 of 9 in the 400-mg group.

DIM was used in another study of 64 patients with HSIL (biopsy-proven CIN 2 or 3) who were scheduled for LEEP. The patients were randomized to receive either a daily dose of DIM (approximately 2 mg/kg) or a placebo for 12 weeks. Though there was no statistically significant difference in any outcome between the DIM and placebo groups overall, the results with DIM showed an improved Pap smear in 49%, with either a less severe abnormality or a normal result. Colposcopy also improved in 56% of subjects in the DIM group.[40]

Botanical Medicines

Constituents of green tea (*Camellia sinensis*), namely, polyphenol E and epigallocatechin-3-gallate (EGCG), have been effective against HPV-infected cervical cells and lesions in both laboratory and clinical studies. Green tea appears to induce apoptosis of HPV-infected cervical cells and also to arrest cell cycles, modify gene expression, and inhibit tumor formation.[41]

A clinical study confirmed these findings in patients through the use of either topical application via a green tea polyphenol ointment and/or oral ingestion of a green tea polyphenol capsule or an EGCG capsule. Twenty out of 27 patients (74%) under green tea topical therapy showed a response. Six out of 8 patients using the green tea ointment plus EGCG capsule therapy (75%) showed a response, and 6 out of 10 patients (60%) taking the EGCG capsule showed a response. Overall, a 69% response rate was noted for treatment with green tea extracts, as compared with a 10% response rate in untreated controls.[41]

QUICK REVIEW

- **Cervical dysplasia reflects the presence of abnormal cells on the cervix and is usually a precancerous condition.**
- **Severe surgical dysplasia (stage IV Pap smear) requires cone biopsy or a similar procedure.**
- **Risk factors for cervical dysplasia include early age of first intercourse, multiple sexual partners, exposure to viruses, low income, smoking, oral contraceptive use, and many nutritional factors.**
- **Women who have low vitamin C levels are 6.7 times more likely to develop cervical cancer than women with sufficient vitamin C levels.**
- **The higher the intake of dietary sources of beta-carotene, the lower the rate of cervical dysplasia.**
- **Many abnormal Pap smears reflect folic acid deficiency rather than true dysplasia.**
- **Folic acid supplementation (10 mg per day) has resulted in improvement or normalization of Pap smears in patients with cervical dysplasia.**
- **Selenium levels are significantly lower in patients with cervical dysplasia.**

TREATMENT SUMMARY

Proper medical evaluation and monitoring are required. The basic strategy is to eliminate all factors known to be associated with cervical dysplasia and to optimize the patient's nutritional status regardless of current staging. In patients with HSIL a colposcopy with endocervical curettage is recommended.

Diet

Follow the guidelines in the chapter "A Health-Promoting Diet." Try to achieve the recommended intake of fruits and vegetables, especially those green, yellow, and orange in color. Eat vegetables from the brassica family on a regular basis.

Nutritional Supplements

- A high-potency multiple vitamin and mineral formula as described in the chapter "Supplementary Measures"
- Key individual nutrients:
  - Beta-carotene (mixed carotenes preferred): 50,000 to 150,000 IU per day
  - Vitamin B_6: 25 to 50 mg per day
  - Folic acid: 800 to 2,000 mcg per day
  - Vitamin B_{12} (methylcobalamin): 1,000 mcg per day
  - Vitamin C: 500 to 1,000 mg per day
  - Vitamin E (mixed tocopherols): 100 to 200 IU per day multiple vitamin and mineral formula
  - Selenium: 100 to 200 mcg per day
  - Zinc: 30 to 45 mg per day
  - Vitamin D_3: 2,000 to 4,000 IU per day (ideally, measure blood levels and adjust dosage accordingly)
- Fish oils: 1,000 mg EPA + DHA per day
- One of the following:
  - Grape seed extract (>95% procyanidolic oligomers): 100 to 300 mg per day
  - Pine bark extract (>95% procyanidolic oligomers): 100 to 300 mg per day
  - Some other flavonoid-rich extract with a similar flavonoid content, super greens formula, or another plant-based antioxidant that can provide an oxygen radical absorption capacity (ORAC) of 3,000 to 6,000 units or more per day
- One of the following:
  - I3C: 200 to 400 mg per day
  - DIM: 2.2 mg/kg per day

Botanical Medicines

- Green tea extract (>90% total polyphenol content): 150 to 300 mg per day

Chronic Fatigue Syndrome

· ·

- Some combination of the following symptoms:
    - Recurrent fatigue
    - Mild fever
    - Recurrent sore throat
    - Painful lymph nodes
    - Muscle weakness
    - Muscle pain
    - Recurrent headache
    - Migratory joint pain
    - Depression
    - Sleep disturbance (hypersomnia or insomnia)

Chronic fatigue syndrome (CFS) includes varying combinations of the symptoms listed above. Although relatively newly defined, CFS is not a new disease. References to a similar condition in the medical literature go back as far as the 1860s. In addition, symptoms of CFS mirror symptoms of neurasthenia, a condition first described in 1869. In the past, CFS has also been known by various other names, including chronic mononucleosis-like syndrome, chronic Epstein-Barr virus (EBV) syndrome, yuppie flu, postviral fatigue syndrome, postinfectious neuromyasthenia, chronic fatigue and immune dysfunction syndrome (CFIDS), Iceland disease, and Royal Free Hospital disease.

In 1988 the Centers for Disease Control and Prevention (CDC) established a formal (and controversial) set of diagnostic criteria for CFS (see the first list below).[1] One of the major complaints from physicians about the CDC definition is that it appears better suited for research than for clinical purposes. Another problem with the CDC criteria is that they ignore many of the common symptoms reported by patients with CFS (described in the second list).

The British and Australian criteria for the diagnosis of CFS are less strict than those of the CDC.[2] In particular, the minor diagnostic criteria are not required and the major diagnostic criteria are not as strict. For example, in the Australian definition the major criterion is simply fatigue at a level that causes disruption of everyday activities in the absence of other medical conditions associated with fatigue.

On the basis of the CDC criteria, the prevalence of CFS in individuals suffering from chronic fatigue in the United States is thought to be about 11.5%. On that of the British criteria, it is about 15%; and on that of the Australian criteria, it is about 38%.[2]

Centers for Disease Control and Prevention Diagnostic Criteria for Chronic Fatigue Syndrome
Major criteria (both required)

- New onset of fatigue causing 50% reduction in activity for at least six months

- Exclusion of other illnesses that can cause fatigue

Minor criteria (8 of the 11 symptoms listed below, or 6 of 11 symptoms and 2 of 3 signs)

- Symptoms
  - Mild fever
  - Recurrent sore throat
  - Painful lymph nodes
  - Muscle weakness
  - Muscle pain
  - Prolonged fatigue after exercise
  - Recurrent headache
  - Migratory joint pain
  - Neurological or psychological complaints:
      - Sensitivity to bright light
      - Forgetfulness
      - Confusion
      - Inability to concentrate
      - Excessive irritability
      - Depression
  - Sleep disturbance (hypersomnia or insomnia)
  - Sudden onset of symptom complex
- Signs:
  - Low-grade fever
  - Nonexudative pharyngitis
  - Palpable or tender lymph nodes

Frequency of Chronic Fatigue Syndrome Symptoms Reported by Patients	
SYMPTOM/SIGN	FREQUENCY (%)
Fatigue	100
Low-grade fever	60–95
Muscle pain	20–95
Sleep disorder	15–90
Impaired mental function	50–85
Depression	70–85
Headache	35–85
Allergies	55–80
Sore throat	50–75
Anxiety	50–70
Muscle weakness	40–70
Postexercise fatigue	50–60
Premenstrual syndrome (women)	50–60
Stiffness	50–60
Visual blurring	50–60
Nausea	50–60
Dizziness	30–50
Joint pain	40–50
Dry eyes and mouth	30–40
Diarrhea	30–40
Cough	30–40
Decreased appetite	30–40
Night sweats	30–40
Painful lymph nodes	30–40

Causes

Owing in part to its similarity to acute or chronic infection, chronic fatigue syndrome was initially thought to be caused by a virus (such as EBV). It now seems clear that CFS is not caused by any single recognized infectious agent. A CDC study found no association between CFS and infection by a wide variety of organisms, including EBV, human retroviruses, herpes virus, rubella, *Candida albicans*, and others. However, the possibility remains that CFS may have multiple causes leading to a common end point, in which case some viruses or other infectious agents may be contributing factors.

There is little doubt that a disturbed immune system plays a central role in CFS. A variety of immune system abnormalities have been reported in CFS patients, with the most common one being decreased number or activity of natural killer (NK) cells.[3–6] NK cells received their name because of their ability to destroy cells that have become cancerous or infected by viruses. In fact, for a time, CFS was also referred to as low natural killer cell syndrome (LNKS).

Other consistent findings include a reduced ability of lymphocytes, a type of white blood cell that is key in the battle against viruses, to respond to stimuli.[7] One reason for this lack of response may be reduced activity or decreased production of interferon—a natural antiviral compound. Although both low and high levels of interferon have been reported in CFS, levels are low in most cases. When interferon levels are low, reactivation of latent viral infection is likely. On the other hand, when interferon levels are high, the condition can produce many of the symptoms observed in CFS.

Immunological Abnormalities Reported for Chronic Fatigue Syndrome

Elevated levels of antibodies to viral proteins

Decreased natural killer cell activity

Low or elevated antibody levels

Increased or decreased levels of circulating immune complexes

Increased cytokine (e.g., interleukin-2) levels

Increased or decreased interferon levels

Altered ratio of T helper cells to T suppressor cells

Two conditions similar to CFS are fibromyalgia (FM) and multiple chemical sensitivities (MCS).[3,4,7,8] In fact, the only difference in the diagnostic criteria for FM and CFS is the requirement of musculoskeletal pain in

fibromyalgia and fatigue in CFS. The likelihood of being diagnosed as having fibromyalgia or CFS depends on the type of physician consulted. Specifically, if a rheumatologist or orthopedic specialist is consulted, the patient is much more likely to be diagnosed with fibromyalgia. (The box below presents the diagnostic criteria for fibromyalgia.)

One group of researchers carefully compared the symptom picture of 90 patients who had been diagnosed as having CFS, MCS, or FM (30 in each category).[8] They used the same questionnaire for all 90 patients and found that 70% of the patients diagnosed with FM and 30% of those diagnosed with MCS met the CDC criteria for CFS. Particularly significant was the observation that 80% of both the FM and the MCS patients met the CFS criteria of fatigue lasting more than six months with a 50% reduc-

---

DIAGNOSTIC CRITERIA FOR FIBROMYALGIA

MAJOR CRITERIA (ALL THREE REQUIRED)
- Generalized aches or stiffness of at least three anatomical sites for at least three months
- Six or more typical reproducible tender points
- Exclusion of other disorders that can cause similar symptoms

MINOR CRITERIA (FOUR OR MORE REQUIRED)
- Generalized fatigue
- Chronic headache
- Sleep disturbance
- Neurological and psychological complaints
- Joint swelling
- Numbness or tingling sensations
- Irritable bowel syndrome
- Variation of symptoms in relation to activity, stress, and weather changes

---

tion in activity. More than 50% of the CFS and FM patients reported adverse reactions to various chemicals.

In addition to CFS, chronic fatigue can be caused by various physical and psychological factors. The following list shows the major causes of chronic fatigue; the order represents how common the cause is among sufferers of chronic fatigue. The list is based on the findings of several large studies as well as the authors' clinical experience.

Causes of Chronic Fatigue

Preexisting physical condition

Diabetes

Heart disease

Lung disease

Rheumatoid arthritis

Chronic inflammation

Chronic pain

Cancer

Liver disease

Multiple sclerosis

Prescription drugs

Antihypertensives

Anti-inflammatory agents

Birth control pills

Antihistamines

Corticosteroids

Tranquilizers and sedatives

Depression

Stress and/or low adrenal function

Impaired liver function, environmental illness, or both

Impaired immune function

Chronic candida infection

Other chronic infections

Food allergies

Hypothyroidism

Hypoglycemia

Anemia and nutritional deficiencies

Sleep disturbances

Mitochondrial dysfunction

Diagnostic Considerations

The importance of a thorough medical exam cannot be overstated. The goal is to identify and eliminate or deal with as many factors as possible that may be contributing to the feeling of fatigue. Undiagnosed disease is surprisingly common. For example, 50% of diabetics in the United States have not yet been diagnosed.

A detailed medical history and a review of body systems go a long way toward identifying important factors, but in many cases of chronic fatigue, further evaluation is necessary. The next steps can include a complete physical examination and laboratory studies. In particular, low thyroid function (hypothyroidism) is a common cause of chronic fatigue and is often overlooked. In the physical examination, it is important to look for clues that may point to the cause of chronic fatigue. For example, swollen lymph nodes may indicate a chronic infection, and the presence of a diagonal crease on both earlobes usually indicates impaired blood flow to the brain, a significant cause of fatigue in the elderly.

Therapeutic Considerations

Because chronic fatigue is generally a multifactorial condition, the therapeutic approach typically involves multiple therapies that address different facets of the disease. A person's energy level, as well as his or her emotional state, is determined by an interplay between two primary factors—internal focus and physiology. Many people with chronic fatigue focus on how tired they are. They repeatedly reaffirm their fatigue to themselves and to anyone who will listen. Their physiology includes not only the chemicals and hormones circulating in the body but also the way they hold their bodies (usually slouched) and the way they breathe (shallowly). In most patients with chronic fatigue, both the mind and the body must be addressed. The most effective treatment is a comprehensive program designed to help people use their mind, attitudes, and physiology to fuel higher energy levels.

Lifestyle Practices Associated with Higher Natural Killer Cell Activity

Not smoking

Increased intake of green vegetables

Regular meals

Proper body weight

More than seven hours of sleep a night

Regular exercise

A vegetarian diet

Depression

The mind and attitude play a critical role in determining the status of the immune system and energy levels. Many patients with chronic fatigue (including CFS) either are depressed or just seem to have lost enthusiasm for life. Of course, it is not easy to have much enthusiasm when you do not have much energy, but the two usually go hand in hand. Depression is one of the major causes of chronic fatigue, and it is a common feature of CFS. In the absence of a preexisting physical condition, depression is generally regarded as the most common cause of chronic fatigue. However,

it is often difficult to determine whether the depression preceded the fatigue or vice versa. (Depression is fully discussed in the chapter "Depression").

One interesting finding is that CFS patients tend to lack social support.[9] An open question is whether the lack of energy affects the CFS patient's ability to maintain a relationship or vice versa, or possibly both.

Cognitive behavioral therapy has shown some effective results in clinical use.[10,11] The first step is for CFS patients to understand that they can get better. Many patients with CFS are told that this is "something they will have to live with" and that "there is no cure." A positive mental attitude is critical to good health and high energy levels, especially in patients with CFS. In order to achieve a positive mind-set, a person must exercise or condition the attitude, much as one would condition the body. Mental exercises such as visualizations, goal setting, affirmations, and empowering questions, as detailed in the chapter "A Positive Mental Attitude," should be performed every day.

Stress and Low Adrenal Function

Stress and low adrenal function are other factors to consider in CFS. Stress can be an underlying factor in patients with depression, low immune function, or another cause of chronic fatigue. The adrenal glands are very much involved in the body's energy level and ability to deal with stress. Low adrenal function and adrenal exhaustion were first proposed as causes of chronic fatigue more than 50 years ago.[12] Laboratory tests of adrenal function now confirm that low function is common in CFS.[13,14] However, whether the low adrenal function is the cause of the illness or an effect is not yet known.[15] Either way, one of the major symptoms of adrenal hormone deficiency is debilitating fatigue. In particular, suspect insufficient cortisol when a stressful event is followed by feverishness, joint and muscle pain, swollen lymph glands, post-exertional fatigue, worsening of allergic responses, and disturbances of mood and sleep (i.e., the typical presentation of CFS). There is also significant evidence that a drop in adrenal hormone secretion is a factor in the development of many of the biological and behavioral features of CFS.[16] For complete information on supporting the adrenal glands, see the chapter "Stress Management."

Impaired Liver Function, Environmental Toxin Overload, or Both

Enhancing detoxification processes is another important goal in CFS. Exposure to food additives, solvents (cleaners, formaldehyde, toluene, benzene), pesticides, herbicides, heavy metals (lead, mercury, cadmium, arsenic, nickel, aluminum), and other toxins can greatly stress the liver and detoxification processes and produce CFS-like symptoms.[17–19] Specifically, people who have impaired detoxification processes or who have been exposed to toxic chemicals often complain of fatigue along with the following:

- Depression
- General malaise
- Headaches
- Digestive disturbances
- Allergies and chemical sensitivities
- Premenstrual syndrome
- Constipation

For a complete discussion of detoxification processes, see the chapter "Detoxification and Internal Cleansing." A couple of studies using a comprehensive detoxification program featuring a hypoallergenic diet along with a dietary food supplement rich in nutri-

ents that assist liver detoxification has shown good results in CFS. In one of these studies, 52% of patients reported a reduction in symptoms after 10 weeks.[19] In the other, the clinical improvement in CFS was paralleled by improved liver detoxification function.[20]

The hypoallergenic diet appears to be quite useful, because excessive gastrointestinal permeability and food allergies are important considerations in CFS. In fact, as far back as 1930, chronic fatigue was recognized as a key feature of food allergies.[21] Originally, the term *allergic toxemia* was used to describe a syndrome that included the symptoms of fatigue, muscle and joint aches, drowsiness, difficulty in concentration, nervousness, and depression. Around the 1950s, this syndrome began to be referred to as the "allergic tension-fatigue syndrome."[22] With the popularity of CFS as a diagnosis, many physicians and others are forgetting that food allergies can lead to chronic fatigue. Furthermore, between 55% and 85% of individuals with CFS have allergies. For more information on food allergies, see the chapter "Food Allergy." Another important consideration is gastrointestinal overgrowth of *Candida albicans* (see the chapter "Candidiasis, Chronic").

Diet

Energy levels appear to be directly related to the quality of foods routinely ingested. We recommend the dietary guidelines in the chapter "A Health-Promoting Diet." It is especially important to eliminate or restrict caffeine and refined sugar. Hypoglycemia can produce significant fatigue and other symptoms associated with CFS.

Although occasional use of caffeine can give you a boost, regular caffeine intake may actually lead to chronic fatigue. Mice fed one dose of caffeine demonstrated significant increases in their swimming capacity, but when the dose of caffeine was given repeatedly for six weeks, a significant decrease in the mice's swimming capacity was observed.[23]

Several studies have found caffeine intake to be extremely high in individuals with psychiatric disorders. Another interesting finding is that the degree of fatigue experienced is often related to the quantity of caffeine ingested. In one survey of hospitalized psychiatric patients, 61% of those ingesting at least 750 mg per day of caffeine (the amount found in about five cups of coffee) complained of fatigue, compared with 54% of those ingesting 250 to 749 mg per day and only 24% of those ingesting less than 250 mg per day.[24] Of course, this is not necessarily causative, as those who are fatigued may try to cope by consuming large amounts of caffeine.

In patients who routinely drink coffee, abrupt cessation of coffee drinking will probably result in symptoms of caffeine withdrawal, including fatigue, headache, and an intense desire for coffee.[25,26] Fortunately, this withdrawal period does not last more than a few days.

Nutritional Supplements

Nutritional supplementation is essential in the treatment of CFS. A deficiency of virtually any nutrient can produce the symptoms of fatigue as well as render the body more susceptible to infection. Individuals with chronic fatigue require, at the bare minimum, a high-potency multiple vitamin and mineral formula along with extra vitamin C (1,000–3,000 mg per day in divided doses) and magnesium (500 to 1,200 mg per day in divided doses). Fish oil supplements have also been shown to be quite beneficial.[27,28]

Magnesium
An underlying magnesium deficiency, even if very mild, can result in chronic fatigue and symptoms similar to those of CFS. In addition, low red blood cell magnesium levels, a more accurate measure of magnesium status than routine blood analysis, have been found in many patients with chronic fatigue and CFS. The literature demonstrates that magnesium deficiency is not necessarily due to low dietary intake,[29] and several studies have shown good results with supplementation with improvements in magnesium stores.

For example, in one double-blind, placebo-controlled trial, 32 CFS patients received an intramuscular injection of either magnesium sulfate (1 g) or a placebo for six weeks. At the end of the study, 12 of the 15 patients receiving magnesium reported, on the basis of strict criteria, significantly improved energy levels, improved emotional state, and less pain. In contrast, only 3 of the 17 placebo patients reported that they felt better and only 1 reported improved energy levels.[30]

This study seems to confirm some impressive results obtained in clinical trials during the 1960s on patients suffering from chronic fatigue.[31–34] These studies used oral magnesium and potassium aspartate (1 g each) rather than injectable magnesium. Between 75 and 91% of the nearly 3,000 patients studied experienced relief of fatigue during treatment with the magnesium and potassium aspartate. In contrast, the proportion of patients responding to a placebo was between 9 and 26%. The beneficial effect was usually noted after only 4 to 5 days, but sometimes it took as long as 10 days to achieve results. Patients usually continued treatment for four to six weeks; afterward, fatigue frequently did not return.

Injectable magnesium is not necessary to restore magnesium status.[35] Studies indicate that magnesium is easily absorbed orally when it is bound to aspartate or citrate. In addition, both of these compounds may also help to fight fatigue. Aspartate feeds into the

Krebs cycle, the final common pathway for the conversion of glucose, fatty acids, and amino acids to chemical energy, while citrate is itself a component of the Krebs cycle. Krebs cycle components (including aspartate, citrate, fumarate, malate, and succinate) usually provide a better mineral chelate: evidence suggests that these chelates are better absorbed, used, and tolerated compared with inorganic or relatively insoluble mineral salts (such as magnesium chloride, oxide, or carbonate).[35,36]

Carnitine

Carnitine is an essential nutrient for the transport of long-chain fatty acids into the mitochondria, the energy-producing compartments in cells of the body. In 30 CFS patients, carnitine or the drug amantadine was given. Amantadine was poorly tolerated and produced no statistically significant difference in any of the clinical indicators. With carnitine, there was a statistically significant clinical improvement in 12 of the 18 studied indicators after eight weeks of treatment, with none of the clinical indicators showing any deterioration.[37] Carnitine is extremely safe, with no significant side effects having been reported in any of the human clinical studies.

Coenzyme Q_{10} (CoQ_{10})

CoQ_{10} also plays a role in mitochondrial function and acts as an essential cofactor for the cellular production of energy. Low blood levels of CoQ_{10} have been found in CFS patients compared with normal subjects, suggesting that supplementation may be useful.[38]

Other Therapies

Breathing, Posture, and Bodywork

Proper care of the body is critical to the achievement of high levels of energy. Breathing with the diaphragm, good posture, and bodywork (e.g., massage, spinal manipulation) are all important in helping to relieve the stress that is a common contributor to fatigue.

Exercise

Exercise alone has been demonstrated to have a tremendous impact on mood and the ability to handle stressful life situations.[39,40] Regular exercise has also been shown to lead to improved immune status. For CFS patients, regular exercise has been shown to lead to a significant increase (up to 100%) in natural killer cell activity.[41,42] Although relatively strenuous exercise is required to benefit the cardiovascular system, light to moderate exercise may be best for the immune system. One study found that immune function was significantly increased by the practice of tai chi exercises.[43] Tai chi is a martial art technique that features movement from one posture to the next in a flowing motion that resembles dance. Gradual increases in exercise intensity (for example, begin with gradual walking and weight exercises and increase duration and intensity over time as is comfortable) may be the best approach.[44,45]

Botanical Medicines

Several botanical medicines support adrenal function and may offer significant benefits in CFS. Most notable are adaptogens such as Chinese ginseng (*Panax ginseng*), Siberian ginseng (*Eleutherococcus senticosus*), rhodiola (*Rhodiola rosea*), and ashwaganda (*Withania somnifera*). The adaptogenic effects of these herbs were discussed in the chapter "Stress Management." Of these herbal adaptogens, both Siberian ginseng and rhodiola have shown effects specific to CFS.

Siberian Ginseng

In addition to supporting adrenal function and acting as a nonspecific adaptogen, Siberian ginseng (*E. senticosus*) has been shown to exert a number of beneficial effects on immune function that may be useful in the treatment of CFS. In one double-blind study, 36 healthy subjects received either 10 ml of a fluid extract of Siberian ginseng or a placebo per day for four weeks.[46] The group receiving the ginseng demonstrated significant improvements in various immune system indicators. Most notable were a significant increase in T-helper cells and an increase in NK cell activity, both of which are of value in the treatment of CFS.

Rhodiola rosea

Rhodiola rosea (Arctic root) is a popular plant in traditional medical systems in Eastern Europe and Asia, where it has traditionally been recommended to help combat fatigue and restore energy. In one randomized, placebo-controlled trial of 60 patients with stress-related fatigue, rhodiola was found to have an antifatigue effect that increased mental performance, particularly the ability to concentrate, as well as decreased the cortisol response to stress.[47]

. . . .

QUICK REVIEW

- **A disturbed immune system plays a central role in chronic fatigue syndrome (CFS).**
- **Fibromyalgia and multiple chemical sensitivity disorder have symptoms similar to those of CFS.**
- **Chronic fatigue can be caused by a variety of physical and psychological factors other than CFS.**
- **The importance of a thorough medical exam cannot be understated. The goal is to identify and eliminate or deal with as many factors as possible that may be contributing to the feeling of fatigue.**
- **A person's energy level and emotional state are determined by the interplay between internal focus and physiology.**
- **Enhancing detoxification processes is another important goal in CFS.**
- **As far back as 1930, chronic fatigue was**

- **recognized as a key feature of food allergies.**
- **The mind and attitude play a critical role in determining the status of the immune system and energy levels.**
- **Energy levels appear to be directly related to the quality of foods routinely ingested.**
- **A deficiency of virtually any nutrient can produce the symptoms of fatigue and render the body more susceptible to infection.**
- **An underlying magnesium deficiency, even if very mild, can result in chronic fatigue and symptoms similar to those of CFS.**
- **Carnitine and coenzyme Q_{10} are essential cofactors in the manufacture of energy within the mitochondria.**
- **Breathing with the diaphragm, good**

posture, and bodywork are all important in helping to relieve the stress that is a common contributor to fatigue.

- In CFS patients regular exercise has been shown to lead to a significant increase (up to 100%) in natural killer cell activity.

- Siberian ginseng has been shown to exert a number of beneficial effects that may be useful in the treatment of CFS.

TREATMENT SUMMARY

Successful treatment of CFS requires a comprehensive diagnostic and therapeutic approach. Especially important is identifying underlying factors that may be affecting the patient's energy levels or immune system. The strong correlation between CFS, FM, and MCS suggests that all three conditions may respond to liver detoxification, food allergy control, and a gut-restoration diet. Special attention should be paid to the advice in the chapter "Immune System Support."

Diet

Identify and control food allergies. Increase water consumption, and stop consuming caffeine-containing drinks and alcohol. The diet should be rich in whole, organically grown foods. Hypoglycemia should be controlled through the elimination of sugar and other refined foods and the regular consumption of small meals and snacks.

Lifestyle

Key practices include diaphragmatic breathing exercises, proper posture, and a regular exercise program focusing on low-intensity activities. For other recommendations see the chapter "A Health-Promoting Lifestyle."

Nutritional Supplements

- A high-potency multiple vitamin and mineral formula as described in the chapter "Supplementary Measures"
- Key individual nutrients:
  - Vitamin B_6: 25 to 50 mg per day
  - Folic acid: 800 to 2,000 mcg per day
  - Vitamin B_{12}: 800 mcg per day
  - Vitamin C: 500 to 1,000 mg per day
  - Vitamin E (mixed tocopherols): 100 to 200 IU per day
  - Magnesium (bound to aspartate, citrate, fumarate, malate, or succinate): 200 to 300 mg three times per day
  - Selenium: 100 to 200 mcg per day
  - Zinc: 30 to 45 mg per day
  - Vitamin D_3: 2,000 to 4,000 IU per day (ideally, measure blood levels and adjust dosage accordingly)
- Fish oils: 1,000 mg EPA + DHA per day
- One of the following:
  - Grape seed extract (>95% procyanidolic oligomers): 100 to 300 mg per day

- Pine bark extract (>95% procyanidolic oligomers): 100 to 300 mg per day
- Or some other flavonoid-rich extract with a similar flavonoid content, super greens formula, or another plant-based antioxidant that can provide an oxygen radical absorption capacity (ORAC) of 3,000 to 6,000 units or more per day
- Specialty supplements:
  - Carnitine: 900 to 1,500 mg per day
  - Coenzyme Q_{10}: 100 to 200 mg per day
  - SAM-e: 200 mg twice per day

Botanical Medicines

- Siberian ginseng (*E. senticosus*):
  - Dried root: 2 to 4 g three times per day
  - Fluid extract (1:1): 2 to 4 ml three times per day
  - Solid (dry powdered) extract (20:1 or standardized to contain more than 1% eleutheroside E): 100 to 200 mg three times per day
- *Rhodiola rosea:* The therapeutic dose varies according to the rosavin content. The typical daily dosage is 200–300 mg per day of an extract standardized to contain 3% rosavins and 0.8 to 1% salidroside.

Chronic Obstructive Pulmonary Disease

....

- Cough, with or without mucus
  - Fatigue
  - History of repeated respiratory infections
  - Shortness of breath (dyspnea) that gets worse with mild activity
  - Trouble catching one's breath
  - Wheezing

Chronic obstructive pulmonary disease (COPD) has two main forms: chronic bronchitis, which involves a long-term cough with mucus; and emphysema, which involves destruction of the lungs over time.

Although chronic bronchitis and emphysema are distinct conditions, people with COPD often have aspects of both. In chronic bronchitis, the linings of the bronchial tubes are inflamed and thickened, leading to a chronic, mucus-producing cough and shortness of breath. In emphysema, the alveoli (tiny air sacs in the lungs) are damaged, also leading to shortness of breath. COPD is generally irreversible and may even be fatal.

Symptoms of COPD usually develop gradually and may initially include shortness of breath during exertion, wheezing (especially during exhaling), and frequent coughing that produces variable amounts of mucus. In more advanced stages, people may experience rapid changes in the ability to breathe, shortness of breath at rest, fatigue, depres-

sion, memory problems, confusion, and frequent waking during sleep.

Causes

Smoking is the leading cause of COPD. The more a person smokes, the more likely it is that he or she will develop COPD. However, some people smoke for years and never get COPD. In rare cases, nonsmokers who lack a protein called alpha-1 antitrypsin can develop emphysema. Other risk factors for COPD are:

- Exposure to certain gases or fumes in the workplace
- Exposure to heavy amounts of secondhand smoke and pollution
- Frequent use of cooking fire without proper ventilation

Therapeutic Considerations

Obviously, people with COPD must stop smoking and/or exposure to lung irritants, as this is the best way to slow down the lung damage.[1]

The natural approach to COPD involves three primary goals: (1) stimulation of normal processes that promote the expectoration (removal) of mucus, (2) thinning the mucus to aid expectoration, (3) enhancement of immune function, and (4) decreasing the chronic inflammation in the lungs. The approaches described in the chapter "Bronchitis and Pneumonia" are appropriate here as well, because from a naturopathic perspective the aims are very similar. The major difference is that in COPD the focus is definitely more on the use of expectorants and mucolytics, especially if the problem is emphysema.

In addition, as COPD progresses it generally requires complementary conventional medical care. Therefore, the goal should also be to try to address any nutrient depletions caused by drug therapy. Medications used to treat COPD include:

- Inhalers (bronchodilators) to open the airways, such as ipratropium (Atrovent), tiotropium (Spiriva), salmeterol (Serevent), formoterol (Foradil), or albuterol

- Inhaled steroids to reduce lung inflammation

- Anti-inflammatory medications such as montelukast (Singulair) and roflumilast (Daliresp) are sometimes used

An especially useful therapy for COPD is the use of oral NAC (N-acetylcysteine); in more serious cases it can be inhaled with the addition of glutathione. The NAC acts as a mucolytic, helping clear mucus from the bronchioles, and the glutathione substantially decreases inflammation in the lungs.[2]

In severe cases or during flare-ups, even more aggressive therapy may be necessary, including oral steroids, oxygen therapy, and antibiotics.

An often unrecognized consequence of many prescription drugs commonly taken by people with COPD is a magnesium deficiency produced by the drugs.[3] That is potentially very serious, as magnesium is needed for normal lung function. One group of researchers reported that 47% of people with COPD had a magnesium deficiency.[4] In this study, magnesium deficiency was also linked to increased hospital stays.

Just as in the treatment of an acute asthma attack, intravenous magnesium has improved breathing capacity in people experiencing an acute worsening of COPD.[5] In one double-blind study, the need for hospitalization was also reduced in the magnesium group (28% vs. 42% with a placebo), but this difference was not statistically significant. Intravenous

· ·

QUICK REVIEW

- **Chronic obstructive pulmonary disease (COPD) has two main forms: chronic bronchitis and emphysema.**
- **Smoking is the leading cause of COPD.**
- **The natural approach to COPD involves four primary goals: (1) stimulation of normal processes that promote the expectoration of mucus, (2) thinning**

the mucus to aid expectoration, (3) enhancement of immune function, and (4) reduction of lung inflammation.

- **As COPD progresses it generally requires complementary conventional medical care.**
- **Oral magnesium supplementation is strongly indicated.**

magnesium is known to be a powerful bronchodilator.

Given that many people with COPD may be magnesium deficient and that magnesium may also improve lung and airway function, oral magnesium supplementation in people with COPD is very much indicated.

TREATMENT SUMMARY

As described above, the basic approach is to use an expectorant, a mucolytic, and immune-supportive nutrients. We also recommend the use of a salt pipe or bottle blowing (see the chapter "Bronchitis and Pneumonia").

Diet

Follow the general guidelines in the chapter "A Health-Promoting Diet." Especially important are foods with high antioxidant content, such as dark leafy vegetables, berries, and legumes.

Nutritional Supplements

- A high-potency multiple vitamin and mineral formula as described in the chapter "Supplementary Measures"
- Key individual nutrients:
  - Vitamin C: 500 to 1,000 mg per day
  - Vitamin E (mixed tocopherols): 100 to 200 IU per day
  - Magnesium (bound to aspartate, citrate, fumarate, malate, or succinate): 200 to 300 mg three times per day
  - Selenium: 100 to 200 mcg per day
  - Vitamin D_3: 2,000 to 4,000 IU per day (ideally, measure blood levels and adjust dosage accordingly)
- Fish oils: 1,000 mg EPA + DHA per day

- One of the following:
  - Grape seed extract (>95% procyanidolic oligomers): 100 to 300 mg per day
  - Pine bark extract (>95% procyanidolic oligomers): 100 to 300 mg per day
  - Some other flavonoid-rich extract with a similar flavonoid content, super greens formula, or another plant-based antioxidant that can provide an oxygen radical absorption capacity (ORAC) of 3,000 to 6,000 units or higher per day

Expectorants

- Take one or both:
  - *Lobelia inflata:*
    - Dried herb: 0.2 to 0.6 g three times per day
    - Tincture: 15 to 30 drops three times per day.
    - Fluid extract: 8 to 10 drops three times per day
  - *Hedera helix* (ivy leaf), available as tincture, fluid extract, and dry powdered extract in capsules and tablets; typical dosage for adults and children over 12 years of age for a 4:1 dry powdered extract is 100 mg per

day (the equivalent of 420 mg dried herbal substance); for children 1–5 years old, dosage is the equivalent of 150 mg dried herbal substance; for children 6–12 years old, the equivalent of 210 mg dried herbal substance

Mucolytics

- Take one or more of the following:
  - ○ Guaifenesin:
    - – Adults and children 12 years of age and older: 200 to 400 mg every four hours. Do not take more than 2,400 mg in a two-hour period.
    - – Children age 6 to 11: 100 to 200 mg every four hours, with no more than 1,200 mg in a 24-hour period. For children age 2 to 5, the dosage is 50 to 100 mg every four hours, with no more than 600 mg in 24 hours.
    - – Guaifenesin is not recommended for children under 2 years of age.
  - ○ N-acetylcysteine: 200 mg three times per day
  - ○ Bromelain (1,200 to 1,800 MCU or GDU): 500 to 750 mg three times per day between meals

Common Cold

- Nasal discomfort with watery discharge and sneezing
- Dry, sore throat
- Red, swollen nasal passages
- Swollen lymph nodes on the neck

The common cold can be caused by a wide variety of viruses that are capable of infecting the upper respiratory tract—the nasal passages, sinuses, and throat. We are all constantly exposed to many of these viruses, yet the majority of us experience the discomfort of a cold only once or twice a year. This situation implies that a decrease in resistance or immune function is the major factor in catching a cold.

In general, the individual with a cold will experience a general malaise, fever, headache, and upper respiratory tract congestion. Initially there is usually a watery nasal discharge with sneezing followed by thicker secretions containing mucus, white blood cells, and dead organisms. The throat may be red, sore, and quite dry.

Usually a cold can be distinguished from other conditions with similar symptoms (influenza and allergies for example) by some common sense. Influenza is much more severe and usually occurs in epidemics. Allergies may be an underlying factor in decreasing resistance and allowing a virus to infect the upper airways, but usually allergies can be differentiated from the common cold by the fact that no fever occurs with allergies, there is usually a history of seasonal allergic episodes, and there is no evidence of infection.

Therapeutic Considerations

Maintaining a healthy immune system is the primary way of protecting against an excessive number of colds. If you catch more than one or two colds a year, you may have a weak immune system. To strengthen the immune system, follow the recommendations in the chapter "Immune System Support."

What to Do Once You Catch a Cold

Once a cold develops, there are several things that can speed up recovery. It should be noted, however, that in people with a healthy, functioning immune system, a cold should not last more than three or four days. Even if you utilize a wide variety of natural healing methods, once a cold is well under way it is very difficult to completely throw it off in two days. Do not expect immediate relief in most instances when using natural substances. In fact, since most natural therapies for colds involve assisting the body rather than suppressing symptoms, as drugs do, often the symptoms of the cold temporarily worsen.

Many of the symptoms of a cold are a result of our body's defense mechanisms. For example, the potent immune-stimulating compound interferon, released by our blood cells and other tissues during infections, is responsible for many flu-like symptoms. Another example is the fever. While an elevated body temperature can be uncomfortable, suppression of fever is thought to counteract a major defense mechanism and prolong the infection. In general, fever should not be suppressed during an infection unless it is dangerously high (>104°F).

Rest

The immune system functions better when the parasympathetic nervous system (a part of our autonomic nervous system) assumes control over bodily functions, as happens during periods of rest, relaxation, visualization, meditation, and sleep. During the deepest levels of sleep, potent immune-enhancing compounds are released and many immune functions are greatly increased. The value of sleep and rest during a cold cannot be overemphasized.

Liquids

Drink lots of fluids, particularly water and unsweetened herbal teas. Increased fluid consumption offers several benefits. When the membranes that line the respiratory tract get dehydrated, they provide a much more hospitable environment for cold viruses. Drinking plenty of liquids and using a vaporizer help maintains a moist respiratory tract, which repels viral infection. Drinking plenty of liquids will also improve the function of white blood cells by decreasing the concentration of solutes in the blood.

It should be noted that the type of liquids you drink is very important. Studies have shown that consuming concentrated sources of sugars such as glucose, fructose, sucrose, honey, or orange juice greatly reduces the ability of white blood cells to kill bacteria.[1–3] If you want to drink fruit juices, dilute them with water. Drinking concentrated orange juice or other sweet juice during a cold probably does more harm than good.

Avoid Sugar

As mentioned above, sugar, even if derived from natural sources such as fruit juices and honey, can impair immune function.[1–3] This impairment appears to be due to the fact that glucose (blood sugar) and vitamin C compete for transport sites into the white blood cells. Excessive sugar consumption may decrease vitamin C levels and result in a significant reduction in white blood cell function.

Vitamin C

Many claims have been made about the role of vitamin C (ascorbic acid) in the prevention and treatment of the common cold. It has been more than 40 years since Linus Pauling wrote the book *Vitamin C and the Common Cold.*[4] Pauling based his opinion on several studies showing that vitamin C was very effective in reducing the severity of symptoms as well as the duration of the common cold. This makes sense, as vitamin C is not only critical for immune system function but also directly antiviral. There have now been more than 30 clinical trials involving 11,350 study participants that have been designed to judge the effectiveness of vitamin C in the prevention or treatment of the common cold. A very detailed analysis of these studies has concluded that vitamin C can be quite beneficial in reducing the risk of developing a cold in high-stress situations, and it may also reduce the duration of a cold by a day or so. In six trials involving a total of 642 marathon runners, skiers, and soldiers on subarctic exercises, the risk of developing a cold was reduced by 50% in the vitamin C group compared with a placebo group. While vitamin C can reduce the duration of a cold slightly, it does not seem to have any effect on reducing symptoms.[5]

Zinc Lozenges

One of the most popular natural approaches to the common cold is the use of zinc lozenges. There are good scientific data to support this practice, as several studies have now shown that zinc lozenges provide relief of a sore throat due to the common cold. Zinc is a critical nutrient for optimal immune system function and, like vitamin C, also exerts direct antiviral activity.[6]

Thirteen placebo-controlled comparisons have examined the therapeutic effect of zinc lozenges on the common cold. Three trials used zinc acetate in daily doses of over 75 mg, with pooled results indicating a 42% reduction in the duration of colds. Five trials used zinc salts other than acetate in daily doses of over 75 mg, with a 20% reduction in the duration of colds. Five of the trials used a total daily zinc dose of less than 75 mg and uniformly found no effect.[7]

Good results were seen in one study with zinc gluconate; it may have been due to the formulation of the lozenge. In the study, 100 patients experiencing early signs of the common cold were provided a lozenge that contained either 13.3 mg zinc (from zinc gluconate) or a placebo.[8] They took the lozenges as long as they had symptoms. The subjects kept track of symptoms such as cough, headache, hoarseness, muscle ache, nasal drainage, nasal congestion, scratchy throat, sore throat, sneezing, and fever. The time to complete resolution of symptoms was significantly shorter in the zinc group than in the placebo group. Complete recovery was achieved in 4.4 days with zinc compared with 7.6 days for the placebo. The zinc group also had significantly fewer days with coughing (2.0 days compared with 4.5 days), headache (2.0 days vs. 3.0 days), hoarseness (2.0 days vs. 3.0 days), nasal congestion (4.0 days vs. 6.0 days), nasal drainage (4.0 days vs. 7.0 days), and sore throat (1.0 day vs. 3.0 days).

The formulation in this study differed from those in the studies that did not show much benefit from zinc lozenges; the lack of benefit in the latter group of studies may have been due to an ineffective lozenge formulation. The explanation for this can be found in an interesting study that evaluated the actual amount of ionized zinc released into the saliva by various lozenges. It appears that in order for zinc to be effective it must be ionized in saliva. The study showed that sucking on hard candy lozenges containing zinc gluconate and citric acid delivered an insignificant amount of ionized zinc.[9] It was found that saliva completely suppresses the ionization of zinc in the presence of citric acid. Certain sweetening agents such as mannitol and sorbitol also prevent the ionization of zinc. The best zinc lozenges are those that provide zinc acetate or gluconate and do not contain citric acid, mannitol, or sorbitol. They may be sweetened with the amino acid glycine. In contrast to citric acid, mannitol, or sorbitol, glycine—even in excessively large amounts—was found not to interfere with ionization of zinc. In fact, 90% of the zinc was ionized in this study.

So what does all this mean? In order for a zinc lozenge to be effective, it must be free from sorbitol, mannitol, and citric acid. Use lozenges supplying 15 to 25 mg elemental zinc. Dissolve in the mouth every two waking hours after an initial double dose. Continue for up to seven days.

Echinacea

There have been more than 300 scientific investigations on the immune-enhancing effects of echinacea—one of the most popular herbs in the treatment of the common cold. Mixed results from clinical studies with echinacea are most likely due to lack of or insufficient quantity of active compounds. The effectiveness of any herbal product depends on its ability to deliver an effective dosage of active compounds. If the product had sufficient levels of active compounds, it would be effective. If not, it would probably be no more effective than a placebo. For example, in one double-blind study 160 subjects were given either echinacea or a placebo and then exposed to a common cold virus. Infection occurred in 44 and 57% of the echinacea- and placebo-treated subjects, respectively, and illness occurred in 36 and 43%. However, the preparation lacked the active components of echinacea—it contained no echinacosides or alkamides and only 0.16% cichoric acid.[10]

In contrast, a clinical trial using a well-defined echinacea extract containing alkamides, cichoric acid, and polysaccharides at concentrations of 0.25, 2.5, and 25 mg/ml, respectively, prepared from freshly harvested *E. purpurea* plants (commercially available as Echinilin or Echinamide), showed excellent results.[11] In this randomized, double-blind, placebo-controlled trial, 282 subjects 18 to 65 years old with a history of two or more colds in the previous year, but otherwise in good health, were randomly assigned to receive either echinacea extract or a placebo. They were instructed to start the echinacea or placebo at the onset of the first symptom related to a cold, consuming 10 doses the first day and 4 doses per day on subsequent days for seven days. Severity of symptoms was recorded each day, and a nurse examined the subjects on the mornings of days three and eight. A total of 128 subjects contracted a common cold (59 echinacea, 69 placebo). The total daily symptom scores were found to be 23.1% lower in the echinacea group than in the placebo group. Throughout the treatment period, the response rate to treatments was greater in the echinacea group.

Again, to highlight the issue of quality control and source of preparation, several studies with less well-defined echinacea products showed little benefit, especially in experimentally induced rhinovirus infections.[12] For example, in one double-blind study, 302 volunteers from four military institutions and one industrial plant in Germany were given either a placebo or alcohol-based tinctures from either *E. purpurea* or *E. angustifolia* dried root for 12 weeks. The main outcome measure was time until the first upper respiratory tract infection. The secondary outcome measures were the number of participants with at least one infection, global assessment, and adverse effects. The time until occurrence of the first upper respiratory tract infection was 66 days in the *E. angustifolia* group, 69 days in the *E. purpurea* group, and 65 days in the placebo group. In the placebo group 36.7% had an infection, while in the *E. angustifolia* group the proportion was 32% and in the *E. purpurea* group it was 29.3%. These results indicate that there was no significant benefit with either form of echinacea, although there was an approximately 20% reduced risk of infection in the echinacea groups.

In one of the most detailed clinical trials, 719 patients were assigned to one of four groups: no pills, placebo pills (blinded), echinacea pills (blinded), or echinacea pills (unblinded). Echinacea groups received 8 tablets on the first day and 4 tables on the subsequent four days. Each tablet contained the equivalent of 675 mg alcoholic extract of dried *Echinacea purpurea* root and 600 mg alcoholic extract of *Echinacea angustifolia* root; the placebo group received the same number of tablets. The results showed only a statistically insignificant trend in reduction of the cold duration (half a day) and a reduction of severity of approximately 10%.[13]

The result from this trial indicates that a major issue with some of the echinacea research may be the echinacea preparations used—weak ethanol-based tinctures derived from dried root. Clinical studies of upper respiratory tract infections treated with extracts of fresh *Echinacea purpurea* whole plant or aerial plant, especially in liquid form, are consistently positive compared with those using dried echinacea extracts or powdered herbs, especially in solid forms (tablets or capsules). It is possible that echinacea may exert direct local effects and that contact with lymphatic tissue in the mouth and throat is extremely important in an upper respiratory tract infection. Reasonably large and well-designed, double-blind, placebo-controlled studies have found that preparations of echinacea from the aerial portion of the plant produce modest effects in staving off colds as well as reducing symptoms and duration.[12,14]

Another study showed good results when 108 patients with initial symptoms suggesting a cold received an extract of the freshly pressed juice of *E. purpurea* (EchinaGuard) at a dosage of 4 ml twice per day or a placebo for eight weeks.[15] In the echinacea group, 35.2% of patients remained healthy, compared with 25.9% in the placebo group. The length of time between infections was 40 days with echinacea, 25 days with the placebo. When infections did occur in patients receiving echinacea, they were less severe and resolved more quickly. Patients showing evidence of a weakened immune system (CD4:CD8 ratio <1.5) benefited the most from echinacea.

The results from another trial were especially encouraging, as they suggested that echinacea can not only make colds shorter and less severe but also sometimes stop a cold that is just starting.[16] In this study, 120 people were given a preparation from the freshly pressed juice of *E. purpurea* or a placebo as soon as they started showing signs of getting a cold. Participants took either echinacea or the placebo at a dosage of 20 drops every two hours the first day, then 20 drops three

times a day for nine more days. Fewer people in the echinacea group felt that their initial symptoms actually developed into "real" colds (40% of those taking echinacea vs. 60% taking the placebo). Also, among those who did come down with real colds, improvement in the symptoms started sooner in the echinacea group (after four days instead of eight days). Both results were statistically significant. However, echinacea's ability to shorten the duration of colds was more dramatic.

Not all studies using the freshly pressed juice of *E. purpurea* or EchinaGuard have shown positive effects in reducing duration of upper respiratory infections, severity, or both. For example, a study of children 2 to 11 years old was particularly disappointing, as the results indicated not only that it was ineffective but also that its use was associated with an increased risk of rash.[17] In another double-blind trial, 128 patients received 100 mg freeze-dried pressed juice from the aerial portion of *E. purpurea* or a placebo three times per day until cold symptoms were relieved or until the end of 14 days, whichever came first.[18] No statistically significant difference was observed between treatment groups for either total symptom scores or mean individual symptom scores. The time to resolution of symptoms was also not statistically different. The failure in this trial may have been due to the above-mentioned lack of direct contact with the oral cavity's lymphatic system.

Clearly, more research using well-characterized echinacea preparations at appropriate dosages in well-designed trials is necessary. Currently, the gold standard for evaluating cold remedies involves inoculating healthy individuals with rhinovirus. Though the concentration of viral assault is much greater than what one might encounter in the real world, any substance showing efficacy in this model is regarded as being highly efficacious. In one study, 48 healthy adults received the freshly pressed juice of *E. pur-purea* (EchinaGuard) or a placebo, 2.5 ml three times a day, for seven days before and seven days after intranasal inoculation with rhinovirus (RV-39).[19] A total of 92% of echinacea recipients and 95% of placebo recipients were infected. Colds developed in 58% of echinacea recipients compared with 82% of placebo recipients. Although administration of echinacea before and after exposure to rhinovirus did not decrease the rate of infection, it did appear to reduce the clinical development of a cold. However, because of the small sample size, it was not possible to detect statistically significant differences in the frequency and severity of illness.

South African Geranium (*Pelargonium sidoides*)

The common name for this plant, *Umck-aloaba*, is a close approximation of the word in the Zulu language that means "severe cough" and is a testimony to its effect in bronchitis (see the chapter "Bronchitis and Pneumonia"). In addition to showing significant benefits in bronchitis and sinusitis, it has also shown benefit in treating the common cold. In one study, 103 adult patients were randomly assigned to receive either 30 drops (1.5 ml) of an extract of *P. sidoides* (EPs 7630 or Umcka) or a placebo three times a day. From baseline to day five, symptom intensity improved by 14.6 points in the EPs 7630 group compared with 7.6 points in the placebo group. After 10 days, 78.8% of those in the EPs 7630 group vs. 31.4% in the placebo group were clinically cured. The mean duration of inability to work was significantly lower in the EPs 7630 treatment group (6.9 days) than in the placebo group (8.2 days). EPs 7630 significantly reduces the severity of symptoms and shortens the duration of the common cold by a little more than a day compared with a placebo.[20]

- -

QUICK REVIEW

- **Many of the symptoms of a cold are a result of our body's defense mechanisms.**

- **With a healthy, functioning immune system, a cold should not last more than three or four days.**

- **The value of sleep and rest during a cold cannot be overemphasized.**

- **Consuming plenty of liquids and using a vaporizer will maintain a moist respiratory tract that helps repels viral infection.**

- **Vitamin C can help prevent the common cold and can also help reduce the duration by about one full day.**

- **Zinc lozenges can be effective in reducing the duration of symptoms if they are properly prepared and taken in dosages of 75 mg per day.**

- **Mixed results from clinical studies with echinacea are most likely due to insufficient quantity of active compounds.**

- **Clinical trials of an extract from freshly harvested *E. purpurea* plants have shown excellent results.**

- **In addition to showing significant benefits in bronchitis and sinusitis, an extract of *Pelargonium sidoides* has also shown benefit in treating the common cold.**

TREATMENT SUMMARY

Although the focus of this chapter was on the use of natural methods to assist the body in recovering from the common cold, prevention is by far the best medicine. The old adage "An ounce of prevention is worth a pound of cure" is true for the common cold as well as the majority of other conditions afflicting human health. For more information on supporting the immune system, see the chapter "Immune System Support."

General Recommendations

- Rest (bed rest is best).
- Drink large amount of fluids (preferably diluted vegetable juices, soups, and herb teas).
- Limit simple sugar consumption (including fruit sugars) to less than 50 g a day.

Nutritional Supplements

- Vitamin C: 500 to 1,000 mg every two hours (decrease if it produces excessive gas or diarrhea) along with 1,000 mg mixed bioflavonoids per day
- Zinc lozenges: The best lozenges are those that utilize glycine as the sweetener. Those that use citric acid, mannitol, or sorbitol should be avoided. Use lozenges supplying 15 to 25 mg elemental zinc. Dissolve in the mouth every two waking hours after an initial double dose. Continue for up to seven days. Prolonged supplementation (more than one week) at this dose is not recom-

mended, as it may lead to suppression of the immune system.

Botanical Medicines

- Take one of the following:
  - Echinacea (first two forms are preferred):
    - Fluid extract of the fresh aerial portion of *E. purpurea* (1:1): 2 to 4 ml (½ to 1 tsp) three times a day (preferred)
    - Juice of aerial portion of *E. purpurea* stabilized in 22% ethanol: 2 to 4 ml (½ to 1 tsp) three times a day (preferred)
    - Dried root (or as tea): 1 to 2 g three times a day
    - Freeze-dried plant: 325 to 650 mg three times a day
    - Tincture (1:5): 2 to 4 ml (½ to 1 tsp) three times a day
    - Fluid extract (1:1): 2 to 4 ml (½ to 1 tsp) three times a day
    - Solid (dry powdered) extract (6.5:1 or 3.5% echinacosides): 150 to 300 mg three times a day
  - *Pelargonium sidoides* (EPs 7630 or equivalent preparation):
    - Adults: 1.5 ml three times per day or 20 mg tablets three times per day for up to 14 days
    - Children: age 7–12 years, 20 drops (1 ml) three times per day; under age 6, 10 drops (0.5 ml) three times per day

Congestive Heart Failure

- Left-side heart failure: shortness of breath on exertion, cough, fatigue, enlargement of the heart
  - Right-side heart failure: elevated venous pressure, enlargement of the liver, whole-body edema
  - Both left and right ventricular failure: combinations of the above

Congestive heart failure (CHF) is an inability of the heart to effectively pump enough blood. Chronic CHF is most often due to long-term effects of high blood pressure, previous heart attack, disorder of a heart valve, disorder of the heart muscle (cardiomyopathy), or chronic lung disease. Factors that precipitate or worsen CHF are listed below.

One of the most serious consequences of CHF is reduction in blood flow to the kidneys. This results in a reduced filtration rate by the kidneys, which in turn leads to sodium and fluid retention. Adding more stress to the situation is the secretion of hormones by the kidneys to try to raise blood pressure by constricting blood vessels and increasing the fluid volume in the blood. In an attempt to compensate for the reduced output by the heart, the heart beats faster (tachycardia), the force of contraction increases, and the heart enlarges from the stress. Ultimately these factors severely worsen the picture.

Factors That Precipitate or Worsen Congestive Heart Failure

Low levels of essential fatty acids

Increased demand on the heart

Anemia

Fever

Infection

Fluid overload

High sodium intake

High environmental temperature

Kidney failure

Liver failure

Chronic respiratory disease (such as asthma)

Emotional stress

Pregnancy

Obesity

Arrhythmias

Pulmonary embolism

Alcohol ingestion

Nutrient deficiency

Uncontrolled hypertension

Drugs:

- Beta-adrenergic blockers
- Antiarrhythmic drugs
- Sodium-retaining drugs
- Steroids
- Nonsteroidal anti-inflammatory drugs

Therapeutic Considerations

CHF is most effectively treated by natural measures in the early stages. Hence early diagnosis and prevention are imperative. The first symptom of CHF is usually shortness of breath. A chronic, nonproductive cough may also be the first presenting symptom. Anyone suspected of having CHF should have an extensive cardiovascular evaluation including a complete physical examination to look for the characteristic signs of CHF (e.g., peripheral signs of heart failure, enlarged and sustained left ventricular impulse, diminished first heart sound, gallop rhythm), electrocardiogram, and echocardiogram.

In the initial stages of CHF, natural measures designed to address the underlying cause (e.g., high blood pressure) or improve the metabolic functions of the heart muscle (described later, as well as measures described in the chapter "Angina") are often quite effective. In later stages, however, medical treatment involving the use of diuretics, angiotensin-converting enzyme (ACE) inhibitors, or digitalis glycosides is indicated in most cases. The measures described here can be used as adjunctive therapy in these more severe cases. The New York Heart Association (NYHA) staging system for CHF (see the table below) can be used to help determine which patients are likely to respond to natural therapy alone. In general, excellent clinical results can be expected in stages (or classes) I and II with the use of the natural measures described below.

Nutritional Supplements

The natural approach focuses on improving energy production within the heart muscle (myocardium), as CHF is always characterized by impaired energy production within the myocardium. This impaired energy production is often the result of nutrient or coenzyme deficiency (e.g., magnesium, thiamine, coenzyme Q_{10}, or carnitine deficiency). The dietary recommendations given in the chapter "High Blood Pressure" are appropriate for most patients with CHF, especially if the CHF is due to long-term high blood pressure (hypertension). Of particular importance is a diet low in sodium and high in potassium. A high intake of sodium greatly worsens CHF. Sodium intake should be restricted to less than 1.8 g per day. Furthermore, CHF patients are likely to have a low dietary intake of several nutrients, most notably magnesium, calcium, zinc, copper, manganese, energy, thiamine, riboflavin, and folic acid.[1] A high-potency multivitamin and mineral formula is critical, especially if a person is on a diuretic.

Stages of Congestive Heart Failure as Defined by the New York Heart Association	
STAGE	**SYMPTOMS**
Stage I	Patient is symptom free at rest and with treatment.
Stage II	Patient experiences impaired heart function with moderate physical effort. Shortness of breath with exertion is common. There are no symptoms at rest.
Stage III	Even minor physical exertion results in shortness of breath and fatigue. There are no symptoms at rest.
Stage IV	Symptoms such as shortness of breath and signs such as lower-extremity edema are present when the patient is at rest.

Magnesium

Low magnesium level (particularly white blood cell magnesium) is a common finding in patients with CHF. This association is extremely significant, as magnesium levels have been shown to correlate directly with survival rates. In one study, CHF patients with normal levels of magnesium had one- and two-year survival rates of 71% and 61%, respectively, compared with rates of 45% and 42%, respectively, for patients with lower magnesium levels.[2] In other words, magnesium level was a strong predictor of survival. These results are not surprising, considering that magnesium deficiency is associated with cardiac arrhythmias, reduced cardiovascular prognosis, worsened angina, lower mitochondrial energy production (critical for heart muscle health), and increased mortality due to heart attack (myocardial infarction).

The magnesium deficiency is probably due to a combination of inadequate intake and overactivation of the kidneys' attempt to increase blood flow. It can also be the result of diuretics such as furosemide (Lasix).

In addition to providing benefits of its own in CHF, magnesium supplementation also prevents the magnesium depletion caused by conventional drug therapy for CHF (i.e., digitalis, diuretics, and vasodilators such as beta-blockers and calcium-channel blockers). Magnesium supplementation has even been shown to produce positive effects in CHF patients receiving conventional drug therapy, even if serum magnesium levels are normal.[3] However, magnesium supplementation is not indicated in patients with kidney failure, as this condition predisposes them to elevations in magnesium in the blood (hypermagnesemia), which is a significant risk factor for death in these patients.[4,5]

Typical dosages are 200 to 300 mg one to three times per day of magnesium in the citrate form. Oral magnesium can be effective in raising white blood cell magnesium (and potassium) levels.[6] Monitoring blood (serum) magnesium levels is critical to preventing hypermagnesemia in patients with kidney failure, as well as those on drugs such as digoxin. Magnesium significantly reduces the frequency and complexity of ventricular arrhythmias in digoxin-treated patients with CHF even without the presence of digoxin toxicity, but too much magnesium may interfere with digoxin.[7]

Thiamine

Interest has recently risen regarding the potential role of thiamine deficiency in CHF. Thiamine was the first B vitamin discovered, hence its designation as vitamin B_1. It is well established that thiamine deficiency can result in "wet beriberi," sodium retention, peripheral vasodilation, and heart failure. It is also well established that furosemide (Lasix), the most widely prescribed diuretic, has been shown to cause thiamine deficiency in animals and patients with CHF.

Although severe thiamine deficiency is relatively uncommon (except in alcoholics), many Americans do not consume the recommended dietary intake of 1.5 mg, especially elderly patients in hospitals or nursing homes. In an attempt to gauge the prevalence of thiamine deficiency in the geriatric population, 30 people visiting a university outpatient clinic in Tampa, Florida, were tested for thiamine levels. Depending on how the thiamine was measured, low levels were found in 57% and 33%, respectively.[8]

These results highlight the growing body of evidence that a significant percentage of the geriatric population is deficient in one or more of the B vitamins. Given the essential role of thiamine and other B vitamins in normal human physiology, especially cardiovascular and brain function, routine B vitamin supplementation appears to be worthwhile in this age group.

The association between thiamine deficiency and long-term furosemide use was discovered in 1980 when it was shown that after only four weeks of furosemide use, thiamine concentrations and the activity of the thiamine-dependent enzyme transketolase were significantly reduced. The first study looking at thiamine as a potential support aid in the treatment of CHF showed only modest benefits. However, several subsequent studies have shown that daily doses of 80 to 240 mg thiamine per day resulted in a 13% to 22% increase of left ventricular ejection fraction—a marker that tells us that thiamine improved the heart's ability to perform.[9,10] This increase is quite significant, as an increase in ejection fraction is associated with a greater survival rate in patients with CHF. In one study, biochemical evidence of severe thiamine deficiency was found in 98% of patients receiving at least 80 mg per day of furosemide and in 57% of patients taking 40 mg furosemide per day.[11]

Given the possible benefit, lack of risk, and low cost of thiamine supplementation, administration of 200 to 250 mg thiamine per day appears to be a wise recommendation in patients with CHF, especially if they are on furosemide.

Carnitine

Normal heart function is critically dependent on adequate concentrations of carnitine and CoQ_{10} (discussed later). These compounds are essential in the transport of fatty acids into the myocardium and mitochondria for energy production. Although the normal heart stores more carnitine and CoQ_{10} than it needs, if the heart does not have a good supply of oxygen, carnitine and CoQ_{10} levels quickly decrease. Both of these agents have shown benefit in the treatment of CHF.

Several double-blind clinical studies have shown carnitine supplementation to improve cardiac function in patients with CHF.[12–14] In one double-blind study, only one month of treatment (500 mg three times per day) was needed to cause significant improvement in heart function.[13] The longer carnitine was used, the more dramatic the improvement. After six months of use, the carnitine group demonstrated a 25.9% increase in maximum exercise time and a 13.6% increase in ventricular ejection fraction. In another double-blind study of similar patients, at the end of six months of treatment maximum exercise time on the treadmill increased by 16.4% and the ejection fraction increased by 12.1%.[14]

Even more obvious benefits were seen in a three-year study of 80 patients with moderate to severe heart failure (NYHA classification III to IV) caused by a condition known as dilated cardiomyopathy. After a period of stable cardiac function of up to three months, patients were randomly assigned to receive either carnitine (2 g per day orally) or a placebo. After a mean of 33.7 months of follow-up (range 10 to 54 months), 70 patients were in the study: 33 in the placebo group and 37 in the carnitine group. At the time of analysis, 63 patients were alive. Six deaths occurred in the placebo group, and one death in the carnitine group. Survival analysis showed that patients' survival was statistically significant in favor of the carnitine group.[15]

Coenzyme Q$_{10}$ (COQ$_{10}$)

Numerous studies have shown CoQ_{10} supplementation to be extremely effective in the treatment of CHF. Most of these studies used CoQ_{10} as an adjunct to conventional drug therapy. In one of the early studies, 17 patients with mild CHF received 30 mg per day of CoQ_{10}.[16] All patients improved, and nine (53%) became asymptomatic after four weeks. In another early study, 20 patients with congestive heart failure due to either atherosclerosis or high blood pressure were treated with CoQ_{10} at a dosage of 30 mg per day for one to two months.[17] Of these patients, 55% reported subjective improvement, 50% showed a decrease in NYHA classification, and 30% showed a "remarkable" decrease in chest congestion as seen on chest X-rays. Patients with mild disease were more likely to improve than those with more severe disease. Subjective improvements in how the patients felt were confirmed by various objective tests, including increased cardiac output, stroke volume, cardiac index, and ejection fraction. These results were consistent with CoQ_{10} producing an increased force of contraction similar to but less potent than that produced by digitalis.[18,19]

Three more studies have also shown CoQ_{10} to be effective in significantly improving heart function in patients with CHF. In a double-blind Scandinavian study of 80 patients, participants were given either CoQ_{10} (100 mg per day) or a placebo for three months and then crossed over to the other treatment. The improvements noted with CoQ_{10} were found to be more positive than those obtained from conventional drug therapy alone.[20] In another double-blind study, 641 patients with CHF received either CoQ_{10} (2 mg/kg) or a placebo for one year.[21] The number of patients requiring hospitalization or experiencing serious consequences due to CHF was significantly reduced in the CoQ_{10} group compared with the placebo group.

In the largest study to date, a total of 2,664 patients in NYHA classes II and III were enrolled in an open study in Italy.[22] The daily dosage of CoQ_{10} was 50 to 150 mg orally for 90 days, with the majority of patients (78%) receiving 100 mg per day. After three months of CoQ_{10} treatment, the proportions of patients with improvement in clinical signs and symptoms were as follows:

- Cyanosis (extremities turning blue): 78.1%
- Edema (fluid retention): 78.6%
- Pulmonary edema: 77.8%
- Enlargement of liver area: 49.3%
- Venous congestion: 71.81%
- Shortness of breath: 52.7%
- Heart palpitations: 75.4%
- Sweating: 79.8%
- Subjective arrhythmia: 63.4%
- Insomnia: 66.2%
- Vertigo: 73.1%
- Nocturnal urination: 53.6%

Improvement of at least three symptoms occurred in 54% of patients, indicating a significantly improved quality of life with CoQ_{10} supplementation. The results also showed a low incidence of side effects—only 36 patients (1.5%) reported mild side effects attributed to CoQ_{10}.

These positive results with CoQ_{10}, however, were not seen in one clinical trial. In this double-blind study, 55 patients with CHF NYHA class III and IV, ejection fraction less than 40%, and peak oxygen consumption less than 50% during standard therapy were randomly assigned to receive CoQ_{10} (200 mg) or a placebo. Analysis indicated that there were no changes in ejection fraction, peak oxygen consumption, or exercise duration in either group. Possible explanations for failure to achieve a therapeutic benefit in this study may be that the CoQ_{10} was not strong enough to produce significant effects in more severe stages of CHF or that blood levels of CoQ_{10} did not reach sufficient values. Though the mean serum concentration of CoQ_{10} increased from 0.95 mcg/ml to 2.2 mcg/ml in 19 of 22 patients on CoQ_{10}, blood levels were below the suggested threshold of 2.5 mcg/ml.[23]

An important consideration in patients

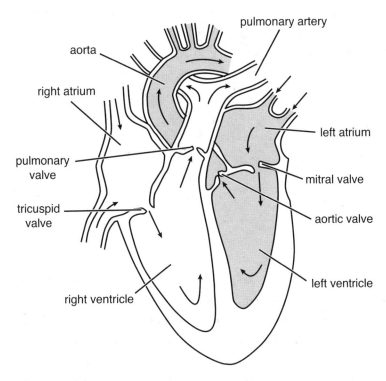

aorta

pulmonary artery

right atrium

left atrium

pulmonary
valve

mitral valve

tricuspid
valve

aortic valve

right ventricle

left ventricle

Cross Section of the Heart

with CHF, especially at the more advanced stages, is that they often fail to achieve adequate plasma CoQ_{10} levels (>2.5 mcg/ml) on supplemental ubiquinone (the common form of CoQ_{10}) even at dosages up to 900 mg per day. These patients may respond better to highly absorbed forms of CoQ_{10} such as ubiquinol or emulsified ubiquinone. In one study, seven patients with advanced CHF who had average plasma CoQ_{10} levels of 1.6 mcg/ml on an average dose of 450 mg ubiquinone per day (range: 150–600 mg per day) were changed to an average of 580 mg per day of ubiquinol (range: 450–900 mg per day) with follow-up plasma CoQ_{10} levels, clinical status, and ejection fraction measurements by echocardiography. Average plasma CoQ_{10} levels increased from 1.6 mcg/ml to 6.5 mcg/ml. The average ejection fraction improved from 22% (10–35%) to 39% (10–60%) and NYHA

class improved from a mean of IV to a mean of II (range: I to III). In this study, ubiquinol dramatically improved absorption in patients with severe heart failure, and the improvement in plasma CoQ_{10} levels was correlated with both clinical improvement and improvement in measurement of left ventricular function.[24]

Arginine

Another amino acid of value in CHF is arginine, although its effects come by means of a totally different mechanism from other nutrients. One of the experimental findings in patients with CHF is that they are less able to achieve peripheral dilation of blood vessels during exercise due to dysfunction of the lining of the blood vessels (endothelium). Since the cells that line blood vessels make the natural blood vessel dilating compound nitric acid from arginine, several researchers have evaluated arginine's effect in improving CHF. The first study of orally administered arginine showed promising results. In a randomized, double-blind, placebo-controlled study of 5.6 to 12.6 g per day of oral L-arginine, peripheral blood flow was found to increase by 29%, 6-minute walking distance increased by 8%, and arterial flexibility (compliance) increased by 19%.[25] Subsequent studies have shown arginine supplementation to improve endothelial cell function and kidney function in patients with CHF.[26,27] However, use of arginine requires caution in survivors of a heart attack, because in one study supplementation with arginine (9 g per day for six months) was associated with an increase in mortality compared with that in the placebo group (8.6% vs. 0%).[28]

QUICK REVIEW

- In the early stages of CHF, natural measures designed to address the underlying cause (e.g., high blood pressure) or improve the metabolic functions of the heart are often quite effective.
- In later stages, however, medical treatment involving the use of diuretics, angiotensin-converting enzyme (ACE) inhibitors, or digitalis glycosides is indicated in most cases.
- CHF is always characterized by impaired energy production within the heart muscle, often the result of nutrient or coenzyme deficiency (e.g., magnesium, thiamine, coenzyme Q_{10}, carnitine).
- The level of magnesium is a strong predictor of survival in CHF.
- Magnesium supplementation has been shown to produce positive effects in CHF patients receiving conventional drug therapy, even if serum magnesium levels are normal.
- Studies have shown that doses of 80 to 240 mg thiamine per day produced a 13 to 22% increase in the heart's ability to perform.
- Several double-blind clinical studies have shown carnitine supplementation to improve cardiac function in patients with CHF.
- Numerous studies have also shown CoQ_{10} supplementation to be extremely effective in the treatment of CHF.
- Patients with severe CHF may respond better with highly absorbable forms of CoQ_{10} such as ubiquinol or emulsified ubiquinone.
- Arginine supplementation improves blood vessel and kidney function in patients with CHF.
- Preparations of hawthorn appear to be quite useful in CHF, especially in the early stages as a sole agent and in the latter stages in combination with conventional medicines such as digitalis.
- *Terminalia arjuna*, a traditional ayurvedic medicine for cardiac failure, has recently been shown to be effective in a controlled clinical study.

Botanical Medicines

Hawthorn

Preparations of hawthorn (*Crataegus oxyacantha*) appear to be quite useful in CHF, in the early stages as a sole agent and in the latter stages in combination with conventional medicines such as digitalis. The effectiveness of hawthorn in CHF has been repeatedly demonstrated in double-blind studies.[29–31] In one recent study, 30 patients with CHF (NYHA stage II) were assessed in a randomized, double-blind format.[29] Treatment consisted of a hawthorn extract standardized to contain 15 mg proanthocyanidin oligomers per 80 mg capsule, taken twice a day. Treatment duration was eight weeks. The group receiving the hawthorn extract showed a statistically significant advantage over the group taking a placebo in terms of changes in heart function as determined by standard testing procedures. Systolic and diastolic blood pressures were also mildly reduced. As in all other studies with hawthorn extracts, no adverse reactions occurred.

In another study, 78 patients with CHF (NYHA stage II) were given either 600 mg standardized hawthorn extract or a placebo per day.[30] The indicator used to measure effectiveness was the patient's working capacity on a stationary bicycle. After 56 days of treatment, the hawthorn group had a mean increase of 25 watts compared with the placebo group's increase of only 5 watts. In addition, the hawthorn group also experienced a mild but significant reduction in systolic blood pressure (from 171 to 164 mm Hg) and heart rate (115 to 110 beats/min). There was no change in blood pressure or heart rate with the placebo group.

In patients with NYHA stage III, hawthorn may not be sufficient to produce clinical effects. In a randomized, double-blind, placebo-controlled trial involving 120 ambulatory patients with NYHA class II-III CHF, all patients received conventional medical therapy, as tolerated, and were randomly assigned to receive either hawthorn 450 mg twice per day or a placebo for six months. The primary outcome was a change in the six-minute walk distance at six months and no significant effect was noted.[31]

Arjun Tree (*Terminalia arjuna*)

A traditional ayurvedic medicine for cardiac failure has recently been shown to be effective in a controlled clinical study. Twelve patients with severe refractory congestive heart failure (class IV NYHA) received an extract (500 mg every eight hours) from the bark of *Terminalia arjuna* or a placebo for two weeks. Those receiving the medicinal plant experienced, according to echocardiogram evaluation, statistically significant improvement in several indicators of cardiac function, such as end-systolic volume and left ventricular ejection fractions. A second, uncontrolled phase of the study using a combination of *T. arjuna* with conventional medication found that after two years, nine patients showed a remarkable improvement to NYHA class II, with the other three improving to class III.[32]

TREATMENT SUMMARY

Treatment with diet and the natural agents mentioned earlier is effective in early stages of CHF (i.e., NYHA stages I and II). In later stages, adjunct drug therapy is usually necessary. Treatment is designed to address the underlying disease process and to improve heart function through improved energy production.

Diet

It is essential to achieve and maintain ideal body weight, restrict sodium intake (to below 1.8 g per day), increase consumption of plant foods, reduce the intake of saturated fat, and follow the other dietary guidelines for lowering blood pressure in the chapter "High Blood Pressure."

Nutritional Supplements

- A high-potency multiple vitamin and mineral formula as described in the chapter "Supplementary Measures"
- Key individual nutrients:
  - Thiamine (vitamin B_1): 200 to 250 mg per day
  - Vitamin B_6: 25 to 50 mg per day
  - Folic acid: 800 to 2,000 mcg per day
  - Vitamin B_{12}: 800 mcg per day
  - Vitamin C: 500 to 1,000 mg per day
  - Vitamin E (mixed tocopherols): 100 to 200 IU per day
  - Magnesium (bound to aspartate, citrate, fumarate, malate, or succinate): 200 to 300 mg three times per day
  - Vitamin D_3: 2,000 to 4,000 IU per day (ideally, measure blood levels and adjust dosage accordingly)
- Fish oils: 1,000 mg EPA + DHA per day
- Specialty supplements:
  - L-carnitine: 500 to 1,000 mg three times per day
  - CoQ_{10}: 100 to 200 mg three times per day
  - Arginine: 1,000 to 2,000 mg three times per day

Botanical Medicines

- Hawthorn (*Crataegus* species) extract (1.8% vitexin-4-rhamnoside or 10% proanthocyanidin content): 200 to 300 mg three times per day
- *T. arjuna* extract: 500 mg three times per day

Constipation

- Infrequent bowel movements (typically three times or fewer per week)
- Difficulty during defecation (straining during more than 25% of bowel movements or a subjective sensation of hard stools)
- The sensation of incomplete bowel evacuation
- Two or fewer bowel movements in a week.

Constipation is the most common digestive complaint in the United States, as more than 4 million Americans have frequent constipation, accounting for 2.5 million physician visits a year. In addition, over $725 million is spent on laxative products each year in America.

How often a person should have a bowel movement is debatable. It is highly individualized, but in general a daily bowel movement should be considered normal (though some people eating a particularly high-fiber diet may have bowel movements three times a day). Going longer than three days without a bowel movement is of definite concern, as after three days the stool or feces become harder and more difficult to pass.

Causes

There are a number of possible causes of constipation, as noted below, but by far the most common cause of constipation is a low-fiber diet.

Causes of Constipation

- Not enough fiber in the diet
- Inadequate fluid intake
- Lack of physical activity (especially in the elderly)
- Medications:
  - Pain medications (especially narcotics)
  - Antacids that contain aluminum and calcium
  - Blood pressure medications (calcium-channel blockers)
  - Anti–Parkinson's disease drugs
  - Antispasmodics
  - Antidepressants
  - Iron supplements
  - Diuretics
  - Anticonvulsants
- Milk
- Irritable bowel syndrome
- Pregnancy
- Abuse of laxatives
- Ignoring the urge to have a bowel movement
- Specific diseases or conditions:
  - Stroke
  - Multiple sclerosis
  - Low potassium stores
  - Diabetes
  - Kidney disease

○ Hypothyroidism

○ Pituitary disorders

- Problems with the colon and rectum:

○ Diverticulosis

○ Irritable bowel syndrome (alternating diarrhea and constipation)

○ Colon cancer

Therapeutic Considerations

Constipation will often respond to a high-fiber diet, plentiful fluid consumption, and exercise. There is absolutely no argument from anyone in the medical community that these recommendations should constitute the first step in the treatment of chronic constipation.

Especially important is the recommendation to increase dietary fiber. High levels of dietary fiber increase both the frequency and the quantity of bowel movements, decrease the transit time of stools, decrease the absorption of toxins from the stool, and appear to be a preventive factor in several diseases. The recommended daily intake is 25–35 g fiber from dietary sources. However, higher amounts may be optimal for health, as the diet humans evolved with contained approximately 100 g fiber per day. Most Western diets provide only 10 to 15 g.

Foods particularly effective in relieving constipation are bran and prunes. The typical daily recommendation for bran is ½ cup of bran cereal, increasing over several weeks to 1½ cups. When using bran, make sure to consume enough liquids. Drink at least six to eight glasses of water per day. Whole prunes as well as prune juice also exert good laxative effects. Four to 8 fl oz prune juice or 5 to 10 prunes will usually be an effective dose.

If you need additional support, consider using fiber formulas. These formulas act as bulking agents. They can be composed of natural soluble fiber derived from psyllium seed, kelp, agar, pectin, and plant gums such as karaya and guar, or they can be purified semisynthetic polysaccharides such as methylcellulose and carboxymethyl cellulose sodium. Psyllium-containing laxatives are the most popular and usually the most effective. Psyllium is derived from the seed of the plant *Plantago ovago*, native to Iran and India. The laxative properties of psyllium are due to the swelling of the husk when it comes in contact with water. This forms a gelatinous mass and keeps the feces hydrated and soft. The resulting bulk stimulates a reflex contraction of the walls of the bowel, followed by emptying. Bulk-forming fiber supplements such as psyllium are the laxatives that approximate most closely the natural mechanism that promotes a bowel movement. They are both safe and effective in the treatment of chronic constipation.[1] That said, prunes may be more effective, based upon the results of one study.[2] Subjects suffering from chronic constipation received either prunes (50 g per day, providing 6 g fiber; about 10 prunes) or psyllium (11 g per day, providing 6 g fiber) for three weeks each, in a crossover trial with a one-week washout period. Subjects maintained a daily symptom and stool diary. The number of complete spontaneous bowel movements per week and stool consistency scores improved significantly with prunes when compared with psyllium. However, straining and global constipation symptoms did not differ significantly between treatments.

Constipation in Children

Constipation in children usually occurs at three distinct points in time: in infancy, after starting formula or processed foods; during toilet training in toddlerhood; and soon after

Types of Laxatives

TYPE OF LAXATIVE	HOW IT WORKS	SIDE EFFECTS
Bulk-forming fibers (psyllium, guar, methylcellulose)	Absorb water to form soft, bulky stool, prompting normal contraction of intestinal muscles	Bloating, gas, cramping, choking, or increased constipation if not taken with enough water
Oral osmotics (magnesium hydroxide)	Draw water into colon from surrounding body tissues to allow easier passage of stool	Bloating, cramping, diarrhea, nausea, gas, increased thirst
Oral stool softeners (docusate)	Add moisture to stool to allow strain-free bowel movements	Throat irritation, cramping
Oral stimulants (senna and cascara)	Trigger rhythmic contractions of intestinal muscles to eliminate stool	Belching, cramping, diarrhea, nausea, urine discoloration
Rectal stimulants (glycerin suppositories)	Trigger rhythmic contractions of intestinal muscles to eliminate stool	Rectal irritation, stomach discomfort, cramping

starting school (e.g., kindergarten). There are many factors to consider, but just as with adults, increasing fiber content usually produces the desired result. In addition, for children with a history of constipation, the first thing we recommend is eliminating milk and other dairy products from the diet. It is well accepted that cow's milk intolerance (either allergy or lactose intolerance) can produce diarrhea. What is not as well known is that cow's milk intolerance can also lead to constipation and is a major cause of childhood constipation.[3] About 70% of cases of childhood constipation are cured by eliminating cow's milk from the diet and substituting soy, nut (e.g., almond), or rice milk. Children with constipation who respond to milk elimination also experience a decreased frequency of allergy symptoms, including runny nose, eczema, and asthma. Our recommendation is that if a child is constipated, start by eliminating cow's milk and other dairy products while increasing the intake of high-fiber foods, especially pears, apples, and other whole fruit. If this approach is not successful, try barley malt syrup or powder. Definitely avoid mineral oil as well as stimulant laxatives unless absolutely necessary.

Laxatives

Bulk-forming fiber supplements are preferred to other forms of laxatives. However, occasional use of other types of laxatives definitely has its place. In general, stimulant laxatives, even natural ones such as cascara sagrada (*Rhamnus purshiana*) or senna (*Cassia senna*) should not be used long-term. If they are, the bowels will need to be "retrained." The list below offers a plan for reestablishing bowel regularity; the recommended procedure will take four to six weeks.

Rules for Bowel Retraining

- Find and eliminate known causes of constipation.
- Never repress an urge to defecate.

PRUNES: NOT JUST A LAXATIVE

A prune is a dried plum, just as a raisin is a dried grape. Prunes are well known for their ability to prevent and relieve constipation. In addition to providing bulk and decreasing the transit time of fecal matter, prunes' insoluble fiber also provides food for the "friendly" bacteria in the large intestine. When these helpful bacteria ferment prunes' insoluble fiber, they produce a short-chain fatty acid called butyric acid, which serves as the primary fuel for the cells of the large intestine and helps maintain a healthy colon. These helpful bacteria also create two other short-chain fatty acids, proprionic acid and acetic acid, which are used as fuel by the cells of the liver and muscles.

Prunes contain large amounts of phenolic compounds (184 mg/100 g), mainly as neochlorogenic and chlorogenic acids. As well as aiding in the laxative action, these compounds inhibit free radical damage to LDL cholesterol and might serve to protect against heart disease and osteoporosis. Eating five prunes or drinking 4 fl oz prune juice is all that is required to help relieve constipation in many sufferers.

- Eat a high-fiber diet, particularly fruits and vegetables.

- Drink six to eight glasses of fluid per day.

- Sit on the toilet at the same time every day (even when the urge to defecate is not present), preferably immediately after breakfast or exercise.

- Exercise at least 20 minutes three times per week.

- Stop using laxatives (except as discussed below to reestablish bowel activity) and enemas.

  - Week one: Every night before bed take a stimulant laxative containing either cascara or senna. Take the lowest amount necessary to reliably ensure a bowel movement every morning.

  - Weekly: Each week decrease dosage of the laxative by half. If constipation recurs, go back to the previous week's dosage. Decrease dosage if diarrhea occurs.

When a stimulant laxative is required, we prefer senna. The laxative components are compounds known as sennosides. Senna relieves constipation by increasing the strength of contraction of the intestinal muscles. Like other stimulant laxatives, it should be limited to occasional use, as long-term use of senna can lead to dependence.

Stimulant laxatives, such as senna, are likely to cause abdominal cramping, nausea, and increased mucus secretion. Less common side effects are associated with chronic use and are usually related to loss of potassium and other electrolytes (e.g., muscle spasms, weakness, and fatigue). Call your doctor right away if you have any of these side effects: a sudden change in bowel habits that persists over a period of two weeks, rectal bleeding, or failure to have a bowel movement after use.

A benign blackish-brown pigmentation of the lining of the colon (pseudomelanosis coli) may occur with prolonged use (at least four months) of senna, owing to the anthraquinones it contains. This condition gener-

---

CAUTIONS AND WARNINGS

- Do not use senna for more than seven days unless directed by your doctor.
- Stimulant laxatives should not be used by patients with abdominal pain, nausea or vomiting, intestinal obstruction, inflammatory bowel disease, or appendicitis, or by women who are pregnant or lactating.
- Do not take more than the recommended amount. Excessive laxative use or inadequate fluid intake may lead to significant fluid and electrolyte imbalance.

ally disappears within 4 to 15 months after discontinuation.

Senna and other stimulant laxatives may decrease the absorption of drugs that pass through the gastrointestinal tract. If you are currently taking an oral medication, talk to your pharmacist or doctor before self-medicating with senna.

Senna may potentiate the action of digoxin and other heart medications, owing to potassium depletion. The use of senna with thiazide diuretics and corticosteroids may further decrease potassium levels.

Generally, take senna on an empty stomach. Drink six to eight glasses of liquid per day while taking senna or any other laxative.

QUICK REVIEW

- **Constipation is a common problem in Western societies.**
- **The most common causes are inadequate consumption of dietary fiber and fluids and/or a sedentary lifestyle.**

- **Treatment involves addressing the cause and helping with supplemental fiber and herbal laxatives as needed.**

TREATMENT SUMMARY

Keep in mind that constipation is a symptom, not a disease. Determining the cause is the first step in treatment. In most cases constipation is not serious and responds quickly to dietary and supplement strategies.

Diet

Follow the guidelines in the chapter "A Health-Promoting Diet." In particular, try to consume 25 to 35 g fiber from dietary sources each day and drink at least six to eight glasses of water per day. Bran cereal can be helpful; start with ½ cup daily, increasing over several weeks to 1½ cups. Whole prunes and prune juice also possess good laxative effects. Four to 8 fl oz prune juice or 5 to 10 prunes will usually be an effective dose.

Nutritional Supplements

- **Soluble fiber supplement (e.g., psyllium): 5 g in at least 8 fl oz water, followed by another 8 fl oz of water, one to two times per day**
- **Probiotic (active lactobacillus and bifidobacteria cultures): a minimum of 5 billion to 10 billion colony-forming units per day**

Botanical Medicines

- **Senna: Follow label instructions (usual dosage recommendation is based upon sennoside content: 15–30 mg sennosides at bedtime); use only on an occasional basis.**

Crohn's Disease and Ulcerative Colitis (Inflammatory Bowel Disease)

- Crohn's disease:
  - Intermittent bouts of diarrhea, low-grade fever, and pain in the lower right abdomen
  - Loss of appetite, weight loss, flatulence, and malaise
  - Abdominal tenderness, especially in the lower right part of the abdomen
  - X-rays show abnormality of the terminal portion of the small intestine
- Ulcerative colitis:
  - Bloody diarrhea with cramps in the lower abdomen
  - Mild abdominal tenderness, weight loss, and fever
  - Rectal examination may show fissures, hemorrhoids, fistulas, and abscesses
  - Diagnosis confirmed by X-ray and sigmoidoscopy (examination of the colon with a fiber-optic tube)

Inflammatory bowel disease (IBD) is a general term for a group of chronic inflammatory disorders of the intestines. It is divided into two major categories: Crohn's disease (CD) and ulcerative colitis (UC). Clinically, IBD is characterized by recurrent inflammation of specific intestinal segments. In the United States, about 1.4 million people have IBD, with the number equally split between CD and UC. IBD may occur at any age, but it most often occurs between the ages of 15 and 35. Females are affected slightly more frequently than males. Caucasians have the disease two to five times more often than African-Americans or Asian-Americans, and those with a Jewish heritage have a three- to sixfold higher incidence than non-Jews.

Crohn's Disease

CD is characterized by an inflammatory reaction throughout the entire thickness of the bowel wall. In approximately 40% of cases, however, the inflammatory lesions (granulomas) are either poorly developed or totally absent. The original description in 1932 by Crohn and colleagues localized the disease to segments in the ileum, the terminal portion of the small intestine. However, it is now known that the same granulomatous process may involve the mucosa of the mouth, esophagus, stomach, duodenum, jejunum, and colon.

Ulcerative Colitis

In UC, there is a nonspecific inflammatory response, limited largely to the lining of the colon. CD and UC do share many common features and, where appropriate, will be discussed together. Otherwise they will be discussed as separate entities.

Features Shared by Crohn's Disease and Ulcerative Colitis

- The colon is frequently involved in Crohn's disease and is invariably involved in ulcerative colitis.

- Although this is rare, patients with ulcerative colitis who have total colon involvement may develop so-called backwash ileitis. Thus, both Crohn's disease and ulcerative colitis may cause changes in the small intestine.

- Patients with Crohn's disease often have close relatives with ulcerative colitis, and vice versa.

- When there is no granulomatous reaction in Crohn's disease of the colon, the two lesions may resemble each other in both the clinical picture and the biopsy result.

- The many epidemiological similarities between the two diseases include age, race, sex, and geographic distribution.

- Both conditions are associated with similar manifestations outside the gastrointestinal tract (extraintestinal).

- The causative factors appear to be parallel for the two conditions.

- Both conditions are associated with an increased frequency of colon cancer.

Causes

Genetic Predisposition

There is a very strong genetic component in IBD.[1,2] As already mentioned, IBD is two to four times more common in white than nonwhite people, and about four times more common in those with a Jewish heritage. In addition, multiple members of a family have CD or UC in 15% to 40% of cases. CD is among the best-known of complex genetic disorders. Several genetic pathways involving the maintenance of the integrity and immune function of the lining of the intestinal tract have been found for an increased susceptibility for CD, while only one gene (ECM1) has been reported for UC. Nonetheless, dietary and environmental factors appear to be required for the expression of IBD.

Infections

Many microorganisms have been hailed as putative causes of IBD, but in spite of numerous attempts to confirm a bacterial, mycobacterial, fungal, or viral etiology, the idea that a transmissible agent is responsible for IBD is still hotly debated. Viruses—rotavirus, Epstein-Barr virus, cytomegalovirus, measles virus, and an uncharacterized RNA intestinal virus—and mycobacteria continue to be favored candidates. Gastrointestinal infections with various microbes and the yeast *Candida albicans* can trigger a flare-up of disease, and all patients with IBD should be tested for gastrointestinal infections at the start and during the course of their illness.

The development of IBD probably reflects a nonspecific abnormal host-microbe interaction, rather than infection by any single responsible organism. The ability of microbes to coexist within the human intestinal tract involves host genetic factors, barrier function, and immune function, as well as the number and type of health-promoting gut bacteria. Microbes with virulence factors that allow them to breach the intestinal barrier and induce chronic inflammation are probably responsible for triggering IBD in many cases, hence the long list of implicated microorganisms.[3]

Exposure to Antibiotics

Exposure to antibiotics is being linked to IBD and probably is a factor in causing disruption of the intestinal lining in some cases. Subjects diagnosed with IBD were more likely to have been prescribed antibiotics two to five years before their diagnosis. A dose-dependent relationship was shown: the more prescriptions for antibiotics, the greater the risk for IBD.[4]

Before the 1950s, CD was found in selected groups with a strong genetic component. Since this time there has been a rapid climb in incidence in developed countries, particularly the United States, and in countries that previously had virtually no reported cases. In fact, IBD has spread like an epidemic since 1950. Are antibiotics to blame? Penicillin and tetracycline have been available in oral form since 1953. The annual increase in prescriptions of antibiotics parallels the rise in the annual incidence of IBD. Comparative statistics have shown that wherever antibiotics have been used early and in large quantities, the incidence of IBD is now quite high. Considering the critical importance of having the right bacteria in the gut, it is not surprising that the disruption of bacterial balance caused by antibiotics may be a causative factor in IBD.

Over the years researchers have sought to identify IBD as an infectious process. The problem may be that the infectious agent is a component of the normal intestinal flora that suddenly produces immune-stimulatory toxins or becomes invasive as a direct result of sublethal doses of antibiotics. When microbes are not given a full lethal dose, their usual response is to adapt and become even more virulent and numerous. Other medications that have been implicated as well include nonsteroidal anti-inflammatory drugs such as ibuprofen and most recently the acne medication Accutane.

Immune Mechanisms

An overwhelming amount of evidence points to an association of immunologic disturbances with IBD, but whether they cause the disease or are the result of it remains unclear. Theories about immune mechanisms as a cause of IBD have been proposed, but the current evidence seems to indicate that the immune system abnormalities seen in IBD are probably secondary to the disease process.

Dietary Factors

Despite the fact that a dietary cause of CD is barely considered (if mentioned at all) in most standard medical and gastroenterology texts, there is considerable scientific evidence supporting the notion that dietary factors are the most important triggers for IBD.[5-7] The incidence of IBD increased in cultures consuming the Western diet, but it is virtually nonexistent in cultures consuming a more primitive diet. Food is the major factor in determining the intestinal environment, so the considerable change in dietary habits over the last century could explain the rising incidence of IBD. Several studies that analyzed the pre-illness diet of patients with IBD have found that they habitually ate more refined sugar, chemically modified fats and fast food, and meat while consuming less raw fruit, vegetables, omega-3 fatty acids, and dietary fiber than healthy people.[5-11]

Another important dietary factor is the role of food allergies. Studies have shown that an elemental diet or an allergy exclusion diet can be very successful in the treatment of IBD. The role of food allergy is discussed in greater detail later in the chapter, as is the effect of dietary fiber in the etiology and treatment of IBD.

A reduced intake of omega-3 oils and an increased intake of omega-6 oils are also being linked to the growing rise of IBD. Recently this link was shown in a study in Japan. Because the genetic background of the Japanese is relatively homogeneous, this higher incidence is most likely due to the incorporation of Western foods in the diet. The analysis showed that the greater incidence of CD was strongly correlated with increased dietary intake of total fat, animal fat, omega-6 fatty acids, animal protein, milk protein, and the ratio of omega-6 to omega-3 fatty acids.[12] Multivariate analysis showed that higher intake of animal protein was the strongest independent factor, followed by an increased ratio of omega-6 to omega-3 fatty acids. Correction of this increased ratio by reduction of omega-6 oil intake and increase of omega-3 oil intake may lead to significant clinical benefit through an effect on eicosanoid metabolism (discussed later).

Therapeutic Considerations

Inflammatory bowel disease is the end result of a complex interplay of several factors. This section discusses the key nutritional, microbial, and toxic issues that must be addressed for the successful management of this difficult disease.

Little is known about the natural course of CD, because virtually all patients with the disease undergo standard medical care (drugs and/or surgery) or alternative therapy. The only exceptions are patients in clinical trials who are assigned to the placebo group.[13,14] However, even these patients do not represent the natural course of the disease, because they are seen frequently by physicians and other members of a health care team and are taking medication, even if it is only in the form of a placebo. If proper evaluation of therapies for IBD is to occur, there must be a greater understanding of its natural history. This is particularly important for natural medicine practitioners, because it is commonly believed that standard medical care often interferes with the normal efforts of the body to restore health. Some aspects of the natural course of CD support this idea, especially when coupled with the limited efficacy of current medications and surgery and their known toxicity. However, conventional measures do have their place in many instances and should be used when appropriate.

Researchers in the National Cooperative Crohn's Disease Study (NCCDS) reviewed 77 patients who received placebo therapy in part one of the 17-week study.[13,14] They all had active disease, as defined by a Crohn's disease activity index (CDAI) higher than 150. Of the patients completing the study:

- None died.
- Only seven (9%) suffered a major worsening of their disease (i.e., either a major fistula developed or the patient required abdominal surgery).
- Twenty-five (32%) suffered a less serious worsening (increase in the CDAI to >450 or presence of fever of 100°F for two weeks).
- Treatment was considered to have failed in 25 (32%), because their CDAI remained higher than 150.
- Twenty (26%) achieved clinical remission.

On at least one occasion during the 17 weeks of therapy, 49% of the patients on the placebo treatment were found to have a CDAI lower than 150. The patients who showed favorable response to the placebo continued to be observed with placebo therapy for up to two years. It is interesting to note that none of these patients' intestinal X-rays showed worsening during the study, and 18% showed improvement. Of the patients whose disease responded to the placebo (20 of 77; 26%), the majority (70%) remained in remission at one year, and a fair number (45%) remained in remission at two years. These results indicate that many patients undergo spontaneous remission, approximately 20% at one year and 12% at two years. However, when another factor is considered, the success of placebo therapy rises dramatically. Of patients in the placebo group who had no previous history of steroid therapy, 41% achieved remission after 17 weeks. In addition, 23% of this group continued in remission after two years, compared with only 4% of the group with a history of steroid use.

The European Cooperative Crohn's Disease Study (ECCDS), although different in some methodological details, is quite similar to the NCCDS.[13,15] In the ECCDS, 110 patients constituted the placebo group: 68 patients with prior treatment and 42 patients with no prior treatment. The results of the study showed that 55% of the total placebo group achieved remission by 100 days, 34% remained in remission at 300 days, and 21% remained in remission at 700 days. Like the NCCDS, the ECCDS demonstrated that patients with no prior drug therapy have a greater likelihood of remission.

Although the researchers did not advocate placebo therapy, they did carefully point out that once remission is achieved, 75% of the patients continue in remission at the end of one year and up to 63% at two years, regardless of the maintenance therapy used. These results would suggest that the key is achieving remission, which, once attained, can be maintained by conservative nondrug therapy.[13]

Eicosanoid Metabolism in Inflammatory Bowel Disease

Patients with IBD show greatly increased levels of inflammatory chemicals in the lining of the intestines, serum, and stool samples. These compounds are produced by white blood cells (neutrophils) to amplify the inflammatory process and cause smooth muscle contraction. The formation of these inflammatory compounds can be decreased by reducing or eliminating consumption of omega-6-rich foods (corn, beef, liver, pork, lamb, milk/dairy products, and soy, safflower, sunflower, and corn oil) and increasing consumption of the longer-chain omega-3 fatty acids eicosapentaenoic acid (EPA) and docosahexaenoic acid (DHA) through higher intake of cold-water fish such as anchovies, sardines, salmon, small mackerel, herring, and halibut as well as fish oil supplements.[16]

Detailed analyses of double-blind studies with fish oil supplements (2.7 to 5.1 g total omega-3 oils per day) have demonstrated an ability to prevent or delay relapses in both CD and UC.[16,17] In one study an omega-3 fatty acid supplement reduced the one-year relapse rate by half with an absolute risk reduction of 31%.[18] Much larger studies have asked whether omega-3 fatty acids could sustain remission once it is achieved, but these studies failed to show an advantage of fish oils over a placebo. These results indicate that other factors are not being adequately addressed when fish oils are used as the sole therapy.[19]

Mucin Defects in Ulcerative Colitis

Mucins are sticky protein compounds that line and protect the intestinal lining. Alterations in mucin composition and content in the colonic mucosa have been reported in patients with UC.[20–22] The factors responsible for these changes appear to be a dramatic drop in the mucus content of the goblet cells that produce the mucin (proportional to the severity of the disease) and a decrease of the major sulfomucin subfraction. In contrast, these abnormalities are not found in patients with CD. It is significant that although the mucin content of the goblet cells returns to normal during remission, the sulfomucin deficiency does not. The specific components of the sulfomucin and the cause of its lower concentration have not yet been determined. These mucin abnormalities are also thought to be a major factor in the higher risk of colon cancer in patients with UC. The mucin abnormalities may be the result of lack of dietary fiber.

Intestinal Microflora

The intestinal microflora is extraordinarily complex and contains more than 400 distinct microbial species. In an effort to describe a nonspecific alteration (qualitative or quantitative) in the intestinal flora, the term *dysbiosis* is often used. Dysbiosis is a common feature in many patients with IBD. For example, the fecal flora of many patients with IBD has been found to contain higher numbers of gram-positive anaerobic bacteria and *Bacteroides vulgatus*, a gram-negative rod bacterium.[23] Alterations in the metabolic activity of the various bacteria are thought to be more important than alterations in the number of bacteria per se. In addition, specific bacterial cell components (which vary even within the same species) are thought to be responsible for promoting cell destruction activity against the cells that line the colon (the colonic epithelial cells).[3]

It is very interesting to note that researchers investigating the intestinal flora of UC often use carrageenan (a sulfated polymer of galactose and d-anhydrogalactose extracted from red seaweed, principally *Eucheuma spinosum* and *Chondrus crispus*) to experimentally induce the disease in animals.[24] In its natural state, this polymer has a molecular weight of 100,000 to 800,000, but in the studies it was degraded by mild acidic hydrolysis to yield products with weights in the vicinity of 30,000. These smaller molecules are thought to be responsible for inducing the ulcerative damage seen in the animal studies. Carrageenan compounds are used by the food industry as stabilizing and suspending agents (for example, in products that contain milk, such as cottage cheese, ice cream, and milk chocolate), with polymers of different molecular weights being used for a variety of purposes.

As suggestive as the animal studies are in linking UC with carrageenan, no lesions of IBD were observed in healthy human subjects and primates fed enormous quantities of degraded carrageenan.[25,26] However, differences in intestinal bacterial flora are probably responsible for this discrepancy, as germ-free animals do not display carrageenan-induced damage either.

The bacteria linked to facilitating the carrageenan-induced damage in animals are a strain of *Bacteroides vulgatus*.[23] This organism is found in much higher concentrations (six times as high) in the fecal cultures of patients with UC. The data imply that while carrageenan can be metabolized into nondamaging components in most human subjects, individuals with an overgrowth of

Bacteroides vulgatus may be at risk. Strict avoidance of carrageenan appears warranted at this time for individuals with IBD until further research clarifies its safety for them. Read food labels carefully.

Complications of IBD

There are more than 100 systemic complications of IBD (known as extraintestinal lesions, or EILs). The most common EIL in adults is arthritis, which is found in about 25% of patients. Two types are typically described, the more common being peripheral arthritis affecting the knees, ankles, and wrists. Arthritis is more frequently found in patients with colon involvement. Severity of symptoms is typically proportional to disease activity.

Less frequently, the arthritis affects the spine. Symptoms are low back pain and stiffness with eventual limitation of motion. This EIL occurs predominantly in males and is difficult to distinguish from typical ankylosing spondylitis (rheumatoid arthritis of the spine). In fact, it may precede the bowel symptoms by several years. There is probably a consistent underlying factor in both the progression of ankylosing spondylitis and IBD.

Skin lesions are also common, being seen in approximately 15% of patients. The skin lesions can be quite severe, including gangrene and/or painful, red lumps (e.g., erythema nodosum and pyoderma gangrenosum), but are usually simply annoying, like canker sores. In fact, recurrent canker sores occur in approximately 10% of patients with IBD.

Serious liver disease (i.e., sclerosing cholangitis, chronic active hepatitis, cirrhosis, etc.) is also a common EIL, affecting 3 to 7% of people with IBD. Individuals with liver enzyme abnormalities should take silymarin, a group of flavonoid compounds derived from milk thistle (*Silybum marianum*). These compounds have a tremendous protective effect on the liver and enhance detoxification processes (see the chapter "Hepatitis").[27] The standard dosage for silymarin is 70 to 210 mg three times per day.

Other common EILs are inflammation of blood vessels, impaired blood flow to the fingers or toes, inflammatory eye manifestations (episcleritis, iritis, and uveitis), kidney stones, gallstones, and, in children, failure to grow, thrive, and mature normally.

Nutritional Considerations

A decreased food intake is the most significant cause of nutritional deficiency in patients with IBD. It is the most common nutritional deficit in patients who require hospitalization. Often the IBD patient feels pain, diarrhea, nausea, or other symptoms after a meal, resulting in a subtle decrease in dietary intake. Weight loss and protein-calorie malnutrition are prevalent in 65 to 75% of IBD patients.[28]

Malabsorption—lack of absorption of food and nutrients—can be anticipated in patients with extensive involvement of the small intestine and in patients who have had surgical resection of segments of the small intestine. Particularly common is fat malabsorption, resulting in significant caloric loss as well as loss of fat-soluble vitamins and minerals. Involvement or resection of the ileum of that area typically results in bile acid malabsorption. The laxative effect of bile acids on the colon may result in a chronic watery diarrhea.

Patients with a history of chronic diarrhea may develop electrolyte and trace mineral deficiency, while chronic fat malabsorption (steatorrhea) may result in calcium and magnesium deficiency.

Increased secretion of tissue components and nutrient loss often occur, owing to the inflammatory nature of IBD. In particular, there is a significant loss of blood proteins across the damaged and inflamed mucosa. The loss of protein may exceed the ability of the liver to replace blood proteins, even with a high protein intake. The chronic loss of blood often leads to iron depletion and anemia.

The most common drugs used in the conventional treatment of IBD are corticosteroids (e.g., prednisone) and sulfasalazine, both of which increase nutritional needs. Corticosteroids are known to stimulate protein breakdown (catabolism); depress protein synthesis; decrease the absorption of calcium and phosphorus; increase the urinary excretion of vitamin C, calcium, potassium, and zinc; increase levels of blood glucose, serum triglycerides, and serum cholesterol; increase the requirements for vitamin B_6, vitamin C, folate, and vitamin D; decrease bone formation; and impair wound healing. Sulfasalazine inhibits the absorption and transport of folate, decreases serum folate and iron, and increases the urinary excretion of ascorbic acid.

A chronic inflammatory and/or infectious disease such as IBD also leads to nutritional deficiency because of increased nutritional needs. For example, patients with IBD typically require as much as 25% more protein than usual (and sometimes even more), especially if a significant amount of protein is being lost.

Causes of Malnutrition in Inflammatory Bowel Disease

- Decreased oral intake
  - Disease-induced (pain, diarrhea, nausea, anorexia)
  - Iatrogenic (restrictive diets without supplementation)
- Malabsorption
  - Decreased absorptive surface due to disease or resection

- Bile salt deficiency after resection
- Bacterial overgrowth
- Drugs (e.g., corticosteroids, sulfasalazine, cholestyramine)
- Increased secretion and nutrient loss
  - Protein-losing enteropathy
  - Electrolyte, mineral, and trace mineral loss in diarrhea
- Increased utilization and increased requirements
  - Inflammation, fever, infection
  - Increased intestinal cell turnover

The importance of correcting nutritional deficiencies in patients with IBD cannot be overstated. Nutrient deficiencies, both macro and micro, lead to altered gastrointestinal function and structure, which may result in the patient's entering a vicious circle. That is, the secondary effects of malnutrition on the gastrointestinal tract may lead to a further increase in malabsorption, further decreasing nutrient status.

The majority of individuals with IBD suf-

Frequency of Nutritional Deficiency in Patients with Inflammatory Bowel Disease	
DEFICIENCY	**PREVALENCE (%)**
Protein	25–80
Anemia	60–80
Iron deficiency	40
Low serum vitamin B_{12}	48
Low serum folate	54–64
Low serum magnesium	14–33
Low serum potassium	6–20
Low serum retinol	21
Low serum vitamin C	12
Low serum vitamin D	25–65
Low serum zinc	40–50

fer from nutritional deficiencies. Providing adequate caloric intake is the most important aspect of nutritional therapy. The next step in dietary treatment involves the use of either an elemental or an elimination diet.

Elemental and Elimination Diets

An elemental diet is often an effective nontoxic alternative to corticosteroids as the primary treatment of acute IBD. An elemental diet is one that contains all essential nutrients, with protein being provided only in the form of predigested or isolated amino acids. However, the improvements seen in patients on an elemental diet are probably not primarily related to nutritional improvement; rather, the elemental diet is probably serving as an allergen-elimination diet. Some improvement may also be the result of alterations in the fecal flora that have been observed in patients consuming an elemental diet.[29,30]

Hospitalization is often required for satisfactory administration of elemental diets, and relapse is common when patients resume normal eating. An elimination diet may be a more acceptable alternative in the treatment of IBD, particularly chronic cases.

Elimination (oligoantigenic) diets are described in detail in the chapter "Food Allergy." Basically they are diets consisting of foods that have a lower tendency to produce allergic reactions.

Food allergy has long been considered an important causative factor in the development of IBD, and studies have shown an elimination diet produces considerable benefit in the treatment of IBD.[31–34] In fact, these studies demonstrate that an elimination diet should be the primary therapy in the treatment of chronic IBD. The most common offending foods were found to be wheat and dairy products. Hence, a gluten-free and dairy-free diet may also be effective.

An alternative approach is to determine the actual food allergens by laboratory methods, preferably a method that measures both IgG- and IgE-mediated reactions, such as the ELISA test (see the chapter "Food Allergy"). The allergens can then be avoided, or a diversified rotation diet may be appropriate.

High-Fiber Diet

Treatment with a high-fiber diet has been shown to have a favorable effect on the course of CD and UC.[35] This is in direct contrast to one of the oldest conventional medical dietary treatments of IBD: a low-fiber diet. Although some foods, such as wheat bran, may be too difficult to handle, the dietary treatment of IBD should involve foods rich in fiber and unrefined carbohydrates, combined with a diet that avoids known food allergens or a diversified rotation diet. The combination is much more effective than a high-fiber diet alone.

Dietary fiber has a profound effect on the intestinal environment and is thought to promote a more optimal intestinal flora composition. However, considering the high degree of intolerance to wheat found in patients with IBD and the known roughness of wheat bran, supplemental wheat bran is not a good choice for these patients.

Nutritional Supplements

Multiple Vitamin and Mineral Formula
It is absolutely essential that patients with IBD take a high-quality multiple vitamin and mineral supplement that provides all of the known vitamins and minerals. Use the recommendations in the chapter "Supplementary Measures" to select a high-quality multiple.

Along with taking a high-potency multiple vitamin and mineral formula, individuals with IBD will need to take additional antioxidants, especially vitamin C and either grape seed, pine bark, or green tea extract, as individuals with IBD show increased oxidative stress and decreased antioxidant defenses in the lining of the intestines.[36] Flavonoid-rich extracts such as grape seed, pine bark, and green tea are showing considerable benefits in preliminary studies and animal models of IBD.[37]

Zinc, Folic Acid, and Vitamin B$_{12}$ in IBD

Three nutrients deserve special mention in the treatment of IBD: zinc, folic acid, and vitamin B$_{12}$. Zinc deficiency is a well-known complication of CD, due to low dietary intake, poor absorption, and excess fecal losses.[38] Evidence of zinc deficiency occurs in approximately 45% of CD patients, and in similar proportions of patients with UC. Low zinc concentrations in the blood, low zinc levels in the hair, malabsorption of zinc, altered urinary excretion of zinc, and impaired taste acuity are commonly found in CD patients. In addition, many of the complications of the disease may be a direct result of zinc deficiency: poor healing of fissures and fistulas, skin lesions, decreased sexual development (hypogonadism), growth retardation, retinal dysfunction, depressed immunity, and loss of appetite.[39]

Many IBD patients may not respond to oral or even intravenous zinc supplementation; there appears to be a defect in tissue transport. Supplying zinc in the form of zinc picolinate may be more advantageous, possibly improving both intestinal absorption and tissue transport. Picolinate is a zinc-binding molecule secreted by the pancreas and appears to be better absorbed and utilized than other forms of zinc in certain situations.

Like zinc deficiency, folic acid deficiency is quite common in IBD. The reason for this deficiency, in many cases, is the drug sulfasalazine.[40] Correction of folate deficiency is absolutely essential because folate deficiency promotes further malabsorption and diarrhea due to altered structure of the intestinal mucosal cells.[41] These cells have a very rapid turnover (one to four days) and need to have a constant supply of folic acid.

Since vitamin B$_{12}$ is absorbed at the portion of the intestine most commonly affected with CD (the terminal ileum), deficiency of this vitamin is also quite common. Overall, abnormal B$_{12}$ absorption is found in almost half of patients with CD.[42] Often the terminal ileum of a CD patient has been surgically removed (resected). If the length of the resection is less than 60 cm, or the extent of the inflammatory lesion is less than 60 cm, adequate absorption may occur. Otherwise, intake of active vitamin B$_{12}$ (methylcobalamin) in a daily sublingual tablet or a monthly injection (1,000 mcg intramuscularly) is recommended.

Vitamin D

There is evidence that vitamin D deficiency is quite common in IBD, with laboratory evidence in 75% of CD and 35% of UC patients.[43] This is probably a result of decreased absorption of vitamin D. Patients with IBD are at an increased risk for the development of metabolic bone diseases such as osteoporosis and osteomalacia. Vitamin D plays an important role is supporting proper immune regulation and has also been shown to dampen pro-inflammatory cytokines produced in animal models of IBD. Early research with supplemental vitamin D is encouraging, with 1,200 IU per day resulting in a reduction of relapse rate from 29 to 13% in one study after a year of treatment.[44]

Prebiotics

Prebiotics are non-digestible food ingredients that stimulate the growth or modify the metabolic activity of intestinal bacterial species that have the potential to improve the health of their human host. Prebiotic food ingredients include bran, psyllium husk, resistant (high-amylose) starch, inulin (a polymer of fructofuranose), lactulose, and various natural or synthetic oligosaccharides, which consist of short-chain complexes of sucrose, galactose, fructose, glucose, maltose, or xylose. Bacterial fermentation of prebiotics yields short-chain fatty acids such as butyrate. Several studies have shown significant benefits of various prebiotics for the treatment of patients with UC. When oat bran at 60 g per day (supplying 20 g dietary fiber) was given to UC patients, fecal butyrate increased by 36% and abdominal pain improved.[45]

A dietary supplement containing fish oil and two types of indigestible carbohydrate, FOS and xanthan gum, allowed reduction of glucocorticoid dosage when compared with a placebo, in patients with steroid-dependent UC.[46] In a trial, a Japanese germinated barley foodstuff containing hemicellulose-rich fiber at a dose of 20 to 30 g per day was found to increase stool butyrate concentration,[47] decrease the clinical activity index of patients with active disease,[48] and induce prolonged remission in patients with inactive disease.[49] In another trial, a mixture of *Bifidobacterium longum* and inulin-derived FOS administered for one month as monotherapy to patients with UC produced improvement in sigmoidscopic appearance and several biochemical indices of tissue inflammation when compared with a placebo.[50]

Probiotics

Probiotics are the beneficial bacteria and yeast that can be administered orally to achieve a therapeutic benefit. Over the last 20 years there have been numerous studies demonstrating the benefits of probiotic supplementation. For the most part, they are of little if any benefit during an active flare-up of disease; however there is significant benefit of probiotics for maintaining remissions. Several different probiotic organisms have shown benefit, including the beneficial yeast *Saccharomyces boulardii* and the bacteria *Lactobacillus rhamnosus* and *Bifidobacterium* species.[50–58]

Psychological Support

Mental and emotional stress can promote exacerbation of IBD, so stress management techniques may prove useful for some patients. Psychological counseling to help deal with the stress of IBD was shown to also help reduce recurrences.[59]

Botanical Medicines

Curcumin

Turmeric (*Curcuma longa*) contains the active anti-inflammatory compound curcumin. Studies have demonstrated that curcumin administration in animal models of IBD produced significant improvement and decreased inflammatory cytokine production.[60–63]

In a pilot study involving open-label administration of curcumin preparation to five patients with UC and five patients with CD, 9 of the 10 patients reported improvement at the conclusion of the two-month study.[64] Four of the five patients with UC were able to decrease or eliminate their medications. In a larger, randomized, double-blind multicenter trial involving 89 patients with UC, administration of 1 g curcumin twice per day resulted in both clinical improvement and a statistically significant decrease in the rate of relapse.[65] Given its excellent safety profile, its defined mechanism for affecting inflammation, and the results above, curcumin appears to have an important role in the management of IBD.

Indian Frankincense

The ayurvedic herb *Boswellia serrata* (Indian frankincense) contains boswellic acids, which inhibit the production of inflammatory compounds involved in IBD.[66] During a small six-week trial, 350 mg three times a day of boswellia gum resin was as effective as the drug sulfasalazine (1,000 mg three times a day) in reducing symptoms or laboratory abnormalities of patients with active UC.[67] The rate of remission was 82% with boswellia and 75% with sulfasalazine.[68] In another double-blind study, boswellia extract was found to be as effective as mesalazine is improving symptoms of active CD.[69]

Aloe Vera

Aloe vera gel inhibits the production of reactive oxygen metabolites and inflammatory mediators by human colon epithelial cells grown in tissue culture.[70] When administered orally, aloe vera gel at 100 ml twice a day for four weeks produced a clinical response significantly more often than a placebo in patients with UC.[71] Remission occurred in 30% of patients taking aloe vera gel and 7% of patients receiving the placebo. In this clinical trial, aloe also reduced objective measures of disease activity, whereas the placebo did not. Acemannan, an extract of aloe vera, at a mucopolysaccharide concentration of 30% of solid weight, has also been demonstrated to reduce symptoms and indices of inflammation in controlled studies of patients with UC.[72]

Therapeutic Monitoring

Calprotectin

Calprotectin is a protein secreted into the intestinal lumen in direct proportion to inflammation. Measurement of calprotectin in stool samples has been shown to be a sensitive and specific noninvasive assessment for inflammation in patients with IBD, and the test is helpful for distinguishing IBD from other, noninflammatory gastrointestinal conditions, such as irritable bowel syndrome.[73]

Crohn's Disease Activity Index (CDAI)

The CDAI provides a consistent numerical index for monitoring IBD.[74] The CDAI is calculated by adding together eight variables (see the table below). It incorporates both subjective and objective information in determining relative disease activity. In general, CDAI scores below 150 indicate a better prognosis than higher scores. The CDAI is a very useful way to monitor progress of therapy.

Monitoring of the Pediatric Patient

Pediatric patients with IBD present a particularly difficult problem, in that it is often very difficult for them to achieve normal growth and development. Growth failure occurs in 75% of children with CD and in 25% of children with UC. The pediatric patient with IBD should receive an evaluation at least twice yearly by a knowledgeable physician, including detailed body and weight measurements and appropriate laboratory testing.

The list below outlines the necessary components of a comprehensive twice-yearly nutritional evaluation of pediatric patients with IBD. An aggressive nutritional program should be instituted, including supplements (it may be necessary to use injectable methods for some patients), that is similar to the approach outlined for the adult patient, with the doses adjusted as appropriate.

Parents of children who have IBD need to know the components necessary to monitor their children. They need not understand the significance of each component, but they do need to make sure that their children are being properly evaluated.

Independent Variables and Formula Used to Calculate the Crohn's Disease Activity Index (CDAI)*	
X_1	Number of liquid or very soft stools in 1 week
X_2	Sum of seven per day abdominal pain ratings: 0 = none 1 = mild 2 = moderate 3 = severe
X_3	Sum of seven per day ratings of general well-being: 0 = well 1 = slightly below par 2 = poor 3 = very poor 4 = terrible
X_4	Symptoms or findings presumed related to Crohn's disease. Add 1 point for each category corresponding to patient's symptoms: • Arthritis or arthralgia • Iritis or uveitis • Erythema nodosum, pyoderma gangrenosum, aphthous stomatitis • Anal fissure, fistula, or perirectal abscess • Other bowel-related fistula • Episode of fever >100° F during past week
X_5	Taking diphenoxylate HCl/atropine sulfate tablets (Lomotil) or opiates for diarrhea: 0 = no 1 = yes
X_6	Abdominal mass: 0 = none 0.4 = questionable 1 = present
X_7	47—hematocrit value, males 42—hematocrit value, females
X_8	100 (standard weight—body weight) π standard weight

* CDAI = $2\yen X_1 + 5\yen X_2 + 7\yen X_3 + 20\yen X_4 + 30\yen X_5 + 10\yen X_6 + 6\yen X_7 + X_8$.

Source: Adapted from Ford-Hutchinson AW. *J Allergy Clin Immunol* 1984;74:437–440.

Monitoring of the Pediatric Patient with Inflammatory Bowel Disease
History

- Appetite, extracurricular activities
- Type and duration of inflammatory bowel disease, frequency of relapses
- Severity and extent of ongoing symptoms
- Medication history
- Three-day diet diary

Physical examination

- Height, weight, arm circumference, triceps skinfold measurements
- Loss of subcutaneous fat, muscle wasting, edema, pallor, skin rash, hepatomegaly

Laboratory tests

- Complete blood count and differential, reticulocyte and platelet count, sedimentation rate, urinalysis
- Serum total proteins, albumin, globulin, retinol-binding protein
- Serum electrolytes, calcium, phosphate, ferritin, folate, carotenes, tocopherol, vitamin B_{12}
- Leukocyte ascorbate, magnesium, and zinc
- Creatinine height index, blood urea nitrogen/creatinine ratio

QUICK REVIEW

- Antibiotic exposure is being linked to Crohn's disease.
- Over 100 disorders, known as extraintestinal lesions (EIL), constitute a diverse group of systemic complications of IBD.
- Clinical studies that have utilized an elemental diet, intravenous nutrition, or an exclusion diet have produced great success in the treatment of Crohn's disease and ulcerative colitis.
- Treatment with a high-fiber diet has been shown to have a favorable effect on the course of CD and UC.

- Nutritional complications occur during the course of IBD.
- Foremost in nutritional therapy is providing adequate caloric intake.
- Elemental and elimination diets have been shown to be an effective nontoxic primary treatment of acute and chronic IBD.
- Treatment with a high-fiber diet has been shown to have a favorable effect on the course of Crohn's disease.
- The majority of individuals with IBD suffer from nutritional deficiencies.

TREATMENT SUMMARY

It is important to recognize that in some patients CD and UC are life-threatening diseases that at times require emergency treatment. A small percentage of patients who have severe UC may experience exacerbations requiring hospitalization.

Typically, IBD is a chronic disease requiring long-term therapy and follow-up. The first step is to identify and remove all factors that may be initiating or aggravating the inflammatory reaction, such as food allergens and low levels of omega-3 fatty acids or dietary antioxidants.

A broad-based nutritional supplementation plan is necessary for all patients with IBD. Particularly important are the nutrients zinc, folic acid, vitamin B_{12},

magnesium, vitamin A, and possibly vitamin D. Nutritional supplements are used as appropriate to correct deficiencies, normalize the inflammatory process, and promote healing of the damaged mucosa. Botanical medicines are used to promote healing and normalize the intestinal flora.

Diet

The recommendations given in the chapter "A Health-Promoting Diet" are appropriate in IBD. All allergens, wheat, corn, and dairy products, and carrageenan-containing foods should be eliminated. The diet should be high in dietary fiber and low in sugar and refined carbohydrates.

Nutritional Supplements

- A high-potency multiple vitamin and mineral formula as described in the chapter "Supplementary Measures"
- Key individual nutrients:
  - Vitamin A: 2,500 to 5,000 IU per day (Note: dosages in excess of 3,000 IU per day should not be used in women who are or may become pregnant.)
  - Vitamin B_6: 25 to 50 mg per day
  - Folic acid: 800 mcg per day
  - Vitamin B_{12}: 800 mcg per day
  - Vitamin C: 500 to 1,000 mg two to three times per day
  - Vitamin E (mixed tocopherols): 100 to 200 IU per day
  - Selenium: 100 to 200 mcg per day
  - Zinc (picolinate form recommended): 30 to 45 mg per day
  - Vitamin D_3: 2,000 to 4,000 IU per day (ideally, measure blood levels and adjust dosage accordingly)
  - Fish oils: 1,000 mg EPA + DHA per day
- One of the following:
  - Grape seed extract (>95% procyanidolic oligomers): 100 to 300 mg per day
  - Pine bark extract (>95% procyanidolic oligomers): 100 to 300 mg per day
  - Green tea extract (>90% polyphenol content): 300 to 450 mg per day
  - Some other flavonoid-rich extract with a similar flavonoid content, super greens formula, or another plant-based antioxidant that can provide an oxygen radical absorption capacity (ORAC) of 3,000 to 6,000 units or more per day
- Probiotic (active lactobacillus and bifidobacteria cultures): a minimum of 5 billion to 10 billion colony-forming units per day
- Prebiotics (inulin, fructose oligosaccharides, etc.): 5 g per day

Botanical Medicines

- Curcumin (*Curcuma longa*): 1,000 mg two to three times per day before meals
- Boswellia extract: equivalent of 400 mg boswellic acids three times per day
- Aloe vera, one of the following:
  - Aloe vera gel: 100 ml per day orally
  - Aloe vera juice: a variety of different preparation types and concentrations make accurate dosage recommendations difficult, but it can be consumed orally as a beverage or tonic
  - Acemannan: 400 to 800 mg per day

Cystitis and Interstitial Cystitis/Painful Bladder

- One or more of the following signs or symptoms:
  - Increased urinary frequency, urgency, nocturia (waking up to urinate at night)
  - Burning pain on urination
  - Turbid, foul-smelling, or dark urine
  - Lower abdominal pain
  - Chronic pelvic pain
  - A persistent, urgent need to urinate
  - Pain during sexual intercourse

Irritation of the bladder (cystitis) is a very common condition, especially in women. It is estimated that 10 to 20% of all women have urinary tract discomfort at least once a year, 37.5% of women with no history of urinary tract infection (UTI) will have one within 10 years, and 2% to 4% of apparently healthy women have elevated levels of bacteria in their urine, indicative of an unrecognized UTI. Women with a history of recurrent UTIs will typically have an episode at least once a year. Recurrent bladder infections can be a significant problem for some women because 55% will eventually involve the kidneys, and recurrent kidney infection can have serious consequences, including abscess formation, chronic progressive kidney damage, and kidney failure.

UTIs are much less common in males than females, except infants, and in general indicate an anatomical abnormality, a prostate infection, or rectal intercourse.

Chronic interstitial cystitis or painful bladder syndrome (IC/PBS) is a persistent form of bladder irritation not due to infection. In addition to the general measures given below, the therapeutic focus is on enhancing the integrity of the tissue (interstitium) along with the lining of the bladder wall. The symptoms of IC/PBS can overlap with such conditions as endometriosis, recurrent urinary tract infection, chronic pelvic pain, overactive bladder, and vulvodynia. Studies have indicated that interstitial cystitis affects 52 to 67 per 100,000 people in the United States.[1] Some investigators believe these numbers are vastly underestimated owing to lack of proper diagnosis.

Diagnostic Considerations

The diagnosis is usually made according to signs and symptoms and urinary findings. Microscopic examination of the infected urine shows high levels of white blood cells (WBCs) and bacteria. Culturing the urine determines the quantity and type of bacteria involved. The bacteria *Escherichia coli* is by far the most common. The presence of fever, chills, and low back pain can indicate involvement of the kidneys.[2]

IC/PBS can also be difficult to diagnose, as the symptoms overlap with a variety of other disorders, including endometriosis, UTI, chronic pelvic pain, overactive bladder, and vulvodynia. Because there is no definitive diagnostic test, IC/PBS remains a diagnosis of exclusion. The presence of additional symptoms caused by other conditions can confuse the diagnosis even further. Patients may not receive an accurate diagnosis for years. The average time between the development of IC/PBS symptoms and the diagnosis is approximately five years.[3]

Therapeutic Considerations

Although most bladder infections are not serious, it is important that you be properly diagnosed, treated, and monitored. If you have symptoms suggestive of a bladder infection, consult a physician. That is especially true if you are also experiencing fever, abdominal or flank pain, or nausea and vomiting. If a urine culture indicates the presence of bacteria, it is appropriate to follow up with another culture 7 to 14 days after treatment is started to ensure it has been resolved. Most physicians will want to prescribe antibiotics. However, please discuss your desire to utilize a more natural approach. Notify your physician if any change occurs in your condition (fever, more painful urination, low back pain, etc.).

For most bladder infections, especially those that are chronic or recurrent, the best treatment appears to be the natural approach. There is a growing concern that antibiotic therapy actually promotes recurrent bladder infection by disturbing the bacterial flora of the vagina and by giving rise to antibiotic-resistant strains of *E. coli*. One of the body's most important defenses against

bacterial colonization of the bladder is a protective shield of healthful bacteria that line and protect the external portion of the urethra. When antibiotics are used, this normal protective shield can be stripped away or replaced by less effective organisms.

If a woman tends to suffer from recurrent bladder infections, or if antibiotics have been used, it is appropriate to reintroduce friendly bacteria into the vagina. The best way to do this is to use commercially available *Lactobacillus acidophilus* products. Use a product that is a capsule or tablet, and simply place one or two in the vagina before going to bed, every other night for two weeks. In addition, oral supplementation with a probiotic is recommended (5 billion to 10 billion live bacteria per day).

The primary goal in the natural approach to treating infectious cystitis is enhancing normal host protective measures against UTI. Specifically, this refers to enhancing the flow of urine by achieving and maintaining proper hydration, promoting a pH that inhibits the growth of infectious organisms, preventing bacterial adherence to the endothelial cells of the bladder, and enhancing the immune system. In addition, several botanical medicines with antimicrobial activity can be employed.

In IC/PCP the therapeutic focus is also on enhancing the integrity of the tissue along with the lining of the bladder wall—the interstitial tissue. Eliminating food allergens appears to be a valid goal, as food allergies have been shown to produce cystitis in some patients. Repeated ingestion of a food allergen could easily explain the chronic nature of interstitial cystitis. In addition, certain foods are notorious for producing symptoms.[4] For example, one study found that 90% of IC patients experience an increase in symptoms when they consume certain foods and beverages, especially coffee, tea, soda, alcoholic beverages, citrus fruits and juices, artificial sweeteners, and hot peppers.[5]

The herbs gotu kola (*Centella asiatica*) and aloe vera appear to address some of the other features of chronic IC. Specifically, gotu kola extracts have been shown to heal ulcerations of the bladder and to improve the integrity of the connective tissue that lines the bladder wall.[6,7] Aloe vera may also be of benefit.

Pentosan polysulfate sodium (PPS), sold under the name Elmiron, is an FDA-approved drug that is thought to replenish the defective bladder lining. It is very similar to natural hyaluronic acid (HA), a key component of the interstitial tissue. Supplementation with HA (100 to 200 mg per day) may be of similar value, as it has been shown to improve the connective tissue matrix of the interstitium of the skin.

Increasing Urine Flow

Increasing urine flow can be easily achieved by increasing the amount of liquids consumed. Ideally, the liquids should be in the form of water, herbal teas, and fresh fruit and vegetable juices diluted with at least an equal amount of water. Drink at least 64 fl oz from this group, with at least half of this amount being water. Avoid soft drinks, concentrated fruit drinks, coffee, and alcoholic beverages.

Acidify or Alkalinize?

Although many practitioners believe acidifying the urine is the best approach in addressing cystitis, several arguments can be made for alkalinizing the urine. First, it is often difficult to acidify the urine. Many popular methods of attempting to acidify the urine, such as vitamin C supplementation and cranberry juice, have little effect on pH at commonly prescribed doses.

Alkalinizing the urine is easily achieved with the use of citrate salts (e.g., potassium citrate, sodium citrate). These salts are rapidly absorbed and metabolized without affecting gastric pH or producing a laxative effect. They are excreted partly as carbonate, thus raising the pH of the urine.

Potassium citrate and sodium citrate have long been employed in the treatment of lower UTIs. They are often used for temporary relief until the results of a urine culture are available. Some clinical studies support this practice. For example, in one study, women presenting with symptoms of a UTI were given 4 g sodium citrate every 8 hours for 48 hours.[8] Of the 64 women evaluated, 80% of the women had relief of symptoms, 12% had deterioration of symptoms, and 91.8% of the women rated the treatment as acceptable. Of the 64 women, 19 were shown to have positive bacterial cultures. There was more variation in response to treatment in the group of women with proven bacterial infection, with those having symptoms of urethral pain (7 of 10) and dysuria (13 of 18) improving more than those with symptoms of frequency (9 of 17) and urgency (6 of 13). These results were similar to those of a previous study that demonstrated significant symptomatic relief in 80% of the 159 women who did not have bacteria in their urine.[9]

One more possible advantage to alkalizing rather than acidifying the urine is that many herbs used to treat UTIs, such as *Hydrastis canadensis* and *Arctostaphylos uva ursi*, contain antibacterial components that work most effectively in an alkaline environment.

Botanical Medicines

Cranberry

Based on extensive experimental research and positive clinical results, cranberry (*Vaccinium macrocarpon*) has gained a lot of attention as a possible alternative to antibiotics in the prevention and treatment of UTIs.[10] For many years it was thought that the action of cranberry juice was due to acidifying the urine and to the antibacterial effects of a cranberry component, hippuric acid. However, these are probably not the major mechanisms of action. Rather than its action as an antibiotic or acidifying the urine, the most likely explanation for cranberry's beneficial effects are that components known as proanthocyanidins interfere with the adherence of bacteria to the cells that line the urinary tract. In order to cause an infection in the urinary tract, bacteria must first attach to these cells. So when the bacteria are blocked from attaching, an infection can be prevented. And, in the case of an active infection, the proanthocyanidins can make it too "slippery" for the bacteria to maintain their hold. In the studies looking at cranberry and bacterial adherence, cranberry was found to decrease adherence in more than 60% of the strains of bacteria tested.[11-14]

The scientific support for the positive effect of cranberry preparations in the prevention and treatment of UTIs is somewhat inconsistent.[10] However, that may be because it does not prevent adhesion of all bacteria to the bladder cells. So while many women (and men) with a history of UTIs will gain benefit from cranberry, some will not. The effectiveness of cranberry may be enhanced by using well-defined preparations standardized for proanthocyanidin content rather than commercial cranberry juice. Most cranberry juices on the market contain one-third cranberry juice mixed with water and sugar. Since sugar has such a detrimental effect on the immune system (see the chapter "Immune System Support"), use of sweetened cranberry juice cannot be recommended. Fresh cranberry juice (sweetened with blueberry juice) or blueberry juice is preferred. For tough cases, we recommend using cranberry extracts instead.

One study did compare the efficacy and cost of taking a cranberry extract (CranMax) in tablet form vs. cranberry juice in the prevention of UTI in 150 women over the course of one year. Both cranberry juice and cranberry tablets significantly decreased the number of patients experiencing at least one symptomatic infection per year (20% and 18%, respectively) compared with a placebo (32%). The average annual cost of cranberry tablets was $624, whereas the juice cost $1,400.[15]

To illustrate just how effective cranberry juice can be in preventing a bladder infection, in one study 300 ml (about 8 fl oz) of cranberry juice per day dramatically decreased the level of bacteria in the urine and the frequency of recurrence of infection in 153 women (average age 78.5).[16] However, in another study, involving 319 college women, no significant effect was seen. In this double-blind study participants were followed up until a second UTI or for 6 months, whichever came first. The study concluded that 8 fl oz low-calorie cranberry juice twice per day gave no greater protection against the risk of recurring UTI among college-age women compared with a placebo juice.[17] Lack of active compounds is probably not the reason the study failed, as the juice used in the study was standardized to provide 112 mg per day of proanthocyanidins. The possible explanation again is that since cranberry proanthocyanidins do not prevent the adhesion of all types of bacteria to the urinary tract lining, cranberry may not be effective in all cases.

The bottom line is that cranberry is very safe and can be quite effective, so it is worth using. One sure benefit is that cranberry ingestion can significantly reduce strong urinary odor—a common problem in elderly people, especially those in nursing homes or assisted living facilities.[18,19]

Uva Ursi

Uva ursi (upland cranberry or bearberry, *Arctostaphylos uva ursi*) is another popular herbal medicine for UTIs. It has been used by women for centuries, with the first recorded use in the thirteenth century. It exerts urinary antiseptic activity by means of its component arbutin, which typically makes up 6.3 to 9.6% of the leaves.[20] Once ingested, arbutin is broken down into hydroquinone and excreted into the urine. It is the hydroquinone that prevents bacterial growth, and it is most effective in an alkaline urine. The preventive effect of a standardized uva ursi extract on recurrent cystitis was evaluated in a double-blind study of 57 women.[21] At the end of one year, 5 of 27 women in the placebo group had a recurrence, while none of the 30 women receiving the uva ursi extract had a recurrence. No side effects were reported in either group. These impressive results indicate that regular use of uva ursi, like cranberry, may prevent bladder infections. Uva ursi has also been shown to be helpful in increasing the susceptibility of antibiotic-resistant bacteria to antibiotics.

Care must be taken to avoid excessive dosages of uva ursi—as little as 15 g (0.5 oz) of the dried leaves has been shown to produce toxicity in susceptible individuals. Early signs of toxicity include ringing in the ears, nausea, and vomiting.[22]

Goldenseal

Goldenseal (*Hydrastis canadensis*) is one of the most effective of the herbal antimicrobial agents. Its long history of use by herbalists and naturopathic physicians for the treatment of infections is well documented in the scientific literature. Of particular importance here is its efficacy against *E. coli, Proteus*

· ·

QUICK REVIEW

- **If you have symptoms suggestive of a bladder infection, consult a physician.**
- **There is a growing concern that antibiotic therapy actually promotes recurrent bladder infections.**
- **The primary goal in the natural approach to treating infectious cystitis is enhancing normal host protective measures against urinary tract infection.**
- **Drink at least 64 fl oz water per day.**
- **Alkalinize the urine with citrate.**
- **Cranberry juice has been shown to be quite effective in several clinical studies.**

- **Uva ursi is effective in the acute treatment of bladder infections as well as a preventive measure.**
- **In interstitial cystitis the therapeutic focus is on enhancing the integrity of the tissue along with the lining of the bladder wall.**
- **Gotu kola extracts have been shown to heal ulcerations of the bladder and to improve the integrity of the bladder lining.**

species, *Klebsiella* species, *Staphylococcus* spp., *Enterobacter aerogenes* (requires large dosage), and *Pseudomonas* species.[22,23] Its active ingredient, berberine, like hydroquinone from uva ursi, works better in alkaline urine.

Immune Support

See the chapter "Immune System Support," for a complete discussion on how to optimize the functioning of your immune system.

. . . .

TREATMENT SUMMARY

Although most cases of cystitis are relatively benign, it is extremely important to seek medical care for proper diagnosis and monitoring. Owing to the possibility of a kidney infection, it is imperative to consult a physician if there is fever, low back pain, nausea, or vomiting. Kidney infections (e.g., pyelonephritis) require immediate antibiotic therapy and sometimes hospitalization.

Although the occasional acute bladder infection is easily treated, dealing with chronic cystitis can be a challenge. Long-term success requires determining the underlying cause, such as loss of the probiotic urethral shield, structural abnormalities, excessive sugar consumption, food allergies, nutritional deficiencies, or chronic vaginitis.

General Recommendations

- Drink large quantities of fluids (at least 64 fl oz per day), including at least 16 fl oz unsweetened cranberry juice or 8 fl oz blueberry juice per day. Or, take a clinically proven cranberry extract.
- Urinate after intercourse.

Diet

- Follow the guidelines in the chapter "A Health-Promoting Diet."
- Avoid all simple sugars, refined carbohydrates, full-strength fruit juice (diluted fruit juice is acceptable), and food allergens.

Nutritional Supplements

- A high-potency multiple vitamin and mineral formula as described in the chapter "Supplementary Measures"
- Key individual nutrients:
  - Vitamin C: 500 to 1,000 mg per day
  - Magnesium (bound to aspartate, citrate, fumarate, malate, or succinate): 200 to 300 mg three times per day
  - Vitamin D_3: 2,000 to 4,000 IU per day (ideally, measure blood levels and adjust dosage accordingly)
- Fish oils: 1,000 mg EPA + DHA per day
- One of the following:
  - Grape seed extract (>95% procyanidolic oligomers): 100 to 300 mg per day

○ Pine bark extract (>95% procyanidolic oligomers): 100 to 300 mg per day

- During acute cystitis:
  ○ Citrate: dosage can be based on the level of elemental mineral such as potassium, magnesium, or calcium; recommendation is 125 to 250 mg three to four times per day
  ○ Vitamin C: 500 mg every two hours
  ○ Zinc: 30 mg per day

Botanical Medicines

For symptoms associated with a bladder infection, choose one of the following; dosages can be taken three times per day with a large glass of water. (Neither uva ursi nor goldenseal is recommended during pregnancy.)

- Uva ursi (*Arctostaphylos uva ursi*):
  ○ Dried leaves or as a tea: 1.5 to 4.0 g (1 to 2 tsp)
  ○ Freeze-dried leaves: 500 to 1,000 mg
  ○ Tincture (1:5): 4 to 6 ml (1 to 1.5 tsp)
  ○ Fluid extract (1:1): 0.5 to 2.0 ml (¼ to ½ tsp)
  ○ Powdered solid extract (10% arbutin): 250 to 500 mg

- Goldenseal (*Hydrastis canadensis*):
  ○ Dried root (or as tea): 1 to 2 g
  ○ Freeze-dried root: 500 to 1,000 mg
  ○ Tincture (1:5): 4 to 6 ml (1 to 1.5 tsp)
  ○ Fluid extract (1:1): 0.5 to 2.0 ml (¼ to ½ tsp)
  ○ Powdered solid extract (8% alkaloids): 250 to 500 mg

For symptoms associated more with nonbacterial interstitial cystitis or painful bladder, one of the following:

- Gotu kola (*Centella asiatica*): 60 to 120 mg per day of an extract standardized to contain 40% asiaticoside, 29 to 30% asiatic acid, 29 to 30% madecassic acid, and 1 to 2% madecassoside
- Aloe vera juice: up to 32 fl oz per day as a beverage

Depression

....

The official definition of clinical depression is based on the following eight primary criteria:

- Poor appetite accompanied by weight loss, or increased appetite accompanied by weight gain
- Insomnia or excessive sleep habits (hypersomnia)
- Physical hyperactivity or inactivity
- Loss of interest or pleasure in usual activities, or decrease in sexual drive
- Loss of energy; feelings of fatigue
- Feelings of worthlessness, self-reproach, or inappropriate guilt
- Diminished ability to think or concentrate
- Recurrent thoughts of death or suicide

The presence of five of these eight symptoms definitely indicates clinical depression; an individual with four is probably depressed. The symptoms must be present for at least one month to be called clinical depression.

Depression reflects a disturbance in mood. Used in this context, *mood* means a prolonged emotional tone that dominates an individual's outlook. Normal moods (sadness, grief, elation, etc.), which are typically transient, are a part of everyday life, making the demarcation between "normal" and "abnormal" often difficult to determine. Depression is the most common mood disorder.

Obviously, there is a spectrum of clinical depression, ranging from mild feelings of depression to serious consideration of suicide.

Mild depression is also known as *dysthymia*. Like clinical depression, dysthymia is diagnosed according to certain criteria. In order to be officially diagnosed as dysthymic, a person must be depressed most of the time for at least two years (one year for children or adolescents) and have at least three of the following symptoms:

- Low self-esteem or lack of self-confidence
- Pessimism, hopelessness, or despair
- Lack of interest in ordinary pleasures and activities
- Withdrawal from social activities
- Fatigue or lethargy
- Guilt or ruminating about the past
- Irritability or excessive anger
- Lessened productivity
- Difficulty concentrating or making decisions

Approximately 20 million Americans suffer from true clinical depression each year, and more than 30 million Americans take antidepressant drugs. The obvious question is: "Why are so many people depressed?" From a nonphysiological standpoint, several basic theoretical models of depression attempt to answer this question:

- **The "aggression-turned-inward" construct.** Although this behavior is apparent in many clinical cases, the theory has no substantial proof.

- **The "loss model."** This model postulates that depression is a reaction to the loss of a person, a thing, status, self-esteem, or even a habit.

- **The "interpersonal relationship" model.** This theory holds that depression is an extension or outgrowth of behaviors used to control others, such as pouting, silence, or ignoring something or someone. The initial behaviors fail to serve the need, and so the problem worsens.

- **The "learned helplessness" model.** This theorizes that depression is the result of habitual feelings of pessimism and hopelessness.

- **The "biogenic amine" hypothesis.** This stresses biochemical derangement characterized by imbalances of biogenic amines.

- **The analytical (or adaptive) rumination hypothesis.** In this model, the ruminative thinking processes of a person with depression facilitate complex, social problem solving.

Of the various psychological theories of depression, the one that may have the most merit is the learned helplessness model, developed by Martin Seligman, Ph.D. During the 1960s, Dr. Seligman discovered that animals could be trained to be helpless. His animal model provided a valuable clue to human depression, as well as serving as the research model to test antidepressant drugs.[1]

The "Learned Helplessness" Model

Seligman's early experiments were performed on three groups of dogs. The first group of dogs received an escapable electrical shock. The dogs could turn off the shock by simply pressing a panel with their noses. This group of dogs would thus have control. The dogs in the second group were "yoked" to the first group. They got exactly the same shocks as the first group but could not turn off the shock. The shock would cease only when the "yoked" dog in the first group would press its nose to the panel. Thus the second group of dogs had no control over the degree of shock they received. The third group of dogs received no shocks at all.

Once the dogs went through this first part of the experiment, they were placed in a "shuttle box," a box separated in the middle by a small barrier that the dogs could jump over. The dogs would be electrically shocked but could escape the shock by simply jumping over the barrier to the other side. Seligman hypothesized that the first and third groups would quickly figure this out but that the second group of dogs would have learned to be helpless in that they would believe nothing they could do mattered. Seligman thought that the dogs in the second group would simply lie down and accept the shock.

As predicted, the first and third groups of dogs learned within seconds that they could avoid the shock by jumping over the barrier, while the dogs in the second group would simply lie down and not even make an effort to jump over the barrier, though they could see the other side of the shuttle box. Seligman and his colleagues went on to show that many humans react in a fashion identical to that of animals in these experiments.

The adoption of Seligman's model was revolutionary in psychopharmacology, as it became an effective experiment to test antidepressant drugs. Basically, when animals that had learned to be helpless were given antidepressants, they would unlearn helplessness and start exerting control over their environment. Researchers discovered that when animals learned to be helpless, this resulted in alteration of brain monoamine content. The drugs would restore proper monoamine balance and alter the animals' behavior. Researchers also discovered that when animals with learned helplessness were taught how to gain control over their environment, their brain chemistry also normalized. The alteration in brain monoamine content in the animals with learned helplessness mirrors the altered monoamine content in human depression.

Although most physicians look quickly to drugs to alter brain chemistry, helping patients to gain greater control over their lives actually produces even greater biochemical changes. One of the most powerful techniques to produce the necessary biochemical changes in the brains of depressed individuals is to teach them to be more optimistic.

Outside the laboratory setting, Seligman discovered that the determining factor in how a person would react to uncontrollable events, either "bad" or "good," was his or her explanatory style—the way in which the person explained events. Optimistic people were immune to becoming helpless and depressed.

However, individuals who were pessimistic were extremely likely to become depressed when something went wrong in their lives. Seligman and other researchers also found a direct correlation between an individual's level of optimism and the likeliness of developing not only clinical depression but other illnesses as well.[2] In one of the longer studies, patients were followed for a total of 35 years. Optimists rarely got depressed, but pessimists were extremely likely to battle depression and other psychological disturbances.

For more information, see the chapter "A Positive Mental Attitude."

Depression as a Result of Low Serotonin Level

Serotonin is an important neurotransmitter—a chemical messenger responsible for transmitting information from one nerve cell to another. Serotonin has been referred to as the brain's own mood-elevating and tranquilizing drug. There is a lot of support for

The Effects of Different Levels of Serotonin	
OPTIMAL LEVEL OF SEROTONIN	**LOW LEVEL OF SEROTONIN**
Hopeful, optimistic	Depressed
Calm	Anxious
Good-natured	Irritable
Patient	Impatient
Reflective and thoughtful	Impulsive
Loving and caring	Abusive
Able to concentrate	Short attention span
Creative, focused	Blocked, scattered
Able to think things through	Flies off the handle
Responsive	Reactive
Does not overeat carbohydrates	Craves sweets and high-carbohydrate foods
Sleeps well with good dream recall	Insomnia and poor dream recall

this sentiment. Because the manufacture of serotonin in the brain is dependent upon how much tryptophan is delivered to the brain, in experimental studies researchers can feed human volunteers or animals diets lacking tryptophan and note the effects of such a diet. The results from these sorts of studies have contributed greatly in our understanding on just how vital proper levels of serotonin are to a positive human experience. The table opposite contrasts optimal and low serotonin levels.

The lower the level of serotonin, the more severe the consequences. For example, low levels of serotonin are linked to depression, with the lowest levels being observed in people who have committed or attempted suicide.

Therapeutic Considerations

Modern psychiatry primarily focuses on manipulating neurotransmitter levels in the brain rather than identifying and eliminating the psychological, nutritional, and environmental factors that are responsible for producing the imbalances in serotonin, dopamine, GABA, and other neurotransmitters.

Most of the commonly used antidepressant drugs work primarily by increasing the effects of serotonin. Once serotonin is manufactured in the brain it is stored in nerve cells waiting for release. Upon release, the serotonin carries a chemical message by binding to receptor sites on the neighboring nerve cell. Almost as soon as the serotonin is released enzymes are at work that will either break down the serotonin or work to uptake the serotonin back into the brain cells. Either event results in stopping the serotonin effect. It is at this point that various drugs typically work to either inhibit the reuptake

of serotonin or prevent its breakdown. Most popular drugs are referred to as SSRIs (selective serotonin reuptake inhibitors). Because serotonin reuptake is inhibited, there is more serotonin hanging around, capable of binding to receptor sites.

The effectiveness of antidepressant drugs has been the subject of several reviews. The results indicate that they have not been shown to work any better than a placebo in cases of mild to moderate depression, the most common reason for prescription medication, and claims that antidepressants are more effective in more severe conditions have little evidence to support them.[3,4] In fact, the research indicates that SSRIs and other antidepressant drugs might actually increase the likelihood of suicide in adults and children.[5]

An additional alarming finding is that 25% of patients taking antidepressants do not even have depression or a diagnosable psychiatric problem.[6] So the bottom line is that millions of people are using antidepressants for a problem they do not have, and for the people who have a diagnosable condition, these medications do not work in most cases anyway and may cause significant side effects. As one group of researcher concluded, "Given doubt about their benefits and concern about their risks, current recommendations for prescribing antidepressants should be reconsidered."[3] This statement is a clear mandate to consider natural medicine to deal with the causes of these mood disorders.

While antidepressant drugs are only marginally successful at best in alleviating depression, they do produce many side effects. Approximately 20% of patients experience nausea, 20% headaches, 15% anxiety and nervousness, 14% insomnia, 12% drowsiness, 12% diarrhea, 9.5% dry mouth, 9% loss of appetite, 8% sweating and tremor, and 3% rash. SSRIs also definitely inhibit sexual function. In studies where sexual side effects were thoroughly evaluated, 43% of men and women taking SSRIs reported loss of libido or diminished sexual response. There is also a significant risk for weight gain and the development of type 2 diabetes (see the box below).

There are effective alternatives to antidepressant drugs. For example, there are a number of lifestyle and dietary factors that lead to reduced serotonin levels. Chief among these factors are cigarette smoking, alcohol abuse, a high sugar intake, too much protein, blood sugar disturbances (hypoglycemia and diabetes), and various nutrient deficiencies. All of these factors have one thing in common: they lower serotonin levels by impairing the conversion of tryptophan to serotonin. A health-promoting lifestyle and diet go a long way in restoring optimal serotonin levels and relieving depression. But in the interim, natural agents such as 5-HTP, Saint-John's-wort, lavender, or saffron extract can provide the necessary boost in mood to help make important changes in diet and lifestyle easier to accomplish.

Possible Underlying Causes

Depression can often have an underlying organic (chemical) or physiological cause. Identification and elimination of the underlying cause is a critical step in most cases. Failure to address an underlying cause will make any antidepressant therapy less successful. It is important to rule out simple organic factors that are known to contribute to depression, such as nutrient deficiency or excess, drugs (prescription, illicit, alcohol, caffeine, nicotine, etc.), hypoglycemia, excessive consumption of alcohol, hormonal derangement, allergy, environmental toxins, and microbial factors. Each of these is discussed below. Regardless of any underlying organic cause, counseling is always recommended for the depressed individual.

Organic and Physiological Causes of Depression

- Preexisting physical conditions
  - Diabetes
  - Heart disease
  - Lung disease
  - Rheumatoid arthritis
  - Chronic inflammation
  - Chronic pain
  - Cancer
  - Liver disease
  - Multiple sclerosis
- Prescription drugs
  - Anti-inflammatory agents
  - Birth control pills

SSRIS, WEIGHT GAIN, AND DIABETES

A little-appreciated side effect of SSRIs is weight gain. Statistics show that once weight gain begins in a patient taking these medications it usually does not stop. These drugs induce weight gain because they alter an area of the brain that regulates both serotonin levels and the utilization of glucose.[7] While the human brain will usually make up 2% of our overall body mass, it is so metabolically active that it uses up to 50% of the glucose in the body for energy. Evidently the SSRIs disrupt the utilization of glucose in the brain in such a way that the brain senses that it is low in glucose. That sets in motion very powerful signals to eat. And, typically if a person has had sugar cravings or other food urges, those cravings will be dramatically enhanced by the drug. Other changes produced by the drug will lead to insulin resistance, setting the stage for inevitable weight gain and perhaps even type 2 diabetes. Studies have shown that individuals predisposed to diabetes are two to three times more likely to become diabetic if they use an antidepressant medication.[8]

- ○ Blood pressure lowering drugs
- ○ Antihistamines
- ○ Corticosteroids
- ○ Tranquilizers and sedatives
- Premenstrual syndrome
- Stress/low adrenal function
- Heavy metals
- Food allergies
- Hypothyroidism
- Hypoglycemia
- Nutritional deficiencies
- Sleep disturbances

Counseling

There are a number of counseling techniques that can be quite useful. The therapy that has the most merit and support in the medical literature is cognitive therapy. In fact, cognitive therapy has been shown to be as effective as antidepressant drugs in treating moderate depression.[9,10] However, while there is a high rate of relapse of depression when drugs are used, the relapse rate for cognitive therapy is much lower. People taking drugs for depression tend to have to stay on them for the rest of their lives. That is not the case with cognitive therapy because the patient is taught new skills to deal with the psychological factors that cause depression.[11]

Psychologists and other mental health specialists trained in cognitive therapy seek to change the way the depressed person consciously thinks about failure, defeat, loss, and helplessness. Cognitive therapists employ five basic tactics.

First, they help patients recognize the negative automatic thoughts that flit through consciousness at the times when the patient feels the worst. The second tactic is disputing the negative thoughts by focusing on contrary evidence. The third is teaching patients a different explanation to dispute the negative automatic thoughts. The fourth involves helping patients learn how to avoid rumination (the constant churning of a thought in one's mind) by better controlling their own thoughts. The final tactic is questioning depression-causing negative thoughts and beliefs and replacing them with empowering positive thoughts and beliefs.

Cognitive therapy does not involve the long-drawn-out process of psychoanalysis. It is a solution-oriented psychotherapy designed to help patients learn skills to improve the quality of their lives.

Hormonal Factors

Many hormones are known to influence mood; however, it is beyond the current scope of this chapter to address all of them. Instead, the focus will be on the effects of the thyroid and adrenal hormones.

Low Thyroid Function

Depression is often a first or early manifestation of thyroid disease, as even subtle decreases in available thyroid hormone are suspected of producing symptoms.[12,13] The link between low thyroid function (hypothyroidism) and depression is well known in medical circles, but whether the low thyroid function is a result of depression or the depression is a result of low thyroid function remains to be answered. It is probably a combination. Please see the chapter "Hypothyroidism" for more information on determining thyroid function and promoting function when needed.

Stress and Adrenal Function

As with the thyroid gland, altered function of the adrenal gland is closely associated with depression. Often this dysfunction is the result of chronic stress—a major factor to consider in depression. It is critical to develop a positive way of dealing with the stress of modern life. See the chapter "Stress Management" for more information.

A laboratory technique that many nutritionally oriented physicians use to assess a patient's level of and response to stress is the adrenal stress index. This test measures the level of the adrenal hormones cortisol and dehydroepiandrosterone (DHEA) in the saliva. The typical pattern found in depression is an elevated morning cortisol level and a decreased DHEA level.

The elevations in cortisol reflect a disturbance in the control mechanisms for adrenal function that reside in the hypothalamus and pituitary gland located at the center of the brain. Defects in adrenal regulation seen in affective disorders include excessive cortisol secretion (independent of stress responses) and abnormal release of cortisol. Defects in control mechanisms for adrenal hormones and thyroid function are hallmark features of depression.

The brain effects of increased release of natural cortisol by the adrenal gland mirror the effects of synthetic cortisones such as prednisone: depression, mania, nervousness, insomnia, and, at high levels, schizophrenia. The effects of cortisol on mood is related to its activation of tryptophan oxygenase. This activation results in shunting of tryptophan to the kynurenine pathway at the expense of serotonin and melatonin synthesis.[14] The significance of this shunting is described below.

Environmental Toxins

Heavy metals (lead, mercury, cadmium, arsenic, nickel, and aluminum) as well as solvents (cleaning materials, formaldehyde, toluene, benzene, etc.), pesticides, and herbicides have an affinity for nervous tissue, where they are particularly damaging. As a result, a variety of psychological and neurological symptoms can occur, including depression, headaches, mental confusion, mental illness, tingling in extremities, abnormal nerve reflexes, and other signs of impaired nervous system function.[15–17]

History of exposure and urinary challenge testing are good screening mechanisms for environmental toxicity. Challenge testing employs a chelating agent—such as DMSA (meso-2,3-dimercaptosuccinic acid), which binds to lead; or DMPS (2,3-dimercapto-1-propane sulfonate), which binds to mercury—and promotes its excretion in the urine. These mobilization tests measure the level of toxic metal excreted in the urine for a period of 6 hours after taking the chelating agent.

For more information on dealing with environmental toxins, see the chapter "Detoxification and Internal Cleansing."

Diet and Lifestyle

A health-promoting lifestyle and diet are important in the treatment of depression. It is particularly important to stop smoking and decrease the consumption of alcohol, sugar, and caffeine. These lifestyle changes, coupled with regular exercise and a healthful diet, are more than likely to produce better clinical results than antidepressant drugs, with no side effects.

Alcohol

Alcohol is a brain depressant that increases adrenal hormone output, interferes with many brain cell processes, and disrupts normal sleep cycles. Chronic alcohol ingestion will deplete a number of nutrients, all of which will disrupt mood. Alcohol ingestion also leads to hypoglycemia. The resultant drop in blood sugar produces a craving for sugar because it can quickly elevate blood sugar. Unfortunately, increased sugar consumption ultimately aggravates the hypoglycemia. Hypoglycemia aggravates the mental and emotional problems of the alcoholic. Treatment options that can address both the depression and the addiction of the individual simultaneously are best.[18] Supplementation with selenium in alcoholics can improve mood stability and help change drinking habits as well (see the section below on selenium).

Caffeine

Although caffeine is a well-known stimulant, the intensity of response to caffeine varies greatly, with people who are prone to feeling depressed or anxious tending to be especially sensitive to caffeine. The term *caffeinism* is used to describe a clinical syndrome similar to generalized anxiety and panic disorders; its symptoms include depression, nervousness, palpitations, irritability, and recurrent headache.[19]

Several studies have looked at caffeine intake and depression. For example, one study found that among healthy college students, those who drank moderate or high amounts of coffee scored higher on a depression scale than did low users. Interestingly, the moderate and high coffee drinkers also tended to have significantly lower academic performance.[20] Several other studies have shown that depressed patients tend to consume fairly high amounts of caffeine (e.g., >700 mg per day).[21,22] In addition, caffeine intake has been positively correlated with the degree of mental illness in psychiatric patients.[23,24]

The combination of caffeine and refined sugar seems to be even worse than either substance consumed alone. Several studies have found an association between this combination and depression. In one of the most interesting studies, 21 women and 2 men responded to an advertisement requesting volunteers "who feel depressed and don't know why, often feel tired even though they sleep a lot, are very moody, and generally seem to feel bad most of the time."[25] After baseline psychological testing, the subjects were placed on a caffeine- and sucrose-free diet for one week. The subjects who reported substantial improvement were then challenged in a double-blind fashion. The subjects took either a capsule containing caffeine and a Kool-Aid drink sweetened with sugar or a capsule containing cellulose and a Kool-Aid drink sweetened with NutraSweet. Each challenge lasted up to six days. About 50% of test subjects taking caffeine and sucrose became depressed during the test period.

Another study using a format similar to the Kool-Aid study described earlier found that 7 of 16 depressed patients were depressed with the caffeine and sucrose challenge but symptom free during the caffeine- and sucrose-free diet and cellulose and NutraSweet test period.[26]

The average American consumes 150 to 225 mg caffeine per day, or roughly the amount of caffeine in one to two cups of coffee. Although most people appear to tolerate this amount, some people are more sensitive to the effects of caffeine than others. Even small amounts of caffeine, as found in decaffeinated coffee, are enough to affect some people adversely. Anyone with depression or any psychological disorder should avoid caffeine completely.

Exercise

Regular exercise may be the most powerful natural antidepressant available. In fact, many of the beneficial effects of exercise noted in the prevention of heart disease may be related just as much to its ability to improve mood as to its improvement of cardiovascular function.[27] Furthermore, obesity is associated with depression.[28] Various clinical studies have clearly indicated that exercise has profound antidepressant effects.[29] These studies have shown that increased participation in exercise, sports, and physical activities is strongly associated with decreased symptoms of anxiety, depression, and malaise. Furthermore, people who participate in regular exercise have higher self-esteem, feel better, and are much happier than people who do not exercise.

Much of the mood-elevating effect of exercise may be attributed to the fact that regular exercise has been shown to increase the level of endorphins, which are directly correlated with mood.[30] One of the most interesting studies that examined the role of exercise and endorphins in depression compared the beta-endorphin levels and depression profiles of 10 joggers with those of 10 sedentary men of the same age. The 10 sedentary men tested were more depressed, perceived greater stress in their lives, and had a higher level of cortisol and lower levels of beta-endorphins. As the researchers stated, this "reaffirms that depression is very sensitive to exercise and helps firm up a biochemical link between physical activity and depression."[31]

At least 100 clinical studies have now evaluated the efficacy of an exercise program in the treatment of depression. In an analysis of 64 studies conducted before 1980, physical fitness training was shown to relieve depression and improve self-esteem and work behavior.[32] In fact, exercise can be as effective as other antidepressants, including drugs and psychotherapy.[33–35]

The best exercises are either strength training (weight lifting) or aerobic activities such as walking briskly, jogging, bicycling, cross-country skiing, swimming, aerobic dance, and racket sports.

Diet

The dietary guidelines for depression are identical to the dietary guidelines for optimal health (see the chapter "A Health-Promoting Diet"). It is now a well-established fact that certain dietary practices cause a wide range of diseases, while others prevent them. Quite simply, a health-promoting diet provides optimal levels of all known nutrients and low levels of food components that are detrimental to health, such as sugar, saturated fats, cholesterol, salt, and food additives. A health-promoting diet is rich in whole, unprocessed foods. It is especially high in plant foods such as fruits, vegetables, grains, beans, seeds, and nuts, as these foods contain not only valuable nutrients but also additional compounds that have remarkable health-promoting properties. Although no one diet is a perfect fit for everyone, a four-and-a-half-year study of more than 10,000 people reported that those who ate a healthful Mediterranean diet were about half as likely to develop depression as those who said they did not stick to the diet.[36]

Elements of the Mediterranean Diet

High ratio of monounsaturated fatty acids to saturated fatty acids*

Moderate alcohol intake

High intake of legumes*

High intake of cereal (such as bread)

High intake of fruits and nuts*

High intake of vegetables

Low intake of meat and meat products

Moderate intake of milk and dairy products

High fish intake

* Elements mostly correlated with low depression risk

Stabilizing Blood Sugar Levels

One of the key dietary goals is to ensure blood sugar stability, as the brain requires a constant supply of glucose. In particular, hypoglycemia (low blood sugar) must be avoided. Symptoms of hypoglycemia can range from mild to severe and can include the following:

- Depression, anxiety, irritability, and other psychological disturbances
- Fatigue
- Headache
- Blurred vision
- Mental confusion

Several studies have shown hypoglycemia to be common in depressed individuals.[37–39] A study of six countries showed a highly significant correlation between sugar consumption and the annual rate of depression.[39] Simply eliminating refined carbohydrate from the diet is occasionally all that is necessary for effective therapy in patients who have depression due to reactive hypoglycemia.

Nutrition

A deficiency of any single nutrient can alter brain function and lead to depression, anxiety, and other mental disorders. However, the role of nutrient deficiency is just the tip of the iceberg with regard to the effect of nutrients on the brain and mood. Melvin Werbach, M.D., author of *Nutritional Influences on Mental Illness*, wrote:[40]

It is clear that nutrition can powerfully influence cognition, emotion, and behavior. It is also clear that the effects of classical nutritional deficiency diseases upon mental function constitute only a small part of a rapidly expanding list of interfaces between nutrition and the mind. Even in the absence of laboratory validation of nutritional deficiencies, numerous studies

Behavioral Effects of Some Vitamin Deficiencies	
DEFICIENT VITAMIN	**BEHAVIORAL EFFECTS**
Thiamine	Korsakoff's psychosis, mental depression, apathy, anxiety, irritability
Riboflavin	Depression, irritability
Niacin	Apathy, anxiety, depression, hyperirritability, mania, memory deficits, delirium, organic dementia, emotional lability
Biotin	Depression, extreme lassitude, somnolence
Pantothenic acid	Restlessness, irritability, depression, fatigue
B_6	Depression, irritability, sensitivity to sound
Folic acid	Forgetfulness, insomnia, apathy, irritability, depression, psychosis, delirium, dementia
B_{12}	Psychotic states, depression, irritability, confusion, memory loss, hallucinations, delusions, paranoia
Vitamin C	Lassitude, hypochondriasis, depression, hysteria
Vitamin D	Depression, fatigue, seasonal affective disorder, cognitive impairment, memory loss
Omega-3 fatty acids	Depression, poor concentration, memory loss

utilizing rigorous scientific designs have demonstrated impressive benefits from nutritional supplementation.

A high-potency multiple vitamin and mineral supplement provides a good nutritional foundation on which to build. In selecting a formula, it is important to make sure that it provides the full range of vitamins and minerals. Deficiencies of a number of nutrients are quite common in depressed individuals. The most common deficiencies are folic acid, vitamin B_{12}, and vitamin B_6. The significance of these deficiencies is discussed below.

Folic Acid and Vitamin B_{12}

Folic acid and vitamin B_{12} function together in many biochemical processes. Folic acid deficiency is the most common nutrient deficiency in the world. In studies of depressed patients, 31 to 35% have been shown to be deficient in folic acid.[41–44] In elderly patients this percentage may be even higher. Studies have found that among elderly patients admitted to a psychiatric ward, the proportion with folic acid deficiency ranges from 35 to 92.6%.[45,46] Depression is the most common symptom of a folic acid deficiency. In the past, vitamin B_{12} deficiency has been less common than folic acid deficiency; nonetheless, it can also cause depression, especially in the elderly.[47,48] The fortifying of the food supply with folic acid has reduced the incidence of deficiency and may actually accentuate the effects of vitamin B_{12} deficiency. Correcting folic acid and vitamin B_{12} deficiencies results in a dramatic improvement in mood.

Folic acid, vitamin B_{12}, and a form of the amino acid methionine known as SAM-e (S-adenosyl-methionine) function as "methyl donors"—they carry and donate methyl molecules to important brain compounds including neurotransmitters. SAM-e is the major

methyl donor in the body. The antidepressant effects of folic acid appear to be a result of raising brain SAM-e content.

One of the key brain compounds dependent on methylation is tetrahydrobiopterin (BH4). This compound functions as an essential coenzyme in the activation of enzymes that manufacture monoamine neurotransmitters such as serotonin and dopamine from their corresponding amino acids. Patients with recurrent depression have been shown to have reduced BH4 synthesis, probably as a result of low SAM-e levels. BH4 supplementation has been shown to produce dramatic results in these patients.[49] Unfortunately, BH4 is not currently available commercially. However, since BH4 synthesis is stimulated by folic acid, vitamin B_{12}, and vitamin C, it is possible that increasing these vitamin levels in the brain may stimulate BH4 formation and the synthesis of monoamines such as serotonin.[50]

Some evidence supports the contention that supplementing the diet with folic acid, vitamin C, and vitamin B_{12} can increase BH4 levels. In addition, the folic acid supplementation and the promotion of methylation reactions have been shown to increase the serotonin content.[51–53] The serotonin-elevating effects are undoubtedly responsible for much of the antidepressant effects of folic acid and vitamin B_{12}.

One review of three folate trials involving 247 depressed patients has been published.[54] Two of the studies involving 151 people assessed the use of folate in addition to other treatment and found that adding folate reduced Hamilton Depression Scale (HDS) scores on average by a further 2.65. One of the studies, involving 96 people, assessed the use of folate instead of the antidepressant trazodone. This study did not find a significant benefit from the use of folate. Although the authors of this analysis considered these data "limited," they acknowledged the potential role of folate as a supplement to treat depression. No side effects or toxicities were noted in any of the studies reviewed.

Typically the daily dosages of folic acid in the antidepressant clinical studies have been high: 15 to 50 mg.[55] We do not recommend this dosage level. A dosage of 800 mcg of folic acid and 800 mcg of vitamin B_{12} should be sufficient in most circumstances to prevent deficiencies. Folic acid supplementation should always be accompanied by vitamin B_{12} supplementation to prevent folic acid from masking or aggravating a vitamin B_{12} deficiency.

Vitamin B_6

B_6 levels are typically quite low in depressed patients, especially women taking birth control pills or on hormone replacement therapy for menopausal symptoms.[56–60] Considering the many functions of vitamin B_6 in the brain, including the fact that it is absolutely essential in the manufacture of all monoamines, it is likely that many of the many people taking antidepressants may be suffering depression simply as a result of low vitamin B_6. Patients with low B_6 status usually respond well to supplementation. The typical effective dosage is 50 to 100 mg.

Zinc

Zinc serves as the mineral cofactor in more than 70 enzymes in the body.[61] Not surprisingly, a growing body of evidence implicates low levels of zinc in mood disorders. Interestingly, it has been shown that depressed patients who have low baseline levels of zinc experience increases in these concentrations in the hippocampus and other brain regions after being given prescription antidepressant therapies.[62,63]

One small, placebo-controlled, double-blind pilot study of zinc supplementation in antidepressant therapy was conducted with patients who were diagnosed with major depression. Six patients received 25 mg zinc supplementation per day, while eight patients took a placebo. These patients were also treated with standard antidepressant therapy such as tricyclic antidepressants and selective serotonin reuptake inhibitors (SSRIs). Using standard scales to assess the efficacy of these antidepressant therapies, the researchers found that zinc supplementation significantly reduced depression scores after 6 and 12 weeks of supplementation when compared with a placebo.[64] Although this was a small trial, it seems reasonable to use zinc as part of a multiple vitamin and mineral supplement.

Selenium

Low selenium status contributes to depressed mood, whereas high dietary or supplementary selenium has been shown to improve mood. Research has consistently reported that low selenium status was associated with a significantly increased incidence of depression, anxiety, confusion, and hostility.[65,66]

Chromium

Chromium functions in helping insulin as well as serotonin work properly. A small double-blind study of chromium picolinate was conducted in 15 patients with unusual types of major depressive disorder. Ten patients started with a dose of 400 mcg per day, which was increased to 600 mcg for the remainder of the study.[67] The other five patients took a placebo. Of the patients on chromium, 70% responded positively to the treatment, vs. 0% of the placebo patients. Other outcomes were consistent with greater effect of chromium. Three patients on chromium failed to show any improvement. The chromium picolinate was well tolerated. Another successful study of eight patients with depression found some improvements as well.[68]

Vitamin D

Low levels of vitamin D could be involved in depression in several ways given this vitamin's importance in the human brain.[69] In a study of 441 overweight people vitamin D levels were strongly associated with depression.[70] Those with vitamin D levels below 16 mcg/dl were shown to be more depressed than people with higher vitamin D levels. When these subjects with low vitamin D levels were given vitamin D (20,000 IU or 40,000 IU per week) or a placebo, those given 40,000 IU had a 33% reduction in depression scores, those given 20,000 IU had a 20% reduction, and the placebo group had a 5% decrease. In another study, involving more than 12,000 subjects, low vitamin D levels were associated with depression.[71] We recommend determination of vitamin D levels for people with a history of depression.

With the significant epidemiological evidence documenting a strong association between vitamin D deficiency and depression (as well as dementia, memory loss, and a whole host of other indications of impaired brain function) it was inevitable that researchers would try supplemental vitamin D for depression. While the research is still early, several studies have now shown success. In general, the lower the person's vitamin D level, the more improvement is experienced with supplementation.[72] In addition, the greater the increase, the greater the benefit. Typical effective dosages were in the range of 50,000 IU per week, with low levels of supplementation showing inconsistent results. A single dose of 50,000 IU once a year was not found effective.[73]

Omega-3 Fatty Acids

An insufficiency of the long-chain omega-3 fatty acids eicosapentaenoic acid (EPA) and docosahexaenoic acid (DHA) has been linked to depression.[74] Studies have also reported that countries with high rates of fish oil consumption have low rates of depressive disorder. This may be related to the impact of dietary fatty acids on the phospholipid composition of brain cell membranes. Although it is thought that the cell is programmed to selectively incorporate the different fatty acids it needs to maintain optimal function, a lack of essential fatty acids (particularly the omega-3 oils) and an excess of saturated fats and animal fatty acids lead to the formation of cell membranes that have much less fluidity than normal.

A relative deficiency of essential fatty acids in cellular membranes substantially impairs cell membrane function. Because the basic function of the cell membrane is to serve as a selective barrier that regulates the passage of molecules into and out of the cell, a disturbance of structure or function disrupts homeostasis. The medical literature has demonstrated that there are changes in fatty acid levels in the red blood cells of depressed patients and in serum fatty acid composition in depressive disorder.[75]

Because the brain is the richest source of fats in the human body and proper nerve cell function is critically dependent on proper membrane fluidity, alterations in membrane fluidity affect behavior, mood, and mental function. Studies have shown that the physical properties of brain cell membranes (including fluidity) directly influence neurotransmitter synthesis, signal transmission, uptake of serotonin and other neurotransmitters, neurotransmitter binding, and the activity of monoamine oxidase. All of these factors have been implicated in depression and other psychological disturbances.

In one small study, 20 patients diagnosed with major depressive disorder participated in a four-week, double-blind evaluation of either a placebo or EPA added to their ongoing antidepressant therapy. The effect of EPA was significant from week two of treatment, similar to the time course for effectiveness of antidepressant medications. The effect of the placebo was minimal. Item analysis showed that EPA also reduced core depressive symptoms such as depressed mood, guilt feelings, and feelings of worthlessness, as well as insomnia.[76]

Omega-3 fatty acids may reduce the development of depression just as they reduce the development of coronary artery disease.[77] The evidence supporting this statement includes:

- The quantity and type of dietary fats consumed influence serum lipids and alter the biophysical and biochemical properties of cell membranes.

- Epidemiological studies in various countries and the United States have indicated that decreased consumption of omega-3 fatty acids correlates with increasing rates of depression.

- A consistent association between depression and coronary artery disease also exists.

S-adenosyl-methionine (SAM-e)
SAM-e is involved in the methylation of important brain chemicals, including neurotransmitters and phospholipids such as phosphatidylcholine and phosphatidylserine. Normally, the brain manufactures all the SAM-e it needs from the amino acid methionine. However, SAM-e synthesis is impaired in depressed patients. Supplementing the diet with SAM-e in depressed patients results in increased levels of serotonin, dopamine, and phosphatidylserine, and improved binding of neurotransmitters to receptor sites. This produces increased serotonin and dopamine activity and improved brain cell membrane fluidity, and thus significant clinical improvement.[78–80]

The results of a number of clinical studies suggest that SAM-e is one of the most effective natural antidepressants. Unfortunately, its use is still limited, owing to its high price. Many clinical trials used injectable SAM-e. However, more recent studies using a new oral preparation at a dosage of 400 mg four times per day (1,600 mg total) have demonstrated that SAM-e is just as effective orally. SAM-e is better tolerated and has a quicker onset of antidepressant action than typical antidepressant drugs. Overall, in double-blind studies comparing SAM-e with antidepressant drugs, 76% of the SAM-e group showed significant improvements in mood compared with only 61% in the drug group.[81–90]

No significant side effects have been reported with oral SAM-e. However, because SAM-e can cause nausea and vomiting in some people, it is recommended that it be started at a dosage of 200 mg twice per day for the first day, and increased to 400 mg twice per day on day 3, then to 400 mg three times per day on day 10, and finally to the full dosage of 400 mg four times per day after 20 days.

Individuals with bipolar (manic) depression should not take SAM-e. Because of SAM-e's antidepressant activity, these individuals are susceptible to experiencing hypomania or mania. This effect is exclusive to some individuals with bipolar depression.

Food Allergies

Depression and fatigue have been linked to food allergies for more than 65 years. In 1930, Rowe coined the term *allergic toxemia* to describe a syndrome that included the symptoms of depression, fatigue, muscle and joint aches, drowsiness, difficulty in concentration, and nervousness.[91] Although the term is not used anymore, food allergies still play a major role in many cases of depression.[92]

Tryptophan

For more than 30 years, L-tryptophan was used by millions of people in the United States and around the world safely and effectively for insomnia and depression. But in October 1989, some people taking tryptophan started reporting strange symptoms to physicians—severe muscle and joint pain, high fever, weakness, swelling of the arms and legs, and shortness of breath.[93] It was dubbed *eosinophilia-myalgia syndrome* (EMS).

Laboratory studies showed that the blood of subjects with EMS contained a high level of eosinophils. In patients with EMS, eosinophil levels rose to greater than $1,000/mm^3$, roughly double the normal level, and the proportion of eosinophils often increased to levels above 30% of white cells, whereas the normal level is below 5%.

The problem with such severe elevations in eosinophils is that these white blood cells contain packets that have high levels of histamine and other allergic and inflammatory compounds. When the eosinophils release these compounds, this leads to intense symptoms of an allergic and inflammatory nature (e.g., severe muscle and joint pain, high fever, weakness, swelling of the arms and legs, skin rashes, and shortness of breath)—the same symptoms as those experienced by people with EMS. It was suspected that one or more newly introduced contaminants that activated eosinophils and other white blood cells had to be the reason behind EMS because L-tryptophan had been used successfully by more than 30 million people worldwide without side effects.

Detailed analysis of all evidence by the Centers for Disease Control and Prevention (CDC) led to the conclusion that the cause of the EMS epidemic could be traced to one Japanese manufacturer, Showa Denko.[94,95] Of the six Japanese companies supplying L-tryptophan to the United States, Showa Denko was the largest, supplying 50% to 60%. The L-tryptophan was used not only as a nutritional supplement but also in infant formulas and nutrient mixtures used for intravenous feeding.

The L-tryptophan produced from October 1988 to June 1989 by Showa Denko became contaminated with substances now linked to EMS owing to changes in the filtration process. Examination of the pre-filtered material indicated that it had no detectable levels of the impurities linked to EMS. Somehow the filtration process produced the contaminants.

Although the epidemic of EMS during the last half of 1989 was clearly related to the contaminated L-tryptophan produced by Showa Denko, there have been a handful of other reported cases of EMS in people who never took L-tryptophan and in people who took L-tryptophan before the contaminated batch manufactured by Showa Denko hit the shelves. It is likely that in these earlier reports of EMS-like illnesses among L-tryptophan users, the subjects were also using contaminated L-tryptophan and they also had a predisposition to EMS (discussed later).[96,97] This conclusion is based on the fact that uncontaminated tryptophan has never produced EMS. Clearly, it is absolutely essential that uncontaminated L-tryptophan be used to avoid the possibility of EMS.

The total number of reported cases of EMS in the United States eventually reached 1,511, with 36 deaths.[94–97] An interesting aspect of the entire L-tryptophan catastrophe is that it did not affect more people. Based on very detailed studies, it was concluded that EMS affected 144 out of every 100,000 men and 268 out of every 100,000 women taking L-tryptophan.[98] If 50% of these L-tryptophan users were taking Showa Denko's L-tryptophan, we can assume that EMS affected 72 of every 100,000 men and

134 of every 100,000 women taking contaminated L-tryptophan. In other words, roughly 1 of every 250 people who took the contaminated L-tryptophan developed EMS.

The obvious question is why not everyone taking the contaminated L-tryptophan experienced EMS. The answer appears to be that only those with an abnormal activation of the kynurenine pathway reacted to the contaminant.[99] Kynurenine and its metabolites (especially quinolic acid) are linked to other EMS-related illnesses as well, including toxic oil syndrome, one of the largest food-related epidemics to date. This syndrome occurred in Spain during May 1991. It affected more than 20,000 people and caused more than 12,000 hospitalizations. It was caused by the ingestion of canola oil contaminated with a compound similar to one found in the contaminated Showa Denko L-tryptophan.[100]

An interesting finding from studies conducted by researchers from the Centers for Disease Control was that people who took a multivitamin preparation were extended some protection against EMS.[101] When regular vitamin users did develop EMS, it was less severe than the EMS experienced by those who didn't use vitamins. A likely explanation for this occurrence is that either the vitamins (particularly vitamin B_6 and niacin) shunted tryptophan metabolism away from the kynurenine pathway or the contaminants were somehow metabolized by vitamin-dependent enzymes.

Tryptophan in Depression

Uncontaminated L-tryptophan eventually returned to the marketplace, though we prefer 5-HTP (discussed below). The basic theory of tryptophan supplementation in depression (and insomnia) is that it will increase the level of serotonin and melatonin in the brain. This theory is supported by considerable evidence that many depressed individuals have low tryptophan and serotonin levels. Unfortunately, supplementation with L-tryptophan in depressed patients has produced mixed results in published clinical trials. In only two out of eight studies comparing L-tryptophan with a placebo was L-tryptophan shown to be more effective than the placebo. But, interestingly, 9 of 11 studies comparing L-tryptophan with conventional antidepressant drugs showed no difference.[102–107]

Among the many factors to consider when looking at these studies are study size, severity of depression, duration, and dosage. In addition, a number of factors such as hormones (e.g., estrogen and cortisol), as well as tryptophan itself, stimulate the activity of tryptophan oxygenase, with the result that tryptophan is converted to kynurenine and less tryptophan is delivered to the brain.

In summary, L-tryptophan is only modestly effective in the treatment of depression when used alone.[108] In order to gain any real benefit from L-tryptophan, it must be used along with vitamin B_6 and the niacinamide form of vitamin B_3 to help block the kynurenine pathway to provide better results. Better yet is the use of 5-HTP.

5-Hydroxytryptophan (5-HTP)

Tryptophan must be converted to 5-hydroxytryptophan before it is metabolized to serotonin. Unlike tryptophan, 5-HTP cannot be converted to kynurenine and easily crosses the blood-brain barrier. As a result, while only 3% of an oral dose of L-tryptophan is converted to serotonin, more than 70% of an oral dose of 5-HTP is converted to serotonin. In addition to increasing serotonin levels, 5-HTP causes an increase in endorphin and catecholamine levels. Numerous double-blind studies have shown that 5-HTP is as effective as SSRIs and tricyclic antidepressants and is less expensive, better tolerated, and associated with fewer and much milder side effects.[109–113]

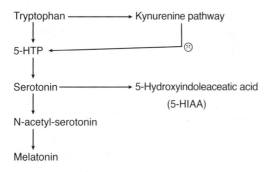

Tryptophan Metabolism

Some of the first clinical studies on 5-HTP for the treatment of depression began in the early 1970s in Japan. These patients received 5-HTP at dosages ranging from 50 to 300 mg per day. The researchers observed a quick response (within two weeks) in more than half of the patients. More than 70% of the patients either experienced complete relief or were significantly improved, and none experienced significant side effects. An interesting aspect in two of these studies was the fact that 5-HTP was shown to be effective in some patients (50% in one study, 35% in another) who had not responded positively to any other antidepressant.[114,115]

The most detailed of the Japanese studies was conducted in 1978.[116] The study enrolled 59 patients with depression: 30 male and 29 female. The groups were mixed in that both unipolar and bipolar depressions were included, along with a number of other subcategories of depression. The severity of the depression in most cases was moderate to severe. Patients received 5-HTP in dosages of 50 or 100 mg three times per day for at least three weeks. The antidepressant activity and clinical effectiveness of 5-HTP were determined by using a rating scale developed by the Clinical Psychopharmacology Research Group in Japan. Results indicated that 5-HTP was helpful in 14 out of 17 patients with unipolar depression and 12 out of 21

patients with bipolar depression. The degree of improvement in most cases ranged from excellent to very good. The results achieved in this study were quite impressive given how rapidly they were achieved. Thirty-two of the 40 patients who responded to 5-HTP did so within the first two weeks of therapy. Typically, in most studies with antidepressant drugs, the benefits are not apparent until after two to four weeks of use. For this reason, the length of a study assessing antidepressant drugs should be at least six weeks because it may take that long to significantly affect brain chemistry in a positive manner. In contrast, many of the studies with 5-HTP were shorter than six weeks because statistically significant results were achieved so soon. However, the longer 5-HTP is used, the better the results. Some people may need to be on 5-HTP for at least two months before experiencing benefits.

The only major side effect noted in this study was mild nausea. The occurrence of nausea due to 5-HTP is actually less frequent than that experienced with other antidepressant drugs (roughly 10% of subjects taking 5-HTP at a dose of 300 mg per day experience nausea compared with about 23% taking Prozac) and about the same as that which occurs with a placebo. Nonetheless, mild nausea may be a natural consequence of elevated serotonin levels with 5-HTP. About 30% of the 5-HTP taken orally is converted to serotonin in the intestinal tract. This can lead to a mild case of nausea. Fortunately, this effect wears off after a few weeks of use.

A 5-HTP dosage of 150 to 300 mg per day is sufficient in most cases. For example, in one study it was shown that 13 out of 18 subjects with depression given 5-HTP at a level of 150 or 300 mg per day experienced good to excellent results.[117] This percentage of responders is quite good, but if the level of serotonin in the blood is viewed as a rough

Level of Serotonin in Blood (ng/ml): Controls, Responders, and Nonresponders		
	BEFORE	**AFTER 1 WEEK** (150 OR 300 MG/DAY 5-HTP)
Normal subjects	150	NA
Responders	78	148
Nonresponders	56	77

indicator of brain serotonin levels, some interesting conclusions can be made (see the table above). In some cases a higher dosage may be necessary.

The measurements above suggest that serotonin levels in depressed individuals are considerably lower than those found in normal subjects and that individuals who respond to 5-HTP show a rise in serotonin to levels consistent with normal subjects. The level of serotonin in those who do not respond to 5-HTP remained quite low. These results imply that nonresponders may require higher dosages to raise serotonin levels or that additional support may be necessary. When higher doses are prescribed, it is important that the 5-HTP be taken in divided dosages not only to reduce the problem with nausea but also because the rate of brain cell uptake of 5-HTP is limited.

The antidepressant effects of 5-HTP were compared with L-tryptophan in the early 1970s.[118] In one study, 45 subjects with depression were given L-tryptophan (5 g per day), 5-HTP (200 mg per day), or a placebo. The patients were matched in clinical features (e.g., age, sex) and severity of depression. The main outcome measure was the Hamilton Depression Scale, the most widely used assessment tool in clinical research on depression.

The HDS score is determined by having the test subject complete a series of questions in which he or she rates the severity of symptoms on a numerical basis, as follows:

0: Not present

1: Present but mild

2: Moderate

3: Severe

4: Very severe

Symptoms assessed by the HDS include depression, feelings of guilt, insomnia, bodily symptoms of depression (gastrointestinal disturbance, headaches, muscle aches, heart palpitations), and anxiety. The HDS is popular in research because it provides a good assessment of the overall symptoms of depression. The table below shows the results of the study.

A review of head-to-head comparison studies showed that 5-HTP, at a dosage of 200 mg per day, produced therapeutic improvement on a par with tricyclic antidepressant drugs. Research has also shown that

Hamilton Depression Scale Scores from a Comparative Study of 5-HTP, Tryptophan, and Placebo			
	5-HTP	**TRYPTOPHAN**	**PLACEBO**
Score at beginning of study	26	25	23
Score at end of 30-day study	9	15	19

combining 5-HTP with clomipramine and other types of antidepressant drugs produces better results than any of the compounds given alone.[110] For example, in one study, 5-HTP combined with a monoamine oxidase (MAO) inhibitor demonstrated significant advantages compared with the MAO inhibitor alone.[118] This line of research suggests that 5-HTP might also be used in conjunction with Saint-John's-wort extract and ginkgo biloba extract, two herbal medicines with proven antidepressant activity.

Because 5-HTP was expensive in 1972, researchers developed a test to determine who was most likely to respond to it, so that it would not be wasted on people who were unlikely to respond. The patients in the test first had a spinal tap to measure the level of 5-hydroxyindoleacetic acid (5-HIAA, the breakdown product of serotonin) in the cerebrospinal fluid (CSF). The drug probenecid, which prevents the transport of 5-HIAA from the CSF to the bloodstream, was given for the next three days. As a result of this blocking action, the amount of serotonin produced over a four-day period could be calculated by a repeat spinal tap. Since the 5-HIAA could not leave the CSF, it accumulated and provided a measure of serotonin manufacture.[119,120]

The researchers discovered that the average level of 5-HIAA after three days of probenecid was significantly lower in depressed individuals than in controls matched for age, sex, and weight. This low level of serotonin reflected a decreased rate of manufacture within the brain. They also found that 5-HTP was most effective in patients with a low 5-HIAA response to three days of probenecid. In other words, 5-HTP is most effective as an antidepressant when the amount of serotonin manufactured in the brain is reduced.

As stated earlier, 5-HTP often produces good results in patients who are unresponsive to antidepressant drugs. One of the more impressive studies involved 99 patients described as suffering from "therapy-resistant" depression.[109] These patients had not responded to any previous therapy, including all available antidepressant drugs and electroconvulsive therapy. These therapy-resistant patients received 5-HTP at dosages averaging 200 mg per day (range: 50 to 600 mg). Complete recovery was seen in 43 of the 99 patients, and significant improvement was noted in 8 more. Such significant improvement in patients suffering from long-standing, unresponsive depression is quite impressive, prompting the author of another study to note:[121]

> 5-HTP merits a place in the front ranks of antidepressants instead of being used as a last resort. I have never in 20 years used an agent that (1) was effective so quickly; (2) restored patients so completely to the persons they had been and their partners had known; and (3) was so entirely without side effects.

A 1987 review article on 5-HTP in depression highlighted the need for well-designed, double-blind, head-to-head studies of 5-HTP vs. standard antidepressant drugs.[110] Although 5-HTP was viewed as an antidepressant agent with few side effects, the authors of this review felt that the big question to answer was how 5-HTP compared with the new breed of antidepressant drugs, SSRIs such as Prozac, Paxil, and Zoloft. In 1991 a double-blind study comparing 5-HTP with an SSRI, fluvoxamine (Luvox), was conducted in Switzerland.[112] Fluvoxamine is used primarily in the United States as a treatment for obsessive-compulsive disorder, an anxiety disorder that affects an estimated 5 million Americans. Fluvoxamine exerts antidepressant activity comparable to (if not better than) other SSRIs such as Prozac, Zoloft, and Paxil.

In the study, subjects received either 5-HTP (100 mg) or fluvoxamine (50 mg) three times per day for 6 weeks. The assessment methods used to judge effectiveness included the HDS, a self-assessment depression scale, and a physician's assessment. As seen in the data below, the percentage decrease in depression was slightly better in the 5-HTP group (60.7 vs. 56.1%). 5-HTP was quicker-acting than the fluvoxamine, and a higher percentage of patients responded to 5-HTP than to fluvoxamine.

One of the most important advantages of 5-HTP may be its ability to not just reduce insomnia but improve the quality of sleep. By contrast, antidepressant drugs greatly disrupt sleep processes.

The data clearly show that 5-HTP is equal to or better than standard antidepressant drugs, and the side effects are much less severe. In the study comparing 5-HTP with fluvoxamine, the two treatment groups did not differ significantly in the number of patients experiencing adverse events, but the degree of severity was highly significant: fluvoxamine predominantly produced moderate to severe side effects, while 5-HTP produced primarily mild side effects. The most common side effects with 5-HTP were nausea, heartburn, and gastrointestinal problems (flatulence, feelings of fullness, and rumbling sensations).

Botanical Medicines

Saint-John's-Wort

Extracts of Saint-John's-wort (*Hypericum perforatum*) standardized for hypericin are the most thoroughly researched natural antidepressants. More than 30 double-blind, randomized trials involving more than 2,200 patients with mild to moderately severe depression have shown that standardized Saint-John's-wort extracts yield excellent results with far fewer side effects than standard antidepressant medications, lower cost, and greater patient satisfaction.[122–126]

In these studies, Saint-John's-wort extract was shown to produce improvements in many psychological symptoms:

- Depression
- Anxiety
- Apathy
- Sleep disturbances
- Insomnia
- Anorexia
- Feelings of worthlessness

Ginkgo Biloba Extract (GBE)

GBE exerts good antidepressant effects, especially in patients older than 50. Researchers became interested in the antidepressant effects of GBE as a result of the improvement in mood reported by patients suffering from cerebrovascular insufficiency who were

Improvement in Specific Depression Symptoms		
SYMPTOM	**5-HTP (%)**	**FLUVOXAMINE (%)**
Depressed mood	65.7	61.8
Anxiety	58.2	48.3
Physical symptoms	47.6	37.8
Insomnia	61.7	55.9

THE DEATH OF AN HERBAL SHINING STAR

In the late 1990s the brightest star in herbal medicine was without question Saint-John's-wort extract. In fact, in Germany it was estimated that in 1996 physicians prescribed Saint-John's-wort extract eight times more frequently than the drug Prozac for the treatment of depression. In the United States, on June 27, 1997, the television news show *20/20* aired a segment called "Nature's Rx: Using Herb St. John's Wort to Treat Depression." This airing brought considerable attention to not only Saint-John's-wort extract but also the entire herbal medicine category. The increased popularity of this safe and effective natural product certainly did not go unnoticed by drug manufacturing executives.

In April 2001, however, a blaring headline on the cover of *Time* magazine stated "St. John's What?" The article went on to highlight the results of a study demonstrating that Saint-John's-wort didn't work any better than a placebo.[127] However, this particular study featured 200 patients who had had severe depression for at least two years, not the typical mild to moderate depression in which other studies had clearly demonstrated significant benefits from Saint-

John's-wort. Many experts felt that the entire study seemed as if the researchers were stacking the deck against Saint-John's-wort. Interestingly, funding for the study came from the giant drug company Pfizer, the maker of Zoloft—the number one antidepressant drug at the time. Also interesting is that usually a study of this type would have compared the Saint-John's-wort group and the placebo group with a third group taking a well-known antidepressant drug. The failure to include that third group indicated to many that the researchers knew that this patient group was not likely to respond to the antidepressant drug either.

Since then, there have been several double-blind studies of Saint-John's-wort extract comparing it with standard SSRIs including Zoloft in mild to moderate depression.[122,128,129] These studies have shown that Saint-John's-wort is more effective and has fewer side effects. The message from all of this research is that for severe cases of depression, Saint-John's-wort may not be strong enough. These patients may be better off focusing on cognitive therapy and other means to improve their mood.

---

treated with ginkgo in double-blind studies.[130–133] In a recent double-blind study, 40 older patients (ranging in age from 51 to 78) with depression who had not benefited fully from standard antidepressant drugs were given either 80 mg GBE three times per day or a placebo.[134] By the end of the fourth week of the study, the total score on the HDS was reduced on average from 14 to 7. At the end of the 8-week study, the total score in the GBE group had dropped to 4.5. In comparison, the placebo group's score dropped only from 14 to 13. This study indicates that GBE can be used with standard antidepressants and may enhance their effectiveness, particularly in older patients.

In addition to human studies, GBE has also demonstrated antidepressant effects in a number of animal models. The most

interesting of these studies demonstrated that GBE was able to counteract one of the major changes in brain chemistry associated with aging—the reduction in the number of serotonin receptor sites.[135] Because of this reduction, the elderly are typically more susceptible to depression, impaired mental function, insomnia, and sleep disturbances. The study was designed to determine whether GBE could alter the number of serotonin receptors in old (24-month-old) and young (4-month-old) rats. At the beginning of the study, the older rats had 22% fewer serotonin binding sites compared with the younger rats. The results of treatment with GBE for 21 consecutive days demonstrated that there was no change in receptor binding in young rats, but in the older rats there was a statistically significant increase (33%) in the number of serotonin binding sites. These results suggest that GBE may counteract at least some, if not all, of the age-dependent decline in serotonin binding sites in the aging human brain as well.

Saffron

Saffron (*Crocus sativus*) is the world's most expensive spice because the stigma (the portion of the flower used for cooking) must be hand-picked off the flower. To obtain one pound of saffron, at least 50,000 flowers are needed. Iran is the world's largest producer of saffron and has been investing in research into its potential medicinal uses. In Persian traditional medicine, saffron is used for depression. Studies have shown that saffron is safe and effective for mild to moderate depression, and one study showed efficacy equal to Prozac.[136,137] The petal of the saffron crocus is much less expensive than the stigma and has also recently been shown to be effective in the treatment of mild to moderate depression. In the first double-blind study, 40 patients with mild depression received 30 mg per day of extract of saffron petals or a placebo for 6 weeks.[138] Results showed a significant reduction in depression with the saffron extract. In another study, 40 patients with mild to moderate depression were randomly assigned to receive saffron petal extract (15 mg morning and evening) or fluoxetine (Prozac, 10 mg morning and evening) in an eight-week study.[139] At the end of trial, the saffron was found to be as effective as the drug.

Lavender

Lavender (*Lavender officinalis*) has long been used by herbalists as a treatment for anxiety, nervous exhaustion, and depression. Recently, this historical use has been verified in a detailed double-blind clinical trial.[140] The findings of the study indicated that taking a moderate amount of lavender can reduce feelings of depression, anxiety, and helplessness. In the study, 45 adults between the ages of 18 and 54 who were diagnosed with depression were assigned to one of three groups. The groups received either (1) lavender extract plus a placebo tablet, (2) a placebo extract plus 100 mg per day of the antidepressant drug imipramine, or (3) lavender extract and 100 mg per day of imipramine. The study lasted for four weeks, and scores on a depression rating scale were evaluated initially and then weekly after the start of treatment. What the results indicated was that the lavender extract was just as effective as the drug, but lavender was without the side effects common in drug treatment for depression (dry mouth, weight loss or weight gain, low blood pressure, arrhythmias, and decreased sexual function).

QUICK REVIEW

- **Approximately 17 million Americans suffer true clinical depression each year and over 28 million Americans take antidepressant drugs or anxiety medications.**
- **One of the most powerful techniques to produce the necessary biochemical changes in the brain of depressed individuals is teaching them to be more optimistic.**
- **Low levels of serotonin contribute to depression.**

- It is important to rule out the simple organic factors that are known to contribute to the depression, i.e., nutrient deficiency or excess, drugs (prescription, illicit, alcohol, caffeine, nicotine, etc.), hypoglycemia, consumption, hormonal derangement, allergy, environmental factors, and microbial factors.
- Cognitive therapy has been shown to be as effective as antidepressant drugs in treating moderate depression.
- Depression is often a first or early manifestation of thyroid disease.
- Increased cortisol levels are common in depression.
- Elimination of sugar and caffeine has been shown to produce significant benefits in clinical trials.
- Increased participation in exercise, sports, and physical activities is strongly associated with decreased symptoms of anxiety, depression, and malaise.
- A deficiency of any single nutrient can alter brain function and lead to depression, anxiety, and other mental disorders.
- Hypoglycemia can cause depression.
- An insufficiency of omega-3 oils in the diet has been linked to depression.
- Several double-blind studies have shown 5-hydroxytryptophan (5-HTP) to be as effective as antidepressant drugs but better tolerated and associated with fewer and much milder side effects.
- Extracts of Saint-John's-wort standardized for hypericin (usually 0.3%) are the most thoroughly researched natural antidepressants.
- Over 25 double-blind studies have shown Saint-John's-wort to produce equally good or better results compared with standard antidepressant drugs, but with signficantly fewer side effects.

TREATMENT SUMMARY

Treatment of depression is largely dependent on a few central elements: balancing of errant neurotransmitter levels and optimizing nutrition, lifestyle, and psychological health.

If you wish to discontinue any antidepressant drug, we recommend that you work with your physician on this goal. In general, discontinuing a SSRI has to be done gradually. Stopping too quickly is associated with symptoms such as dizziness, loss of coordination, fatigue, tingling, burning, blurred vision, insomnia, and vivid dreams. Less often, there may be nausea or diarrhea, flu-like symptoms, irritability, anxiety, and crying spells.

To help support patients as they wean themselves off SSRIs, either 5-HTP or Saint-John's-wort extract can be used. A concern when antidepressant drugs are mixed with Saint-John's-wort or 5-HTP is producing what is referred to as "serotonin syndrome," characterized by confusion, fever, shivering, sweating, diarrhea, and muscle spasms. Although it is theoretically possible that combining Saint-John's-wort or 5-HTP with standard antidepressant drugs could produce this syndrome, to our knowledge no one has experienced this syndrome with simultaneous use of Saint-John's-wort extract or 5-HTP and an SSRI. Nonetheless, our recommendation is that when using Saint-John's-wort or 5-HTP in combination with standard antidepressant drugs, you should be closely monitored by your doctor for any symptoms suggestive of the serotonin syndrome. If these symptoms appear, elimination of one of the therapies is indicated.

In mild cases of depression, we recommend using either 5-HTP (50 mg per day) or Saint-John's-wort extract (900 mg per day) while you work with your doctor to reduce the drug to half the daily dosage for two to four weeks. After four weeks, the drug can be discontinued. For more severe cases, keep the dosage of the antidepressant as it is and add the Saint-John's-wort extract. Evaluate at the end of one month and begin tapering off the drug if sufficient mood-elevating effects have been noted. If additional support is necessary, add 5-HTP at a dosage of 50 mg three times per day.

Psychological Support

Individuals with depression should consider seeing a psychotherapist for help in developing a positive, optimistic attitude. This can be accomplished by helping them set goals, use positive self-talk and affirmations, identify self-empowering questions, and find ways to inject humor and laughter into their lives. For more information, see the chapter "A Positive Mental Attitude."

Diet

The recommendations in the chapter "A Health-Promoting Diet" are important in depression. It is very important to eat a low-glycemic Mediterranean-style diet, increase consumption of fiber-rich plant foods (fruits, vegetables, grains, legumes, and raw nuts and seeds), and avoid caffeine and alcohol. Food allergies must be identified and controlled (see the chapter "Food Allergy").

Lifestyle and Attitude

- Exercise at least 30 minutes at least three times a week, but preferably every day.
- Spend 10 to 15 minutes per day on relaxation/stress reduction techniques.
- Follow the recommendations in the chapter "A Positive Mental Attitude."

Nutritional Supplements

- A high-potency multiple vitamin and mineral formula as described in the chapter "Supplementary Measures"
- Key individual nutrients:
  ○ Vitamin B$_6$: 25 to 50 mg per day
  ○ Folic acid: 800 mcg to 2,000 mcg per day
  ○ Vitamin B$_{12}$: 800 mcg per day
  ○ Vitamin C: 500 to 1,000 mg per day
  ○ Magnesium (bound to aspartate, citrate, fumarate, malate, or succinate): 150 to 250 mg two times per day

- ○ Vitamin D$_3$: 2,000 to 4,000 IU per day (ideally, measure blood levels and adjust dosage accordingly)
- Fish oils: 1,000 mg EPA + DHA per day
- One of the following:
  - ○ Grape seed extract (>95% procyanidolic oligomers): 100 to 300 mg per day
  - ○ Pine bark extract (>95% procyanidolic oligomers): 100 to 300 mg per day
  - ○ Some other flavonoid-rich extract with a similar flavonoid content, super greens formula, or another plant-based antioxidant that can provide an oxygen radical absorption capacity (ORAC) of 3,000 to 6,000 units or higher per day
- Consider one of the following:
  - ○ 5-HTP: 50 to mg three times per day
  - ○ SAM-e: 200 mg twice a day up to 400 mg three times a day

Botanical Medicines

- One of the following:
  - ○ Saint-John's-wort extract (0.3% hypericin content): 900 to 1,800 mg per day (probably the best choice for people younger than 50); in severe cases, can be used in combination with 5-HTP 50 to 100 mg three times per day
  - ○ Ginkgo biloba extract (24% ginkgo flavonglycosides content): 240 to 320 mg per day (perhaps the best choice for people older than 50); in severe cases, can be used in combination with Saint-John's-wort, 5-HTP, or both
  - ○ Saffron petal extract: 15 mg twice per day
  - ○ Lavender extract (4:1): 150 mg twice per day

Diabetes

- Fasting (overnight) blood glucose concentration greater than or equal to 126 mg/dl on at least two separate occasions

- Following ingestion of 75 g glucose, blood glucose concentration greater than or equal to 200 mg/dl two hours after ingestion and at least one other sample during the four-hour test

- A random blood glucose level of 200 mg/dl or more, plus the presence of suggestive symptoms

- Classic symptoms: increased urination, thirst, and hunger

- Fatigue, blurred vision, poor wound healing, periodontal disease, and frequent infections (often presenting symptoms with type 2 diabetes as well)

Diabetes is a chronic disorder of carbohydrate, fat, and protein metabolism characterized by fasting elevations of blood sugar (glucose) levels and a greatly increased risk of heart disease, stroke, kidney disease, and loss of nerve function. Diabetes can occur when the pancreas does not secrete enough insulin or if the cells of the body become resistant to insulin. Hence, the blood sugar cannot get into the cells, and this condition then leads to serious complications.

Major Complications of Diabetes

- **Cardiovascular disease.** Adults with diabetes have death rates from cardiovascular disease about two to four times higher than adults without diabetes.

- **Hypertension.** About 75% of adults with diabetes have high blood pressure.

- **Retinopathy.** Diabetes is the leading cause of blindness among adults.

- **Kidney disease.** Diabetes is the leading reason for dialysis treatment, accounting for 43% of new cases.

- **Neuropathy.** About 60 to 70% of people with diabetes have mild to severe forms of nervous system damage. Severe forms of diabetic nerve disease are a major contributing cause of lower-extremity amputations.

- **Amputations.** More than 60% of lower-limb amputations in the United States occur among people with diabetes.

- **Periodontal disease.** Almost one-third of people with diabetes have severe periodontal (gum) disease.

- **Pain.** Many diabetics fall victim to chronic pain due to conditions such as arthritis, neuropathy, circulatory insufficiency, or muscle pain (fibromyalgia).

- **Depression.** This is a common accompaniment of diabetes. Clinical depression may begin years before diabetes is fully evident. It is difficult to treat in poorly controlled diabetics.

- **Autoimmune disorders.** Thyroid disease, inflammatory arthritis, and other diseases of the immune system commonly add to the suffering of diabetes.

Diabetes is divided into two major categories: type 1 and type 2. About 10% of all diabetics are type 1 and about 90% are type 2. Type 1 is associated with complete destruction of the beta cells of the pancreas, which manufacture the hormone insulin. Type 1 patients require lifelong insulin for the control of blood sugar levels. Type 1 results from injury to the insulin-producing beta cells, coupled with some defect in tissue regeneration capacity. In Type 1, the body's immune system begins to attack the pancreas. Antibodies for beta cells are present in 75% of all individuals with type 1 diabetes, compared with 0.5 to 2% of nondiabetics. It is probable that the antibodies to the beta cells develop in response to cell damage due to other mechanisms (chemical, free radical, viral, food allergy, etc.). It appears that normal individuals either do not develop as severe an antibody reaction or are better able to repair the damage once it occurs.

Type 2 diabetes historically has had an onset after 40 years of age in overweight individuals but today is seen even in children,

owing to the obesity epidemic present in all age groups in America as well as those exposed to high levels of persistent organic pollutants (POPs). Initially, insulin levels are typically elevated in type 2, indicating a loss of sensitivity to insulin by the cells of the body. Obesity is a major factor contributing to this loss of insulin sensitivity. Approximately 90% of individuals categorized as having type 2 are obese. Achieving ideal body weight in these patients is associated with restoration of normal blood glucose levels in many cases. Even if type 2 has progressed to the point where insulin deficiency is present, weight loss nearly always results in significant improvements in blood glucose control and dramatic reductions in other health risks such as cardiovascular disease.

Type 2 is a disease characterized by progressive worsening of blood sugar control. It starts with mild alterations in after-meal (postprandial) glucose elevations, followed by an increase in fasting plasma glucose and often ultimately a lack of production of insulin and the need for insulin therapy.

There are other types of diabetes, such as gestational diabetes—a type of diabetes that affects about 4% of all pregnant women.

Differences Between Type 1 and Type 2 Diabetes		
FEATURES	**TYPE 1**	**TYPE 2**
Age at onset	Usually younger than 40	Usually older than 40
Proportion of all diabetics	<10%	>90%
Family history	Uncommon	Common
Appearance of symptoms	Rapid	Slow
Obesity at onset	Uncommon	Common
Insulin levels	Decreased	Normal-high initially, decreased after several years
Insulin resistance	Occasional	Often
Treatment with insulin	Always	Usually not required until later in the disease

About 135,000 cases of gestational diabetes occur each year in the United States. Gestational diabetes occurs more frequently among African-Americans, Hispanic/Latino-Americans, and American Indians. It is also more common among obese women and women with a family history of diabetes. After pregnancy, 5 to 10% of women with gestational diabetes develop type 2; that increases to a 20 to 50% chance of developing diabetes in the 5 to 10 years after pregnancy.

Prediabetes and Metabolic Syndrome

Prediabetes (also called impaired glucose tolerance) is categorized by a fasting glucose of 100–125 mg/dl and/or postprandial glucose of 140–199 mg/dl. It is the first step in insulin resistance and is estimated to affect 57 million Americans. Many people with prediabetes will go on to develop full-blown type 2 despite the fact that prediabetes is usually reversible and, in most cases, diabetes can be completely avoided through dietary and lifestyle changes. Factors implicated in prediabetes, insulin resistance, and the progression to type 2 include a diet high in refined carbohydrates, particularly high-fructose corn syrup; elevated saturated fat intake; overeating due to increased portion sizes of food; increase in inflammatory markers; lack of exercise; industrial pollution; abdominal weight gain; hormonal imbalances; inadequate sleep; and nutrient deficiencies.

Research increasingly indicates that prediabetes is accompanied by serious health risks, especially an increased risk for cardiovascular disease (CVD). Prediabetics often meet the criteria of metabolic syndrome, a cluster of factors that together carry a significantly greater risk for CVD and developing type 2. These factors include:

- Greater waist-to-hip ratio
- Two of the following:
  ○ Triglycerides higher than 150 mg/dl
  ○ HDL less than 40 mg/dl for men, less than 50 mg/dl for women
  ○ Blood pressure above 130/85 mm Hg
  ○ Fasting blood glucose above 100 mg/dl

By this definition, and on the basis of data from the Third National Health and Nutrition Examination Survey (NHANES III), the prevalence of metabolic syndrome in the United States is 39% among men and women older than 20.[1] Among adolescents, and according to a similar definition, approximately 5.8% meet the established criteria.[2] In addition to an elevated risk for cardiovascular disease and diabetes, individuals with metabolic syndrome report poorer health-related quality of life, both physically and mentally.[3]

Diagnostic Considerations

The classic symptoms of type 1 are frequent urination, weight loss, impaired wound healing, infections, and excessive thirst and appetite. In type 2, because the symptoms are generally milder, they may go unnoticed. For that reason and others, many people with type 2 do not even know they have the disease. Excess abdominal weight, fatigue, blurred vision, poor wound healing, periodontal disease, and frequent infections are often presenting symptoms of type 2.

Blood Glucose Levels

The standard method for diagnosing diabetes involves the measurement of blood glucose levels. The initial measurement is generally a fasting blood glucose level taken after avoiding food for at least 10 hours but not more

Glucose Tolerance Test Response Criteria	
TYPE	**CRITERIA**
Normal	No elevation >160 mg/dl (9 mmol/l); <150 mg/dl (8.3 mmol/l) at the end of the first hour, below 120 mg/dl (6.6 mmol/l) at the end of the second hour
Flat	No variation more than ± 20 mg/dl (1.1 mmol/l) from fasting value
Prediabetic	Blood glucose level of 140 mg/dl (7.8 mmol/l) to 180 mg/dl (10 mmol/l) at the end of the second hour
Diabetic	>180 mg/dl (10 mmol/l) during the first hour; 200 mg/dl (11.1 mmol/l) or higher at the end of the first hour; and 150 mg/dl (8.3 mmol/l) or higher at the end of the second hour

than 16. The normal reading is between 70 and 99 mg/dl. If a person has a fasting blood glucose measurement greater than 126 mg/dl (7 mmol/L) on two separate occasions, the diagnosis is diabetes. As mentioned above, a fasting glucose greater than 100 but less than 126 mg/dl is classified as prediabetes.

Postprandial and random glucose determinations are also quite helpful in diagnosing diabetes. A postprandial measurement is usually made one to two hours after a meal, while a random measurement is one that is made anytime during the day without regard for the time of the last meal. Any reading greater than 200 mg/dl (11 mmol/l) is considered indicative of diabetes.

Glycosylated Hemoglobin

A valuable laboratory test for evaluating long-term blood glucose levels is measuring glycosylated HbA1C. Proteins that have glucose molecules attached to them (glycosylated peptides) are elevated severalfold in diabetics. Normally, about 4.6 to 5.7% of hemoglobin is combined with glucose. An A1C from 5.7 to 6.4% indicates prediabetes; an A1C of 6.5% or higher can be used to diagnose diabetes. A1C measurements are particularly helpful in patients with unclear results from fasting blood sugar levels. They can be coupled with a fasting blood glucose level and a two-hour postprandial glucose level for a more accurate diagnosis.[4] Because the average life span of a red blood cell (RBC) is 120 days, the A1C assay represents time-averaged values for blood glucose over the preceding two to four months. An A1C of 5% indicates that the median blood glucose level for the last three months has been around 100 mg/dl; each point of elevation in the percentage means roughly a 35 mg/dl higher average blood sugar level. Thus, an A1C

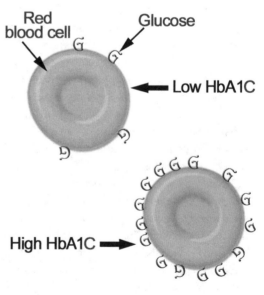

Glycosylation of Red Blood Cells

of 7% means that on average over the last three months the patient's blood glucose was 170 mg/dl. The A1C test is extremely valuable in providing a simple, useful method for assessing treatment effectiveness and should be checked every three to six months.

Type 1 Diabetes

Causes

We know that in type 1 diabetes ultimately the insulin-producing cells of the pancreas are destroyed, in most cases by the body's own immune system, but what triggers this destruction can vary from one person to another. Genetic factors may predispose the insulin-producing cells to damage through either impaired defense mechanisms, immune system oversensitivity, or some defect in tissue regeneration capacity. The entire set of genetic factors linked to type 1 has been termed "susceptibility genes," as they modify the risk of diabetes but are neither necessary nor sufficient for disease to develop.[5] Rather than acting as the primary cause, the genetic predisposition simply sets the stage for the environmental or dietary factor to initiate the destructive process.[6] The very term *predisposition* clearly indicates that something else needs to occur: less than 10% of those with increased genetic susceptibility for type 1 actually develop the disease.[7]

In detailed studies, the concordance rate for developing type 1 in identical twins was only 23% in one study[8] and 38% in another.[9] If one twin develops type 1 after age 24 years, then the rate in the second twin drops all the way down to 6%. These results and others indicate that environmental and dietary factors are more important than a true genetic predisposition in most cases.[10]

There is additional evidence supporting the need to focus on dietary and environmental triggers:

- There has been a three- to tenfold increase in the number of people with type 1 throughout the world over the past 40 years. Such a rise simply cannot be explained by an increased number of people genetically predisposed to type 1. Changes to the human genetic code across large populations take much more than one generation to occur.[11]

- The rate of type 1 can increase dramatically when children in areas where type 1 is relatively rare move to developed countries.[12] For example, the rate of type 1 increased by nearly fourfold in one 10-year period in children of Asian origin moving to Great Britain, and the rate increased more than sevenfold in Polynesians migrating to New Zealand.[13,14] Genetic factors cannot explain such a rapid change.

- There is a strong inverse correlation between maternal vitamin D levels and a child's risk of developing type 1 diabetes.

Environmental and Dietary Risk Factors
Accumulating data indicate that abnormalities of the gut's immune system may play a fundamental role in the immune attack on beta cells and the subsequent development of type 1.[15] The intestinal immune system serves a vital role in processing the many food and microbial antigens, to protect the body from infection or allergy. What appears to happen in the development of some cases of type 1 is the development by the gastrointestinal immune system of antibodies that ultimately attack the beta cells.

It is interesting to consider that poor protein digestion may contribute to type 1. Poorly digested dietary proteins can cross-react with proteins on or within the beta cells of the pancreas. In humans, two dietary proteins that may be incriminated are those found in milk (which contains bovine serum albumin and bovine insulin) and wheat (which contains gluten). For example, dietary bovine insulin differs from human insulin by only three amino acids. If a person develops antibodies to bovine insulin, there is a good chance that these antibodies will also attack the person's own insulin. In addition to causing antibody-mediated destruction of the beta cells, bovine insulin is able to activate T cells in those predisposed to diabetes in a manner that can lead to beta cell destruction by direct attack by T killer cells.

Strong evidence implicates dietary factors such as cow's milk and gluten as important triggers of the autoimmune process that lead to type 1. In contrast, breastfeeding has been identified as an important factor in establishing proper intestinal immune function and reducing the risk of type 1. It is well known that breastfeeding confers a reduction in the risk of food allergies, as well as better protection against both bacterial and viral intestinal infections. In case-controlled studies, patients with type 1 were more likely to have been breastfed for less than three months and to have been exposed to cow's milk or solid foods before four months of age. A critical review and analysis of all relevant citations in the medical literature indicated that early cow's milk exposure may increase the risk about 1.5-fold.[16] In addition, although the risk of diabetes associated with exposure to cow's milk was first thought to relate only to intake during infancy, further studies showed that ingestion at any age may increase the risk of type 1.

There is also considerable evidence that sensitivity to gluten—the major protein component of wheat, rye, and barley—may also play a role. Gluten sensitivity produces celiac disease, another autoimmune disorder. Celiac disease, like type 1 diabetes, is associated with intestinal immune function abnormalities. And, as with diabetes, breastfeeding appears to have a preventive effect, while the early introduction of cow's milk is believed to be a major causative factor. The risk of developing type 1 diabetes is higher in children with celiac disease. Not surprisingly, the highest levels of antibodies to cow's milk proteins are found in people with celiac disease.[17]

Enteroviruses and Type 1 Diabetes

Recent studies have strengthened the hypothesis that type 1 diabetes can be the result of viral infection.[18,19] A working theory is that the immune system has become slightly confused as to which proteins to attack—food-based ones such as those from dairy products or gluten, or similar proteins on the pancreatic beta cells. (Part of this confusion may be due to vitamin D deficiency, as discussed below.) When the person then has a viral infection, the increase in immune system activation sets off the production of more antibodies and sensitized white cells, and those confused immune cells then begin to damage the pancreas. Gastrointestinal infections due to enteroviruses (e.g., coxsackieviruses, echoviruses) and rotavirus are quite common, especially in children. All of these viruses replicate in the gut and cause stimulation of the intestinal immune system; this may activate the insulin-specific immune cells to seek out and destroy beta cells. These viruses and others are also capable of infecting pancreatic beta cells, causing the leukocytes to attack and destroy the beta cells in an attempt to kill the virus. Another possibility is that gastrointestinal virus infections may increase intestinal permeability, leading to absorption of the intact protein; this then enhances the antibody response to dietary bovine insulin. The severe "leaky gut" or increased small-intestine permeability that occurs during and for some time following rotavirus infections (one of the most common causes of acute diarrheal illness in children) exposes the gut-associated immune cells to large quantities of intact proteins.

Vitamin D Deficiency

Emerging evidence indicates that vitamin D supplementation from cod liver oil and other sources during early childhood can prevent type 1 diabetes.[20] In the most extensive studies of vitamin D and type 1, all pregnant women in northern Finland who were due to give birth in 1966 were enrolled (more than 12,000 women) and their children were monitored until December 1997.[21] Final analysis of 10,366 enrollees demonstrated that children who regularly took vitamin D, primarily from cod liver oil, had an 80% reduced risk of developing type 1, while those with a vitamin D deficiency had a 300% increased risk of developing the disease. One study found

that the use of vitamin D from cod liver oil during pregnancy significantly reduced the frequency of type 1 in their children.[22] Furthermore, vitamin D levels are much lower in the blood of people with newly diagnosed type 1 than in healthy controls. Because vitamin D can be produced in the body by the action of sunlight on the skin, lack of sun exposure during childhood may also play a role and partially explain the higher type 1 rates in northern countries. In recent observational studies, vitamin D has been shown to prevent the development of autoimmune conditions, including attacks on beta cells; the degree of protection is dose dependent.[23]

Omega-3 Fatty Acid Deficiency

A strong case can be made for the benefits of omega-3 fatty acids in protecting against the development of type 1 diabetes. In human studies, giving essential fatty acids (EFAs) significantly reduced the onset of type 1;

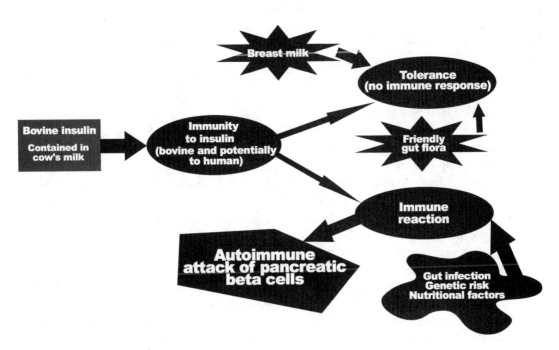

Proposed Triggers of Type I Diabetes

higher red blood cell omega-3 levels are also associated with reduced risk.[24] Cod liver oil provides both EPA and DHA, two vital EFAs. Other studies support the benefit of supplementing EFA in mothers and children. The mechanisms responsible for this effect may be related to improved cell membrane function, leading to enhanced antioxidant status and suppression of the formation of inflammatory compounds known as cytokines.[25]

Nitrates

Clear links have been established between increased levels of nitrate from dietary sources and water and an increased rate for type 1. Nitrates are produced by agricultural runoff from fertilizers; they are also used in cured or smoked meats such as ham, hot dogs, bacon, and jerky to keep the food from spoiling. Nitrates react within the body to form compounds known as nitrosamines. Nitrates and nitrosamines are known to cause diabetes in animals. Infants and young children are believed to be particularly vulnerable to the harmful effects of nitrate exposure.

One of the most alarming features of type 1 is that it is becoming much more prevalent, with a current growth rate of 3% per year worldwide.[11] Some areas have been hit particularly hard, such as Finland, Great Britain, Canada, and the United States. Increased nitrate exposure may be a key factor; nitrate levels in ground and surface waters of agricultural regions have increased over the past 40 years. Nitrate contamination occurs in geographic patterns related to the amount of nitrogen contributed by fertilizers, manure, and airborne sources such as automobile and industrial emissions. Nitrate exposure may explain why some geographic pockets have a substantially higher rate of type 1.[26,27]

Circumstantial evidence from population-based studies also suggests that a higher dietary intake of nitrate from smoked or cured meats is associated with a significantly higher risk for type 1. These foods severely stress body defense mechanisms and should be avoided. Parents would do well to break the habit of feeding children hot dogs, cold cuts, and ham. Health food stores now carry nitrate-free alternatives to these rather toxic food choices. Also, investing in a high-quality water purifier is good insurance against ingesting nitrate-contaminated drinking water.

Early Treatment and Possible Reversal of Type 1 Diabetes

Early intervention in type 1 designed to affect the autoimmune or oxidative process theoretically may be capable of lengthening the "honeymoon" phase (the time before insulin becomes absolutely necessary) or even completely reversing the damage. Two substances that may have some benefit in this regard are niacinamide and epicatechin.

Niacinamide

The niacinamide form of vitamin B_3 has been shown to prevent some of the immune-mediated destruction of pancreatic beta cells and may actually help to reverse the damage.[28,29] Observations that niacinamide can prevent the development of type 1 in experimental animals led to several pilot clinical trials that initially confirmed these observations and suggested that if given soon enough after the onset of diabetes, niacinamide could help restore beta cells or at least slow down their destruction. In a study of newly diagnosed type 1 diabetics, seven patients were given 3 g niacinamide per day and nine were given a placebo. After six months, five patients in the niacinamide group and two in the placebo group were still not taking insulin and had normal blood glucose and hemoglobin A1C. At 12 months, three patients in the niacinamide group but none in the placebo group were in clinical remission.[30]

The results of this pilot study and others suggested that niacinamide can help restore beta cells and prevent type 1 from progressing in some patients if given soon enough at the onset of diabetes. As of 2004, there had been 12 studies of niacinamide treatment in patients with recent-onset type 1, or type 1 of less than five years' duration, and who still had some functional beta cells. Of 10 double-blind, placebo-controlled studies, 5 showed a positive effect compared with a placebo in terms of prolonging the period in which insulin was not yet required, lower insulin requirements when the hormone was required, improved metabolic control, and increased beta cell function as determined by secretion of a substance known as C-peptide. In the 5 studies that showed a positive result, patients had a higher baseline fasting C-peptide level, and patients were generally older than in the negative studies.[31–34]

Despite these positive results, it is important to point out that two large studies designed to evaluate the effectiveness of niacinamide in preventing the development of type 1 in high-risk individuals—such as siblings of children who developed type 1, or individuals who already show elevations in antibodies directed against the beta cells—did not show niacinamide to be effective. The first of these studies, the Deutsche Nicotinamide Intervention Study, did not show much of an effect with 1.2 g niacinamide per day; and results from the larger study, the European Nicotinamide Diabetes Intervention Trial (ENDIT), did not show benefit with dosages as high as 3 g per day.[35,36] A possible shortcoming of these studies was the choice of a timed-released niacinamide. It is possible that such a formulation did not allow for sufficient peak levels of niacinamide to block autoimmune mechanisms.[37]

In the best-case scenario, niacinamide will be likely to work for only a few recent-onset type 1 patients. Nonetheless, the fact that some patients have had a complete reversal of their disease makes its use certainly worth the effort, especially since there is currently no other reasonable alternative.

The dosage recommendation is based on body weight: 25 to 50 mg niacinamide per kg of body weight, up to a maximum dosage of 3 g per day, in divided doses. Niacinamide is generally well tolerated and without side effects. In fact, no side effects have been reported in clinical trials involving type 1. It does not cause the skin flushing typical with high doses of niacin. However, because large doses of niacinamide could possibly harm the liver, a blood test for liver enzymes should be performed every three months to rule out liver damage.

Epicatechin

The second natural compound that may offer benefit is epicatechin. The line of research on its potential role in recent-onset type 1 diabetes began with examining the bark from the Malabar kino tree (*Pterocarpus marsupium*). This botanical medicine has a long history of use in India as a treatment for diabetes. Initially, epicatechin extracted from the bark was shown to prevent beta cell damage in rats. Further research indicated that both epicatechin and a crude alcohol extract of *P. marsupium* were actually able to assist in the regeneration of functional pancreatic beta cells in diabetic animals.[38] Green tea (*Camellia sinensis*) extract appears to be a better choice than extracts of *P. marsupium*, as the epicatechin content is higher in a high-quality green tea extract than in extracts of *P. marsupium*. Second, green tea extract exerts a broader range of beneficial effects. Another reason is that green tea polyphenols exhibit significant antiviral activity against rotaviruses and enteroviruses, two types of virus suspected of being involved in the development of type 1.[39] Last, green tea is considerably easier to find commercially than *P. marsupium*. Recommended dosage for green tea extract in children younger than age 6 is 50 to 150 mg; for children 6 to 12 years old, it is 100 to 200 mg; for children over 12 and adults, it is 150 to 300 mg. The green tea extract should have a polyphenol content of at least 80% and be decaffeinated.

Type 2 Diabetes

Causes

The major risk factor for type 2 diabetes is obesity or, more precisely, excess body fat. Approximately 80 to 90% of individuals with type 2 are obese (body mass index greater than 30). When fat cells (adipocytes), particularly those around the abdomen, become full of fat, they secrete a number of biological molecules (e.g., resistin, leptin, tumor necrosis factor, free fatty acids, cortisol) that dampen the effect of insulin, impair glucose utilization in skeletal muscle, promote glucose production by the liver, and impair insulin release by pancreatic beta cells. Also important is that as the number and size of adipocytes (fat cells) increase, this leads to a reduction in the secretion of compounds that promote insulin action, including adiponectin, a protein produced by fat cells. Not only is adiponectin associated with improved insulin sensitivity, but it also has anti-inflammatory activity, lowers triglycerides, and blocks the development of atherosclerosis (hardening of the arteries). The net effect of all of these actions is that fat cells severely stress blood glucose control mechanisms, as well as lead to the development of the major complication of diabetes, atherosclerosis. Be-

cause of all these newly discovered hormones secreted by adipocytes, many experts now consider adipose tissue to be part of the endocrine system, joining glands such as the pituitary, the adrenals, and the thyroid.[40,41] Measuring blood levels of adiponectin or other hormones secreted by fat cells may turn out to be the most meaningful predictor of the likelihood of developing type 2.[42,43]

In the early stages of the increased metabolic stress produced by the various secretions of adipocytes and the lack of adiponectin, blood glucose levels remain normal despite the insulin resistance because pancreatic beta cells compensate by increasing insulin output. As metabolic stress increases and insulin resistance becomes more significant, eventually the pancreas cannot compensate and elevations in blood glucose levels develop. As the disease progresses from insulin resistance to full-blown diabetes, the pancreas starts to "burn out" and produces less insulin. Fortunately, the pancreas can recover and continue to secrete insulin for the rest of a person's lifetime if ideal body weight is achieved and steps to improve insulin sensitivity are taken.

Risk Factors for Type 2 Diabetes

Family history of diabetes (i.e., parent or sibling with type 2 diabetes)

Obesity

Increased waist-to-hip ratio

Age (increasing age is associated with increased risk beginning at 45)

Race/ethnicity (e.g., African-American, Hispanic-American, Native American/Canadian, Native Australian or New Zealander, Asian-American, Pacific Islander)

Previously identified impaired fasting glucose or impaired glucose tolerance

History of gestational diabetes or delivery of baby weighing more than 9 lb

Hypertension (blood pressure greater than 140/90 mm Hg)

Triglyceride level higher than 250 mg/dl

Low adiponectin levels; elevated fasting insulin levels

Polycystic ovary syndrome (consider in any adult woman who is overweight, has acne, and has fertility problems)

Genetics of Type 2 Diabetes and Obesity

In studies of identical twins, the proportion of both twins having the disease (the concordance rate) was between 70 and 90% for type 2. This high concordance points to a strong genetic relationship. Data from family studies also provide additional support: children who have one parent with type 2 have an increased risk of diabetes in their lifetime, and if both parents have the disease, the risk in offspring is nearly 40%.[44] However, even with the strongest predisposition, diabetes can be avoided in most cases.

The Case of the Pima Indians

The Pima Indians of Arizona have the highest rate of type 2 and obesity anywhere in the world. Research has demonstrated a strong genetic predisposition, but even with this strong tendency it is extremely clear that the high rate of type 2 in this group is almost totally due to diet and lifestyle. The Pima Indians living traditionally in Mexico still cultivate corn, beans, and potatoes as their main staples, plus a limited amount of seasonal vegetables and fruits such as zucchini, tomatoes, garlic, green peppers, peaches, and apples. The Pimas of Mexico also make heavy use of wild and medicinal plants in their diet. They work hard, have no electricity or running water in their homes, and walk long distances to bring in drinking water or to wash their clothes. They use no modern household devices; consequently, food preparation and household chores require extra effort by the women. In contrast, the Pima Indians of Arizona are largely sedentary and follow the dietary practices of typical Americans. The results are astounding. Although roughly 16% of Native Americans in general in the United States have type 2, 50% of Arizona Pimas have type 2, and 95% of those diabetics are overweight or obese. By contrast, type 2 is a rarity among Mexican Pimas and only about 10% could be classified as obese. The average difference in body weight between the Arizona and Mexican Pima men and women is more than 60 lb.[45]

Further evidence that diet and lifestyle appear to be able to overcome even the strongest genetic predisposition is shown by some of the intervention studies with Pima Indians. When patients are placed on a more traditional diet along with physical exercise, blood glucose levels improve dramatically and weight loss occurs. The focus right now by various medical organizations such as the National Institutes of Health is to educate children on the importance of exercise and dietary choices to reduce diabetes risk.

Other Genetic and Racial Factors

Racial and ethnic groups besides Pima Indians that have a higher tendency for type 2 include other Native Americans, African-Americans, Hispanic-Americans, Asian-Americans, Australian Aborigines, and Pacific Islanders. In all of these higher-risk groups, again, it is important to point out that when they follow traditional dietary and lifestyle practices, the rate of diabetes is extremely low. It appears that these groups are simply sensitive to the Western diet and lifestyle.

Diet, Exercise, Lifestyle, and Diabetes Risk

Findings from the U.S. government's Third National Health and Nutrition Examination Survey (NHANES III) make it quite clear that diabetes is a disease of diet and lifestyle. Of individuals with type 2, 69% did not exercise at all or did not engage in regular exercise; 62% ate fewer than five servings of fruits and vegetables per day; 65% obtained more than 30% of their daily calories from fat, with more than 10% of total calories from saturated fat; and 82% were either overweight or obese.[46]

Insights into the role of modern lifestyle in the development of type 2 can be gleaned from the Old Order Amish. These 30,000 or so individuals, whose ancestors arrived on U.S. shores in the 18th century, maintain religious and cultural beliefs that preclude regular use of modern conveniences such as electrical appliances, telephones, and cars, and they have a physically active lifestyle. By comparison, the 300 million typical Americans living alongside them have, over the past 250 years, willingly adopted advances of modern technology, making life less physically demanding.

Although the typical Amish person's diet is not very different from the average American's and the rates of obesity are very similar as well, the rate of diabetes is about 50% lower. Although the percentage of Amish with impaired glucose tolerance (prediabetes) is about the same as the rate among other white populations in America, apparently not as many Amish go on to develop diabetes. This trend suggests that physical activity has a protective effect against type 2, independent of obesity.[47,48]

Results from other studies corroborate this hypothesis. Lifestyle changes alone are associated with a 58% reduced risk of developing diabetes in people at high risk (those with impaired glucose tolerance), according to results from the Diabetes Prevention Program, a large intervention trial of more than 1,000 subjects. The two major goals of the program were achieving and maintaining a minimum of 7% weight loss and a minimum of 150 minutes per week of physical activity similar in intensity to brisk walking.[49]

A Diet High in Refined Carbohydrates

Dietary carbohydrates play a central role in the cause, prevention, and treatment of type 2. In an effort to qualify carbohydrate sources as acceptable or not, two tools have been developed: the glycemic index and glycemic load. The glycemic index is a numerical value that expresses the rise of blood glucose after a particular food is eaten. The standard value of 100 is based on the rise seen with the ingestion of glucose. The glycemic index of foods ranges from about 20 for fructose and whole barley to about 98 for a baked potato. The insulin response to carbohydrate-containing foods is similar to the rise in blood sugar. The glycemic index is often used as a guideline for dietary recommendations for people with either diabetes or hypoglycemia. In addition, eating foods with a lower glycemic index is associated with a reduced risk for obesity and diabetes.[50-52]

One of the shortcomings of the glycemic index is that it tells us only about the quality of the carbohydrates, not the quantity. Obviously, quantity matters too, but the measurement of a food's glycemic index is not related to portion size. That is where the glycemic load comes into play. The glycemic load takes the glycemic index into account but provides much more accurate information than the glycemic index alone. The glycemic load is calculated by multiplying the amount of carbohydrate in a serving of food by that food's glycemic index, then dividing it by 100. The higher the glycemic load, the greater the stress on insulin. In Appendix B, we provide the glycemic index and glycemic load for many common foods.

Research studies are just starting to use glycemic load as a more sensitive marker for the role of diet in chronic diseases such as diabetes and heart disease. Preliminary results are showing that the glycemic load of a person's food intake is a stronger predictor of diabetes than glycemic index.[50,52] Researchers are also showing that a high-glycemic-load diet is associated with an increased risk for heart disease. For example, when researchers from the Nurses Health Study used glycemic load measures to assess the impact of carbohydrate consumption on women, they found that high-glycemic-load diets correlated with a significantly greater risk for heart disease because of their association with lower levels of protective HDL cholesterol and higher triglyceride levels.[53] Increased risk for diabetes and heart disease started, on average, at a daily glycemic load of 45. Therefore we recommend using the information in Appendix B to help determine how to prevent the total daily GL from exceeding 150. Keep in mind that the GL is directly related to serving size: the larger the serving size, the greater the GL.

The Importance of Dietary Fiber in Reducing the Risk of Diabetes

Population studies, as well as clinical and experimental data, show diabetes to be one of the diseases most clearly related to inadequate dietary fiber intake. Different types of dietary fiber act differently in the body. The type of fiber that exerts the most beneficial effects on blood sugar control is the soluble form. Included in this class are hemicelluloses, mucilages, gums, and pectin substances. These are capable of slowing down the digestion and absorption of carbohydrates, thereby preventing rapid rises in blood sugar. They are also associated with increasing the sensitivity of tissues to insulin and improving the uptake of glucose by the muscles, liver, and other tissues, thereby preventing a sustained elevation of blood sugar.[54,55]

Particularly good sources of soluble fiber are legumes, oat bran, nuts, seeds, psyllium seed husks, pears, apples, and most vegetables. Although even the simple change from white-flour products to whole-grain versions is associated with a reduced risk for type 2,[56,57] our recommendation is to consume at least 35 g fiber a day from various food sources, especially vegetables. Fiber supplements can also be taken to help lower the glycemic load of a food or meal.

The Wrong Types of Fats

Dietary fat plays a central role in the likelihood of developing type 2. Large controlled trials have shown that a reduction of fat intake as part of a healthful lifestyle, combined with weight reduction and exercise, reduces the risk of type 2. However, more important than the *amount* of fat in the diet is the *type* of fat.[58] The dietary fat profile linked to type 2 is an abundance of saturated fat (mostly found in animal sources) and trans-fatty acids (mostly found in hydrogenated vegetable oils) along with a relative insufficiency of monounsaturated and omega-3 fatty acids.

One of the key factors behind this linkage is the fact that dietary fat determines cell membrane composition. High consumption of saturated and trans fats leads to reduced membrane fluidity, which in turn decreases the binding of insulin to receptors on cellular membranes, decreases insulin action, or both. Trans-fatty acids, found in margarine, shortening, and other foods that are made with partially hydrogenated vegetable oils, are particularly problematic, as they interfere with the body's ability to use important essential fatty acids. One study estimated that substituting polyunsaturated vegetable oils for margarine would reduce the likelihood of developing type 2 by 40%.[59]

In contrast to the dampening of insulin sensitivity caused by trans and saturated fats, clinical studies have shown that monounsaturated fats and omega-3 oils improve insulin action.[60] Adding further support are population studies showing that frequent consumption of monounsaturated fats (found in, for example, olive oil, raw or lightly roasted nuts and seeds, and nut oils) and omega-3 fatty acids (found in cold-water fish such as wild salmon, trout, anchovies, sardines, halibut, and herring, for example) protect against the development of type 2.

Nuts are particularly helpful in reducing the risk of type 2. Studies have shown that consumption of nuts is inversely associated with risk of type 2, independent of known risk factors for type 2 such as age, obesity, family history of diabetes, physical activity, smoking, and other dietary factors.[61] In addition to providing beneficial monounsaturated and polyunsaturated fats that improve insulin sensitivity, nuts are also rich in fiber and magnesium and have a low glycemic index. Higher intakes of fiber, magnesium, and foods with a low glycemic index have been associated with reduced risk of type 2 in several population-based studies.

Low Intake of Antioxidant Nutrients

Cumulative free radical damage leads to cellular aging and is a major factor contributing to type 2, as well as many other chronic degenerative diseases. Several large population-based studies have shown that the higher the intake of fruit and vegetables, the better blood glucose levels are controlled and the lower the risk for type 2.[62] Many factors could explain this inverse correlation. Fruits and vegetables are good sources of fiber, have a high nutrient content, and contain high levels of antioxidants. Even something as simple as regular salad consumption is associated with a reduced risk for type 2.[63] Studies looking at individual antioxidants have also shown similar inverse correlations—the higher the level of vitamin C, vitamin E, or carotenes, for example, the lower the risk for type 2.[64–66]

Likewise, the lower the levels of antioxidants and the higher the levels of fats that have been damaged by free radicals (lipid peroxides), the greater the risk for developing type 2.[67] In one study 944 men, ages 42 to 60, were followed closely for four years. None of these men had diabetes at the beginning of the study. At the end of this time, 45 men had developed diabetes. What researchers found was that a low vitamin E concentration was associated with a 390% increase in risk of type 2.[68]

Free Radicals and Diabetes

One of the hallmarks of type 2 is the presence of higher levels of free radicals and pro-oxidants,[69] and in particular an increased production of reactive oxygen species and reactive nitrogen species.[70] These are associated with high blood glucose and elevated saturated fat levels, and, as already mentioned, they are produced in abdominal fat cells. These compounds oxidize cellular components such as DNA, proteins, and cell membrane fatty acids. In addition to their ability to directly inflict damage on these structures, reactive oxygen and nitrogen species indirectly induce damage to tissues by activating a number of inflammatory compounds that ultimately lead to both insulin resistance and impaired insulin secretion.

Persistent Organic Pollutants (POPs)

These compounds include such chemicals as polychlorinated dibenzo-p-dioxins (PCDDs), polychlorinated dibenzofurans (PCDFs), hexachlorobenzene (HCB), organophosphates, DDE, and bisphenyl A. These compounds have been linked to development of type 2. In addition, research indicates that the body load of POPs not only is a significant predictor of type 2 but may be a more significant risk factor than obesity.[71] People with the highest levels of organochlorine pesticides have a five times greater risk for metabolic syndrome.[72]

Unfortunately, direct measurement of POP levels is difficult and very expensive. However, a good indirect measure is blood levels of gamma-glutamyltransferase (GGTP), a common test to gauge liver function. Individuals with levels above 40 mcg/l have a 20-fold increased risk.[73] Interestingly, the level of POPs is a better predictor of diabetes risk than weight.

Environmental Toxins

Environmental pollutants can increase the risk of developing type 2. Reducing chemical exposure by choosing organic food when possible, by using natural cleaners at home, and by not using chemical pesticides is a valid step to help prevent environmental toxins from negatively affecting insulin regulation in the body.

Clinical Monitoring

Knowledge and awareness are the greatest allies for people with diabetes. An individual with diabetes who makes a strong commitment to learning about his or her condition and who accepts the lead role in a carefully supervised monitoring program greatly improves the likelihood of living a long and healthy life. On the other hand, individuals who remain blissfully ignorant about their disease and who refuse to undergo regular testing or self-monitoring are far more likely to face years of unnecessary suffering and, more often than not, catastrophic health problems.

Diabetes can be viewed as a state of biochemical and hormonal anarchy that, unless properly managed and supervised, will lead to organ injury and accelerated aging. Many of the complex control systems that faithfully govern and protect the body are damaged in the diabetic. In order to regain control, a diabetic must learn how to maintain intimate awareness of blood sugar levels, risk factors for atherosclerosis (hardening of the arteries), blood pressure, body mass index, level of fitness, and other factors that determine the risk of developing diabetic complications and eroding quality of life.

Fortunately, diabetics who do pay atten-

LIFESTYLE CHANGES VS. DRUGS TO PREVENT TYPE 2 DIABETES

Several well-designed, large trials have shown that lifestyle and dietary modifications can be used to effectively prevent type 2. That fact has not dissuaded drug companies from developing drugs to do the same thing. However, the degree of prevention available from drugs pales in comparison with the effectiveness of diet and lifestyle. For example, in one of the most celebrated studies 3,234 subjects with impaired glucose tolerance (prediabetes) were randomly assigned to either a placebo, the blood-glucose-lowering drug metformin (850 mg twice per day), or a lifestyle modification program, with the goals of at least a 7% weight loss and at least 150 minutes of physical activity per week. The average follow-up was 2.8 years. The incidence of diabetes was 11, 7.8, and 4.8 cases per 100 person-years in the placebo, metformin, and lifestyle groups, respectively. Compared with the placebo, the lifestyle intervention reduced the incidence of diabetes by 58%, and metformin reduced it by 31%. Clearly the lifestyle intervention was significantly more effective than metformin—a drug with sometimes serious side effects.[74]

tion to these risk factors through regular testing and a properly supervised self-monitoring program are also those who are much more likely to benefit from changes in lifestyle and diet, supplements, and, when necessary, medications.

Self-Monitoring of Blood Glucose Levels

Since its introduction, self-monitoring of blood glucose has revolutionized the management of diabetes.[75,76] The publication of the landmark Diabetes Control and Complications Trial,[77] which examined intensive glucose control in type 1 diabetics, and the United Kingdom Prospective Diabetes Study,[78] which examined intensive glucose control in type 2 diabetics, scientifically proved that the most important factor in determining the long-term risk of serious diabetic complications in both type 1 and type 2 diabetics is blood glucose control. Diabetics who do not remain aware of their blood glucose and who do not make every effort to keep their blood sugar under tight control can expect a significant increase in their risk of serious health problems such as eye, kidney, and heart disease, as well as a number of other problems such as depression, fatigue, impotence, and chronic infections. Self-monitoring of blood glucose is important for various reasons:[79]

- Modifications of treatment to achieve appropriate blood glucose control

- Detection and diagnosis of hypoglycemia

- The ability to adjust care in response to shifts in daily life circumstances (e.g., food intake, exercise, stress, illness)

- Detection and treatment of severe hyperglycemia

- Increased compliance with therapy (self-monitoring helps to combat apathy and denial, which are factors in noncompliance)

- Improvement in motivation because of immediate positive and negative feedback

Type 1 Diabetes and Self-Monitoring of Blood Glucose Levels

Without a doubt, all type 1 diabetics must monitor their blood glucose frequently if they want to achieve and maintain good health. In the absence of diabetes, the pancreas monitors blood glucose continuously and adjusts its insulin output moment by moment in response to changes in blood glucose. In order to achieve blood glucose levels that are consistently as close to normal as possible, type 1 diabetics must replicate this natural function as closely as possible. This means that they need to monitor their blood glucose frequently, and they must learn to use this information to make ongoing adjustments to their insulin injections, diet, and exercise.

Intensive insulin therapy allows a diabetic to achieve near-normal levels of blood glucose while enjoying improved lifestyle flexibility. With conventional, infrequent insulin injections, the diabetic must structure meals and other aspects of lifestyle around these injections or face serious abnormalities of blood glucose. On the other hand, with intensive insulin therapy that relies on rapid-acting, short-duration insulin or the use of an insulin pump (an electronic device that provides a continuous injection of short-acting insulin with extra boosts before meals), the timing and size of doses can be adjusted to suit the events of the day.[80] Even though it may involve multiple injections (usually before each meal and often at bedtime) and blood glucose measurements six times or more each day, intensive insulin therapy results in a higher quality of life and near nondiabetic blood glucose control, which is vital for long-term health.

Type 2 Diabetes and Self-Monitoring of Blood Glucose Levels

Self-monitoring of blood glucose has an important place in the management of type 2 diabetes as well. Each type 2 diabetic lies somewhere on a spectrum, with one end of the spectrum being mild glucose intolerance (accompanied by insulin resistance and higher-than-normal levels of insulin) and the other end of the spectrum being more advanced forms (with more severe insulin resistance, the potential for high blood glucose and ketoacidosis, and partial or nearly complete pancreatic failure with an accompanying lack of insulin). Self-monitoring of blood glucose plays a varying role depending on the severity of the disease. Every type 2 diabetic should own a blood glucose monitor and become familiar with its use. Even those diabetics whose blood glucose is well controlled through diet, lifestyle, and supplements should measure their blood glucose regularly.

Numerous dietary factors, supplements, exercise, stress, and illness can all have a significant impact on blood glucose control. Becoming aware of how all these factors influence diabetes will help motivate type 2 diabetics to make positive changes, and monitoring will provide immediate feedback about the results of any changes.

Diabetics who have a more serious case of disease, with diminished pancreatic insulin production, may benefit from efforts to establish consistently near-normal blood glucose control using intensive insulin therapy similar to that of type 1 diabetics.[81] A C-peptide blood test can provide an estimate of how much insulin type 2 diabetics are producing and is one way to help determine the appropriateness of using insulin (discussed below). If diabetics are placed on an intensive insulin therapy program, they must self-monitor their blood glucose as frequently as type 1 diabetics on intensive insulin therapy (usually before and two hours after each meal).

One way to achieve optimal blood glucose in these individuals is to give a daily injection of long-acting insulin (Lantus), which provides a smooth, continual release of insulin for 24 hours, in addition to diet and medication. Diabetics on this type of program definitely need to measure blood glucose frequently.

Guidelines for Self-Monitored Blood Glucose

- Test on awakening and just before each meal. Ideal blood sugar before meals is <120 mg/dl (6.7 mmol/l).

- Test two hours after each meal. Ideal blood sugar two hours after meals is <140 mg/dl (7.7 mmol/l).

- Test at bedtime. Ideal blood sugar level at bedtime is <140 mg/dl (7.7 mmol/l).

C-Peptide Determination

Often it is important to know if the pancreas of a diabetic is making insulin, and if so, how much. This assessment can greatly influence treatment, especially in a diabetic hoping to avoid or cease using insulin. The level of pancreatic insulin production can also partially determine the types of medication or natural health products that are more likely to be effective. Once it is known how well the pancreas is producing insulin, the focus may be shifted toward replacing deficiencies in insulin production, stimulating insulin production, preserving pancreatic function, reducing insulin resistance, or a combination of these therapeutic efforts.

One way to determine the level of insulin production is by measuring C-peptide. The pancreas manufactures a large protein called *proinsulin* first. A piece of this protein

Interpreting C-peptide levels	
C-PEPTIDE RESULTS	**INTERPRETATION**
Normal	Insulin production is at normal levels
Less than normal	A. Newly diagnosed type 1 diabetic B. Long-term type 2 diabetic
Greater than normal	A. Newly diagnosed type 2 diabetic B. Insulinoma (a benign tumor of the pancreas); rare
Undetectable	A. Long-term 1 diabetic B. Post–surgical removal of pancreas; rare

(C-peptide) is then snipped off by enzymes, and both C-peptide and the remaining insulin are released into the bloodstream. Injected insulin has no C-peptide. Measuring C-peptide can be helpful in both type 1 and type 2, but generally is more so for type 2. In type 1, measuring C-peptide can uncover how much insulin the pancreas is making, which may help indicate how much of the pancreas is still active. In type 2, high C-peptide levels confirm that the patient is very insulin resistant. Low C-peptide levels may indicate that enough damage has occurred to the pancreas that the patient needs to be put on some manner of insulin therapy.

Urine Ketone Testing

In any circumstance when the body must derive its primary source of energy from fat, ketones are produced as a by-product. If the level of ketone production is high enough, ketones appear in the urine. In general this is associated only with type 1 diabetic patients, as the vast majority of type 2 patients do not develop ketoacidosis. Ketoacidosis can occur if an insulin-dependent diabetic forgets to take insulin or deliberately avoids taking it. It can also occur when a diabetic becomes ill or injured or is given high doses of cortisone-type drugs. All of these phenomena may result in a severe loss of insulin effectiveness,

with the cells unable to take up and use glucose. In such circumstances, blood glucose rises to extraordinarily high levels, large amounts of fat are used by cells that cannot take in glucose, and the blood becomes polluted with toxic levels of acidic ketones. Severe dehydration occurs rapidly because the kidneys are unable to conserve water in the presence of such high levels of blood glucose. This dangerous state is referred to as *diabetic ketoacidosis*, and it must be treated as a medical emergency, usually necessitating intravenous insulin, high amounts of IV fluids, and careful monitoring, usually in an intensive care unit. Ignoring ketoacidosis can rapidly lead to death.

Because of this, testing the urine for ketones (or, even better, testing the blood for ketones, by use of a special glucometer that has this extra testing capability) remains an important part of monitoring for type 1 patients with no pancreatic function left at all. The presence of urine or blood ketones, accompanied by high blood sugar readings, can help determine how far along the ketoacidosis has developed and what type of medical attention is required. For this reason, all type 1 diabetics should frequently test their urine for ketones during acute illness or severe stress, especially when blood glucose levels are consistently elevated (>300 mg/dl [16.7 mmol/l]), regularly during pregnancy, or when symptoms suggestive of ketoacidosis, such as nausea, vomiting, or abdominal pain, are present.

Monitoring by a Physician

Although diabetics must take charge of their condition, controlling diet, managing lifestyle, and monitoring blood glucose, they are rarely successful without professional guidance. Numerous studies have determined that physician monitoring of diabetics through laboratory measurements of blood glucose control can have a major impact on a diabetic's long-term health.

One of the key determinants of blood glucose control is the A1C test, discussed earlier. Unlike direct measurements of blood glucose, which detect the level of blood glucose at the moment of testing, the A1C test reflects the average level of blood glucose over the preceding three months. Studies have shown that the level of A1C closely correlates with the level of risk for diabetic complications. However, an A1C test has a certain potential level of inaccuracy in it. A patient may have steady, well-regulated blood sugars, producing an A1C of 6%, or may have a combination of very high blood sugars and hypoglycemic events, which can also produce the same A1C of 6%.[4] Big changes in blood sugar, even if the average is good, are very damaging. Having an A1C of 5.5% or less is ideal, as it reflects that blood glucose levels have averaged in a range that is essentially nondiabetic and no damage is occurring in the body as a result of elevated glucose. All diabetics, type 1 and type 2, should have their A1C level measured every three to four months, depending on the stability of their condition.

Although it is clear that optimal blood glucose control is critical to the health of diabetics, several other risk factors need to be carefully monitored as well. Early detection of problems through a program of regular screening and monitoring will allow for preventive efforts and treatments to be put in place before serious complications or catastrophic problems occur.

Complications of Diabetes

While acute complications of diabetes are relatively rare with proper medical care, long-term complications are extremely common. Elevated blood glucose levels cause inflammatory and oxidative damage that unfortunately leads to chronic disease progression and the development of numerous complications.

Acute Complications

The acute complications of diabetes may represent a medical emergency and a possible life-or-death situation. Any diabetic experiencing any symptom even remotely suggestive of an acute complication of diabetes should obtain medical care immediately. The major acute complications of diabetes are hypoglycemia and diabetic ketoacidosis.

Hypoglycemia

Hypoglycemia is usually seen in type 1. Hypoglycemia is the result of injection of too much insulin, decreased or delayed food ingestion, use of alcohol or drugs that interfere with the liver's production of glucose, or an unusual increase in exercise. Severe hypoglycemia can also occur unpredictably in patients with brittle type 1 or in any diabetic on insulin or sulfonylurea drugs who neglects the need for proper monitoring of blood glucose. Daytime hypoglycemic episodes are usually recognized by their symptoms: sweating, nervousness, tremor, and hunger. Nighttime hypoglycemia may be without symptoms or

Clinical Management of the Patient with Diabetes		
	QUARTERLY	**ANNUALLY**
Review management plan:		
Blood glucose self-monitoring results	x	
Medication/insulin regimen	x	
Nutritional plan	x	
Exercise program	x	
Psychosocial support	x	
Physical examination:		
Weight	x	
Height (for child/adolescent)	x	
Sexual maturation (for child/adolescent)	x	
Skin, including insulin injection sites	x	
Feet: pulses, capillary refill, color, sensation, nails, skin, ulcers	x	
Neurological: reflexes, proprioception, vibratory sensation, touch (distal temperature sensation, distal pinprick or pressure sensation, standardized monofilament)		x
Regular retinal examination	x	
Dilated retinal examination		x
Electrocardiogram		x
Laboratory tests:		
Fasting or random plasma glucose	x	
(target range: 80–120 mg/dl before meals)		
Glycosylated hemoglobin (A1C)	x	
(target range: <7% in adults, <7.5% in children)		
Urinalysis	x	
Glucose, ketones, microalbumin, protein, sediment		
Complete cardiovascular profile		x
Cholesterol (target: <200 mg/dl)		
Triglycerides (target: <200 mg/dl)		
LDL (target: <130 mg/dl)		
HDL (target: <35 mg/dl)		
Lipoprotein (a) (target: <40 mg/dl)		
C-reactive protein (target: <1.69 mg/l)		
Fibrinogen (target: <400 mg/l)		
Homocysteine (target: <16 mmol/l)		
Ferritin (target: 60–200 mcg/l)		
Lipid peroxides (target: <normal; note: will vary depending upon the laboratory		
Serum creatinine (in adults; in children only if protein is present in urine)	x	

may be manifested as night sweats, unpleasant dreams, or early-morning headache.

Treatment of hypoglycemia follows the "15-15 rule," whereby patients are told to have 15 g carbohydrates, then recheck their glucose in 15 minutes. If the glucose is still less than 80 mg/dl, ingest another 15 g and check glucose in an hour. When glucose sinks below 55 mg/dl, it is likely that a diabetic will need help from another person; and when glucose is under 20 mg/dl, a seizure is highly likely and is a medical emergency. Any hypoglycemic event should be recorded and reported to a physician.

Diabetic Ketoacidosis

Diabetic ketoacidosis (DKA) is most commonly seen in newly diagnosed type 1 diabetics; in type 1 diabetics with infections (including dental abscesses); in cases of deliberate or accidental omission of insulin; in cases of trauma, heart attack, or stroke; during surgery; and in other miscellaneous situations. The lack of insulin leads to extremely high blood glucose and a buildup of acidic ketone molecules in the body as a result of the burning of fat stores for energy. If progressive, ketoacidosis can result in numerous metabolic problems and even coma or death. Since ketoacidosis is a medical emergency, prompt recognition is imperative. Patients should be taught to check for ketones in their urine or blood when their glucose is above 250 mg/dl for more than a few hours; if they are feverish or have an infection; if they do not feel well; and regularly during pregnancy, as ketoacidosis is usually fatal to the fetus. The symptoms of diabetic ketoacidosis include fruity breath, disorientation, abdominal tenderness, excessive urination and thirst, hyperventilation, and signs of dehydration. Treatment of DKA depends on the severity of the situation and where the glucose level is—it can require insulin injection, insulin injection plus food, or a visit to the emergency room.

Chronic Complications

Much more common than the acute complications of diabetes are certain long-term complications. The main four areas of the body affected most by diabetic complications are the eyes, the kidneys, the nerves, and the lining of blood vessels and organs. These four areas of the body do not require insulin to absorb glucose into their cells, in contrast to the liver, muscle and fat cells, so when glucose levels are elevated in uncontrolled diabetes, glucose floods those cells and causes significant damage.

Atherosclerosis

Atherosclerosis and other vascular lesions are the underlying factors in the development of many chronic complications of diabetes. Individuals with diabetes have a four- to sixfold higher risk of dying prematurely of heart disease or stroke than a nondiabetic individual, and 55% of deaths in diabetes patients are caused by cardiovascular disease.

Retinopathy

Diabetic retinopathy is the leading cause of blindness in the United States for people between the ages of 20 and 64. In diabetic retinopathy, the retina is damaged by microscopic hemorrhages, scarring, and the attachment of glucose molecules (glycosylation) to structural proteins in the retina. Studies have shown that 20 years after the diagnosis of diabetes, 80% of type 1 and 20% of type 2 diabetics have significant retinopathy. Diabetics are also prone to cataracts.

Neuropathy

Neuropathy usually refers to the loss of peripheral nerve function and is characterized by tingling sensations, numbness, loss of function, and a characteristic burning pain. It commonly occurs noticeably in the feet, but if it progresses it can also spread elsewhere in the body, such as in the autonomic nerves of the gastrointestinal tract, causing diarrhea, constipation, and disturbances in stomach emptying. If it progresses, then impaired heart function, alternating bouts of diarrhea and constipation, and inability to empty the bladder may occur. Approximately 60% of all people with diabetes eventually develop neuropathy. The main problem of peripheral neuropathy is that lack of feeling in the feet can lead to sores and lesions that patients do not notice and that then ulcerate, leading to gangrene and the need for amputation.

Kidney Disease (Nephropathy)

Nephropathy due to diabetes accounts for 40% of the cases of severe kidney disease and is the most common reason for end-stage kidney disease, dialysis, and kidney transplant in patients in America. ACE inhibitors or angiotensin receptor blockers are part of standard care, as they have been shown to protect the kidneys from diabetic damage.

Poor Wound Healing and Foot Ulcers

Poor wound healing is common in diabetes for several reasons, such as functional nutrient deficiencies and microvascular changes that lead to poor circulation. For these reasons and others (peripheral neuropathy, immune system dysfunction leading to chronic infections), foot ulcers are common in individuals with diabetes. Except for trauma, diabetic wounds are the leading cause of limb amputations in the United States. More than 50% of lower limb amputations in the United States (70,000 each year) are due to diabetic foot ulcers.

Immune System Dysfunction

Immune system dysfunction often begins to occur long before a diagnosis of diabetes is made. In fact, in many cases a recurrent vaginal or skin yeast infection is the clue that leads to the detection of diabetes. Immune system problems are made worse by poor glucose control, and this puts the diabetic at risk for serious infections or complications of simple infections. Susceptibility to chronic, hidden infections in the oral cavity, blood, or respiratory tract may be a primary reason for increased risk of cardiovascular disease in diabetics.

Depression and Cognitive Difficulties

Depression and cognitive difficulties are common in diabetics. In fact, depression may begin to occur decades before the onset of type 2 diabetes, when the individual first develops insulin insensitivity. The brain has a greater need for glucose than any other organ, and it appears that the brain cells may suffer from some degree of glucose deprivation when insulin resistance occurs.[82] Depression is also much more common in overweight and obese individuals, probably owing to a combined effect from insulin resistance and diminished self-esteem. Cognitive changes begin to occur after the first severe hypoglycemic episode in diabetics. Hypoglycemia is profoundly stressful to the brain, and if severe hypoglycemia occurs many times, significant cognitive impairment is possible. Uncontrolled diabetes is also associated with an increased risk of developing Alzheimer's disease.

Contributors to Long-Term Complications of Diabetes

The major factors contributing to the long-term complications of diabetes are listed here, followed by a brief description of each, along with coping measures:

- Poor glucose control
- Glycosylation of proteins (by means of an action similar to glycosylation of hemoglobin)

- Intracellular accumulation of sorbitol
- Increased oxidative damage
- Nutrient deficiency
- Elevated homocysteine levels
- Hypertension
- Changes in blood vessel linings

Poor Glucose Control

A large body of evidence indicates that good blood glucose control significantly reduces the development of complications. Maintaining hemoglobin A1C levels near normal (less than 7%) can dramatically help reduce the risk of eye problems (up to 76%), nerve damage (up to 60%), and kidney disease (up to 56%).

As described previously, *glycosylation* refers to the binding of glucose to proteins. The poorer the glucose control, the greater the binding of glucose molecules to proteins. This binding leads to changes in the structure and function of the protein. Among the adverse effects of excessive glycosylation are inactivation of enzymes, inhibition of regulatory molecule binding, and formation of abnormal protein structures. For example, when glucose molecules bind to cholesterol-carrying LDL molecules, they block LDL from binding to receptors on the liver that signal the liver to cease manufacturing cholesterol. As a result, the liver "thinks" there is a shortage of cholesterol in the body and continues to produce more and release it into the blood. This is one reason diabetes is almost always associated with high cholesterol levels.

In addition to keeping blood glucose levels as close to ideal as possible, high intakes of antioxidants—especially vitamins C and E, flavonoids, and alpha-lipoic acid (discussed later)—help to reduce glycosylation.

Intracellular Accumulation of Sorbitol

Sorbitol is a sugar molecule that is formed from glucose within cells. In people without diabetes, once sorbitol is formed it is quickly broken down into fructose. This conversion to fructose is critical because the intact sorbitol molecule cannot exit the cell, and if sorbitol levels continue to increase within a cell, the cell leaks small molecules such as amino acids, inositol, glutathione, niacin, vitamin C, magnesium, and potassium to maintain osmotic balance. Because these compounds function to protect cells from damage, their loss results in increased susceptibility to damage.

Intracellular accumulation of sorbitol is a major factor in the development of most complications of diabetes, as evidenced by the fact that elevated sorbitol levels are found in high concentrations in the tissues commonly involved in the major diabetic complications: the lens of the eye, nerve cells, kidney cells, and the cells that line blood vessels.

In addition to controlling blood glucose levels, vitamin C and flavonoids such as quercetin, grape seed extract, and bilberry extract can help lower intracellular sorbitol levels. (Sorbitol accumulation, by the way, has nothing to do with eating foods that contain sorbitol.)

Increased Oxidative Damage

Individuals with diabetes typically have elevated levels of free radicals and oxidative compounds.[83] These highly reactive compounds bind to and destroy cellular compounds, cause damage all over the body, and increase insulin resistance. They also greatly increase the inflammatory process by increasing the formation of inflammatory mediators such as C-reactive protein.[84] One of the critical goals in diabetes prevention and treatment is to flood the body with a high level of antioxidant compounds to counteract the negative effects of free radicals and pro-oxidants. In addition to a basic supplementation program, supplementing the diet with antioxidants such as alpha-lipoic acid and flavonoid-rich extracts is often useful.

Nutrient Deficiency

A deficiency of any one of several nutrients has been shown to contribute to several chronic complications of diabetes. Nutrient supplementation has been found in studies to help diabetic patients with glucose control, to lower blood pressure, and to protect the body from diabetic complications. In general, the risk of long-term complications of diabetes is inversely proportional to micronutrient status. Sometimes the symptoms of nutrient deficiency can mimic closely a chronic complication of diabetes. For example, vitamin B_{12} deficiency is characterized by numbness, pins-and-needles sensations, or a burning feeling in the hands or feet—symptoms virtually identical to those of diabetic neuropathy. Although vitamin B_{12} supplementation has been used with some success in treating diabetic neuropathy, it is really not clear if this success is due to correction of a B_{12} deficiency state or the normalization of the deranged vitamin B_{12} metabolism seen in diabetics.

High-potency multiple vitamin and mineral supplementation is critical to the management of diabetes. Supplying the diabetic with additional key nutrients improves blood glucose control and reduces the development of the major long-term complications of diabetes.

Elevated Homocysteine Levels

Elevated homocysteine levels are an independent risk factor for dementia, heart attack, stroke, and peripheral vascular disease. In addition, recent research has implicated elevations of homocysteine in the develop-

ment of long-term complications of diabetes, especially diabetic retinopathy.[85]

Hypertension

Blood pressure control is essential in preventing the complications of diabetes, especially kidney disease, retinopathy, and stroke. Maintaining blood pressure in the normal range (120–140/80 mm Hg) can reduce the risk of heart disease and stroke by approximately 33 to 50% and reduce microvascular disease (eye, kidney, and nerve disease) by approximately 33% in patients with diabetes.

Changes in Blood Vessel Linings

A single layer of endothelial cells lines all blood vessels and acts as a metabolically active barrier between the components of blood and the blood vessel. These cells regulate many important aspects of blood flow, coagulation and clot formation, and the formation of key regulating compounds, including those that control blood pressure. Endothelial cells are susceptible to damage by oxidized LDL cholesterol and other free radicals—hence the importance of high dietary antioxidant intake, flavonoids, and key supplemental antioxidants such as vitamins C and E and alpha-lipoic acid. All of these factors have been shown to improve endothelial cell function and are critical in the battle against vascular disease in diabetes.[86–89]

Therapeutic Considerations

Diet

The optimal diet for the treatment of diabetes is virtually the same as the program we have presented in the chapter "A Health-Promoting Diet." The difference is that there often needs to be an even stricter avoidance of foods with a high carbohydrate concentration. What determines how strict the diet needs to be with regard to the intake of carbohydrates is based on the ability to get blood glucose measurements and A1C levels under control and achieve and maintain ideal body weight. Obviously, the poorer the control, the more the carbohydrate intake must be restricted. Initially, some people with diabetes—especially those who have poorly controlled blood glucose levels—may need to avoid meals with a total glycemic load of more than 20 (see Appendix B) and space these meals at least three hours apart. Meals with a higher glycemic load can be consumed if a natural product designed to slow gastric emptying and blunt after-meal blood glucose levels is used (these compounds are discussed later).

Clinical Studies of Diet Therapy in Type 1 Diabetes

Numerous clinical studies have shown impressive results in improving blood glucose control when diets high in fiber and low in glycemic load are followed. This holds for children and pregnant women as well.[90–94] We have taken the proven diet to a much higher level by also considering the impact of fats on insulin action.

Clinical Studies of Diet Therapy in Type 2 Diabetes

Diet can often be effective as the sole factor in treating and reversing type 2. Other lifestyle factors and supplements are important, but treatment of type 2 begins with diet. And, just as in type 1, there is considerable evidence from clinical trials that a low-glycemic-load diet is emerging as the most scientifically proved approach, especially when we consider not only its effect on blood glucose levels but also its ability to reduce consequences of diabetes such as high

cholesterol levels, cardiovascular disease, hypertension, and other complications.[95] One of the key goals is to get the total fiber intake from foods up to at least 25 to 40 g per day. High fiber intake has been shown to lower average daily glucose levels as well as insulin concentrations and total cholesterol levels.[96] There is no debate that a low-glycemic-load diet shows significant advantages.[97,98]

Psychological Support

Helping people with diabetes deal with their diagnosis, develop a sense of empowerment, and make important lifestyle changes is an extremely important aspect of proper medical care. Counseling is especially effective in helping adolescents with type 1 cope with their disease, leading to improvements in both mood and blood glucose control.[99]

Stress

Stress adversely affects blood glucose control, as higher stress levels are associated with higher blood glucose levels in both type 1 and type 2.[100] There is a simple explanation for this phenomenon. Exposure to stress, whether it be physical, mental, or emotional, leads to activation of the body's stress response and causes increases in the adrenal gland hormones adrenaline and cortisol. Among other things, these hormones cause blood glucose levels to rise and blunt the response to insulin. They also negatively affect the immune system. Because stress seems to be an inevitable part of modern living, it is critical to develop effective methods to deal with it. Some studies have shown that positive methods for dealing with stress, such as relaxation training, can improve blood glucose control, especially in individuals who are anxious or experiencing significant stress in their lives.[101,102]

Exercise

Exercise is absolutely essential in the prevention and management of diabetes. Exercise directly improves insulin sensitivity and blood glucose control because of a combination of increased lean muscle mass and improvement in muscle cell metabolism.[103] Exercise also has profound benefits for the cardiovascular system directly, as well as indirectly, through improvements in blood lipids (especially an improvement in HDL or "good" cholesterol). Exercise decreases symptoms of anxiety and depression, improves sexual functioning, and improves confidence and self-esteem. It is important to note that exercise has been shown to help people attain and sustain weight loss.[104] Three types of exercise are important for people with diabetes: aerobic, strength training, and stretching.

Nutritional Supplements

The treatment of diabetes with natural medicine involves trying to achieve ideal blood glucose control and metabolic targets, as well as reducing the risk of the complications of diabetes by focusing on the following four areas:

1. Providing optimal nutritional status

2. Reducing after-meal elevations in blood glucose levels

3. Improving insulin function and sensitivity

4. Preventing nutritional and oxidative stress

Even though natural products can have significant effects on their own, the proper and effective treatment of diabetes requires the careful integration of diet and lifestyle changes along with any required medication and then natural medicines. Furthermore, all type 1 diabetics and many type 2 diabetics also require conventional medical treatments (oral drugs or insulin), depending on the adequacy of pancreatic insulin production (this can be determined by the C-peptide level) and the response of the diabetic to dietary and lifestyle measures. The most important factor determining whether or not the diabetic needs to be managed by drugs or insulin is the adequacy of blood glucose control.

Providing Optimal Nutritional Status

In addition to a nutrient-dense diet, a high-potency multiple vitamin and mineral formula is an absolute must for people with diabetes. Follow the guidelines given in the chapter "Supplementary Measures." The individual with diabetes has such an increased need for many nutrients that supplementation is critical. Supplying the diabetic with additional key nutrients has been shown to improve blood glucose control, as well as help prevent or reduce the development of the major complications of diabetes. Taking a multivitamin and mineral supplement has also been shown to boost immune function and reduce infections in diabetics.[105] Whenever a diabetic patient adds significant nutrient, fiber, or botanical medicines to his or her protocol, glucose monitoring is recommended, as oral or injectable medicines may need to be reduced.

Chromium. Chromium is vital to proper blood glucose control because it functions in the body as a key constituent of what is known as glucose tolerance factor—a molecule that facilitates the action of insulin. As a result, chromium works closely with insulin in assisting the uptake of glucose into cells. Without chromium, insulin's action is blocked and glucose levels are elevated. Evidence indicates that marginal chromium status is quite common in the United States. A chromium deficiency may be an underlying contributing factor in the tremendous number of Americans who have diabetes and hypoglycemia and are obese.

More than 20 clinical studies have focused on chromium supplementation in diabetes. In some of these studies involving type 2 diabetics, supplementing the diet with chromium has been shown to decrease fasting glucose levels, improve glucose tolerance, lower insulin levels, and decrease total cholesterol and triglyceride levels while increasing HDL cholesterol levels. Although there are also studies that have not shown chromium to exert much effect in improving glucose tolerance in diabetes, there is no argument that chromium is an important mineral in blood glucose metabolism. At this time, however, it appears, not unexpectedly, that chromium supplementation is likely to produce meaningful improvements in glycemic control only in people who are deficient in this essential trace element.[106]

Although there is no recommended dietary intake (RDI) for chromium, it appears that at least 200 mg each day in the diet is required. People with diabetes need to supplement this with 400–600 mg per day. Chromium polynicotinate and chromium picolinate may offer the best results, as chromium-rich yeast failed to produce any significant benefit in recent trials.[107] In contrast, several recent studies with 600 mcg chromium picolinate in combination with 2 mg biotin showed considerable benefit in helping patients with type 2 improve blood sugar control, as fasting glucose levels dropped 10 mg/dl and A1C levels dropped 0.54%.[108] Improvements in blood lipids were also noted in other studies.[109]

Vitamin C. Because the transport of vitamin C into cells is enhanced by insulin,[110] many people with diabetes suffer from a relative deficiency of vitamin C inside their cells even if they consume an adequate amount of vitamin C in their diet. As a result, the individual with diabetes needs to take extra vitamin C.

In addition to its role as an antioxidant, vitamin C is required in immune system function and the manufacture of collagen, the main protein substance of the human body. Because collagen is such an important protein for the structures that hold our body together (connective tissue, cartilage, tendons), vitamin C is vital for wound repair, healthy gums, and prevention of easy bruising. A chronic, latent vitamin C deficiency leads to a number of problems for the diabetic, including an increased capillary permeability, poor wound healing, elevations in cholesterol levels, and a depressed immune system. Vitamin C supplementation has been shown to exert a mild effect in improving glucose control, as evidenced by a slightly lower A1C in the vitamin C group (8.5%) compared with a placebo (9.3%) in one double-blind study.[111] Probably more important than any significant effect on improving blood glucose control is the fact that vitamin C supplementation has been shown to reduce the formation of compounds linked to the development of diabetic complications.

In one double-blind study of vitamin C supplementation in type 2, 30 patients who were 45 to 70 years old and had not only type 2 but also hypertension were randomly assigned to take either 500 mg ascorbic acid or a placebo for four weeks. Vitamin C supplementation decreased systolic blood pressure from 142.1 to 132.3 mm Hg and diastolic pressure from 83.9 to 79.5. Additional analytic methods designed to measure vascular resistance also demonstrated significant improvements in arterial flexibility. These results indicate that vitamin C supplementation is effective in improving the elasticity and function of blood vessels in patients with type 2.[112]

Vitamin C can also prevent sorbitol accumulation (see above). In one study of young adults with type 1, the baseline measurement of sorbitol in RBCs was nearly double in these patients despite adequate dietary intakes of vitamin C. Vitamin C supplementation at a dosage of either 100 mg or 600 mg normalized RBC sorbitol within 30 days. This correction of sorbitol accumulation was independent of changes in diabetic control as monitored by fasting glucose or hemoglobin A1C. In fact, overall diabetic control during the study was moderate to poor, indicating that vitamin C's effect was not dependent on glucose concentration. Vitamin C inhibits the enzyme aldose reductase, which converts glucose to sorbitol.[113]

Although vitamin C supplementation is necessary, patients should not rely exclusively on it to meet all of their vitamin C requirements. Foods rich in vitamin C are also good sources of compounds such as flavonoids and carotenes, which work to enhance the effects of vitamin C, as well as exert favorable effects of their own.

Vitamin E. Vitamin E functions primarily as an antioxidant in protecting against damage to the cell membranes. Without vitamin E, the cells of the body would be quite susceptible to damage. Nerve cells are particularly vulnerable. Diabetics appear to have an increased requirement for vitamin E. Vitamin E not only improves insulin action but when taken at dosages ranging from 400 to 800 IU exerts a number of beneficial effects that may aid in preventing the long-term complications of diabetes:

- Prevents free radical damage to LDL cholesterol and the vascular lining[114–116]
- Improves the functioning of blood vessels and cells that line the blood vessels[117,118]

- Increases the concentration of magnesium within cells[119,120]
- Decreases the level of C-reactive protein and other inflammatory compounds[121,122]
- Increases the level of glutathione—an important intracellular antioxidant—within cells[123]
- Improves the rate of conduction of the electrical impulse through the nervous system[124]
- Improves blood flow to the eye and improves diabetic retinopathy
- Improves kidney function and normalizes creatinine clearance—an indicator of kidney function—in diabetics with mild elevations[125]

Vitamin E supplementation may be particularly helpful for patients with a specific genetic marker—the haptoglobin (Hp) 2-2 genotype—associated with an increased risk for atherosclerosis. In a large study of more than 1,400 diabetics with the Hp 2-2 genotype, those given vitamin E (400 IU per day) for 18 months showed a 50% decrease in the rate of heart attacks, stroke, and death from cardiovascular factors.[126]

It should be noted that in one study in patients with type 2, treatment with either 500 mg alpha-tocopherol or mixed tocopherols significantly increased systolic blood pressure (approximately 6–7 mm Hg), vs. a placebo, indicating that some patients may have a hypertensive reaction.[127] Blood pressure should be monitored in patients taking higher dosages of vitamin E to rule out this negative effect. We suspect this effect was due to the heart's becoming stronger in response to the vitamin E supplementation.

Niacin and Niacinamide. Enzymes containing niacin (vitamin B$_3$) play an important role in energy production; fat, cholesterol, and carbohydrate metabolism; and the manufacture of many body compounds, including sex and adrenal hormones. Niacin, like chromium, is an essential component of glucose tolerance factor, and therefore is a key nutrient for hypoglycemia and diabetes.

In addition to offering possible benefits in type 1, niacinamide may also help in type 2. Eighteen normal-weight patients with type 2 diabetes who had failed to respond to oral diabetes drugs were randomly assigned to one of three treatments for six months: (1) insulin plus niacinamide (500 mg three times per day); (2) insulin plus a placebo; or (3) an oral diabetes drug plus niacinamide (500 mg three times per day). The indicators assessed included C-peptide, A1C, and fasting and mean daily blood glucose levels. With detailed analysis, niacinamide administration was the only significant factor accountable for the improvement of C-peptide release. The data indicated that niacinamide improved C-peptide release and blood glucose control in type 2 diabetic patients who had previously failed to respond to oral diabetes drugs alone.[128]

Vitamin B6. Vitamin B6 supplementation appears to offer significant protection against the development of diabetic neuropathy.[129] Diabetics with neuropathy have been shown to be deficient in vitamin B6 and to benefit from supplementation.[130] The neuropathy of a vitamin B6 deficiency is indistinguishable from diabetic neuropathy. Individuals who have long-standing diabetes or who are developing signs of peripheral nerve abnormalities should definitely supplement their diets with vitamin B6. Vitamin B6 is also important in preventing other diabetic complications.

Vitamin B6 supplementation can be a safe and effective treatment for gestational diabetes (diabetes caused by pregnancy). One study of 14 women with gestational diabetes given 100 mg vitamin B6 per day for two weeks resulted in eliminating the diagnosis in 12 of the 14 women.[131]

Magnesium. Like chromium, magnesium is involved in glucose metabolism. Considerable evidence indicates that diabetics should take supplemental magnesium, the reasons being that more than half of all people with diabetes show evidence of magnesium deficiency and magnesium may prevent some of the complications of diabetes such as retinopathy and heart disease. Magnesium levels are usually low in diabetics and lowest in those with diabetic complications such as retinopathy and neuropathy. Clinical studies have shown that magnesium supplementation (usually 400 to 500 mg per day) improves insulin response and action, glucose tolerance, and the fluidity of the RBC membrane in patients with diabetes.[132,133]

The RDI for magnesium is 420 mg per day for adult males and 320 mg per day for adult females. Diabetics may need twice this amount because they tend to lose excessive magnesium through their kidneys.[134] Most of the magnesium should be derived from the diet. The average intake of magnesium by healthy U.S. adults ranges from 143 to 266 mg per day. This is obviously far below the RDI. Food choices are the main reason. Although magnesium occurs abundantly in whole foods, food processing refines out a large portion of a food's magnesium. The best dietary sources of magnesium are tofu, seeds, nuts, and green leafy vegetables. Fish, meat, milk, and the most commonly eaten fruits are low in magnesium. Most Americans consume a low-magnesium diet because their diet is high in refined foods, meat, and dairy products.

In addition to eating a diet rich in magnesium, diabetics should supplement their diet with 300 to 500 mg magnesium daily. For best results, highly absorbable sources of magnesium such as magnesium aspartate or citrate should be taken. Diabetics should also be sure to get at least 25 mg vitamin B_6 per day, as the level of vitamin B_6 inside the cells of the body appears to be intricately linked to the magnesium content of the cell. In other words, without vitamin B_6 (as well as vitamin E), magnesium will not get inside the cell and will therefore be useless.

Zinc. Zinc functions in more enzymatic reactions than any other mineral, as it is a cofactor in more than 200 different enzymes. Although severe zinc deficiency is rare in developed countries, many individuals in the United States have marginal zinc deficiency. This is particularly true of the elderly population, as well as of people with diabetes. Low levels of zinc in the body are associated with increased susceptibility to infection, poor wound healing, a decreased sense of taste or smell, or skin disorders. It has also been suggested that zinc deficiency, like chromium deficiency, plays a role in the development of diabetes.[135]

Zinc is involved in virtually all aspects of insulin metabolism: synthesis, secretion, and utilization. Zinc also has a protective effect against beta cell destruction and has well-known antiviral effects. Diabetics typically excrete too much zinc in the urine and therefore require supplementation. Diabetics should take at least 30 mg zinc per day. Zinc is also found in good amounts in nuts and seeds.

Manganese. Manganese functions in many enzyme systems, including those involved in blood glucose control, energy metabolism, and thyroid hormone function. Manganese also functions in the antioxidant enzyme superoxide dismutase (SOD). In guinea pigs, a deficiency of manganese results in diabetes and an increase in the number of offspring that develop pancreatic abnormalities or

have no pancreas at all. Diabetics have been shown to have only one-half the manganese of normal individuals. A good daily dose of manganese for a diabetic is 3 to 5 mg.

Biotin. Biotin is a member of the B vitamin family and functions in the manufacture and utilization of carbohydrates, fats, and amino acids. Without biotin, sugar metabolism is severely impaired. Biotin supplementation has been shown to enhance insulin sensitivity and increase the activity of glucokinase, the enzyme responsible for the first step in the utilization of glucose by the liver. Glucokinase concentrations in diabetics are low. Evidently, supplementing the diet with high doses of biotin improves glucokinase activity and glucose metabolism in diabetics. In one study, 16 mg biotin per day resulted in significant lowering of fasting blood glucose levels and improvements in blood glucose control in type 1 diabetics. In another study, involving type 2 diabetics, similar effects were noted with 9 mg biotin per day.[136] Biotin therapy has also been shown to be quite helpful in the treatment of diabetic neuropathy.[137]

Omega-3 Fatty Acids from Fish Oil. Omega-3 fatty acids are vital supplements for diabetic patients to take. They offer significant protection against heart disease in diabetes, helping to lower lipids and blood pressure. They are anti-inflammatory and promote insulin sensitivity. Omega-3 oils are usually nearly completely lacking in the basic diet of a diabetic patient. Foods that contain omega-3s include oily fishes such as wild salmon, anchovies, sardines, herring, trout, and mackerel; walnuts; grass-fed beef; wild game meat; omega-3 eggs; and ground flax, hemp, and chia seeds. Initially there were concerns that omega-3 fatty acid supplementation might adversely affect blood glucose control, but two intensive investigations, one conducted at Oxford University and the other at the Mayo Clinic, analyzed data from 18 double-blind clinical trials involving 823 participants followed for an average of 12 weeks.[138,139] Both evaluations came to the same conclusions: fish oil supplementation has no adverse effect on blood sugar control, but it does appears to offer the same protection against cardiovascular disease in people with diabetes that it does in people without diabetes.[140] Importantly, many studies of patients with diabetes were conducted with lower-quality fish oil products that contained significant amounts of cholesterol and lipid peroxides. As a result, in some of these studies an elevation in LDL cholesterol was noted. It is important for diabetic patients to ingest a high-quality fish oil product. The combined total EPA + DHA level should be approximately 1,000 mg per day.

Reducing After-Meal Elevations in Blood Glucose Levels

Elevations of blood glucose levels after a meal can wreak biochemical havoc in both type 1 and type 2 diabetics. In fact, an elevation in postprandial blood glucose levels is the major contributor to the development of diabetic complications, especially cardiovascular disease and diseases of the microvasculature (retinopathy, neuropathy, and nephropathy). For example, patients who have a normal fasting blood glucose measurement but an average 2-hour postprandial glucose level greater than 200 mg/dl (11 mmol/l) have a threefold increase in the incidence of diabetic retinopathy.[141] Therefore, blunting the after-meal increase in blood glucose levels is an important goal.

In addition to low-glycemic-load meals, several natural products can be used to reduce postprandial blood glucose levels. The best supplements to use in this regard are fiber supplements and natural glucosidase inhibitors.

Fiber Supplements. Fiber supplements have been shown to enhance blood glucose control, decrease insulin levels, and reduce the number of calories absorbed by the body. The best fiber sources for these purposes are those that are rich in soluble fiber, such as glucomannan (from konjac root), psyllium, guar gum, defatted fenugreek seed powder or fiber, seaweed fiber (alginate and carrageenan), and pectin.

Clinical studies have repeatedly shown that after-meal blood glucose levels decrease as soluble fiber viscosity increases.[142,143] This relationship has also been shown to hold true for the other physiological benefits produced by soluble fiber, including increased insulin sensitivity, diminished appetite, significant weight control, improved bowel movements, and decreased serum cholesterol.[144]

When taken with water before meals, these fiber sources bind to the water in the stomach and small intestine to form a gelatinous, viscous mass that not only slows down the absorption of glucose but also induces a sense of satiety (fullness) and reduces the absorption of calories.

One of the most viscous naturally occurring dietary fibers is glucomannan, a soluble fiber obtained from the root of konjac, a plant that has been used as a food and remedy for thousands of years in Asia. Highly refined glucomannan possesses the greatest viscosity of any single dietary fiber. It is three times more viscous than guar and approximately seven times more viscous than psyllium. Konjac fiber is now easily available in noodles made with konjac root.

PGX is a novel natural polysaccharide matrix composed of three natural compounds (glucomannan, alginate, and xanthan gum) that are combined in a proprietary process that leads them to coalesce to form the most viscous fiber ever discovered.[145,146] When glucomannan is bonded with alginate and xanthan gum, its viscosity can be amplified three to five times. PGX reduces the glycemic index of any food or beverage by 15% to 70% and also reduces postprandial glucose levels when added to or taken with foods.[147,148] In a double-blind study with an earlier version of PGX, three weeks of supplementation with meals lowered postprandial blood glucose by approximately 20% and lowered insulin secretion by approximately 40% to produce a whole-body insulin-sensitivity index improvement of nearly 50%.[149] It was also shown to reduce total cholesterol (by 12.4%), LDL cholesterol (by 22.3%), the ratio of LDL to HDL (by 15%), and serum fructosamine (by 5%).[149] In another study involving similar patients, postprandial blood glucose (27%), postprandial insulin levels (41%), and insulin resistance were estimated to be improved by 56%.[150] Typical dosage for PGX is 2.5 to 5 g before meals. PGX is discussed further in the chapter "Obesity and Weight Management."

Natural Glucosidase Inhibitors. Starches, complex carbohydrates, and even simple sugars (disaccharides) such as sucrose are broken down in the digestive tract into glucose by the action of certain enzymes. Among the most important enzymes are the alpha-glucosidases, found in the intestines. Because these enzymes are essential for the breakdown of starches, complex carbohydrates, maltose, and sucrose into absorbable glucose molecules, their inhibition can diminish the after-meal rise in both glucose and insulin.

Acarbose (Precose) and miglitol (Glyset) are approved drugs for treating diabetes by inhibiting alpha-glucosidase. Although clinical studies have shown them to be quite effective, they are also characterized by a high frequency of mild to moderate gastrointestinal side effects such as flatulence, diarrhea, and abdominal discomfort. Although these side effects generally diminish in frequency

and intensity with time, few patients are willing to put in the necessary time to get over them.

Instead of the drug acarbose, we recommend trying extracts of either touchi or mulberry, which are natural and superior to their drug counterparts. Touchi is a fermented soybean product that has been used in China and Japan for more than 3,000 years. Touchi extract is concentrated to possess high levels of naturally occurring alpha-glucosidase inhibitors. Several clinical studies have documented its effectiveness in reducing postprandial elevations in blood glucose levels.[151] Longer-term studies have also shown benefit.[152,153] For example, when type 2 patients took 300 mg touchi extract before each meal for six months, there were moderate changes in fasting blood glucose and hemoglobin A1C levels. The effects were apparent after only one month of use. After six months, fasting blood glucose dropped more than 10 mg/dl in nearly 80% of the patients, and hemoglobin A1C levels fell by more than 0.5% in 60% of patients. Surprisingly, touchi extract also had a mild effect in lowering triglyceride and cholesterol levels, probably through a decrease in insulin resistance. With touchi extract—unlike the drug alpha-glucosidase inhibitors—no side effects have ever been seen and no one in the clinical trials has ever complained of the gastrointestinal side effects that are so characteristic of acarbose.

The mulberry plant (*Morus indica*) is probably best known as food for silkworms, but it has also been highly regarded in traditional Chinese and Japanese medicine. It has been shown to have significant hypoglycemic effects in animal studies, and it contains an effective alpha-glucosidase inhibitor, along with other compounds that appear to improve blood glucose control.[154,155] Mulberry extract has been studied in type 2, and the results are excellent. In one study, researchers decided to investigate its effect on blood and RBC lipids, as well as compare its blood-glucose-lowering actions with the oral diabetes drug glyburide.[156] Patients were given either dried mulberry leaves at a dose of 3 g per day or one tablet of glyburide (5 mg per day) for four weeks. Mulberry therapy significantly improved diabetic control in type 2 diabetic patients (see the table below). The results clearly show that the fasting blood glucose concentrations were significantly lowered with mulberry therapy, suggesting that it is effective in controlling diabetes. Mulberry therapy significantly reduced fasting blood glucose concentration of diabetic patients by 27% compared with glyburide, which reduced it by only 8%. Mulberry extract was also superior to glyburide in its ability to decrease hemoglobin A1C, total cholesterol, LDL, and triglycerides. It also resulted in an increase in HDL, the "good" cholesterol. Although these changes were not statistically significant, there are strong suggestions that this natural product is clearly superior to an established drug treatment for type 2 diabetes.

In addition to the beneficial effects on blood glucose levels and blood lipids, mulberry therapy was also shown to reduce the amount of lipid peroxidation in the cell membranes of RBCs, indicating a significant antioxidant effect. Additionally, mulberry therapy significantly decreased membrane cholesterol of type 2 diabetic patients.

Improving Insulin Function and Sensitivity

The first step in improving insulin function and sensitivity is achieving ideal body weight and following the dietary and lifestyle recommendations given earlier, including taking a high-potency multiple vitamin and mineral formula to ensure the body has all of the necessary essential vitamins and minerals that proper insulin sensitivity requires. If additional support is necessary to bring blood glucose levels under control, we would recommend using in isolation or in scientifically formulated combinations one or more of the following: *Gymnema sylvestre* extract, bitter melon, *Panax quinquefolius* (American ginseng) or *Panax ginseng* (Chinese ginseng), and fenugreek seed extract. We also recommend increasing the intake of onions and garlic.

Gymnema sylvestre. Gymnema is a plant from India that has long been used as a treatment for diabetes. Recent scientific investi-

Influence of Mulberry and Glyburide Treatments on Blood Glucose, Glycosylated Hemoglobin, and Serum Lipids of Patients with Type 2 Diabetes						
VARIABLE	**GLYBURIDE**			**MULBERRY**		
	BEFORE	**AFTER**	**CHANGE (%)**	**BEFORE**	**AFTER**	**CHANGE (%)**
Fasting blood glucose (mg/dl)	154.4	141.8	−8	152.7	110.5	−27
A1C (%)	12.5	12.4	0	12.5	11.2	−10
Cholesterol (mg/dl)	190	182	−4	193.7	170.3	−12
LDL (mg/dl)	102.5	95.5	−7	102.1	78.7	−23
HDL (mg/dl)	49.8	51.3	+3	50.1	59.2	+18
Triglycerides (mg/dl)	199.5	180	−10	200.4	168	−16
Free fatty acids (pmol/dl)	589.8	580	−2	590.1	520	−12

gation has upheld its effectiveness in both type 1 and type 2. Gymnema extracts have been shown to enhance glucose control in diabetic dogs and rabbits. Interestingly, in animals that have their pancreas removed, gymnema has no apparent effects, suggesting that it enhances the production or activity of insulin. There is evidence in animal studies that gymnema promotes the regeneration of insulin-producing beta cells in the pancreas. Studies with humans also seem to support the possibility of pancreas regeneration.[157]

An extract of the leaves of *G. sylvestre* given to 27 patients with type 1 on insulin therapy was shown to reduce insulin requirements and fasting blood glucose levels, as well as to improve blood glucose control.[158] These results indicate that gymnema enhances the action of insulin, as these diabetics were not recently diagnosed. Clinical experience also shows that gymnema has a significant benefit in decreasing sugar cravings and enabling patients to follow a lower-carbohydrate diet.

In type 2 diabetes, gymnema extract appears to work by enhancing the action of insulin. In one study, 22 type 2 diabetics were given gymnema extract along with their oral diabetes drugs.[159] All patients demonstrated improved blood glucose control; 21 of the 22 were able to reduce their drug dosage considerably, and 5 were able to discontinue their medication and maintain blood glucose control with the gymnema extract alone.

The dosage for gymnema extract (standardized to contain 24% gymnemic acid) can range between 200 mg twice a day and 2,400 mg per day. No side effects have been reported from gymnema extract.

Bitter Melon. In addition to being eaten as a vegetable in Asia, unripe bitter melon (*Momordica charantia*) has been used extensively in folk medicine as a remedy for diabetes.

The blood-glucose-lowering action of the fresh juice or extract of the unripe fruit has been clearly established in modern scientific studies in both type 1 and type 2.

Bitter melon contains several compounds with confirmed blood-glucose-lowering properties. Charantin, extracted by alcohol, is a hypoglycemic agent composed of mixed steroids that is more potent than the oral hypoglycemic drug tolbutamide. Bitter melon also contains an insulin-like polypeptide, polypeptide-P, which lowers blood glucose levels when injected like insulin into type 1 diabetics. Because it appears to have fewer side effects than insulin, it has been suggested as a replacement for insulin in some patients, although the likelihood that this application will ever be developed is extremely remote. Fortunately, taking as little as 2 fl oz of the juice has shown good results in clinical trials.[160,161]

Unripe bitter melon is available primarily at Asian grocery stores. Health food stores may have bitter melon extracts, but the fresh juice is probably the best to use, as this was what was used in the studies. Bitter melon juice is difficult to make palatable. As its name implies, it is quite bitter, so we recommend that patients hold the nose and take a 2-fl-oz shot of the juice. The dosage of other forms should approximate this dose.

American Ginseng. Research conducted at the University of Toronto's Risk Factor Modification Center has uncovered important properties of some ancient natural medicines. In a study at the center, 3 g whole powdered American ginseng (*Panax quinquefolius*) root taken before each meal reduced postprandial blood glucose significantly in type 2 diabetics.[162–166] American ginseng is now considered by authorities to be the herbal therapy with the strongest evidence of efficacy in type 2.[167]

Panax ginseng (Chinese ginseng) can also be helpful. In a double-blind, controlled study, 36 non-insulin-dependent diabetic patients were treated for eight weeks with ginseng extract at 100 or 200 mg or with a placebo. Ginseng elevated mood, improved both physical and mental performance, and reduced fasting blood glucose and body weight. The 200-mg dose improved A1C levels and physical activity.[168]

Fenugreek. Fenugreek seeds have demonstrated significant antidiabetic effects in experimental and clinical studies. The active principles are the special soluble fiber of fenugreek, along with the alkaloid trigonelline and 4-hydroxyisoleucine. Fenugreek appears to be helpful in both type 1 and type 2 diabetes. Defatted fenugreek seed powder given to type 1 diabetics twice per day at a 50-g dose resulted in a significant reduction in fasting blood glucose and improved glucose tolerance test results.[169] A 54% reduction in two-hour urinary glucose excretion and significant reductions in LDL and VLDL cholesterol and triglyceride values also occurred. In type 2 diabetics, the addition of 15 g powdered fenugreek seed soaked in water significantly reduced postprandial glucose levels during the meal tolerance test.[170] However, that is a very large dose and impractical for daily supplementation. In another study, however, 25 patients with type 2 were randomly assigned to receive 1 g per day of fenugreek seed extract or placebo capsules for 2 months.[171] Complex analysis of the data produced an interesting finding. The group taking the fenugreek seed extract had improved blood glucose measurements (e.g., fasting blood glucose levels dropped from 148.3 to 119.9 mg/dl), but there was a significant decrease in insulin output. This finding indicates that there was a significant improvement in insulin sensitivity. This effect is most likely due to the 4-hydroxyleucine.

Onions and Garlic. Onions (*Allium cepa*) and garlic (*Allium sativum*) appear to have significant blood-glucose-lowering action. The active principles are believed to be the sulfur-containing compounds allyl propyl disulfide (APDS) and diallyl disulphide oxide (allicin), respectively, although other constituents such as flavonoids may play a role as well.

Although garlic generally has more potent effects, onions can be given at higher dosages and the active compounds appear to be more stable than allicin. Graded doses of onion extracts (1 ml extract = 1 g whole onion) at levels sometimes found in the diet (i.e., 1 to 7 oz onion) reduced blood glucose levels during an oral glucose tolerance test in a dose-dependent manner. The effects are similar with both raw and boiled onion extracts, indicating that the active components are probably stable.[172]

Garlic has a wide range of additional well-documented effects useful for the diabetic, including helping to improve blood glucose control, lower cholesterol and blood pressure, and inhibit some of the factors associated with increased risk for vascular complications of diabetes such as increased fibrinogen levels.

Preventing Nutritional and Oxidative Stress

Diabetes is characterized by increased nutritional and oxidative stress. Individuals with diabetes typically have elevated levels of free radicals and oxidative compounds. These highly reactive compounds bind to and destroy cellular compounds. They also greatly increase the inflammatory process by increasing the formation of inflammatory mediators such as C-reactive protein.

One of the critical goals in nutritionally supporting individuals with diabetes is to flood the body with a high level of antioxidant compounds to counteract the negative effects of free radicals and pro-oxidants. The implementation of this goal is achieved by using the recommendations given earlier, along with taking a flavonoid-rich extract and alpha-lipoic acid.

Flavonoids. Recent research suggests that flavonoids may be useful in treating diabetes, as well as in preventing long-term complications. Flavonoids such as quercetin promote insulin secretion and are potent inhibitors of glycosylation and sorbitol accumulation, while flavonoid-rich extracts such as bilberry and hawthorn have been shown to be helpful in diabetic retinopathy and microvascular abnormalities.[173]

The beneficial effects of flavonoids in battling the complications of diabetes are numerous and include the fact that flavonoids are generally more potent and effective against a broader range of oxidants than the traditional antioxidant nutrients vitamins C and E, beta-carotene, selenium, and zinc. Other beneficial effects include increasing

Flavonoids for the Treatment of Diabetes and Diabetic Complications

EXTRACT	DAILY DOSE	INDICATION
Bilberry extract (25% anthocyanidins)	160–320 mg	Best choice in diabetic retinopathy or cataracts.
Ginkgo biloba extract (24% ginkgo flavonglycosides)	120–240 mg	Best choice for most people older than 50. Protects brain and vascular lining. Very important in improving blood flow to the extremities (useful for neuropathy and foot ulcers).
Grape seed extract or pine bark extract (>95% procyanidolic oligomers)	150–300 mg	Systemic antioxidant; best choice for most people younger than 50, especially if retinopathy, hypertension, easy bruising, and poor wound healing exist. Also specific for the lungs, varicose veins, and protection against cardiovascular disease.
Green tea extract (>80% total polyphenols)	150–300 mg	Best choice in the early stage of type 1 diabetes or if there is a family history of cancer.
Hawthorn extract (10% proanthocyanidins)	450–600 mg	Best choice in cardiovascular disease or hypertension.
Milk thistle extract (70% silymarin)	210–350 mg	Best choice if there are signs of impaired liver function.
Mixed citrus flavonoids	1,000–2,000 mg	Least expensive choice but may not provide same level of benefit; OK if no complications currently present.

intracellular vitamin C levels, decreasing the leakiness and breakage of small blood vessels (preventing easy bruising), promoting wound healing, and providing immune system support. Good dietary sources of flavonoids include citrus fruits, berries, onions, parsley, legumes, green tea, and red wine.

For individuals with diabetes who are already showing signs of long-term complications, it is extremely important to take a flavonoid-rich extract. Because certain flavonoids concentrate in specific tissues, it is possible to take flavonoids that target specific body tissues. For example, because the flavonoids of bilberry (*Vaccinium myrtillus*) have an affinity for the eye, including the retina, bilberry is probably the best choice for a diabetic already exhibiting signs of diabetic retinopathy. Identify which flavonoid or flavonoid-rich extract is most appropriate and take it according to the recommended dosage (see the table opposite). There is tremendous overlap among the mechanisms of action and benefits of flavonoid-rich extracts; the key point here is to take the one that is most specific to your needs.

Alpha-lipoic Acid. Alpha-lipoic acid is a vitamin-like substance that is often described as "nature's perfect antioxidant." First of all, alpha-lipoic acid is a small molecule that is efficiently absorbed and easily crosses cell membranes. Unlike vitamin E, which is primarily fat soluble, and vitamin C, which is water soluble, alpha-lipoic acid can quench either water- or fat-soluble free radicals both inside the cell and outside in the intracellular spaces. Furthermore, alpha-lipoic acid extends the biochemical life of vitamin C and E, as well as other antioxidants such as glutathione, the most important intracellular antioxidant.

Alpha-lipoic acid is an approved drug in Germany for the treatment of diabetic neuropathy and has been successfully used there for more than 30 years. The beneficial effects of alpha-lipoic acid in diabetic neuropathy have been confirmed in several double-blind studies at a dosage of 400 to 600 mg per day.[174,175] Although the primary effect of alpha-lipoic acid in improving diabetic neuropathy is thought to be the result of its antioxidant effects, it has also been shown to lead to an improvement in blood glucose metabolism, improve blood flow to peripheral nerves, and actually stimulate the regeneration of nerve fibers. Its importance in treating diabetic neuropathy cannot be overstated.

Recommendations for Specific Chronic Complications

Following are additional recommendations for dealing with specific complications of diabetes. The most important method for reducing the risk of all these complications is achieving optimal blood glucose control.

Elevated Cholesterol Levels

Key natural products to lower cholesterol levels in diabetes are soluble fiber, garlic, and niacin. These agents are discussed fully in the chapter "High Cholesterol and/or Triglycerides." Because taking niacin at higher dosages (3,000 mg or more) can impair glucose tolerance, many physicians have avoided using niacin therapy for diabetics, but newer studies with slightly lower dosages (1,000 to 2,000 mg) of niacin have not shown it to adversely affect blood glucose regulation.[176] For example, during a 16-week, double-blind, placebo-controlled trial, 148 type 2 patients were randomly assigned either to a placebo or to 1,000 or 1,500 mg per day of niacin; in the niacin-treated groups there was no significant loss in glycemic control, and the favorable effects on blood lipids were still apparent.[177] Other studies have actually shown hemoglobin A1C to drop, indicating improvement in glycemic control.[178]

The most common blood lipid abnormalities in type 2 diabetic patients are elevated triglyceride levels, decreased HDL cholesterol levels, and a preponderance of smaller, denser LDL particles—the worst type. Niacin has been shown to address all of these areas much more significantly than the statin or other lipid-lowering drugs. However, one reason that niacin may not be as popular as it should be is the side effect of skin flushing—like a prickly heat rash—that typically occurs 20 to 30 minutes after the niacin is taken and disappears after about the same amount of time. Other occasional side effects of niacin include gastric irritation, nausea, and liver damage. The liver damage risk is very pertinent. Diabetic patients who are overweight frequently have developed a fatty liver (see the chapter "Non-Alcoholic Fatty Liver Disease [NAFLD]/Non-Alcoholic Steatohepatitis [NASH]"). Fatty liver is now considered to be as damaging as the effects of alcohol dependence and hepatitis C, and can also lead to fibrosis and cirrhosis of liver tissue. Taking niacin may put extra stress on that vital organ. With overweight diabetic patients, therefore, high-dose niacin is to be used only under a physician's recommendation. To reduce the side effect of skin flushing, use intermediate-release niacin, which is identical in dissolution pattern to the prescription niacin product Niaspan. Taking an intermediate-release product just before going to bed is recommended, as most people sleep right through any flushing reaction if one should occur. Another approach to reduce flushing is to use inositol hexaniacinate. This form of niacin has long been used in Europe to lower cholesterol levels and also to improve blood flow in intermittent claudication, a peripheral vascular disease that is quite common in diabetes.[179] If inositol hexaniacinate does not work, regular niacin can be tried.

If regular niacin or inositol hexaniacinate is being used, a dose of 500 mg should be given at night, before bed, for 1 week. The dosage should be increased to 1,000 mg the next week and 1,500 mg the following week. The 1,500 mg dosage should be given for two months before checking the response; the dosage can be adjusted up or down depending on the response. Intermediate-release niacin products such Niaspan can be used at the full dosage of 1,000 to 2,000 mg at night from the beginning. Regardless of the form of niacin being used, periodic checking (minimum every three months) of cholesterol, A1C, and liver function is strongly indicated.

Retinopathy and Cataracts

Diabetic retinopathy has two forms: (1) simple retinopathy, with bursting of blood vessels, hemorrhages, and swelling; and (2) proliferative retinopathy, with newly formed vessels, scarring, more serious hemorrhage, and retinal detachment. The development of laser photocoagulation therapy is an important treatment for the more severe proliferative retinopathy but is not indicated in milder forms of retinopathy, because the risk of visual loss usually outweighs the benefits.

Extremely important in the battle against retinopathy are flavonoid-rich extracts, especially bilberry, pine bark, or grape seed extract. Flavonoids increase intracellular vitamin C levels, decrease the leakiness and breakage of capillaries, prevent easy bruising, and exert potent antioxidant effects. These effects are of particular value in dealing with the microvascular abnormalities of diabetes. Because the flavonoids in bilberry, pine bark, and grape seed extract have an affinity for the blood vessels of the eye and improve circulation to the retina, they are particularly helpful in slowing the progression of diabetic retinopathy, as evidenced by positive results in more than a dozen clinical trials.[180,181]

Neuropathy

In addition to alpha-lipoic acid and the basic supplementation program, three natural medicines along with acupuncture deserve mention:

- **Gamma-linolenic acid (GLA)** has been shown to improve and prevent diabetic neuropathy. Diabetes is associated with a substantial disturbance in essential fatty acid metabolism. One of the key disturbances is the impairment in the process of converting linoleic acid to GLA. As a result, providing GLA in the form of borage, evening primrose, or black currant oil can bypass some of this disturbance. In the GLA Multicenter Trial, 111 patients with mild diabetic neuropathy were given either GLA at a dose of 480 mg per day or a placebo for one year. Sixteen different variables were assessed, including conduction velocities, hot and cold thresholds, sensation, tendon reflexes, and muscle strength. After one year, all 16 of these improved, 13 of them to a statistically significant degree. Treatment was more effective in patients with relatively well-controlled diabetes than in those with poorly controlled disease.

- **Benfotiamine** is a fat-soluble form of thiamine (vitamin B_1) that is more effective in raising blood thiamine levels (up to 120–240% vs. regular thiamine). In studies of diabetics, benfotiamine decreased advanced glycosylated end-product formation, decreased sorbitol accumulation, and reduced oxidative cellular damage.[182] However, results in the treatment of diabetic neuropathy and nephropathy in small clinical trials with benfotiamine alone show modest to no benefit.[183,184] It is possible that benfotiamine should be combined with alpha-lipoic acid. In a small study of patients with type 1, treatment with 600 mg benfotiamine with 300 mg alpha-lipoic acid produced better results in reducing the effects of hyperglycemia than benfotiamine alone.[185]

- **Capsaicin** is the active component of cayenne pepper (*Capsicum frutescens*), which stimulates and then blocks the small nerve fibers that transmit the pain impulse by depleting these fibers of a transmitting substance known as substance P.[186] Topically applied capsaicin has been shown to be of considerable benefit in relieving the pain of diabetic neuropathy in numerous double-blind studies. Roughly 80% of people with diabetic neuropathy experience tremendous pain relief.[187] Commercial ointments containing 0.025% or 0.075% capsaicin are available over the counter. Apply the 0.075% cream twice per day to the affected area (cover the hand with plastic wrap or use disposable gloves to avoid the chance that the capsaicin will come into contact with the eyes or mucous membranes). It may take a few days for the cream to start working, and it will continue to work only with regular application.

- **Acupuncture** can also be helpful in improving neuropathy. The scientific investigation of acupuncture in diabetes includes both experimental and clinical studies. For example, animal experiments have shown that acupuncture can act on the pancreas to enhance insulin synthesis, increase the number of receptors on target cells, and accelerate the utilization of glucose, resulting in lowering of blood glucose.[188] However, the best-documented use for acupuncture is in treating chronic painful diabetic neuropathy. In one clinical study, 77% of patients treated with acupuncture noted significant improvement in their symptoms, with 21% noting that their symptoms were completely eliminated.[189]

That success rate is excellent considering the long-standing nature of the condition in most of the patients and the fact that no side effects were observed.

Nephropathy

Particularly important for kidney protection in diabetics is dietary fiber. Dietary fiber (especially soluble fiber) is fermented in the colon to produce short-chain fatty acids. These by-products are the primary fuel for the cells of the colon, and if present in high amounts, they greatly increase the colon's waste removal capabilities. It has been shown that in the presence of a high-fermentable-fiber diet, the colon turns into a "second kidney," collecting nitrogenous wastes from the blood and disposing of them in the feces. This has been shown to greatly reduce stress on the kidneys.[190]

Highlighting just how important some of the basic supplement recommendations are in halting the progression of diabetic nephropathy are the results of a study of 30 type 2 patients with elevated albumin in their urine. The patients received vitamin C (1,250 mg) and vitamin E (680 IU) per day or a placebo for four weeks, followed by a three-week washout period before being switched to the other treatment.[191] The results were that the vitamins were successful in reducing urinary albumin levels by an average of nearly 20%, indicating that antioxidant therapy may slow or halt the progression of kidney disease in diabetics.

If a diabetic has developed serious kidney failure, then following a low-protein, low-potassium diet is necessary; unfortunately, that does not aid good glucose control, which can then promote worse kidney functioning. The main goal is to prevent end-stage renal disease from developing in the first place.

If drugs are necessary, the angiotensin-converting enzyme (ACE) inhibitors and ACE receptor blockers offer the greatest benefits in dealing with diabetic nephropathy.[192] They are now often prescribed in low doses to help prevent nephropathy, even in the absence of high blood pressure. Alternatively, a special preparation of bonito peptides has been shown to exert similar anti-ACE activity (see the chapter "High Blood Pressure" for more information) and may prevent the need for actual ACE inhibitors.

Poor Wound Healing

A deficiency of virtually any essential nutrient can lead to impaired wound healing. Key nutrients include vitamin C and zinc, both of which are often deficient in the diabetic. Taking a high-potency multiple vitamin and mineral formula should improve nutritional status and promote proper wound healing. For topical application pure (100%) aloe vera gel can be used. Aloe vera contains a number of compounds necessary for wound healing, including vitamin C, vitamin E, and zinc, and has been shown to stimulate many factors important to wound repair. Apply it to affected areas (not severe open wounds) two or three times per day. Another option is a proprietary product called Amerigel, a topical ointment featuring an oak extract (*Quercus rubra*) that contains quercitannic acid, catechin, ellagitannin, and proanthocyanidin, readily absorbed into damaged skin.

Foot Ulcers

Lack of blood supply, poor wound healing, and peripheral neuropathy are key factors in the development of diabetic foot ulcers. Key strategies in prevention and treatment are proper foot care (including care of nails and calluses), preferably by a podiatrist; regular examination of the feet by a physician; avoidance of injury; avoidance of tobacco in any form; and methods to improve local cir-

QUICK REVIEW

- Diabetes is divided into two major categories: type 1 and type 2.
- Type 2 diabetics, who are not dependent upon insulin, account for 90% of all cases of diabetes.
- Although genetic factors appear important in susceptibility to diabetes, environmental factors are required to trigger diabetes.
- Obesity is a major factor in type 2 diabetes, as 90% of type 2 diabetics are obese.
- Exposure to a protein in cow's milk (bovine albumin peptide) in infancy may trigger the autoimmune process and subsequent type 1 diabetes.
- The trace mineral chromium plays a major role in the sensitivity of cells to insulin.
- To reduce the risk of developing the complications of diabetes, it is important to control against elevations in blood sugar by careful monitoring.
- Dietary modification and dietary treatment are fundamental to the successful treatment of diabetes, whether it be type 1 or 2.
- The treatment of diabetes requires nutritional supplementation, as diabetics have a greatly increased need for many nutrients.
- Since the transport of vitamin C into cells is facilitated by insulin, many diabetics do not have enough intracellular vitamin C.
- Some newly diagnosed type 1 diabetics have experienced complete reversal of their diabetes with niacinamide supplementation.
- Vitamin B_6 supplementation appears to offer significant protection against the development of diabetic nerve disease.
- Diabetics appear to have an increased requirement for vitamin E and benefit from high-dose supplementation.
- Flavonoid-rich extracts such as bilberry, grape seed, or pine bark are extremely important in protecting against the long-term complications of diabetes.
- Onions and garlic have demonstrated blood-sugar-lowering action in several studies and help reduce the risk of cardiovascular disease.
- The oral administration of bitter melon preparations has shown good results in clinical trials in patients with both type 1 and type 2 diabetes.
- Recent scientific investigation has upheld the effectiveness of *Gymnema sylvestre* in treating both type 1 and type 2 diabetes.

culation. Proper foot care includes keeping the feet clean, dry, and warm and wearing well-fitting shoes. Tobacco use in any form constricts the peripheral blood vessels and can lead to more serious peripheral vascular disease with severe arterial blockages. Circulation can be improved by exercising regularly, avoiding sitting cross-legged or in other positions that compromise circulation, and massaging the feet lightly upward. Ginkgo biloba or grape seed extract can also be used to support optimal circulation.

TREATMENT SUMMARY

Effective treatment of the diabetic patient requires the careful integration of wide-ranging therapies and a willingness to substantially improve diet and lifestyle. Type 2 is usually the end result of many years of chronic metabolic insult, and although it is treatable with the natural approach presented here, resolving it will take persistence.

The first step in the therapy of either type 1 or type 2 is a thorough diagnostic workup. Of particular importance is identifying any of the complications of diabetes. Diet, environment, and lifestyle need to be carefully studied to rule out any exposure to agents that may be inducing glucose intolerance. Then a diet, exercise, and supplement program that meets your personal needs must be developed. For maximum efficacy, ideal body weight must be achieved (see the chapter "Obesity and Weight Management").

Monitoring—both by the diabetic and by a physician—is very important in diabetes. Home glucose monitoring and the HbA1C test are essential. It is important to recognize that as the natural therapies described in this chapter take effect, drug dosages must be altered, and so a good working relationship with the prescribing doctor is required. The ultimate goal is to reestablish normal blood sugar control and prevent the development of (or ameliorate) the complications of diabetes.

WARNING: Under no circumstances should a person suddenly stop taking medications for diabetes, especially insulin, unless under direct medical supervision.

Diet

The optimal diet detailed in the chapter "A Health-Promoting Diet" is clearly the diet of choice. Avoid all simple, processed, and concentrated carbohydrates. A low-glycemic diet rich in high-fiber foods should be stressed, and sources of healthful fats should be ingested. Low-glycemic vegetables, including onions and garlic, are particularly useful.

Nutritional Supplements for Type 1 Diabetes

The recommended supplementation program depends on the existing degree of blood glucose control, as indicated by self-monitored blood glucose and A1C levels.

Recently Diagnosed Type 1 Diabetes

- High-potency multiple vitamin and mineral formula as described in the chapter "Supplementary Measures"
- Fish oils: 1,000 mg EPA + DHA per day
- Vitamin C: 500 to 1,500 mg per day
- Vitamin E (mixed tocopherols): 100 to 200 IU per day
- Vitamin D: 4,000 to 10,000 IU per day (ideally, determine dosage according to blood levels)
- Niacinamide: 25 to 50 mg/kg body weight
- Green tea extract: Recommended dosage for children under 6 years is 50 to 150 mg; for children age 6 to 12, 100 to 200 mg; for children older than 12 and adults, 150 to 300 mg. The green tea extract should have a polyphenol content of >90% and be decaffeinated.

Level 1 (Achievement of Targeted Blood Glucose Levels, A1C Levels Less than 7%, No Lipid Abnormalities, No Signs of Complications)

- A high-potency multiple vitamin and mineral formula as described in the chapter "Supplementary Measures"
- Key individual nutrients:
  - Vitamin B_6: 25 to 50 mg per day
  - Folic acid: 800 mcg per day
  - Vitamin B_{12}: 800 mcg per day
  - Vitamin C: 500 to 1,000 mg three times per day

  - Vitamin E (mixed tocopherols): 400 to 800 IU per day
  - Selenium: 100 to 200 mcg per day
  - Zinc: 30 mg per day
  - Vitamin D_3: 4,000 to 10,000 IU per day (ideally, measure blood levels and adjust dosage accordingly)
- Fish oils: 1,000 mg EPA + DHA per day
- Alpha-lipoic acid: 400 to 600 mg per day
- One of the following:
  - Grape seed extract (>95% procyanidolic oligomers): 100 to 300 mg per day
  - Pine bark extract (>95% procyanidolic oligomers): 100 to 300 mg per day
  - Green tea extract (>80% polyphenol content): 150–300 mg per day

Level 2 (Failure to Achieve Targeted Blood Glucose Levels, A1C Above 7%)

- Level 1 supplements
- *Gymnema sylvestre* extract (24% gymnemic acid): 200 mg twice per day
- Biotin: 8 mg twice per day
- Bitter melon juice (optional): 2 to 4 fl oz per day

Nutritional Supplements for Type 2 Diabetes

The recommended supplementation program depends on the degree of blood glucose control, as evidenced by self-monitored blood glucose and A1C levels.

Level 1 (Achievement of Targeted Blood Glucose, A1C Levels Less than 7%, No Lipid Abnormalities, No Signs of Complications)

- Same recommendations as for Level 1 for type 1 diabetes, with the addition of PGX, glucomannan, or another source of soluble fiber, 2,500 to 5,000 mg before meals

Level 2 (Failure to Achieve Targeted Blood Glucose Levels, A1C Above 7%)

- Level 1 supplements
- One of the following insulin enhancers:
  - *Gymnema sylvestre* extract (24% gymnemic acid): 200 mg twice per day
  - Fenugreek extract: 1 g per day
  - Garlic: minimum 4,000 mcg of allicin per day
- One of the following glucosidase inhibitors:
  - Touchi extract: 300 mg three times per day with meals
  - Mulberry extract: equivalent of 1,000 mg dried leaf three times per day

If self-monitored blood glucose levels do not improve after four weeks of following the recommendations for the current level, move to the next highest level. If you are already at Level 2, the next step is to add a prescription medication (either an oral hypoglycemic drug or insulin).

Additional Supplements for the Prevention and Treatment of Diabetic Complications

- For high cholesterol levels and other cardiovascular risk factors:
  - Total cholesterol greater than 200 mg/dl or LDL cholesterol greater than 135 mg (100 mg if history of heart attack); HDL cholesterol below 45 mg/dl; lipoprotein (a) above 40 mg/dl; or triglycerides above 150 mg/dl
  - Niacin (or Niaspan or inositol hexaniacinate): 1,000–2,000 mg at night at bedtime
  - Garlic: minimum of 4,000 mcg of allicin per day
- For hypertension:
  - Garlic: minimum of 4,000 mcg of allicin per day
  - CoQ_{10}: 100 to 200 mg per day
  - One of the following:
    - Hawthorn extract (10% proanthocyanidins or 1.8% vitexin-4¢-rhamnoside): 100 to 250 mg three times per day
    - Olive leaf extract (17% to 23% oleuropein content): 500 mg two times per day
    - Hibiscus: three 240-ml servings/day or an extract providing 10–20 mg anthocyanidins per day
- For diabetic retinopathy:
  - Bilberry extract: 160 to 320 mg per day or grape seed extract: 150 to 300 mg per day
- For diabetic neuropathy:
  - Gamma-linolenic acid from borage,

evening primrose, or blackcurrant oil: 480 mg per day

○ Benfotiamine: 600 mg per day

○ Capsaicin (0.075%) cream: apply to affected area twice per day

- For diabetic nephropathy:

    ○ Follow recommendations for high blood pressure, above, unless kidney function falls below 40% of normal; seek a physician's advice regarding magnesium and potassium supplements

    ○ Benfotiamine: 600 mg per day

- For poor wound healing:

    ○ Aloe vera gel: Apply to affected areas twice per day.

- For diabetic foot ulcers, one of the following:

    ○ *Gingko biloba* extract: 120 to 240 mg per day

    ○ Grape seed extract: 150 to 300 mg per day

Diarrhea

- Increase in frequency, fluidity, and volume of bowel movements

Diarrhea is a common symptom that usually indicates a mild, temporary event. However, it may also be the first suggestion of a serious underlying disease or infection. Severe bloody diarrhea, diarrhea in a child less than six years of age, or diarrhea that lasts more than three days should not be taken lightly; its cause must be determined and it must be treated appropriately.

Diarrhea is divided into four major types: osmotic, secretory, exudative, and inadequate-contact. *Osmotic diarrhea* is caused by an excess of water-soluble molecules in the stool, which results in increased fluid retention. *Secretory diarrhea* results from excessive secretion of ions into the bowel, with the same result of excessive water retention in the stools.

Types of Diarrhea	
TYPE	**CAUSES**
Osmotic	Saline laxatives that contain magnesium, phosphate, or sulfate
	Carbohydrate malabsorption (e.g., lactose intolerance)
	Antacids that contain magnesium salts
	Excess consumption of polyols, such as sorbitol
	Excessive vitamin C intake
	Excessive magnesium intake
Secretory	Toxin-producing bacteria
	Hormone-producing tumors
	Fat malabsorption (e.g., lack of bile output)
	Laxative abuse
	Surgical resection of the small intestine
Exudative	Inflammatory bowel disease (Crohn's disease or ulcerative colitis)
	Pseudomembranous colitis (a post-antibiotic diarrhea caused by an overgrowth of the bacterium *Clostridium difficile*)
	Invasive bacteria
Inadequate-contact	Surgical removal of sections of the intestine
	Short bowel syndrome

Exudative diarrhea is usually due to infections and inflammatory bowel diseases, resulting in abnormal intestinal permeability and intestinal loss of serum proteins, blood, mucus, and pus. Frequent small, painful evacuations are usually a result of disease in the rectum or at the end of the colon. *Inadequate-contact diarrhea* is the result of inadequate contact between the intestinal contents and the absorbing surfaces, resulting in inadequate absorption.

Causes

Diarrhea can have many causes. Again, it is important to consult a physician for an accurate determination.

Viruses are the most common cause of infectious diarrhea, accounting for at least 75% of cases. Viruses are suspected when vomiting is prominent, the incubation period is longer than 14 hours, and the entire illness is over in less than 72 hours. A virus is likely to be the cause if there are no warning signs of bacterial infection (such as high fever, bloody diarrhea, severe abdominal pain, or more than six stools in 24 hours) and there are no epidemiological clues from the history (i.e., travel, sexual contact, antibiotic use). One of the most common causes of viral gastroenteritis, especially in children, is rotavirus. It can be an extremely serious infection, especially in developing countries, where it is estimated to cause more than 800,000 annual deaths among young children.

Besides infectious diarrhea, common causes of chronic diarrhea include lactose intolerance, food allergies, celiac disease (gluten sensitivity), and inflammatory bowel disease (Crohn's disease and ulcerative colitis).

Lactose intolerance is due to a deficiency in the enzyme lactase, responsible for digest-ing the lactose found in dairy products; it is common worldwide. It has been estimated that 70 to 90% of adults of Asian, black, American Indian, and Mediterranean ancestry lack this enzyme. The frequency of deficiency is 10 to 15% among adults of northern and western European descent. While almost all infants are able to digest milk and other dairy products, many children lose their lactase enzyme by three to seven years of age. Symptoms range from minor abdominal discomfort and bloating to severe diarrhea in response to even small amounts of lactose. Symptoms occur because unabsorbed lactose passes through the small intestine and into the colon.

Chronic diarrhea is also one of the most common symptoms of irritable bowel syndrome, a functional disorder of the intestines that can include chronic loose stools (see the chapter "Irritable Bowel Syndrome"), and food allergies, as ingestion of an allergenic food can result in the release of histamine and other allergic-reaction compounds that can produce a powerful laxative effect (see the chapter "Food Allergy").

Celiac disease (see the chapter "Celiac Disease") is caused by sensitivity to gluten, a protein in many grains. One of the hallmark features of celiac disease is chronic diarrhea.

Inflammatory bowel disease (see the chapter "Crohn's Disease and Ulcerative Colitis") is characterized by recurring bouts of often painful and bloody diarrhea.

Therapeutic Considerations

Since most causes of acute diarrhea, such as mild infections due to food poisoning or viral gastroenteritis, are self-limiting and will resolve on their own, only some general recommendations may be needed. If the diarrhea

Causes of Diarrhea	
CAUSE	**MOST COMMON EXAMPLES**
Functional disorders	Irritable bowel syndrome
Intestinal viral infections	Enterovirus, rotavirus
Intestinal bacterial infections	*Campylobacter jejuni, Shigella* species, *Salmonella* species, *Yersinia enterocolitica*
Intestinal bacterial toxins	*Clostridium difficile,* pathogenic *Escherichia coli, Staphylococcus* species. *Vibrio parahaemolytica, Vibrio cholerae*
Parasitic infections	*Giardia lamblia, Entamoeba histolytica, Cryptosporidium* species, *Isospora* species
Inflammatory bowel disease	Crohn's disease, ulcerative colitis, diverticulitis
Antibiotic therapy	Tetracycline, amoxicillin, others
Inadequate bile secretion	Hepatitis, bile duct obstruction
Malabsorption states	Celiac disease, short small bowel, lactose intolerance
Pancreatic disease	Pancreatic insufficiency, pancreatic tumor
Reflex from other areas	Pelvic inflammatory disease
Neurological disease	Diabetic neuropathy, multiple sclerosis
Metabolic disease	Hyperthyroidism
Malnutrition	Severe protein and/or calorie malnutrition Food allergy Laxative abuse Heavy metal poisoning
Miscellaneous	Fecal impaction, cancer

is severe or bloody, or if it involves a child under the age of six years, contact a physician immediately. A physician should also be consulted if any diarrhea lasts for more than three days.

Therapy for any chronic diarrhea requires identification of the underlying cause and treatment designed to restore normal bowel function. The discussion in this chapter will focus on general support for all diarrheas. Other chapters discuss treatments for some other causes of diarrhea, such as inflammatory bowel disease (see "Crohn's Disease and Ulcerative Colitis"), celiac disease (see "Celiac Disease"), and impaired digestion (see "Digestion and Elimination").

General Recommendations

There are several measures that can be used as general support during any case of diarrhea:

- Focus on liquids and follow the BRAT diet
- Replace electrolytes
- Avoid dairy products
- Take carob powder or pectin
- Take probiotics

Focus on Liquids and Follow the BRAT Diet

During the acute phase of diarrhea, the focus should be on liquids and the BRAT diet. The components of this diet are bananas, white rice, apples, plain white toast or bread (consider bread made with rice flour instead of wheat flour), and tea. These foods are easy on the digestive system and tend to slow down the rhythmic contractions of the intestines.

Replace Electrolytes

With diarrhea, a person loses much water and a great deal of electrolytes, such as potassium, sodium, and chloride. It is important to replace these lost items. This replacement can be in the form of herbal teas, vegetable broths, fruit juices, and electrolyte replacement drinks. An old naturopathic remedy is to sip a drink made of equal parts of sauerkraut juice and tomato juice.

When there are young children in the household, it is a good idea to have electrolyte replacement drinks on hand as a precautionary measure. In addition to the well-known Pedialyte and Gatorade brands, electrolyte replacement drinks with healthier ingredients are now available at health food stores.

Avoid Dairy Products

Acute intestinal illnesses, such as viral or bacterial intestinal infections, will frequently injure the cells that line the small intestine. This results in a temporary deficiency of lactase, the enzyme responsible for digesting milk sugar (lactose) from dairy products. Avoid dairy products (with the possible exception of yogurt with live cultures) while experiencing diarrhea.

Take Carob Powder or Pectin

Since the early 1950s, there have been several reports in the medical literature indicating that brewed teas of roasted carob powder are effective and without side effects in the treatment of acute-onset diarrhea.[1,2] Carob is rich in dietary fiber and compounds known as polyphenols. These two components are thought to be responsible for the beneficial effects.

Carob powder is particularly helpful in treating diarrhea in young children. One study involved 41 infants from 3 to 21 months of age, with acute diarrhea of bacterial and viral origin. The infants were treated in a hospital setting with oral rehydration fluid (e.g., Pedialyte) and randomly received either carob powder (a daily dose of 1.5 g/kg) or an equivalent placebo for up to six days.[1] The powders were diluted either in the oral rehydration solution or in milk (which we do not recommend; see "Avoid Dairy Products," above). The duration of diarrhea in the carob group was 2 days, compared with 3.75 days in the placebo group. Normalizations in defecation, body temperature, and weight, plus cessation of vomiting, were also reached more quickly in the carob group. No side effects from carob were reported.

An alternative approach to carob is the use of pectin, a fiber found in citrus fruits, apples, and many other fruits and vegetables.

Take Probiotics

The term *probiotics* refers to bacteria in the intestine considered beneficial to health. The most important healthful bacteria are *Lactobacillus acidophilus* and *Bifidobacterium bifidum*. Probiotics have a protective effect against acute diarrheal disease and have been shown to be successful in the treatment or prevention of various types of infectious diarrhea, including rotavirus, *Clostridium difficile*, and traveler's diarrhea. There is absolutely no question that probiotic supplementation shortens the duration of acute infectious diarrhea and reduces stool frequency, as numerous clinical studies now document this benefit. Probiotic supplementation is especially important in helping children susceptible to infectious diarrhea.

Furthermore, probiotics exert immune-enhancing effects.[3–6]

Probiotic supplementation is also well documented to prevent antibiotic-induced diarrhea as well as promote recovery from it. Although it is commonly believed that acidophilus supplements are not effective if taken during antibiotic therapy, the research actually supports usage of *L. acidophilus* during antibiotic administration.[3–9] Reduc-

PARASITES

Parasites are microorganisms that live off their host (in this case, a human being) and ultimately cause damage to the host. There are about 500 normal microbial inhabitants of the human digestive tract; whether any of them will become parasitic depends on whether they are living in harmony with the host or growing out of balance. *Candida albicans* is an example of an organism that, under normal circumstances, lives in harmony with the host. But if candida overgrows and is out of balance with other gut microbes, it can result in problems. In general, parasites cause most of their problems by interfering with digestion and/or damaging the intestinal lining, either of which can lead to diarrhea.

Diarrheal diseases caused by parasites that are not part of the normal gastrointestinal tract still constitute the single greatest worldwide cause of illness and death. The problem is magnified in underdeveloped countries that have poor sanitation, but even in the United States diarrheal diseases are the third leading cause of sickness and death. Furthermore, the ease and frequency of worldwide travel and increased migration to the United States are resulting in growing numbers of parasitic infections.

There are many types of microbes that can be classified as parasites, but usually when physicians refer to parasites they mean the organisms known as *protozoa* (one-celled organisms) and *helminths* (worms).

Common Parasites
- Common protozoa
  - Amoeba (primarily *Entamoeba histolytica*)
  - Giardia
  - Trichomonas
  - Cryptosporidium
  - *Dientamoeba fragilis*
  - *Iodamoeba butschlii*
  - Blastocystis
  - *Balantidium coli*
  - Chilomastix
- Helminths
  - Roundworms (*Ascaris lumbricoides*)
  - Pinworms (*Enterobius vermicularis*)
  - Hookworms (*Necator americanus*)
  - Threadworms (*Strongyloides stercoralis*)
  - Whipworms (*Trichuris trichiura*)
- Tapeworms (various species)

Detection of parasites involves collecting multiple stool samples at two- to four-day intervals. The stool sample is analyzed under a microscope after it has been prepared with specialized staining techniques and fluorescent antibodies (the antibodies attach to any parasites present and fluoresce when exposed to a certain wavelength of light).

There are a number of natural compounds that can be useful in helping the body get rid of parasites. However, before selecting a natural alternative to an antibiotic, try to discern what factors may have been responsible for setting up the internal terrain for a parasitic infection—decreased output of hydrochloric acid, decreased pancreatic enzyme output, and so on. Proper treatment with either an antibiotic or a natural alternative requires monitoring by repeating multiple stool samples two weeks after therapy.

Popular natural treatments for parasitic infections include high dosages of pancreatic enzymes (8–10X USP; 750 to 1,000 mg 10 to 20 minutes before meals) and berberine-containing plants such as goldenseal (*Hydrastis canadensis*), barberry (*Berberis vulgaris*), Oregon grape (*Berberis aquifolium*), and goldthread (*Coptis chinensis*).

tions of friendly bacteria or superinfection with antibiotic-resistant flora, or both, may be prevented by administering *L. acidophilus* products during antibiotic therapy. For example, in one double-blind study of 740 patients undergoing cataract surgery, the patients were given an antibiotic containing ampicillin (250 mg) and cloxacillin (250 mg) and either a placebo or a probiotic supplement. The incidence of diarrhea in patients receiving the antibiotic alone was 13.3% compared with 0% in patients receiving the antibiotic with the probiotic.[9]

Antibiotics often cause diarrhea by altering the type of bacteria in the colon or by promoting the overgrowth of *Candida albicans*. Antibiotic use can result in a severe form of diarrhea known as pseudomembranous enterocolitis. This condition is attributed to an overgrowth of one type of bacteria (*Clostridium difficile*) that results from the death of the bacteria that normally keep it under control. We recommend a dosage of at least 15 billion to 20 billion organisms during antibiotic therapy; leave as much time as possible between the dose of antibiotic and the probiotic supplement. If pseudomembranous enterocolitis develops, in addition to *Lactobacillus* and *Bifidobacter* species we also recommend supplementing with *Saccharomyces boulardi* (also known as *S. cerevisiae*), a nonpathogenic probiotic yeast shown to be very helpful alone or in combination with the antibiotic vancomycin for pseudomembranous enterocolitis.[10] Although *Saccharomyces boulardi* is generally safe, a few case reports have demonstrated that it should not be used in patients with impaired immune function (such as those with AIDS, cancer patients going through chemotherapy, or people taking immune-suppressing drugs).

Botanical Medicines

Berberine

Plants that contain the alkaloid berberine such as goldenseal (*Hydrastis canadensis*), barberry (*Berberis vulgaris*), Oregon grape (*Berberis aquifolium*), and goldthread (*Coptis chinensis*) have a long history of use in infectious diarrhea. Clinical studies with pure berberine have shown significant success in the treatment of acute diarrhea. It has been found effective against diarrheas caused by *E. coli* (traveler's diarrhea), *Shigella dysenteriae* (shigellosis), *Salmonella paratyphi* (food poisoning), *Klebsiella pneumoniae*, *Giardia lamblia* (giardiasis), *Entamoeba histolytica* (amebiasis), and *Vibrio cholerae* (cholera).[11–17]

Berberine appears to be effective in treating the majority of common gastrointestinal infections. Clinical studies have shown berberine comparable to standard antibiotics in most cases; in fact, results were better in several studies. For example, one study focused on 65 children under five years of age who had acute diarrhea caused by *E. coli*, *Shigella*, *Salmonella*, *Klebsiella*, or *Faecalis aerogenes*. The children who were given berberine tannate (25 mg every six hours) responded better than those who received standard antibiotic therapy.[15]

Another study involved 40 children, ages 1 through 10 years, who were infected with giardia. The children received daily divided doses of either berberine (5 mg/kg per day), the drug metronidazole (10 mg/kg per day), or a placebo of vitamin B syrup.[16] After six days, 48% of the children treated with berberine were symptom-free, and upon stool analysis 68% were found to be giardia-free. In the metronidazole group, 33% of the children were without symptoms and, upon stool analysis, all were found to be giardia-free. In comparison, 15% of the children who took the placebo were without symptoms and, upon stool analysis, 25% were found to be giardia-free. These results indicate that berberine was actually more effective than metronidazole in relieving symptoms at half the dose, but less effective than the drug in clearing the organism from the intestines.

Finally, in a study of 200 adult patients with acute diarrhea, the subjects were given standard antibiotic treatment with or without berberine hydrochloride (150 mg per day). Results of the study indicated that the patients who received berberine recovered more quickly.[17] An additional 30 cases of acute diarrhea were treated with berberine alone. Berberine arrested diarrhea in all of these cases, with no mortality or toxicity.

Despite these results, owing to the serious consequences of an ineffectively treated infectious diarrhea, the best approach may be to use berberine-containing plants along with standard antibiotic therapy. Much of berberine's effectiveness is undoubtedly due to its direct antimicrobial activity. However, it also has an effect in blocking the action of toxins produced by certain bacteria.[18–20] This toxin-blocking effect is most evident in diarrheas caused by the enterotoxins *Vibrio cholerae* (cholera) and *E. coli* (traveler's diarrhea).

Cholera is a serious disorder that needs standard therapy. However, traveler's diarrhea is usually self-limiting. Good results have been obtained using berberine in the

- -

QUICK REVIEW

- **Severe bloody diarrhea, diarrhea in a child under six years of age, or diarrhea that lasts more than three days should not be taken lightly; its cause must be determined and it must be treated appropriately.**

- **The therapy for any chronic diarrhea requires identification of the underlying cause and then treatment designed to restore normal bowel function.**

- **Replace lost water and electrolytes by drinking herbal teas, vegetable broths, fruit juices, or electrolyte replacement drinks.**

- **Avoid dairy products (with the possible exception of yogurt with live cultures) while experiencing diarrhea.**

- **Carob powder is particularly helpful in treating diarrhea in young children.**

- **Supplementation with probiotics is cru-** cial in the treatment of diarrhea of any kind, but particularly in antibiotic-associated diarrhea.

- **Chronic diarrhea is one of the most common symptoms of food allergy.**

- **It has been estimated that 70 to 90% of adults of Asian, black, Native American, and Mediterranean ancestry lack the enzyme required to digest milk sugar (lactose).**

- **Diarrheal diseases caused by parasites still constitute the single greatest worldwide cause of illness and death.**

- **Popular natural treatments of parasitic infections include high dosages of pancreatic enzymes and berberine-containing plants, such as goldenseal.**

- **Berberine has shown significant success in the treatment of acute diarrhea in several clinical studies.**

treatment of traveler's diarrhea. In one study, patients with traveler's diarrhea randomly served as controls or received 400 mg berberine sulfate in a single dose.[21] In treated patients, mean stool volumes were significantly less than those of controls during three consecutive eight-hour periods after treatment. Twenty-four hours after treatment, significantly more treated patients than controls stopped having diarrhea (42% vs. 20%).

If you are planning to travel to an underdeveloped country or an area where there is poor water quality or poor sanitation, the prophylactic use of berberine-containing herbs (and probiotic preparations) may be appropriate. Take them one week prior to your trip, during your stay, and one week after visiting.

Tormentil Root

An extract of tormentil root (*Potentilla tormentilla*) has been shown to be useful to treat infectious diarrhea, shorten the duration of rotavirus diarrhea, and decrease the requirement for rehydration solutions.[22] A randomized, double-blinded trial was conducted at a children's hospital in Saint Petersburg, Russia. In this study, 40 children ranging in age from three months to seven years with rotavirus diarrhea were divided into two groups: a treatment group that consisted of 20 children given 3 drops of tormentil root extract per year of life three times per day until discontinuation of diarrhea or a maximum of five days, and a control group of 20 children who received a placebo. The duration of diarrhea was 60% less in the tormentil root extract treatment group than in the placebo group (three days compared with five days in the control group). In the treatment group 8 of 20 children (40%) were diarrhea free 48 hours after admission to the hospital, compared with 1 of 20 (5%) in the control group. Children in the treatment group also needed smaller volumes of parenteral fluids than subjects in the control group.

. . . .

TREATMENT SUMMARY

Since most acute cases of diarrhea are self-limiting, the general recommendations given are often all that are needed. If any of the following apply, a physician should be consulted:

- **Diarrhea in a child under six years of age**
- **Severe or bloody diarrhea**
- **Diarrhea that lasts more than three days**
- **Significant signs of dehydration (sunken eyes, severe dry mouth, strong body odor, etc.)**

After identification of the cause of chronic diarrhea, appropriate treatment can be determined with the help of a physician.

General Recommendations

There are several measures that can be used as general support during any case of diarrhea:

- **Focus on liquids and follow the BRAT diet**
- **Replace electrolytes**
- **Avoid dairy products**
- **Take carob powder or pectin**
- **Take probiotics**

Nutritional Supplements

- A high-potency multiple vitamin and mineral formula as described in the chapter "Supplementary Measures"
- Fish oils: 1,000 mg EPA + DHA per day
- One of the following:
  - Grape seed extract (>95% procyanidolic oligomers): 100 to 300 mg per day
  - Pine bark extract (>95% procyanidolic oligomers): 100 to 300 mg per day
  - Some other flavonoid-rich extract with a similar flavonoid content, super greens formula, or another plant-based antioxidant that can provide an oxygen radical absorption capacity (ORAC) of 3,000 to 6,000 units or more per day
- Probiotic supplement: For prevention of antibiotic-induced diarrhea, a dosage of at least 15 billion to 20 billion organisms, with as much time as possible between the dose of antibiotic and the probiotic supplement; in children younger than age six experiencing antibiotic-induced diarrhea, the probiotic should be taken every day of the antibiotic dose and continued for 1 week after the antibiotic is discontinued.
- *Saccharomyces boulardi*: to treat *Clostridium difficile*, 500 mg twice per day for at least four weeks; can be used to support the antibiotic vancomycin

Botanical Medicines

- Berberine-containing plants: Dosage of any berberine-containing plant should be based on berberine content, to equal 25 to 50 mg berberine three times per day for adults, 5 to 10 mg/kg daily for children (standardized extracts preferred); doses listed below are for goldenseal.
  - Dried root or as infusion (tea), 2 to 4 g three times per day
  - Tincture (1:5), 6 to 12 ml (1.5 to 3 tsp), three times per day
  - Fluid extract (1:1), 2 to 4 ml (0.5 to 1 tsp), three times per day
  - Solid (dry powdered) extract (4:1 or 8% to 12% alkaloid content), 250 to 500 mg three times per day
- Tormentil liquid extract:
  - For adults: 2–4-ml drops three times per day until discontinuation of diarrhea or a maximum of five days
  - For children: 3 drops per year of life three times per day until discontinuation of diarrhea or a maximum of five days

Ear Infection (Otitis Media)

- Acute otitis media:
  - Earache or irritability
  - History of recent upper respiratory tract infection or allergy
  - Red, opaque, bulging eardrum with loss of the normal features
  - Fever and chills
- Chronic or serous otitis media:
  - Painless hearing loss
  - Dull, immobile tympanic membrane

An acute ear infection is usually preceded by an upper respiratory infection or allergy. The organisms most commonly cultured from middle ear fluid during acute otitis media include *Streptococcus pneumoniae* (40–50%), *Haemophilus influenzae* (30–40%), and *Moraxella catarrhalis* (10–15%).

Chronic ear infection—also known as serous, secretory, or nonsuppurative otitis media; chronic otitis media with effusion; and "glue ear"—is a constant swelling and fluid accumulation in the middle ear.

Nearly two-thirds of American children have a bout of acute otitis media by two years of age, and chronic otitis media affects two-thirds of children younger than the age of six. Otitis media is the most common diagnosis in children and is the leading cause of all visits to pediatricians. It is the main reason for antibiotic and surgical interventions during childhood. Children diagnosed with otitis media during infancy are also at greater risk for developing allergic eczema and asthma during school age. The more frequent the ear infections, the stronger these associations.[1] A conservative estimate is that approximately $4 billion to $8 billion is spent annually on medical and surgical treatment of otitis media in the United States.

Standard Medical Treatment

The standard medical approach to an ear infection in children is antibiotics, pain relievers (acetaminophen or ibuprofen), and/or antihistamines. If the ear infection is long-standing and unresponsive to the drugs, surgery is performed. The surgery involves the placement of a tiny plastic myringotomy tube through the eardrum to assist the normal drainage of fluid into the throat via the eustachian tube. It is not a curative procedure, as children with myringotomy tubes in their ears are in fact more likely to have further problems with otitis media.

Myringotomies are currently performed on nearly 1 million American children each year. It appears that the unnecessary surgery of the past, the tonsillectomy, has been replaced by this new procedure. In fact, there is a direct correlation between the decline of the tonsillectomy and the rise of the myringotomy. More than 2 million myringotomy tubes are inserted into children's ears each

year, and 600,000 tonsillectomies and ad-
enoidectomies are done. These surgeries are
unnecessary for most children.

A 1994 evaluation of the appropriateness
of myringotomy tubes for children younger
than 16 years of age in the United States
found that only 42% were judged as being
appropriate.[2] These results mean that several
hundred thousand children are subjected to
a procedure that will do them little good and
possibly significant harm.

A number of well-designed studies have
demonstrated that there were no significant
differences in the clinical course of acute otitis
media when conventional treatments were
compared with a placebo. Specifically, no differences were found between treatment other
than antibiotics, ear tubes, ear tubes with antibiotics, and antibiotics alone.[3–7] Interestingly,
in some studies, children not receiving antibiotics had fewer recurrences than those receiving antibiotics. This reduced recurrence rate
is undoubtedly a reflection of the suppressive
effects antibiotics have on the immune system,
and of the fact that they disturb the normal
flora of the upper respiratory tract.[8]

Since in most children with acute otitis
media (70 to 90%) the infection clears up by
itself within 7 to 14 days, antibiotics should
not routinely be prescribed initially for all
children.[7] Extensive review of the scientific
literature on the value of antibiotics in the
treatment of otitis media over the past 30
years has led to the following conclusions:

- The benefit of routine antibiotic use for
  otitis media, judged by either short-term
  or long-term outcomes, is unproved.

- Existing research offers no compelling
  evidence that children with acute otitis
  media routinely given antibiotics have a
  shorter duration of symptoms, fewer recurrences, or better long-term outcomes
  than those who do not receive them.

- Antibiotics did not improve outcome at
  two months, and no differences in rates of
  recovery were found for either the type of
  antibiotic given or the duration of treatment with the antibiotic.

While these results have been accepted by
some U.S. pediatricians, others still rely heavily on antibiotics to treat otitis media. Instead
of antibiotics, the recommendation from this
group of experts was to use pain relievers
and have the parent observe the child closely.
Results from clinical trials have shown that
more than 80% of children with acute otitis
media respond to a placebo within 48 hours.
Although pain relievers may help relieve the
child's discomfort, they have their own toxicity profile. Therefore, we recommend other
proven pain-relieving options such as botanical eardrops (discussed later).

In addition to antibiotics' lack of effectiveness in otitis media, the widespread use and
abuse of antibiotics is becoming increasingly
alarming. Risks of antibiotics include allergic
reactions, gastric upset, accelerated bacterial
resistance, and unfavorable changes in the
bacterial flora in the nose and throat. Antibiotics not only fail to eradicate the organisms
but can induce middle ear superinfection.
Moreover, prescribing antibiotics can increase return office visit rates.[9] Additionally,
studies on concomitant antibiotic and steroid
treatment have revealed a lack of long-term
efficacy in chronic otitis media.[10]

Antibiotics are encouraging the near-
epidemic proportion of chronic candidiasis,
as well as the development of "superbugs"
that are resistant to currently available
antibiotics. The American Academy of
Otolaryngology—Head and Neck Surgery
states that there is no evidence to indicate
that systemic antibiotics alone can improve
treatment outcome and recommends that
they should not be used except when there is

an underlying systemic infection.[11] According to many experts, as well as the World Health Organization, we are coming dangerously close to arriving at a "postantibiotic era" in which many infectious diseases will once again become almost impossible to treat because of our overreliance on antibiotics.[12]

The bottom line is that otitis media is normally a self-limiting disease, clearing up on its own, regardless of treatment. Three meta-analyses independently found that approximately 80% of children with acute otitis media had spontaneous relief within 2 to 14 days. Some studies of children younger than two years do suggest a lower spontaneous resolution of about 30% after a few days.[9]

The risks and failure of antibiotics, when coupled with the high rate of spontaneous resolution and the high rate of recurrent otitis media following insertion of ear tubes, suggest that conservative (nonantibiotic, nonsurgical) treatment alone would reduce the frequency rate and decrease the yearly financial costs of otitis media. To examine this concept, in one study the parents of children with acute otitis media were given a "safety prescription" of antibiotics to be filled only if there was no improvement within two days. This wait-and-see method reduced antibiotic use by 31%.[13]

Although standard antibiotic and surgical procedures may not be statistically effective, each child must be evaluated individually, and appropriate follow-up including physician-family communication should be planned before a decision not to use these procedures is made. A special need to prevent hearing-loss-induced developmental delays may indicate a more appropriate use of ear tubes.

Finally, pneumococcal and viral vaccines have been designed but have also shown little benefit, probably owing to the multifactorial nature of this condition.[9] Given the inherent risks and complications, vaccinations do not appear to be warranted at this time.

Causes

The primary risk factors for otitis media are food allergies, day care attendance, wood-burning stoves, parental smoking (or exposure to other sources of secondhand smoke), and not being breastfed. Besides day care, all of the other factors have something in common: they lead to abnormal eustachian tube function, the underlying cause in virtually all cases of otitis media. The eustachian tube regulates gas pressure in the middle ear, protects the middle ear from nose and throat secretions and bacteria, and clears fluids from the middle ear. Swallowing causes active opening of the eustachian tube due to the action of the surrounding muscles. Infants and small children are particularly susceptible to eustachian tube problems since their tubes are smaller in diameter and more horizontal.

Obstruction of the eustachian tube leads first to fluid buildup and then, if the bacteria present are pathogenic and the immune system is impaired, to bacterial infection. Obstruction results from collapse of the tube (due to weak tissues holding the tube in place, an abnormal opening mechanism, or both), blockage by mucus in response to allergy or irritation, swelling of the mucous membrane, or infection.

Diagnostic Considerations

Bottle-feeding

Recurrent ear infection is strongly associated with early bottle-feeding, while breastfeeding for a minimum of three months has a protective effect.[14,15] Whether this is due to cow's milk allergy or to the protective effect of human milk against infection has not yet been conclusively determined. It is probably a combination.

In addition, bottle-feeding while a child is lying on his or her back (bottle-propping) leads to regurgitation of the bottle's contents into the middle ear and should be avoided.

Whatever the causative organism in otitis media—viral (respiratory syncytial virus, rhinovirus, or influenza A) or bacterial (*S. pneumoniae, M. catarrhalis,* or *H. influenza*)—human milk offers protection because of its high antibody content, which helps to inhibit infectious agents.[16] Breastfed infants also have a thymus gland (the major organ of the immune system) roughly 20 times larger than that of formula-fed infants.[17]

Food Allergies

The role of allergies as the major cause of chronic otitis media has been firmly established in the research literature.[18–23] Most studies show that 85 to 93% of these children have allergies: 16% to inhalants only, 14% to food only, and 70% to both.

Another way in which prolonged breastfeeding prevents otitis media may be by the avoidance of food allergies, particularly if the mother avoids sensitizing foods (i.e., those to which she is allergic) during pregnancy and lactation. In addition to breastfeeding, also of value is the exclusion or limited consumption of the foods to which children are most commonly allergic—wheat, egg, peanuts, corn, citrus, chocolate, and dairy products—particularly during the first nine months.

Because a child's digestive tract is quite permeable to food antigens, especially during the first three months, careful control of eating patterns (no frequent repetitions of any food, avoiding the common allergenic foods, and introduction of foods in a controlled manner, one food at a time, while carefully watching for a reaction) will reduce or prevent the development of food allergies.

The allergic reaction causes blockage of the eustachian tube by two mechanisms: inflammatory swelling of the mucous membranes lining the tube and inflammatory swelling of the nose, causing the Toynbee phenomenon (swallowing when both mouth and nose are closed, forcing air and secretions into the middle ear). The middle and inner ear are immunologically responsive, and this responsiveness includes food hypersensitivities.[18] In chronic earaches, an allergic cause should always be considered, and the offending allergens determined and avoided.

One illustrative study of 153 children with earaches demonstrated that 93.3% of the children (according to the RAST test for diagnosis) were allergic to foods, inhalants, or both. The 12-month success rate for 119 of the children, when they were treated with serial dilution titration therapy for inhalant sensitivities and an elimination diet for food allergens, showed that 92% improved. This result is significantly higher than that seen

Food Allergies in Children with Chronic Otitis Media		
FOOD	**NUMBER OF PATIENTS**	**PERCENTAGE OF PATIENTS**
Cow's milk	31	38
Wheat	27	33
Egg white	20	25
Peanut	16	20
Soy	14	17
Corn	12	15
Tomato	4	5
Chicken	4	5
Apple	3	4

in the surgically treated control group (ear tubes and, as indicated, removal of the tonsils and adenoids), which showed only a 52% response.[19]

In another study, a total of 104 children with recurrent otitis media ranging in age from 18 months to 9 years were evaluated for food allergy by means of skin-prick testing, specific IgE tests, and food challenge.[23] Results indicated a statistically significant association between food allergy and recurrent otitis media in 81 of 104 patients (78%). An allergy elimination diet led to a significant improvement of chronic otitis media in 70 of 81 patients (86%) as assessed by detailed clinical evaluation. The challenge diet with the suspected offending food provoked a recurrence of serous otitis media in 66 of 70 patients (94%).

Therapeutic Considerations

The primary treatment goals are to ensure that the eustachian tubes are unobstructed and to promote drainage by identifying and addressing causative factors. Supporting the immune system is also important. The recommendations that follow should be used along with the recommendations given in the chapter "Immune System Support."

Botanical Medicines

Naturopathic Ear Drops

In acute otitis media, naturopathic botanical ear drops have been shown to be as effective as either antibiotic or anesthetic drops[24,25] and offer a much less toxic approach to pain management.

In a double-blind outpatient trial, one group from Israel studied 171 children ages 5 to 18 who were randomly assigned to receive treatment with naturopathic herbal extract ear drops or anesthetic ear drops (amethocaine and phenazone), with or without amoxicillin (a daily dose of 80 mg/kg per day).[24] The plant medicine was a combination of *Calendula officinalis* flowers (marigold, 28%), *Hypericum perforatum* complete herb (Saint-John's-wort, 30%), *Verbascum thapsus* flowers (mullein, 25%), and *Allium sativum* oil (garlic, 0.05%) in olive oil (10%), *Lavendula officinalis* (lavender oil, 5%), and tocopherol acetate oil (vitamin E, 2%) and the dose was 5 drops three times per day. All groups had a statistically significant improvement in ear pain over the course of the three days, with a 95.9% reduction of pain in the group treated with naturopathic drops alone. The group treated with naturopathic drops plus antibiotics had a 90.9% pain diminution. The anesthetic drops alone and anesthetic drops with antibiotics had 84.7% and 77.8% reductions, respectively.

Xylitol

Xylitol is a commonly used natural sweetener derived mainly from birch and other hardwood trees. It has demonstrated inhibition of *S. pneumoniae*. Two double-blind clinical trials illustrated xylitol's ability to reduce acute otitis media incidence by 40%. In one study of 306 children in day care with recurrent acute otitis media, 157 children were given xylitol (8.4 g per day) chewing gum and 149 children were given a sucrose control gum.[26] During the two months, at least one event of acute otitis media was experienced by 20.8% of the children who received sucrose compared with only 12.1% of those receiving xylitol. Significantly fewer antibiotics were prescribed among those receiving xylitol.

In a second randomized and controlled blinded trial,[27] 857 healthy children were randomly assigned to one of five treatment groups to receive control syrup, xylitol syrup, control chewing gum, xylitol gum, or xylitol lozenges for a period of three months. The daily dose of xylitol varied from 8.4 g (chewing gum) to 10 g (syrup). Although at least one event of otitis media was experienced by 41% of the 165 children who received control syrup, only 29% of the 159 children receiving xylitol syrup were affected. Likewise, the occurrence of otitis decreased by 40% compared with control subjects in the children who received xylitol chewing gum and by 20% in the lozenge group. Thus the occurrence of acute otitis media during the follow-up period was significantly lower in those who received xylitol syrup or gum, and these children required antibiotics less often than did controls.

Humidifiers

Humidifiers are popular treatments for otitis media and upper respiratory tract infections in children. This may be justified, according to a 1994 study that evaluated the role of low humidity in this disorder.[28] The study examined the effect of low humidity on the middle ear using a rat model. Twenty-three rats were housed for five days in a low-humidity environment (10 to 12% relative humidity), and 23 control rats were housed at 50 to 55%

QUICK REVIEW

- **Since an ear infection can be quite serious, it is necessary that anyone with symptoms of acute ear infection be seen by a physician.**
- **Ear infections are extremely common in children under the age of six years.**
- **Acute otitis media is usually preceded by an upper respiratory infection or allergy.**
- **A number of well-designed studies have demonstrated that there are no significant differences in the clinical course of acute otitis media when conventional treatments were compared with a placebo.**
- **The primary risk factors for otitis media are food allergies, day care attendance, wood-burning stoves, parental smoking (or exposure to other sources of second-hand smoke), and not being breastfed.**
- **Recurrent ear infection is strongly associated with early bottle-feeding, while breastfeeding (for a minimum of three months) has a protective effect.**
- **The role of food allergy as the major cause of chronic otitis media has been firmly established in the medical literature.**
- **Elimination of food allergens has been shown to produce a dramatic effect in the treatment of chronic otitis media in more than 90% of children in some studies.**
- **In acute otitis media, naturopathic botanical ear drops have been shown to be as effective as either antibiotic or anesthetic drops.**
- **Two double-blind clinical trials illustrated xylitol's ability to reduce acute otitis media incidence by 40%.**

relative humidity. Microscopic ear examinations were graded for otitis media before testing and on test days three and five. The lining of the middle ear and eustachian tube was examined by biopsy. Significantly more effusions (fluid in the eustachian tubes) were observed in the low-humidity group on both day three and day five, but biopsy results were similar in both groups.

This study indicated that low humidity may be a contributing factor in otitis media. Possible explanations are that low humidity may induce nasal swelling and reduce ventilation of the eustachian tube, or that it may dry the eustachian tube lining, possibly leading to an inability to clear fluid, as well as to increased secretions. The mast cells that reside in the lining of the eustachian tube may also come into play by releasing histamine and producing swelling.

Although preliminary, this research indicates that increasing humidity with the use of a humidifier may be helpful in the treatment of otitis media with effusion.

TREATMENT SUMMARY

The key factor in the natural approach to chronic otitis media in children appears to be the recognition and elimination of allergies, particularly food allergies, as well as support for the immune system and healthy digestive function. Because it is usually not possible to determine the exact allergen during acute otitis media, the most common allergic foods should be eliminated from the diet:

- Milk and other dairy products
- Eggs
- Wheat
- Corn
- Oranges
- Peanuts
- Chocolate

The diet should also eliminate concentrated simple carbohydrates (e.g., sugar, honey, dried fruit, concentrated fruit juice) because they inhibit the immune system. These simple dietary recommendations bring relief to most children in a matter of days.

Nutritional Supplements

- A high-potency multiple vitamin and mineral formula as described in the chapter "Supplementary Measures"
- Vitamin C: adults, 500 to 1,000 mg three times per day; children, 50 mg for each year of age every two hours
- Zinc: adults, 15 to 30 mg per day; children, 2.5 mg for each year of age per day (up to 30 mg)
- Xylitol: approximately 8 g per day as either chewing gum chewed throughout the day or 10 g syrup per day in divided doses

Botanical Medicines

- Naturopathic ear drop formula: 5 drops in the affected ear three times per day
- If the otitis media is due to an upper respiratory tract infection, follow the

recommendations in the chapter "Sinus Infections"

Physical Medicine

Local application of heat is often helpful in reducing discomfort. It can be applied as a hot pack, with warm oil (especially mullein oil) dripped into the ear, or by blowing hot air into the ear with the aid of a straw and a hair dryer. These treatments help to reduce pressure in the middle ear and promote fluid drainage.

Endometriosis

- Painful menstruation, painful intercourse, and infertility
- Physical examination by a physician reveals one or more of the following: tenderness of the pelvic area, enlarged or tender ovaries, a uterus that tips backward and lacks mobility, and adhesions (abnormal scarring)
- Pelvic ultrasound detects endometrial tissue outside the uterus
- Definitive diagnosis: laparoscopy or laparotomy visualizing endometrial implants within the pelvic cavity

Endometriosis is a women's health condition in which cells from the lining of the uterus (endometrium) appear and flourish outside the uterine cavity, most commonly on the ovaries. Since the endometrial cells are under the influence of female hormones even when they reside outside the uterine lining, they can produce symptoms that often worsen at specific points during the menstrual cycle. Pelvic pain is a particularly bothersome symptom. Endometriosis lesions react to hormonal stimulation and may "bleed" at the time of menstruation. The blood accumulates locally, causes swelling, and triggers inflammatory responses, including the activation of pain-producing molecules known as cytokines.

Pain can also occur from adhesions (internal scar tissue) binding internal organs to each other, causing organ dislocation. Fallopian tubes, ovaries, the uterus, the bowels, and the bladder can be bound together in ways that are painful on a daily basis, not just during certain times of the menstrual cycle.

Endometriosis affects 10 to 15% of menstruating women between the ages of 24 and 40 years old.

Causes

The predominant theory of the cause of endometriosis is that during menses, blood flows backward and implants endometrial cells in the pelvic cavity. The problem found with this theory is that more than 90% of menstruating women without endometriosis have this backward flow. Typically their immune system is able to prevent implantation and growth of the endometrial cells outside the uterus, so defects in immune function may be responsible for the development of endometriosis. However, in some patients, endometrial tissue transplanted by retrograde menstruation may be able to implant and establish itself as endometriosis. Women with endometriosis typically show alterations in immune function, particularly in those factors that are responsible for proper surveillance in the pelvic area.[1]

Other research suggests that estrogen-mimicking environmental toxins or radiation exposure increases the risk for endometriosis. Substances that have been shown to have estrogenic effects in the body include polychlorinated biphenyls (PCBs), pesticides, herbicides, certain plastics, heavy metals such as lead, and some kinds of household cleaners. However, these compounds are also known to adversely affect the immune system. Particularly incriminating are phthalates, used as plasticizers (substances added to plastics such as polyvinyl chloride to increase their flexibility, transparency, durability, and lon-. gevity).[2] Phthalates are used in a large variety of products, from enteric coatings for pharmaceutical pills and nutritional supplements to viscosity control agents, gelling agents, film formers, stabilizers, dispersants, lubricants, binders, emulsifying agents, and suspending agents. Phthalates are being phased out of many products in the United States, Canada, and the European Union because of health concerns.

Risk factors for endometriosis include family history, lack of exercise from an early age, a high-fat diet, use of intrauterine devices, and increased or unbalanced estrogen levels. Women with a mother or a sister with endometriosis have an increased risk.[1]

Therapeutic Considerations

In most cases, endometriosis will cease after menopause. But in women in their reproductive years, endometriosis is merely managed. The most aggressive treatment is surgery. In younger women who may desire to get pregnant in the future, surgical treatment attempts to remove the stray endometrial tissue and preserve the ovaries. The dominant nonsurgical treatment is the use of hormonal medication that suppresses the natural menstrual cycle, plus pain medication to manage the discomfort. On occasions, naturopathic physicians will use natural progesterone therapy (a form of bioidentical hormone therapy) to help relieve the symptoms of endome-

triosis. Although progesterone creams may be available over the counter, we recommend being treated and monitored by a physician.

The natural approach to endometriosis is designed to achieve the following goals:

- Reduce inflammation
- Enhance detoxification mechanisms
- Reduce bothersome symptoms

The strategies discussed in the chapter "Silent Inflammation" are extremely important in endometriosis. Especially important is eating the right type of fats. The consumption of trans-fatty acids appears to increase the risk of endometriosis, while long-chain omega-3 fatty acids from fish oils appear to be protective. Twelve years of prospective data from the Nurses Health Study II, which began in 1989, were analyzed for the association between dietary fat and many health problems, including endometriosis. Those women who consumed the most trans-fatty acids were 48% more likely to be diagnosed with endometriosis. In contrast, those women with the highest consumption of long-chain omega-3 fatty acids were 22% less likely to be diagnosed with endometriosis.[3]

One study looked directly at the effect of essential fatty acid ratios on production of inflammatory cytokines by endometrial cells.[4] The test tube study took endometrial cells from women with and without endometriosis attending an infertility clinic. The cell cultures were provided with nutrients and supplemented with various ratios of omega-3 polyunsaturated fatty acids and omega-6 polyunsaturated fatty acids (found in meat and dairy products, and in soy, safflower, corn, and sunflower oil). They found that the higher the ratio of omega-6 to omega-3 fatty acids, the greater the secretion of an inflammatory compound, interleukin-8, in cells from women both with and without endometriosis, with the cells from women with endometriosis secreting significantly higher levels.[5]

The importance of a high-fiber diet in enhancing detoxification cannot be overstated. Foods high in fiber are associated with the growth of friendly microorganisms within the large intestine. Studies show that a high intake of fiber and a predominantly vegetarian diet lead to a decrease of biologically active free estrogens in blood plasma.[6] Increasing the intake of high-fiber foods, especially vegetables, also helps clear excess estrogen from the body. Foods that are particularly helpful in this regard are vegetables in the brassica family, such as broccoli, brussels sprouts, cabbage, and cauliflower.[7] Other liver-cleansing foods are beets, carrots, artichokes, lemons, dandelion greens, watercress, and burdock root. Onions, garlic, and leeks contain organosulfur and flavonoid compounds, which enhance the immune system and encourage the production of liver enzymes that have a role in detoxification.[8] See the chapter "Detoxification and Internal Cleansing" for more discussion.

Last, the isoflavones in soy products and the lignans in flaxseed may also be important in a dietary approach to endometriosis. These foods counter the effects of excess estrogen. A Japanese study demonstrated that moderate soy intake was associated with a decreased risk of premenopausal hysterectomy. Since some of the surgeries were due to endometriosis, these results led the authors to conclude that moderate soy intake may decrease the risk for endometriosis.[9]

Foods to decrease include dairy products, red meat, sugar, caffeine, and alcohol. The Environmental Protection Agency estimates that 90% of human pesticide exposure occurs through food, primarily meat and dairy products.[10] Dairy products (except nonfat versions) also tip the ratio of omega-6 to omega-3 fatty acids toward inflammation.

Dietary therapy can be very helpful in endometriosis. In a two-month study of 50 women with endometriosis, a significant reduction in symptoms occurred when the intake of higher-glycemic carbohydrates and caffeine was decreased and the intake of omega-3 and omega-9 fatty acids (e.g., from olive oil) was increased.[11] Caffeine is a particular problem for many women with endometriosis. In one study, women consuming an average of more than 150 to 225 mg of caffeine per day (about the amount in 1 to 1½ cups of coffee) had a 20% increased risk of endometriosis, while those consuming more than 225 mg had a 60% increase.[12]

Nutritional Supplements

Lipotropic Supplements

Historically, naturopaths have used lipotropic factors such as inositol, methionine, and choline in cases of endometriosis. Lipotropic supplements usually are a combination of vitamins and herbs designed to support the liver's functions of removing fat, detoxifying the body's wastes, detoxifying external toxins, and metabolizing and excreting estrogens. These lipotropic products vary in formulation depending on the manufacturer, but they are all similar. Many now contain anticancer phytonutrients found in brassica-family vegetables, such as indole-3-carbinol (I3C), di-indoylmethane (DIM), and sulfurophane. Research has shown that these compounds help to break down cancer-causing forms of estrogens to non-cancer-causing forms, making them especially important for women with endometriosis.[7]

Grape Seed or Pine Bark Extract

Extracts from grape seed and the bark of the maritime pine (Pycnogenol) are rich sources of proanthocyanidins, one of the most beneficial groups of plant flavonoids. Because

Pycnogenol was shown to inhibit inflammation in a test tube study, researchers sought to evaluate its role in a study of 58 women with endometriosis. The women were randomly assigned to receive either Pycnogenol 30 mg twice per day for 48 weeks or an anti-hormonal drug, leuprorelin acetate, given by intramuscular injection every four weeks for 24 weeks. After four weeks on Pycnogenol, patients slowly but steadily improved, with their symptoms decreasing from severe to moderate. Overall, this group experienced a 33% reduction in symptoms of endometriosis. The leuprorelin group had a greater response within the treatment period but relapsed after 24 weeks. The Pycnogenol group maintained regular menses and normal estrogen levels during treatment; in contrast, the leuprorelin group had suppressed menstruation and drastically lowered estrogen levels (which were expected). In addition, five women in the trial taking Pycnogenol became pregnant.[13]

Botanical Medicines

Many traditional herbal medicines used to treat women with endometriosis contain phytoestrogens. However, their activity is certainly less that the effects of dietary phytoestrogens such as soy and flax. So we recommend focusing on dietary phytoestrogens rather than botanical sources.

Vitex or chasteberry (*Vitex agnus-castus*) has traditionally been used as a treatment for hormone imbalances in women. Through action on the pituitary gland, it increases progesterone production by means of an increase in luteinizing hormone, with the effect of making estrogen less available. This herb is useful for fibroids and premenstrual syndrome, and it may also have an effect in endometriosis.[14]

. . . .

QUICK REVIEW

- **Endometriosis is a women's health condition in which cells from the lining of the uterus (endometrium) appear and flourish outside the uterine cavity.**

- **Risk factors for endometriosis include family history, lack of exercise from an early age, a high-fat diet, use of intrauterine devices, and increased or unbalanced estrogen levels.**

- **The natural approach to endometriosis is designed to reduce inflammation, enhance detoxification mechanisms, and reduce bothersome symptoms.**

- **The consumption of trans-fatty acids appears to increase the risk of endometriosis, while long-chain omega-3 fatty acids from fish oils appear to be protective.**

- **Increasing the intake of high-fiber foods, especially vegetables of the brassica family, helps clear excess estrogen from the body.**

- **A significant reduction in symptoms occurs with a decreased intake of higher-glycemic carbohydrates, an increased intake of omega-3 and omega-9 fatty acids, and a decreased intake of caffeine.**

- **Pycnogenol showed an ability to reduce endometriosis symptoms by 33% in one clinical trial.**

- **Vitex extract may reduce estrogen's effect on endometrial tissue.**

TREATMENT SUMMARY

The natural approach to endometriosis is designed to reduce inflammation, enhance detoxification mechanisms, and reduce bothersome symptoms.

Diet

Follow the guidelines in the chapter "A Health-Promoting Diet." Consume a diet low in fat and high in fiber, whole grains, flaxseed, soy foods, and vegetables in the cabbage family, and avoid overconsumption of meat and dairy products, omega-6 fatty acids, saturated fats, sugar, caffeine, and alcohol. Soy isoflavone intake should be approximately 45 mg per day. Ground flaxseed at a dosage of 1 to 2 tablespoons per day is also recommended.

Nutritional Supplements

- A high-potency multiple vitamin and mineral formula as described in the chapter "Supplementary Measures"
- Key individual nutrients:
  - Vitamin B_6: 25 to 50 mg per day
  - Folic acid: 800 to 2,000 mcg per day
  - Vitamin B_{12}: 800 mcg per day
  - Vitamin C: 500 to 1,000 mg per day
  - Vitamin E (mixed tocopherols): 100 to 200 IU per day
  - Magnesium (bound to aspartate, citrate, fumarate, malate, or succinate): 200 to 300 mg three times per day
  - Selenium: 100 to 200 mcg per day
  - Zinc: 30 to 45 mg per day
  - Vitamin D_3: 2,000 to 4,000 IU per day (ideally, measure blood levels and adjust dosage accordingly)
- Flaxseed oil: 1 tbsp per day
- Fish oils: 1,000 mg EPA + DHA per day
- One of the following:
  - Grape seed extract (>95% procyanidolic oligomers): 100 to 300 mg per day
  - Pine bark extract (>95% procyanidolic oligomers): 100 to 300 mg per day
  - Some other flavonoid-rich extract with a similar flavonoid content, super greens formula, or another plant-based antioxidant that can provide an oxygen radical absorption capacity (ORAC) of 3,000 to 6,000 units or more per day
- Specialty supplements, one of the following:
  - Lipotropic formula providing 1,000 mg betaine, 1,000 mg choline, and 1,000 mg cysteine or methionine
  - SAM-e: 200 to 400 mg per day
- One or a combination of the following:
  - Indole-3-carbinol: 300 to 600 mg per day
  - Di-indoylmethane (DIM): 100 to 200 mg per day taken with food

Botanical Medicines

- Vitex (chasteberry): In tablet or capsule form (often standardized to contain 0.5% agnuside), 175 to 225 mg per day; in liquid form, 2 to 4 ml (½ to 1 tsp) per day

Erectile Dysfunction

- Inability to attain or maintain an erection

Erectile dysfunction (ED) is the inability of a man to attain and maintain erection of the penis sufficient to permit satisfactory sexual intercourse. In the past, the term *impotence* was used, but that word may also imply loss of libido, premature ejaculation, or inability to achieve orgasm.[1]

An estimated 20 million to 30 million American men suffer from ED. This number is expected to increase dramatically as the median age of the population increases. Currently, the prevalence of ED is 12% in men younger than 59, 22% in those 60 to 69, and 30% in those older than 69.

Although the frequency of erectile dysfunction increases with age, it must be stressed that aging itself is not a cause of impotence. Although the amount and force of the ejaculate as well as the need to ejaculate decrease with age, the capacity for erection is retained. Men are capable of retaining their sexual virility well into their 80s. ED is now thought to be a major risk factor for cardiovascular disease.[2]

The Stages of the Sexual Act for Men

For men, the sexual act is initiated in most instances by an interplay of psychic and physical stimulation. Simply thinking sexual thoughts or dreaming that the act of sexual intercourse is taking place can lead to an erection and even ejaculation. Most men at some point in their sexual development (usually their teen years) experience nocturnal emissions (wet dreams at night).

Although psychological factors obviously contribute to the male sexual response, it is interesting to note that they are not absolutely necessary in the performance of the male sexual act. Appropriate genital stimulation can lead to an erection and ejaculation without psychic stimuli through an inherent reflex mechanism. For example, some individuals with spinal cord damage that prevents the transmission of nerve impulses from the brain are still capable of achieving an erection and ejaculation.

So either psychic or physical stimulation can initiate the sexual act. Physical stimulation of sensitive tissue, primarily the penis but also the entire pubic region, sends nerve impulses to the spinal cord, causing a reflex impulse to the penis that leads to dilation of the arteries and the filling up with blood of the erectile tissue. In addition, these same nerve impulses cause the glands in the urethra to secrete mucus that lubricates the urethra and also aids in the lubrication of intercourse.

The initial nerve stimulus from the spinal cord during the sexual act is controlled by the parasympathetic nervous system, which also controls bodily functions such as digestion, breathing, and heart rate during periods of rest, relaxation, visualization, meditation, and sleep. In contrast, the sympathetic nervous system is designed to protect us against immediate danger and is responsible for the so-called fight-or-flight reaction. While the parasympathetic nervous system is responsible for an erection and lubrication, the sympathetic nervous system controls emission and ejaculation.

Emission and ejaculation are the culmination of the male sexual act. When sexual stimulation becomes extremely intense, the reflex centers of the spinal cord begin to emit sympathetic nerve impulses to initiate emission, the forerunner of ejaculation.

Emission begins with contraction of the vas deferens, the tubule that transports the sperm from the epididymis to the prostate. This contraction leads to the expulsion of sperm into the ejaculatory duct and urethra. Then contractions of the prostate and seminal vesicles expel prostatic and seminal fluid into the ejaculatory duct, forcing the sperm into the urethra. All of these fluids mix in the internal urethra along with the secretions of the urethral glands to form semen. The process to this point is referred to as emission.

The filling of the urethra then elicits sensory nerve impulses that further excite the rhythmic contractions of the internal organs and also cause the rhythmic contraction of the erectile tissues. Together, these contractions lead to a tremendous increase in pressure that ejaculates the semen from the urethra. Simultaneously, the pelvic muscles and even muscles of the abdomen cause thrusting movements of the pelvis and penis, which also help propel the semen.

The entire process of emission and ejaculation is known as the male orgasm. After ejaculation, the male sexual excitement disappears almost entirely within one or two minutes, and erection disappears.

Causes

Erectile dysfunction may be due to organic or psychogenic factors. In the overwhelming majority of cases the cause is organic, that is, it is due to some physiological dysfunction. In fact, in men over the age of 50, organic causes are responsible for erectile dysfunction in more than 90% of cases.[3] In the past, a man with ED who was able to have nighttime or early morning erections was thought to have psychogenic impotence. However, it is now recognized that this is not a reliable indicator. Common causes of ED are listed immediately below, and discussed in greater detail later in the chapter.

Causes of Erectile Dysfunction
Organic (90%)

- Vascular insufficiency
  - Atherosclerosis
  - Pelvic surgery
  - Pelvic trauma
- Drugs
  - Antihistamines
  - Antihypertensives
  - Anticholinergics
  - Antidepressants
  - Antipsychotics
  - Tranquilizers
  - Others
- Alcohol and tobacco use
- Endocrine disorders
  - Diabetes
  - Hypothyroidism
  - Decreased male sex hormones
  - Elevated prolactin levels
  - High serum estrogen levels

- Diseases of or trauma to the sexual organs
  - Diseases of the penis
  - Prostate disorders
- Neurological diseases
- Pelvic trauma
- Pelvic surgery
- Multiple sclerosis

Psychological (10%)

- Psychiatric illness
- Stress
- Performance anxiety
- Depression

Since correction of any underlying organic factor is the first step in restoring sexual function, it is critically important that a proper diagnosis be made. A thorough history and physical exam are most often all that is needed; however, there are special noninvasive tests that can be performed to diagnose the cause of erectile dysfunction. These tests are best performed or supervised by a urologist.

Procedures Used to Evaluate Erectile Dysfunction

- Medical history
- Physical examination
- Laboratory studies
  - Complete blood count and urinalysis
  - Biochemical profile
  - Glucose tolerance test
  - Serum hormone levels
- Psychological evaluation
- Nighttime penile monitoring
- Neurological examination
- Vascular examination

Atherosclerosis of the penile artery is the primary cause of impotence in nearly half the men over the age of 50 who have erectile dysfunction.[1,2] *Atherosclerosis* refers to a process of hardening of the artery walls due to a buildup of plaque containing cholesterol, fatty material, and cellular debris. Atherosclerosis-related erectile dysfunction has been shown to be a risk factor for a heart attack or stroke.[3] The process of atherosclerosis occurs systemically throughout the body, not just in the arteries supplying the heart or penis. Patients with diseased coronary arteries are much more likely to have erectile dysfunction than individuals without coronary disease. If erectile dysfunction is due to vascular insufficiency, especially important are measures to reduce cardiovascular risk factors such as elevated cholesterol and triglyceride levels, high blood pressure, obesity, lack of exercise, and smoking.

The diagnosis of erectile dysfunction due to atherosclerosis can be made with the aid of ultrasound techniques. It is also a good idea to have blood cholesterol and triglyceride levels checked. A total cholesterol level above 200 mg/dl is an indicator that atherosclerosis may be responsible for the decreased blood flow.

In many instances, physicians will inject papaverine or PGE1 into the penis during the clinical evaluation of erectile dysfunction when a vascular cause is suspected. These drugs cause the arteries to dilate, thus delivering more blood to erectile tissues. If the erectile dysfunction is due to arterial insufficiency, the penis will experience a sustained erection. But if the erection cannot be maintained it is a sign of venous leakage. This form of erectile dysfunction is much more difficult to treat and may require surgery.

Drugs

A long list of prescription medications and drugs can interfere with sexual function, including medications such as blood pressure medications (especially beta-blockers), peptic ulcer medications, sleeping pills (sedative hypnotic drugs), antidepressants, and statins to lower cholesterol. If you are on a medication that may be linked to ED, work with your physician to get off the medication. For most common health conditions there are natural measures that will produce safer and better clinical results than these drugs.

Alcohol and Tobacco

Long-term alcohol consumption or tobacco use is often a big contributor to ED. In addition to increasing the risk for atherosclerosis, both of these agents negatively affect sexual function. Alcohol use can produce acute episodes of ED as well as more permanent ED due to testicular shrinkage. Smoking just two cigarettes has been shown to inhibit an erection.[3]

Hormonal Disorders

There are various endocrine and hormonal disorders that can lead to erectile dysfunction. The most common of these disorders is diabetes. Individuals with diabetes are at higher risk for atherosclerosis and nerve damage, both of which can cause ED. If you have diabetes, see the chapter "Diabetes."

Other relatively common endocrine disorders associated with ED include low levels of testosterone and hypothyroidism (see the chapter "Hypothyroidism"). The diagnosis of low testosterone requires a blood test. Symptoms of low testosterone include decreased sexual desire and erectile dysfunction, changes in mood associated with

fatigue, depression and anger, and decreases in memory and spatial orientation ability. It may also produce decreased lean body mass, reduced muscle volume and strength, and increases in abdominal obesity. Decreased or thinning facial and chest hair and skin alterations such as increases in facial wrinkling and pale-appearing skin suggestive of anemia are also common. Sometimes the testicles may have become smaller or softer.

Low testosterone levels are most often treated with prescription testosterone preparations. The most popular choices are transdermal gels, injectables, and transdermal patches. The adrenal hormone DHEA may be helpful (see the chapter "Longevity and Life Extension") but for best results should be used under a physician's guidance for proper monitoring.

Diseases of or Trauma to the Sexual Organs

Diseases of or trauma to the male sexual organs can cause erectile dysfunction. Diseases of the penis, such as Peyronie's disease, and an enlarged prostate (see the chapter "Prostate Enlargement [BPH]") are among the most common findings in this particular category. Peyronie's disease (PD) is a disorder of the penis in which part of the sheath of fibrous connective tissue within the penis thickens, causing the penis to bend at an angle during an erection. Intercourse is often difficult and quite painful. The underlying cause of PD is not well understood, but it is thought to be caused by minor trauma or injury to the penis. PD may also be caused by the use of high blood pressure medications including beta-blockers and calcium channel blockers.

Although PD will sometimes improve without any treatment, coenzyme Q_{10}, the enzyme bromelain, and a concentrated extract of gotu kola (*Centella asiatica*) may be helpful. CoQ_{10} exerts antioxidant effects that are thought to play a role in arresting and possibly reversing PD. In the development of PD an initial inflammatory reaction is followed by fibrous inelastic scar formation. It is thought that CoQ_{10} prevents or reduces the action of a specific mediator of the fibrous scar, a compound known as TGF-b1. In a double-blind clinical trial of 186 patients with chronic early PD, patients were randomly assigned to take either 300 mg CoQ_{10} per day or a placebo for 24 weeks. Erectile function, pain during erection, plaque volume, penile curvature, and satisfaction with treatment were assessed at baseline and every four weeks during the study period. After 24 weeks, significant improvements were noted in all these variables. Average plaque size and penile curvature degree were decreased in the CoQ_{10} group (average reduction approximately 40%), whereas an increase (average 35%) was noted in the placebo group. Only 11 patients in the CoQ_{10} group (13.6%) had disease progression. In contrast, 46 patients (56.1%) in the placebo group experienced disease progression. This study provides compelling evidence that CoQ_{10} at the very least can impair disease progression and in many cases may lead to significant improvements in plaque size, penile curvature, and erectile function.[4]

Bromelain prevents the deposition of fibrin, which is thought to be responsible for the thickening of the fibrous connective tissue in the penis. For PD, take 750 mg bromelain three times per day on an empty stomach (20 minutes before meals is good). The dosage of gotu kola is based upon the concentration of active compounds (triterpenic acids). An effective dosage is 60 mg triterpenic acids twice per day.

Therapeutic Considerations

Although erectile function is largely dependent upon adequate male sex hormones, adequate sensory stimulation, and adequate blood supply to the erectile tissues, a strong case could be made that all of these factors are dependent upon adequate nutrition. Therefore, it can be concluded that nutrition plays a major role in determining virility. Exercise is also critical. The health benefits of regular exercise cannot be overstated. The immediate effect of exercise is stress on the body; however, with a regular exercise program the body adapts. The body's response to this regular stress is that it becomes stronger, functions more efficiently, and has greater endurance. Exercise is a vital component of health, especially sexual health.

Regular exercise improves a man's sexual performance. In one study the effects of nine months of regular exercise on aerobic work capacity (physical fitness), coronary heart disease risk factors, and sexuality were studied in 78 sedentary but healthy men (average age 48 years).[5] The men exercised in supervised groups 60 minutes per day, 3.5 days per week on average. Peak sustained exercise intensity was targeted at 75 to 80% of maximum heart rate (see the chapter "The Healing Power Within"). A control group of 17 men (mean age 44 years) participated in organized walking at a moderate pace 60 minutes per day, 4.1 days per week on average. Each subject maintained a daily diary of exercise, diet, smoking, and sexuality during the first and last months of the program. Like many other studies, this one showed the beneficial effects of regular exercise on fitness and coronary heart disease risk factors. Analysis of diary entries revealed significantly greater sexuality enhancements in the exercise group

BICYCLE SEATS AND ERECTILE DYSFUNCTION

While exercise is good for sexual function, riding a bike can be very detrimental to erectile function. The problem is not in the activity but in the design of the seat. Several studies have shown that cyclists experience more erectile dysfunction, groin and penile numbness, and problems urinating than noncyclists. Riding on a hard bicycle seat too long can compress the vital arteries and nerves necessary for normal sexual functioning. Studies done with bicycle seats designed to shift the rider's weight off the vital blood vessels and nerves show a dramatic reduction in complaints.[6]

If you are an enthusiastic cyclist, we recommend utilizing one of the newly designed seats that solve the problem. There are several on the market. One that we like is the RideOut (see www.rideout.com for more information).

(frequency of various intimate activities, reliability of adequate functioning during sex, percentage of satisfying orgasms, etc.). Moreover, the degree of sexuality enhancement among exercisers was correlated with the degree of their individual improvement in fitness. In other words, the better physical fitness the men were able to attain, the better their sexuality.

Diet

Optimal sexual function requires optimal nutrition. The diet and nutritional supplementation program in the chapters "A Health-Promoting Diet" and "Supplementary Measures," respectively, provide the factors men need to function at their best. A diet rich in whole foods, particularly vegetables, fruits, whole grains, and legumes, is extremely important. Adequate protein is also a must; it is better to get high-quality protein from fish, chicken, turkey, and lean cuts of beef (preferably hormone free) than from

fat-filled sources such as hamburgers, roasts, and pork.

Special foods often recommended to enhance virility include liver, oysters, and various types of nuts, seeds, and legumes. All of these foods are good sources of zinc, which is perhaps the most important nutrient for sexual function. Zinc is concentrated in semen, and frequent ejaculation can greatly diminish body zinc stores. If a zinc deficiency exists, the body appears to respond by reducing sexual drive as a mechanism by which to hold on to this important trace mineral.

Other key nutrients for sexual function include essential fatty acids, vitamin A, vitamin B_6, and vitamin E. A high-potency multiple vitamin and mineral formula ensures adequate intake of these nutrients as well as others important for health and sexual function.

Atherosclerosis and Diabetes

Since atherosclerosis and diabetes are primary causes of erectile dysfunction, it is especially important to address these underlying issues if they are present. For atherosclerosis, follow the dietary recommendations in the chapter "A Health-Promoting Diet" along with the additional recommendations given in the chapter "Heart and Cardiovascular Health"; for help in lowering cholesterol levels, see the chapter "High Cholesterol and/or Triglycerides." These recommendations will prevent as well as possibly reverse atherosclerosis. For information on diabetes, see the chapter "Diabetes."

Arginine and Procyanidolic Oligomers

Arginine increases the formation of nitric oxide within blood vessels, and higher levels of nitric oxide may improve blood flow to erectile tissue—the same net effect as that of drugs such as Viagra and Cialis. In one double-blind study, 31% of patients taking L-arginine reported a significant improvement in sexual function compared with only 11% of the control subjects.[7] Even more effective is combining arginine with procyanidolic oligomers from either grape seed or pine bark extract. Three double-blind studies have shown that a combination of pine bark extract (Pycnogenol) and arginine dramatically increases the benefits of arginine, presumably by enhancing the production of nitric oxide within erectile tissues even more than with arginine alone.[8–10] In a more recent study, Japanese patients with mild to moderate erectile dysfunction were instructed to take a supplement (Pycnogenol 60 mg per day, L-arginine 690 mg per day, and aspartic acid 552 mg per day) or a placebo for eight weeks.[10] Results were assessed using the five-item erectile domain of the International Index of Erectile Function (IIEF-5). Eight weeks of supplement intake improved the total score on the IIEF-5. In particular, a marked improvement was observed in hardness of erection and satisfaction with sexual intercourse. A decrease in blood pressure and a slight increase in salivary testosterone were observed in the supplement group.

In another double-blind study, involving 124 patients age 30 to 50 with moderate ED, the effects of the Pycnogenol-arginine combination were significant compared with the placebo. In addition, total plasma testosterone levels increased significantly, from 15.9 to 18.9 nmol/l, after six months of treatment with the combination.[10]

Recently, L-citrulline has been proposed as an alternative to arginine. The rationale is that it is efficiently converted to arginine where needed. In one study, 50% of men with mild ED taking 1.5 g L-citrulline per day for one month had an improvement in the erection hardness score, while that improvement was noted in only 8.3% of the men taking a placebo.[11]

Botanical Medicines

Improving sexual desire and function is possible with the use of herbs that (1) improve the activity of the male glandular system, (2) improve the blood supply to erectile tissue, and (3) enhance the transmission or stimulation of the nerve signal.

Yohimbe

The first FDA-approved medicine for ED was yohimbine, an alkaloid isolated from the bark of the yohimbe tree (*Pausinystalia johimbe*), native to tropical West Africa. Yohimbine hydrochloride increases libido, but its primary action is to increase blood flow to erectile tissue. Contrary to popular belief, yohimbine has no effect on testosterone levels. The use of yohimbine as a prescription for ED has been supplanted by newer medications.

When used alone, yohimbine is successful in 34 to 43% of cases.[12] If combined with strychnine and testosterone it is much more effective. However, side effects often make yohimbine very difficult to utilize. Yohimbine can induce anxiety, panic attacks, and hallucinations in some individuals. Other side effects include elevations in blood pressure and heart rate, dizziness, headache, and skin flushing. Yohimbine should not be used by individuals with kidney disease, women, or individuals with psychological disturbances.

Because of the yohimbine content of yohimbe bark, the FDA classifies yohimbe as an unsafe herb. We think there is some validity to this classification. Nonetheless, it is available without a prescription. It is our opinion that yohimbe and yohimbine are best used under the supervision of a physician. In addition to the problem of side effects with the use of commercial yohimbe preparations, consumers should be very suspicious of the quality of yohimbe products that are sold in health food stores. A 1995 analysis showed that while crude yohimbe bark typically contains 6% total alkaloids, most commercial products contained virtually no yohimbine.[13] Compared with authentic yohimbine bark, which contained yohimbine in concentrations of 7,089 parts per million (ppm), concentrations in the commercial products ranged from less than 0.1 to 489 ppm. Of the 26 samples, 9 were found to contain absolutely zero yohimbine and 7 contained only trace amounts (0.1 to 1 ppm). The remaining 10 products contained negligible amounts of yohimbine. In other words, none of the products tested was of acceptable quality. If you elect to use yohimbine, choose products marketed by reputable companies that clearly state the level of yohimbine per dose. If the content of yohimbine is unknown, it is virtually impossible to prescribe an effective and consistent dosage or attain any consistent benefit.

Potency Wood or Muira Puama

Muira puama (*Ptychopetalum olacoides*) is a shrub native to Brazil that has long been used as an aphrodisiac in South American folk medicine. At the Institute of Sexology in Paris, France, under the supervision of one of the world's foremost authorities on sexual function, Dr. Jacques Waynberg, a clinical study with 262 patients complaining of lack of sexual desire and the inability to attain or maintain an erection demonstrated muira puama extract to be effective in many cases. Within two weeks, at a dose of 1 to 1.5 g per day, 62% of patients with loss of libido claimed that the treatment had a dynamic effect, while 51% of patients with erection failure felt that muira puama was of benefit.[14]

At present, the mechanism of action of muira puama is unknown. From preliminary information, it appears that it enhances both psychological and physical aspects of sexual function.

Ginseng

In animal studies, ginseng (*Panax ginseng*) has been shown to promote the growth of the testes, increase sperm formation and testosterone levels, and increase sexual activity and mating behavior. These results seem to support ginseng's use as a fertility and virility aid, but human studies have been somewhat inconsistent. In regard to ED, a meta-analysis of existing studies concluded that there is suggestive evidence to indicate benefit with *Panax ginseng*, but more research is needed.[15] In the study with the highest-quality research methods, 45 men diagnosed with ED were randomized and received either 900 mg *Panax ginseng* or a placebo three times per day for eight weeks.[16] Results showed significant improvements in indexes of erectile function, but there were no changes in serum testosterone.

Longjack

In Southeast Asia, longjack (*Eurycoma longifolia Jack*) is a traditional remedy for preventing or treating ED. Several experimental studies of rodents were performed, showing the ability of longjack to improve sexual behavior, and including impressive results with sluggish and impotent rats—regarded as the most meaningful animal model of human ED.[17,18] The only human study was a small pilot study of 14 men randomly selected to consume either 100 mg per day longjack extract or a placebo.[19] The results indicated that water-soluble extract of *Eurycoma longifolia Jack* increased lean body mass, reduced body fat, and increased muscle strength and size.

Tribulus

Tribulus (*Tribulus terrestris*) has been used traditionally to energize, vitalize, and improve sexual function and physical performance in men. Based upon animal studies, it is believed that tribulus affects testosterone levels.[20] However, studies of humans have not found any consistent effect on levels of testosterone or testosterone precursor.[21] Nonetheless, it has demonstrated sexual enhancement in primates.

Fenugreek

Fenugreek (*Trigonella foenigracum*) contains a number of active plant steroids, most notably fenuside and protodioscin. A proprietary fenugreek extract, Testofen, has shown promising results in improving libido and testosterone levels in human clinical studies. In a recent double-blind study, the group taking 600 mg Testofen per day reported improved libido (81.5%), shortened recovery time (66.7%), and improved quality of sexual performance (63%).[22]

Ginkgo biloba

The idea that ginkgo biloba extract (GBE) may benefit ED started with the observation that male geriatric patients taking GBE for memory enhancement reported improved erections. This observation led to several studies in men with ED due to insufficient penile blood flow. In the first study, 60 patients with proven erectile dysfunction were treated with GBE at a dose of 60 mg per day for 12 to 18 months.[23] Penile blood flow was reevaluated by ultrasound every four weeks. The first signs of improved blood supply were seen after six to eight weeks; after six months of therapy 50% of the patients had fully regained potency. In a follow-up study, 50 patients with erectile dysfunction due to arterial insufficiency were divided into two groups: the first group (20 subjects) responded to injection of a drug that improves blood flow to erectile tissue prior to taking the ginkgo, and the second group did not respond to injection therapy.[24] After six months of treatment, all 20 patients in the first group regained the ability to attain and maintain a rigid erection. In the second group, 19 out of 30 responded positively to ginkgo in that they were able to attain and maintain an erection with the help of a drug injected into the erectile tissue.

Initial research also suggested that GBE can offset sexual dysfunction caused by antidepressant drugs. An open trial of GBE to alleviate antidepressant-induced sexual dysfunction found it to be 76% effective in alleviating symptoms related to all phases of the sexual response cycle in men, including erectile function.[25] Subsequent trials, including a double-blind study, have not shown much benefit with GBE in this application.[26]

Other Measures

Psychotherapy

Psychological therapies for ED are useful in some cases, but it must be kept in mind that in men over the age of 50, psychological factors are rarely the cause of erectile dysfunction. Nonetheless, ED itself can lead to psychological disturbances. Even in men with clear-cut organic erectile dysfunction, repeated inability to attain or sustain an erection leads to frustration, anxiety, and anticipation of failure. Learning stress reduction techniques such as relaxation exercises, biofeedback, and deep-breathing exercises may help when anxiety is present. Also, for ED in men with depression, psychological treatment may be especially beneficial.

Drugs for Erectile Dysfunction

Viagra, Cialis, Levitra, and Staxyn are popular drug treatments for ED that work by inhibiting an enzyme called phosphodiesterase. The end result is increased production of nitric oxide and hence increased blood supply to the erectile tissue of the penis. Interestingly, men who do not respond to phosphodiesterase inhibitors are apparently the ones who are most likely to benefit from citrulline—a precursor to arginine, which in turn is the precursor to nitric oxide.

There are certain situations in which these drugs may not be safe to take. If you have suffered a heart attack, stroke, or life-threatening arrhythmia (irregular heartbeat) or are currently taking medications for angina, then these drugs are not for you. These drugs also have significant side effects. Common side effects include headache, painful or prolonged erection (longer than four hours), upset stomach or heartburn, flushing (feeling warm), nasal congestion, changes in vision (color, glare), rash, itching or burning during urination, and back pain. Occasionally men experience even more serious side effects, including hearing loss, fainting, chest pain, and heart attacks.

Penile Prosthesis

One medical treatment of erectile dysfunction is the surgical insertion of a penile prosthesis. Three forms are available: semi-rigid, malleable, and inflatable. Effectiveness, complications, and acceptability vary among the three types. The main problems are mechanical failure, infection, erosions, and irreversible damage to erectile tissue.

Obviously, insertion of a penile prosthesis should be viewed not as a first step in the treatment of erectile dysfunction but rather as the very last step, after all other attempts have proved futile.

QUICK REVIEW

- **An estimated 10 million to 20 million American men suffer from impotence.**
- **Men are capable of retaining their sexual virility well into their 80s.**
- **Atherosclerosis of the penile artery is the primary cause of impotence in nearly half the men over the age of 50 who have erectile dysfunction.**
- **Alcohol or tobacco use decreases sexual function.**
- **Nutrition plays a major role in determining virility.**
- **Low levels of testosterone and hypothyroidism can lead to erectile dysfunction.**
- **Regular exercise improves a man's sexual performance.**
- **A combination of pine bark extract (Pycnogenol) and arginine dramatically increases the benefits of arginine.**
- **A meta-analysis of existing studies concluded that there is sufficient evidence to indicate that *Panax ginseng* has benefit in ED.**
- **Ginkgo biloba extract can be helpful in cases that are due to a lack of blood flow.**
- **In men over the age of 50, psychological factors are rarely the cause of erectile dysfunction.**
- **Another treatment for erectile dysfunction is the surgical insertion of a penile prosthesis.**

Vacuum-Constrictive Devices

Vacuum-constrictive devices are used to literally pump blood into the erectile tissue. Most of these devices consist of a vacuum chamber, a pump, connector tubing, and penile constrictor bands. The vacuum chamber is large enough to fit over the erect penis. A connector tube runs to the pump from a small opening at the closed end of the container. An elastic constrictor band is placed around the base of the chamber. Water-soluble lubricant is applied to the open end of the cylinder and to the entire penis. The chamber is placed over the flaccid penis, and an airtight seal is obtained.

Vacuum is applied with the pump (some pumps are battery operated) to create negative pressure within the chamber. The suction produced draws blood into the penis to produce an erection-like state. The constrictor band is then guided from the vacuum chamber onto the base of the penis. An erection is maintained because the blood is essentially trapped in the penis.

Although manufacturers and many physicians have stated that vacuum devices have revolutionized the management of erectile dysfunction, patient acceptance does not match this enthusiasm. Vacuum constrictive devices are generally effective and are extremely safe, but for some reason they have a significant rate of patient dropout. The reason may be that they are somewhat uncomfortable, cumbersome, and difficult to use; it takes patience and persistence to master the process. Most vacuum devices require both hands or the assistance of the sexual partner. Other patients quit using these devices because they may impair ejaculation and thus lead to some discomfort; some patients and partners complain about the lack of spontaneity. Despite these shortcomings, vacuum constrictive devices have been used successfully by many men with erectile dysfunction.

TREATMENT SUMMARY

It is normal for a man to retain sexual function well into his 80s. However, erectile dysfunction is an extremely common condition. Restoring potency requires addressing the underlying cause. In the majority of cases, organic factors are the cause. The chief cause is decreased blood flow (vascular insufficiency) due to atherosclerosis.

There are a variety of medical treatments for erectile dysfunction, but each treatment has its drawbacks. The natural approach to ED involves the use of diet, exercise, nutritional supplements, and botanical measures designed to address underlying issues. This combined approach is designed to restore potency by restoring normal physiology.

Diet

Follow the recommendations given in the chapter "A Health-Promoting Diet." Maintaining ideal body weight and blood sugar control is an important consideration for long-term male sexual vitality. A diet rich in whole foods, particularly vegetables, fruits, whole grains, and legumes, is also extremely important. Adequate protein is a must, and it is better to get high-quality protein from fish, chicken, turkey, and lean cuts of beef (preferably hormone free) than from fat-filled sources such as hamburgers, roasts, and pork.

Special foods often recommended to enhance virility include liver, oysters, nuts, seeds, and legumes. All of these foods are good sources of zinc.

Lifestyle

Avoid health-destroying practices such as smoking or excessive consumption of alcohol. Develop a regular exercise program according to the guidelines in the chapter "A Health-Promoting Lifestyle."

Nutritional Supplements

- A high-potency multiple vitamin and mineral formula as described in the chapter "Supplementary Measures"
- Fish oils: 1,000 to 3,000 mg EPA + DHA per day
- L-arginine or L-citrulline: 1,600 to 3,200 mg per day
- Grape seed extract or pine bark extract (>95% procyanidolic oligomers): 150 to 300 mg per day

Botanical Medicines

- One or more of the following:
  - *Panax ginseng:* Dose depends on ginsenoside content, with a goal of 5 mg ginsenosides with a 2:1 ratio of Rb1 to Rg1, one to three times a day; for example, for a high-quality ginseng root powder or extract containing 5% ginsenosides, the dose would be 100 mg.
  - Muira puama *(Ptychopetalum olacoides)* extract (6:1): 250 mg three times per day
  - Longjack *(Eurycoma longifolia Jack)*: 100 mg water-soluble extract per day
  - Tribulus *(Tribulus terrestris)*: 85 to 250 mg three times per day
  - Fenugreek *(Trigonella foenigracum)*: equivalent of 600 mg Testofen per day
- For arterial insufficiency, ginkgo biloba extract (24% ginkgo flavonglycosides): 240 to 320 mg per day
- For supportive therapy, the herbs described in the chapter "Prostate Enlargement (BPH)," especially *Pygeum africanum,* may be helpful.

Eczema (Atopic Dermatitis)

- Chronic itchy, inflamed skin
- Skin is very dry, red, and scaly
- Scratching and rubbing lead to darkened and hardened areas of thickened skin with accentuated furrows, most commonly seen on the front of the wrist and elbows and the back of the knees
- Personal or family history of allergy

Eczema, also called *atopic dermatitis*, is a common condition that affects approximately 2 to 7% of the population. Current research indicates that eczema is, at least partially, an allergic disease because:

- Levels of serum IgE (an allergic antibody) are elevated in 80% of eczema patients
- All eczema patients have positive allergy tests
- There is a family history in two-thirds of eczema patients
- Many eczema patients eventually develop hay fever and/or asthma
- Most eczema patients improve with a diet that eliminates common food allergens

Eczema is also characterized by a variety of physiological and anatomical abnormalities of the skin. The major abnormalities are:

- A greater tendency to itch
- Dry, thickened skin that has decreased water-holding capacity
- An increased tendency to thickening of the skin in response to rubbing and scratching
- A tendency of the skin to be overgrown by bacteria, especially *Staphylococcus aureus*

Causes

The underlying abnormalities leading to eczema originate primarily in the immune system and structural components of the skin. For example, the allergy-related antibody IgE is elevated in up to 80% of patients with eczema due to increased activation of a specific type of white blood cell (type 2 T helper cells). In addition, mast cells (specialized white blood cells) from the skin of patients with eczema have abnormalities that cause them to release higher amounts of histamine and other allergy-related compounds compared with people without eczema. Histamine and other allergy-related compounds result in the inflammation and itching characteristic of eczema.

Another immune-system abnormality is a defect in the ability to kill bacteria. This defect in immune function, coupled with scratching and the predominance of the bacteria *Staphylococcus aureus* in the skin flora in 90% of eczema patients, leads to an increased susceptibility to potentially severe staph infections of the skin. There are also other immune defects in patients with eczema that lead to increased susceptibility to other infections of the skin, including infections caused by a herpesvirus and by common wart viruses.

A genetic basis for eczema has long been recognized. A family history of allergic disease such as eczema and asthma is a major risk factor. In addition to possible defects in immune function, one of the major genetic defects appears to be in the manufacture of filaggrin, a protein that facilitates proper integrity and moisture content of the skin.[1]

Therapeutic Considerations

Numerous studies have documented the major role that food allergy plays in eczema (see the chapter "Food Allergy"). Studies have also shown that breastfeeding offers significant protection against developing eczema as well as allergies in general.[2,3] Interestingly, studies suggest that mothers of breastfed infants with allergies should avoid the common food allergens (especially milk, eggs, and peanuts and, to a lesser extent, fish, soy, wheat, citrus, and chocolate) themselves, to prevent traces of food antigens from appearing in their breast milk.[4,5] Maternal avoidance of these common allergens is associated with complete resolution in the majority of cases.

In older or formula-fed infants, milk, eggs, and peanuts appear to be the most common food allergens that lead to eczema. In one study, these three foods were implicated in 81% of all cases of childhood eczema,[6] while in another study 60% of children with severe eczema had a positive food challenge to one or two of the following: eggs, cow's milk, peanuts, fish, wheat, or soybeans. One randomized, controlled trial found that in individuals with a positive reaction to eggs on a radioallergosorbent test, an egg-free diet was associated with improvement in the severity of eczema, with the greatest effect seen in those most severely affected.[7] Although eggs are a major suspect, virtually any food can be the offending agent.[8]

Diagnosis of food allergy is usually best achieved by the elimination diet and challenge method. This approach is especially useful in childhood eczema. Elimination of milk products, eggs, peanuts, tomatoes, and artificial colors and preservatives results in significant improvement in at least 75% of cases.[6-9] Laboratory tests used to identify food allergies in eczema are described in the chapter "Food Allergy."

Some offending foods will have to be avoided indefinitely; others can be added back to the diet after 6 to 12 months. After one year, 26% of patients with eczema were no longer allergic to the five major allergens (egg, milk, wheat, soy, and peanut), and 66% were no longer allergic to other food allergens.[10]

Candida

An overgrowth of the common yeast *Candida albicans* in the gastrointestinal tract has been implicated as a causative factor in allergic conditions including eczema. Elevated levels of antibodies against candida are common in atopic individuals, indicating an active infection. Furthermore, the severity of lesions tends to correlate with the level of antibodies to candidal antigens. The bottom line is that elimination of candida results in significant clinical improvement of eczema in some patients.[11,12] See the chapter "Candidiasis, Chronic" for information on how to prevent the overgrowth of candida.

Probiotics

Because the intestinal flora plays a major role in the health of the host, especially regarding eczema, probiotic therapy is particularly indicated. Studies show that administration of the probiotic *Lactobacillus rhamnosus* alone or in conjunction with *Lactobacillus reuteri* to infants with eczema and cow's milk allergy demonstrates significant reduction of the severity of eczema.[13–16]

Essential Fatty Acids

In the past it was thought that supplementing the diet of eczema patients with evening primrose, borage, or blackcurrant oil (commercial sources of gamma-linolenic acid) might prove helpful. In fact, several double-blind studies with evening primrose oil (typically using dosages of at least 3,000 mg daily, providing 270 mg of gamma-linolenic acid) did show benefit.[17–19] However, overall the therapeutic results appear to be more favorable with omega-3 oil supplementation from fish oils than with evening primrose oil. Several studies with evening primrose oil failed to demonstrate any therapeutic benefit over a placebo. In the largest of these studies and the one with the highest-quality methods, no benefit could be demonstrated for evening primrose oil.[20] Similarly, one study of 140

people, including 69 children, showed few beneficial effects of borage oil.[21]

In contrast, fish oil supplements providing EPA and DHA are showing significant protective effects against allergy development as well as therapeutic effects in double-blind clinical trials.[22,23] The difference in response is probably due to several factors. One is that fish oils contain primarily long-chain omega-3 fatty acids, which are further down the anti-inflammatory pathway, while evening primrose oil contains both omega-6 and omega-3 fatty acids and gamma-linolenic acid is at the beginning of the omega-3 anti-inflammatory chain. Some people, such as those with atopic disease, have poorer-functioning enzymes for the conversion to the anti-inflammatory prostaglandins.

Botanical Medicines

The use of botanical medicines in eczema can be generally divided into two categories: internal and external. Licorice (*Glycyrrhiza glabra*) appears to be useful in either application. Internally, licorice preparations can

. . . .

QUICK REVIEW

- **Eczema is an allergic disease.**
- **The underlying abnormalities leading to eczema originate primarily in the immune system and structural components of the skin.**
- **A genetic basis for eczema has long been recognized. A family history of allergic disease such as eczema and asthma is a major risk factor.**
- **Food allergy in susceptible individuals is the major cause of eczema.**

- **Allergies to milk, eggs, and peanuts account for roughly 81% of all cases of childhood eczema.**
- **Fish oils offer greater treatment benefits than evening primrose oil.**
- **Glycyrrhetinic acid, from licorice root, applied topically has shown advantages over corticosteroid creams.**

exert significant anti-inflammatory and anti-allergic effects. These benefits are perhaps best exemplified in several double-blind studies featuring a licorice-containing Chinese herbal formula.[24] Interest in this formula by a group of researchers began after a patient with eczema experienced tremendous improvement after taking a decoction prescribed by a Chinese doctor. In one study, 40 adult patients with long-standing, refractory, widespread eczema were randomized to receive two months' treatment consisting of either the active formula or a placebo decoction, followed by a crossover to the other treatment after a four-week washout period.[25] The treatment group demonstrated significant improvement over the placebo group in clinical evaluation. In addition, of the 31 patients completing the study, 20 preferred the active formula, while only 4 preferred

· ·

TREATMENT SUMMARY

Effective management requires relief from and prevention of itching while the underlying abnormalities are being treated. Addressing food allergies is the first step. Follow the recommendations in the chapter "Food Allergy."

Scratching is extremely detrimental because it breaks the skin, and this can lead to hardening of the skin as well as bacterial infection. The topical preparations mentioned below can be helpful in reducing itching.

Supplements

- High-potency multiple vitamin and mineral formula
- Vitamin E: 400 international units daily (mixed tocopherols)
- Fish oils: 1,000 to 3,000 mg EPA + DHA daily
- Probiotics: 5 to 10 billion viable lactobacillus and bifidobacteria cells per day
- Choose one of the following:
  - Enzymatically modified isoquercetin (EMIQ): 50–100 mg before meals
  - Grape seed or pine bark extract (>95% procyanidolic oligomers): 50–100 mg before meals

Topical Treatments

- Ceramide-containing moisturizers can be used to reduce water loss from the skin.
- Glycyrrhetinic-acid-containing commercial preparations may be helpful. Chamomile and oatmeal preparations are also popular. In particular, commercially available colloidal oatmeal products (e.g., Aveeno) contain starches and beta-glucans that have protective and water-holding effects, and their polyphenols (avenanthramides) are antioxidant and anti-inflammatory.
- Wash clothing with mild soaps only and rinse thoroughly.
- Avoid exposure to chemical irritants and any other agent that might cause skin irritation.

the placebo. There was also a subjective improvement in itching and sleep during the active treatment phase. No side effects were reported, although many subjects complained about the poor palatability of the decoction. Similar results were demonstrated in a double-blind study of children.[26]

With regard to using licorice topically, the best results are likely to be obtained by using commercial preparations featuring pure glycyrrhetinic acid. Several studies have shown glycyrrhetinic acid to exert an effect similar to that of topical hydrocortisone in the treatment of eczema, contact and allergic dermatitis, and psoriasis. In one study, 9 of 12 patients with eczema unresponsive to other treatments noted marked improvement, and two noted mild improvement when an ointment containing glycyrrhetinic acid was applied topically. In another study, 93% of the patients with eczema who applied glycyrrhetinic acid demonstrated improvement compared with 83% using cortisone.[27]

Fibrocystic Breast Disease

· ·

- Characteristically cyclic and bilateral, with multiple cysts of varying sizes giving the breast a nodular consistency
- Pain or premenstrual breast pain and tenderness common, although condition is often without symptoms
- Occurs in 20 to 40% of premenopausal women

Benign fibrocystic breast disease (FBD), also known as *diffuse cystic mastopathy*, is usually a component of premenstrual syndrome (PMS). It is also considered a risk factor for breast cancer, though not as significant as the classic breast cancer risk factors: family history, early onset of menstruation, and late first pregnancy or no pregnancy.

FBD cannot be definitively differentiated from breast cancer on clinical criteria alone. Although pain, cyclic variations in size, high mobility, and multiplicity of nodules are indicative of FBD, you should see a physician immediately if you notice a lump of any kind. Noninvasive procedures, such as ultrasound, can help in differentiation, but at this time definitive diagnosis depends upon biopsy.

Causes

FBD is apparently the result of an increased estrogen-to-progesterone ratio. However, other hormones are also important. For example, the changes within the breast in FBD may be due to the hormone prolactin. Typi-

cally, significantly elevated levels of prolactin are found in women with FBD, though the levels are not so high as to cause menstruation to cease. The increase in prolactin is thought to be the result of higher estrogen levels.[1]

Therapeutic Considerations

For a more comprehensive discussion of the many factors involved in FBD, read the chapter "Premenstrual Syndrome" as well. The factors discussed here were chosen because they are not covered in depth in the PMS chapter and are particularly relevant to FBD.

Caffeine and Other Methylxanthines

According to population-based studies,[2] experimental evidence,[3–5] and clinical studies,[3–5] there is strong evidence supporting an association between caffeine consumption and FBD. The methylxanthines caffeine, theophylline, and theobromine elevate the levels of compounds that promote overproduction within breast tissue of cellular products linked to FBD, such as fibrous tissue and cyst fluid.[3–5]

In one study, limiting methylxanthines (coffee, tea, cola, chocolate, and caffeinated medications) resulted in improvement in 97.5% of the 45 women who completely abstained and in 75% of the 28 who limited their consumption. Those who continued with little change in their methylxanthine consumption showed little improvement.[3] According to this study, women may have varying thresholds of response to methylxanthines. However, three other studies have shown no association between methylxanthines and FBD.[6,7,8] Stress may also play an important role.

Fiber

A comparison between the diets of 354 women with benign proliferative epithelial disorders of the breast and those of 354 matched controls and 189 unmatched controls found an inverse association between dietary fiber and the risk of such disorders.[9] An increased intake of dietary fiber may be associated with a reduced risk of both benign breast disease and breast cancer.

Breast disease has been linked to a low-fiber diet and constipation. There is an association between abnormal cell structure in nipple aspirates of breast fluid and the frequency of bowel movements.[10] Women having fewer than three bowel movements per week have a risk of FBD 4.5 times greater than women having at least one bowel movement a day. The cause of this association is probably that the bacterial flora in the large intestine transform estrogen into various toxic metabolites, including carcinogens and mutagens. Fecal microorganisms are capable of synthesizing estrogens as well as breaking the bond between excreted estrogen and glucuronate, resulting in absorption of bacteria-derived estrogens and reabsorption of previously excreted estrogen as free estrogen. Diet plays a major role in colon microflora, transit time, and concentration of absorbable metabolites.

Vegetarian Diet

Women on a vegetarian diet excrete two to three times more conjugated estrogens than women on an omnivorous diet.[11] Furthermore, omnivorous women have a 50% higher average level of free estrogen reabsorbed from the intestinal tract. Bacterial beta-glucuronidase is a bacterially produced enzyme that breaks the bond between excreted estrogen and glucuronic acid. Not surprisingly, excess beta-glucuronidase activity is associated with an increased risk of estrogen-dependent breast cancer and may be a factor in FBD as well. Probiotic supplementation has been shown to lower fecal beta-glucuronidase and may help improve bowel function as well.[12]

Dietary Fat

Reducing the total fat content of the diet is also important. Reducing the total fat intake to 15% of total calories while increasing consumption of high-fiber foods has been shown to reduce the severity of premenstrual breast tenderness and swelling, as well as reducing the actual breast swelling and nodules in some women.[13] Reducing the dietary fat intake to 20% of total calories has also been shown to result in significant decreases in circulating estrogens in women with benign breast disease.[14]

Nutritional Supplements

Because FBD is so often linked to PMS, the nutritional supplements recommended in the chapter "Premenstrual Syndrome" are appropriate here. It is especially important to promote the excretion of excess estrogen. FBD may be related to an increased sensitivity to estrogen, and because the liver is the primary site for estrogen clearance, adequate levels of

B vitamins and lipotropic factors are necessary. Historically, naturopaths have used lipotropic factors such as inositol and choline to support the excretion of estrogen. Lipotropic factors promote the removal of fat from the liver. Lipotropic supplements usually are a combination vitamin-and-herbal formulation designed to support the liver's functions of removing fat, detoxifying the body's wastes, detoxifying external toxins, and metabolizing and excreting estrogens. These lipotropic products vary in formulation depending on the manufacturer, but they are all similar. Many now contain anticancer phytonutrients found in brassica-family vegetables, such as indole-3-carbinol (I3C), di-indoylmethane (DIM), and sulfurophane. These compounds help to break down cancer-causing forms of estrogens to non-cancer-causing forms, making them especially important in women with FBD.

Evening Primrose Oil

The only essential fatty acid to be studied in relation to fibrocystic breasts is evening primrose oil. When 291 women with cyclic and noncyclic breast pain were given 3,000 mg evening primrose oil for six months, almost half of the 92 women with cyclic breast pain experienced improvement, compared with one-fifth of the patients who received the placebo. For those women who experienced breast pain throughout the month, 27% (of 33 women) improved with evening primrose oil, compared with 9% on the placebo.[15] In another study, 73 women with breast pain randomly received 3 g per day of EPO or a placebo. After three months, pain and tenderness were significantly reduced in both the women with cyclic breast pain and those with noncyclic pain. The women who took the placebo did not significantly improve.[16] Other seed oils with gamma-linolenic acid should also be considered, including black-

currant oil and borage oil. However, fish oils would probably be most effective. One study showed that red blood cells with higher levels of EPA and DHA—the two primary omega-3 fatty acids in fish—were associated with a significantly reduced risk for FBD.[17]

Vitamin E

Vitamin E (alpha-tocopherol) has been shown to relieve many PMS symptoms, particularly FBD, as evidenced by several double-blind clinical studies.[18] Two studies demonstrated that vitamin E is clinically useful in relieving pain and tenderness, whether it is cyclical or noncyclical.[19,20] The mode of action remains unclear. When larger numbers of women were studied, vitamin E did not fare so well, showing no significant effects either subjectively or objectively.[21,22]

Vitamin E may work best when part of a more comprehensive antioxidant plan. In one study, 66 women with FBD were given a combination of beta-carotene, vitamin E, vitamin C, and garlic powder. There was a reduction in the severity of breast pain, premenstrual syndrome, infrequent menses, and menstrual cramping as well as a reduction in symptoms of FBD in 75% of the women taking the combination, compared with 45% of women on a placebo.[23]

The Thyroid and Iodine

Experimentally induced iodine deficiency in rats results in mammary changes similar to human FBD.[24] This suggests that iodine (specifically iodine caseinate) may be an effective treatment for FBD.[25] It is theorized that an absence of iodine renders the epithelium more sensitive to estrogen stimulation. This hypersensitivity can produce excessive amounts of secretions, distending the breast ducts and producing small cysts and later fibrosis (hardening of the tissue due to the deposition of fibrin, similar to the formation of scar tissue). Iodine may help to arrest this process.[26]

Since 1975, three clinical trials with iodine have been performed on women with FBD. Results from these studies indicate that although treatment with high doses of iodides was effective in about 70% of subjects, it was associated with a high rate of side effects (altered thyroid function in 4%, iodinism in 3%, and acne in 15%).[26] The dosage of iodine was quite high. We recommend that patients take iodine only under strict medical supervision, as taking too much iodine can lead to altered levels of thyroid hormone.

In addition to iodine, there is research showing that thyroid hormone replacement therapy may result in clinical improvement.[27] Thyroid supplementation (0.1 mg Synthroid per day) decreases breast pain, serum prolactin levels, and breast nodules in supposedly normal thyroid patients. These results suggest that subclinical hypothyroidism, iodine deficiency, or both may be etiologic factors in FBD. For more information on subclinical hypothyroidism, see the chapter "Hypothyroidism."

Botanical Medicines

Chasteberry

A large open study (that is, a study without a control group) of 1,634 women with FBD as part of their premenstrual syndrome demonstrated that after three months of treatment, 81% of the patients being treated rated chasteberry (*Vitex agnus-castus*) as a good or very good treatment for FBD.[28] In a double-blind study, 97 women with FBD had twice the decrease in intensity of pain after one or two treatment cycles as compared with a placebo.[29] In another double-blind study comparing chasteberry with fluoxetine (Prozac) in PMS, 58% of patients being treated with chasteberry had an improvement in their FBD and 68% of patients had improvements in their psychological symptoms.[30] And in the largest double-blind study, 170 women with PMS were given chasteberry or a placebo for three consecutive cycles. The improvement in breast pain was greater in the chasteberry group (52%) compared with the placebo group (24%).[31]

· ·

QUICK REVIEW

- **Fibrocystic breast disease is most often a component of premenstrual syndrome.**
- **Elevated estrogen-to-progesterone ratio or both increased prolactin levels are thought to play a role in FBD.**
- **Eliminating caffeine and similar compounds has produced improvements in as many as 97% of women in clinical trials.**
- **Hypothyroidism and/or iodine deficiency may be a causative factor in fibrocystic breast disease.**
- ***Vitex* extract has been shown in several clinical trials to produce significant benefits in improving breast pain and FBD.**
- **Women who have fewer than three bowel movements per week have a 4.5-fold greater rate of fibrocystic breast disease than women who have at least one bowel movement a day.**

TREATMENT SUMMARY

Given the close association of FBD with PMS, we encourage you to also see the chapter "Premenstrual Syndrome."

Diet

Follow the guidelines in the chapter "A Health-Promoting Diet." Consume a diet low in fat and high in fiber, whole grains, flaxseed, and soy foods and avoid saturated fats, sugar, caffeine, and alcohol. Soy isoflavone intake should be between 45 and 90 mg per day. Ground flaxseed at a dosage of 1 to 2 tbsp per day is also recommended.

Nutritional Supplements

- A high-potency multiple vitamin and mineral formula as described in the chapter "Supplementary Measures"
- Key individual nutrients:
  - Vitamin B_6: 25 to 50 mg two times per day
  - Folic acid: 800 mcg per day
  - Vitamin B_{12}: 800 mcg per day
  - Vitamin C: 500 to 1,000 mg per day
  - Vitamin E (mixed tocopherols): 100 to 200 IU per day
  - Magnesium (bound to aspartate, citrate, fumarate, malate, or succinate): 200 to 300 mg three times per day
  - Zinc: 15 to 30 mg per day
  - Vitamin D_3: 2,000 to 4,000 IU per day (ideally, measure blood levels and adjust dosage accordingly)
- Fish oils: 1,000 mg EPA + DHA per day
- Evening primrose oil: 3,000 mg per day
- Specialty supplements, one of the following:
  - Lipotropic formula providing 1,000 mg betaine, 1,000 mg choline, and 1,000 mg cysteine or methionine
  - SAM-e: 200 to 400 mg per day
- One or a combination of the following:
  - Indole-3-carbinol: 300 to 600 mg per day
  - Di-indoylmethane: 100 to 200 mg per day taken with food

Botanical Medicines

- *Vitex* (chasteberry): Usual dosage of chasteberry extract (often standardized to contain 0.5% agnuside) in tablet or capsule form is 175 to 225 mg per day; for liquid extract, typical dosage is 2 to 4 ml (½ to 1 tsp) per day.

Food Allergy

- Significant improvement in symptoms and signs of a disease linked to food allergy while on an allergy-elimination diet
- Positive test result from an acceptable food allergy test
- Typical signs of allergy:
  - Dark circles under the eyes (allergic shiners)
  - Puffiness under the eyes
  - Horizontal creases in the lower eyelid
  - Chronic (noncyclic) fluid retention
  - Chronic swollen glands

A food allergy occurs when there is an adverse reaction to the ingestion of a food. The reaction may or may not be mediated (controlled and influenced) by the immune system. The reaction may be caused by a protein, a starch, or another food component, or by a contaminant found in the food (a coloring, a preservative, etc.).

A classic food allergy occurs when an ingested food molecule acts as an *antigen*—a substance that can be bound by an antibody. Antibodies are the protein molecules made by white blood cells that bind to foreign substances, in this case various components of foods. The food antigen is bound by antibodies known as IgE (immunoglobulin E) for immediate reactions and IgG and IgM for delayed reactions. The IgE antibodies are specialized immunoglobulins (proteins) that bind to specialized white blood cells known as *mast cells* and *basophils*. When the IgE and

food antigen bind to a mast cell or basophil, the binding causes a release of *histamines*, substances that in turn cause swelling and inflammation. The mechanisms that lead to allergy symptoms are further discussed below.

Other terms often used to refer to food allergy include *food hypersensitivity, food anaphylaxis, food idiosyncrasy, food intolerance, pharmacological* (drug-like) *reaction to food, metabolic reaction to food*, and *food sensitivity*.

The recognition of food allergy was first recorded by the Greek physician Hippocrates, who observed that milk could cause gastric upset and hives. He wrote, "To many this has been the commencement of a serious disease when they have merely taken twice in a day the same food which they have been in the custom of taking once."[1]

Food allergies have been implicated in a wide range of medical conditions affecting virtually every part of the body—from mildly uncomfortable symptoms such as indigestion and gastritis to severe illnesses such as multiple sclerosis, rheumatoid arthritis, and chronic infection. Allergies have also been linked to numerous disorders of the central nervous system, including depression, anxiety, and chronic fatigue. The actual symptoms produced during an allergic response depend on the location of the immune system activation, the mediators of inflammation involved, and the sensitivity of the tissues to specific mediators. As is evident in the table opposite, food allergies have been linked to

Common Symptoms and Diseases Associated with Food Allergy/Sensitivity	
SYSTEM	**SYMPTOMS AND DISEASES**
Gastrointestinal	Canker sores, celiac disease, chronic diarrhea, duodenal ulcer, gastritis, irritable bowel syndrome, malabsorption, ulcerative colitis
Genitourinary	Bed-wetting, chronic bladder infections, nephrosis
Immune	Chronic infections, frequent ear infections
Mental/emotional	Anxiety, depression, hyperactivity, inability to concentrate, insomnia, irritability, mental confusion, personality change, seizures
Musculoskeletal	Bursitis, joint pain, low back pain
Respiratory	Asthma, chronic bronchitis, wheezing
Skin	Acne, eczema, hives, itching, skin rash
Miscellaneous	Arrhythmia, edema, fainting, fatigue, headache, hypoglycemia, itchy nose or throat, migraines, sinusitis

many common symptoms and health conditions.

Scope of the Problem

The frequency of food allergies has increased dramatically in recent times. It is estimated that 6% of children and 4% of adults in America have IgE-mediated food allergies[2] and that 20% of the population have altered their diet owing to adverse reactions to foods.[3,4] Some physicians believe that food allergies are the leading cause of undiagnosed symptoms and that at least 60% of Americans suffer from symptoms associated with food reactions.

The primary causes of the increased frequency of food allergy appear to be excessive regular consumption of a limited number of foods (often hidden as ingredients in commercially prepared foods) and the high level of preservatives, stabilizers, artificial colorings, and flavorings now added to foods.[5] Some researchers and clinicians believe that the increased chemical pollution in our air, water, and food is to blame. For example,

foods can easily become contaminated following the use of pesticides in farming.

Other possible reasons for the increased occurrence of food allergy include earlier weaning and earlier introduction of solid foods to infants; genetic manipulation of plants, resulting in food components with greater allergenic properties; and impaired digestion (especially lack of hydrochloric acid and/or pancreatic enzymes). Finally, incomplete digestion and excessive permeability of the intestinal lining significantly contribute to the risk of becoming allergic to foods.

Causes

It is well documented that food allergy is often inherited. When both parents have allergies, there is a 67% chance that the children will also have allergies. When only one parent is allergic, the chance that a child will be prone to allergies is still high but drops from 67 to 33%. The theory is that individuals with a tendency to develop food allergies have abnormalities in the number and ratios of special white blood cells known as T lymphocytes or T cells. Specifically, these individuals have nearly 50% more helper T cells than nonallergic persons. These cells help other white blood cells make antibodies.

Individuals prone to food allergies have a lower allergic set point because they have more helper T cells in circulation. Therefore, the level of insult required to trigger an allergic response is lowered. The actual expression of an allergy can be triggered by a variety of stressors that can disrupt the immune system, such as physical or emotional trauma, excessive use of drugs, immunization reactions, frequent consumption of a specific food, and/or environmental toxins.

Improper digestion and poor integrity of the intestinal barrier are other factors that can lead to the development of food allergy. When properly chewed and digested, 90% of ingested proteins are completely broken down and then absorbed as amino acids and small peptides. However, partially digested dietary proteins can cross the intestinal barrier and be absorbed into the bloodstream. These larger molecules can cause an allergic response that can occur either directly at the intestinal barrier, at distant sites, or throughout the body.

People with food allergies often need supplements of hydrochloric acid and/or pancreatic enzymes (see the chapter "Digestion and Elimination"). Incompletely digested proteins can impair the immune system, leading to long-term allergies and frequent infections.

Stress

During stressful times, food allergies tend to develop or become worse. This situation probably results from a stress-induced decrease in secretory IgA levels. IgA plays an important role in the lining of the mucosal membrane of the intestinal tract, where it helps protect against the entrance of foreign substances into the body. In other words, IgA acts as a barricade against the entry of food antigens. When there is a lack of IgA lining the intestines, the absorption of food allergens and microbial antigens increases dramatically. Even a relatively short-term IgA deficiency predisposes a person to the development of food allergy. People with food allergies typically have unusually low levels of IgA, making them particularly susceptible.

The Immune System and Food Allergies

Most food allergies are mediated by the immune system as a result of interactions between ingested food, the digestive tract, white blood cells, and food-specific antibodies such as IgE, IgG, and IgM. Food represents the largest antigenic challenge that confronts the human immune system, whether a person suffers from food allergies or not. When food antigens activate the immune system, white blood cells and antibodies cooperate in an immune response that, under certain circumstances, can have negative effects.

There are five major families of antibodies: IgE, IgD, IgG, IgM, and IgA. IgE is involved primarily in the classic immediate reaction, while the others seem to be involved in delayed reactions, such as those seen in the cyclical type of food allergy (one that comes and goes). Although the function of the immune system is to protect a person from infections and cancer, abnormal immune responses can lead to tissue injury and disease; food allergy reactions are just one expression.

There are four distinct types of immune-mediated reactions: type I, immediate hypersensitivity; type II, cytotoxic; type III, immune-complex-mediated; and type IV, T-cell-dependent.

Type I: Immediate Hypersensitivity Reactions

Type I reactions occur less than two hours after consumption of an allergenic food. This quick reaction makes it easy to identify the offending foods—getting hives after eating strawberries makes the connection obvious. Antigens bind to preformed IgE antibodies, which are attached to the surface of the mast cell or the basophil, and cause the release of mediators such as histamines and leukotrienes. A variety of allergic symptoms may result, depending on the location of the mast cell: in the nasal passages, this causes sinus congestion; in the bronchioles, constriction (asthma); in the skin, hives and eczema; in the synovial cells that line the joints, arthritis; in the intestinal mucosa, inflammation with resulting malabsorption and possibly diarrhea; and in the brain, headaches, loss of memory, and "spaciness." It is estimated that 10 to 15% of all food allergies are type I reactions.

Oral allergy syndrome is an immediate type I reaction in which symptoms are usually limited to the lips and oral cavity. It occurs in sensitive individuals upon ingestion of proteins in pollens and raw fruits, nuts, or vegetables. Symptoms usually occur within five minutes of eating the food and commonly include itching, tingling, redness, and swelling of the lips, mouth, and throat. Cooked foods rarely induce the same response, because the protein shapes are changed when food is heated or digested.

Type II: Cytotoxic Reactions

Cytotoxic reactions involve the binding of either IgG or IgM antibodies to cell-bound antigens. Antigen-antibody binding activates factors that cause the destruction of the cell to which the antigen is bound. Most often this reaction is seen in antibiotic or other drug reactions when IgG antibodies attach to red blood cells, ultimately destroying them (hemolysis); this can lead to anemia. The same process can occur in intestinal cells.

Type III: Immune-Complex-Mediated Reactions

Immune complexes are formed when antigens bind to antibodies. They are usually cleared from the circulation by white blood cells (macrophages) located in the liver and the spleen. However, if there are increased quantities of circulating immune complexes or if histamines and other amines that increase vascular permeability are present, these immune complexes may be deposited in tissues, producing tissue injury.

These responses are of the delayed type, often occurring more than two hours or even days after exposure. This type of allergy has been shown to involve IgG and IgG4 immune complexes. It is estimated that 80% of food allergy reactions involve IgG and IgG4.

Type IV: T-Cell-Dependent Reactions

These delayed reactions are mediated primarily by white blood cells known as T lymphocytes. The reaction results when an allergen comes into contact with the skin, respiratory tract, or gastrointestinal tract, or another body surface, stimulating sensitized T cells and causing inflammation within 36 to 72 hours. Type IV reactions do not involve any antibodies. Examples include poison ivy (contact dermatitis), allergic colitis, and regional ileitis.

Other Mechanisms That Trigger Food Allergies

Many adverse reactions to foods are not triggered by the immune system. Instead, the reaction is caused by inflammatory mediators (histamine, prostaglandins, leukotrienes, SRS-A, serotonin, platelet-activating factor, kinins, etc.) released by mast cells and other white blood cells. In addition, foods with high histamine content or histamine-releasing effects may produce allergy-like reactions.

Cyclical vs. Fixed Food Allergies

From a clinical perspective, naturopathic and other nutrition-oriented physicians recognize two basic types of food allergies: cyclical and fixed.

Cyclical allergies develop slowly through repeated eating of a food. If the allergenic food is avoided for a period of time (typically more than four months), it may be reintroduced and tolerated unless it is again eaten too frequently. Cyclic allergies account for 80 to 90% of food allergies.

Fixed allergies occur whenever a food is eaten, no matter what the time span is between episodes of ingestion. In other words, in fixed allergies the person remains allergic to the food throughout life.

Diagnostic Considerations

There are two basic categories of tests commonly used: (1) food challenge methods and (2) laboratory methods. Each has its advantages and disadvantages. Food challenge methods require no additional expense, but they do require a great deal of motivation; also, detection is subjective and thus prone to error and confounding factors like stress or environmental exposure. Laboratory procedures such as blood tests can provide immediate identification of suspected allergens, but they are more expensive and report only on the specific antibodies measured.

Elimination Diet and Food Challenge

Many physicians believe that oral food challenge is the best way to diagnose food sen-

> **WARNING:** Food challenge testing should *not* be used by people who have potentially life-threatening symptoms such as airway constriction or severe allergic reactions.

sitivities. There are two broad categories of food challenge testing: (1) an elimination diet (also known as an *oligoantigenic* diet) followed by food reintroduction, and (2) a water fast followed by food challenge.

In the elimination diet method, the patient is put on a limited diet. Commonly eaten foods are eliminated and replaced with either hypoallergenic foods or special hypoallergenic meal-replacement formulas.[6–8] The fewer allergenic foods eaten, the greater the ease of establishing a diagnosis using an elimination diet.

The standard elimination diet consists of lamb, chicken, potatoes, rice, bananas, apples, and vegetables in the brassica family (cabbage, brussels sprouts, broccoli, etc.). There are also other suitable variations of the elimination diet. However, it is extremely important that no allergenic foods be consumed. The individual stays on this limited diet for at least one week, and up to one month. If the symptoms are related to food sensitivity, they will typically disappear by the fifth or sixth day of the diet. If the symptoms do not disappear, it is possible that a reaction to a food in the elimination diet is responsible. In that case, an even more restricted diet must be utilized.

After the elimination diet period, individual foods are reintroduced every two days. Methods range from reintroducing a single food every two days to reintroducing a food every one or two meals. Usually, after the "cleansing" period, the patient will develop an increased sensitivity to offending foods. Reintroduction of allergenic foods will typically produce a more severe or recognizable symptom than appeared before. A careful, detailed record must be maintained, describing when foods were reintroduced and what symptoms appeared upon reintroduction.[9]

For many people, elimination diets offer the most feasible means of detection. Because the effects of food reactions can be dramatic, motivation to eliminate the food may be high. The downside of this procedure is that it is time-consuming and requires discipline and motivation.

Laboratory Methods

There are two popular types of laboratory test used to diagnose food allergies: the skin-prick test and blood tests that measure the levels of antibodies relative to food antigens.

The Skin-Prick Test

The skin-prick test or skin-scratch test is commonly employed by many allergists but tests only for IgE-mediated allergies. Since just 10 to 15% of all food allergies are mediated by IgE, this test is of little value in diagnosing most food allergies. Nevertheless, skin tests are often performed and can provide good information if the food allergy is mediated by IgE.

In this type of test, a small scratch is made on the patient's skin and a food extract is applied to the scratched area. If the patient has elevated levels of IgE with regard to the food, a welt will form immediately as the allergen reacts with IgE-sensitized cells in the patient's skin.

Blood Tests

Most nutritionally oriented physicians now employ blood tests to diagnose food allergies. These tests are convenient, but they can range in cost from a modest $130 to an extravagant $1,200. The ELISA (enzyme-linked immunosorbent assay) test appears to be the best and most popular laboratory method currently available, as well as the most reasonably priced. This test can measure IgE, IgG, IgG4, IgM, and IgA antibodies, therefore identifying both immediate and delayed allergic reactions.

One of the key advantages of the ELISA over other laboratory methods is its ability to measure IgG4 antibodies. This subclass of antibody was initially thought to act as a blocking antibody, thereby exerting protective effects against allergy. However, it is now established that IgG4 antibodies are actually involved in producing allergic symptoms.[10] For example, in a study of asthmatics it was demonstrated that attacks in these patients could be produced in response to inhaled antigens that did not bind to IgE antibodies but did bind to IgG4.[11] These results suggested that IgG4 antibodies act as allergic antibodies, especially to food antigens.[12] Nonetheless, the combination of IgE and IgG4 provides the best answers, especially when compared with skin testing.[13]

Newer ELISA assays—ImmunoCAP (from Phadia), Immulite (from Siemens), and Turbo RAST (from Hycor)—are available and are very sensitive, but as of 2012 they identify only IgE antibodies.[14–16]

Other Methods

Energetic methods of food sensitivity testing (electroacupuncture according to Voll, Vega testing, Carroll testing, applied kinesiology, electrodermal screening, and bioresonance therapy), cytotoxic food allergy testing, and Nambudripad's allergy elimination techniques (NAET) are some of the ways alternative medicine practitioners test for food sensitivities or intolerances, but scientific studies either have not been done to verify the clinical relevance of these methods or have shown these methods to be unreliable and clinically questionable.[17–24]

Therapeutic Considerations

The simplest and most effective method of treating food allergies is through avoidance of allergenic foods. Elimination of offending antigens from the diet will begin to alleviate associated symptoms after the body has cleared itself of the antigen/antibody complexes and after the intestinal tract has eliminated any remaining food (usually three to five days). Avoidance means avoiding the food not only in its most identifiable state (e.g., eggs in an omelet), but also in its hidden state (e.g., eggs in bread). For severe reactions, it may also be necessary to eliminate closely related foods with similar antigenic components (e.g., rice and millet, for patients with severe wheat allergy). Avoiding allergenic foods may not be simple or practical, for several reasons:

- Common allergenic foods, such as wheat, corn, and soy, are found as components of many processed foods.

- When patients are eating away from home, it is often difficult to determine what ingredients are used in purchased foods and prepared meals.

- There may have been a dramatic increase in the number of foods to which a given individual is allergic.

It is often difficult (psychologically, socially, and nutritionally) to eliminate a large number of common foods from a person's diet. But it is often the best approach.

Rotation Diversified Diet

Many experts believe that the key to dietary control of food allergies is the rotation diversified diet. The diet was first developed by Dr. Herbert J. Rinkel in 1934.[25] The diet consists of a highly varied selection of foods that are eaten in a definite rotation, in order to prevent the formation of new allergies and to control preexisting ones.

Tolerated foods are eaten at regularly spaced intervals of four to seven days. For example, a person who has wheat on Monday will have to wait until Friday to have anything with wheat in it again. This approach is based on the principle that infrequent consumption of tolerated foods is not likely to induce new allergies or exacerbate mild allergies, even in highly sensitized and immune-compromised individuals. As tolerance for eliminated foods returns, they may be added back into the rotation schedule without reactivating the allergy (this, of course, applies only to cyclic food allergies; foods involved in fixed allergies may never be eaten again).

It is not simply a matter of rotating tolerated foods; food families must also be rotated. Foods, whether animal or vegetable, come in families. The reason it is important to rotate food families is that allergenic foods can cross-react with other foods from the same family. In other words, people who are allergic to wheat produce antibodies that can react with other grains in the wheat family. Overconsumption or too frequent consumption of foods from the same family can lead to allergies. Food families need not be as strictly rotated as individual foods, though the usual recommendation for people prone to food allergies is to avoid eating members of the same food family two days in a row.

Digestive Support

Insufficient release of pancreatic enzymes as well as low secretion of stomach acid (hypochlorhydria) may play a major role in many cases of food allergies, particularly if a person has multiple allergies. While starch and fat digestion can be carried out satisfactorily

Edible Plant and Animal Kingdoms Taxonomic List

VEGETABLES

Legume	Mustard	Parsley	Potato	Grass	Lily
Bean	Broccoli	Anise	Chili	Barley	Asparagus
Cocoa bean	Brussels sprouts	Caraway	Eggplant	Corn	Chive
Lentil	Cabbage	Carrot	Pepper	Oat	Garlic
Licorice	Cauliflower	Celery	Potato	Rice	Leek
Peanut	Mustard	Coriander	Tomato	Rye	Onion
Pea	Radish	Cumin	Tobacco	Wheat	
Soybean	Turnip	Parsley			
Tamarind	Watercress				
Laurel	**Sunflower**	**Beet**	**Buckwheat**		
Avocado	Artichoke	Beet	Buckwheat		
Camphor	Lettuce	Chard	Rhubarb		
Cinnamon	Sunflower	Spinach			

FRUITS

Gourd	Plum	Citrus	Cashew	Nut	Beech
Cantaloupe	Almond	Grapefruit	Cashew	Brazil nut	Beechnut
Cucumber	Apricot	Lemon	Mango	Pecan	Chestnut
Honeydew	Cherry	Lime	Pistachio	Walnut	Chinquapin nut
Other melon	Peach	Mandarin			
Pumpkin	Plum	Orange			
Squash	Persimmon	Tangerine			
Zucchini					
Banana	**Palm**	**Grape**	**Pineapple**	**Rose**	**Birch**
Arrowroot	Coconut	Grape	Pineapple	Blackberry	Filbert
Banana	Date	Raisin		Loganberry	Hazelnut
Plantain	Date sugar			Raspberry	
				Rose hip	
				Strawberry	
Apple	**Blueberry**	**Pawpaw**			
Apple	Blueberry	Papaya			
Pear	Cranberry	Pawpaw			
Quince	Huckleberry				

(continued on next page)

Edible Plant and Animal Kingdoms Taxonomic List

ANIMALS					
Mammal (Meat/Milk)	**Bird (Meat/Egg)**	**Fish**	**Fish**	**Crustacean**	**Mollusk**
Beef	Chicken	Catfish	Salmon	Crab	Abalone
Goat	Duck	Cod	Sardine	Crayfish	Clam
Pig	Goose	Flounder	Snapper	Lobster	Mussel
Rabbit	Pheasant	Halibut	Trout	Prawn	Oyster
Sheep	Turkey	Mackerel	Tuna	Shrimp	Scallop

Simplified Four-Day Rotation Diet Plan

FOOD FAMILY	FOOD
Day 1	
Citrus	Lemon, orange, grapefruit, lime, tangerine, kumquat, citron
Banana	Banana, plantain, arrowroot
Palm	Coconut, date, date sugar
Parsley	Carrot, parsnip, celery, celery seed, celeriac, anise, dill, fennel, cumin, parsley, coriander, caraway
Spices	Black and white pepper, peppercorn, nutmeg, mace
Subucaya	Brazil nut
Bird	All poultry and game birds (chicken, turkey, duck, goose, guinea, pigeon, quail, pheasant), eggs
Juices	Juices (preferably fresh) may be made from any fruits and vegetables listed above, and used in any combination desired, without adding sweeteners
Day 2	
Grape	Grape, raisin
Pineapple	Packed in juice or water, or fresh
Rose	Strawberry, raspberry, blackberry, loganberry, rose hip
Gourd	Watermelon, cucumber, cantaloupe, pumpkin, squash, other melon, zucchini, pumpkin seed, squash seed
Beet	Beet, spinach, chard
Legume	Pea, black-eyed pea, dry bean, green bean, carob, soybean, lentil, licorice, peanut, alfalfa
Cashew	Cashew, pistachio, mango
Birch	Filbert, hazelnut
Flaxseed	Flaxseed

Simplified Four-Day Rotation Diet Plan	
FOOD FAMILY	**FOOD**
Day 2 (cont.)	
Swine	Pork products
Mollusks	Abalone, snail, squid, clam, mussel, oyster, scallop
Crustaceans	Crab, crayfish, lobster, prawn, shrimp
Juices	Juices (preferably fresh) may be made from any fruits, berries, or vegetables listed above, and used without added sweeteners in any combination desired
Day 3	
Apple	Apple, pear, quince
Gooseberry	Currant, gooseberry
Buckwheat	Buckwheat, rhubarb
Aster	Lettuce, chicory, endive, escarole, globe artichoke, dandelion, sunflower seed, tarragon
Potato	Potato, tomato, eggplant, bell pepper, chili pepper, paprika, cayenne, ground cherries
Lily (onion)	Onion, garlic, asparagus, chive, leek
Spurge	Tapioca
Herb	Basil, savory, sage, oregano, horehound, catnip, spearmint, peppermint, thyme, marjoram, lemon balm
Walnut	English walnut, black walnut, pecan, hickory nut, butternut
Pedalium	Sesame
Beech	Chestnut
Saltwater fish	Herring, anchovy, cod, sea bass, sea trout, mackerel, tuna, swordfish, flounder, sole
Freshwater fish	Sturgeon, salmon, whitefish, bass, perch
Juices	Juices (preferably fresh) may be made from any fruits and vegetables listed above, and used without added sweeteners in any combination desired
Day 4	
Plum	Plum, cherry, peach, apricot, nectarine, almond, wild cherry
Blueberry	Blueberry, huckleberry, cranberry, wintergreen
Pawpaw	Pawpaw, papaya, papain
Mustard	Mustard, turnip, radish, horseradish, watercress, cabbage, Chinese cabbage, broccoli, cauliflower, brussels sprouts, kale, kohlrabi, rutabaga
Laurel	Avocado, cinnamon, bay leaf, sassafras, cassia bud or bark
Sweet potato	Sweet potatoes (including those referred to as yams)

(continued on next page)

Simplified Four-Day Rotation Diet Plan	
FOOD FAMILY	**FOOD**
Day 4 (cont.)	
Grass	Wheat, corn, rice, oats, barley, rye, wild rice, millet, sorghum, bamboo shoot
Orchid	Vanilla
Protea	Macadamia nut
Conifer	Pine nut
Fungus	Mushrooms and yeast (brewer's yeast, etc.)
Bovid	Milk products: butter, cheese, yogurt, beef and milk products, margarine, lamb
Juices	Juices (preferably fresh) may be made from any fruits and vegetables listed above, and used without added sweeteners in any combination desired

without the help of pancreatic enzymes, the enzymes called proteases are critical to proper protein digestion. Incomplete digestion of proteins creates a number of problems for the body, including the development of food allergies.

In order for a food molecule to produce an allergic response it must be fairly large. In studies performed in the 1930s and 1940s, pancreatic enzyme supplementation was shown to be quite effective in preventing food allergies.[26] In a more recent study, 10 patients with food allergy documented by double-blind, placebo-controlled food challenges underwent further double-blind food challenges through a nasogastric tube with a known offending food, with or without the addition of an enteric-coated pancreatic enzyme preparation.[27] Compared with no enzymes, administration of pancreatic enzymes markedly reduced the severity of food-induced symptoms in all 10 patients. All 10 patients in the study suffered from postprandial abdominal symptoms, whereas fewer experienced allergic sinusitis (6 did), skin reactions (5 did), or asthma (2 did). Other protein-digesting enzymes may be of benefit as well.

Quercetin

Quercetin consistently demonstrates the greatest antiallergy activity among the flavonoids studied in experimental models, particularly in test tube studies. In particular, it prevents the release of histamine from mast cells and basophils. Unfortunately, regular quercetin is not very well absorbed. Recently a highly bioavailable enzymatically modified form of isoquercitrin (EMIQ) has been developed. This form has shown significant ability to improve some of symptoms of hay fever in double-blind clinical studies and may show some effect in other allergic conditions as well (see the chapter "Hay Fever" for more information).

Apple Polyphenols

As with EMIQ, two double-blind studies showed apple polyphenols (AP) to reduce hay fever symptoms. In animal models AP has also reduced allergic reactions to food.[28,29] Similar results may be achieved with other polyphenol-rich extracts such as grape seed, pine bark, or green tea extract.

QUICK REVIEW

- Food allergies have been linked to many common symptoms and health conditions.
- Some physicians believe that at least 60% of the American population suffers from symptoms associated with food reactions.
- When both parents have allergies, there is a 67% chance that the children will also have allergies.
- It is often necessary to support the individual who has food allergies with supplemental levels of hydrochloric acid and/or pancreatic enzymes.
- During stressful times, food allergies tend to develop or become worse.
- Many physicians believe that oral food challenge is the best way to diagnose food sensitivities.
- The skin-prick test or skin-scratch test commonly employed by many allergists is of little value in diagnosing most food allergies.
- There are now effective blood tests to identify food allergies.
- The simplest and most effective method of treating food allergies is through avoidance of allergenic foods.
- Many experts believe that the key to the dietary control of food allergies is the rotation diversified diet.
- Pancreatic enzyme preparations, quercetin, and apple polyphenols may be helpful in lessening food allergy symptoms.

TREATMENT SUMMARY

While there is no known simple cure for food allergies, there are a number of measures that will help avoid and lessen symptoms and correct the underlying causes. First, all allergenic foods should be identified using one of the methods discussed in this chapter. After the problematic foods have been identified, the best approach is clearly avoidance of all major allergens, and rotation of all other foods for at least the first few months. As you begin to see improvement, the dietary restrictions can be relaxed, although some people may re-quire a rotation diet indefinitely. If there is a food to which you are strongly allergic, all members of that food family should be avoided.

Nutritional Supplements

- A high-potency multiple vitamin and mineral formula as described in the chapter "Supplementary Measures"
- Vitamin D$_3$: 2,000 to 4,000 IU per day (ideally, measure blood levels and adjust dosage accordingly)
- Fish oils: 1,000 mg EPA + DHA per day

- One of the following:
  - ○ EMIQ: 50 to 100 mg before meals
  - ○ Apple polyphenols extract: 100 to 250 mg before meals
  - ○ Grape seed or pine bark extract (>95% procyanidolic oligomers): 50 to 100 mg before meals
- Pancreatin (8–10X USP) or fungal protease formula: 350 to 1,000 mg per day before meals

Gallstones

- May be without symptoms or may be associated with periods of intense pain in the abdomen that radiates to the upper back
- Ultrasound provides definitive diagnosis

Gallstones are definitely another example of a Western-diet-induced disease.[1] Conservative estimates suggest that about 20 million Americans (10% of the U.S. adult population) and 5 to 22% of the population in the Western world have gallstones.[2] Each year in the United States another 1 million people develop gallstones, and more than 300,000 gallbladders are removed owing to the presence of gallstones. While often considered a nuisance, gallstones are a serious health concern. Persons with gallstone disease or a history of gallbladder removal (cholecystectomy) have a shorter life span, primarily due to increased mortality from cardiovascular disease and cancer, particularly gallbladder cancer.[3,4] Of course, obesity, type 2 diabetes, and insulin resistance are primary risk factors for gallstones and also carry with them the risk of early death.

Bile has many components, including bile salts, bilirubin, cholesterol, phospholipids, fatty acids, water, electrolytes, and other organic and inorganic substances. Bile also contains toxins the body is trying to eliminate, such as persistent organic pollutants (POPs) and mercury. The following table shows the characteristics of the major bile components. Gallstones arise when the concentration of a normal bile component becomes too high.

Gallstones can be divided into four major categories:

- Pure cholesterol
- Pure pigment (calcium bilirubinate)
- Mixed, containing cholesterol and its derivatives along with varying amounts of bile salts, bile pigments, and inorganic salts of calcium
- Stones composed entirely of minerals

Pure stones, either cholesterol or calcium bilirubinate, are uncommon in the United States. Recent studies indicate that in the United States, approximately 80% of stones are of the mixed variety. The remaining 20% of stones are composed entirely of minerals, principally calcium salts, although some stones contain oxides of silicon and aluminum.

The formation of gallstones occurs in three steps:

1. Increase in the concentration of a bile component
2. Formation of a small solid mass (the gallstone)
3. Enlargement of the gallstone by accretion

The requisite step in cholesterol and mixed stone formation is the increased concentration of cholesterol within the gallbladder. Because free cholesterol is insoluble in water, it must be incorporated into a lecithin-bile salt emulsion. Either an increase in cholesterol secretion or a decrease in bile acid

Characteristics of the Major Bile Components			
COMPONENT	**% OF BILE**	**WATER SOLUBILITY**	**PHYSIOCHEMICAL PROPERTIES**
Cholesterol	5	Very poor	Will precipitate from aqueous solutions
Bile salts	65–90	Soluble; have polar and nonpolar regions	Capable of solubilizing cholesterol and phospholipids in aqueous phase
Phospholipids	2–25	Poor	Fit between bile salt molecules, thus increasing their capacity to solubilize cholesterol

or lecithin secretion will result in too much free cholesterol in the bile. Once that has occurred, stone formation is initiated by factors such as decreased bile flow, infection, and increased mucin secretion by the gallbladder lining. Once the stone begins to form, it becomes larger year by year. Symptoms typically occur an average of eight years after formation begins. Gallstones are present in 95% of patients with gallbladder pain and inflammation.

Causes

The major risk factors for the development of cholesterol and mixed gallstones include the following:

- Diet
- Obesity
- Gender
- Race
- High caloric intake
- Estrogens
- Gastrointestinal tract diseases (especially Crohn's disease and cystic fibrosis)
- Drugs
- Age

The role of a low-fiber, high-fat diet in the development of gallstones, as well as other dietary factors, is discussed later; the remaining factors are briefly discussed here.

Obesity

Obesity, type 2 diabetes, insulin resistance, and elevated blood triglyceride levels are well-known risk factors for gallstones. Obesity causes increased cholesterol manufacture in the liver with increased secretion of cholesterol in the bile. Therefore obesity is associated with a significantly increased incidence of gallstones.

Important to note is that during active weight reduction, changes in body fat and diet can actually promote gallstone problems.[5] During the first stages of weight loss, the amount of cholesterol in the bile initially increases, because the secretion of bile acids decreases more than the secretion of cholesterol. Once weight is stabilized, bile acid output returns to normal levels, while the cholesterol output remains low. The net effect is a significant reduction in cholesterol concentration in the bile. Obese patients with a high risk of gallstones should realize that prolonged dietary fat reduction can also promote a condition called biliary stasis, thus contributing to the risk of gallstone formation.[1] Studies show that at least 10 g fat per day is necessary in order to ensure proper gallbladder emptying.[6]

Gender

The frequency of gallstones is two to four times greater in women than in men. Women are thought to be predisposed to gallstones because of either increased cholesterol synthesis or suppression of bile acids by estrogens. Pregnancy, use of oral contraceptives or other causes of elevated estrogen levels, and the chemotherapy drug tamoxifen greatly increase the incidence of gallstones.

Genetic and Ethnic Factors

The prevalence of gallstones appears to have some genetic aspects. Gallstones are most common in Native American women older than 30. Nearly 70% of the women in this group have gallstones. In contrast, only 10% of black women older than 30 have gallstones.

The difference in the prevalence rate between different ethnic and genetic groups reflects the concentration of cholesterol in the bile. The extent to which dietary factors affect this value probably outweighs genetic factors.

Gastrointestinal Tract Diseases

Malabsorption of bile acids from the small intestine disturbs the natural circulation of excreted bile acids back to the liver, thereby reducing the bile acid pool and the rate of secretion of bile. Diseases associated with this phenomenon include Crohn's disease and cystic fibrosis.

Drugs

Tamoxifen treatment in postmenopausal breast cancer patients greatly increases gallstones. One study of 703 women demonstrated that after five years, the incidence of stone formation in the tamoxifen-treated patients was 37.4%, whereas it was 2% in patients who did not receive tamoxifen.[7] Most gallstones became apparent after three years.

In addition to oral contraceptives and other estrogens, as discussed earlier, drugs that increase the risk of gallstones include ceftriaxone, octreotide, statins, and possibly other lipid-lowering drugs.

Age

Gallstones have been reported in fetuses and extremely old people and at all ages in between, but the average patient is 40 to 50 years old. Decline in the activity of enzymes that manufacture bile acids with age leads to an increase in biliary cholesterol hypersecretion and thus cholesterol saturation with accelerated formation of gallstones. Aging itself appears to be a risk factor for gallstones.[8]

Risk Factors for Pigmented Gallstones

Risk factors for pigmented gallstones are not related to diet as much as they are to geography, sun exposure, and severe diseases. Pigmented gallstones are more common in Asia, owing to the higher incidence of parasitic infection of the liver and gallbladder by various organisms including the liver fluke *Clonorchis sinensis*. Bacteria and protozoa can cause stagnation of bile flow or initiate the process of stone formation. In the United States, pigmented stones are usually caused by chronic hemolysis or alcoholic cirrhosis of the liver.

Therapeutic Considerations

Gallstones are easier to prevent than to reverse. Primary treatment, therefore, involves reducing the controllable risk factors discussed earlier. Once gallstones have formed, therapeutic intervention involves avoiding aggravating foods and employing measures that increase the solubility of cholesterol in bile and possibly help dissolve the stones. If symptoms persist or worsen, surgery may be required.

A number of dietary factors are important in the prevention and treatment of gallstones. Foremost is the elimination of foods that can produce symptoms. Also important are increasing dietary fiber, eliminating food allergies, and reducing the intake of refined carbohydrates and animal protein. Vegetables and fruits have a protective effect against gallbladder cancer, while red meat was found to be associated with increased risk of gallbladder cancer.[9] Because gallstones are a risk factor for gallbladder cancer, a healthful diet will protect against both cancer and development of gallstones.

Other treatment measures involve the use of nutritional lipotropic compounds, herbal choleretics, and other natural compounds in an attempt to increase the solubility of bile.

Biliary cholesterol concentration and serum cholesterol levels do not seem to correlate.[10] However, there is a link between high triglyceride levels and gallstone formation.[11,12] Drugs to lower triglycerides actually worsen the situation by reducing bile acid content, while fish oils produce the exact opposite effect.[12] In general, the higher the level of triglycerides the more saturated the bile is and the more likely it is that a stone will form.

Silent Gallstones

The natural history of silent or asymptomatic gallstones supports the contention that elective gallbladder removal is not warranted. There is a cumulative chance of developing symptoms—10% at 5 years, 15% at 10 years, and 18% at 15 years—but if controllable risk factors are eliminated or reduced, a person should never experience discomfort and require surgery.

Diet

Dietary Fiber
The theory that the main cause of gallstones is the consumption of fiber-depleted, refined foods has considerable research support.[1] Gallstones are clearly associated with the Western diet in population studies. Such a diet, high in refined carbohydrates and fat and low in fiber, leads to a reduction in the synthesis of bile acids by the liver and a lower bile acid concentration in the gallbladder.

Another way in which fiber may prevent gallstone formation is by reducing the absorption of deoxycholic acid. This compound is produced from bile acids by bacteria in the intestine. Deoxycholic acid greatly lessens the solubility of cholesterol in bile. Dietary fiber has been shown both to decrease the formation of deoxycholic acid and to bind deoxycholic acid and promote its excretion in the feces. This greatly increases the solubility of cholesterol in the bile. A diet high in fiber, especially soluble fiber, which is capable of binding to deoxycholic acid, is extremely important in both the prevention and the reversal of gallstones.

Interestingly, diets rich in legumes, which are high in soluble fiber, are associated with an increased risk for gallstones in some populations.[13] Specifically, Chileans, Pima Indians, and other North American Indians have the highest prevalence rates for cholesterol gallstones, and all typically consume a diet rich in legumes. Evidently legume intake may increase biliary cholesterol saturation in these populations. A study conducted in the Netherlands showed just the opposite, as legume intake was shown to offer significant protection against gallstones.[14] Until this issue is clarified, it might be best to restrict legume intake in individuals with existing gallstones.

Vegetarian Diet

A vegetarian diet has been shown to be protective against gallstone formation.[15] A recent study in England compared a large group of healthy nonvegetarian women with a group of vegetarian women. Ultrasound diagnosis showed that gallstones occurred significantly less frequently in the vegetarian group.

Although this may simply be a result of the increased fiber content of the vegetarian diet, other factors may be equally important. Animal proteins, such as casein from dairy products, have been shown to increase the formation of gallstones in animals, while vegetable proteins such as soy were shown to be preventive against gallstone formation.[16]

Food Allergies

In 1948 Dr. J. C. Breneman, author of *Basics of Food Allergy*, began to use a therapeutic regimen that proved very successful in preventing prevent gallbladder attacks: allergy elimination diets. The idea that food allergies cause gallbladder pain has some support in the scientific literature.[17–20] A 1968 study revealed that 100% of a group of patients were free from symptoms while they were on a basic elimination diet (beef, rye, soybean, rice, cherry, peach, apricot, beet, and spinach).[17] Foods inducing symptoms were as follows (those that most frequently caused symptoms are listed first):

- Eggs
- Pork
- Onion
- Poultry
- Milk
- Coffee
- Citrus fruits
- Corn
- Beans
- Nuts

Adding eggs to the diet caused gallbladder attacks in 93% of the patients.

Several mechanisms have been proposed to explain the association of food allergy and gallbladder attacks. Dr. Breneman believes the ingestion of allergy-causing substances causes swelling of the bile ducts, resulting in impairment of bile flow from the gallbladder.

Buckwheat

Buckwheat is a well-known alternative for those avoiding wheat for hypoallergenic purposes. Giving three groups of eight hamsters a buckwheat-, soy-, or casein-based diet, one Japanese research group demonstrated that buckwheat can significantly decrease gallstone formation and reduce the concentration of cholesterol in the gallbladder, plasma, and liver of hamsters, compared with the casein diet.[21] Even though soy itself prevents gallstones,[22] these researchers found that the positive effects of buckwheat were far stronger than those of soy. Gallstones were clearly visible in all eight hamsters fed the casein diet, whereas two of seven hamsters fed the soy diet (29%) and none of the buckwheat-fed animals had gallstones. Studies of rats have corroborated these findings.[23] The hypothesis is that buckwheat can enhance bile acid synthesis and fecal excretion of steroidal compounds. Buckwheat may be useful to treat patients with both high cholesterol and gallstones and may reduce colon cancer cell proliferation.[24] It is also possible that higher levels of arginine and glycine may play a role in buckwheat's protective function.

Sugar

Diets high in refined carbohydrates and sugar have been found to be associated with increased cholesterol concentration in the bile and an increased risk for both gallstones and gallbladder cancer.[25–30]

Caloric Restriction

Rapid weight loss[31] and fasting[32] increase the risk of gallstones (see the section "Obesity" earlier in the chapter). For example, in 179 obese patients, 9% of whom had preexisting gallstones, a low-calorie diet (605 calories) resulted in 11% of the patients developing gallstones either while on the diet or within six months of completing it.[31] A study of a 925-calorie diet found that 12.8% of the 47 women patients had ultrasound evidence of gallstones at week 17. Those who developed gallstones had significantly higher baseline triglyceride and total cholesterol levels than those who did not. They also had a significantly greater rate of weight loss.[33]

Coffee

Although coffee can exacerbate the symptoms of gallstones, it may also inhibit their formation. In one interesting study, 400 ml regular coffee and 165 ml regular and decaffeinated coffee were assessed for their effect on cholecystokinin secretion. Regular coffee at both dosages and decaffeinated coffee caused significant gallbladder contractions in six healthy regular coffee drinkers.[34] Another study, of 80,898 female nurses between the ages of 34 and 59, found that drinking four cups of caffeinated coffee per day lowered the risk of developing symptoms of gallstones by 28%. Even one to three cups seemed to have some protective effect, though not as great.[35] It may be that the gallbladder contractions from coffee consumption were able to either inhibit the development of stones or clear small ones. In women who already have large stones, the increased contractions produced by coffee may worsen their condition.

Nutritional Supplements

Lecithin (Phosphatidylcholine)

Because lecithin is the main cholesterol solubilizer in bile, a low lecithin concentration may be a causative factor for many people with gallstones. Studies have shown that ingestion of lecithin can have a direct effect on cholesterol solubilization.[36] Taking as little as 100 mg lecithin three times per day will increase the concentration of lecithin in the bile, while larger doses (up to 10 g) produce even greater increases.[37,38] This effect is significant, as an increased lecithin content of bile usually increases the solubility of cholesterol. However, no significant effects on gallstone dissolution have been obtained using lecithin supplementation alone. Therefore, moderate dosages are recommended as supportive therapy.

Vitamins E and C

A deficiency of either vitamin E or vitamin C has been shown to cause gallstones in experimental studies of animals.[39,40]

Olive Oil Liver Flush

A popular remedy for gallstones is the so-called olive oil liver flush. There are several variations. A typical one involves drinking 1 cup of unrefined olive oil with the juice of two lemons in the morning for several days.

Many people tell tales of passing huge stones while on the liver flush. However, what they think are gallstones are simply a complex of minerals, olive oil, and lemon juice produced within the gastrointestinal tract.[41]

The olive oil liver flush is potentially dangerous for people with gallstones for several reasons. First, consuming a large quantity of any oil results in contraction of the gallbladder, which may increase the likelihood of a stone blocking the bile duct. This may result in inflammation of the gallbladder (cholecystitis), requiring immediate surgery to prevent death. Second, in animal studies high doses of olive oil have been shown to increase the development of gallstones by increasing the content of cholesterol in the gallbladder.[42–44] Although this effect has not yet been observed in humans, common sense and the animal research suggest it is unwise to use an olive oil liver flush as a treatment for gallbladder disease.

Fish Oils

In animal studies, fish oil supplementation has been shown to reduce gallstone formation.[45,46] In human studies, fish oil supplementation improves bile acid content and increases the solubility of cholesterol in the bile in obese women losing weight.[12,47,48] As mentioned above, fish oils increase bile acid content of the bile and lower triglycerides; this effect makes them a very important recommendation in gallstone prevention and treatment.

Lipotropic Factors and Botanical Choleretics

The naturopathic approach to the treatment of gallstones has typically involved the use of lipotropic and choleretic formulas. Lipotropic factors are, by definition, substances that hasten the removal of fat from, or decrease the deposit of fat in, the liver through their interaction with fat metabolism. Compounds commonly employed as lipotropic agents include choline, methionine, betaine, folic acid, and vitamin B_{12}.

Often these nutritional factors are used with herbal cholagogues and choleretics. Cholagogues stimulate gallbladder contraction to promote bile flow, while choleretics increase bile secretion by the liver.

Herbal choleretics that are appropriate to use in the treatment of gallstones include dandelion (*Taraxacum officinale*), milk thistle (*Silybum marianum*) and its active ingredient silymarin, artichoke (*Cynara scolymus*), turmeric (*Curcuma longa*) and its active ingredient curcumin, and boldo (*Peumus boldo*).

One study of rats given a diet that promoted gallstones demonstrated that the animals given supplemental curcumin for 10 weeks had only a 26% incidence of gallstone formation, compared with a 100% incidence in the group fed the stone-forming diet alone.[49] This effect was found to be dose-dependent.

Chemical Dissolution of Gallstones

As described above, the formation of gallstones depends on either increased accumulation of cholesterol or reduced levels of bile acids or lecithin. So decreasing gallbladder cholesterol levels or increasing bile acid or lecithin levels should result in dissolution of the stone over time. Chemical dissolution is especially indicated in the treatment of gallstones in children, elderly patients who cannot withstand the stress of surgery, and other cases where surgery is contraindicated.[50,51]

Several successful nonsurgical alternatives for the treatment of gallstones now exist. For example, use of prescription bile acids such as ursodeoxycholic acid and tauroursodeoxycholic acid are effective in dissolving small, uncalcified cholesterol gallstones. About 15% of all patients with cholesterol gallstones would meet this criterion. Treatment with bile acids will lead to complete dissolution in about 90% of cases after six months of therapy. Once the stones have been dissolved, it is important to follow the recommendations given here for gallstone prevention in order to reduce the risk of recurrence. The typical daily dosage of prescription bile acids is 12 mg/kg.

In several studies, gallstone dissolution has also been accomplished with Rowachol, a proprietary combination of natural terpenes such as menthol, menthone, pinene, borneol, cineol, and camphene.[52–56] Although terpenes are effective alone, the best results appear to be achieved when plant terpene complexes are used in combination with bile acid therapy.[56–58] This combined approach offers better results than either bile acids or plant terpenes used alone.[57,58] Furthermore, when plant terpenes are used, a lower dose of bile acids can be taken, significantly reducing the risk of complications or side effects and the cost of bile acid therapy. As menthol is the major component of this formula, peppermint oil, especially enteric-coated capsules, may offer similar results and is more readily available.

. . . .

QUICK REVIEW

- **Gallstones can be prevented through diet and lifestyle measures.**
- **Obesity, type 2 diabetes, insulin resistance, and elevated blood triglyceride levels are well-known risk factors for gallstones.**
- **Fasting or severe calorie restriction can lead to gallstone formation.**
- **Food allergies can lead to gallbladder symptoms. A 1968 study revealed that 100% of a group of patients were free from symptoms while they were on a basic elimination diet.**
- **Biliary cholesterol concentration and serum cholesterol levels do not seem to correlate.**
- **There is a link between high triglyceride levels and gallstone formation.**
- **Coffee can aggravate symptoms of gallstones by causing the gallbladder to contract, but it may also help prevent formation.**
- **A low lecithin concentration in the bile may be a causative factor for many individuals with gallstones.**
- **Diets high in refined carbohydrates and sugar have been associated with increased cholesterol concentration in the bile and an increased risk for both gallstones and gallbladder cancer.**
- **Vitamin C supplementation (2,000 mg per day) has been shown to produce positive effects on bile composition and reduces cholesterol stone formation.**
- **Milk thistle extract and other herbal choleretics may help dissolve gallstones through their ability to increase the solubility of the bile.**
- **Bile acids such as ursodeoxycholic acid and tauroursodeoxycholic acid are effective in dissolving small, uncalcified cholesterol gallstones in about 90% of cases after six months of therapy.**
- **A complex of plant terpenes alone or, preferably, in combination with oral bile acids can help dissolve gallstones.**

TREATMENT SUMMARY

As is typical of most diseases, gallstones are much easier to prevent than reverse. The risk factors and causes of gallstones are well known, and in most cases a healthful diet rich in dietary fiber, moderate in calories, and low in saturated fats is adequate prevention.

Once gallstones have developed, measures to avoid gallbladder attacks and increase the solubility of the bile are necessary. To limit the incidence of symptoms, avoid allergenic foods (see the chapter "Food Allergy") and fatty foods.

Diet

Follow the general guidelines given in the chapter "A Health-Promoting Diet." Definitely increase the intake of vegetables, fruits, dietary fiber (especially soluble fiber, found in, for example, flaxseed, oat bran, guar gum, and pectin), and buckwheat. Reduce the consumption of saturated fats, refined carbohydrates, cholesterol, sugar, and animal proteins. Avoid fried foods.

An allergy elimination diet can be used to reduce gallbladder attacks (see the chapter "Food Allergy").

Drink six to eight glasses of water each day to maintain the water content of the bile.

Nutritional Supplements

- A high-potency multiple vitamin and mineral formula as described in the chapter "Supplementary Measures"

- Key individual nutrients:
  - Vitamin C: 500 to 1,000 mg three times per day
  - Vitamin E (mixed tocopherols): 100 to 200 IU per day
  - Vitamin D_3: 2,000 to 4,000 IU per day (ideally, measure blood levels and adjust dosage accordingly)
  - Fish oils: 1,000 mg EPA + DHA per day
- Take one of the following:
  - Grape seed extract (>95% procyanidolic oligomers): 100 to 300 mg per day
  - Pine bark extract (>95% procyanidolic oligomers): 100 to 300 mg per day
  - Some other flavonoid-rich extract with a similar flavonoid content, super greens formula, or another plant-based antioxidant that can provide an oxygen radical absorption capacity (ORAC) of 3,000 to 6,000 units or higher per day
- One of the following:
  - Lipotropic formula providing 1,000 mg betaine, 1,000 mg choline, and 1,000 mg cysteine or methionine
  - SAM-e: 200 to 400 mg per day
- Phosphatidylcholine: 500 mg per day
- Fiber supplement (guar gum, pectin, psyllium, or PGX): 2.5 to 5 g per day

Botanical Medicines

- One or more of the following:
  - ○ Dandelion (*Taraxacum officinale*):
    - – Dried root: 4 g three times per day
    - – Fluid extract (1:1): 4 to 8 ml three times per day
    - – Solid extract (4:1): 250 to 500 mg three times per day
  - ○ *Pneumus boldo*:
    - – Dried leaves (or by infusion): 250 to 500 mg three times per day
    - – Tincture (1:10): 2 to 4 ml three times per day
    - – Fluid extract (1:1): 0.5 to 1 ml three times per day

  - ○ Milk thistle (*Silybum marianum*): sufficient dosage to yield 70 to 210 mg silymarin, three times per day
  - ○ Artichoke (*Cynara scolymus*) extract (15% cynarin): 500 mg three times per day
  - ○ Curcumin: 200 to 400 mg three times per day
  - ○ One of the following:
    - – Rowachol (proprietary gallstone-dissolving formula): 1 capsule three times per day with meals
    - – Peppermint oil: 1 to 2 enteric-coated capsules (0.2 ml per capsule) three times per day between meals

Glaucoma

- Acute glaucoma:
  - ○ Severe throbbing pain in eye with markedly blurred vision
  - ○ Pupil moderately dilated and fixed
  - ○ Absence of pupillary light response
  - ○ Increased intraocular pressure, usually in just one eye
  - ○ Nausea and vomiting are common
- Chronic glaucoma:
  - ○ Persistent elevation of intraocular pressure associated with pathological cupping of optic discs
  - ○ No symptoms in the early stages
  - ○ Gradual loss of peripheral vision resulting in tunnel vision
  - ○ Insidious onset in older individuals
- Normotensive glaucoma:
  - ○ Normal intraocular pressure with no pathological cupping of optic discs
  - ○ Asymptomatic in the early stages
  - ○ Gradual loss of peripheral vision resulting in tunnel vision
  - ○ Insidious onset in older individuals, more common in women than men
  - ○ Low blood pressure a common underlying feature

Glaucoma most often refers to the vision loss caused by increased intraocular pressure as a result of greater production than outflow of the fluid of the eye (the aqueous humor).

The normal intraocular pressure is about 10 to 21 mm Hg. In chronic glaucoma, the intraocular pressure is usually mildly to moderately elevated (22 to 40 mm Hg). In acute glaucoma, the intraocular pressure is greater than 40 mm Hg. Acute glaucoma is a medical emergency; fortunately, it is the rarest form of glaucoma.

Chronic open-angle glaucoma[1] is by far the most common form. It accounts for about 70 to 75% of the approximately 3 million cases of glaucoma in the United States.

In some cases glaucoma develops in people with normal intraocular pressure. Referred to as *low-tension glaucoma* or *normotensive glaucoma*, this form accounts for approximately 25 to 30% of all glaucoma cases in the United States. Normotensive glaucoma is more common in women than in men and in adults around 60. A common risk factor for normotensive glaucoma is low blood pressure.

Since many patients with glaucoma have no symptoms, it is important that regular eye exams be included in annual checkups for those over the age of 60. Glaucoma is a serious condition that requires strict attention.

Causes

There is a strong correlation between the composition of collagen and chronic glaucoma.[2] Collagen is the most abundant protein in the body, including the eye, where it provides strength and integrity to tissues.

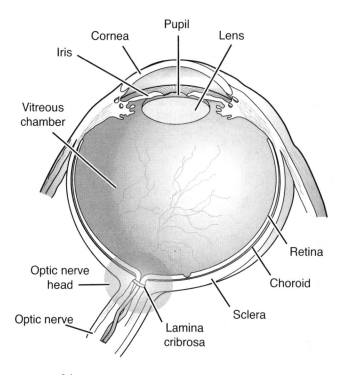

Iris **Cornea** **Pupil** **Lens**

Vitreous chamber

Retina

Choroid

Optic nerve head

Sclera

Optic nerve

Lamina cribrosa

Anatomy of the Eye

Inborn errors of collagen metabolism (e.g., osteogenesis imperfecta, Ehlers-Danlos syndrome, and Marfan's syndrome) are often associated with glaucoma and other eye disease.[3] Structural changes in the eye involving the connective tissue network (through which aqueous humor must pass to reach the canal of Schlemm) and blood vessels in the eye have all been observed in glaucoma.[2,4–6] These changes may result in elevated intraocular pressure or, perhaps more significantly, lead to the progression of peripheral vision loss. Changes in collagen structure would explain the following:[2,4–6]

- The visual loss in normal-tension glaucoma
- Cupping of the optic disc even at low intraocular pressures
- No apparent anatomical reason for decreased aqueous outflow in chronic or normal-tension glaucoma

Furthermore, since elevated intraocular pressure is not a factor in normal-tension glaucoma, other factors have been suggested that may also have significance in chronic glaucoma:

- Reduced blood flow
- Early nerve cell death
- Nerve irritation
- Excessive glutamate production
- Autoimmune disease

Therapeutic Considerations

Prevention and treatment of chronic glaucoma are dependent on reduction of intraocular pressure and improvement of collagen metabolism. The role of collagen destruction

WARNING: Acute closed-angle glaucoma is a medical emergency. Unless it is adequately treated within 12 to 48 hours, a person will become permanently blind within two to five days. Individuals with a narrow anterior chamber angle may spontaneously develop acute glaucoma. The process can be precipitated by anything that dilates the pupil, such as atropine and epinephrine-like drugs. Typical signs and symptoms include extreme pain, blurring of vision, redness, and a fixed and dilated pupil. Agents that dilate the pupils must be strictly avoided in anyone suspected of having glaucoma.

in the etiology of glaucoma is apparent in corticosteroid-induced glaucoma, in which corticosteroids inhibit the manufacture of collagen in the eye.[2] Glaucoma patients should not use corticosteroids.

Allergies

The successful treatment of chronic glaucoma by antiallergy measures has been reported in the literature.[7] In one study, many of the 113 patients demonstrated an immediate rise in intraocular pressure of up to 20 mm Hg (in addition to other typical allergic symptoms) when challenged with the appropriate allergen, whether foodborne or environmental. The author speculated that the known allergic responses of altered vascular permeability and vasospasm could result in the congestion and edema characteristic of glaucoma.

Nutritional Supplements

Vitamin C

Optimal tissue concentrations of vitamin C are central to achieving collagen integrity. Furthermore, supplemental vitamin C has been demonstrated to lower intraocular pressure in many clinical studies.[8–12] For example, in one study a daily dose of 500 mg/kg vita-

min C, whether in single or divided doses, reduced intraocular pressure in glaucoma patients by an average of 16 mm Hg.[12] Using vitamin C, significant improvements have been achieved in some patients who were unresponsive to common glaucoma drugs.[12]

The ability of vitamin C to reduce intraocular pressure lasts only as long as supplementation is continued. Although vitamin C therapy is effective orally, intravenous administration results in an even greater reduction.[8,10–12] Monitoring of intraocular pressure is required to determine the appropriate individual dose, as some patients respond to as little as 2 g per day, while others will respond only to extremely high doses (35 g per day).[8–12] Abdominal discomfort is common with high doses but usually tapers off after three to four days.[12] We feel that lower dosages of vitamin C may be possible if supplemental flavonoids are also used to further aid normal collagen metabolism. It is important to understand that the short-term benefits of high doses of vitamin C are primarily due to an osmotic effect, while long-term use of moderate doses is necessary to promote improved collagen strength and integrity of eye tissues.

Flavonoid-Rich Extracts

The most beneficial flavonoids are the anthocyanosides and proanthocyanosides—the blue-red pigments found in many fruits and plant extracts. These compounds elicit a vitamin-C-sparing effect, improve capillary integrity, and stabilize the collagen matrix by preventing free radical damage, inhibiting enzymatic cleavage of collagen, and cross-linking with collagen fibers directly.[13–15] *Vaccinium myrtillus* (European bilberry) extract is particularly rich in anthocyanoside compounds and has been used with good results in improving night vision and diabetic retinopathy. Grape seed and pine bark extract have also shown benefits in several

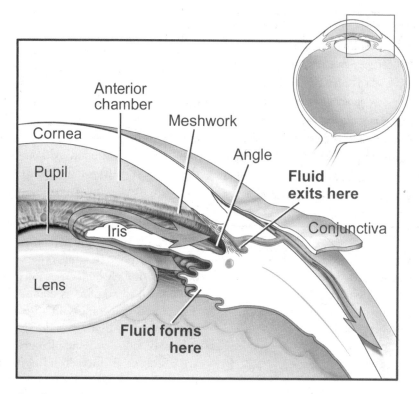

Cornea

Pupil

Anterior chamber

Meshwork

Angle

Fluid exits here

Iris

Lens

Conjunctiva

Fluid forms here

Flow of Aqueous Humour

eye disorders. In one study, a combination of bilberry anthocyanoside extract (160 mg) and pine bark extract (80 mg) was studied in 38 asymptomatic subjects with increased intraocular pressure.[16] After two months of supplementation with the flavonoids, mean intraocular pressure decreased from a baseline of 25.2 mm Hg to 22.2 mm Hg. After an additional three months of treatment, 19 of the 20 patients taking the flavonoids showed decreased intraocular pressure. No side effects were observed. In addition, the blood flow to eye structures including the retina improved as measured by ultrasound.

Rutin, a common citrus flavonoid, has also been demonstrated to lower intraocular pressure when used as an adjunct in patients unresponsive to drug therapy alone.[17]

Ginkgo biloba extract is rich in flavonoids and may be helpful in normotensive glaucoma, based upon the results of two double-blind studies. In the first study, involving healthy human volunteers, ginkgo biloba extract (120 mg per day) significantly increased end diastolic velocity in the ophthalmic artery (23% change), while no change was seen with a placebo. Ginkgo did not alter arterial blood pressure, heart rate, or intraocular pressure.[18] In the second study, patients with normotensive glaucoma received either 40 mg ginkgo biloba extract or a placebo three times per day for four weeks, followed by a washout period of eight weeks, then four weeks of the other treatment. After ginkgo treatment, a significant improvement in visual field indicators was recorded, showing that ginkgo improves preexisting visual field damage in some patients with normotensive glaucoma.[19]

Magnesium

Since calcium-channel-blocking drugs benefit some glaucoma patients, a group of researchers in Switzerland decided to evaluate the effect of supplemental magnesium, which has been referred to as "nature's physiological calcium-channel blocker." Ten glaucoma patients (six with chronic glaucoma, four with normotensive glaucoma) participated in the trial. Magnesium was given at a modest dose of 121.5 mg twice a day for one month. After four weeks of treatment, the visual fields improved, and measures of blood flow showed improvement. These results demonstrate that magnesium supplementation improves peripheral circulation and seems to have a beneficial effect on the visual field in patients with glaucoma.[20]

To evaluate the effect of oral magnesium therapy on blood flow to the eye and visual function, 15 patients with normotensive glaucoma received 300 mg oral magnesium citrate for one month, while 15 patients received no treatment. In the magnesium group, significant improvements were noted in visual field measurements. There was no change in ocular blood flow, so the exact mechanism of magnesium's effect is not known.[21]

Chromium

A case-controlled study of 400 eye patients, 52 of whom had chronic glaucoma, found that chronic glaucoma was strongly associated with a deficiency of chromium and low vitamin C intake.[22]

Fish Oil

In an interesting speculative study, feeding rabbits food soaked with cod liver oil resulted in a 25 mm Hg drop in intraocular pressure, to 11 mm Hg. Intramuscular injections of cod liver oil produced a dose-dependent reduction in intraocular pressure. When the animals were taken off cod liver oil, their intraocular pressure returned to baseline. Control animals given liquid lard or safflower oil experienced no change in intraocular pressure.[23] Preliminary studies of the omega-3 fatty acid DHA with human subjects are encouraging.[24]

Caffeine

Many physicians instruct patients with glaucoma to avoid coffee and other caffeinated beverages, and research seems to support this recommendation. Consumption of regular coffee (180 mg caffeine in 200 ml coffee)

· ·

QUICK REVIEW

- **Acute glaucoma is a medical emergency.**
- **Prevention and treatment of chronic glaucoma are dependent on reduction of intraocular pressure and improvement of collagen metabolism.**
- **The most beneficial flavonoids are the anthocyanosides and proanthocyanosides— the blue-red pigments found in many fruits and plant extracts.**
- **Ginkgo biloba extract may be helpful in normotensive glaucoma.**
- **Magnesium supplementation improves both chronic and normotensive glaucoma.**
- **Caffeine intake should be avoided by individuals with glaucoma.**
- **Exercise is very effective in lowering intraocular pressure.**

and decaffeinated coffee (3.6 mg caffeine in 200 ml coffee) was compared in patients with normotensive or chronic glaucoma in a double-blind crossover study.[25] Intraocular pressure was monitored in both groups at 30, 60, and 90 minutes after coffee ingestion. In patients with normotensive glaucoma who drank regular coffee, increases in intraocular pressure at 30, 60, and 90 minutes were 0.9, 3.6, and 2.3 mm Hg, respectively; in those who drank decaffeinated coffee, increases were 0.75, 0.70, and 0.4 mm Hg, respectively. The corresponding values in patients with chronic glaucoma were as follows: after regular coffee, increases of 1.1, 3.4, and 3 mm Hg; and after decaffeinated coffee, increases of 0.6, 0.9, and 0.5 mm Hg. This study showed quite clearly that subjects who drank regular coffee demonstrated a greater elevation in intraocular pressure whether they had normotensive or chronic glaucoma.

Exercise

Exercise can lead to immediate and prolonged reduction in intraocular pressure. Intraocular pressure initially increases within five minutes of starting exercise, then gradually decreases, reaching its lowest level one hour following exercise. The drop in intraocular pressure is approximately 23% in normal individuals, while people with glaucoma usually experience a greater drop and longer duration of postexercise recovery.[26] Specifically, the drop in intraocular pressure for glaucoma patients after walking/jogging and running was 7.2% and 12.7%, respectively, more than the decrease experienced by those with normal eyes. Similarly, the mean duration of the pressure drop following running was approximately 84 minutes in those with glaucoma and 63 minutes in those with normal eyes. The lowering of intraocular pressure is independent of systemic blood pressure.

Exercise appears to be effective in lowering intraocular pressure in sedentary subjects engaging in moderate to heavy exercise but is somewhat less effective in physically fit subjects.[27] However, it must be pointed out that individuals who are more physically fit tend to have lower intraocular pressure. If one stops exercising, the effect wears off in three weeks. Although exercise may not be effective in lowering intraocular pressure in everyone, it can lead to significant improvements in many. One study found a postexercise intraocular pressure drop of at least 2 mm Hg in 34% of subjects; however, 57% had no change, while 9% had an elevation in pressure.[28]

. . . .

TREATMENT SUMMARY

Take general measures to improve overall health. In particular, engage in regular physical exercise and follow the guidelines in the chapter "A Health-Promoting Diet."

Nutritional Supplements

- A high-potency multiple vitamin and mineral formula as described in the chapter "Supplementary Measures"

- Key individual nutrients:
  ○ Vitamin C: 500 to 1,000 mg three times per day
  ○ Magnesium (bound to aspartate, citrate, fumarate, malate, or succinate): 200 to 300 mg three times per day
  ○ Chromium: 200 to 400 mcg per day
  ○ Zinc: 30 to 45 mg per day
  ○ Vitamin D$_3$: 2,000 to 4,000 IU per

day (ideally, measure blood levels and adjust dosage accordingly)

- Fish oils: 1,000 mg EPA + DHA per day
- One of the following:
  - Grape seed extract (>95% procyanidolic oligomers): 100 to 300 mg per day
  - Pine bark extract (>95% procyanidolic oligomers): 100 to 300 mg per day
  - Some other flavonoid-rich extract with a similar flavonoid content, super greens formula, or another plant-based antioxidant that can provide an oxygen radical absorption capacity (ORAC) of 3,000 to 6,000 units or more per day

Botanical Medicines

- For chronic glaucoma:
  - *Vaccinium myrtillus* (European bilberry) extract (25% anthocyanidin content): 160 to 240 mg per day
- For normotensive glaucoma:
  - Ginkgo biloba extract: 240 to 320 mg per day

Gout

· ·

- Acute onset of intense joint pain, typically involving the first joint of the big toe (about 50% of cases)

- Elevated serum uric acid level

- Periods without symptoms between acute attacks

- Identification of urate crystals in joint fluid

- Aggregated deposits of urate crystals in and around the joints of the extremities, but also in subcutaneous tissue, bone, cartilage, and other tissues

- Uric acid kidney stones

Gout is a common type of arthritis caused by an increased concentration of uric acid (the final breakdown product of the metabolism of purine, one of the units of DNA and RNA) in biological fluids. In gout, uric acid crystals (monosodium urate) are deposited in joints, tendons, kidneys, and other tissues, where they cause considerable inflammation and damage.[1,2] The uric acid deposits around the joints and tendons may lead to pain. Excessive uric acid deposits in the kidneys may result in kidney failure.

The first attack of gout is characterized by intense pain, usually involving only one joint. The first joint of the big toe is affected in nearly half of first attacks and is at some time involved in more than 90% of individuals with gout. If the attack progresses, fever and chills will appear. The first attacks usually occur at night and are usually preceded by a specific event, such as dietary excess, alcohol ingestion, trauma, certain drugs (mainly chemotherapy drugs, certain diuretics, and high doses of niacin), or surgery.

The classic description of gout was written by an English physician, Thomas Sydenham, who suffered from it in 1683.[1] Little has changed in the clinical picture of gout in more than 300 years. This is Sydenham's classic description:

> The victim goes to bed and sleeps in good health. About two o'clock in the morning he is awakened by a severe pain in the great toe; more rarely in the heel, ankle, or instep. The pain is like that of a dislocation, and yet parts feel as if cold water were poured over them. Then follows chills and shivers, and a little fever. The pain which at first was moderate, becomes more intense. With its intensity the chills and fever increase. After a time this comes to a height, accommodating itself to the bones and ligaments of the tarsus and metatarsus. Now it is a violent stretching and tearing of the ligaments, now it is a gnawing pain, and now a pressure and tightening. So exquisite and lively meanwhile is the feeling of the part affected, that it cannot bear the weight of bedclothes nor the jar of a person walking in the room. The night is passed in torture, sleeplessness, turning the part affected, and perpetual change of posture; the tossing about of the body being as incessant as the pain of the tortured joint, and being

worse as the fit comes on. Hence the vain effort by change of posture, both in the body and the limb affected, to obtain an abatement of pain.

Subsequent attacks are common, with the majority of gout patients having another attack within one year. However, nearly 7% never have a second attack. Chronic gout is extremely rare these days, owing to the advent of dietary therapy and drugs that lower uric acid levels. Some degree of kidney dysfunction occurs in almost 90% of subjects with gout as a result of uric acid deposits, and there is a higher risk of kidney stones.

Causes

Gout is divided into two major categories: primary and secondary. Primary gout accounts for about 90% of all cases, while secondary gout accounts for only 10%. The cause of primary gout is usually unknown. There are, however, several genetic defects in which the exact cause of the elevated uric acid is known.

The increased serum uric acid level observed in primary gout can be divided into three categories:

1. Increased synthesis of uric acid, found in a majority of gout patients
2. Reduced ability to excrete uric acid, found in about 30% of gout patients
3. Overproduction and underexcretion of uric acid, found in a small minority of gout patients

Although the exact metabolic defect is not known in the majority of cases, gout is one of the most controllable metabolic diseases.

Secondary gout refers to those cases in which the elevated uric acid level is a result of some other disorder, such as excessive breakdown of cells or some form of kidney disease. Diuretic therapy for high blood pressure and low-dose aspirin therapy are also important causes of secondary gout, since they cause decreased uric acid excretion.

Causes of Gout

- Increased purine intake
- Increased production of purines (primary causes):
  - Idiopathic (unknown causes)
  - Due to specific enzyme defects
- Increased production of purines (secondary to another factor)
- Increased turnover of purines due to:
  - Cancer
  - Chronic hemolytic anemia
  - Chemotherapy drugs
  - Psoriasis
- Increased synthesis of purines
- Increased breakdown of purines due to:
  - High fructose intake
  - Exercise
- Impaired kidney function:
  - Decreased kidney clearance of uric acid (primary)
  - Intrinsic kidney disease
  - Decreased kidney clearance of uric acid (secondary)
  - Functional impairment of kidney function
    - Drug-induced (e.g., thiazides, salicylates, etc.)
    - Increased lactic acid (e.g., lactic acidosis, alcoholism, toxemia of pregnancy, etc.)
    - Increased ketoacid levels (e.g., diabetic ketoacidosis)
    - Chronic lead intoxication

About 200 to 600 mg uric acid is excreted per day in the urine of an adult male, and another 100 to 300 mg is excreted in the bile and other gastrointestinal tract secretions. The dietary contribution to the level of uric acid in the blood is usually only 10 to 20% of the total, but purines and uric acid obtained through the diet can increase crystal formation in tissues nonetheless.

Uric acid is a highly insoluble molecule, and at a blood pH of 7.4 and normal body temperature, the serum (blood minus the blood cells) is saturated with uric acid at 6.4 to 7.0 mg/100 ml. Although higher concentrations do not necessarily result in the deposit of uric acid crystals in tissues (some unknown factor in serum appears to inhibit crystal precipitation), the chance of an acute attack of gout is greater than 90% when the level is above 9 mg/100 ml.

Lower body temperatures decrease the saturation point of uric acid, and this may explain why uric acid deposits tend to form in areas such as the top of the ear, where the temperature is lower than the average body temperature. Uric acid is even less soluble when the blood pH is below 6.0; this condition can lead to kidney stones.

Therapeutic Considerations

The current standard medical treatment of acute gout is administration of colchicine, an anti-inflammatory drug originally isolated from the plant *Colchicum autumnale* (autumn crocus, meadow saffron). Colchicine has no effect on uric acid levels; rather, it stops the inflammatory process by inhibiting neutrophil migration into areas of inflammation.

More than 75% of patients with gout show major improvement in symptoms within the first 12 hours after receiving colchicine. However, up to 80% of patients are unable to tolerate an optimal dose because of gastrointestinal side effects.

Colchicine may also cause bone marrow suppression, hair loss, liver damage, depression, seizures, respiratory depression, and even death. Other anti-inflammatory agents used in acute gout include various nonsteroidal anti-inflammatory drugs (NSAIDs) such as indomethacin, phenylbutazone, naproxen, and fenoprofen.

Once the acute episode has resolved, a number of measures are taken to reduce the likelihood of recurrence:

- Drugs such as allopurinol or febuxostat to keep uric acid levels within a normal range
- Controlled weight loss in obese individuals
- Avoidance of known precipitating factors such as heavy alcohol consumption or a diet rich in purines or refined carbohydrates
- Low doses of colchicine to prevent further acute attacks

Several dietary factors are known to lead to the development of gout or trigger an attack: alcohol, especially beer and hard liquor; high-purine foods (e.g., organ meats, meat, yeast, poultry); fats; refined carbohydrates, particularly high amounts of fructose; and overconsumption of calories. Individuals with gout are typically obese; prone to hypertension, metabolic syndrome,[3] and diabetes;[4] and at a greater risk for cardiovascular disease. Obesity is probably the most important factor. Thiazide and loop diuretics also are associated with a higher risk of incident gout and a higher rate of gout flares.[5]

The naturopathic approach to chronic gout focuses on dietary and herbal measures to keep uric acid levels within the normal range. The conventional medical treatment of gout often relies excessively on drugs that inhibit xanthine oxidase. The drug allopurinol, a structural isomer of hypoxanthine (a naturally occurring purine in the body), has been the mainstay treatment for decades. However, in February 2009 the FDA approved febuxostat (Uloric), another xanthine oxidase inhibitor, which is more effective at lowering and maintaining serum urate levels and is beginning to supplant allopurinol.[6] Agents that increase uric acid excretion (probenecid, sulfinpyrazone, and benzbromarone) are used as second-line therapy for patients with underexcretion of uric acid.

Lead Toxicity

A secondary type of gout, sometimes called saturnine gout, can result from lead toxicity. Historically, saturnine gout was caused by the consumption of alcoholic beverages stored in containers with lead in them. An unexpected and fairly common source of lead appears to be leaded crystal; port wine, for example, takes on lead when stored in a crystal decanter.[7] Lead concentration increases with storage time, reaching toxic levels after several months. Even a few minutes in a crystal glass results in a measurable increase in the level of lead in wine. While lead levels in the general population have decreased substantially since it was banned from gasoline, those working with aviation fuel are still exposed. The mechanism of action is related to a decrease in excretion of uric acid by the kidneys.

Dietary Considerations

The dietary treatment of gout involves the following guidelines:

- Decreasing purine intake
- Eliminating alcohol

- Achievement of ideal body weight
- Liberal consumption of complex carbohydrates
- Low fat intake
- Low protein intake
- Liberal fluid intake

Low-Purine Alkaline-Ash Diet

A low-purine diet has been the mainstay of the dietary therapy of gout for decades. Today, however, many physicians prefer to lower uric acid levels by prescribing potent drugs rather than subjecting the patient to the inconvenience and deprivation associated with a purine-free diet. However, dietary restriction of purines is still recommended to reduce metabolic stress. Foods with high purine levels should be entirely omitted. These include organ meats, yeast (brewer's and baker's), and smaller fish such as sardines, herring, and anchovies. Foods with moderate levels of purine should be curtailed as well. These include dried legumes, spinach, asparagus, fish, meat, poultry, shellfish, and mushrooms.

An alkaline-ash diet is recommended in the dietary treatment of gout because a more alkaline pH increases uric acid solubility. An alkaline-ash diet was shown to increase uric acid excretion from 302 mg per day at pH 5.9 to 413 mg per day at pH 6.5.[8] For information on the acid-alkaline effect of common foods, see Appendix C.

High-Purine Foods

- Anchovies
- Consommé
- Meat extracts
- Organ meats (brain, kidney, liver, sweetbreads)
- Roe (fish eggs)

- Sardines (and other small fish such as herring and mackerel)
- Yeast

Moderate-Purine Foods

- Asparagus
- Fish (larger species)
- Legumes
- Meat
- Mushrooms
- Peas (dried)
- Poultry
- Shellfish
- Spinach

Low-Purine Foods

- Eggs
- Fruit
- Grains
- Milk
- Pasta
- Nuts
- Olives

Alcohol

Alcohol consumption increases uric acid production by accelerating purine nucleotide degradation and reduces uric acid excretion by increasing lactate production, which impairs kidney function. The net effect is a significant increase in serum uric acid levels. This explains why alcohol consumption is often a precipitating factor in acute attacks of gout. In many individuals, eliminating alcohol is all that is necessary to reduce uric acid levels and prevent gout.

Excess Weight

Excess weight is associated with an increased incidence of gout. Weight reduction in obese individuals significantly reduces serum uric acid levels.[9] See the chapter "Obesity and Weight Management" for more information.

Carbohydrates, Fats, and Protein

Refined carbohydrates and saturated fats should be kept to a minimum, as the former increase uric acid production while the latter increase uric acid retention. In addition, one of the key dietary goals in the treatment of gout appears to be to enhance insulin sensitivity.[9]

Protein intake should not be excessive (i.e., more than 0.8 g/kg per day), as it has been shown that uric acid synthesis may be accelerated in both normal and gouty patients by a high protein intake.[5]

Fluid Intake

Liberal fluid intake keeps the urine dilute and promotes the excretion of uric acid. Furthermore, dilution of the urine reduces the risk of kidney stones.

Nutritional Supplements

Fish Oils

Fish oil supplementation may prove useful in the treatment of gout. The omega-3 fatty acids EPA and DHA limit the production of leukotrienes, which contribute to much of the inflammation and tissue damage observed in gout.

Folic Acid

Folic acid has been shown to inhibit xanthine oxidase, the enzyme responsible for producing uric acid.[10] Research has demonstrated that a derivative of folic acid is an even greater inhibitor of xanthine oxidase than allopurinol, suggesting that folic acid at pharmacological doses may be an effective treatment in gout.[11] Positive results in the treatment of gout have been reported, but the data are incomplete and uncontrolled.[12]

Quercetin

The bioflavonoid quercetin has demonstrated several effects in experimental studies that indicate its possible benefit to individuals with gout.[13–15] Quercetin may offer significant protection by inhibiting the following:

- Xanthine oxidase in a fashion similar to the drug allopurinol
- Leukotriene synthesis and release
- White blood cell accumulation and enzyme release

However, since the absorption of quercetin is quite poor, we recommend using the highly bioavailable enzymatically modified form of isoquercitrin (EMIQ) instead.

Vitamin C

Megadoses of vitamin C should be avoided by individuals with gout, as vitamin C may increase uric acid levels in a small number of individuals.[16]

Niacin

High doses of niacin (i.e., above 100 mg per day) are probably contraindicated in the treatment of gout, as niacin competes with uric acid for excretion.[17]

Botanical Medicines

Cherries and Other Dark Red and Blue Fruits

Consuming ½ lb fresh or canned cherries per day has been shown to be effective in lowering uric acid levels and preventing attacks of gout.[18] One study measured plasma uric acid and antioxidant and inflammatory markers in 10 healthy women who consumed 280 g cherries after an overnight fast.[19] Blood and urine samples were taken before the cherry dose and at 1.5, 3, and 5 hours afterward. Five hours after cherry consumption, plasma uric acid levels had decreased by an average of 30 mmol/l. This reduction correlated with increased urinary excretion of urate. Inflammatory markers (plasma C-reactive protein and nitric oxide concentrations) decreased slightly after the 1.5-hour mark.

Cherries, hawthorn berries, blueberries, and other dark red and blue fruits are rich sources of anthocyanidins and proanthocyanidins. These compounds are flavonoid molecules, which give these fruits their deep red-blue color and are remarkable in their ability to prevent collagen destruction. Anthocyanidins and other flavonoids affect collagen metabolism in many ways:

· ·

QUICK REVIEW

- **Gout is caused by uric acid crystals deposited in joints.**
- **Several dietary factors are known to be causes of gout: alcohol, high-purine foods, fats, and refined carbohydrates.**
- **Elimination of alcohol consumption reduces uric acid levels and prevents gouty arthritis in many individuals.**
- **Liberal fluid intake dilutes the urine and promotes the excretion of uric acid.**
- **Consuming ½ lb fresh or canned cherries per day has been found effective in lowering uric acid levels and preventing attacks of gout.**

- They have the unique ability to actually cross-link collagen fibers, resulting in reinforcement of the natural cross-linking of collagen that forms the collagen matrix of connective tissue.

- They prevent free radical damage through their potent antioxidant and free-radical-scavenging action.

- They inhibit enzymatic cleavage of collagen by enzymes secreted by leukocytes during inflammation.

- They prevent the release and synthesis of compounds that promote inflammation, such as histamine, serine proteases, prostaglandins, and leukotrienes.

Celery Seed Extract

The compound 3-n-butylphthalide (3nB) is unique to celery and is responsible for its characteristic flavor and odor. A celery seed extract standardized to contain 85% 3nB and other celery phthalides has shown benefit in the treatment of rheumatism—the general term used for arthritic and muscular aches and pain.[20,21] In studies that included gout sufferers, subjects had for approximately 10 years been experiencing lack of joint mobility and intermittent or continual pain, interfering with household duties, hobbies, and job-related activities. Subjects noted significant pain relief after three weeks of use, with an average 68% reduction in pain scores and some subjects experiencing complete relief from pain. Most subjects achieved maximum benefit after six weeks of use, although some did notice improvements the longer the extract was used. Celery seed extract appears to be particularly helpful for sufferers of gout, as 3nB lowers the production of uric acid by inhibiting the enzyme xanthine oxidase.[22]

TREATMENT SUMMARY

The naturopathic approach to the prevention and treatment of gout involves the following:

- **Dietary and herbal measures that maintain uric acid levels within the normal range**

- **Controlled weight loss in obese individuals**

- **Avoidance of known precipitating factors (such as heavy alcohol consumption and a high-purine diet)**

- **The use of nutritional substances to prevent further acute attacks**

- **The use of herbal and nutritional substances to inhibit the inflammatory process**

Diet

Follow the general guidelines given in the chapter "A Health-Promoting Diet." Eliminate alcohol intake, avoid high-purine foods, increase consumption of complex carbohydrates, decrease consumption of simple carbohydrates, maintain a low fat intake, optimize protein intake (under 0.8 g/kg per day), and consume liberal quantities of fluid.

In addition, liberal amounts (4 to 8 oz per day) of cherries, blueberries, and other anthocyanoside-rich red or blue berries should be consumed; their extracts can be substituted. See Appendix C, "Acid-Base Values of Selected Foods."

Nutritional Supplements

- A high-potency multiple vitamin and mineral formula as described in the chapter "Supplementary Measures"
- Vitamin D_3: 2,000 to 4,000 IU per day (ideally, measure blood levels and adjust dosage accordingly)
- Fish oils: 1,000 mg EPA + DHA per day
- One of the following:
  - Cherry fruit extract (10:1): 500 to 1,000 mg three times per day
  - Grape seed extract (>95% procyanidolic oligomers): 100 to 300 mg per day
  - Pine bark extract (>95% procyanidolic oligomers): 100 to 300 mg per day
  - Enzymatically modified isoquercitrin (EMIQ): 100 mg twice per day

Botanical Medicines

- Celery seed extract (85% 3nB content): 75 mg two to three times per day

Hair Loss in Women

- Hair loss of any type: diffuse or focal, chronic or acute

Many women experience excessive hair loss. In fact, it is one of the most common complaints from female patients. In most cases the hair loss is not severe; rather, the patient perceives that hair loss is occurring at an increasing rate. Unfortunately, these complaints are often dismissed by many physicians. Hair loss is difficult to quantify, and it is certainly not a life-threatening disorder. Nonetheless, the complaint should not be dismissed.

Physiology of the Hair Cycle

The human scalp has between 100,000 and 350,000 hair follicles, which undergo cyclical phases of growth and rest. During the anagen phase, the hair is actively growing. As the hair matures, it enters into a resting (telogen) phase. Then the hair bulb migrates outward and eventually is sloughed off. It is during this migratory phase that the stage is set for new hair to come in after the original hair is lost. Age, various diseases, and a wide variety of nutritional and hormonal factors influence the duration of the hair cycle.

Generally speaking, hair loss is a normal part of aging. By the age of 40 or so, the rate of hair growth slows down. New hairs are not replaced as quickly as old ones are lost.

The hair pull test can help determine the relative formation of new hair. It involves taking a few strands between the thumb and forefinger and pulling on them gently. Hairs in the anagen phase should remain rooted in place, while hairs in the telogen phase should come out easily. Knowing approximately how many hairs were pulled, and the number that came out, indicates the percentage of hair follicles in a telogen state. For example, if 20 hairs were pulled and 2 came out, then the frequency of telogen hair follicles is 10%. As a very rough guide, a 10% telogen frequency is excellent, up to 25% is typical, and over 35% is problematic.

Types of Hair Loss

Hair loss—the medical term is *alopecia*—can be broadly divided into two types: focal (small patches) or diffuse (all over the head). Diffuse hair loss is most often due to metabolic or hormonal stress or to medications. It can vary from mild thinning to complete hair loss (e.g., as seen with chemotherapy drugs). Generally, recovery occurs when precipitating factors are dealt with. Women can also experience either male- or female-pattern hair loss. Focal hair loss is most often secondary to an underlying disorder, and it may be of two types, nonscarring or scarring alopecia. Nonscarring focal alopecia is usually caused by tinea capitis (a fungal infection) or alopecia areata (which is autoimmune-

Types of Hair Loss	
TYPE OF HAIR LOSS	**DISTINGUISHING CHARACTERISTICS**
Diffuse	
Female-pattern hair loss	Presents with hair thinning; frontal hairline intact; negative pull test
Male-pattern hair loss	Presents with hair thinning; loss of frontal hair; negative pull test
Diffuse alopecia areata	Distribution more patchy; positive pull test
Alopecia totalis or universalis	Total hair loss on the scalp and/or body
Telogen effluvium	Sudden hair loss of 30 to 50% three months after precipitating event; positive pull test
Anagen effluvium	Sudden hair loss of up to 90% two weeks following chemotherapy
Focal	
Nonscarring	
Alopecia areata	Normal scalp with surrounding exclamation-point- shaped hairs on microscopic examination
Tinea capitis	Scaly scalp with fungus visible on potassium hydroxide examination
Traction alopecia	Patchy; related to hair-styling practices; may have some scarring
Trichotillomania	Patchy; related to pulling of hair; may be some scarring; may have associated psychological disturbance
Scarring	
Scarring (cicatricial)	Scarring and atrophy of scalp (e.g., discoid lupus erythematosus)

related), although there are other causes. Scarring alopecia is rare and has a number of causes, but the most common is lupus, an autoimmune disorder.[1]

Causes of Hair Loss in Women and Therapeutic Considerations

Female-Pattern Hair Loss

Women can suffer from hormone-related hair loss just like men.[1–4] Female-pattern hair loss, however, is more diffuse than characteristic male-pattern baldness.[1,4] It is a relatively common condition affecting approximately 30% of women before the age of 50. Al-though genetic factors are clearly significant, testosterone excess, insulin resistance, poly-cystic ovarian syndrome, and low antioxidant status are also associated with female-pattern hair loss.[2–8] Three recommendations that may help slow down this genetically predisposed process are: (1) improve blood sugar regula-tion through diet, lifestyle measures, and supplements; (2) increase antioxidant intake; and (3) consider saw palmetto extract.

Free radical damage has been shown to play a central role (along with testosterone) in male-pattern baldness. Higher levels of these damaging compounds are found in the hair follicles in men (and presumably women) with male-pattern hair loss.[5] This appears owing to lower levels of glutathione. The use of glutathione-sparing antioxidants such as vitamin C, N-acetylcysteine, alpha-lipoic acid, and flavonoids may help slow down the process.

The potent androgen dihydrotestosterone (DHT) is formed from testosterone by the action of the enzyme 5-alpha-reductase. The activity of this enzyme is increased in both male- and female-pattern hair loss.[6] Saw palmetto extract can inhibit the formation and transport of DHT. This is the same mechanism as that of the drug finasteride (Propecia), which is often used in female-pattern hair loss.[9] The dosage for saw palmetto extract standardized to contain 85 to 95% fatty acids and sterols is 320 mg per day.

Drug-Induced Hair Loss

A long list of drugs can cause hair loss, but they are not always the sole cause of hair loss in a woman who is taking one of them. Of course, some drugs, most notably chemotherapy agents such as fluorouracil, are obviously the cause because they are such powerful inhibitors of hair growth. When medically appropriate, natural alternatives to suspected culprits of hair loss should be employed.

Nutritional Deficiencies

A deficiency of any number of nutrients can lead to significant hair loss. Zinc, vitamin A, essential fatty acids, and iron are the most important.

If the fingernails have horizontal white lines, these may indicate poor wound healing of the nail bed even with the most minor trauma, which may be a sign of low zinc levels. If the backs of the arms are bumpy and rough, that may represent hyperkeratosis, a common sign of vitamin A deficiency. If the elbows are very dry and cracked, the condition may be due to essential fatty acid deficiency.

For evaluating iron status, a blood test for serum ferritin is recommended. If the serum ferritin is less than 30 mg/l, iron intake must be increased via diet and supplementation. When serum ferritin levels fall below this level, hair growth and regeneration are impaired, as the body seeks to conserve iron.[10] There is a very strong association between low body iron stores and diffuse hair loss in women.[11,12] For more information, see the chapter "Anemia."

Classes of Drugs That Can Cause Hair Loss	
CLASS	**EXAMPLES**
Antibiotics	Gentamycin, chloramphenicol
Anticoagulants	Warfarin, heparin
Antidepressants	Fluoxetine, desipramine, lithium
Antiepileptics	Valproic acid, phenytoin
Cardiovascular drugs	Angiotensin-converting enzyme inhibitors, beta-blockers
Chemotherapy drugs	Adriamycin, vincristine, etoposide
Endocrine drugs	Bromocriptine, clomiphene, danazol
Gout medications	Colchicine, allopurinol
Lipid-lowering drugs	Gemfibrozil, fenofibrate
Nonsteroidal anti-inflammatory drugs	Ibuprofen, indomethacin, naproxen
Ulcer medications	Cimetidine, ranitidine

Typically, women with noticeable generalized hair loss suffer from apparent deficiencies of all of these nutrients. Treatment of hair loss due to nutritional deficiency is straightforward—increase dietary intake of these nutrients and supplement appropriately. One caveat is that many of these women may not be secreting enough stomach acid. In these cases, hydrochloric acid supplementation at meals may be all that is necessary. (See the chapter "Digestion and Elimination" for more information.) A general recommendation for women with hair loss related to nutritional status is to take a high-potency multivitamin and mineral formula that contains iron, along with 1 tbsp flaxseed oil per day.

Another general recommendation for hair loss is to take a special form of silicon, an essential trace element required for the normal growth and development of hair. Studies show that choline-stabilized orthosilicic acid (ch-OSA or BioSil), a highly bioavailable and stabilized form of silicon, increases levels of hydroxyproline, the key amino acid required for the production of collagen and elastin—compounds that are essential to the strength, thickness, and elasticity of hair. In one double-blind study, 48 women with fine hair were given 10 mg silicon as ch-OSA per day for nine months. Oral intake of Ch-OSA had a positive effect on tensile strength, including elasticity and break load, and resulted in thicker hair.[13]

Hypothyroidism

It is a well-known fact that hair loss is one of the cardinal signs of hypothyroidism. The prevalence of hypothyroidism in American women is estimated to be as high as 20%. For more information, see the chapter "Hypothyroidism."

Antigliadin Antibodies

The protein gluten and its polypeptide derivative gliadin are found primarily in wheat, barley, and rye. It appears that antibodies to gliadin can lead to cross-reacting anti-

QUICK REVIEW

- **Although some hair loss is a natural part of the aging process, excessive or accelerated hair loss should be investigated and treated appropriately.**
- **Hair loss can be broadly divided into two types: focal (small patches) or diffuse (all over the head).**
- **Five common causes of hair loss in women are female-pattern hair loss, drugs, nutritional deficiencies, hypothyroidism, and the presence of antigliadin antibodies.**
- **Deficiencies of zinc, vitamin A, essential fatty acids, and iron are the most important nutrition-related causes of hair loss in women.**
- **Oral intake of a special preparation of silicon had a positive effect on tensile strength including elasticity and break load and resulted in thicker hair.**
- **Antibodies to gliadin can lead to cross-reacting antibodies that attack the hair follicles.**

bodies that attack the hair follicles, leading to alopecia areata—an autoimmune disease characterized by areas of virtually complete hair loss.[14]

Celiac disease is characterized by malabsorption and an abnormal small intestine structure that reverts to normal on removal of dietary gluten. Evidence is growing that many people with gluten intolerance do not have overt gastrointestinal symptoms. Instead, they may demonstrate gluten intolerance in less obvious ways, including hair loss. Rather than testing for antigliadin antibodies in patients with general hair loss or alopecia areata, the test for human antitissue transglutaminase antibodies (IgA anti-tTG) is recommended, as it has a greater sensitivity compared with antigliadin antibodies (see the chapter "Celiac Disease"). This recommendation is especially important if there are any gastrointestinal symptoms that might indicate celiac disease.

Key Diagnostic Features of Celiac Disease

- Bulky, pale, frothy, foul-smelling, greasy stools with increased fecal fat
- Weight loss and signs of multivitamin and mineral deficiencies
- Increased levels of serum gliadin antibodies
- Diagnosis can be confirmed by biopsy of the small intestine

....

TREATMENT SUMMARY

Hair loss in a woman should not be dismissed, and a thorough clinical evaluation can be very valuable. Clinical studies have investigated the psychological impact of hair loss in women and found that is a significant source of anxiety, fear, and depression.[1,4]

Diet

- **Follow the recommendations in the chapter "A Health-Promoting Diet"**
- **Rule out gluten sensitivity; see the chapter "Celiac Disease"**

Nutritional Supplements

- **Follow the general recommendations in the chapter "Supplementary Measures"**
- **If serum ferritin levels are below 30 mg/l, take iron bound to either pyrophosphate, succinate, glycinate, or fumarate, at a dosage of 30 mg twice per day between meals (if this recommendation results in abdominal discomfort, take 30 mg with meals three times per day).**
- **Choline-stabilized orthosilicic acid (ch-OSA or BioSil): 10 mg per day**

Hay Fever

∙∙

- Watery nasal discharge, sneezing, itchy eyes and nose
- Usually associated with a particular season

Hay fever (also known as allergic rhinitis and pollinosis) is an allergic inflammation of the nasal airways and eyes. It occurs when an allergen, such as pollen or dust, is inhaled by an individual with a sensitized immune system. In sensitized people the allergen triggers the production of the allergic antibody immunoglobulin E (IgE), which binds to specialized white blood cells known as mast cells and basophils, causing them to release histamine and other mediators of the allergic reaction. These chemicals can cause itching, swelling, and mucus production. Symptoms vary in severity between individuals. Some may have symptoms limited to red, itchy eyes, while extremely sensitive individuals can experience hives or other rashes along with the typical hay fever symptoms. About 25% of the adult U.S. population will experience hay fever symptoms each year.

Causes

In the United States, allergy to ragweed pollen accounts for about 75% of cases of hay fever. Other significant pollens inducing hay fever include various grass and tree pollens. In northern latitudes in the United States birch is considered to be the most important allergenic tree pollen, with an estimated 15 to 20% of hay fever sufferers sensitive to birch pollen. If the hay fever develops in the spring, it is usually due to tree pollens. If it develops in the summer, grass and weed pollens are usually the culprits. Hay fever symptoms that persist year-round (perennial allergic rhinitis) may be due not to pollen but rather to some other allergen, such as a food or mold.

The reason ragweed is a major cause of hay fever is that it produces a huge amount of pollen. A single ragweed plant can produce up to 1 billion pollen grains and each grain can travel more than 100 miles from its source. Ragweed allergy generally surfaces between August and October in many parts of the country.

Allergy testing may identify specific allergens. Skin testing is the most common method of allergy testing. This may include intradermal, scratch, patch, or other tests. An alternative to skin testing is the RAST blood test.

Therapeutic Considerations

The first step in the natural approach to hay fever is reducing exposure.

- Track the pollen count in your area and try to stay indoors when pollen counts are highest.
- At home and in the car, keep the windows closed and the air conditioner on. Air con-

ditioners filter the air as well as cool it. Just make sure to change or clean the filters every three months or so.

- Shower before bed to remove pollen, especially from your face and hair.
- Try nasal irrigation. Get a neti pot and wash nasal passages with a saline solution twice per day.
- Equip your home with HEPA filters, which can be attached to central heating and air-conditioning systems.

If you suffer from perennial hay fever, removing dogs and cats and any surfaces where allergens can collect (carpets, rugs, upholstered furniture) is ideal. If this can't be done entirely, make sure that the bedroom is as allergy-proof as possible. Encase the mattress in allergen-proof plastic; wash sheets, blankets, pillowcases, and mattress pads every week in hot water with additive- and fragrance-free detergent; consider using bedding material made with Ventflex, a special hypoallergenic synthetic material; and install an air purifier. Search the house for areas of constant moisture. Such moisture can result in the growth of a black mold that is highly sensitizing to some people.

Immunotherapy

A popular treatment for hay fever is immunotherapy. In the classic form of this therapy the patient receives a series of injections of the allergy-causing agent into the skin (subcutaneous immunotherapy) until the body no longer mounts an immune response. The injections are usually given for several months before the effectiveness of the treatment can be determined. Typically, at the end of three years, one-third of patients will be cured of their allergies, one-third will have a significant reduction in symptoms, and one-third

will show little or no benefit. With subcutaneous immunotherapy there is a small but definite risk of inducing a systemic allergic reaction. This reaction occurs in less than 0.1% of those treated (1 in 1,000), but it may be life-threatening.

In recent years, sublingual (under the tongue) immunotherapy has shown efficacy at least on a par with allergy shots. Drops of liquid containing minute quantities of the offending pollen(s) are placed under the tongue. Sublingual immunotherapy can be more convenient than traditional subcutaneous immunotherapy—there is no need to come in for shots—and it takes less time. Permanent results are often seen within weeks or months.[1,2] We recommend physician supervision with the initial use of sublingual immunotherapy; although it is much safer than subcutaneous immunotherapy, allergic reactions may still occur, and though they are usually restricted to the upper airway and gastrointestinal tract, rare anaphylactic episodes (but no deaths) have been reported.[1,2]

Quercetin

Quercetin consistently demonstrates the greatest activity among the flavonoids studied in experimental models, particularly in test tube studies. In these studies, quercetin has been shown to exert significant antiallergy effects. In particular, it prevents the release of histamine from mast cells and basophils. Unfortunately, regular quercetin is not very well absorbed.[3,4] Recently, a highly bioavailable enzymatically modified form of isoquercitrin (EMIQ) has been developed. This form has shown significant effects in improving some of symptoms of hay fever in double-blind clinical studies. In one of these studies, 20 subjects with hay fever took two capsules per day of 100 mg EMIQ or a placebo for eight weeks during the pollen season.[5] During the entire study period, total ocular score and ocular itching score were significantly lower for the EMIQ group than for the placebo group. In another study, 24 subjects with hay fever took 100 mg EMIQ or a placebo for eight weeks, starting four weeks prior to the onset of pollen release.[6] During the entire study period, ocular symptom scores for the EMIQ group were significantly lower than those of the placebo group. When limited to the pollen release period, ocular symptom scores and ocular congestion scores for the EMIQ group were significantly lower than those for the placebo group, while other scores for the EMIQ group, such as ocular itching scores, lacrimation scores, and ocular congestion scores, all tended to be lower. However, no significant differences were found in nasal symptoms between the two groups. These results indicate that EMIQ is useful in reducing ocular symptoms of hay fever, especially ocular congestion.

Apple Polyphenols

Two double-blind studies showed apple polyphenols to reduce hay fever symptoms. The first study was conducted on patients with allergy to cedar pollen.[7] The results showed that the sneezing score was significantly lower for the AP group than for the placebo group during the early and main periods of pollen dispersion. The second study was of patients with persistent allergic rhinitis due to house dust mites.[8] Patients were treated with a low dose of apple polyphenols (50 mg per day), or with a high dose of apple polyphenols (250 mg per day); controls received none. Significant improvements were observed in sneezing attacks and nasal discharge in the high-dose group and in sneezing attacks in the low-dose group. There was also a significant improvement observed in swelling of the nasal passages in the treated groups. Similar results may be achieved with other polyphenol-rich extracts such as grape seed, pine bark, or green tea extract.

- -

QUICK REVIEW

- **Hay fever (seasonal allergic rhinitis) is an allergic reaction of the nasal passages and airways to windborne pollens that shares many features with asthma.**
- **In the United States allergy to ragweed pollen accounts for about 75% of the cases of hay fever.**
- **The first step in the natural approach to hay fever is to reduce exposure.**
- **In recent years, sublingual immuno-** **therapy has shown efficacy at least on a par with allergy shots.**
- **A highly bioavailable enzymatically modified form of isoquercitrin (EMIQ) has shown significant effects in improving some of symptoms of hay fever in double-blind clinical studies.**
- **Two double-blind studies showed apple polyphenols to reduce hay fever symptoms.**

TREATMENT SUMMARY

If a specific allergen can be identified, immunotherapy (preferably sublingual) may offer the best long-term solution. Otherwise, allergen avoidance and supporting the body's antiallergy mechanisms appear to offer some benefit.

Diet

Eliminate all food allergens and food additives to reduce the allergic threshold. If you have multiple food allergies, utilize a four-day rotation diet, as described in the chapter "Food Allergy." Otherwise, follow the general guidelines detailed in the chapter "A Health-Promoting Diet."

Nutritional Supplements

- A high-potency multiple vitamin and mineral formula as described in the chapter "Supplementary Measures"

- Vitamin D_3: 2,000 to 4,000 IU per day (ideally, measure blood levels and adjust dosage accordingly)
- Fish oils: 1,000 mg EPA + DHA per day
- EMIQ: 100 mg twice per day
- One of the following:
  - Apple polyphenols extract: 100 to 250 mg twice per day
  - Grape seed or pine bark extract (>95% procyanidolic oligomers): 150 to 300 mg per day
  - Green tea extract (90% polyphenols): 150 to 300 mg per day

Headache, Nonmigraine Tension Type

- Gradual onset of a mild, steady, or dull aching in the head
  - Pain often described as vise-like squeezing or heavy pressure around head
  - Constant headache (does not throb)

Although a headache may be associated with a serious medical condition, most headaches are not serious. Headaches can be caused by a wide variety of factors, but the overwhelming majority that require medical attention are either tension or migraine headaches. A quick way to differentiate between the two is the nature of the pain. Tension headaches usually have a steady, constant, dull pain that starts at the back of the head or in the forehead and spreads over the entire head, giving the sensation of pressure or a feeling that a vise grip has been applied to the skull. In contrast, migraine headaches are vascular headaches characterized by a throbbing or pounding sharp pain. For more information on migraines, see the chapter "Migraine Headache."

Causes

A tension headache is usually caused by tightening in the muscles of the face, neck, or scalp as a result of stress or poor posture. The other most important causes are drug reactions and magnesium insufficiency. The tightening of the muscles results in pinching of the nerve or its blood supply, which results in the sensation of pain and pressure. Relaxation of the muscles usually brings about immediate relief. Often the headache can be worsened (or improved) by applying hand pressure to *trigger points* on neck muscles. A trigger point is the central area of tension in the muscle. A tension headache only rarely mimics other types of headaches of a more serious nature, such as those associated with a stroke or brain tumor. Consult a physician immediately if a headache feels different from a tension headache or migraine, or if the headache is unrelenting.

Therapeutic Considerations

Modern drug treatment of headache, whether migraine or tension, is ultimately doomed because it fails to address the underlying cause and as a result produces significant risk for side effects. Rather than focusing on identifying and eliminating the precipitating factor, the goal with headache medications is simply to provide symptomatic relief. Particularly interesting are several clinical studies estimating that approximately 70% of patients with chronic headaches suffer from drug-induced headaches, a result of the medications they are taking to suppress the symptoms of headache. In other words, the headache medications are giving them headaches, and if they quit taking the drugs their headaches go away. In one study of 200 patients suffering from analgesic rebound headache, discontinuation of these medications resulted in a 52% improvement in the total headache index. Specific improvements occurred in headache frequency and severity, general well-being, and sleep patterns, and there were also reductions in irritability, depression, and lethargy.[1]

Tension headaches have been shown to respond to a number of natural therapies. Particularly helpful are physical treatments such as massage, chiropractic, and other forms of bodywork (discussed later in this chapter). *Bodywork* is the term often used to describe healing techniques that work with the structure of the body. Most of these therapies involve hands-on work, such as massage. Virtually all bodywork techniques may be helpful in the treatment of both acute and chronic tension headaches. However, rather than simply getting a massage whenever a headache appears, we recommend seeking out physical therapies that teach people to become aware of body tension and posture.

Chiropractic care can be quite helpful when misalignment of the spine creates muscular tension in the neck. In 1996, the RAND Corporation analyzed all of the scientific evidence from 1966 to 1996 on chiropractic treatment of tension headaches.[2] Their conclusion was that chiropractic care probably provides at least short-term benefits for some patients with neck pain and headaches. A follow-up analysis provided additional support for the value of chiropractic care.[3] Our feeling is that it is definitely worth a try. However, if you do not get relief within a few sessions, either this is not what you

need or you should find another practitioner. We also do not agree with some chiropractors' recommendation that treatments be continued indefinitely. The best chiropractors not only adjust your neck or other areas of the spine needing attention but also provide you with postural and muscle exercises to correct the causes of the underlying imbalance.

An alternative to chiropractic care involves getting a referral to a conventional physical therapist from your primary care doctor. Clinical studies have shown that conventional physical therapy (consisting of education for posture at home and in the workplace, home exercise, massage, and stretching of the cervical spine muscles) can reduce the frequency and severity of tension headaches.[4,5] For example, in one study 20 patients with a diagnosis of tension headache were treated for pain relief in a physical therapy clinic once a week for six weeks.[4] The previous three-week period of no treatment served as a control period during which patients recorded their headache frequency, duration, and intensity using a numeric pain scale. Results indicated that the frequency of headaches and activity scores were significantly improved over the course of treatment. These benefits were maintained after 12 months. Given the problems associated with chronic use of aspirin and other pain relievers, this study provides evidence that addressing the cause rather than suppressing symptoms is clearly the better approach.

The next goal is to learn how to relax the tight muscles by alternating tension and then relaxation in the muscle. See the exercise for progressive relaxation in the chapter "Stress Management." Learning how to relax has been shown in clinical studies to provide exceptional benefits without side effects. One of the more interesting studies compared the effectiveness of school-based, nurse-administered relaxation training vs.

no treatment for chronic tension headache in children (10 to 15 years old).[6,7] After six weeks and at the six-month follow-up, 69% and 73%, respectively, of the students who received relaxation training had achieved at least a 50% reduction in headaches as compared with 8% and 27%, respectively, of those in the control group. So teaching children with chronic tension headaches how to relax can be quite effective, and it is without side effects. What we really like about this therapy is that the children get a better message: rather than seeking relief from a drug, they learn how to control the headache themselves.

If these treatments are not effective, the next step is to follow the recommendations given in the chapter "Migraine Headache." Those recommendations are also appropriate in the treatment of chronic tension headaches, which share the following features with migraine headaches:

- Both can be the result of chronic use of aspirin and other pain relievers.

- Tension and migraine headaches are often triggered by food allergies.
- Magnesium supplementation can help both.
- 5-hydroxytryptophan (5-HTP) has been shown to help both.

Finally, occasional use of aspirin (or willow bark extracts standardized for salicin, the natural form of aspirin) or acetaminophen is safe and effective in the treatment of an acute headache. The key is not to rely too heavily on these medications. After all, a headache is not caused by a lack of aspirin or acetaminophen. But chronic headaches may be due to low magnesium. A study in Italy showed just how effective magnesium supplementation can be for children with chronic or episodic tension-type headaches.[8,9] Supplementation with 180 mg magnesium twice per day produced a symptom reduction of 87.5%, with 100% of the patients experiencing at least a 50% reduction in symptoms. Analgesic consumption also decreased a remarkable 65.4%.

QUICK REVIEW

- **A tension headache is usually caused by tightening in the muscles of the face, neck, or scalp as a result of stress or poor posture.**
- **The first therapeutic goal in treating the chronic tension headache sufferer is to address any structural problem that may trigger a tension headache.**
- **Regularly taking drugs for acute headaches often causes chronic headaches.**

- **Learning how to relax and defuse tension goes a long way in the treatment and prevention of tension headache.**
- **Migraine and tension headaches share many features.**
- **Magnesium insufficiency is common in tension headaches.**

TREATMENT SUMMARY

The primary therapy should be addressing the factors that trigger tension in the neck muscles. Since the neck is an area of the body that often holds tension produced by psychological stress, it is especially important to learn to relax neck muscles through techniques such as progressive relaxation. In addition, it is important to address any structural factors that may be triggering tension headaches. Chiropractic care, physical therapy, and bodywork are important treatments.

Nutritional Supplements

- A high-potency multiple vitamin and mineral formula as described in the chapter "Supplementary Measures"
- Key individual nutrients:
  - Vitamin B$_6$: 25 to 50 mg three times per day
  - Magnesium (bound to aspartate, citrate, fumarate, malate, or succinate): 150 to 250 mg two to three times per day
  - Vitamin D$_3$: 2,000 to 4,000 IU per day (ideally, measure blood levels and adjust dosage accordingly)
- Fish oils: 1,000 mg EPA + DHA per day
- One of the following:
  - Grape seed extract (>95% procyanidolic oligomers): 100 to 300 mg per day
  - Pine bark extract (>95% procyanidolic oligomers): 100 to 300 mg per day
  - Some other flavonoid-rich extract with a similar flavonoid content, super greens formula, or another plant-based antioxidant that can provide an oxygen radical absorption capacity (ORAC) of 3,000 to 6,000 units or more per day

Heart Arrhythmias

- Shortness of breath, especially with exertion
- Fatigue
- Sensation of palpitations
- Signs of reduced blood flow (blue extremities, swelling of the ankles)
- Abnormal finding with electrocardiograph and/or echocardiograph evaluation

Arrhythmia is a disturbance in the rhythm of the heartbeat. Some arrhythmias are very mild and nothing to worry about (such as mild atrial fibrillation and premature ventricular contractions); others are potentially life-threatening (ventricular tachycardia and severe ventricular arrhythmias). While atrial fibrillation may not be immediately life-threatening, over time it can result in congestive heart failure and increases the risk of stroke.

Each heartbeat originates as an electrical impulse from a small area of tissue in the right atrium of the heart called the sinus node (or sinoatrial node, or SA node). The impulse initially causes both atria to contract, then activates the atrioventricular (AV) node, which is normally the only electrical connection between the atria and the ventricles (main pumping chambers). The impulse then spreads through both ventricles, causing a synchronized contraction of the heart muscle.

In adults the normal resting heart rate ranges from 60 to 80 beats per minute. A slow rhythm (less than 60 beats per minute) is called bradycardia. It may be caused by a slowed signal from the sinus node (sinus bradycardia), by a pause in the normal activity of the sinus node (sinus arrest), or by blocking of the electrical impulse on its way from the atria to the ventricles (AV block or heart block). Bradycardias may also be present in the normally functioning heart of endurance athletes or other well-conditioned people.

In adults and children over 15, a resting heart rate faster than 100 beats per minute is labeled tachycardia. Tachycardia may result in palpitations—an awareness of one's heartbeat. Not always is tachycardia an arrhythmia. Increased heart rate is a normal response to physical exercise or emotional stress.

One of the most common arrhythmias is atrial fibrillation, a minor arrhythmia in which the atria (the upper chambers of the heart) beat irregularly and very rapidly (up to 300 to 500 beats per minute). An atrial fibrillation is usually minor because the atrium's job is simply to fill the ventricle—the lower chamber. Atrial fibrillation is more common with age and is found in about 8% of those over the age of 80. Premature ventricular contractures simply reflect an occasional irregular heartbeat; the heartbeat itself is normal. In contrast, in ventricular tachycardia the beat is too fast (120 to 200 per minute). Other ventricular arrhythmias tend to be even more serious, such as ventricular fibrillation—rapid, uncontrolled, and ineffective contractions of the heart.

Diagnostic Considerations

If you feel that your heartbeat is irregular, you should see your doctor for evaluation. Your doctor will check you for heart disease, which may require a complete physical exam to look for signs of poor blood flow, an electrocardiogram to assesses the electrical function of the heart, and an echocardiogram to assess the mechanical function of the heart and determine the heart's shape and size.

Minor arrhythmias, like other types of heart diseases, are most effectively treated with natural measures in the early stages. Hence, early diagnosis and prevention by addressing causative factors is imperative. The first symptom of significant heart disease of any type is usually shortness of breath. A chronic cough may also be the first presenting symptom.

Therapeutic Considerations

The therapeutic goals in the treatment of arrhythmias are quite similar to those given in the chapter "Angina": improve energy metabolism within the heart and increase the blood supply to the heart. Not surprisingly, the natural measures used to achieve these goals are also similar to those used in the treatment of angina. In addition, natural therapies can ensure normal nerve functioning.

Diet

The guidelines given in the chapter "A Health-Promoting Diet" are appropriate here. In addition, consult the chapter "Heart and Cardiovascular Health." Many people with arrhythmias, mitral valve prolapse, or cardiomyopathy may be on the drug warfarin (Coumadin). This drug is used to prevent the formation of blood clots. It works by blocking the action of vitamin K. Since green leafy vegetables and green teas contain high levels of vitamin K, you should avoid increasing your intake of these foods while taking Coumadin. You can eat the same levels you're accustomed to—just don't increase your consumption. Your physician will monitor your blood using a test known as the international normalized ratio (INR) and will adjust your dose of Coumadin as needed.

In addition to high-vitamin-K foods, other natural remedies may interact with warfarin. For example, coenzyme Q_{10} and Saint-John's-wort (*Hypericum perforatum*) may reduce the efficacy of Coumadin, while proteolytic enzymes and several herbs, including Chinese ginseng (*Panax ginseng*), devil's claw (*Harpagophytum procumbens*), and dong quai (*Angelica sinensis*), can increase its effects. It's likely that you can continue using these products, but don't change the dosage from what your body is accustomed to. INR values must be monitored appropriately.

Garlic (*Allium sativum*) and ginkgo (*Ginkgo biloba*) extracts may reduce the ability of platelets to stick together, increasing the likelihood of bleeding. However, neither appears to interact directly with Coumadin. We generally tell people taking Coumadin to avoid these products at higher dosages (more than the equivalent of one clove of garlic per day or more than 240 mg per day of ginkgo extract) but not to worry if they are just on the typical support dose.

Iron, magnesium, and zinc may bind with Coumadin, potentially decreasing its absorption and activity. Take Coumadin at least two hours before or after any product that contains iron, magnesium, or zinc.

Nutritional Supplements

Magnesium

The level of magnesium in the blood correlates with the ability of the heart muscle to manufacture enough energy to beat properly. Also, low levels of magnesium can make the nerves overly sensitive. Not surprisingly, many disorders of heart rhythm are related to an insufficient level of magnesium in the heart muscle. Magnesium was first shown to be of value in the treatment of cardiac arrhythmias in 1935. More than 75 years later, there are now many clinical studies that show magnesium supplementation to be of benefit in treating many types of arrhythmias, including atrial fibrillation, ventricular premature contractions, ventricular tachycardia, and severe ventricular arrhythmias.[1–3] The current understanding is that magnesium depletion within the heart muscle leads to potassium depletion as well. Given the importance of these two electrolytes for proper nerve and muscle firing, it is little wonder that low levels of these substances can produce arrhythmias.

According to the results from one double-blind, placebo-controlled study, magnesium supplementation may offer significant benefit in the treatment of new-onset atrial fibrillation.[4] The drug of choice for this condition is digoxin; unfortunately, it has been shown to offer no better results than a placebo for facilitating proper heart rhythm. Because of the benefits noted in several studies of patients with atrial fibrillation who were taking magnesium, researchers decided to conduct a study to determine if magnesium and digoxin were better than digoxin alone in controlling ventricular response.

Eighteen people with atrial fibrillation of less than seven days' duration received either digoxin plus a placebo or digoxin plus magnesium, both intravenously. Those who received magnesium were given 20% of a magnesium solution during the initial 15 minutes, with the rest infused over the next six hours. The benefit of magnesium was obvious within the first 15 minutes, as heart rate decreased immediately from an average of 130 to 120 beats per minute. After 24 hours, the group that received the magnesium had an average heart rate of roughly 80, while the group that received only digoxin had an average heart rate of 105. In the magnesium group, 6 of 10 patients (60%) converted to normal rhythm, whereas just 3 of 8 in the digoxin-only group (37.5%) converted.

The recommended intake for oral magnesium in arrhythmia appears to be approximately 6 to 10 mg/kg per day. Be sure to use a form that is easily absorbed, such as citrate, as other forms can cause diarrhea at these dosages.

Coenzyme Q_{10} (CoQ_{10})

Coenzyme Q_{10} plays a critical role in the cellular production of energy. As the heart is among the most metabolically active tissues in the body, a CoQ_{10} deficiency can lead to serious problems there. A good analogy is that the role of CoQ_{10} is similar to the role of a spark plug in a car engine. Just as the car cannot function without that initial spark, the human body cannot function without CoQ_{10}. Because of its safety and possible benefit, CoQ_{10} supplementation is indicated in any condition affecting the heart.

Botanical Medicines

Hawthorn

Hawthorn (*Crataegus* species) preparations have a long history of use in minor arrhythmias. The benefits in congestive heart failure have been repeatedly demonstrated in double-blind studies (see the chapter "Congestive Heart Failure").

QUICK REVIEW

- Individuals suspected of having any heart disease should have an extensive cardiovascular evaluation.
- The therapeutic goals in the treatment of arrhythmias are to improve energy metabolism within the heart and to improve the blood supply to the heart.
- The level of magnesium in the blood correlates with the ability of the heart muscle to manufacture enough energy and with the neurological activity necessary for the heart to beat properly.
- Many disorders of heart rhythm may be related to an insufficient level of magnesium in the heart muscle.
- The recommended intake for magnesium in arrhythmia appears to be approximately 6 to 10 mg/kg per day.
- CoQ_{10} is an important natural prescription for all types of heart disease.

TREATMENT SUMMARY

The primary goals of therapy for arrhythmia are to improve the blood supply to the heart and to improve energy production within the heart muscle. Follow the general guidelines on diet and lifestyle in the chapter "Heart and Cardiovascular Health."

Diet

Follow the guidelines given in the chapter "A Health-Promoting Diet." If you are taking Coumadin (warfarin), follow the guidelines in the "Diet" section (above) in this chapter.

Nutritional Supplements

- A high-potency multiple vitamin and mineral formula as described in the chapter "Supplementary Measures"

- Key individual nutrients:
  - Vitamin B_6: 25 to 50 mg per day
  - Magnesium (bound to aspartate, citrate, fumarate, malate, or succinate): 200 to 300 mg three times per day
  - Vitamin D_3: 2,000 to 4,000 IU per day (ideally, measure blood levels and adjust dosage accordingly)
  - CoQ_{10}: 150 to 300 mg per day

Botanical Medicines

- Hawthorn (*Crataegus* species) extract (1.8% vitexin-4'-rhamnoside or 10% proanthocyanidin content): 100 to 250 mg three times per day

Hemorrhoids

· ·

- Abnormally large or painful conglomerates of vessels, supporting tissues, and overlying mucous membrane or skin of the rectal area
- Bright red bleeding on the surface of the stool, on the toilet tissue, and/or in the toilet bowl

In the United States and other industrialized countries, hemorrhoids are extremely common. Estimates have indicated that 50% of those over 50 years of age have symptomatic hemorrhoidal disease, and up to one-third of the total U.S. population has hemorrhoids to some degree. Although most individuals may begin to develop hemorrhoids in their 20s, hemorrhoidal symptoms usually do not become evident until the 30s.

Causes

The causes of hemorrhoids are similar to the causes of varicose veins (see the chapter "Varicose Veins"): genetic weakness of the veins and/or excessive pressure on the veins.

Because the venous system that supplies the rectal area contains no valves, factors that increase venous congestion in the region can lead to hemorrhoid formation. These factors include increased intra-abdominal pressure (caused by defecation, pregnancy, coughing, sneezing, vomiting, physical exertion, or portal hypertension due to cirrhosis); an increase in straining during defecation due to a low-fiber diet; diarrhea; and standing or sitting for prolonged periods of time.

Classification of Hemorrhoids

Hemorrhoids are typically classified according to location and degree of severity. External hemorrhoids occur below the anorectal line—the point in the 3-cm-long anal canal where the skin lining changes to mucous membrane. They may be full of either blood clots (thrombotic hemorrhoids) or connective tissue (cutaneous hemorrhoids). A thrombotic hemorrhoid is produced when a hemorrhoidal vessel has ruptured and formed a blood clot (thrombus), while a cutaneous hemorrhoid consists of fibrous connective tissue covered by anal skin. Cutaneous hemorrhoids can be located at any point on the circumference of the anus. Typically, they are caused by the resolution of a thrombotic hemorrhoid: that is, the thrombus becomes organized and replaced by connective tissue.

Internal hemorrhoids occur above the anorectal line. Occasionally, an internal hemorrhoid enlarges to such a degree that it prolapses and descends below the anal sphincter. Internal hemorrhoids are graded by the degree of prolapse:

Grade I: No prolapse

Grade II: Prolapses upon defecation but spontaneously reduces

Grade III: Prolapses upon defecation and must be manually reduced

Grade IV: Prolapsed and cannot be manually reduced

Internal-external, or mixed, hemorrhoids are a combination of contiguous external and internal hemorrhoids that appear as baggy swellings. The following types of mixed hemorrhoids can occur:

- Without prolapse: Bleeding may be present, but there is no pain.
- Prolapsed: Characterized by pain and possibly bleeding.
- Strangulated: The hemorrhoid has prolapsed to such a degree and for so long that its blood supply is occluded by the anal sphincter's constricting action; strangulated hemorrhoids are very painful and usually become filled with blood clots (thrombosed).

Diagnostic Considerations

The symptoms most often associated with hemorrhoids include itching, burning, pain, inflammation, irritation, swelling, bleeding, and seepage. Itching is caused when there is mucous discharge from prolapsing internal hemorrhoids; tissue trauma resulting from excessive use of harsh toilet paper; *Candida albicans;* parasitic infections; and food allergies. Pain occurs when there is acute inflammation of external hemorrhoids. However, as there are no sensory nerve endings above the anorectal line, uncomplicated internal hemorrhoids rarely cause pain. Bleeding is almost always associated with internal hemorrhoids and may occur before, during, or after defecation. When bleeding occurs from an external hemorrhoid, it is due to rupture of an acute thrombotic hemorrhoid. Bleeding

hemorrhoids can produce severe anemia due to chronic blood loss.

Therapeutic Considerations

Conventional Medical Treatment

Conventional medical treatment of acute hemorrhoids may be appropriate.

- Rubber band ligation is a procedure in which elastic bands are applied to an internal hemorrhoid to cut off its blood supply. Within a week the hemorrhoid simply falls off. This technique is inexpensive, is simple, and has a cure rate of about 87%.
- Sclerotherapy involves the injection of a scar-forming agent into the hemorrhoid, causing the vein walls to collapse and the hemorrhoid to shrivel up. The success rate four years after treatment is 70%.
- A number of cautery methods (electrocautery, infrared radiation, laser, and cryosurgery) have been shown to be effective for hemorrhoids.
- Hemorrhoidectomy is surgical excision of the hemorrhoid. It is used only in severe cases because it is associated with significant postoperative pain and usually requires two to four weeks for recovery.

Diet

Hemorrhoids are rarely seen in parts of the world where diets rich in high-fiber, unrefined foods are consumed. A low-fiber diet, high in refined foods, like that common in the United States, contributes greatly to the development of hemorrhoids.[1]

Individuals who consume a low-fiber diet tend to strain more during bowel movements,

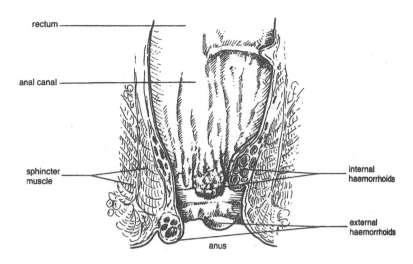

Hemorrhoids

since their smaller, harder stools are more difficult to pass. This straining increases the pressure in the abdomen, which obstructs venous blood flow. The intensified pressure increases pelvic congestion and may significantly weaken the veins, causing hemorrhoids to form.

A high-fiber diet is perhaps the most important component in the prevention of hemorrhoids. A diet rich in vegetables, fruits, legumes, and grains promotes rapid transit of the feces through the intestine. Furthermore, many fiber components attract water and form a gelatinous mass that keeps the feces soft, bulky, and easy to pass. The net effect of a high-fiber diet is significantly less straining during defecation. The importance of fiber is discussed in more detail in the chapter "A Health-Promoting Diet."

Bulking Agents

Natural bulking compounds can also be used to reduce fecal straining. These fibrous substances, particularly psyllium seed husks and guar gum, possess mild laxative action, owing to their ability to attract water and form a ge-

latinous mass. They are generally less irritating than wheat bran and other cellulose-fiber products. Several double-blind clinical trials have demonstrated that supplementing the diet with bulk-forming fiber can significantly reduce the symptoms of hemorrhoids (bleeding, pain, itching, and prolapse) and improve bowel habits.[2,3] A meta-analysis of seven studies showed that the use of fiber helps relieve overall symptoms and bleeding in the treatment of symptomatic hemorrhoids.[2]

Hydrotherapy

A warm sitz bath (a partial-immersion bath of the pelvic region) is an effective noninvasive therapy for uncomplicated hemorrhoids. The temperature of the water should be between 100 and 105°F. The warm sitz bath is soothing, but as with creams and ointments, its relief is short-lived.

Topical Treatments

Topical treatments, in most circumstances, will provide only temporary relief, but even temporary relief is better than no relief at all. Topical treatments include suppositories, ointments, and anorectal pads. Many over-the-counter products for hemorrhoids contain primarily natural ingredients, such as witch hazel, aloe vera gel, shark liver oil, cod liver oil, cocoa butter, Peruvian balsam, zinc oxide, live yeast cell derivative, and allantoin.

Flavonoids

Flavonoid preparations have been shown to relieve hemorrhoids by strengthening the veins. Early studies featured rutin. More-recent and much more extensive studies have been performed using hydroxyethylrutoside (HER). Rutin and citrus bioflavonoid preparations can be viewed as providing effects similar to those of HER, but probably not as potent.

In several double-blind clinical studies, HER has been found helpful in the treatment of varicose veins and hemorrhoids.[4,5] Some of the studies involved pregnant women; HER was shown to be of great benefit in improving venous function and helping relieve hemorrhoidal signs and symptoms during pregnancy. In one study, 90% of the women who were given HER (1,000 mg per day for four weeks) experienced relief from symptoms, compared with only 12% in the placebo group. Similar results have been reported for the use of HER to treat hemorrhoids not associated with pregnancy.

Micronized diosmin and flavonoid-rich extracts such as those from grape seed or pine bark are also suitable choices.

Botanical Medicines

Any of the botanicals described in the chapter "Varicose Veins," and particularly butcher's broom (*Ruscus aculeatus*), are useful for enhancing the integrity of the veins of the rectum. In one multicenter study of 124 patients with hemorrhoids, 69% of the patients and 75% of the treating physicians rated a formula containing butcher's broom extract as having good or excellent efficacy, and 92% of physicians rated the treatment as safe and well tolerated.[6] Significant positive effects were observed after seven days of treatment.

. . . .

QUICK REVIEW

- **The veins in the rectal area contain no valves, so factors that increase congestion of blood flow or pressure in the region can lead to hemorrhoid formation.**
- **Common causes of anal itching include tissue trauma from excessive use of harsh toilet paper, *Candida albicans*, parasitic infections, and food allergies.**
- **A high-fiber diet is perhaps the most important component in the prevention of hemorrhoids.**
- **Flavonoid preparations have been helpful in relieving hemorrhoids by strengthening the veins.**

TREATMENT SUMMARY

As with all diseases, the primary treatment for hemorrhoids is prevention. This goal involves reducing the factors that may be responsible for increasing pelvic congestion: straining during defecation, sitting or standing for prolonged periods of time, or underlying liver disease. A high-fiber diet is crucial for the maintenance of proper bowel activity. Fiber supplements, flavonoids, and various botanical medicines such as butcher's broom are appropriate supplementary measures.

Warm sitz baths and topical preparations help relieve the discomfort but have only temporary effects.

Diet

The recommendations in the chapter "A Health-Promoting Diet" are very important in preventing and treating hemorrhoids. The diet should contain liberal amounts of soluble dietary fiber and flavonoid-rich foods, such as blackberries, citrus fruits, cherries, and blueberries, to strengthen vein structures.

Nutritional Supplements

- A high-potency multiple vitamin and mineral formula as described in the chapter "Supplementary Measures"

- Psyllium seed husk: 5 g at bedtime with 6 to 8 ounces of water
- Vitamin C: 500 to 1,000 mg three times per day
- Flavonoids, one or more of the following:
  - HER: 1,000 to 3,000 mg per day
  - Citrus bioflavonoids, rutin, and/or hesperidin: 3,000 to 6,000 mg per day
  - Micronized diosmin: 500 to 1,000 mg per day
  - Grape seed extract (>95% procyanidolic oligomers): 150 to 300 mg per day
  - Pine bark extract: 150 to 300 mg per day.

Botanical Medicines

- Butcher's broom (*Ruscus aculeatus*) extract (9%% to 11% ruscogenin content): 100 mg three times per day

Physical Medicine

- Hydrotherapy: warm sitz baths to relieve uncomplicated hemorrhoids

Hepatitis

· ·

- Prodrome of loss of appetite, nausea, vomiting, fatigue, and flu-like symptoms that can occur two weeks to one month before liver involvement, depending upon the incubation period of the virus

  - Symptoms may occur abruptly or rather insidiously

  - Fever; enlarged, tender liver; jaundice (yellow appearance of the skin and whites of the eye)

  - Dark urine

  - Normal to low white blood cell count; markedly elevated liver enzymes (aminotransaminases) in the blood; elevated bilirubin levels

Hepatitis (inflammation of the liver) can be caused by many drugs and toxic chemicals, but in most instances it is caused by a virus. Viral types A, B, and C are the most common. Hepatitis A occurs sporadically or in epidemics, and is transmitted primarily through fecal contamination. Hepatitis B is transmitted through infected blood or blood products as well as through sexual contact (the virus is shed in saliva, semen, and vaginal secretions). Hepatitis C (formerly known as non-A, non-B hepatitis) can be transmitted through blood transfusions or intravenous drug use, but in some cases the source of infection is unclear; the mortality rate (1% to 12%) is much higher than that for the other forms. Other viral causes of hepatitis include hepatitis viruses D, E, and G, as well as herpes simplex, cytomegalovirus, and Epstein-Barr virus.

Acute viral hepatitis can be an extremely debilitating disease requiring bed rest. Recovery can take anywhere from 2 to 16 weeks. Most patients recover completely (usually by 9 weeks in type A and 16 weeks in B, C, D, and G). However, about 1 out of 100 people infected with hepatitis dies, and 10% of hepatitis B cases and 10 to 40% of hepatitis C cases develop into chronic viral hepatitis forms (hepatitis C contracted from a transfusion is associated with a 70 to 80% rate of development of chronic hepatitis). The symptoms of chronic hepatitis vary: they can be virtually nonexistent or they can lead to chronic fatigue, serious liver damage, and even death due to cirrhosis of the liver or liver cancer.

Diagnostic Considerations

Diagnosis is based on the appearance of the typical signs and symptoms (listed in the table opposite) along with blood tests showing elevation in liver enzymes (such as SGPT, GGPT, SGOT, and alkaline phosphatase, which leak out into the blood when liver cells are damaged) and the presence of viral antigens (compounds recognized as being foreign to the body and resulting in the formation of antibodies against them) or the antibodies that bind antigens. The type of virus involved is determined by identifying viral antigens or specific antibodies in the blood.

Incidence of Symptoms in Viral Hepatitis[1]	
SYMPTOM	**% OF PATIENTS SUFFERING FROM IT**
Dark urine	94
Fatigue	91
Loss of appetite	90
Nausea	87
Fever	76
Vomiting	71
Headache	70
Abdominal discomfort	65
Light stools	52
Muscle pain	52
Drowsiness	49
Irritability	43
Itching	42
Diarrhea	25
Joint pain	21

In cases of chronic hepatitis B or C it is necessary to perform continued blood evaluation to monitor progression or clearance of the infection. In addition to liver enzymes, hepatitis C is monitored by the presence of hepatitis C viral RNA by polymerase chain reaction (HCV-RNA[PCR]). The higher the level of HCV-RNA, the more aggressive the chronic infection.

Prevention Strategies

Hepatitis A

For primary prevention of hepatitis A, the Centers for Disease Control (CDC) recommends vaccination for three categories of people: (1) children living in areas with high rates of hepatitis A; (2) people at increased risk, such as travelers to endemic regions, men having sex with men, illegal drug users, employees in research laboratories who work with hepatitis A, and individuals with clotting factor disorders needing blood components; (3) people with chronic liver disease, especially chronic hepatitis B or C. Vaccination is also advised during outbreaks in communities with higher rates of hepatitis A.[2,3] Postexposure prevention consists of injections of specific hepatitis A immune globulins (antibodies) during the first two weeks after an individual has been exposed.[4]

Hepatitis B

Vaccination is prudent for those in high-risk occupations, such as members of the medical and dental fields who regularly encounter blood and other body fluids. In the case of exposure to the hepatitis B virus (HBV), hyperimmune globulin is administered in a series of two injections within two weeks of exposure. It is said to confer adequate protective immunity to 75% of exposed individuals, though the protection lasts for only three months.

Newborns whose mothers are positive for hepatitis B surface antigen (HBsAg) should also receive the vaccine shortly after birth and again at ages three and six months.

Hepatitis C

As there is currently no vaccine for hepatitis C, prevention entails minimizing routes of infection. Because 50 to 80% of IV drug abusers get infected during the first year,[4] cessation of IV drug use or using only previously unused, clean, sterile needles is recommended. Similarly, modifying or ceasing intranasal cocaine use decreases risk. Accepting blood transfusions only from blood sources known to be uncontaminated also curtails a major risk factor.

Health care workers should practice strict occupational safety and health standards, especially when dealing with blood products, and should never recap used needles, to avoid needle stick transmission.

Although sexual transmission is an inefficient method of transfer, the risk is higher in male homosexuals, patients with multiple sexual partners, and those with sexually transmitted diseases.[4] Someone in a monogamous heterosexual relationship with a hepatitis C patient has a low risk of infection unless the patient is coinfected with hepatitis C and human immunodeficiency virus (HIV).

Therapeutic Considerations

Natural therapies can be of great benefit in hepatitis, but the disease requires proper medical care and supervision. Several nutrients and herbs have been shown to inhibit viral reproduction, improve immune system function, and greatly stimulate regeneration of damaged liver cells. General therapies to protect and support the liver are discussed in more detail in the chapter "Detoxification and Internal Cleansing." Those recommendations can be used in conjunction with the more specific recommendations given in this chapter.

It is absolutely essential to be aggressive in the treatment of chronic hepatitis due to the increased risk for liver cancer and cirrhosis. If cirrhosis is present in chronic hepatitis B, for example, the five-year survival rate is just 50 to 60%.

The best available conventional drug treatment for chronic hepatitis is the combination of pegylated interferon and ribavirin. Unfortunately, this regimen is costly, is fraught with side effects, and eradicates hepatitis C in only 50% to 70% of patients at best.[1] However, patients with hepatitis can greatly benefit from natural therapies.

Diet

During the acute hepatitis phase, the focus should be on replacing fluids through consumption of vegetable broths, vegetable juices diluted with an equal amount of water, and herbal teas. Solid foods should be restricted to brown rice, steamed vegetables, and moderate intake of lean protein sources.

In chronic cases, follow the dietary recommendations in the chapter "A Health-Promoting Diet." The diet should definitely be low in saturated fats, simple carbohydrates (e.g., sugar, white flour, fruit juice, honey), oxidized fatty acids (oils used for frying), and animal products. A diet that focuses on plant foods (i.e., a high-fiber diet) has been shown to increase the elimination of bile acids, drugs, and toxic bile substances from the system. Alcohol should be completely avoided.

Nutritional Supplements

Vitamin C

According to nutritional medicine pioneer Robert Cathcart, M.D., acute hepatitis is one of the easiest diseases for vitamin C to cure.[5,6] Cathcart demonstrated that high dosages of vitamin C (40 to 100 g orally or intravenously per day) were able to greatly improve acute viral hepatitis in two to four days and to clear jaundice within six days.[6] Other studies demonstrated similar benefits.[7–9] A controlled study found that 2 g per day or more of vitamin C was able to dramatically prevent hepatitis B in hospitalized patients. Although 7% of the control patients (receiving less than 1.5 g per day of vitamin C) developed hepatitis, none of the treated patients did.[10]

Selenium

Selenium is a trace element required for the activity of the antioxidant enzyme glutathione peroxidase. Selenium deficiency is associated with immune system dysfunction, cancer, and liver damage. Whole blood and plasma selenium levels in 59 patients with chronic liver disease including alcoholic and viral liver cirrhosis were found to be significantly lower when compared with those in healthy controls.[11] Another study revealed that liver cancer cells are able to acquire a selective survival advantage that is prominent under conditions of selenium deficiency and oxidative stress.[12] Oxidative stress is a well-known feature in late-stage cirrhotic liver disease, but subsequent study has found that this type of oxidant stress actually occurs much earlier than previously believed.[13] Given this information and the safety of selenium when used in doses under 400 mcg, it is reasonable to employ selenium for treatment of hepatitis.

Alpha-Lipoic Acid

Alpha-lipoic acid is a sulfur-containing compound produced by the cells of the body. It has a role in energy metabolism and is also a valuable antioxidant. Alpha-lipoic acid has been successfully used to treat a number of conditions relating to liver disease, including alcohol-induced damage, metal intoxication, carbon tetrachloride poisoning, and amanita mushroom poisoning, as well as hepatitis C.[14–16]

Vitamin D

New research is showing that vitamin D not only is directly antiviral—specifically against hepatitis C—but also promotes immune function that is critical to helping the body eliminate the virus.[17] Several studies have now used vitamin D in conjunction with conventional antiviral drugs, resulting in improved outcomes.[18] People with low blood vitamin D levels are much more likely to have more serious cases of hepatitis that progress to chronic hepatitis, as well as to develop cirrhosis.[19] One study found that more than 90%

of patients with chronic hepatitis C had low levels of vitamin D.[20]

Botanical Medicines

Although long-term clinical trials have yet to confirm the efficacy of plant medicines, several have been investigated for their effects in viral hepatitis. The two with the greatest amount of positive documentation are licorice (*Glycyrrhiza glabra*) and silymarin (the flavonoid complex from milk thistle, *Silybum marianum*). A third, *Phyllanthus amarus*, sparked considerable excitement on the basis of preliminary results, but detailed follow-up studies showed it to provide no benefit.[21]

Licorice Root

Licorice (*Glycyrrhiza glabra*) exerts many actions beneficial in the treatment of acute and chronic hepatitis, including protecting the liver, enhancing the immune system, potentiating interferon (the body's own antiviral and immune-enhancing agent), and promoting the flow of bile and fat to and from the liver. In addition, licorice root is directly antiviral. Clinical studies with a product in Japan containing glycyrrhizin—the key component of licorice—have shown excellent results in the treatment of acute and chronic hepatitis. The product, Stronger Neominophagen C (SNMC), consists of 200 mg glycyrrhizin, 100 mg cysteine, and 2,000 mg glycine in 100 ml physiological saline solution. It is administered intravenously, though oral administration may be just as effective, as discussed below.[22–26]

SNMC has demonstrated impressive results in treating chronic hepatitis B or C. Approximately 40% of patients will have complete resolution—a proportion that compares quite favorably with alpha-interferon's 40 to 50% clearance rate. Like SNMC, alpha-interferon administration has been shown to lead to dramatic reductions in the risk for liver cancer. However, it is expensive and causes side effects (primarily fever, joint pain, nausea, and flu-like symptoms) in all patients.

In a recent study of 453 patients diagnosed with chronic hepatitis C at a hospital in Japan between 1979 and 1984, 84 patients were treated with SNMC at a dosage of 100 ml per day for eight weeks followed by treatments two to seven times weekly for periods up to 16 years.[26] The 15th-year cumulative rates of liver cancer and cirrhosis were 7% and 12%, respectively. The numbers are consistent with alpha-interferon's success rates in both patients at early stages of the disease (0.6% per year progression to liver cancer with alpha-interferon and 0.7% for SNMC) and those at advanced stages (1.5% per year progression to liver cancer in alpha-interferon-treated patients compared with 1.3% for those treated with SNMC).

Although the studies with SNMC utilized injectable glycyrrhizin, injection may not be necessary, as glycyrrhizin is readily absorbed from licorice. The goal is to achieve a high level of glycyrrhizin in the blood without producing side effects. The dosages given in the "Treatment Summary" section below provide roughly half the dosage of glycyrrhizin used in the studies with SNMC. Over longer periods, licorice root (more than 3 g per day for more than six weeks) or glycyrrhizin (more than 100 mg per day) may cause sodium and water retention, leading to high blood pressure. Monitoring blood pressure, increasing dietary potassium intake, and following a low-sodium diet are suggested.[27] There is great individual variation in susceptibility to the blood-pressure-elevating effects of licorice. While adverse effects are quite common at levels above 400 mg per day, they are rarely observed at levels below 100 mg per day.[27] Nonetheless, licorice should probably not be used by patients with a history of

hypertension or renal failure, or by patients currently using digitalis preparations.

Milk Thistle

Milk thistle (*Silybum marianum*) contains silymarin, a mixture of flavonolignans consisting chiefly of silybin, silidianin, and silichristine. Silymarin is one of the most potent liver-protecting substances known. Silymarin inhibits hepatic damage by doing the following:

- Acting as a direct antioxidant and free radical scavenger
- Increasing the content of the protective compounds glutathione and superoxide dismutase within the liver cells
- Inhibiting the formation of inflammatory compounds that can damage liver cells
- Stimulating liver cell regeneration

Silymarin is effective in both acute and chronic viral hepatitis. In one study of acute viral hepatitis, 29 patients treated with silymarin showed a reduction in serum levels of bilirubin and liver enzymes after five days compared with a placebo group.[28] The number of patients attaining normal liver values after three weeks of treatment was significantly higher in the silymarin group than in the placebo group.

In a study of chronic viral hepatitis, silymarin was shown to result in dramatic improvement. High doses (420 mg per day) of silymarin for periods of 3 to 12 months resulted in a reversal of liver cell damage (as noted by biopsy), an increase in protein level in the blood, and a lowering of liver enzymes. Common symptoms of hepatitis (e.g., abdominal discomfort, decreased appetite, fatigue) all improved.[29]

Silymarin phytosome is a newer form of silymarin, bound to phosphatidylcholine, that may provide even greater benefit. A growing body of scientific research indicates that phosphatidylcholine-bound silymarin is better absorbed and produces better clinical results than unbound silymarin.[30–35] These benefits were demonstrated in one study involving 232 patients with chronic hepatitis (viral, alcohol-related, or chemically induced) treated with silymarin phytosome at a dose of either 120 mg twice per day or 120 mg three times per day for up to 120 days.[35] An additional 49 patients were treated with a commercially available unbound silymarin, while 117 were untreated or given a placebo. Liver function returned to normal faster in all patients given silymarin phytosome, compared with those given the commercially available silymarin and those who received the placebo.

Silymarin has low toxicity and is well tolerated. However, because it stimulates bile flow, it may produce a looser stool. If higher doses are used, it may be appropriate to use bile-sequestering fiber compounds (e.g., guar gum, pectin, psyllium, oat bran) to prevent mucosal irritation and loose stools. Because of silymarin's lack of toxicity, long-term use is appropriate.

QUICK REVIEW

- **Hepatitis is a serious disease requiring the care of a physician.**
- **Several nutrients and herbs have been shown to inhibit viral reproduction, improve immune system function, and greatly stimulate regeneration of damaged liver cells.**
- **In the case of acute exposure to the hepatitis B virus, hyperimmune globulin is administered by injection.**
- **During the acute phase, the focus should be on replacing fluids through consumption of vegetable broths, diluted vegetable juices, and herbal teas.**
- **In chronic cases, the diet should be low in saturated fats, simple carbohydrates, oxidized fatty acids, and animal products.**
- **High dosages of vitamin C (40 to 100 g orally or intravenously) are able to greatly improve acute viral hepatitis in two to four days.**
- **Licorice exerts many actions beneficial in the treatment of acute and chronic hepatitis, including protecting the liver, enhancing the immune system, and potentiating interferon.**
- **Silymarin, the flavonoid complex from milk thistle, is effective in both acute and chronic viral hepatitis.**
- **A growing body of scientific research indicates that silymarin phytosome is better absorbed and produces better clinical results than unbound silymarin.**

TREATMENT SUMMARY

In cases of hepatitis, natural medicine's therapeutic goals are to prevent further damage to the liver by supporting the immune system, decrease viral load, and protect the liver. Bed rest is important during the acute phase of viral hepatitis, with slow resumption of activities as health improves. Strenuous exertion, alcohol, and other liver-toxic drugs and chemicals should be avoided. During the contagious phase (two to three weeks before symptoms appear to three weeks after), there is not much that can be done unless there is prior knowledge of infection, in which case careful hygiene and avoiding close contact with others is important. Once diagnosis is made at any point, work that involves public contact, such as work in day care centers, restaurants, and similar places, is not recommended.

Diet

During the acute phase, the focus should be on replacing fluids through consumption of vegetable broths, vegetable juices diluted with an equal amount of water, and herbal teas.

In the chronic phase, follow the guidelines in the chapter "A Health-Promoting Diet." Certain foods are particularly helpful because they contain the nutrients your body needs in order to produce and activate the dozens of enzymes involved in the various phases of detoxification. These foods include:

- Garlic, legumes, onions, eggs, and other foods with a high sulfur content
- Good sources of water-soluble fiber, such as pears, oat bran, apples, and legumes
- Vegetables in the brassica family, especially broccoli, brussels sprouts, and cabbage
- Artichokes, beets, carrots, dandelion greens, and many herbs and spices such as turmeric, cinnamon, and licorice
- Green foods such as wheatgrass juice, dehydrated barley grass juice, chlorella, and spirulina

Nutritional Supplements

- A high-potency multiple vitamin and mineral formula as described in the chapter "Supplementary Measures"
- Fish oils: 1,000 mg EPA + DHA
- Vitamin C: 500 to 1,000 mg three times per day
- Vitamin D: 2,000 to 4,000 IU per day (ideally, measure blood levels and adjust dosage accordingly)
- One of the following:
  ○ Grape seed extract (>95% procyanidolic oligomers): 150 to 300 mg per day
  ○ Pine bark extract (>95% procyanidolic oligomers): 150 to 300 mg per day

Botanical Medicines

- Licorice *(Glycyrrhiza glabra)*:
  - Powdered root: 1 to 2 g three times a day
  - Fluid extract (1:1): 2 to 4 ml three times a day
  - Solid (dry powdered) extract (5% glycyrrhetinic acid content): 250 to 500 mg three times a day

Note: If licorice is to be used over a long period of time, it is necessary to increase the intake of potassium-rich foods.

- Milk thistle *(Silybum marianum)*: Dosage is based on silymarin content (standardized extracts are preferred), and the best results are achieved at higher dosages, i.e., 140 mg to 210 mg silymarin three times per day; dosage for silymarin phytosome is 120 mg two to three times per day between meals.

Herpes

. . . .

- Recurrent viral infection of the skin or mucous membranes characterized by the appearance of single or multiple clusters of small blisters on a reddened base, frequently occurring about the mouth, lips, genitals, and eye (conjunctiva and cornea)

- Incubation period 2 to 12 days, averaging 6 to 7

- Regional lymph nodes may be tender and swollen

- Outbreak recurrences may follow minor infections, trauma, stress (emotional, dietary, and environmental), and sun exposure

There are more than 70 members in the herpes family of viruses. Here we will be considering herpes simplex, in which two types of viruses are involved: HSV-1 and HSV-2. Current estimates are that 20 to 40% of people in the United States have recurrent HSV infections.[1] Previously, HSV-1 was isolated primarily from sites other than the genitals, while genital infections were caused primarily by HSV-2; by the year 2000, however, HSV-1 had replaced HSV-2 as the primary cause of genital lesions.[2] In 2001, HSV-1 accounted for 78% of all cases of genital herpes, compared with 31% of cases in 1993.[3]

The risk of clinical herpes infection after sexual contact with an individual who has active lesions is estimated to be 75%. Although 80% of individuals who have been infected do not have clinically apparent recurrences, they can still shed a virus even if they have no symptoms.

HSV-1 is frequently acquired in early childhood, with evidence of past exposure in nearly 90% in adults. After the initial infection, in most people the virus becomes dormant in the nerve cells. In others, however, it can be reactivated. This reactivation causes recurring outbreaks. HSV-1 genital lesions have a recurrence rate of 14%, while the HSV-2 recurrence rate is 60%. Men seem more susceptible to recurrences.

Recurrences develop at or near the sites of primary infection and may be precipitated by many different stimuli:

- Sunburn or sun exposure
- Sexual activity
- Menses
- Stress
- Food allergy
- Drugs
- Certain foods

Therapeutic Considerations

Because not everyone exposed to HSV develops recurrent clinical infection, it appears that the body's defense mechanisms are paramount in protecting against active infection.

Chronic, persistent herpes infections are seen in immune-suppressed individuals. The cell-mediated immune system is undoubtedly the major factor in determining whether herpes exposure leads to resistance, latent infection, or clinical disease.

The goals of natural medicine are to decrease the number and severity of outbreaks, reduce viral shedding, and prevent transmission to a partner. Enhancement of immune function is key in the control of herpes infection. Following the recommendations in the chapter "Immune System Support" is a good start. Other specific measures are discussed below.

Nutritional Supplements

Zinc

Oral supplementation with zinc (50 mg per day) has been shown to be effective in clinical studies.[4] Although zinc is an effective inhibitor of HSV replication in test tube studies, its effect in the human body is probably related to its role in enhancing cell-mediated immunity. Topical application of a 0.01 to 0.025% zinc sulfate solution has also been shown to be effective in both reducing symptoms and inhibiting recurrences of HSV infection.[5]

Vitamin C

Both the oral consumption and the topical application of vitamin C increase the rate of healing of herpes ulcers. In a randomized, double-blind study, an ascorbic-acid-containing pharmaceutical formulation (Ascoxal) was applied with a soaked cotton wool pad three times per day for two minutes. Patients reported fewer days with scabs and fewer cases of worsening of symptoms. Cultures yielded herpes complex viruses significantly less frequently in the treatment group.[6]

In another study, 20 episodes of cold sores were treated with a complex of 200 mg water-soluble bioflavonoids and 200 mg vitamin C given orally three times per day; 20 episodes were treated with a complex of 200 mg water-soluble bioflavonoids and 200 mg vitamin C five times per day; and 10 episodes were treated with a lactose preparation. This approach was maintained for three days after the recognition of symptoms. The bioflavonoid–vitamin C complex was shown to reduce herpes blisters and to prevent the blisters from rupturing. The therapy was most beneficial when it was initiated at the beginning of symptoms. Those treated with bioflavonoids and vitamin C three times per day saw remission of symptoms in 4.2 days, while those treated five times per day saw their blisters heal in 4.4 days; those on the placebo did not heal until after 10 days.[7]

Vitamin C has also been given intravenously with benefit in the treatment of patients with HSV infection, including AIDS patients.[8]

Lysine and Arginine

A diet rich in lysine and low in arginine has become a popular treatment for HSV infections. This approach came from research showing that lysine has antiviral activity in vitro, owing to its antagonism of arginine metabolism (the two amino acids compete for intestinal transport mechanisms).[9] HSV replication requires the synthesis of arginine-rich proteins, and so it has been suggested that arginine is required for the virus to replicate.[10] Rats fed a lysine-rich diet displayed a 60% decrease in brain arginine levels, although there was no change in blood levels.[9] Because HSV is believed to reside in the nerve root (ganglia) during latency, lysine supplementation and avoidance of high-arginine foods have been suggested as appropriate. How-

Arginine and Lysine Content of Selected Foods

FOOD	SERVING SIZE	ARGININE (MG)	LYSINE (MG)
Almonds	70 nuts	2,730	580
Beans, green	¾ cup	80	80
Beans, lima	3.5 oz	1,170	1,470
Beans, mung	3.5 oz	1,320	1,930
Beans, red	⅓ cup	340	420
Beef chuck	3.5 oz	1,600	2,200
Brazil nuts	3.5 oz	2,250	470
Bread, whole wheat	4 slices	510	290
Buckwheat	3.5 oz	1,200	460
Carob	3.5 oz	710	340
Cashews	40 nuts	1,990	740
Cheese, cheddar	3.5 oz	850	1,700
Chicken	3.5 oz	1,930	2,700
Chocolate	3.5 oz	4,500	2,000
Clams	½ cup	830	840
Coconut	3.5 oz	470	148
Crustaceans	3.5 oz	1,330	1,260
Eggs	2 large	840	820
Fish sticks, breaded	4–5 sticks	940	1,400
Flaxseeds	3.5 oz	2,030	810
Garbanzo beans	3.5 oz	1,900	1,380
Halibut	3.5 oz	140	2,220
Hazelnuts	3.5 oz	3,510	690
Lentils	3.5 oz	2,100	1,740
Liver, beef	3.5 oz	1,590	1,950
Milk, whole	3.5 oz	130	280
Millet	3.5 oz	410	260
Oatmeal, cooked	⅓ cup	130	70
Oysters	5–8 medium	310	280
Peanuts, without skins	3.5 oz	3,240	1,090
Peas, green	⅝ cup	420	220
Pecans	3.5 oz	2,030	810
Pork, lean	3.5 oz	1,510	1,850
Rice, brown	⅔ cup	120	100
Salmon	3.5 oz	1,530	2,350

Arginine and Lysine Content of Selected Foods			
Sardines	7 medium	190	1,850
Sesame seeds	3.5 oz	2,590	580
Shrimp	3.5 oz	1,360	2,130
Soybeans, boiled	⅔ cup	620	620
Sunflower seeds	3.5 oz	1,190	540
Tuna	⅝ can	1,530	2,530
Turkey	3.5 oz	1,700	2,450
Walnuts, English	27 whole	2,250	490
Yeast	3.5 oz	1,940	3,510

ever, double-blind studies of the effectiveness of lysine supplementation with uncontrolled avoidance of arginine-rich foods have shown inconsistent results.[10–13] This inconsistency may be due to the relatively low levels of lysine used (1,200 mg per day) and the severity of the cases in some of the studies (placebo and treated groups had lesions for 40% of the time in one negative study).[10,11] In one study, lysine was given at a larger dosage (1,000 mg three times per day) along with the dietary restriction of nuts, chocolate, and gelatin.[12] At six months, lysine was rated as effective or very effective by 74% of those receiving it; only 28% of those receiving the placebo gave similar ratings. The average number of outbreaks was 3.1 in the lysine group compared with 4.2 in the placebo group.

In some patients, withdrawal from lysine is followed by relapse within one to four weeks.[14]

. . . .

QUICK REVIEW

- **Current estimates indicate that 20 to 40% of people in the United States have recurrent HSV infections.**
- **Enhancement of the immune status is key to the prevention and control of herpes infection.**
- **A diet that avoids arginine-rich foods while promoting lysine-rich foods can be quite effective.**
- **Oral supplementation with zinc has been shown to be effective in reducing the frequency, duration, and severity of herpes in clinical studies.**
- **Both oral consumption and topical application of vitamin C increase the rate of healing of herpes ulcers.**
- **One of the most widely used and effective topical preparations in the treatment and prevention of herpes outbreaks is a concentrated extract of *Melissa officinalis* (lemon balm).**

Topical Treatments

Lemon Balm

One of the most widely used topical preparations in the treatment and prevention of herpes outbreaks is a concentrated extract (70:1) of lemon balm (*Melissa officinalis*). Rather than a single antiviral chemical, lemon balm contains several components that work together to prevent the virus from infecting human cells. When lemon balm cream was used in patients with an initial herpes infection, results from comprehensive trials in three German hospitals and a dermatology clinic demonstrated that there was not a single recurrence.[15] In other words, with use of the cream, not a single patient with a first herpes outbreak developed another cold sore.

Furthermore, it was noted in these studies that the lemon balm cream produced an interruption of the infection and promoted healing of the herpes blisters much faster than normal. The control group receiving other topical creams had a healing period of 10 days, while the group receiving the cream healed completely within 5 days. The cream was also studied in patients suffering from recurrent cold sores. Researchers found that if subjects used this cream regularly, they would either stop having recurrences or experience a tremendous reduction in the frequency of recurrences (an average cold-sore-free period of more than 3.5 months).[16]

The lemon balm cream should be applied fairly thickly (1 to 2 mm) to the lips two to four times per day during an active recurrence. Detailed toxicology studies have demonstrated that it is extremely safe and suitable for long-term use. Extracts of other species of the mint family have also shown in vitro efficacy against the adhesion but not replication of HSV-1 and HSV-2, including peppermint (*Mentha piperita*), rosemary (*Rosmarinus officinalis*), and thyme (*Thymus vulgaris*).[17]

Licorice

Another popular ingredient for the topical treatment and prevention of herpes outbreaks is glycyrrhetinic acid. This triterpenoid component of licorice (*Glycyrrhiza glabra*) root inhibits both the growth and the cell-damaging effects of herpes simplex and other viruses.[18] Topical glycyrrhetinic acid has been shown in clinical studies to be helpful in reducing the healing time and pain associated with cold sores and genital herpes.[19–21]

· ·

TREATMENT SUMMARY

The goals of natural medicine are to shorten the current attack and prevent recurrences. Support of the immune system is of primary importance, necessitating control of food allergens and optimizing nutrients necessary for cell-mediated immunity. Inhibition of HSV replication by increasing the lysine/arginine ratio in the diet has been found useful. Strengthening the immune system can be effective at reducing the frequency, duration, and severity of recurrences.

Diet

A diet that avoids major food allergens and limits arginine-rich foods while promoting lysine-rich foods is recommended (refer to the table above). The foods with the worst arginine-to-lysine ratio are chocolate, peanuts, and almonds.

Nutritional Supplements

- A high-potency multiple vitamin and mineral formula as described in the chapter "Supplementary Measures"
- Key individual nutrients:
  - Vitamin C: 500 to 1,000 mg two to three times per day
  - Vitamin D_3: 2,000 to 4,000 IU per day (ideally, measure blood levels and adjust dosage accordingly)
- Fish oils: 1,000 mg EPA + DHA per day
- One of the following:
  - Grape seed extract (>95% procyanidolic oligomers): 100 to 300 mg per day
  - Pine bark extract (>95% procyanidolic oligomers): 100 to 300 mg per day
  - Some other flavonoid-rich extract with a similar flavonoid content, super greens formula, or another plant-based antioxidant that can provide an oxygen radical absorption capacity (ORAC) of 3,000 to 6,000 units or more per day
  - Lysine: 1,000 mg three times per day

Topical Treatments

- Zinc sulfate solution: apply 0.025% solution three times a day
- Lemon balm cream: apply at least twice a day
- Glycyrrhetinic acid: apply at least twice a day

High Blood Pressure

- Borderline high blood pressure (prehypertension): 130–139/85–89 mm Hg
- Mild high blood pressure (stage 1): 140–159/90–99 mm Hg
- Moderate high blood pressure (stage 2): 160–179/100–109 mm Hg
- Severe high blood pressure (stage 3): 180 or over/110 or over mm Hg

Elevated blood pressure (hypertension) is a major risk factor for a heart attack or stroke. In fact, it is generally regarded as the most significant risk factor for a stroke. More than 60 million Americans have high blood pressure (high BP), including more than half (54.3%) of all Americans ages 65 to 74 and almost three-quarters (71.8%) of all American blacks in the same age group.

Individuals with a normal diastolic pressure (under 85 mm Hg) but significantly elevated systolic pressure (over 158 mm Hg) have what is termed *isolated systolic hypertension*. It is usually an indication of significant hardening of the aorta and carries with it a twofold increase in cardiovascular death rates when compared with a systolic pressure under 130 mm Hg).

Causes

High BP is most often the result of factors that affect the degree of blood vessel constriction and fluid volume. Although genetic factors play a role, there is little debate that dietary, lifestyle, psychological, and environmental factors are the underlying causes in most cases of high BP. Dietary factors include excessive calorie consumption; high sodium-to-potassium ratio; low-fiber, high-sugar diet; high consumption of saturated fat and low consumption of omega-3 fatty acids; and a diet low in calcium, magnesium, and vitamin C. Important lifestyle factors that may cause high BP include stress, lack of exercise, and smoking. The dietary factor that has received the greatest attention is salt intake. Between 40 and 60% of people with high blood pressure are salt-sensitive (as discussed later).

Exposure to heavy metals such as lead, mercury, cadmium, and arsenic may also be a significant factor in some patients. The kidneys take the primary role in the elimination of heavy metals, so these metals concentrate there and disrupt the kidneys' ability to regulate the body's fluid volume; this disruption results in sodium and water retention. Although studies of blood lead levels have not consistently shown an association with high blood pressure, it is important to point out that blood lead levels reflect primarily acute exposure.[1–3] Studies looking at bone lead levels, for example, have clearly documented that exposure to heavy metals is associated with an increased risk for high BP.[4]

Classification of Blood Pressure

- Optimal: systolic under 120, diastolic under 80 mm Hg

- Normal: systolic 120–129, diastolic 80–85 mm Hg
- Borderline high blood pressure (prehypertension): systolic 130–139, diastolic 85–89 mm Hg
- Mild high blood pressure (stage 1): systolic 140–159, diastolic 90–99 mm Hg
- Moderate high blood pressure (stage 2): systolic 160–179, diastolic 100–109 mm Hg
- Severe high blood pressure (stage 3): systolic 180 or over, diastolic 110 mm Hg or over

"White-Coat Hypertension"

"White-coat hypertension" has been defined as the elevation of blood pressure in a clinic or doctor's office only. The prevalence of white-coat hypertension may be as high as 20 to 45% of people diagnosed as having high BP.[5] It appears to be more frequent in women and older patients. The current conventional wisdom among naturopathic physicians is to treat white-coat hypertension as if it were real, as results from recent studies suggest that it is not an innocent phenomenon.[6,7] To rule out white-coat hypertension a patient wears a device to measure blood pressure continuously (ambulatory blood pressure monitoring).[8] In patients with confirmed white-coat hypertension, drug treatment is usually not indicated; instead, treatment should consist of counseling for better stress management, lifestyle and dietary modification, weight reduction, regular exercise, smoking cessation, and correction of blood sugar and cholesterol elevations.

Therapeutic Considerations

Because more than 80% of patients with high BP are in the borderline-to-moderate range, most cases of high BP can be brought under control through changes in diet and lifestyle. In fact, in head-to-head comparisons, many nondrug therapies such as diet, exercise, and relaxation therapies have proved superior to drugs in cases of borderline to mild high BP. For moderate through severe hypertension, drug therapy may be necessary. Ideally, drug treatment should be used only until the dietary, lifestyle, and supplement strategies take hold. However, sometimes long-term drug therapy is required.

Lifestyle

High BP is closely related to lifestyle and dietary factors. The important lifestyle factors include smoking, stress, and lack of exercise. The most important dietary factors include excessive calorie intake; high sodium-to-potassium ratio; low-fiber, high-sugar diet; high consumption of saturated fat and low consumption of essential fatty acids; a diet low in calcium, magnesium, or vitamin C; and excessive alcohol or caffeine intake.

In addition to the following discussions, several of these dietary and lifestyle factors are also discussed in the chapter "Heart and Cardiovascular Health," because the health of the arteries is critical to maintaining normal blood pressure.

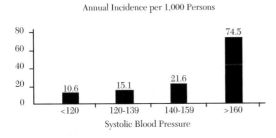

Annual Incidence per 1,000 Persons

High Blood Pressure

Stress

Stress can be the cause of high BP in many instances, although, as in other health conditions, this has more to do with the response to and processing of stress than with stress itself. Relaxation techniques such as deep breathing exercises, biofeedback, transcendental meditation, yoga, progressive muscle relaxation, and hypnosis have all been shown to have some value in lowering blood pressure.[9] Although the effect may be only modest in some cases, a stress reduction technique is nonetheless a necessary component in a natural blood-pressure-lowering program.

One of the most powerful ways to manage stress and have more energy is diaphragmatic breathing. Regular, short sessions of slow and regular diaphragmatic breathing have also been shown to lower blood pressure in several studies.[10–12] In one study, volunteers with normal blood pressure were taught shallow breathing. Measurement of the amount of sodium and potassium excreted in the urine indicated that shallow breathing led to the retention of sodium in the body. It was suggested that this breathing pattern may play a causative role in some cases of high BP.[13] In contrast, deep, slow breathing (six breaths per minute) has been shown to improve oxygen saturation, exercise tolerance, and blood pressure monitoring by the body's pressure sensors.[14]

RESPeRATE is a medical device that interactively guides the user toward slow and regular breathing by voluntarily synchronizing respiration to musical tones. When used for 15 minutes per day, this device can lead to significant reduction in blood pressure. In one eight-week study, systolic BP was reduced by 10.0 mm Hg and diastolic BP by 3.6 mm Hg in the subjects who used RESPeRATE, but not in the controls; greater BP reduction was observed with increased compliance with device usage.[15]

Exercise

Population-based studies have consistently demonstrated an inverse association between physical activity (or fitness) and blood pressure. The more fit a person is, the less likely he or she is to have high BP. In addition, clinical trials involving hypertensive patients have clearly established regular exercise as an effective treatment for high BP.[16–20] Although it is generally thought that the greater the intensity of aerobic exercise, the greater the blood-pressure-lowering effect, recently it was shown that even as little as 20 minutes of mild to moderate aerobic exercise three times per week can lower blood pressure.[20] The degree of blood pressure reduction achieved by adopting a regular exercise program is typically in the range of 5 to 10 mm Hg for both the systolic and the diastolic readings. Patients with borderline and mild hypertension typically can bring blood pressure readings into the normal range with regular exercise.

Diet

The most important dietary goal for most patients with any form of high BP is achieving normal body weight. Weight loss can lead to significant improvement in and even complete elimination of the problem; it can also reduce the number of prescription drugs a person needs to take.[21,22]

Next to attaining ideal body weight, perhaps the most important dietary recommendation is to increase the proportion of plant foods in the diet. Vegetarians generally have lower blood pressure and a lower incidence of high BP and other cardiovascular diseases than nonvegetarians.[23] Although dietary levels of sodium do not differ significantly between these two groups, a vegetarian's diet typically contains more potassium, complex carbohydrates, beneficial oils, fiber, calcium, magnesium, and vitamin C and less saturated fat and refined carbohydrate; all of these factors have a favorable influence on blood pressure.

Increasing fruit and vegetable intake has been shown to lower blood pressure.[24] This effect may be the result of increasing antioxidant concentrations. People with high BP have been shown to have increased oxidative stress, and dietary antioxidants have been shown to produce some benefits in high BP.[25,26]

The most useful foods for people with high BP include the following:

- Celery
- Garlic and onions
- Nuts and seeds or their oils
- Cold-water fish (e.g., salmon, mackerel)
- Green leafy vegetables, for their rich content of calcium and magnesium
- Whole grains and legumes
- Foods rich in vitamin C, such as broccoli and citrus fruits
- Foods rich in flavonoids, including berries, cherries, grapes, and red kidney beans

Celery is a particularly interesting recommendation for high BP. It contains 3-n-butylphthalide, a compound that has been found to lower blood pressure. In animals, a small amount of this compound lowered blood pressure by 12 to 14% and cholesterol by about 7%.[27] The equivalent dose in humans can be supplied by about four to six ribs of celery. The research was prompted by the father of one of the researchers, who, after eating ¼ lb of celery per day for one week, observed that his blood pressure had dropped from 158/96 to 118/82.

Garlic and onions are also important foods for lowering blood pressure. Although most recent research has focused on the cholesterol-lowering properties of garlic and onions, both have been shown to lower blood pressure in people with high BP. In addition, commercial garlic supplements may be of benefit. In a meta-analysis of published clinical trials of garlic preparations that included a total of 415 subjects, subjects who were given a dried garlic powder standardized to contain 1.3% alliin at a dosage of 600 to 900 mg per day (corresponding to 7.8 or 11.7 mg alliin, the equivalent of approximately 1.8 to 2.7 g fresh garlic per day) saw a typical drop of 11 mm Hg in systolic blood pressure and 5 mm Hg in diastolic blood pressure over a period of one to three months.[28]

The Dietary Approaches to Stop Hypertension (DASH) Diet

The Dietary Approaches to Stop Hypertension (DASH) clinical studies were funded by the National Heart, Lung, and Blood Institute to fully evaluate the efficacy of a system of dietary recommendations in the treatment of high BP. The DASH diet is rich in fruits, vegetables, and low-fat dairy foods and low in saturated and total fat. It is also low in cholesterol; high in dietary fiber, potassium, calcium, and magnesium; and moderately high in protein.

The first study showed that a diet rich in fruits, vegetables, and low-fat dairy products can reduce blood pressure in the general population and people with high BP.[29] The original DASH diet did not require either sodium restriction or weight loss—the two traditional dietary tools to control blood pressure—to be effective.[30] The second study from the DASH research group found that coupling the original DASH diet with sodium restriction is more effective than either the DASH diet alone or restricting sodium alone.[31] In the first trial, the DASH diet produced a net blood pressure reduction of 11.4 and 5.5 mm Hg systolic and diastolic, respectively, in patients with high BP. In the second trial, sodium intake was also quantified at a "higher" intake of 3,300 mg per day,

Components of the DASH Eating Plan				
FOOD GROUP	**SERVINGS PER DAY**	**SERVING SIZE**	**EXAMPLES**	**SIGNIFICANCE OF EACH FOOD GROUP IN THE DASH DIET**
Vegetables	4–5	1 cup raw leafy vegetables ½ cup cooked vegetables 6 fl oz vegetable juice	Tomatoes, potatoes, carrots, peas, squash, broccoli, turnip greens, collards, kale, spinach, artichokes, sweet potatoes, beans	Rich sources of potassium, magnesium, and fiber
Fruits	4–5	6 fl oz fruit juice 1 medium fruit ¼ cup dried fruit ½ cup fresh, frozen, or canned fruit	Apricots, bananas, dates, oranges, orange juice, grapefruit, grapefruit juice, mangoes, melons, peaches, pineapples, prunes, raisins, strawberries, tangerines	Important sources of potassium, magnesium, and fiber
Low-fat or nonfat dairy foods	2–3	8 fl oz milk 1 cup yogurt 1.5 oz cheese	Skim or 1% milk, skim or low-fat buttermilk, nonfat or low-fat yogurt, part-skim mozzarella cheese, nonfat cheese	Major sources of calcium and protein
Meats, poultry, and fish	2 or less	3 oz cooked meats, poultry, or fish	Select only lean; trim away visible fats; broil, roast, or boil, instead of frying; remove skin from poultry	Rich sources of protein and magnesium
Nuts, seeds, and legumes	4–5 per week	1.5 oz or ⅓ cup nuts ½ oz or 2 tbsp seeds ½ cup cooked legumes	Almonds, filberts, mixed nuts, peanuts, walnuts, sunflower seeds, kidney beans, lentils	Rich sources of energy, magnesium, potassium, protein, and fiber

an "intermediate" intake of 2,400 mg per day, and a "lower" intake of 1,500 mg per day. Compared with the control diet, the DASH diet was associated with a significantly lower systolic blood pressure at each sodium level. The DASH diet with the lower sodium level led to a mean systolic blood pressure that was 7.1 mm Hg lower in participants without hypertension and 11.5 mm Hg lower in participants with hypertension. These results are clinically significant and indicate that a sodium intake below 1,500 mg per day can significantly and quickly lower blood pressure.

Potassium and Sodium

Considerable evidence indicates that a diet low in potassium and high in sodium is associated with high BP and plays a major role in the development of cancer and heart disease.[32,33] There is overwhelming evidence that dietary sodium chloride (salt) is a major cause of raised blood pressure, and that a modest reduction in salt intake lowers blood pressure; this is predicted to reduce cardiovascular disease, as there is a direct relation between salt intake and cardiovascular risk.[34] Conversely, a diet high in potassium and low in sodium is protective against these diseases. In the case of high BP, as evident in the second DASH study and others, this type of diet can be therapeutic.

It is a well-established fact that excessive consumption of dietary sodium chloride, coupled with diminished dietary potassium, is a common cause of high BP in many people. Some people are sensitive to salt and others are not, but as of 2012 there is no way to identify those who are salt sensitive except by restricting salt intake and seeing the effect. However, while salt restriction is important, numerous studies have shown that sodium restriction alone does not significantly improve blood pressure control in many cases—it must be accompanied by a high potassium

intake. In a typical Western diet only 5% of sodium intake comes from the natural constituents in food. Prepared foods contribute 45% of the sodium intake, 45% is added during cooking, and another 5% is added as a condiment.

Most Americans have a potassium-to-sodium (K:Na) ratio of less than 1:2. Epidemiological and experimental research suggests that a dietary K:Na ratio greater than 5:1 is necessary to maintain health. However, even this level may not be optimal. A natural diet rich in fruits and vegetables can produce a K:Na ratio greater than 100:1, as most fruits and vegetables have a K:Na ratio of at least 50:1.

Many studies have now shown that increasing dietary potassium intake can lower blood pressure.[35] In addition, several studies have shown that potassium supplementation alone can produce significant reductions in blood pressure in hypertensive subjects. In a meta-analysis of 33 randomized, controlled trials totaling 2,609 participants, potassium supplementation was associated with a reduction in mean systolic and diastolic blood pressure of 4.44 and 2.45 mm Hg, respectively. The effects of potassium supplementation appeared to be enhanced in subjects who had a high intake of sodium, indicating that potassium is important for prevention and treatment of high BP in those who are unable to reduce their intake of sodium. The dosage of potassium typically used in the studies ranged from 2.5 to 5 g per day.

In one study, 37 adults with mild hypertension received either 2.5 g per day of potassium, 2.5 g per day of potassium plus 480 mg per day of magnesium, or a placebo for eight weeks, and then were crossed over to receive one of the other treatments for another eight weeks and then crossed over again to receive the third treatment for an additional eight weeks.[36] The potassium supplementation lowered systolic blood pressure an average of 12 mm Hg and diastolic blood pressure an average of 16 mm Hg. Interestingly, the addition of magnesium offered no further reduction in blood pressure; nonetheless, other studies have showed magnesium supplementation to be helpful (this is discussed later).

Potassium supplementation may be especially useful in the treatment of high BP in people older than 65, who often do not fully respond to BP-lowering drugs. In one double-blind study, 18 untreated elderly patients (average age 75 years) with a systolic blood pressure greater than 160 mm Hg or a diastolic blood pressure greater than 95 mm Hg, or both, were given either potassium chloride (2.5 g potassium) or a placebo each day for four weeks.[37] After this relatively short treatment period, the group receiving the potassium experienced a drop of 12 mm Hg in systolic blood pressure and 7 mm Hg in diastolic blood pressure. These results compare quite favorably with the reduction of blood pressure produced by drug therapy, but without the side effects.[38]

Potassium supplements are available by prescription as well as over the counter. However, the FDA restricts the amount of potassium available in over-the-counter potassium supplements to a mere 99 mg per dose because of problems associated with high-dosage prescription potassium salts. Yet salt substitutes such as the popular brands NoSalt and Nu-Salt are, in fact, potassium chloride and provide 530 mg potassium per ⅙ tsp. Potassium salts are commonly prescribed in the dosage range of 1.5 to 3 g per day, but at these high dosages they can cause nausea, vomiting, diarrhea, and ulcers when given in pill form. These effects are not seen when potassium levels are increased through the diet or through the use of potassium-based salt substitutes. This difference highlights the advantages of using foods or food-based potassium supplements rather than pills to meet the human body's high potassium requirements.

Potassium supplementation is relatively safe, except for patients with kidney disease. Their inability to excrete excess potassium may result in heart arrhythmias and other consequences of potassium toxicity. Potassium supplementation is also contraindicated when a patient is using any of a number of prescription medications including digitalis, potassium-sparing diuretics, and the ACE inhibitor class of antihypertensive drugs.

Caffeine

Caffeine consumption from coffee, tea, and other sources can produce an immediate, short-lived increase in blood pressure, and regular coffee drinking has been associated with a slight increases in blood pressure, but it is generally thought that habitual coffee or tea drinkers develop a tolerance to the hypertensive effects of caffeine.[39-41] However, some studies showed that repeated administration of caffeine produced a persistent blood-pressure-increasing effect. For example, in 11 short-term trials looking at the effect of caffeine consumption (ranging from 14 to 79 days), average consumption was five cups of coffee per day, and this was associated with an increase of 2.4 mm Hg in systolic blood pressure and 1.2 mm Hg in diastolic blood pressure.[42] Although the overall benefit of long-term avoidance of caffeine (from coffee, tea, chocolate, cola drinks, and some medications) on blood pressure is unclear, it appears that because some patients seem to respond quite favorably to caffeine avoidance, it should at least be attempted in patients with hypertension.

Nutritional Supplements

Magnesium

Potassium interacts in many body systems with magnesium, and low intracellular potassium levels may be the result of low magnesium intake. It is therefore appropriate to use supplemental magnesium (400 mg to 1,200 mg per day in divided dosages) along with potassium. This supplementation may also lower blood pressure.

A meta-analysis of 14 clinical trials that tested the effects of magnesium supplementation on high BP demonstrated clear dose-dependent blood pressure reductions—a drop of 4.3 mm Hg systolic and 2.3 mm Hg diastolic for each 10 mmol/day increase in magnesium dose.[43]

In one double-blind clinical study 21 male patients with high BP were given 600 mg per day of magnesium (as magnesium oxide) or a placebo.[44] Mean blood pressure (the average between systolic and diastolic) decreased from 111 to 102 mm Hg. The patients who responded the best were those with reduced red blood cell potassium. After therapy with magnesium, the levels of intracellular sodium, potassium, and magnesium normalized, suggesting that one of the ways magnesium lowers blood pressure is through activation of the cellular membrane pump, which pumps sodium out of, and potassium into, the cell.

Considerable evidence indicates that in population studies a high intake of magnesium is associated with lower blood pressure. The principal source of magnesium in early studies was water. Water that is high in minerals such as magnesium is often referred to as "hard." Numerous studies have demonstrated an inverse correlation between water hardness and high BP.[45]

These early studies gave way to more extensive dietary studies looking at the association of magnesium with high BP. These dietary studies found the same results as the studies of hard water. In one of the most extensive studies—the Honolulu Heart Study—systolic blood pressure was 6.4 mm Hg lower and diastolic blood pressure 3.1 mm Hg lower in the highest magnesium intake group compared with the lowest magnesium intake group.[46]

The studies of magnesium supplementation in the treatment of high BP have yielded mixed results. Although the overall results in a very detailed analysis of the data are quite favorable, the hypertensive patients who respond best appear to be those taking a diuretic, those with low RBC magnesium, or those with elevated intracellular sodium or decreased intracellular potassium.

The recommended intake for magnesium in cases of high BP appears to be approximately 6 to 10 mg/kg per day. Magnesium is available in several different forms. Although most are equally well absorbed, magnesium bound to organic compounds (aspartate, malate, succinate, fumarate, or citrate) is usually preferable to magnesium bound to mineral salts (oxide, gluconate, sulfate, or chloride).[47,48] In addition, magnesium aspartate, malate, succinate, fumarate, or citrate may also help with fatigue, as the binding compounds are involved in the Krebs cycle, the final common pathway for the conversion of glucose, fatty acids, and amino acids to chemical energy. Minerals chelated to the Krebs cycle intermediates are better absorbed, used, and tolerated compared with inorganic mineral salts. In addition, although inorganic magnesium salts often cause diarrhea at higher dosages, organic forms of magnesium usually do not.

Like potassium, magnesium supplementation must be used with great care in patients with kidney disease.

Calcium

Population-based studies have suggested a link between high BP and a low intake of calcium. However, the association is not as strong as the one for magnesium and potassium. In addition to the epidemiological data, several clinical studies have demonstrated that calcium supplementation can lower blood pressure in cases of high BP, but the results have been inconsistent.[49]

To clarify the effectiveness of calcium supplementation for patients with high BP, one double-blind, placebo-controlled study was performed on 46 patients with either salt-sensitive or salt-resistant hypertension.[50] During the calcium supplementation phase, patients received 1.5 g per day of calcium (as calcium carbonate) for eight weeks. The calcium supplementation was found to effectively reduce blood pressure in blacks and in patients who were salt-sensitive, but not in patients who had salt-resistant hypertension. Better results have been found for calcium citrate vs. calcium carbonate.[51]

Another group that appears to respond to calcium supplementation is the elderly with high BP. One study used monitoring of blood pressure to evaluate the effect of calcium supplementation on mild to moderate hypertension in elderly hospitalized patients. The mean systolic and diastolic blood pressures over a period of 24 hours declined by 13.6 mm Hg and 5 mm Hg, respectively, in patients whose diets were supplemented with 1 g elemental calcium.[52]

Vitamin C

Population-based and clinical studies have shown that the higher the intake of vitamin C, the lower the blood pressure. The results from several preliminary studies showing a modest blood-pressure-lowering effect with vitamin C supplementation in people with mild elevations of blood pressure have been confirmed in two recent double-blind trials.[53,54] One of the key findings of these studies was that a daily dosage of 500 mg produced the same benefit as higher dosages (1,000 and 2,000 mg per day). Vitamin C supplementation can produce decreases of up to 4.5 mm Hg in systolic pressure and 2.5 mm Hg for diastolic pressure.

One of the ways vitamin C exerts this antihypertensive effect is by promoting the excretion of lead. Chronic exposure to lead from environmental sources including drinking water is associated with hypertension and increased cardiovascular mortality. Areas with a soft water supply often have an increased lead concentration in drinking water due to the greater acidity of the water, and people living in these areas may be predisposed to hypertension. It should be noted that soft water is also low in calcium and magnesium, two minerals that have been shown to protect against hypertension.

Vitamin C is likely to be more effective when used with other antioxidant nutrients. The combination of 500 mg vitamin C, 600 mg alpha-tocopherol, 200 mg zinc sulfate, and 30 mg beta-carotene per day produced mild reductions in systolic blood pressure compared with a placebo both in subjects receiving antihypertensive therapy and in those who had normal blood pressure.[55]

Folic Acid and Vitamin B$_6$

Folic acid and vitamin B$_6$ reduce levels of plasma homocysteine, a known contributor to atherosclerosis. A two-year trial of folic acid and B$_6$ therapy to lower homocysteine was associated with a 3.7-mm-Hg lower systolic and a 1.9-mm-Hg lower diastolic blood pressure.[56] Vitamin B$_6$ supplementation alone has also been shown to lower blood pressure. In one study, vitamin B$_6$ supplementation at a single oral daily dosage of 5 mg/kg for four weeks in 20 people with hypertension demonstrated significant reductions in blood pressure (systolic pressure dropped from 167 to 153 mm Hg, and diastolic pressure dropped from 108 to 98 mm Hg) as well as in serum norepinephrine levels.[57]

Omega-3 Fatty Acids

Increasing the intake of omega-3 fatty acids can lower blood pressure. More than 60 double-blind studies have demonstrated that fish oil supplements are effective in lowering blood pressure.[58,59] However, the effect is modest. Typically, fish oils produced a reduction of 2.1 mm Hg for systolic blood pressure and 1.6 mm Hg for diastolic blood pressure at a typical dosage of 3,000 mg EPA + DHA per day. Flaxseed oil may also lower BP. The key to getting results with flaxseed oil may require reducing the intake of saturated fat and omega-6 fatty acids. In one study 1 tbsp per day of flaxseed oil along with a reduction in the intake of saturated fat resulted in a drop of up to 9 mm Hg in both the systolic and the diastolic readings.[60] Another study found that for every absolute 1% increase in body alpha-linolenic acid content, there was a decrease of 5 mm Hg in the systolic, diastolic, and mean blood pressures.[61]

Arginine

Arginine is important for the formation of nitric oxide, a compound that plays a central role in relaxing blood vessels, thereby improving blood flow, and in improving kidney function. Normally, the body makes enough arginine, even when it is lacking in the diet. However, in some instances the body may not be able to keep up with increased requirements, and supplementation may prove useful. In high BP, even in mild cases, there appears to be a problem with nitric oxide production, especially in the kidneys.

Arginine supplementation has been shown to be beneficial in a number of cardiovascular diseases, including hypertension. By increasing nitric oxide levels, arginine supplementation improves blood flow, reduces blood clot formation, and improves blood fluidity. In hypertension, the degree of improvement offered by arginine supplementation can be quite significant in some cases,[62,63] but in general a dosage of 4 g three times per day will produce only modest decreases (e.g., 5 mm Hg) in systolic BP with little meaningful change in diastolic BP.[64] Arginine supplementation may prove to be most beneficial in younger subjects with high BP, as older subjects appear to have less effective nitric-oxide-dependent mechanisms. In a study of younger and older subjects with high BP, intravenous arginine induced a significant increase in kidney blood flow, filtration rate, and sodium excretion in the younger subjects.[65] These effects were not observed in older subjects.

Anti-ACE Peptides

Various naturally occurring peptides have been shown to inhibit angiotensin-converting enzyme (ACE), which plays in role in processes that constrict large blood vessels and cause the kidneys to hold on to more sodium. The most thoroughly studied of these peptides is derived from a fish called bonito (a member of the tuna family).[66–69] Anti-ACE bonito peptides do not appear to produce the side effects typical of ACE inhibitor drugs, according to human safety studies, and do not lower blood pressure in people with normal blood pressure—even when administered at levels 20 times greater than the dosage that reduces blood pressure in people with high BP. A possible reason is that their mechanism of action in inhibiting ACE is different from that of the drugs. Research bears out this theory. ACE converts angiotensin I to angiotensin II by cleaving off a small peptide. Drugs work by directly blocking this action. By contrast, naturally occurring anti-ACE peptides react with the peptides instead of with angiotensin.

Four clinical studies (three with the bonito peptides and one with a dipeptide from sardine) have shown that fish-derived anti-ACE peptides exert significant blood-pressure-lowering effects in people with high BP.[67-70] Systolic blood pressure was typically reduced by at least 10 mm Hg and diastolic by 7 mm Hg in people with borderline and mild hypertension. Greater reductions are seen in people with higher initial blood pressure readings.

Coenzyme Q$_{10}$ (CoQ$_{10}$)

Coenzyme Q$_{10}$, also known as ubiquinone, is an essential component of the mitochondria. Although CoQ$_{10}$ can be synthesized within the body, deficiency states have been reported, especially in those taking statin drugs. CoQ$_{10}$ deficiency has been shown to be present in 39% of patients with hypertension. This finding alone suggests a need for CoQ$_{10}$ supplementation. However, CoQ$_{10}$ appears to provide benefits beyond correction of a deficiency.

The majority of studies exploring CoQ$_{10}$ in the treatment of high BP have been uncontrolled, or have used CoQ$_{10}$ in combination with conventional antihypertensive medical treatments, so these studies are difficult to interpret. A Cochrane review of CoQ$_{10}$ in the treatment of hypertension (12 clinical trials, 362 patients) concluded that in hypertensive patients, CoQ$_{10}$ has the potential to lower systolic and diastolic blood pressure without significant side effects.[71] Among all included studies, decreases in systolic blood pressure ranged from 11 to 17 mm Hg and decreases in diastolic blood pressure from 8 to 10 mm Hg. In 3 of the 12 studies CoQ$_{10}$ was given in addition to existing antihypertensive medication, and in one of these more than 50% of the patients were able to cease taking at least one antihypertensive medication during the trial. These results are consistent with some of the uncontrolled studies. For example, in one uncontrolled study, the dosage of CoQ$_{10}$ was adjusted in 109 patients with high BP according to clinical response and blood CoQ$_{10}$ levels (the aim was to attain blood levels over 2 mcg/ml). The average CoQ$_{10}$ dose was 225 mg per day in addition to the patients' usual antihypertensive regimen. The need for antihypertensive medication declined gradually, and after a mean treatment period of 4.4 months, about half of the patients were able to discontinue between one and three drugs.[72]

It is important to keep in mind that the antihypertensive effect of CoQ$_{10}$ is usually not seen until after 4 to 12 weeks of therapy. Thus CoQ$_{10}$ is not a typical blood-pressure-lowering drug; rather, it seems to correct some metabolic abnormality, which in turn has a favorable influence on blood pressure.[73]

Botanical Medicines

Hawthorn

Extracts of hawthorn (*Crataegus* species) berries, as well as of the flowering tops, are widely used by naturopathic physicians in Europe because of their cardiovascular activity. Several studies including double-blind trials have demonstrated that hawthorn extracts are effective in lowering blood pressure and improving heart function.[74,75] However, the blood-pressure-lowering effect of hawthorn is mild, and the extracts usually need to be taken for at least two to four weeks before any effects are seen.

Olive

The leaves of the olive tree (*Olea europaea*) have been used since ancient times to combat high BP, and recent animal and human studies support their use as an antihypertensive as well as for lowering cholesterol. The active substances are oleuropein (a polyphenolic iridoid glycoside),[76] oleacein, and oleanolic acid, which act as natural calcium-channel-blocking agents to relax constricted large blood vessels. Hydroxytyrusol is a metabolite of oleuropein that exerts antioxidant effects. Often olive extracts are standardized for hydroxytyrusol, but this compound has no significant effect on BP. Oleuropein is also found in the fruit and oil, but in significantly smaller quantities than in the leaf.

In an initial small, double-blind study of patients with essential hypertension—12 who had never been treated and 18 who were currently on antihypertensive drugs—olive leaf extract at a dosage of 400 mg four times per day for three months produced a modest yet statistically significant decrease of blood pressure with no side effects.[77]

More recent studies have utilized an extract standardized for oleuropein (16 to 24%) and polyphenols. In a preliminary clinical study carried out with 10 sets of identical adult twins with mild hypertension, one of the twins received a dose of either 500 or 1,000 mg per day and the other twin took a matching placebo. After eight weeks, systolic blood pressure remained unchanged from baseline in the placebo group and the group

. . . .

QUICK REVIEW

- **Elevated blood pressure is a major risk factor for heart attack and stroke.**
- **Most cases of borderline to mild hypertension can be treated with nondrug therapies.**
- **Vegetarians generally have lower blood pressure levels and a lower incidence of and other cardiovascular diseases than non-vegetarians.**
- **A high ratio of potassium to sodium in the diet is associated with lower blood pressure.**
- **Relaxation techniques have been shown to have some value in lowering blood pressure.**
- **Population-based and clinical studies have shown that the higher the intake of vitamin C, the lower the blood pressure.**

- **Chronic exposure to lead from environmental sources, including drinking water, is associated with high blood pressure and increased cardiovascular mortality.**
- **CoQ$_{10}$ deficiency has been shown to be present in 39% of patients with high blood pressure, and supplementation with CoQ$_{10}$ can lower blood pressure.**
- **More than 60 double-blind studies have demonstrated that either fish oil supplements or flaxseed oil exert some blood-pressure-lowering effect.**
- **Hawthorn, olive leaf, and hibiscus extracts have shown mild blood-pressure-lowering effects in double-blind studies.**

taking 500 mg per day but had significantly decreased for the group taking 1,000 mg per day (137 vs. 126 mm Hg).[78]

In another study, 232 patients with high BP were given either olive leaf extract (500 mg twice per day) or the conventional antihypertensive drug captopril (12.5 mg twice per day). The average reduction in blood pressure was 11.5 mm Hg systolic and 4.8 mm Hg diastolic in the olive group, compared with 13.7 mm Hg systolic and 6.4 mm Hg diastolic in the captopril group.[79]

Hibiscus

Hibiscus tea and extracts prepared from the dried flowers of *Hibiscus sabdariffa* have demonstrated antihypertensive properties in clinical trials. The active components are anthocyanidin glycosides. One double-blind trial was conducted with 65 prehypertensive and mildly hypertensive adults, 30 to 70 years of age, who were not taking antihypertensive medications. They were given either three 240-ml servings per day of brewed hibiscus tea or a placebo beverage. After six weeks, hibiscus tea had lowered systolic BP compared with the placebo (7.2 vs. 1.3 mm Hg). Diastolic BP was also lower, although this change did not differ from that with the placebo. Participants with higher systolic BP at baseline showed a greater response to hibiscus treatment.[80]

In another double-blind study, the effect of hibiscus tea was compared with black tea in 60 diabetic patients who had mild hypertension but were not taking antihypertensive or lipid-lowering drugs. Average systolic BP in the hibiscus group decreased from 134.4 mm Hg at the beginning of the study to 112.7 mm Hg after one month, while it increased from 118.6 to 127.3 mm Hg in the black tea group. The intervention had no statistically significant effect on diastolic BP in either group.[81]

Another study did show that hibiscus tea had an effect on diastolic BP (reduced by 10.7%) as well as systolic BP (reduced by 11.2%) after 12 days of treatment.[82]

Two clinical studies featured a standardized extract of hibiscus in high BP. In one double-blind study, 193 patients with hypertension were given either hibiscus extract (250 mg total anthocyanins per day) or 10 mg lisinopril (control group). Results showed that the hibiscus extract decreased systolic blood pressure by 17.14 mm Hg and diastolic by 11.97 mm Hg with no side effects, though the lisinopril was more effective. Hibiscus treatment lowered plasma ACE activity by 31 percent.[83]

Similar results with BP were shown in another double-blind study. A standardized hibiscus extract (9.6 mg total anthocyanins per day) was compared with another drug (captopril, 50 mg per day). Results showed no significant differences in lowering blood pressure between the two treatments. Hibiscus extract was able to decrease systolic BP from 139.05 to 123.73 mm Hg and diastolic BP from 90.81 to 79.52 mm Hg.[84]

TREATMENT SUMMARY

We recommend a comprehensive program that utilizes lifestyle, dietary, and supplemental strategies to lower blood pressure. Every effort should be made to achieve and maintain ideal body weight.

Borderline, Mild, or White-Coat Hypertension

- Achieve and maintain ideal body weight. See the chapter "Obesity and

Weight Management" for more information.

- Substantially decrease salt intake.

- Follow a healthful lifestyle. Avoid alcohol, caffeine, and smoking. Exercise and use stress-reduction techniques.

- Follow a high-potassium diet rich in fiber and consistent with either the Mediterranean or the DASH Diet and the recommendations given in the chapter "A Health-Promoting Diet."

- Increase dietary consumption of celery, garlic, and onions.

- Reduce or eliminate the intake of animal fats while increasing the intake of monounsaturated vegetable oils.

- Supplement with the following:
  ○ High-potency multivitamin and mineral formula
  ○ Vitamin C: 500 to 1,000 mg three times/day
  ○ Magnesium (preferably citrate): 6 to 10 mg/kg per day, in divided doses
  ○ Garlic: the equivalent of 4,000 mg per day of fresh garlic
  ○ Omega-3 fatty acids, either fish oils (3 g total EPA + DHA content per day) or flaxseed oil (1 tbsp per day)

If you have tried these recommendations for a period of three months but blood pressure has not returned to normal, follow the recommendations below for moderate hypertension.

Moderate Hypertension:

- All the measures mentioned under "Borderline, Mild, or White-Coat Hypertension"

- CoQ_{10}: 200 to 300 mg per day
- Anti-ACE peptides from bonito: 1,500 mg per day
- One of the following:
  ○ Hawthorn extract (10% proanthocyanidins or 1.8% vitexin-4'-rhamnoside): 100 to 250 mg three times per day
  ○ Olive leaf extract (17% to 23% oleuropein content): 500 mg two times per day
  ○ Hibiscus: three cups of tea per day, or an extract providing 10 to 20 mg anthocyanidins per day

These guidelines should be followed for one to three months. If the blood pressure has not dropped below 140/105, medications to lower blood pressure may be required.

Severe Hypertension

Drug intervention is required. All the measures mentioned previously under "Borderline, Mild, or White-Coat Hypertension" and "Moderate Hypertension" should be employed as well. When satisfactory control over the high BP has been achieved, it may be possible to taper off the medication gradually under a physician's supervision.

High Cholesterol and/or Triglycerides

- Elevations in cholesterol and/or triglycerides above accepted levels

The evidence overwhelmingly demonstrates that elevated cholesterol and triglycerides greatly increase the risk of death due to cardiovascular disease. It is currently recommended that total blood cholesterol be less than 200 mg/dl and triglycerides be lower than 150 mg/dl. In addition, low-density lipoprotein (LDL) cholesterol should be less than 130 mg/dl and high-density lipoprotein (HDL) cholesterol greater than 40 mg/dl in men and 50 mg/dl in women.

LDL and HDL are carriers for cholesterol in the blood. The major categories of lipoproteins are very low-density lipoprotein (VLDL), LDL, and HDL. Because VLDL and LDL are responsible for transporting fats (primarily triglycerides and cholesterol) from the liver to body cells, while HDL is responsible for returning fats to the liver, elevations of either VLDL or LDL are associated with an increased risk for developing atherosclerosis (hardening of the arteries), the primary cause of a heart attack or stroke. In contrast, higher levels of HDL are associated with a lower risk of heart attacks. The real problem is oxidized LDL, which fuels the inflammatory process involved in atherosclerosis, coupled with low levels of HDL.

Determining Risk

The ratios of total cholesterol to HDL cholesterol and LDL to HDL are referred to as the *cardiac risk factor ratios* because they reflect whether cholesterol is being deposited into tissues or broken down and excreted. The total cholesterol-to-HDL ratio should be no higher than 4.2, and the LDL-to-HDL ratio should be no higher than 2.5. The risk for heart disease can be reduced dramatically by lowering LDL cholesterol while simultaneously raising HDL cholesterol levels. For every 1% drop in the LDL cholesterol level, the risk for a heart attack drops by 2%. Conversely, for every 1% increase in HDL levels, the risk for a heart attack drops 3% to 4%.[1]

Although LDL cholesterol is referred to as "bad cholesterol," there are some forms that are worse than others. For example, oxidized LDL is a persistent pro-inflammatory trigger for the progression of atherosclerosis and plaque rupture. Also, smaller, higher-density LDL molecules are associated with greater risk than larger, lower-density LDL molecules.[2] In a small trial of nondiabetic subjects, researchers determined that smaller LDL particles are more likely than larger LDL particles to be attached to sugar molecules (glycated or glycosylated), strongly suggesting an explanation for why these particles are more likely to participate in the process of atherosclerosis, and highlighting the importance of avoiding high blood sugar levels and subsequent glycation.[3]

Another marker that deserves mention is Lp(a), a plasma lipoprotein whose structure and composition closely resemble that of LDL but which has an additional molecule of an adhesive protein called apolipoprotein(a) that helps the LDL stick to the walls of the artery. Elevated plasma levels of Lp(a) are an independent risk factor for coronary heart disease, particularly in patients with elevated LDL cholesterol. In fact, in one analysis a high level of Lp(a) was shown to carry with it a 10 times greater risk for heart disease than an elevated LDL cholesterol level alone.[4] Levels of Lp(a) below 20 mg/dl are associated with a low risk for heart disease; levels between 20 and 40 mg/dl are associated with a moderate risk; and levels above 40 mg/dl are associated with an extremely high risk for heart disease.

Elevations of Triglycerides

In the past, the relation between elevations of blood triglycerides (hypertriglyceridemia) and coronary heart disease has been uncertain. However, a large body of accumulating evidence indicates that elevated triglycerides are an independent risk factor for cardiovascular disease.[5,6] When elevated triglycerides are combined with elevations in LDL cholesterol, the result is a recipe for an early heart attack. In one analysis, high triglycerides combined with elevated LDL cholesterol and a high LDL:HDL ratio (greater than 5) increased the risk of coronary heart disease by approximately sixfold.

Inherited Elevations of Cholesterol and Triglycerides

Elevations of blood cholesterol, triglycerides, or both can be due to genetic factors. These conditions are referred to as familial hypercholesterolemia (FH), familial hypertriglyceridemia (FT), and familial combined hyperlipidemia (FCH). Relatively speaking, these disorders are among the most common inherited diseases, as they affect about 1 in every 500 people.

The basic problem in FH is a defect in the receptor protein for LDL in the liver. Under normal situations the LDL receptor is responsible for removing cholesterol from the blood. When the liver cell takes up the LDL after it has bound to the receptor, it signals the liver cell to stop making cholesterol. In FH the result of the defect in the LDL re-

Recommended Cholesterol and Triglyceride Levels		
	LEVEL (MG/DL)	**RESULT**
Total cholesterol	<200	Desirable
	200–239	Borderline
	≥240	High
LDL cholesterol	<100*	Desirable
	100–130	Borderline
	130–159	Borderline high risk
	≥160	High risk
HDL cholesterol	<35	Low (undesirable)
	35–59	Normal
	≥60	Desirable
Triglycerides	<150	Desirable
	150–199	Borderline high
	200–499	High
	>500	Very high

* For very high-risk patients (those having cardiovascular disease with multiple risk factors such as diabetes, severe and poorly controlled risk factors such as continued smoking, or the presence of metabolic syndrome), the goal is <70 mg/dl for LDL.

ceptor is that the liver does not receive the message to stop making cholesterol.

Damage to the LDL receptor occurs with normal aging and in several disease states, with diabetes being chief among them owing to increased glycosylation of the receptor proteins. As a result of LDL receptor damage, cholesterol levels tend to rise with age. In addition, a diet high in saturated fat and cholesterol decreases the number of LDL receptors, thereby reducing the feedback mechanism that tells the liver cell that no more cholesterol is necessary.

Fortunately, lifestyle and dietary changes can increase the function or number of LDL receptors, or both. The most dramatic effects are in people without inherited causes of elevated cholesterol or triglycerides, or both, but even people with FH can benefit.

FCH and FT result in defects similar to those seen in FH. In FCH the basic defect appears to be an accelerated production of VLDL in the liver. People with FCH may have only a high blood triglyceride level, only a high cholesterol level, or both. In FT there is only an elevation in blood triglyceride levels, and HDL cholesterol levels tend to be low. The defect in FT is that the VLDL particles made by the liver are larger than normal and carry more triglycerides. FT is made worse by diabetes, gout, and obesity.

Therapeutic Considerations

Lowering total cholesterol as well as LDL cholesterol and triglycerides is clearly associated with reducing the risk of cardiovascular disease. Most of the benefits noted with lowering LDL are based on a large number of randomized clinical trials involving the use of statin drugs (HMG CoA reductase inhibitors). Statin drugs owe their origin to

red yeast (*Monascus purpureus*) fermented on rice. This traditional Chinese medicine has been used for more than 2,000 years. Red yeast rice is the source of a group of compounds known as monacolins (such as lovastatin, also known as monacolin K). The marketing of an extract of red yeast rice standardized for monacolin content as a dietary supplement in the United States caused controversy in 1997 because it contained a natural source of a prescription drug. The FDA eventually ruled that red yeast rice products could be sold only if they were free of monacolin content. Nonetheless, it appears some red yeast products on the market do contain these compounds.

In high risk patients the data are clear that statin drugs can produce decreases in total mortality, cardiovascular events, hospitalizations, and the need for revascularization procedures. The debate remains whether statin therapy represents the optimal treatment approach to primary prevention of coronary artery disease in patients whose only risk factor is elevated LDL, especially in light of the growing importance of risk factors such as C-reactive protein and nutritional factors.[7,8] For example, one interesting study compared the Portfolio Diet (which emphasizes plant-based cholesterol-lowering foods) with lovastatin.[9] The participants were randomly assigned to a control diet low in saturated fat, the control diet plus 20 mg lovastatin per day, or a diet like the Portfolio Diet (high in plant sterols, soy protein, soluble fiber, and almonds). After one month, the control, statin, and Portfolio Diet groups had mean decreases in LDL of 8%, 30.9%, and 28.6%, respectively. Respective reductions in C-reactive protein were 10%, 33.3%, and 28.2%. This study and subsequent studies show that including a diverse array of cholesterol-lowering components in the diet (as in the Portfolio Diet) increased the effectiveness of diet as a treatment for hypercholesterolemia, producing results comparable to a statin drug but without the side effects.[10,11]

The best clinical approach is not to rely on a single supplement, but rather to incorporate a broad-spectrum dietary approach that has a wide array of components shown to positively affect lipid levels (reducing saturated fat, trans-fatty acids, and cholesterol, as well as increasing monounsaturated fats, soluble fiber, and nuts). For example, while a meta-analysis of 27 randomized, controlled trials demonstrated that soy protein supplementation reduced total cholesterol, LDL, and triglycerides, the effect was greater when the soy protein was used in conjunction with other dietary interventions.[12] In addition, the effects of isolated soy protein appear to be considerably less than those of increasing soy food consumption in general.[13] Much of the cholesterol-lowering effect of soy foods may relate more to soy's isoflavone and soluble fiber content than to the protein.

Despite research documenting the benefits of nondrug approaches, it is unlikely that they will replace the use of statin drugs as a primary therapy anytime soon. In 2011, more than one of every six adults—nearly 40 million people—took a statin drug to lower LDL. Therefore, the focus for many will be on how to support statin therapy. For example, it appears that individuals taking statins need supplemental coenzyme Q_{10}. HMG-CoA reductase is required not only for the synthesis of cholesterol but also for the production of CoQ_{10}. Thus administration of statins might compromise CoQ_{10} status by decreasing its synthesis. Even modest dosages of various statins have been shown to lower blood CoQ_{10} levels. Researchers have concluded that inhibition of CoQ_{10} synthesis by statin drugs could explain the most commonly reported side effects, especially

fatigue and muscle pain, as well as the more serious side effects such as rhabdomyolysis.[14,15] CoQ_{10} supplementation in subjects on statin drugs has also been shown to reduce markers of oxidative damage.

Elevations in cholesterol may be the result of low thyroid function (hypothyroidism); see the chapter "Hypothyroidism."

Dietary Cholesterol

While the liver is the major source of blood cholesterol, dietary cholesterol can be an important contributor. Diets high in cholesterol are associated with an increased risk for heart disease, cancer, and stroke. However, it may turn out that the level of saturated fats in these foods is more relevant than their cholesterol content. This opinion is supported by a statistical analysis of 224 dietary studies carried out over the past 25 years that investigated the relationship between diet and blood cholesterol levels in more than 8,000 subjects.[16] What investigators found was that saturated fat in the diet, not dietary cholesterol, influences blood cholesterol levels most, and that for most people dietary cholesterol has very little effect on blood cholesterol levels. Nonetheless, it is generally recommended that a healthy person should restrict dietary cholesterol intake to 300 mg per day, while someone with high cholesterol or heart disease should consume no more than 200 mg cholesterol per day. In addition, keep saturated fat intake to a bare minimum, certainly no more than 10 to 15 g per day and ideally even less.

The Importance of Soluble Fiber in Lowering Cholesterol

It is well established that the soluble fiber found in legumes, fruit, and vegetables is effective in lowering cholesterol levels.[17] The

Cholesterol and Fat Content of Selected Foods

FOOD	SERVING SIZE	TOTAL FAT (G)	SATURATED FAT (G)	MONOUNSATURATED FAT (G)	POLYUNSATURATED FAT (G)	CHOLESTEROL (MG)
Beef, lean	3 oz	7.9	3.0	3.3	0.3	73
Beef liver, braised	3 oz	4.2	1.6	0.6	0.9	331
Chicken, breast, roasted	3 oz	3.0	0.9	1.1	0.6	72
Chicken, leg, roasted	3 oz	7.2	2.0	2.6	1.7	79
Egg yolk	1 large	5.1	1.6	1.9	0.7	213
Fish, cod	3 oz	0.7	0.1	0.1	0.3	40
Lobster, boiled	3 oz	0.5	0.1	0.1	0.1	61
Pork, lean	3 oz	11.1	3.8	5.0	1.3	79
Shrimp, boiled	3 oz	0.9	0.2	0.2	0.4	166
Turkey, dark, roasted	3 oz	6.1	2.1	1.4	1.8	73
Turkey, light, roasted	3 oz	2.7	0.9	0.5	0.7	59
Cheese, cheddar	1 oz	9.4	6.0	2.7	0.3	30
Ice cream, regular	½ cup	7.2	4.5	2.1	0.3	30
Milk, low-fat (2%)	1 cup	4.7	2.9	1.4	0.2	18
Milk, skim	1 cup	0.4	0.3	0.1	negligible	4
Milk, whole	1 cup	8.2	5.1	2.4	0.3	33
Butter	1 tbsp	11.5	7.2	3.3	0.4	31

greater the degree of viscosity or gel-forming ability, the greater the effect of a particular type of dietary fiber on lowering cholesterol levels; new, highly viscous blends of soluble fiber provide greater effects than single fiber sources.[18,19] The table below shows the effects of various soluble fiber products.[20]

The overwhelming majority of studies have demonstrated that individuals with high cholesterol levels experience significant reductions with frequent oatmeal or oat bran consumption. In contrast, individuals with normal or low cholesterol levels see little change. In individuals with high cholesterol levels (above 200 mg/dl), the daily consumption of the equivalent of 3 g soluble oat fiber typically lowers total cholesterol by 8 to 23%. This is highly significant, as with each 1%

drop in serum cholesterol level there is a 2% decrease in the risk of developing heart disease. One bowl of ready-to-eat oat bran cereal or oatmeal has approximately 3 g fiber. Although oatmeal's fiber content (7%) is less than that of oat bran (15 to 26%), it has been determined that oatmeal's polyunsaturated fatty acids contribute as much to its cholesterol-lowering effects as its fiber content does.

To help lower cholesterol, try to eat 35 g fiber per day from fiber-rich foods (a full listing can be found in Appendix B). Achieving higher fiber intake is associated not only with lower cholesterol levels but also with lower levels of inflammatory mediators such as C-reactive protein.[21]

Impact of Various Sources of Fiber on Serum Cholesterol Levels		
FIBER	DOSAGE (G)	TYPICAL REDUCTION IN TOTAL CHOLESTEROL (%)
Oat bran (dry)	50–100	15–20
PGX	3	10–15
Guar gum	9–15	10
Pectin	6–10	5
Psyllium	10–20	10–20
Vegetable fiber	27	10

The Use of Fish Oils to Lower Triglyceride Levels

The cardiovascular benefits of the long-chain omega-3 fatty acids EPA and DHA have been demonstrated in more than 300 clinical trials and are detailed in the chapter "Heart and Cardiovascular Health." Supplementation with EPA + DHA has little effect on cholesterol levels but does lower triglyceride levels significantly and has a myriad of additional beneficial effects in protecting against cardiovascular disease.[22] In general, for cardiovascular protection the dosage recommendation is 1,000 mg EPA + DHA per day, but for lowering triglycerides the dosage is 3,000 to 5,000 mg EPA + DHA.[23] Lower dosages of EPA + DHA exert only mild effects on triglyceride levels (e.g., intakes of 200 and 500 mg per day lower triglyceride levels by 3.1% and 7.2% respectively).[24] In one double-blind study, after eight weeks of supplementation a daily dosage of 3.4 g EPA + DHA lowered triglycerides by 27%, while a lower dosage of 0.85 g had no significant effect.[25] These results clearly indicate that lowering triglycerides with fish oils requires dosages of 3 g EPA + DHA per day. In patients with triglyceride levels above 500 mg/dl, approximately 4 g per day of EPA + DHA reduced triglyceride levels by 45%. Fish oils work to lower triglyceride levels by reducing the formation of triglycerides while increasing their breakdown into energy.[26]

The Use of Natural Products to Lower Cholesterol Levels

In many cases dietary therapy, while important, is not sufficient alone to reduce lipid levels to the desired ranges. Fortunately, several natural compounds can lower cholesterol levels and other significant risk factors for cardiovascular disease. In fact, when cost, safety, and effectiveness are all considered, the natural alternatives presented here may offer significant advantages over standard drug therapy, especially when used together rather than as isolated therapies.

Niacin

Since the 1950s niacin (vitamin B_3) has been known to be effective in lowering blood cholesterol levels. In the 1970s the famous Coronary Drug Project demonstrated that niacin was the only cholesterol-lowering agent to actually reduce overall mortality. Niacin typically lowers LDL cholesterol by 16 to 23% while raising HDL cholesterol by 20 to 33%. These effects, especially the effect on HDL, compare quite favorably with those of conventional cholesterol-lowering drugs.[27,28]

It is now known that niacin does much more than lower total cholesterol. Specifically, niacin has been shown to lower LDL, the more harmful Lp(a), triglycerides, C-reactive protein, and fibrinogen while simultaneously raising beneficial HDL. Despite the fact that niacin has demonstrated better overall results in reducing risk factors for coronary heart disease compared with other cholesterol-lowering agents, physicians are often reluctant to prescribe it. The reason is a widespread perception that niacin is difficult to work with because of the bothersome flushing of the skin. In addition, because niacin is a widely available generic agent, it does not offer the drug companies the huge profits that the other lipid-lowering agents have enjoyed. As a result, niacin does not benefit from the intensive research and advertising that focus on the statin drugs. Despite the advantages of niacin over other lipid-lowering drugs, it accounts for less than 10% of all cholesterol-lowering prescriptions. Niaspan, a prescription niacin product, accounted for 952,000 prescriptions in 2002, translating to sales of $145.7 million—a dramatic 73% increase from 2001 levels. By 2010, sales had reached over $927 million, with approximately 100,000 prescriptions per week. The increasing sales of niacin reflect physicians' growing awareness of the advantages of niacin over statin drugs.

Several studies have compared niacin with standard lipid-lowering drugs, including statins. These studies have shown significant advantages for niacin. In the first published clinical study, niacin was compared with lovastatin directly in 136 subjects. Some of these subjects had LDL over 160 mg/dl and coronary heart disease or more than two coronary heart disease risk factors, or both; the others

had LDL cholesterol levels greater than 190 mg/dl and did not have coronary heart disease or had fewer than two coronary heart disease risk factors.[29] In the controlled, randomized, open-label, 26-week study, patients were first placed on a 4-week diet run-in period, after which eligible patients were randomly assigned to receive treatment with either lovastatin (20 mg per day) or niacin (1.5 g per day). On the basis of the LDL cholesterol response and patient tolerance, the doses were sequentially increased to 40 and 80 mg per day of lovastatin or 3 and 4.5 g per day of niacin after 10 and 18 weeks of treatment, respectively. In the two patient groups, 66% of those treated with lovastatin and 54% of those treated with niacin reached the maximum dose. The results (see the table below) indicate that while lovastatin produced a greater LDL cholesterol reduction, niacin provided better overall results despite the fact that fewer patients were able to tolerate a full dosage of niacin because of skin flushing. The percentage increase in HDL cholesterol, a more significant indicator for coronary heart disease, was dramatically in favor of niacin (33% vs. 7%). Equally impressive was the percentage decrease in Lp(a) for niacin. Although niacin produced a 35% reduction in Lp(a) levels, lovastatin did not produce any effect. Niacin's effect on Lp(a) in this study confirmed a previous study that showed niacin (4 g per day) reduced Lp(a)

Comparison of Niacin with Lovastatin				
LIPOPROTEIN	**GROUP**	**WEEK 10 (%)**	**WEEK 18 (%)**	**WEEK 26 (%)**
LDL cholesterol (reduction)	Lovastatin	26	28	32
	Niacin	26	28	32
HDL cholesterol (increase)	Lovastatin	6	8	7
	Niacin	20	29	33
Lp(a) lipoprotein (reduction)	Lovastatin	0	0	0
	Niacin	14	30	35

levels by 38%, and a subsequent study that showed similar reductions in Lp(a) in patients with diabetes.[30,31]

Another comparative study evaluated the lipoprotein responses to niacin, gemfibrozil, and lovastatin in patients with normal total cholesterol levels but low levels of HDL cholesterol.[32] The first phase of the study compared lipoprotein responses with lovastatin and gemfibrozil in 61 middle-aged men; gemfibrozil therapy increased HDL cholesterol levels by 10% and lovastatin increased them by 6%. In the second phase, 37 patients agreed to take niacin; 27 patients finished this phase at a dose of 4.5 g per day. In the second phase, niacin therapy was shown to raise HDL cholesterol by 30%.

Another study compared niacin with atorvastatin (Lipitor).[33] The average dosage was 3,000 mg niacin and 80 mg Lipitor. The patients selected had small, dense LDL particles linked to an increased risk for CVD and low levels of HDL2, a specific fraction of HDL associated with a greater protective effect than HDL alone. Although Lipitor reduced total LDL cholesterol levels substantially more than niacin did, niacin was more effective at increasing LDL particle size and raising HDL and HDL2 than Lipitor was (see the table below).

Because taking niacin at higher dosages (e.g., 3,000 mg or more) can impair glucose tolerance, many physicians have avoided niacin therapy with diabetics, but newer studies using slightly lower dosages (1,000 to 2,000 mg) of niacin have not shown it to adversely affect blood sugar regulation.[34] For example, during a 16-week, double-blind, placebo-controlled trial, 148 type 2 diabetes patients were randomly assigned to receive either a placebo or 1,000 or 1,500 mg per day of niacin; in the niacin-treated groups there was no significant loss in glycemic control, and the favorable effects on blood lipids were still apparent.[35] Other studies have actually shown hemoglobin A1C to drop, indicating improvement in blood sugar control.[34]

The most common blood lipid abnormalities in type 2 diabetic patients are elevated triglyceride levels, decreased HDL levels, and a preponderance of smaller, denser LDL particles. Niacin has been shown to address all of these areas much more significantly than the statins or other lipid-lowering drugs.[33–35]

In addition to lowering cholesterol and triglycerides, niacin exerts additional benefits in battling atherosclerosis. Specifically, in patients with coronary artery disease niacin produces beneficial changes in lipid particle

Effects of Atorvastatin (Lipitor) and Niacin on Lipid Profiles						
VARIABLE	**ATORVASTATIN**		**NIACIN**		**ATORVASTATIN + NIACIN**	
	BEFORE	**AFTER**	**BEFORE**	**AFTER**	**BEFORE**	**AFTER**
Total LDL (mg/dl)	110	56	111	89	123	55
LDL peak diameter	251	256	253	263	250	263
Lipoprotein(a) (mg/dl)	45	44	37	23	54	35
HDL (mg/dl)	42	43	38	54	38	54
HDL2 (%)	30	42	29	43	32	37
Triglycerides (mg/dl)	186	100	194	108	235	73

distribution that are not well reflected in typical lipoprotein analysis. Systemic markers of inflammation decrease in patients receiving niacin as well. In one study of 54 subjects with stable coronary artery disease, when a modest dosage of niacin (1,000 mg per day) was added to existing therapy for three months, there was a 32% increase in large-particle HDL2 (protective), an 8% decrease in small-particle HDL (nonprotective), an 82% increase in large-particle LDL (not associated with increased risk for CVD), and a 12% decrease in small-particle LDL (significantly associated with increased risk for CVD).[36] Niacin therapy also decreased lipoprotein-associated phospholipase A2 and CRP levels (20% and 15%, respectively). No significant changes from baseline were seen in any tested variable in subjects who received a placebo. These results indicate that the addition of niacin to existing medical regimens for patients with coronary artery disease and already well-controlled lipid levels favorably improves the distribution of lipoprotein particle sizes and inflammatory markers in a manner expected to improve cardiovascular protection.

While niacin exerts significant benefit on its own, it does not appear to enhance the benefits of statins in patients whose lipid levels are well controlled. A study funded by the National Heart, Lung, and Blood Institute recruited 3,400 patients who were at risk for heart trouble despite the fact that their LDL cholesterol was under control with the use of the statin drug simvastatin (Zocor). The study ended 18 months early because there was no additional cardiovascular benefit in those taking niacin. Nonetheless, other studies are under way to determine the effect of niacin combined with a statin in patients with very low HDL levels and/or poorly controlled LDL levels.

The side effects of niacin are well known.

The most common and bothersome side effect is the skin flushing that typically occurs 20 to 30 minutes after the niacin is taken. Other occasional side effects of niacin include gastric irritation, nausea, and liver damage. In an attempt to combat the acute skin flushing, several manufacturers began marketing sustained-release, timed-release, or slow-release niacin products. These formulations allow the niacin to be absorbed gradually, thereby reducing the flushing reaction. However, although these forms of niacin reduce skin flushing, early versions of timed-release preparations were proved to be more toxic to the liver than regular niacin. In one analysis 52% of the patients taking an early sustained-release niacin preparation developed liver toxicity, while none of the patients taking immediate-release niacin developed liver toxicity.[37] The newer timed-released preparations on the market, referred to as "intermediate-release," appear to have solved this problem, as relatively large clinical trials have shown them to be extremely well tolerated even when combined with statins.[38–41] For example, the safety and tolerability of intermediate-release niacin preparation was evaluated in a multicenter study of 566 patients.[41] The target dose was achieved by 65% of patients. Flushing was the most common side effect (42%), as expected, and 9.7% withdrew because of it. Other drug-related adverse reactions occurred at a low frequency (18.6%), and 8.7% withdrew for an adverse reaction other than flushing. Most adverse reactions were mild or moderate in severity. There was no liver toxicity or serious adverse muscle event.

Another safe form of niacin is inositol hexaniacinate. This form of niacin has long been used in Europe to lower cholesterol levels and also to improve blood flow in intermittent claudication. It yields slightly better clinical results than standard niacin and is much better tolerated, in terms of both flushing and, more important, long-term side effects.[42,43]

Regardless of the form of niacin you choose to use, your doctor should check your cholesterol and liver function periodically (minimum every three months). Niacin should not be used by anyone with pre-existing liver disease or elevation in liver enzymes. For these people, plant sterols, garlic, and pantethine are recommended.

For best results niacin should be taken at night, as most cholesterol synthesis occurs during sleep. If pure crystalline niacin is being used, begin with a dose of 100 mg a day and increase carefully over four to six weeks to the full therapeutic dose of 1.5 to 3 g per day. If you use an intermediate-release product (do not use any other form of time-release niacin) or inositol hexaniacinate, a 500-mg dosage should be taken at night and increased to 1,500 mg after two weeks. If after one month of therapy the dosage of 1,500 mg per day fails to effectively lower LDL cholesterol, the dosage should be increased to 2,000 mg; if that dosage fails to lower lipids, increase the dosage to 3,000 mg before discontinuing owing to lack of efficacy.

Plant Sterols and Stanols

Phytosterols and phytostanols are structurally similar to cholesterol and can act in the intestine to lower cholesterol absorption by displacing cholesterol from intestinal micelles (an aggregate of water-insoluble molecules, such as cholesterol, surrounded by water-soluble molecules that facilitate absorption into the body). Because phytosterols and phytostanols are poorly absorbed themselves, blood cholesterol levels will drop, owing to increased excretion. These compounds are being added to so-called functional foods (e.g., margarine and other spreads; orange juice) and are also available as dietary supplements.[44]

Phytosterols and phytostanols are effective in lowering LDL in some people. A meta-analysis of 41 trials showed that an intake of 2 g stanols or sterols per day reduced LDL by 10%.[44] Taking higher dosages added little additional benefit. Phytosterols and phytostanols can be used in addition to diet or drug interventions, as they provide additional benefits. For example, eating foods low in saturated fat and cholesterol and high in stanols or sterols can reduce LDL by 20%; adding sterols or stanols to statin medication is more effective than doubling the statin dose. The individuals most likely to respond are those who have been identified as having high cholesterol absorption and low cholesterol biosynthesis. Phytosterols and phytostanols have also shown antiplatelet and antioxidant effects.[45–47]

Be aware, however, that at higher dosages, phytosterols or phytostanols may reduce carotenoid absorption. Human subjects consuming 6.6 g per day of phytosterols showed cholesterol-adjusted plasma reduction of alpha- and beta-carotene levels (19 to 23%), lutein (14%), and lycopene (11%). This effect was partially reversed by increased fruit and vegetable intake.[48]

Pantethine

Pantethine is the stable form of pantetheine, the active form of vitamin B_5 (pantothenic acid). Pantothenic acid is the most important component of coenzyme A, which is involved in the transport of fats to and from cells as well as to the energy-producing compartments within the cell. Without coenzyme A, the cell's fats cannot be metabolized to energy.

Pantethine has significant lipid-lowering activity, while pantothenic acid has little if any effect in lowering cholesterol and triglyceride levels. Pantethine at 900 mg per day has been shown to significantly reduce levels

Effects on Blood Lipids of Several Natural Compounds			
	NIACIN	**GARLIC**	**PANTETHINE**
Total cholesterol (% decrease)	18	10	19
LDL cholesterol (% decrease)	23	15	21
HDL cholesterol (% increase)	32	31	23
Triglycerides (% decrease)	26	13	32

of serum triglyceride (32%), total cholesterol (19%), and LDL cholesterol (21%) while increasing HDL cholesterol (23%).[49,50] It appears to be especially useful in diabetics.[51–53]

The lipid-lowering effects of pantethine are especially impressive because it has virtually no toxicity compared with conventional lipid-lowering drugs.

Garlic

Garlic (*Allium sativum*) appears to be an important protective factor against heart disease and stroke for many reasons. Garlic has been shown to lower blood cholesterol levels even in apparently healthy individuals. In numerous double-blind, placebo-controlled studies of patients with initial cholesterol levels greater than 200 mg/dl, daily supplementation with commercial preparations providing at least 10 mg alliin or a total allicin potential of 4,000 mcg can lower total serum cholesterol by about 10 to 12%, LDL cholesterol by about 15%, and triglycerides by around 15%, with HDL cholesterol levels usually increasing by about 10%. However, most trials not using products that can deliver this dosage of allicin fail to produce a lipid-lowering effect.[54–58]

. . . .

QUICK REVIEW

- **Elevated cholesterol levels in the blood are linked to heart attacks and strokes.**
- **Although in most cases high cholesterol is due to dietary and lifestyle factors, it can also be the result of genetic factors.**
- **Elevations in cholesterol may be the result of low thyroid function (hypothyroidism).**
- **The most important approach to lowering high cholesterol is a healthful diet and lifestyle.**
- **Soluble fiber from the diet and/or supplements can lower cholesterol levels.**
- **Fish oils do not significantly lower cholesterol but do exert exceptional triglyceride-lowering action.**
- **Niacin has been shown to both lower cholesterol and reduce overall early mortality.**
- **Niacin has demonstrated better overall results in reducing the risk for coronary heart disease compared with cholesterol-lowering drugs.**
- **Garlic has a positive effect provided that the dosage of allicin is sufficient.**
- **Pantethine improves cholesterol and triglyceride levels as well as normalizes platelet lipid composition and function and blood viscosity.**

Although the effects of supplemental garlic preparations on cholesterol levels are modest, the combination of lowering LDL and raising HDL can greatly improve the HDL-to-LDL ratio, a significant goal in the prevention of heart disease and strokes. Garlic preparations have also demonstrated blood-pressure-lowering effects, inhibition of platelet aggregation, reduction of plasma viscosity, promotion of fibrinolysis, prevention of LDL oxidation, and positive effects on endothelial function, vascular reactivity, and peripheral blood flow.

TREATMENT SUMMARY

Keep in mind that cholesterol levels are just one piece of the puzzle of reducing cardiovascular disease. A comprehensive perspective is very important. Follow the recommendations given in the chapter "Heart and Cardiovascular Health."

Numerous natural compounds can effectively improve cholesterol and triglyceride levels. Of the several described above, niacin produces the best overall effect. However, the others do have a place in the clinical management of high cholesterol and triglycerides. In particular, the benefits of fish oils extend far beyond their effect on blood lipids.

Typically, along with dietary and lifestyle recommendations, niacin (1,000 mg to 3,000 mg at night) reduces total cholesterol by 50 to 75 mg/dl in patients with initial total cholesterol levels above 250 mg/dl within the first two months. In patients with initial cholesterol levels above 300 mg/dl, it may take four to six months before cholesterol levels begin to reach recommended levels. Once cholesterol levels are below 200 mg/dl for two successive blood measurements at least two months apart, the dosage can be reduced to 500 mg three times per day for two months. If the cholesterol levels creep up above 200 mg/dl, then the dosage of niacin should be raised back up to previous levels. If the cholesterol level remains below 200 mg/dl, then the niacin can be withdrawn completely and the cholesterol levels rechecked in two months, with niacin therapy reinstituted if levels have exceeded 200 mg/dl. The same sort of schedule applies to other natural cholesterol-lowering agents as well.

Hives (Urticaria)

- Hives (urticaria): raised and swollen welts with blanched centers (wheals) that may coalesce to become giant welts. Limited to the superficial portion of the skin.
- Angioedema: Eruptions similar to hives, but with larger swollen areas that involve structures beneath the skin.
- Chronic versus acute: Recurrent episodes of urticaria and/or angioedema of less than six weeks' duration are considered acute, while attacks persisting beyond this period are designated as chronic.
- Special forms: Special forms have characteristic features (dermographism, cholinergic urticaria, solar urticaria, cold urticaria).

Hives (urticaria) are an allergic reaction in the skin characterized by white or pink welts or large bumps surrounded with redness. These lesions are known as wheal and flare lesions and are caused primarily by the release of histamine (an allergic mediator) in the skin. About 50% of patients with hives develop angioedema—a deeper, more serious form involving the tissue below the surface of the skin.

Hives and angioedema are relatively common conditions: it is estimated that 15 to 20% of the general population has had hives at some time. Although persons in any age group may experience acute or chronic hives and/or angioedema, young adults (from the end of adolescence through the third decade of life) are most often affected.[1,2]

The basic cause of hives involves the release of inflammatory mediators from mast cells or basophils—white blood cells that play a key role in allergies. Mast cells are widely distributed throughout the body and are found primarily near small blood vessels, particularly in the skin, while basophils circulate in the blood. The classic allergic reaction occurs as a result of complexes of allergic antibodies (IgE) and antigens (foreign molecules) binding to mast cells and basophils and stimulating the release of histamine and other inflammatory compounds. However, other factors appear to be more important in stimulating the release of histamine in hives.

Causes

Physical Conditions

Hives can be produced as a result of reactions to various physical conditions. The most common forms of physical urticaria are dermographic, cholinergic, and cold urticaria. These are briefly described in the table opposite. Less common types of physical urticaria or angioedema include contact, solar, pressure, heat contact, aquagenic, vibratory, and exercise-induced.

Dermographism
Dermographism, or dermographic urticaria, is a readily elicited hive formation that evolves rapidly when moderate amounts of

Clinical Aspects of Physical Urticarias					
TYPE	**ELICITING STIMULUS**	**TIME OF ONSET**	**DURATION OF LESION**	**DIAGNOSTIC TEST**	**ASSOCIATED SYMPTOMS**
Dermographic	Stroking, scratching	2–5 min	1–5 hr	Firm stroking of skin	Headache, malaise
Cholinergic	Physical exercise; overheating; sauna	2–20 min	30–60 min	Bicycling, running	Headache, mental upset, wheezing, salivation, fainting
Cold urticaria	Cold bath, cold air	2–5 min	1–2 hr	Ice cube, cold arm	Wheezing, fainting
Solar urticaria	Exposure to sunlight	2–15 min	0.25–3 hr	Exposure to UV light	Wheezing, dizziness, fainting
Pressure urticaria	Pressure	3–8 hr	8–24 hr	Locally applied weights	Flu-like syndrome, fever, increased white blood cells, joint pain
Heat contact urticaria	Contact with heat	2–15 min	30–60 min	Hot arm bath	Gastrointestinal upset, dizziness, fatigue, wheezing, shortness of breath
Aquagenic urticaria	Contact with water	2–30 min	30–60 min	Bath, compresses	None
Vibratory angioedema	Vibration	0.5–4 min	1 hr	Vibrating motor	Faintness, headache
Exercise-induced	Exercise	2–5 min	10–30 min	Exercise	Faintness, flushing, disorientation, swollen tongue, shortness of breath, headache
Familial cold	Cold wind, change from cold to warm air	0.5–3 hr	48 hr	Cold wind and subsequent rewarming	Tremor, headache, joint pain

pressure are applied. This pressure may occur as a result of simple contact with another human being, furniture, bracelets, watchbands, towels, or bedding.

The frequency of dermographic urticaria has been estimated at 1.5 to 5% in the general population. It is the most common type of physical urticaria and is found twice as frequently in women as in men, with the average age of onset in the third decade. The incidence is much greater among the obese, especially those who wear tight clothing.

Dermographic lesions usually start within one to two minutes of contact as a generalized redness in the area; this effect is replaced within three to five minutes by a welt and surrounding reflex urticaria. Maximal edema usually occurs within 10 to 15 minutes. While the redness (erythema) generally regresses within an hour, the edema can persist for up to three hours.

Dermographism may be associated with other diseases, including parasite infection, insect bites, hormonal changes, thyroid disorders, pregnancy, menopause, diabetes, immunological alterations, other urticarias, drug therapy (during or following), chronic candidiasis, angioedema, and elevated blood levels of eosinophils (another type of white blood cell linked to allergies).

Cholinergic Urticaria

Cholinergic, or heat-reflex, urticaria (commonly referred to as "prickly heat rash") is the second most frequent type of physical urticaria. These lesions, which depend upon stimulation of the sweat gland, consist of pinpoint wheals surrounded by reflex erythema. The wheals arise at or between hair follicles and develop most often on the upper trunk and arms.

The three basic types of stimuli that may produce cholinergic urticaria are passive overheating, physical exercise, and emotional stress. Typical eliciting activities, besides physical exercise, may include taking a warm bath or sauna, eating hot spices, or drinking alcoholic beverages. The lesions usually arise within 2 to 10 minutes after provocation and last for 30 to 50 minutes.

A variety of systemic symptoms may also occur, suggesting a more generalized mast cell release of the mediators than just in the skin. Headache, swelling around the eyes, tearing, and burning of the eyes are common symptoms. Less frequent symptoms include nausea, vomiting, abdominal cramps, diarrhea, dizziness, low blood pressure, and asthma attacks.

Cold Urticaria

Cold urticaria is a hives reaction of the skin when it comes into contact with cold objects, water, or air. Lesions are usually restricted to the area of exposure and develop within a few seconds to minutes after the removal of the cold object and rewarming of the skin. The lower the object's temperature, the faster the reaction.

Widespread local exposure and generalized hives can be accompanied by flushing, headaches, chills, dizziness, rapid heartbeat, abdominal pain, nausea, vomiting, muscle pain, shortness of breath, wheezing, or unconsciousness. Cold urticaria has been observed to accompany a variety of clinical conditions, including viral infections, parasitic infestations, syphilis, multiple insect bites, penicillin injections, dietary changes, and stress.[1]

Drugs

Drugs are the leading cause of hives in adults. In children, hives are usually due to foods, food additives, or infections. Most drugs are composed of small molecules incapable of inducing antigenic/allergenic activity on their own. Typically, they produce allergic effects by binding to larger molecules and inducing the immune system to develop allergic antibodies to the new molecule complex. Alternatively, drugs can interact directly with mast cells to induce the release of histamine. Many drugs have been shown to produce hives. The two most common drugs that produce hives are antibiotics and aspirin.

Antibiotics

Antibiotics, including penicillin and related compounds, are the most common cause of drug-induced hives. At least 10% of the general population is thought to be allergic to penicillin; of these people, nearly 25% react with hives, angioedema, or anaphylaxis.[2]

Penicillin and related contaminants can exist undetected in foods. It is not known to what degree penicillin in the food supply contributes to hives. However, hives and anaphylactic symptoms have been traced to penicillin in milk,[3] soft drinks,[4] and frozen dinners.[5] In one study of 245 patients with chronic hives, 24% had positive skin tests and 12% a positive RAST (a blood test for allergies; see the chapter "Food Allergy" for further information) for penicillin sensitivity.[6] Of the 42 patients who were sensitive to penicillin, 22 improved clinically on a diet free of dairy products, while only 2 out of 40 patients with negative skin tests improved on the same diet. This study would seem to provide indirect evidence that penicillin in the food supply contributes to hives.

In an attempt to provide direct evidence, penicillin-contaminated pork was given to penicillin-allergic volunteers. No significant reactions were noted other than transient itching in two volunteers.[7] Penicillin in milk appears to be more allergenic than penicillin in meat. Presumably this is because penicillin breaks down into more allergenic compounds in the milk.

Aspirin

The frequency of aspirin sensitivity in patients with chronic hives is at least 20 times greater than it is in people without hives.[8–12] Hives is a more common indicator of aspirin sensitivity than is asthma. In addition to exerting direct effects, aspirin and other non-steroidal anti-inflammatory drugs (NSAIDs) have been shown to dramatically increase gut permeability and increase the absorption of allergens from the digestive tract, which may also trigger hives.

Daily administration of 650 mg aspirin for three weeks has been shown to desensitize patients with hives who have aspirin sensitivity. While taking the aspirin, patients also became nonresponsive to foods to which they usually reacted (pineapple, milk, egg, cheese, fish, chocolate, pork, strawberries, and plums).[13]

Food Allergies

Although any food can be the causative agent, the most common offenders are: milk, fish, meat, eggs, beans, and nuts. Individuals with eczema or asthma are most likely to experience hives as a result of classic allergic (IgE-mediated) mechanisms.

A basic requirement for the development of a food allergy is the absorption of the allergen through the intestinal barrier. Several factors are known to significantly increase gut permeability, including compounds called *vasoactive amines* ingested in foods or produced by bacterial action on essential amino acids, alcohol, NSAIDs, and possibly many food additives. In addition, several investigators have reported alterations in gastric acidity, intestinal motility (contractions of the intestine that propel the food through), and other functions of the digestive tract in up to 85% of patients with chronic hives.[14–17] These alterations may in turn temporarily or permanently alter the barrier and immune function of the gut wall and predispose an individual to allergic reactions.

In one study of 77 patients with chronic hives, 24 (31%) were diagnosed as having no gastric acid output, and 41 (53%) were shown to have low gastric acid output.[16] Treatment with a hydrochloric acid supplement and a vitamin B complex gave impressive clinical results, highlighting the importance of correcting any underlying digestive factor in the treatment of chronic hives. (See the chapter "Digestion and Elimination" for further discussion.)

Food Additives

Food additives are a major factor in many cases of chronic hives in children. Colorants (azo dyes), flavorings (salicylates, aspartame), preservatives (benzoates, nitrites, sorbic acid), preservatives (hydroxytoluene, sulfite, gallate), and emulsifiers/stabilizers (polysorbates, vegetable gums) have all been shown to produce hives in sensitive individuals.

The importance of controlling food additives is demonstrated by a study of 64 patients with hives. After two weeks on an additive-free diet, 73% of the patients had a significant reduction in their symptoms.[17]

Tartrazine

Tartrazine (FD & C Yellow #5) is one of the most widely used colorants that can trigger hives.[18] It is added to almost every packaged food and to many drugs, including some antihistamines, antibiotics, steroids, and sedatives. Reactions to this food additive are so common that its use has been banned in some countries (e.g., Sweden).[19]

In the United States, the average daily per capita consumption of certified dyes is 15 mg, of which 85% is tartrazine. Among children, consumption is usually much higher. Tartra-

zine sensitivity has been estimated to occur in 0.1% of the population; however, we think it is much more common.

Tartrazine sensitivity is extremely common (20 to 50%) in individuals who are sensitive to aspirin.[18] Like aspirin, tartrazine is a known inducer of asthma, hives, and other allergic conditions, particularly in children. Both compounds inhibit the enzyme cyclooxygenase; this inhibition results in a higher production of allergic compounds known as leukotrienes in some individuals. These compounds are roughly 100 times more potent than histamine in producing an allergic reaction.

In addition, tartrazine (as well as benzoate and aspirin) increases the production of lymphokine leukocyte inhibitory factor; this effect results in an increase in the number of mast cells throughout the body. Biopsies of patients with hives show that over 95% have more mast cells than individuals without hives.[20]

Diets that eliminate tartrazine, as well as other food additives, have in many cases been shown to be of great benefit to sensitive individuals.

Food Flavorings

Salicylates (Aspirin-like Compounds). A broad range of salicylic acid esters are used to flavor such foods as cake mixes, puddings, ice cream, chewing gum, and soft drinks. The mechanism of action of these agents is thought to be similar to that of aspirin.

Salicylates are also found naturally in many foodstuffs. Most fruits, especially berries and dried fruits, contains salicylates; raisins and prunes have the highest amounts. Salicylates are also found in appreciable amounts in licorice and peppermint candies. Moderate levels of salicylate are found in nuts and seeds. Vegetables, legumes, grains, meat, poultry, fish, eggs, and dairy products typically contain insignificant levels of salicylates. Salicylate levels are especially high in some herbs and condiments, including curry powder, paprika, thyme, dill, oregano, and turmeric. Although intake of these herbs and spices tends to be relatively small, they can make a significant contribution to dietary salicylate intake.

Average salicylate intake from foods is in the range of 10 to 200 mg per day.[21] Dietary salicylates may be a significant factor for aspirin-sensitive individuals.

Other Flavoring Agents. Other flavoring agents, such as cinnamon, vanilla, menthol, and other volatile compounds, may produce hives in some individuals. The artificial sweetener aspartame (NutraSweet) has also been shown to induce hives.[22]

Food Preservatives

Benzoates. Benzoic acid and benzoates are the most commonly used food preservatives. Although the incidence of adverse reactions to these compounds in the general population is thought to be less than 1%, the frequency of reactions in patients with chronic hives varies from 4 to 44%.

Fish and shrimp frequently contain extremely high quantities of added benzoates. This may be one reason adverse reactions to these foods are so common in patients with hives.

BHT and BHA. Butylated hydroxytoluene (BHT) and butylated hydroxyanisol (BHA) are the primary antioxidants used in prepared and packaged foods. Typically, 15% of patients with chronic hives test positive to oral challenge with BHT. The use of chewing gum containing BHT was enough to induce hives in one patient.[23]

Sulfites. Like tartrazine, sulfites have been shown to induce asthma, hives, and angio-edema in sensitive individuals.[24] Sulfites are ubiquitous in foods and drugs. They are typically added to processed foods to prevent microbial spoilage and to keep them from browning or changing color. The earliest known use of sulfites was in the treatment of wines with sulfur dioxide by the Romans.

Sulfites are used to preserve many foods, especially dried fruit, prepared salads, items at salad bars, wine, and beer. Wine and beer drinkers typically consume up to 10 mg sulfites per day even with moderate drinking (two to three glasses of wine or beer). Sulfites are also used as preservatives in many pharmaceuticals. Sulfites can cause asthma as well as hives.

Normally, the enzyme sulfite oxidase metabolizes sulfites to safer sulfates, which are excreted in the urine. Those with a poorly functioning sulfoxidation system, however, have an increased ratio of sulfite to sulfate in their urine. Sulfite oxidase is dependent on the trace mineral molybdenum. Although most nutrition textbooks list molybdenum deficiency as uncommon, an Austrian study of 1,750 patients found that 41.5% were molybdenum deficient.[25] Molybdenum deficiency may produce sulfite sensitivity. If so, supplementation (200 mcg per day) may be beneficial.

Food Emulsifiers and Stabilizers

Various compounds are used to emulsify and stabilize many commercial foods to ensure that the solids, oils, and liquids do not separate out. Most of the foods that contain these compounds contain other additives as well, such as preservatives, and dyes. Polysorbate in ice cream has been reported to induce hives, and vegetable gums such as acacia, gum arabic, tragacanth, quince, and carrageenan may also induce hives in susceptible individuals.[4]

Infections

Infections are a major cause of hives in children. In adults, immunological tolerance to many microorganisms apparently occurs owing to repeated antigen exposure. The role of bacteria, viruses, and yeast *(Candida albicans)* in hives is briefly reviewed below. Chronic trichomonas infections have also been found to cause hives.

Bacterial Infections

Bacterial infections contribute to hives in two major settings: in acute streptococcal tonsillitis in children and in chronic dental infections in adults. In the first setting, acute hives predominate, while in the second, chronic hives predominate.[1]

Viral Infections

Hepatitis B is the most frequent cause of virally induced hives. Hives have also been strongly linked to infectious mononucleosis and may develop several weeks before the disease is manifested clinically. The incidence of hives during infectious mononucleosis is 5%.

Candida

The association between *Candida albicans* and chronic hives has been suggested in several clinical studies. The proportion of patients with chronic hives who react positively to an immediate skin test with candida antigens is 19 to 81%, compared with 10 to 15% of people without hives.[26,27] It appears that sensitivity to *Candida albicans* is an important factor in at least 25% of patients who have chronic hives. Approximately 70% of patients who have a positive skin reaction to *Candida albicans* also react to oral provocation tests using foods prepared with baker's or brewer's yeast.

Treatment with the drug nystatin has shown that elimination of the candida organism can achieve a cure in a number of sensitive individuals. However, in one study more patients (18 of 49) responded to nystatin plus a yeast-free diet than to nystatin alone (9 of 49). The yeast-free diet excluded breads, sausages, wine, beer, cider, grapes, raisins, vinegar, tomato, ketchup, pickles, and prepared foods containing yeast.[27]

Further support for the importance of diet can be found in a study of 36 patients with a positive skin prick test to candida. Only 3 patients became symptom-free from taking nystatin alone, compared with 23 who had diet therapy that included avoiding food allergies and yeast following the nystatin therapy.[28] Obviously the best approach is to focus on both elimination of yeast and avoidance of food allergies.

Stress

In one study involving 236 cases of chronic hives, psychological factors (stressors) were reported to be the most frequent primary cause.[29] Stress appears to play an important role by decreasing intestinal secretory IgA levels.

In one study of 15 patients who had chronic hives, relaxation therapy and hypnosis were shown to provide significant benefit.[30] Patients were given an audiotape and asked to use the relaxation techniques described on the tape at home. At a follow-up examination 5 to 14 months after the initial session, six patients were free of hives and an additional seven reported improvement.

Therapeutic Considerations

The treatment goals in hives are straightforward: identify and eliminate the factors that are causing the release of histamine and other allergic compounds and decrease the body's overreactivity. As noted above, allergy (to foods, food additives, and drugs) and stress are common causes of hives. The best diagnostic test (and therapy) appears to be an elimination diet.

The strictest elimination diets allow only water, lamb, rice, pears, and vegetables. Those foods most commonly associated with inducing hives (milk, eggs, chicken, fruits, nuts, and additives) should definitely be avoided. Foods containing vasoactive amines should be eliminated even if no direct allergy to them is noted. The primary foods to eliminate are cured meat, alcoholic beverages, cheese, chocolate, citrus fruits, and shellfish. Also, the importance of eliminating food additives cannot be overstated. If food additives do, in fact, increase the number of mast cells in the skin, they may also do the same in the small intestine, thereby greatly increasing the risk of developing a leaky gut.

In addition to an elimination diet, there are several other factors that can be helpful, such as ultraviolet light therapy, vitamin C, vitamin B_{12}, fish oils, quercetin, and thyroid hormone. These factors are discussed below.

Ultraviolet Light Therapy

Ultraviolet light (from sunlight or tanning beds) has been shown to be of some benefit to patients with chronic hives.[31,32] Both ultraviolet A (UVA), the non-burning type of sunlight, and ultraviolet B (UVB), the one that causes a sunburn, have been used. Patients with cold, cholinergic, and dermographic hives experience the greatest therapeutic response.

Nutritional Supplements

Vitamin C

High-dose vitamin C therapy may help hives (as well as other allergic conditions) by lowering histamine levels.[33] Vitamin C prevents the secretion of histamine by white blood cells and increases the detoxification of histamine. Dosages of at least 2,000 mg per day appear necessary to produce these effects.

Vitamin B_{12}

Although blood levels of vitamin B_{12} are normal in most patients with hives, additional B_{12} has been anecdotally reported to be of value in the treatment of acute and chronic hives.[34,35]

Fish Oils

Fish oils may be helpful. In one report, three patients with aspirin-induced urticaria experienced alleviation of symptoms following dietary supplementation with omega-3 fatty acids. All three patients had severe urticaria and asthma. They were on oral corticosteroid therapy (i.e., prednisone) but still experiencing some symptoms. After dietary supplementation with fish oils (3,000 mg EPA + DHA per day) for six to eight weeks, all three experienced resolution of symptoms, allowing discontinuation of systemic corticosteroid therapy. Symptoms relapsed after the dose of fish oil was reduced, indicating that higher dosages may have to be maintained to keep symptoms from reappearing.[36] This is not surprising when we consider that the typical diet contains excessive amounts of pro-inflammatory omega-6 fatty acids such as arachidonic acid (see the chapter "Silent Inflammation").

Quercetin

The flavonoid quercetin inhibits both the manufacture and the release of histamine and other allergic/inflammatory mediators by mast cells and basophils. Because of the poor absorption of quercetin, enzymatically modified isoquercitrin (EMIQ) may be a better choice. For more information, see the chapter "Hay Fever."

Thyroid Hormone

The association of low thyroid function and hives has been established since the 1950s. A subset of patients with chronic hives respond to thyroid hormone, especially if they have antibodies to thyroid tissue.[38,39] For example, one study evaluated a group of 624 patients with presumed idiopathic chronic hives and/or angioedema. Of these, 90 patients were found to have thyroid antibodies.[39] Forty-six of these patients were treated with L-thyroxine therapy, and eight of them had a remission within four weeks of therapy. Four patients with high thyroid antibody titers repeatedly experienced worsening when therapy was discontinued and had repeated remissions when therapy with L-thyroxine was resumed. Although L-thyroxine did not always improve the patient's urticaria or angioedema, when it did work the response was dramatic.

QUICK REVIEW

- **Fundamental to the treatment of hives are recognition and control of causative factors.**
- **Drug reactions are the leading cause of hives in adults.**
- **In children, hives are usually due to foods, food additives, or infections.**
- **Antibiotics, including penicillin and related compounds, are the most common cause of drug-induced hives.**
- **Although any food can be the causative agent, the most common offenders are milk, fish, meat, eggs, beans, and nuts.**
- **Several food additives (e.g., tartrazine, benzoate) and aspirin augment production of a compound that increases the number of mast cells throughout the body.**
- **Elimination of food additives leads to tremendous improvement in chronic hives in children.**
- **Chronic candidiasis can be an underlying factor in cases of chronic hives.**
- **Vitamin C prevents the secretion of histamine by white blood cells and increases the breakdown of histamine.**
- **Fish oils have been shown to be helpful in resolving chronic hives in some people.**
- **The flavonoid quercetin inhibits both the manufacture and the release of histamine and other allergic/inflammatory mediators by mast cells and basophils.**
- **It is important to rule out low thyroid function or the presence of antibodies against the thyroid gland in cases of chronic hives.**

TREATMENT SUMMARY

The first goal of treatment is to identify and control all of the factors that promote the hives. Acute hives is usually a self-limiting disease, especially once the eliciting agent has been removed or reduced. Chronic hives also responds to the removal of the eliciting agent.

Diet

An elimination diet is of utmost importance in the treatment of chronic hives (see the chapter "Food Allergy"). The diet should eliminate not only suspected allergens but also all food additives.

Nutritional Supplements

- A high-potency multiple vitamin and mineral formula as described in the chapter "Supplementary Measures"
- Key individual nutrients:
  - Vitamin B$_{12}$ (methylcobalamin): 1,000 mcg per day
  - Vitamin C: 500 to 1,000 mg three times per day
  - Magnesium (bound to aspartate, citrate, fumarate, malate, or succinate): 200 to 300 mg three times per day
  - Vitamin D$_3$: 2,000 to 4,000 IU per day (ideally, measure blood levels and adjust dosage accordingly)

- Fish oils: 3,000 mg EPA + DHA per day
- One of the following:
  - Grape seed extract (>95% procyanidolic oligomers): 100 to 300 mg per day
  - Pine bark extract (>95% procyanidolic oligomers): 100 to 300 mg per day
  - Quercetin: 200 to 400 mg 20 minutes before each meal; or EMIQ, 50–100 mg before each meal

Psychological Measures

Use relaxation techniques regularly. For example, listen to audiotaped relaxation programs.

Physical Medicine

Sunbathe for 15 to 20 minutes per day or use a UVA solarium, especially for chronic physical urticaria. Obviously, sunbathing is contraindicated in cases of solar urticaria.

Hyperthyroidism

- Weakness, sweating, weight loss, nervousness, loose stools, heat intolerance, irritability, fatigue
- Racing heartbeat; warm, thin, moist skin; stare; tremor
- Diffuse enlargement of the thyroid, non-painful goiter
- Increased blood levels of thyroid hormones

Hyperthyroidism is a condition characterized by increased levels of thyroid hormones: thyroxine (T4) and triiodothyronine (T3). The autoimmune disorder Graves' disease accounts for up to 85% of all cases of hyperthyroidism. Although no single immunological abnormality explains all of the clinical features of the disease, the common denominator is the presence of antibodies against receptors in the thyroid for thyroid-stimulating hormone (TSH). TSH receptor antibodies (TSH-R Ab) or thyroid-stimulating immunoglobulins (TSI) are present in 80% of cases of Graves' disease. About 25 to 30% of people with Graves' disease will also suffer from Graves' ophthalmopathy (a protrusion of one or both eyes), in which the eye muscles become inflamed, attacking autoantibodies.

There are definite patterns of susceptibility for Graves' disease. In particular, it is eight times more common in women than in men and typically begins between the ages of 20 and 40. The classic clinical presentation of Graves' disease is a young adult female complaining of nervousness, irritability, sweating, palpitations, insomnia, tremor, frequent bowel movements, and unexplained weight loss.

Physical signs of hyperthyroidism include a smooth, diffuse, nontender goiter in the neck; a racing pulse, especially after exercise; loud heart sounds; and mild protrusion of the eyes with lid retraction. Other signs and symptoms include muscle weakness and fatigue, anxiety, heat intolerance, and fluid retention. The skin can also become moist, warm, and finely textured. Perspiration increases as a response to the increased body temperature. Pigment changes such as vitiligo (areas with loss of pigment) can be associated with Graves' disease, as well as increased pigmentation of areas such as skin creases and the knuckles. Hair may thin or fall out in patches or all over the scalp. Nails may separate prematurely from the nail bed.

Causes

Stress

One of the key causes of hyperthyroidism and/or Graves' disease is recent stress. This association has been recognized as a precipitating factor ever since Graves' disease was first recognized. In fact, the most common precipitating event is an "actual or threatened separation from an individual upon whom the patient is emotionally dependent."[1] Studies now support the long-held observation that the onset of Graves' disease often follows some kind of emotional shock, in particular some sort of loss, such as divorce, death, or difficult separations.[2,3]

The next most common cause of hyperthyroidism is a toxic nodular goiter. Other causes of hyperthyroidism include early Hashimoto's thyroiditis (see the chapter "Hypothyroidism").

Genetics

People with certain types of genetic markers are statistically more prone to develop Graves' disease, while people with other types of markers seem to be less frequently affected. In identical twins, if one twin is affected, the other has a 50% chance of manifesting the disease. In fraternal twins, if one twin is affected, the other has a 9% chance of having it as well.

Smoking

Smoking is known to raise the risk and severity of Graves' ophthalmopathy.[4–6]

Iodine Supplementation

Several studies have shown that dietary iodine supplementation, usually through consumption of iodized salt, in areas where there is already sufficient iodine in the food supply can increase the incidence of hyperthyroidism in susceptible individuals. In one study, the effects of consuming iodized salt were studied in 267,330 inhabitants of Galicia. The incidence of hyperthyroidism increased throughout the study period, with 4.89 new cases per 100,000 people, though the increase was due to larger numbers of both nodular and diffuse goiters rather than Graves' disease. Also, iodine from other

sources in doses above 600 mcg, such as potassium iodide, iodine supplements, medications such as amiodarone, and imaging contrast agents, can trigger Graves' disease and toxic multinodular goiter.[7]

Therapeutic Considerations

Conventional treatment of hyperthyroidism in the United States focuses on destroying the thyroid gland with radioactive iodine (radioactive iodine ablation, RIA). Advantages include the high rate of response and the fact that there is no need for ongoing suppression. Disadvantages include progression to hypothyroidism, elevated risk of nonlocalized cancers, and risk for parathyroid disease. We do not recommend surgery to remove the thyroid unless there are significant extenuating circumstances. It carries with it too many risks compared with RIA.

We feel that prior to RIA a trial of antithyroid drugs should be attempted. This drugs work by entering the thyroid and blocking the formation of thyroid hormones; specifically, they inhibit binding of iodine to tyrosine. In many parts of the world, including Europe and Japan, antithyroid drugs are the first-line treatment for hyperthyroidism, as many cases of hyperthyroidism resolve spontaneously within 18 months. Some people develop hypothyroidism after treatment with antithyroid drugs, and some go on to require RIA.

Naturopathic Care

The chief objective of the natural treatment of Graves' disease and hyperthyroidism is to reduce symptoms while trying to reestablish normal thyroid status. We recommend use of antithyroid drugs to reduce the immediate severity of hyperthyroid symptoms. Recommended dietary and lifestyle measures may lower the required dose or duration of antithyroid drugs, or raise the likelihood of disease remission with conventional treatment.

Practical steps include reduction of risk factors (stress, smoking, excess iodine intake). Stress control is important in normalization of the thyroid, and counseling can prevent a return to stress-generating life strategies. Increase the amount of rest you get, including a nap after lunch and a full night's sleep.

Diet

Patients with autoimmune thyroid disease, either Graves' disease or Hashimoto's thyroiditis (the major cause of low thyroid function), are more likely than the general population to suffer from celiac disease and/or gluten sensitivity. Therefore, these conditions must be ruled out. See the chapter "Celiac Disease" for specific guidance. Also, identify food allergies and avoid problematic foods; see the chapter "Food Allergy." Otherwise, the recommendations given in the chapter "A Health-Promoting Diet" are appropriate here. Keep in mind that the diet may need to be higher in calories to compensate for the increase in metabolism. We also recommend that you avoid caffeine and dietary sources of iodine (especially iodized salt, kelp and other seaweeds, seafood, and nutritional supplements that contain more than 300 mcg of iodine).

Dietary Goitrogens
Some foods contain goitrogens, substances that prevent the utilization of iodine. These compounds—primarily isothiocyanates, which are similar in action and structure to antithyroid drugs such as propylthiouracil—are found in such foods as turnips, cabbage, rutabagas, mustard greens, rapeseed, cassava root, soybeans, peanuts, pine nuts, and millet.

However, these foods cannot reliably be used to treat hyperthyroidism for the following reasons:

- Their goitrogen content is quite low compared with the dosages of propylthiouracil required to treat hyperthyroidism.
- Cooking inactivates the goitrogens.
- No substantial documentation exists that these naturally occurring goitrogens interfere with thyroid function to any significant degree when dietary iodine levels are adequate.

Despite these shortcomings, some natural medicine practitioners may use naturally occurring goitrogens in mild cases instead of propylthiouracil and related drugs. Anecdotally, the typical recommendation is the equivalent of half a head of raw cabbage per day.

Carnitine
Carnitine is manufactured within the body, where it plays an important role in energy metabolism. Carnitine has been shown to be an antagonist of thyroid hormone in peripheral tissues, inhibiting the hormone's entry into the cell nucleus. A six-month, randomized, double-blind, placebo-controlled study evaluated the use of carnitine in patients prescribed high doses of thyroid hormone.[8] During this study, 50 women with benign nodular goiter who already had been prescribed a suppressive dose of thyroxine were randomly assigned to five groups of 10 subjects each. One group was given a placebo for six months. Two groups started with the placebo for two months, then were prescribed 2 or 4 g carnitine per day, then were returned to the placebo for the last two months. The last two groups were started with either 2 or 4 g carnitine per day for the first four months and then were given placebo for the last two

months. Symptoms of hyperthyroidism, bone mineralization markers, and liver indicators were recorded.

In the second and third groups, the symptoms that had worsened while the subjects were on thyroxine plus the placebo returned to baseline once carnitine had replaced the placebo. In the fourth and fifth groups, symptoms remained stable or improved as long as carnitine was given with thyroxine, implying that the carnitine effect prevailed over the T4 effect. For those given supplemental carnitine, liver profiles improved, although cholesterol levels were virtually unaffected. Side effects were minor. Symptoms and biochemical variables only worsened in the placebo group.

Because carnitine has extremely low tox-icity, the authors of this study recommend considering carnitine for Graves' disease–induced thyrotoxicosis during pregnancy, during lactation, or in other conditions in which antithyroid drugs may be unwanted, such as liver disease and blood disorders.

Botanical Medicines

There is a long list of plants used traditionally in the treatment of hyperthyroidism. Unfortunately, these plants have not been adequately evaluated in clinical studies. Rather than discuss these plants here, we would encourage anyone interested to consult a naturopathic physician to allow for proper monitoring.

QUICK REVIEW

- **Hyperthyroidism is a condition characterized by increased levels of thyroid hormones.**
- **Graves' disease accounts for up to 85% of all cases of hyperthyroidism.**
- **One of the key causes of hyperthyroidism and/or Graves' disease is recent stress.**
- **Smoking is known to raise the risk and severity of Graves' ophthalmopathy.**
- **Dietary iodine supplementation in iodine-sufficient areas can increase the incidence of hyperthyroidism in susceptible individuals.**

- **A trial of antithyroid drugs should be attempted before radioactive iodine ablation of the thyroid is considered.**
- **Stress control is important in the treatment of hyperthyroidism.**
- **Patients with autoimmune thyroid disease, either Graves' disease or Hashimoto's thyroiditis, are more likely than the general population to suffer from celiac disease and/or gluten sensitivity.**
- **Carnitine has been shown to counteract the effects of elevated thyroxine.**

TREATMENT SUMMARY

Acute Graves' disease is not easily treated by naturopathic methods. In severe cases, there is no guarantee that natural treatments will alleviate the symptoms adequately. In mild cases, natural therapeutics can manage symptoms well, but patients must be monitored carefully.

Diet

Rule out gluten sensitivity and then follow the guidelines in the chapter "A Health-Promoting Diet." Higher calorie intake may be necessary to meet the hyperthyroid patient's metabolic needs. In mild cases, consumption of large amounts of raw vegetables from the brassica (cabbage) family may be adequate to control symptoms when combined with restricted iodine consumption.

Nutritional Supplements

- Foundation supplement program as described in the chapter "Supplementary Measures"
- Carnitine: 2 to 4 g per day

Hypoglycemia

· ·

- Blood glucose level at or below 40 to 50 mg/dl
- A normal response curve during the first two to three hours of a glucose tolerance test, followed by a decrease of 20 mg or more below the fasting glucose level during the final hours of the test, with symptoms developing during the decrease

Hypoglycemia is low blood sugar (glucose). Normally, the body maintains blood sugar levels within a narrow range through the coordinated effort of several glands. If these control mechanisms are disrupted, hypoglycemia or diabetes (high blood sugar) may result. Americans tend to overstress these control mechanisms because of poor diet and lifestyle habits. As a result, diabetes and hypoglycemia are common diseases.

Hypoglycemia is divided into two main categories: reactive hypoglycemia and fasting hypoglycemia. Reactive hypoglycemia, the more common, is characterized by the development of symptoms of hypoglycemia three to five hours after a meal. Reactive hypoglycemia may also result from drugs used in the treatment of diabetes (see the chapter "Diabetes").

Some experts have recommended that instead of using the term *reactive hypoglycemia*, we should call the syndrome *increased glycemic volatility* or *idiopathic postprandial syndrome* because absolute glucose levels are not reliable indicators of symptoms. Many times people with glucose levels below 50 mg/dl have no symptoms, while people with symptoms of hypoglycemia can have normal or even elevated glucose levels. Symptoms appear to correlate better with rapid drops in blood glucose than with drops below 50 mg/dl (as discussed below).[1–3]

Fasting hypoglycemia is rare, as it usually appears only in severe disease states such as pancreatic tumors, extensive liver damage, prolonged starvation, or various cancers, or as a result of excessive insulin dosages in diabetics. Pregnant diabetic women using insulin or oral diabetes medications often experience hypoglycemia but usually do not have symptoms.[4]

Because glucose is the primary fuel for the brain, low levels affect the brain first. Symptoms of hypoglycemia can range from mild to severe, including headache; depression, anxiety, irritability, and other psychological disturbances; blurred vision; excessive sweating; mental confusion; incoherent speech; bizarre behavior; and convulsions.

Hypoglycemia can promote many detrimental changes in the body, such as increasing the levels of C-reactive protein, a marker for inflammation that is a known risk factor for heart disease.[5]

Diagnosing Hypoglycemia

The most popular method of diagnosing reactive hypoglycemia is the oral glucose tolerance test. After the patient fasts for at least 12 hours, a baseline blood glucose measurement is made. Then the patient drinks a liquid containing glucose (the amount is based on body weight). Blood sugar levels are measured at 30 minutes, at 1 hour, and then hourly for up to 6 hours. Basically, blood sugar levels greater than 200 mg/dl indicate diabetes. Levels below 50 mg/dl indicate reactive hypoglycemia.

Continuous Glucose Monitoring

Continuous glucose monitoring is an electronic diagnostic system that requires the insertion of a tiny sensing catheter under the skin of the abdomen. The sensor measures blood sugar and sends this information to a small receiver worn on the patient's belt for up to one week. A graph showing the average blood sugar reading every five minutes (288 blood sugar readings per day) can then be generated and studied in relationship to food intake, appetite, food cravings, hypoglycemic symptoms, medication, and exercise. This has been shown to be a very useful tool in the diagnosis of, and monitoring of blood sugar control in, diabetes.[6]

Using continuous glucose monitoring, Michael R. Lyon, M.D., has discovered that most people with weight problems and insulin resistance go through their days with remarkable fluctuations in blood sugar. Dr. Lyon has found that symptoms of hypoglycemia occur when blood sugar drops rapidly, even when blood sugar was above the normal range.

Together with Dr. Lyon, we believe that increased glycemic volatility is at the heart of most weight problems. The data indicate that rapidly fluctuating blood sugar levels are generally related to some degree of insulin resistance and are made worse by excessive consumption of foods with a high glycemic impact.[7]

THE HYPOGLYCEMIA QUESTIONNAIRE

When all factors are considered (including cost and convenience), the most useful measure of diagnosing hypoglycemia in many cases remains an assessment of symptoms. In general, when symptoms appear three to four hours after eating and disappear after food is again eaten, hypoglycemia should be considered. The questionnaire below is an excellent screening method for hypoglycemia.

Hypoglycemia Questionnaire

	No	Mild	Moderate	Severe
Crave sweets	0	1	2	3
Irritable if a meal is missed	0	1	2	3
Feel tired or weak if a meal is missed	0	1	2	3
Dizziness when standing suddenly	0	1	2	3
Frequent headaches	0	1	2	3
Poor memory (forgetfulness) or concentration	0	1	2	3
Feel tired an hour or so after eating	0	1	2	3
Heart palpitations	0	1	2	3
Feel shaky at times	0	1	2	3
Afternoon fatigue	0	1	2	3
Vision blurs on occasion	0	1	2	3
Depression or mood swings	0	1	2	3
Overweight	0	1	2	3
Frequently anxious or nervous	0	1	2	3

Total: _____

Scoring:
5 or less: hypoglycemia is not likely to be a factor
6 to 15: hypoglycemia is likely to be a factor
16 or more: hypoglycemia is extremely likely to be a factor

General Considerations

Although all of the symptoms mentioned in the questionnaire above may be due to hypoglycemia, there are obviously other causes in many cases. However, in the 1970s public interest in hypoglycemia and sugar intake was fueled by a number of books including *Sugar Blues* by William Duffy, *Hope for Hypoglycemia* by Broda Barnes, and *Sweet and Dangerous* by John Yudkin. The popularity of these books and the diagnosis of hypoglycemia were met by much skepticism from the medical community. Editorials in the *Journal of the American Medical Association* and the *New England Journal of Medicine* during the 1970s denounced this public interest in hypoglycemia and tried to invalidate the concept of hypoglycemia.[8,9]

Research in the past 30 years has provided an ever-increasing amount of information concerning the role that refined carbohydrates and faulty blood sugar control play in many disease processes. For example, the term *metabolic syndrome* is used to describe a set of cardiovascular risk factors including glucose or insulin disturbances, high blood cholesterol and triglyceride levels, elevated blood pressure, and abdominal obesity, all of which are tied to elevated insulin levels and insulin resistance. There is little doubt about what contributes to these problems: the human body was not designed to handle the amount of refined carbohydrates (and salt, saturated fats, and other harmful food compounds) that feature prominently in the diets of many people in the United States and other Western countries.

A substantial amount of information indicates that hypoglycemia (increased glycemic volatility) is caused by an excessive intake of refined carbohydrates, especially added sugar.[10,11] Although most medical and health organizations, as well as the U.S. government, have recommended that no more than 10% of a person's total caloric intake come from added sugars, in fact they account for roughly 30% of the total calories consumed by most Americans.[12] The average American consumes more than 100 lb of sucrose and 40 lb of high-fructose corn syrup each year. This sugar addiction plays a major role in the high prevalence of chronic disease in the United States.

Consequences of Hypoglycemia

The Brain

The brain depends on glucose as an energy source. The association between hypoglycemia and impaired mental function is well known. What is not as well known is the role that hypoglycemia plays in various psychological disorders. For example, despite numerous studies that show a high incidence of abnormal glucose tolerance tests in depressed individuals, rarely is hypoglycemia considered as a cause of depression, and rarely are depressed individuals prescribed dietary therapy.[13,14] This is despite the fact that dietary therapy (usually simply eliminating refined carbohydrates from the diet) is occasionally all that is necessary for patients who suffer from depression due to reactive hypoglycemia.

Aggressive or Criminal Behavior

A strong yet controversial link exists between hypoglycemia and aggressive or criminal behavior. Several controlled studies have found that reactive hypoglycemia (as determined by an oral glucose tolerance test) is common among psychiatric patients and habitually violent and impulsive criminals.[15,16] Furthermore, abnormal and sometimes emotionally explosive behavior is often observed during the glucose tolerance test itself. In one study, reactive hypoglycemia was shown to induce fire-setting behavior in pyromaniacs.[17]

Several large studies involving more than 6,000 inmates in 10 penal institutions in three states have now evaluated the effect of dietary intervention on antisocial or aggressive behavior.[18,19] In the first study, 174 incarcerated juvenile delinquents were placed on a sugar-restricted diet, while another 102 offenders were placed on a control diet.[18] During the two-year study the number of incidents of antisocial behavior was reduced by 45% in the treatment group. The most significant reductions came in assaults (which dropped by 83%), theft (77%), "horseplay" (65%), and refusal to obey an order (55%). Antisocial behavior changed the most in those charged with assault, robbery, rape, aggravated assault, auto theft, vandalism, child molestation, arson, and possession of a deadly weapon.

In the largest study, 3,999 incarcerated juveniles of both sexes were studied over a period of two years.[19] This study limited the dietary revisions to replacing sugary soft drinks with fruit juices and replacing high-sugar snacks with unrefined-carbohydrate snacks (e.g., replacing a candy bar with popcorn). When 1,121 young men on the sugar-restricted diet were compared with 884 young men on the control diet, there were significant differences: in the first group: suicide attempts were reduced by 100%, the need for restraints to prevent self-injury was reduced by 75%, disruptive behavior was reduced by 42%, and assaults and fights were reduced by 25%. Interestingly, the dietary changes did not seem to affect the behavior of young women, perhaps suggesting that men react to hypoglycemia differently from women. From an anthropological and evolutionary view, this

makes sense. Low blood sugar levels were undoubtedly an internal signal for men to hunt for food.

The link between hypoglycemia and aggressive behavior also extends to men without a history of criminal activity. In one study, a glucose tolerance test was given to a group of men who did not have a history of aggressive behavior or hypoglycemia.[16] In these subjects a significant correlation was found between the tendency to become mildly hypoglycemic and scores on questionnaires used to measure aggression. These results indicated that aggressiveness often coincided with hypoglycemia.

Premenstrual Syndrome

Premenstrual syndrome (PMS) is a recurrent condition characterized by troublesome yet often ill-defined symptoms that usually appear 7 to 14 days before menstruation begins. The syndrome is most common in women between 30 and 40 years of age; it affects nearly one out of three women in this age group, and about 10% of those affected may have a significantly debilitating form.

An authority on PMS, Guy Abraham, M.D., attempted to clarify the different forms by subdividing PMS into four distinct subgroups (A, C, D, and H).[20] Each subgroup is linked to specific symptoms, hormonal patterns, and metabolic abnormalities (see the chapter "Premenstrual Syndrome" for further information). PMS-C is associated with increased appetite, craving for sweets, headache, fatigue, fainting spells, and heart palpitations. Glucose tolerance tests of PMS-C patients during the 5 to 10 days before their menses typically suggested reactive hypoglycemia (the result of excessive secretion of insulin in response to sugar intake), whereas during other parts of the menstrual cycle the same tests were normal. This excessive insulin secretion appears to be hormonally regulated, but other factors may also be involved.[21] Salt enhances the insulin response to sugar, and decreased magnesium levels in the pancreas can result in increased secretion of insulin. Regardless of the cause, women with PMS-C appear to be extremely sensitive to hypoglycemia.

Migraine Headaches

Migraine headaches are probably caused by excessive dilation of a blood vessel in the head (see the chapter "Migraine Headache"). Migraines are a surprisingly common disorder, affecting 15 to 20% of men and 25 to 30% of women at some time in their lives. More than half of patients have a family history of the illness. Hypoglycemia has long been known to be a precipitating factor in migraine headaches.[22]

Several studies have found that eliminating refined sugar from the diet of migraine sufferers with confirmed hypoglycemia results in significant improvement. In one study of 48 migraine sufferers with reactive hypoglycemia, 27 (56%) showed a greater than 75% improvement in symptoms, 17 (35%) showed a greater than 50% improvement, and 4 (8%) showed a greater than 25% improvement.[23]

Atherosclerosis, Intermittent Claudication, and Angina

Substantial evidence indicates that reactive hypoglycemia or impaired glucose tolerance is a significant factor in the development of atherosclerosis. Although a high sugar intake leads to rises in triglycerides and cholesterol, the real culprit may be elevations of insulin.[24] Abnormal glucose tolerance tests and elevations in insulin secretion are common findings in patients with heart disease.[25,26]

In addition to playing a role in atherosclerosis, high sugar consumption and reactive hypoglycemia can be a cause of angina and intermittent claudication, a painful cramp that usually occurs in the calf during walking.[27,28]

Therapeutic Considerations

Diet

Dietary carbohydrates play a central role in the cause, prevention, and treatment of hypoglycemia. Simple carbohydrates such as sugars are quickly absorbed by the body; this absorbtion results in a rapid elevation in blood sugar and stimulates a corresponding elevation in serum insulin.

Problems with carbohydrates begin when they are refined, because refining strips them of associated nutrients and increases their rate of absorption. Virtually the entire vitamin and mineral content has been removed from white sugar, white breads, pastries, and many breakfast cereals. When high-sugar foods are eaten alone, blood sugar levels rise quickly, producing a strain on blood sugar control. Some think that the natural simple sugars in fruits and vegetables have an advantage over sucrose and other refined sugars in that they are balanced by a wide range of nutrients that aid in the utilization of the sugars. Of greater importance, though, is the fact that the sugars in whole, unprocessed foods are more slowly absorbed, as they are contained within cells and are associated with fiber and other food elements. Notably, large amounts of fruit juice and even vegetable juice may be a problem for hypoglycemics, as the cell disruption characteristic of juicing increases the rate of the absorption of sugars in the juices.

Currently, more than half of the carbohydrates consumed in the United States are in the form of sugars added to processed foods as sweetening agents. It is important to read food labels carefully for clues to sugar content. Various words are used to describe refined simple carbohydrates, including *sucrose, glucose, maltose, lactose, fructose, corn syrup,* and *white grape juice concentrate.*

A Closer Look at Simple Carbohydrates

Glucose is not particularly sweet-tasting compared with fructose and sucrose (which is made of glucose plus fructose). It is found in abundant amounts in fruits, honey, sweet corn, and most root vegetables. Glucose is also the primary sugar unit that makes up most complex carbohydrates.

Fructose or fruit sugar is the primary carbohydrate in many fruits, maple syrup, and honey. Fructose is very sweet, roughly 1.5 times sweeter than sucrose. Although fructose has the same chemical formula as glucose, its structure is quite different. In order to be used by the body, fructose must be converted to glucose within the liver. Pure crystalline fructose and fruit can be consumed in moderation, but high-fructose corn syrup should definitely be avoided. High-fructose corn syrup (HFCS), a distant derivative of corn, was created in the late 1960s and has become a hard-to-avoid staple of the American diet. Many different products use HFCS as an ingredient. It provides the sweetness in everything from soft drinks and fruit beverages to most commercial baked goods, including cookies, crackers, and bread; it's even found in ketchup. Food companies use so much HFCS because it is very cheap. A single 12-fl-oz can of Coke or Pepsi has as much as 13 tsp of sugar in the form of high-fructose corn syrup. And because the amount of soda we drink has more than doubled since 1970, to about 56 gallons per person a year, so has the amount of high fructose corn syrup we take in. In 2001, we consumed, per person, almost 63 pounds of it, according to the U.S. Department of Agriculture. That translates to an average of 31 tsp a day, and at 16 calories per tsp, that represents a daily intake of 496 calories.

The Glycemic Index

A helpful method of categorizing food on the basis of its ability to alter blood sugar is the glycemic index, developed in 1981 to express the rise of blood glucose after a particular food is eaten.[29] The standard value of 100 is based on the rise seen with the ingestion of glucose. The glycemic index ranges from about 20 for fructose and whole barley to about 98 for a baked potato. The insulin response to carbohydrate-containing foods is similar to the rise in blood sugar.

The glycemic index is used as a guideline for dietary recommendations for people with either diabetes or hypoglycemia (see Appendix B). People with blood sugar problems are advised to avoid foods with high values and choose carbohydrate-containing foods that have lower values. However, the glycemic index should not be the only thing guiding your food choices. For example, high-fat foods such as ice cream and sausage may have a low glycemic index, but because a diet high in fat has been shown to impair glucose tolerance, these foods are not good choices for people with hypoglycemia or diabetes.

The Importance of Fiber

Population studies as well as clinical and experimental data show that blood sugar disorders are clearly related to inadequate dietary fiber intake (see the chapter "Diabetes"). Although consumption of refined sugars should be curtailed, the amount of complex carbohydrate sources that are rich in fiber should be increased.

The term *dietary fiber* refers to the components of the plant cell wall, as well as the indigestible residues from plant foods. Different types of fiber possess different actions. Soluble fiber has the most beneficial effects on blood sugar control. Included in this class are hemicelluloses, mucilages, gums, and pectin. These types of fiber are capable of the following actions:

- Slowing down the digestion and absorption of carbohydrates, thereby preventing rapid rises in blood sugar

- Increasing cell sensitivity to insulin, and thereby preventing the excessive secretion of insulin

- Improving uptake of glucose by the liver and other tissues, and thereby preventing a sustained elevation of blood sugar

The majority of the fiber in most plant cell walls is soluble. Particularly good sources of water-soluble fiber are legumes, oat bran, nuts, seeds, psyllium seed husks, pears, apples, and most vegetables. Everyone's diet should include large amounts of plant foods to provide adequate amounts of dietary fiber; 50 g of fiber is a healthful goal.

PolyGlycopleX (PGX)

Based upon work with continuous glucose monitoring led by Michael R. Lyon, M.D., many important findings have been uncovered on how to effectively reduce blood sugar volatility. For example, Dr. Lyon confirmed earlier work suggesting that while a low-glycemic-index diet is very important in reducing blood sugar levels, it has little effect on blood sugar volatility.[7] He has found that the most effective method of reducing glycemic volatility is a low-glycemic diet with the addition of a novel soluble fiber product called PolyGlycopleX (PGX), which is more viscous and more gel-forming than any other known fiber. This translates to significantly reducing the glycemic impact of any food or meal. Several double-blind studies have shown that PGX reduces after-meal elevations in blood sugar in a dose-dependent manner, independent of the type of food consumed.[30–32] Typical dosage of PGX is 1,500 to 5,000 mg before meals.

Chromium

Chromium is vital to proper blood sugar control, as it functions in the body as a key constituent of what is called glucose tolerance factor. Without chromium, insulin's action is blocked and glucose levels are elevated. Chromium deficiency may be a factor in the tremendous number of Americans who have hypoglycemia or diabetes or who are obese.[33] Evidence exists that marginal chromium deficiency is quite common in the United States and may be responsible for many cases of reactive hypoglycemia.

In one double-blind, crossover study of eight female patients, 200 mcg chromium (as chromium chloride) given twice per day for three months alleviated hypoglycemic symptoms and the glucose nadir two to four hours after a glucose load.[34] In addition, insulin binding improved and the number of insulin receptors increased.[35,36]

Lifestyle

Alcohol

Alcohol consumption severely stresses blood sugar control and is often a factor contributing to hypoglycemia. Alcohol induces reactive hypoglycemia by interfering with normal glucose utilization, as well as by increasing the secretion of insulin. The resultant drop in blood sugar produces a craving for food, particularly foods that quickly elevate blood sugar, as well as a craving for more alcohol. The increased sugar consumption aggravates the reactive hypoglycemia, particularly in the presence of more alcohol, again owing to alcohol-induced impairment of normal glucose utilization and increased secretion of insulin.

Hypoglycemia is an important complication of acute and chronic alcohol abuse. Hypoglycemia aggravates the mental and emotional problems of the alcoholic. Although acute alcohol ingestion induces hypoglycemia, in the long run it leads to hyperglycemia and diabetes. Eventually the body becomes insensitive to the augmented insulin release caused by the alcohol. In ad-

dition, alcohol itself can cause insulin resistance even in healthy individuals.[37] There is also evidence from large population studies that alcohol intake is strongly correlated with diabetes.[38] The higher the alcohol intake, the more likely it is that an individual will have diabetes.

Exercise

A regular exercise program is an important part of a hypoglycemia prevention and treatment plan. Regular exercise prevents type 2 diabetes and improves many aspects of glucose metabolism, including enhancing insulin

· ·

QUICK REVIEW

- **Hypoglycemia is a complex set of symptoms caused by faulty carbohydrate metabolism, almost always induced by a diet too high in refined sugars.**
- **When all factors are considered (including cost and convenience), assessment of symptoms remains the most useful way to diagnose hypoglycemia in most cases.**
- ***Metabolic syndrome*** **is a term used to describe a cluster of abnormalities that owe their existence largely to a high intake of refined carbohydrates, leading to the development of hypoglycemia, excessive insulin secretion, and glucose intolerance, followed by diminished insulin sensitivity leading to high blood pressure, elevated cholesterol levels, obesity, and ultimately type 2 diabetes.**
- **When blood sugar levels are low or drop rapidly, the condition can result in dizziness, headache, clouding of vi-**

sion, blunted mental acuity, emotional instability, confusion, and abnormal behavior.
- **Several controlled studies show that hypoglycemia is common in psychiatric patients and habitually violent and impulsive criminals.**
- **Hypoglycemia has been shown to be a common precipitating factor in migraine headaches.**
- **Problems with carbohydrates begin when they are refined, because refining strips them of associated nutrients and increases their rate of absorption.**
- **Chromium is vital to proper blood sugar control, as it functions in the body as a key constituent of glucose tolerance factor.**
- **Alcohol consumption severely stresses blood sugar control and is often a contributing factor in hypoglycemia.**

sensitivity. Some of the benefits of exercise may stem from the fact that it increases tissue chromium concentrations.[39] Another key advantage of exercise is that increasing muscle mass improves glucose stabilization.

••

TREATMENT SUMMARY

The primary treatment of hypoglycemia is the use of dietary therapy to stabilize blood sugar levels. Reactive hypoglycemia is not a disease; it is simply a complex set of symptoms caused by faulty carbohydrate metabolism induced by an inappropriate diet.

Diet

Avoid simple, processed, and concentrated carbohydrates, as well as food choices with a high glycemic load. Eat more foods rich in soluble fiber, such as legumes and low-glycemic vegetables. Frequent, small meals may be more effective in stabilizing blood sugar levels. Avoid alcohol, as it can cause hypoglycemia. See the chapter "Diabetes" for further dietary recommendations.

Nutritional Supplements

The recommendations for daily intake of vitamins and minerals given in the chapter "Supplementary Measures" are especially important in hypoglycemia, as many essential nutrients are critical to proper carbohydrate metabolism. In particular, we recommend 200 to 400 mcg chromium per day. Additionally, PGX at a dosage of 1,500 to 5,000 mg should be taken before meals (the higher dosage is recommended for those also wanting to lose weight).

Exercise

Because the beneficial effects of exercise that improve insulin sensitivity decrease within three days after exercise and are no longer evident after one week of rest, it's important to exercise regularly.[40] Choose an exercise program that is appropriate to your fitness level and that interests you; try to elevate your heart rate to at least 60% of maximum for half an hour three times a week.

Hypothyroidism

Signs and symptoms of hypothyroidism:

- Depression
- Difficulty losing weight
- Dry skin
- Headaches
- Hyperlipidemia
- Lethargy or fatigue
- Memory problems
- Menstrual problems
- Recurrent infections
- Sensitivity to cold
- Thinning of head hair
- Voice changes

Hypothyroidism is low thyroid gland function. The thyroid gland is situated in the front of the neck, just below the larynx (voice box). Since the hormones of the thyroid gland regulate metabolism in every cell of the body, a deficiency of thyroid hormones can affect virtually all body functions. The severity of symptoms in adults ranges from very mild deficiency states that are barely detectable (subclinical hypothyroidism) to severe deficiency states that are life-threatening (myxedema).

A deficiency of thyroid hormone may be due to defective hormone synthesis or to lack of stimulation by the pituitary gland. The pituitary gland is responsible for secreting thyroid-stimulating hormone (TSH). When thyroid hormone levels in the blood are low, the pituitary secretes TSH. If a blood test shows that thyroid hormone levels are low and TSH levels are elevated in the blood, it usually indicates defective thyroid hormone synthesis. This situation is termed *primary hypothyroidism.*

If TSH levels are low and thyroid hormone levels are also low, this indicates that the pituitary gland is responsible for the low thyroid function. This situation is termed *secondary hypothyroidism.*

Using blood levels of thyroid hormones as the criterion may exclude a large number of people with mild hypothyroidism, but according to this criterion it is estimated that approximately 5 to 10% of the adult population have hypothyroidism.[1–4] The Colorado Thyroid Disease Prevalence Study suggested that no less than 10% of the adult population is affected, with a rate over 20% in senior citizens.[5]

Overall, thyroid disease of all types is two to eight times more common among women. Hypothyroidism is more prevalent among Caucasians and Mexican Americans, with 5.7% being affected, than among African-Americans, with 1.7% affected.[6]

Some writers of popular books estimate that 40% of adults would be considered hypothyroid when symptoms and basal body temperature are used for diagnosis.[7,8] It is likely that the true rate of hypothyroidism according to these criteria is somewhere near 25% of the adult population and significantly higher in the elderly. This makes hypothyroidism a surprisingly common, usually unrecognized condition.

Symptoms

The degree of severity of symptoms in adults ranges from early, mild deficiency states that are not detectable with standard blood tests (hypothyroid syndrome) to severe deficiency states that can be life-threatening (myxedema).

Psychological

The brain appears to be quite sensitive to low levels of thyroid hormone. Depression, weakness, and fatigue are usually the first symptoms of hypothyroidism.[9–11] Later the hypothyroid individual has difficulty concentrating and is extremely forgetful.

Metabolic

A lack of thyroid hormones leads to a general decrease in the rate of utilization of fat, protein, and carbohydrate. Moderate weight gain combined with sensitivity to cold weather (demonstrated by cold hands or feet) is a common finding. Hypothyroidism often results in swelling of tissue and fluid retention (edema).

Cardiovascular

Hypothyroidism, even in very mild cases, is thought to predispose people to atherosclerosis because of increases in cholesterol and triglycerides as well as homocysteine and C-reactive protein (CRP). Hypothyroidism can also cause high blood pressure, reduce the function of the heart, and reduce heart rate.[9,12–14]

Endocrine

Various hormonal symptoms can exist in hypothyroidism. Perhaps the most common is a loss of libido (sexual drive) in men and menstrual abnormalities in women. Women with mild hypothyroidism have prolonged and heavy menstrual bleeding, with a shorter menstrual cycle. Infertility may also be a problem. If a hypothyroid woman becomes pregnant, miscarriages, premature deliveries, and stillbirths are more common.

Low adrenal function is often a companion to low thyroid function, as patients with thyroid antibodies are likely to also have antibodies that attack the adrenals.

Skin, Hair, and Nails

Dry, rough skin covered with fine superficial scales is seen in most hypothyroid individuals, while the hair is coarse, dry, and brittle. Hair loss can be quite severe and is generally diffuse as opposed to patchy. The nails become thin and brittle and typically show crosswise grooves.

Muscular and Skeletal

Muscle weakness and joint stiffness are predominate features of hypothyroidism.[15] Some individuals with hypothyroidism may also experience muscle and joint pain, as well as tenderness.[16]

Other

Shortness of breath, constipation, and impaired kidney function are some of the other common features of hypothyroidism.

Causes

About 95% of all cases of clinical hypothyroidism are primary. Around the globe the most common cause of hypothyroidism is iodine deficiency. The thyroid gland adds iodine to the amino acid tyrosine to create thyroid hormones. Iodine deficiency leads to hypothyroidism or the development of an enlarged thyroid gland (a goiter), or both.

Goiters are estimated to affect more than 200 million people worldwide. In all but 4% of these cases, the cause is an iodine deficiency. Iodine deficiency is quite rare in the United States and other industrialized countries, owing to the addition of iodine to table salt. Adding iodine to table salt began in Michigan, where in 1924 the goiter rate was an incredible 47%. However, the incidence of deficiency has increased owing to several factors: more people eat out, in places where the salt in food is usually not iodized (many chefs believe iodizing affects the taste of food); iodine compounds are no longer used in commercial bread; and dairy products have less iodine because the udders of cows are no longer sterilized with iodine compounds. The end result is that iodine consumption has decreased 50% in the past 20 years.

Although few people in the United States are now considered iodine deficient, some still develop goiters, and many cases of mild hypothyroidism are simply not recognized. A possible cause of goiters or nodules in patients with adequate but marginal iodine intake is the excessive ingestion of goitrogens—foods that block iodine utilization. These include vegetables in the brassica family (turnips, cabbage, broccoli, brussels sprouts, mustard, kale, cauliflower), cassava root, soybeans, peanuts, pine nuts, and millet. Cooking usually inactivates goitrogens.

Environmental goitrogens include perchlorate, fluoride, and mercury. Medications that induce goiters and suppress thyroid function include supplemental iodine in excess of 1,000 mcg per day, amiodarone, carbamazepine, lithium, phenobarbital, phenytoin, and rifampin. In addition, the bromates now used in commercial bread are iodine antagonists.

Goiters can also be the result of Hashimoto's thyroiditis, an autoimmune disorder that is the most frequent cause of clinical hypothyroidism in the United States. In this disease antibodies that bind to the thyroid prevent the manufacture of sufficient levels of thyroid hormone. In addition to binding to thyroid tissue, these antibodies may also bind to the adrenal glands, pancreas, and acid-producing cells of the stomach (parietal cells).

Hashimoto's thyroiditis can be reasonably assumed to be present when there are signs of autoimmune thyroid disease. These can include any of the following:

- Serum antibodies against thyroid proteins such as thyroglobulin or thyroperoxidase
- Diffuse enlargement of the gland detected by physical exam, ultrasound, or CT scan
- Diffuse iodine uptake and glandular enlargement on radioiodine uptake scan

Other causes of clinical hypothyroidism include thyroid surgery and/or ablation and postpartum hypothyroidism, the last of which is a transient form of hypothyroidism that affects 5 to 10% of women in the United States.

Subclinical Hypothyroidism and Hypothyroid Syndrome

In subclinical hypothyroidism, classically defined, TSH is elevated while serum thyroid hormone levels are normal. According to this criterion, subclinical hypothyroidism is a relatively common finding, affecting 2% to 7% of adults.[9] Symptoms of hypothyroidism in the absence of laboratory findings are more accurately called *hypothyroid syndrome*, and this condition is associated with the following:

- The presence of hypothyroid symptoms
- The absence of other explanatory diseases
- Possible functional thyroid abnormalities such as low basal body temperature or slow Achilles reflex

For clinical hypothyroidism to be diagnosed, patients with hypothyroid syndrome must also have one or more of the following objective findings:

- Suboptimal blood levels of thyroid hormones
- Abnormal thyroid antibody studies
- Abnormal findings on ultrasound
- Abnormal findings on biopsy (fine needle aspiration of the thyroid)

Many people with hypothyroid syndrome may have early Hashimoto's disease, while some cases can be attributed to impaired thyroid hormone synthesis or conversion related to nutritional deficiencies or environmental toxins. With the growing incidence of iodine deficiency, we expect this last cause will become more commonly recognized.

Diagnostic Considerations

Screening for hypothyroidism should include a marker of thyroid regulation (TSH), markers of thyroid output (free T4, free T3), and markers of thyroid inflammation (thy-

roid microsomal antibody, thyroperoxidase antibody, antithyroglobulin antibody). The American Thyroid Association recommends TSH screening every five years beginning at age 35.

The diagnosis of hypothyroidism by laboratory methods is primarily based on the results of total T_4, free T_4, T_3, and TSH levels.

Basal Body Temperature

Before the use of blood measurements, it was common to diagnose hypothyroidism on the basis of basal body temperature (the temperature of the body at rest) and Achilles reflex time (reflexes are slowed in hypothyroidism). With the advent of sophisticated laboratory measurement of thyroid hormones in the blood, these functional tests of thyroid function fell by the wayside. The normal basal body temperature is 97.6 to 98.2°F. Instructions for taking basal body temperature are provided below.

Many consider basal body temperature a specific indicator of thyroid status. Yet it is affected by so many other variables, including adrenal function, body composition, activity levels, menstrual status, and immune function, that it has very little specificity for thyroid function. Nonetheless, it is a good general screening test that is easy to do and virtually without cost.

TAKING YOUR BASAL BODY TEMPERATURE

Your body temperature reflects your metabolic rate, which is largely determined by hormones secreted by the thyroid gland. The function of the thyroid gland can be determined by simply measuring your basal body temperature. All that is needed is a thermometer.

1. Shake down the thermometer to below 95°F and place it by your bed before going to sleep at night.

Normal Blood Levels of Thyroid Hormones	
HORMONE	**BLOOD LEVEL**
T_4	4.8–13.2 mcg/dl
Free T_4	0.9–2 ng/dl
T_3	80–220 ng/dl
Thyroid-stimulating hormone (TSH)	0.35–5.50 mIU/ml

2. On waking, place the thermometer in your armpit for a full 10 minutes. It is important to move as little as possible. Lying and resting with your eyes closed is best. Do not get up until the 10-minute test is completed.
3. After 10 minutes, read and record the temperature.
4. Record the temperature for at least three mornings (preferably at the same time of day) and give the information to your physician. Menstruating women must perform the test on the second, third, and fourth days of menstruation. Men and postmenopausal women can perform the test at any time.

Basal body temperature should be between 97.6 and 98.2°F. Low basal body temperatures are quite common and may reflect hypothyroidism. High basal body temperatures (above 98.6°F) are less common but may be evidence of hyperthyroidism (see the chapter "Hyperthyroidism").

Therapeutic Considerations

The medical treatment of hypothyroidism, in all but its mildest forms, involves the use of desiccated thyroid or synthetic thyroid hormone. Although synthetic hormones have become popular, many physicians (particularly naturopathic physicians) still prefer the use of desiccated natural thyroid, which contains all thyroid hormones, not just thyroxine. At this time, it appears that thyroid hormone replacement is necessary in the majority of people with hypothyroidism. In particular, the use of thyroid replacement is very important in patients with Hashimoto's thyroiditis, as it achieves two objectives: it normalizes thyroid hormone levels and also decreases autoimmune processes. Either desiccated or synthetic thyroid replacement should be used in doses high enough to decrease TSH to between 0.5 and 1.5 mIU/ml. We prefer desiccated thyroid, as it may stimulate blocking antibodies to antithyroid antibodies or act as a decoy for thyroid antibodies. Some patients are found to recover from Hashimoto thyroiditis after an extended treatment time with thyroid hormone and no longer need to be maintained on replacement, but the majority will require lifelong replacement therapy.

The thyroid extracts sold in health food stores are required by the Food and Drug Administration to be thyroxine-free. However, it is nearly impossible to remove all the hormone from the gland. In other words, think of health food store thyroid preparations as milder forms of desiccated natural thyroid. If you have mild hypothyroidism, these preparations may provide enough support to help you with your thyroid problem.

Since it is important to nutritionally support the thyroid gland by ensuring adequate intake of key nutrients required in the body's manufacture of thyroid hormone and avoiding goitrogens (see above), most health food stores' thyroid products also contain supportive nutrients such as iodine, zinc, selenium, and tyrosine.

Iodine and Tyrosine

Thyroid hormones are made from iodine and the amino acid tyrosine. The recommended dietary intake (RDI) for iodine in adults is quite small, 150 mcg. The average intake of iodine in the United States, once estimated to be more than 600 mcg per day, is now less than half that. Vegans, especially those who are pregnant, should be careful to ensure adequate iodine intake, as their levels are typically low.

Too much iodine can actually inhibit thyroid gland synthesis. For this reason, and because the only function of iodine in the body is for thyroid hormone synthesis, it is recommended that dietary levels or supplementation of iodine not exceed 600 mcg per day for any length of time.

Vitamins and Minerals

Zinc, selenium, vitamin E, and vitamin A function together in many body processes, including the manufacture of thyroid hormone. A deficiency of any of these nutrients would result in production of lower levels of active thyroid hormone. Low zinc levels are common in the elderly, as is hypothyroidism.[17] There may be a correlation. Supplementation with zinc has been shown to reestablish normal thyroid function in hypothyroid patients who were zinc deficient, even though they had supposedly normal serum T_4 levels.[18]

Similarly, selenium supplementation may be important, as those living in areas of the world where selenium is deficient have a greater incidence of thyroid disease.[19] Of particular significance is the fact that while a selenium deficiency does not decrease the conversion of T_4 to T_3 in the thyroid or the pituitary, it does result in a great decrease in this conversion in other cells of the body.[20] People with a selenium deficiency have elevated levels of T_4 and TSH. Supplementation with selenium results in a decrease in T_4 and TSH, a normalization of thyroid activity,[21] and decreased thyroid antibody levels in autoimmune thyroid conditions.[22] Inadequate selenium is a common nutritional deficiency.

Vitamin B_2 (riboflavin), B_3 (niacin), B_6 (pyridoxine), and C are also necessary for normal thyroid hormone manufacture.

Dehydroepiandrosterone (DHEA)

DHEA is often low in hypothyroid patients and supplementation has shown benefit in the treatment of autoimmune conditions.[23] Although many clinical studies have employed high dosages (100 to 200 mg per day), if there is no physician supervision we recommend much lower doses: 5 to 15 mg per day in women and 10 to 20 mg per day

- -

QUICK REVIEW

- **Since thyroid hormones affect every cell of the body, a deficiency will usually result in a large number of signs and symptoms.**
- **Depression, weakness, and fatigue are usually the first symptoms of hypothyroidism.**
- **The medical treatment of hypothyroidism, in all but its mildest forms, involves the use of desiccated thyroid or synthetic thyroid hormone.**

- **You can support the thyroid gland by avoiding goitrogens (foods that impair the use of iodine) and ensuring adequate intake of key nutrients that are required for the manufacture of thyroid hormone.**
- **In very mild cases, thyroid products from a health food store may provide benefit.**

in men. Higher dosages require monitoring for DHEA blood levels and clinical symptoms of excess estrogen (men) or testosterone (women). As the long-term effects of DHEA administration are unknown, DHEA should be used with caution, particularly in patients at risk for developing hormone-dependent cancers.

Exercise

Exercise is particularly important in a treatment program for hypothyroidism. Exercise stimulates thyroid gland secretion and increases tissue sensitivity to thyroid hormone. Many of the health benefits of exercise may be a result of improved thyroid function.

The health benefits of exercise are especially important in overweight hypothyroid individuals who are dieting. A consistent effect of dieting is a decrease in the metabolic rate as the body strives to conserve fuel. Exercise has been shown to prevent this decline.[24]

TREATMENT SUMMARY

Natural treatment strategies for normalizing thyroid function vary depending on whether there is an autoimmune hypothyroid condition, clinical hypothyroidism, subclinical hypothyroidism, or hypothyroid syndrome. Below are general recommendations to improve thyroid function.

Diet

The recommendations given in the chapter "A Health-Promoting Diet" are suitable, with the following caveat: the diet should be low in raw goitrogens and high in foods rich in the trace minerals needed for thyroid hormone production and activation. Goitrogens to be limited include brassica-family foods (turnips, cabbage, rutabagas, mustard greens, radishes, horseradishes), cassava root, soybeans, peanuts, pine nuts, and millet. When these foods are eaten, they should be cooked to break down their goitrogenic constituents.

We also recommend ruling out gluten sensitivity, as gluten may lead to the formation of thyroid-related autoantibodies in sensitive individuals.[25]

Nutritional Supplements

- A high-potency multiple vitamin and mineral formula as described in the chapter "Supplementary Measures"
- Key individual nutrients:
  - Copper: 1 to 1.5 mg per day
  - Iodine: 300 mcg per day
  - Selenium: 100 to 200 mcg per day
  - Zinc: 15 to 30 mg per day
  - Vitamin D_3: 2,000 to 4,000 IU per day (ideally, measure blood levels and adjust dosage accordingly)
- Fish oils: 1,000 mg EPA + DHA per day
- One of the following:
  - Grape seed extract (>95% procyanidolic oligomers): 100 to 300 mg per day

○ Pine bark extract (>95% procyanidolic oligomers): 100 to 300 mg per day

○ Some other flavonoid-rich extract with a similar flavonoid content, super greens formula, or another plant-based antioxidant that can provide an oxygen radical absorption capacity (ORAC) of 3,000 to 6,000 units or higher per day

Exercise

• Daily exercise, especially high-intensity activities, can stimulate thyroid function.

Infertility (Female)

- Inability to conceive a child after 12 months of regular, unprotected intercourse at least twice weekly with the same male partner and in the absence of male causes.

It is estimated that one in seven couples in the United States experiences infertility. In about 50% of the cases of infertility the issue is with the woman.

A woman's fertility is usually a reflection of her general health and well-being. Optimal fertility generally occurs between 18 and 31 years of age in women. The normal monthly success rate for couples trying to conceive naturally at age 25 is 25%. This figure decreases with increasing age, particularly after 35 for women. Fecundity is defined as the couple's chance of conception in a single menstrual cycle. A couple's fecundity is generally highest in the first three months of unprotected sex; successful conception rates decline gradually thereafter.[1]

Causes

One of the major causes of female infertility is age, owing to the decreasing quantity and quality of the eggs preserved in the ovary.[2] Population-based and clinical studies have shown that women experience optimal fertility before age 31.[3,4] After 31 the probability of conception starts to drop rapidly. By age 40, half of women will have completely lost their capacity for reproduction. By 45 years of age, the fertility rate is only 1 pregnancy per 100 inseminated women.[5] In addition, the probability of birth defects or an adverse pregnancy outcome increases with age.[6]

Therapeutic Considerations

Diagnosing and treating infertility will often require a very thorough health assessment by a physician and may require seeing a fertility specialist. The general recommendations in this chapter can be used along with conventional medical treatments.

It is important to realize that there are three types of patients suffering from infertility:

- Those who achieve pregnancy by maximizing their fertility
- Those who require assistance in the form of in vitro fertilization and other assisted-reproduction technologies
- Those who simply cannot get pregnant owing primarily to age, genetic disorders, or various health conditions that compromise fertility

The first step to successful conception is timing the attempt of conception during a woman's window of fertility. A widely held misinterpretation is that frequent ejaculations decrease male fertility. A retrospective study

Causes of Female Infertility[7]	
DISORDER	**CAUSE**
Ovulation disorders (40%)	Aging
	Diminished ovarian reserve
	Endocrine disorder (e.g., hyperprolactinemia, thyroid disease, adrenal disease)
	Polycystic ovarian syndrome
	Premature ovarian failure
	Tobacco use
Tubal factors (30%)	Obstruction (e.g., history of pelvic inflammatory disease, tubal surgery)
Endometriosis (15%)	
Other (approximately 10%)	
Uterine/cervical factors (approximately 3%)	Congenital uterine anomaly
	Fibroids
	Endometrial polyps
	Poor cervical mucus quantity/quality (caused by smoking, infection); mucus hostility (sperm antibodies)
	Uterine synechiae or adhesions (Asherman's syndrome)

analyzed 9,489 men with normal semen quality, sperm concentrations, and motility and found that profiles remained normal even with daily ejaculation.[8] Of more importance is the finding that in men with sperm abnormalities, fertility may be improved with more frequent (per day) ejaculation. So, in other words, daily intercourse is probably more important than trying to time it just right.

A recently ovulated egg will survive for only a maximum of 24 hours, while sperm can survive for up to five or six days. Hence, the fertility window is best defined as the six-day interval ending on the day of ovulation.[9] Fertility charting can help identify the fertility window. A useful tool in helping to determine ovulation is an at-home kit that measures luteinizing hormone (LH) in the urine. This hormone increases 24 to 48 hours prior to ovulation. The LH surge triggers ovulation.

Body Fat Percentage

For optimal fertility, women need to ensure that their body fat percentage is between 20 and 25%. A body fat percentage below 17% can result in irregular menstrual cycles, and some research suggests that even after ideal body fat levels have been achieved, it can take as long as two years before regular conception occurs.[10] While being underweight is a concern, obesity poses a similar and significant risk for infertility. Obesity increases the risk for miscarriage, birth defects, and pregnancy complications.[11] Maternal obesity carries an increased risk that the child will be overweight as an adult and have the consequent weight-related diseases.

Environmental Factors

Industrialization and the use of agricultural chemicals has contributed to increased exposure to thousands of chemicals now associated with negative impact on male and female infertility. Exposure to environmental toxins such as radiation, heavy metals, and chemicals can cause oxidative stress and damage, negatively affecting female fertility. These issues are more fully discussed in the chapter "Infertility (Male)" but also apply to female infertility.

Smoking

Cigarette smoking, whether active or passive, reduces both pregnancy rates and long-term ovarian function. Additionally, smokers are more likely to have premature menopause, thus making smoking one of the easiest preventable causes of infertility. Smoking appears to reduce fertility by having a direct effect on the uterus, eggs, and embryo.[12,13] Overall, research indicates that smoking can prematurely age eggs by as much as 10 years. Considering that the average age for conception today is 30 and fertility tends to decline greatly after 38 years of age, it should be obvious that a woman trying to get pregnant needs to stop smoking. Even passive smoking is associated with reduced fertility and decreases the chance of a healthy live birth in both fertile and infertile populations.[14]

Caffeine

Couples trying to conceive may want to avoid caffeine, as frequent consumption been shown to increase time to conception.[15–17] As little as one caffeinated beverage per day is associated with a temporary reduction in conception in a number of studies.[18] For example, women who drink less than one cup of coffee per day are twice as likely to conceive compared with moderate coffee drinkers.[16] Caffeine affects female hormone levels as well as stress homones.[19] Caffeine is also likely to interfere with adrenal function and associated cortisol secretion. In addition, diuretic properties will increase the loss of nutrients that are beneficial to fertility.

Alcohol

The effect of alcohol intake on female fertility is variable from one woman to the next, but there is no question that it can negatively affect fertility in many women. One study estimated that as little as one drink per week could lead to a 50% reduction in conception.[20] Frequent or excessive alcohol consumption is associated with elevations in prolactin and alterations in other hormones that could adversely affect menstrual cycles and fertility.[21,22] There is also a strong association between alcohol intake and miscarriage.[23] Obviously, as with smoking, it is critical that alcohol intake be avoided during the preconception period as well as pregnancy. It is a well-known fact that alcohol intake during pregnancy can produce fetal abnormalities.

Diet and Lifestyle

There is abundant scientific research showing the importance of nutrition and lifestyle to a woman's fertility. Specifically, research clearly indicates that eating a healthful diet improves the chances for ovulation, conception, and the birth of a healthy child.

The strongest evidence in favor of diet and lifestyle to support fertility can be seen in data from the Nurses Health Study II.[24]

The following factors were associated with enhanced fertility:

- Lower intake of trans-fatty acids and greater intake of monounsaturated fats[25]

- Lower intake of animal protein and greater intake of vegetable protein[26]

- Higher intake of high-fiber, low-glycemic carbohydrates

- Higher intake of high-fat dairy products (high-fat dairy products reduced the risk of infertility due to lack of ovulation by more than 50% in contrast to low-fat dairy foods, which actually reduced the risk of successful conception by 11%)

- Higher intake of dietary sources of non-heme iron (green leafy vegetables and other plant foods relatively high in iron)

- Higher frequency of multivitamin use

- Being physically active (30 minutes or more of vigorous activity per day)

- Not smoking

- Not having long menstrual cycles

- BMI between 20 and 25

Just as in many other health conditions, researchers have noted that a diet based upon the principles of the Mediterranean diet (see the chapter "A Health-Promoting Diet") also increases the chance of a successful pregnancy.[27]

Nutritional Supplements

The general guidelines in the chapter "Supplementary Measures" are extremely important in maximizing nutritional status and possibly improving fertility, as they address any nutrient deficiency, protect against oxidative damage, and improve overall health. In particular, it is important to point out that iron deficiency is the most common nutritional deficiency in women and can be a cause of infertility.[28] Iron is required for the formation of red blood cells, subsequent transport of oxygen to the tissues by hemoglobin, and DNA formation, as well as being involved in numerous enzyme systems within the body.[29] Results from the Nurses Health Study II suggested that women who consumed iron supplements had a 60% lower risk of infertility than women who did not.[30] Measuring blood levels of ferritin, an iron-binding storage protein, is critical in assessing causes of infertility. Achieving a level of 70 to 80 ng/ml is recommended prior to conception.

A high antioxidant intake, both dietary and supplemental, improves fertility in women as well as reduces the risk for miscarriage.[31,32] The egg cell has high requirements for antioxidants, and oxidative stress has been shown to increase time to conception, decrease fertilization rates, decrease egg viability, and decrease implantation rates.[33,34]

Carnitine

In animal studies, carnitine has been found to exert a protective effect against egg damage and embryo death associated with endometriosis.[35] Although human studies are required, carnitine appears to be an appropriate recommendation for women with infertility due to endometriosis.

Arginine

Arginine is a precursor to the synthesis of nitric oxide, which is required for the formation of new blood vessels to nourish the developing fetus, as well as other aspects of fertility.[36] In one study, arginine supplementation at a dosage of 16 g per day was evaluated in women who failed to achieve an adequate number of mature follicles and/or adequate serum estradiol levels following hormonal stimulation.[37] Results indicated that supplementation improved ovarian response, endometrial receptivity, and pregnancy rates, with

3 of 17 women conceiving in the arginine group, compared with none in the control group. Arginine is not a panacea, but it may be helpful in some situations.

Probiotics

Alterations in the microflora of the vagina and subsequent genital and intrauterine infections have been linked to reproductive failure and adverse pregnancy outcomes such as preterm labor, miscarriage, and spontane-

ous preterm birth.[38] In one study during the first half of pregnancy, women with altered vaginal flora were four times more likely to have a spontaneous preterm birth.[39]

Botanical Medicines

Chasteberry

The best-documented herb for improving fertility is chasteberry (*Vitex agnus-castus*). Clinical studies have shown it to help pro-

- -

QUICK REVIEW

- A woman's fertility is usually a reflection of her general health and well-being.
- By 45 years of age, the fertility rate is only 1 pregnancy per 100 inseminated women.
- Diagnosis and treatment of infertility often require a very thorough health assessment by a physician and may require referral to a fertility specialist.
- The first step to successful conception is timing the attempt of conception during the fertile window.
- For optimal fertility, women need to ensure that their body fat proportion is between 20 and 25%.
- Exposure to environmental toxins such as radiation, heavy metals, and chemicals can cause oxidative stress and damage to subsequently produce a negative impact on female infertility.
- Active and passive cigarette smoking reduces pregnancy rates and long-term ovarian function.
- Women who drink less than one cup of

coffee per day are twice as likely to conceive compared with moderate coffee drinkers.

- Frequent or excessive alcohol consumption is associated with elevations in prolactin and alterations in other hormones that could adversely affect menstrual cycles and fertility.
- Research clearly indicates that eating a healthful diet improves the chances for ovulation, conception, and the birth of a healthy child.
- Iron deficiency is the most common nutritional deficiency in women and can be a cause of infertility.
- Carnitine appears to be an appropriate recommendation for women with infertility due to endometriosis.
- B-complex vitamins are important for fertility.
- Chasteberry has been shown to improve hormone levels, reestablish menstruation in women with amenorrhea, and help achieve pregnancy in women with fertility problems.

mote healthy menstrual cycles. It seems to be especially useful when there is an elevation in the hormone prolactin, which can disrupt the menstrual cycle and contribute to infertility. Chasteberry can inhibit prolactin secretion and has been shown to correct menstrual irregularities caused by mild elevations of prolactin.[40–42] In one double-blind study, chasteberry was shown to improve hormone levels, reestablish menstruation in women with amenorrhea, and help achieve pregnancy in women with fertility problems.[43]

TREATMENT SUMMARY

The primary goal of natural medicine is to increase overall health through dietary and lifestyle strategies to provide the best chance of conception.

General Recommendations

- Identify and eliminate exposure to environmental hazards, including pesticides, solvents, heavy metals, and other toxins
- Utilize effective stress-reduction techniques (employ psychological counseling if needed)
- Avoid cigarette smoking, alcohol, and recreational drugs
- Avoid douches, vaginal sprays, scented tampons, or other feminine products that change the pH of the vagina and disturb vaginal microecology.
- Ensure that body fat is at a healthful proportion (20 to 25%)
- Avoid medications that affect the quality of cervical fluid and interfere with conception, including antihistamines, some cough mixtures, dicyclomine, progesterone (taken prior to or at ovulation), propantheline, tamoxifen, and others
- Avoid all personal lubricants (unless sperm-friendly types are chosen), as common lubricants kill sperm

Diet

- Follow the guidelines given in the chapter "A Health-Promoting Diet"
- Avoid dietary sources of free radicals, saturated fats, trans-fatty acids, and cottonseed oil (it contains gossypol, a compound that may cause infertility)
- Eat ¼ cup of raw nuts or seeds each day and use olive oil in cooking
- Increase consumption of good dietary sources of carotenes and flavonoids (deep- or brightly colored vegetables and fruits).
- Consume 8 to 10 servings of vegetables and 1 to 2 servings of fresh fruits per day
- Optimize protein intake from both vegetarian and organic animal sources
- Eliminate caffeine, alcohol, sugar, and food additives (such as preservatives and colorings)

Nutritional Supplements

- A high-potency multiple vitamin and mineral formula as described in the chapter "Supplementary Measures"

- Vitamin D$_3$: 2,000 to 4,000 IU per day (ideally, measure blood levels and adjust dosage accordingly)
- Fish oils: 1,000 mg EPA + DHA per day
- One of the following:
  - Grape seed extract (>95% procyanidolic oligomers): 100 to 300 mg per day
  - Pine bark extract (>95% procyanidolic oligomers): 100 to 300 mg per day
  - Some other flavonoid-rich extract with a similar flavonoid content, super greens formula, or another plant-based antioxidant that can provide an oxygen radical absorption capacity (ORAC) of 3,000 to 6,000 units or more per day

- Specialty supplements:
  - L-carnitine: 1,000 to 1,500 mg per day
  - Probiotic (*Lactobacillus* species and *Bifidobacter* species): a minimum of 5 billion to 10 billion colony-forming units

Botanical Medicines

- Chasteberry *(Vitex agnus-castus)*: The usual dosage of chasteberry extract (standardized to contain 0.5% agnuside) in tablet or capsule form is 175 to 225 mg per day. If you are using the liquid extract, the typical dosage is 2 to 4 ml (½ to 1 tsp) per day.

Infertility (Male)

- Inability to conceive a child after six months of unprotected sex at least twice weekly with the same partner in the absence of female causes

- A total sperm count lower than 5 million/ml

- The presence of greater than 50% abnormal sperm

- Inability of sperm to impregnate egg, as determined by the postcoital or hamster-egg penetration tests

Infertility affects about 7.3 million couples in the United States: approximately 12% of the reproductive-age population. It is estimated that one in seven couples in the United States experiences infertility. In about 50% of the cases of infertility the issue is with the female. Current estimates suggest that about 6% of men between the ages of 15 and 50 years are infertile.[1]

Causes

Most male infertility is due to abnormal sperm count or quality. Although it takes only one sperm to fertilize an egg, there are nearly 200 million sperm in an average ejaculation. However, because of the natural barriers in the female reproductive tract, only about 40 sperm will ever reach the vicinity of an egg. There is a strong correlation between fertility and the number of sperm in an ejaculation.

In about 90% of the cases of low sperm count, the reason is deficient sperm production. Unfortunately, in about 9 out of 10 of those cases, the cause of the decreased sperm formation cannot be identified, and the condition is labeled *idiopathic oligospermia* (low sperm count) or *azoospermia* (a complete absence of living sperm).

Causes of Male Infertility

Deficient sperm production

Ductal obstruction

Congenital defects

Postinfectious obstruction

Cystic fibrosis

Vasectomy

Ejaculatory dysfunction

Premature ejaculation

Retrograde ejaculation

Disorders of accessory glands

Infection

Inflammation

Antisperm antibodies

Coital disorders

Defects in technique

Premature withdrawal

Erectile dysfunction

Since the overwhelming majority of men who are infertile suffer from deficient sperm production, that is the major focus of this

731

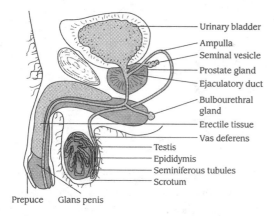

Urinary bladder
Ampulla
Seminal vesicle
Prostate gland
Ejaculatory duct
Bulbourethral gland
Erectile tissue
Vas deferens
Testis
Epididymis
Seminiferous tubules
Scrotum
Prepuce   Glans penis

Anatomy of the Male Sexual System

chapter. Normal sperm are defined as having the following characteristics:

- A smooth, oval-shaped head that is 5 to 6 micrometers long and 2.5 to 3.5 micrometers around (less than the size of a needle point)

- A well-defined cap (acrosome) that covers 40 to 70% of the sperm head

- No visible defect of head, midpiece, or tail

- No fluid droplets in the sperm head that are bigger than one-half the size of the sperm head

Diagnostic Considerations

Semen analysis, which assesses concentration of sperm and sperm quality, is the test most widely used to estimate fertility potential in men. Total sperm count and sperm quality have been deteriorating over the last few decades. In 1940, the average sperm count was 113 million/ml; in 1990, that value had dropped to 66 million/ml; and it is now holding steady at around 60 million/ml. Adding to this problem, the amount of semen in an ejaculation fell almost 20%, from 3.4 ml to 2.75 ml. All together, these changes mean

that men are now supplying about 40% of the number of sperm per ejaculation compared with 1940 levels.

The downward trend in sperm count has led to speculation that environmental, dietary, and/or lifestyle changes in recent decades may be interfering with men's ability to manufacture sperm. Although the theory is controversial, there is substantial supporting evidence.

Possible Causes of Falling Sperm Count

- Increased scrotal temperature
- Tight-fitting clothing and briefs
- Varicoceles (varicose veins that surround the testes)
- Environment
- Increased pollution
- Heavy metals (lead, mercury, arsenic, etc.)
- Organic solvents
- Pesticides (DDT, PCBs, DBCP, etc.)
- Diet
- Increased intake of saturated fats
- Reduced intake of fruits, vegetables, and whole grains
- Reduced intake of dietary fiber
- Increased exposure to synthetic estrogens

As sperm counts in the general population have declined, there has been a parallel reduction in the accepted line between infertile and fertile men, with the minimum sperm count for fertility dropping from 40 million/ml to the current value of 5 million/ml. One of the key reasons these values have dropped so dramatically is that researchers are learning that quality is more important than quantity. A high sperm count means nothing if the percentage of healthy sperm is not also high.

Whenever the majority of sperm are ab-

Semen Terminology	
SYNDROME	**DEFINITION**
Aspermia	An absence of semen despite male orgasm
Azoospermia	A complete absence of sperm in the semen
Oligozoospermia	Reduced number of normal motile sperm cells in the ejaculate
Teratozoospermia	Sperm with abnormal morphology
Asthenozoospermia	Reduced sperm motility
Necrospermia	Death of sperm
Oligoasthenoteratozoospermia	Low sperm count, weak motility, and abnormal morphology

normally shaped or are entirely or relatively nonmotile, a man can be infertile despite having a normal sperm concentration. Conversely, a low sperm count does not always mean that a man is infertile. Numerous pregnancies have occurred involving men with very low sperm counts. For example, in studies at fertility clinics, 52% of couples in which the man's sperm count was below 10 million/ml achieved pregnancy, and 40% of couples in which the man's sperm count was as low as 5 million/ml were able to achieve pregnancy.[1]

Because of these confirmed successes in men with low sperm counts, we recommend that conventional semen analysis be interpreted with caution regarding the likelihood of conception. More sophisticated functional tests should also be used, especially in screening couples for in vitro fertilization.

Causes of Temporary Low Sperm Count

- Increased scrotal temperature
- Infections (common cold, flu, etc.)
- Increased stress
- Lack of sleep
- Overuse of alcohol, tobacco, or marijuana
- Many prescription drugs
- Exposure to radiation
- Exposure to solvents, pesticides, and other toxins

Until recently, pregnancy was the only proof of the ability of sperm to achieve fertilization. Now there are several functional tests in use. The postcoital test measures the ability of the sperm to penetrate the cervical mucus after intercourse. In vitro variants of this test are also available. One of the most encouraging tests is based on the discovery that human sperm, under appropriate conditions, can penetrate hamster eggs. It has been established that fertile men exhibit a range of penetration between 10 and 100%, and that a penetration rate of less than 10% is indicative of infertility. The hamster-egg penetration test is considered to predict fertility in 66% of cases, compared with about 30% for conventional semen analysis.

Another important test in the diagnosis of infertility is the detection of antisperm

Normal Sperm Count	
CRITERION	**VALUE**
Volume	1.5–5.0 ml
Density	>20 million sperm/ml
Motility	>30% motile
Normal forms	>60%

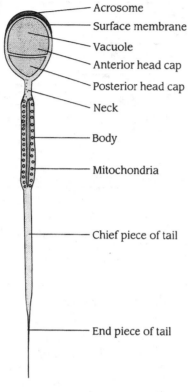

- Acrosome
- Surface membrane
- Vacuole
- Anterior head cap
- Posterior head cap
- Neck
- Body
- Mitochondria
- Chief piece of tail
- End piece of tail

Anatomy of Sperm

antibodies. When produced by the man, these antibodies usually attack the tail of the sperm, thereby impeding the sperm's ability to move and penetrate the cervical mucus. In contrast, the antisperm antibodies produced by women are typically directed against the head of the sperm. The presence of anti-sperm antibodies in semen analysis is usually a sign of past or current infection in the male reproductive tract.

Therapeutic Considerations

The fist step in improving sperm counts, morphology, and function is controlling factors that can damage or impair their formation.

Scrotal Temperature

The scrotal sac normally keeps the testes at a temperature of between 94 and 96°F.[2] At temperatures above 96 degrees, sperm production is greatly inhibited or stopped completely. Typically, the average scrotal temperature of infertile men is significantly higher than that of fertile men. Reducing scrotal temperature in infertile men will often make them fertile. This temperature reduction is best accomplished by not wearing tight-fitting underwear or tight jeans and avoiding hot tubs.

Scrotal temperature can be raised by jogging or the use of rowing machines, simulated cross-country ski machines, or treadmills, especially if a man is wearing synthetic fabrics, tight shorts, or tight underwear. After exercising, a man should allow his testicles to hang free to allow them to recover from heat buildup.

Infertile men should wear boxer-type underwear and periodically take a cold shower or apply ice to the scrotum. They can also choose to use a testicular hypothermia device (also called a testicle cooler) to reduce scrotal temperatures. Still in a primitive stage, the testicle cooler looks like a jock strap from which long, thin tubes extend. The tubes are attached to a small fluid reservoir filled with cold water that attaches to a belt around the waist. The fluid reservoir is also a pump that circulates the water. When the water reaches the surface of the scrotum, it evaporates and keeps the scrotum cool. Because of the evaporation, the reservoir must be filled every six hours or so.

Increased scrotal temperature can be due to the presence of a *varicocele*. (Varicoceles are varicose veins that surround the testes.) A large varicocele can cause scrotum temperatures high enough to inhibit sperm production and motility. Surgical repair may be necessary, but scrotal cooling should be tried first.

Infections

Infections of the male genitourinary tract, including infections of the epididymis, seminal vesicles, prostate, bladder, and urethra, are thought to play a major role in many cases of infertility.[3] The exact extent of the role they play is largely unknown because of the lack of suitable diagnostic criteria coupled with the asymptomatic nature of many infections. If there are no other clinical findings, antisperm antibodies or high levels of debris in a semen sample are considered good indicators of a chronic infection.

There are a large number of bacteria, viruses, and other organisms that can infect the male genitourinary system. It is beyond the scope of this chapter to discuss every type of infection, so the discussion will be limited to *Chlamydia trachomatis.* Chlamydia is now recognized as the most common and the most serious of the infections in the male genitourinary tract.

Chlamydia is considered a sexually transmitted disease. In women, chlamydia infection can lead to pelvic inflammatory disease and scarring of the fallopian tubes. Previous chlamydia infection accounts for a large number of cases of female-factor infertility. In men, chlamydia infection can lead to equally disabling effects. Chlamydia is the major cause of acute nonbacterial prostatitis and urethritis. Typically, the symptoms will be pain or burning sensations upon urination or ejaculation.

More serious is chlamydia infection of the epididymis and vas deferens. The resultant damage to these organs parallels tubal damage in women: serious scarring and blockage can occur. During an acute chlamydia infection, the use of antibiotics is essential. Chlamydia is sensitive to tetracyclines and erythromycin. Unfortunately, because chlamydia lives within human cells, it may be difficult to totally eradicate the organism with antibiotics alone.

While acute chlamydial infections are usually associated with severe pain, chronic infections of the urethra, seminal vesicles, or prostate can occur with few or no symptoms. It is estimated that 28 to 71% of infertile men show evidence of a chlamydial infection. Because of the possible link between chlamydia and low sperm counts, there have been several double-blind studies of the effects of antibiotics on sperm counts. These studies have shown only limited improvements in sperm count and sperm quality. However, there have been isolated cases of tremendous increases in sperm counts and sperm quality after antibiotic treatment. Antibiotics should be used only if there is reason to believe that a chronic infection is present, and both partners should take the antibiotic.

Environmental Estrogen Exposure

According to experts on the impact of the environment and diet on fetal development, we now live in an environment that can be viewed as "a virtual sea of estrogens."[4,5] Increased exposure to environmental estrogens and other environmental pollutants during fetal development, as well as during the reproductive years, is suggested as a major reason for the tremendous rise in disorders of development and function of the male sexual system.[6,7]

One can best view the relationship between estrogens and male sexual development by examining the effects of the synthetic estrogen diethylstilbestrol (DES). Between 1945 and 1971 several million women were treated with DES, which is now recognized to have led to problems in their male offspring. As well as being used in humans, DES and other synthetic estrogens were used for 20 to 30 years in the livestock industry to fatten the animals and help them grow faster. DES exposure has been associated with substantial increases in the number of men suffering from developmental problems of the reproductive tract as well as decreased semen volume and sperm counts.[4] Although DES is now no longer used, poultry and livestock, especially dairy cows, are still hormonally manipulated. Cow's milk contains substantial amounts of estrogen because of modern farming techniques. The rise in consumption of dairy products since the 1940s inversely parallels the drop in sperm counts. Avoidance of meat and milk from animals treated with hormones is important for male sexual vitality, especially in men with low sperm counts or low testosterone levels.

There are reports that estrogens have been detected in drinking water.[4] The source may be estrogens from excreted synthetic estrogens (birth control pills), which are not removed by water treatment plants. These estrogens may be harmful to male sexual vitality. Purified or spring water may be a suitable option to prevent exposure (but ensure that plastic bottles do not contain BPA, which also can have estrogenic effects).

Many of the chemicals that we have contaminated our environment with during the past 50 years are weakly estrogenic. Most of these chemicals, like polychlorinated biphenyls (PCBs), dioxin, and dichlorodiphenyltrichloroethane (DDT), do not easily biodegrade and are recycled in our environment until they accumulate in our bodies. For example, even though DDT has been banned for nearly 30 years, it is still often found in the soil and root vegetables such as carrots and potatoes. These toxic chemicals are known to interfere with spermatogenesis, but their effects during sexual development may be more important.

All of the estrogenic factors previously discussed are thought to have their greatest impact during fetal development. On the basis of animal studies, these estrogens inhibit the multiplication of Sertoli cells. The number of Sertoli cells is directly proportional to the amount of sperm that can be produced, because each Sertoli cell can support only a fixed number of germ cells that will develop into sperm. Sertoli cell multiplication occurs primarily during fetal life and before puberty and is controlled by follicle-stimulating hormone (FSH). In animal studies, estrogens administered early in life inhibit FSH secretion, resulting in a reduced number of Sertoli cells and, in adult life, diminished sperm counts. The impact of environmental estrogens might persist for multiple generations. For example, vinclozolin is a fungicide used in the wine industry. Alarmingly, exposing a pregnant female rat to this fungicide just once was found to disrupt spermatogenesis in more than 90% of male offspring for at least four generations.[8]

Other Environmental Factors

Heavy Metals

Sperm are also particularly susceptible to the damaging effects of heavy metals such as lead, cadmium, arsenic, and mercury.[9] A hair mineral analysis for heavy metals should be performed on all men with reduced sperm counts to rule out heavy metals as a cause. However, a more accurate and sensitive assessment of body load of metals requires challenge testing with a chelating agent. See the chapter "Detoxification and Internal Cleansing."

Radiation

Cell phones operate at between 400 MHz and 2,000 MHz and emit electromagnetic waves that have been linked to DNA damage.[10,11] While the relationship between cell phone use and male infertility remains unclear, there is some evidence that harmful electromagnetic waves emitted from cell phones may interfere with normal spermatogenesis and result in a significant decrease in sperm quality. Specific findings pertaining to sperm motility in humans have also been noted.[12,13]

In one study the use of cell phones decreased sperm count, motility, viability, and normal morphology.[14] The decrease in sperm variables was dependent on the duration of exposure to cell phones and independent of initial semen quality. Of greatest importance was that sperm count, viability, and morphology were reduced as cell phone use increased. Specifically, using the cell phone for more than four hours a day caused a 25% drop in the number of sperm produced, and only 20% of the sperm looked normal.

This preliminary evidence is significant enough for us to discourage cell phone usage, and we definitely recommend that infertile men refrain from storing cell phones in their pockets.

Cigarettes, Alcohol, and Illicit Drugs

Cigarette Smoking

A common source of oxidants is cigarette smoking, which accelerates DNA damage of the sperm and is associated with decreased sperm counts and sperm motility as well as a higher frequency of abnormal sperm.[15–17] Cigarette smoking, as well as the increase in environmental pollution, is thought to be a major contributor to the diminution in sperm counts seen in many industrialized nations during the past few decades.

Alcohol

Excessive alcohol consumption in men is strongly associated with diminished sperm function; however, comprehensive research in this area is limited. Nonetheless, it is prudent to avoid alcohol in the preconception period.

Marijuana and Other Recreational Drugs

The effects of marijuana and other recreational drugs are difficult to determine because their use is illegal. Nevertheless, such drug use generally should be discouraged, particularly because these drugs have well-documented harmful effects on the developing fetus. A known fertility toxicant, marijuana contains cannabinoids, which have been shown to impair signaling pathways, alter hormonal regulation, and cause problems with embryo implantation. In men, cannabinoids have been found to inhibit testosterone production, reduce energy production in human sperm, decrease sperm motility, cause problems with sperm morphology, and decrease sperm function.[18–20] Another factor to consider is that some marijuana is contaminated with herbicides and pesticides. These toxins are very efficiently absorbed into the body when smoked.

Obesity

Obese men are known to have lower sperm counts (up to 50% less), reduced motility, reduced sperm production, increased DNA fragmentation of sperm, and increased levels of erectile dysfunction. Additionally, extra abdominal weight can increase scrotal temperature. Hormonal changes are primarily responsible for the changes in obese men. The level of total and free testosterone is reduced in obese men in proportion to the level of obesity. Estrogen is increased owing to the peripheral aromatization of androgens in adipose tissue. The estrogens produced have a negative feedback effect on gonadotropin production, thereby reducing FSH. This reduction in FSH further reduces testosterone production and sperm production. Additionally, increased body fat and a sedentary lifestyle are associated with raised testicular temperature, which further adversely affects the production of sperm.[21]

Diet

The chapter "A Health-Promoting Diet" provides sound guidance for improving fertility. In particular, it is important to eat the right type of fats. Surrounding the entire sperm is a "shield" of essential fatty acids that protects the sperm, enables movement, and encourages fertilization.[22] Avoid trans fats (found in hydrogenated oils), rancid or oxidized fats, and excessive saturated fat intake.

Studies show that sperm motility strongly correlates with levels of sperm membrane omega-3 fatty acids, in particular DHA.[23] One study noted that excessive omega-6 compared with omega-3 in seminal fluid produced decreased sperm concentration, sperm motility, and sperm morphology.[24] It would be a good idea to restrict the use of popular omega-6 cooking oils such as soy, corn, and safflower. Take omega-3 supplements (optimal dosage is 1,000 to 2,000 mg EPA + DHA); increase consumption of raw nuts and seeds, cold-pressed monounsaturated oils such as olive, canola, and macadamia nut; eat more avocados; and eat more wild and sustainably farmed fish with high levels of essential fatty acids.

In particular, avoid cottonseed oil, as it may contain toxic pesticide residues. Cottonseed also has high levels of gossypol, a substance known to inhibit sperm function. In fact, gossypol is being investigated as the "male birth control pill." Its use as an antifertility agent began after studies demonstrated that men who had used crude cottonseed oil for cooking were shown to have

low sperm counts followed by total testicular failure.[25]

Nutritional Supplements

Antioxidants

A recent Cochrane review assessed the impact of antioxidants on male subfertility by considering 34 trials that involved 2,876 couples.[26] The authors concluded that for subfertile men antioxidant supplementation improves the outcome: live births and pregnancy rates. Important points included these:

- Antioxidant use was associated with a statistically significant increase in pregnancy rate compared with controls.
- No studies reported evidence of harmful side effects of the antioxidant therapy used.
- Up to 80% of male factor subfertility may be due to oxidative stress.
- Subfertile men are confirmed as having lower levels of antioxidants in their semen compared with fertile men.
- Free radical levels are significantly higher in sperm samples from infertile men when compared with healthy controls

Free radicals cause fertility problems by damaging the sperm membrane, thus affecting sperm motility and the ability of sperm to penetrate the egg. They can also alter sperm DNA, which affects fertilization and embryo growth.

In healthy men the seminal plasma is naturally rich in antioxidants that protect it from this damage. Antioxidants are also found in the head of the sperm, where they are responsible for protecting the DNA, promoting the survival and longevity of the sperm, and enabling the sperm to detect chemical signals from the egg.

Free radical or oxidative damage to sperm

is thought to be responsible for many cases of male infertility. High levels of free radicals are found in the semen of approximately 40% of infertile men.[27–29]

Although most free radicals are produced during normal metabolic processes, the environment contributes greatly to the free radical load. Men exposed to higher levels of sources of free radicals are much more likely to have abnormal sperm and sperm counts.[27–29]

Vitamin C. Vitamin C improves all semen variables. A marginal deficiency causes oxidative damage to sperm, resulting in reduced sperm motility and viability. Supplementation leads to improvement in both viability and motility, reduced numbers of abnormal sperm, and reduced sperm agglutination (sperm become agglutinated when antibodies produced by the immune system bind to them; when more than 25% of the sperm are agglutinated, fertility is very unlikely).[30–32]

In infertile men, vitamin C has been found in reduced quantity in the seminal plasma.[33–34] Men with inadequate seminal vitamin C have also been observed to suffer from sperm DNA damage.

When dietary vitamin C was reduced from 250 to 5 mg per day in healthy human subjects, the ascorbic acid content of seminal fluid decreased by 50% and the number of sperm with damage to their DNA rose by 91%.[35]

It is now well documented that cigarette smoking greatly reduces vitamin C levels throughout the body and that smokers require at least twice as much vitamin C as nonsmokers. In one study, men who smoked one pack of cigarettes a day received either 0, 200, or 1,000 mg vitamin C. After one month, sperm quality improved in proportion to the level of vitamin C supplementation.[36]

Nonsmokers appear to benefit from vitamin C as much as smokers. In one study, 30 infertile but otherwise healthy men received either 200 or 1,000 mg vitamin C or a placebo per day.[37] Sperm count, viability, motility, agglutination, abnormalities, and immaturity were measured weekly. After one week, the 1,000-mg group demonstrated a 140% increase in sperm count, the 200-mg group a 112% increase, and the placebo group no change. After three weeks both vitamin C groups continued to improve, with the 200-mg group catching up to the improvement of the 1,000-mg group. At the beginning of the study all three groups had more than 25% agglutinated sperm. After three weeks, the proportion of agglutinated sperm in the vitamin C groups dropped to 11%. Although this result is significant, the most impressive result of the study was that at the end of 60 days, all of the men in the vitamin C groups had impregnated their wives, compared with none in the placebo group.

Vitamin E. Supplementation with vitamin E appears to be especially warranted because it is the main antioxidant in various cell membranes, including those of sperm. Vitamin E has been shown to play an essential role in inhibiting free radical damage to the unsaturated fatty acids of the sperm membrane.[38]

In one study, supplementation with vitamin E was found to decrease malondialdehyde (an indicator of lipid peroxidation) and improve sperm motility.[39] Even more important, however, 11 of 52 treated infertile men (21%) impregnated their spouses, while none did in the placebo group. Following the completion of the study, 26 of the placebo patients were switched to vitamin E, and four were then able to successfully impregnate their spouses.

Supplementation with vitamin E may also be useful for couples undergoing in vitro fertilization. For fertile men with normal sperm who had low fertilization rates, vitamin E (200 mg a day for at least three months) was found to improve the in vitro fertilization rate, possibly by reducing lipid peroxidation.[40]

Vitamin A, Beta-Carotene, and Lycopene. Vitamin A is an antioxidant required for cellular growth and differentiation, gene expression, regulatory functions, and epithelial tissue integrity. It is necessary for the health of the testes and for sperm production. Low concentrations of vitamin A are associated with abnormal semen variables in men,[41] and in animal studies deprivation of vitamin A has been shown to lead to a loss of sperm production.[42]

Beta-carotene levels are significantly reduced in men whose infertility is due to autoimmune issues—conditions in which antibodies form against sperm components. Beta-carotene intake is associated positively with a higher sperm concentration as well as higher quantities of motile sperm.[43] Lycopene may be even more useful than beta-carotene. Lycopene is found in high concentrations in the testes and seminal plasma, and reduced levels have been demonstrated in men with infertility. In one clinical trial, 30 men with fertility problems were administered 2 mg lycopene twice a day for three months. Twenty patients (66%) showed an improvement in sperm concentration, 16 (53%) had improved motility, and 14 (46%) showed improvement in sperm morphology.[44]

Zinc. Zinc is perhaps the most critical trace mineral for male sexual function and is found in high concentrations within the prostate, testes, and semen (approximately 2.5 mg of zinc is lost per ejaculation). It is involved in virtually every aspect of male reproduction, including hormone metabolism, sperm production, and sperm motility.

Zinc plays an important role in all human living cells, where it is involved in RNA transcription, DNA replication, and protein synthesis, all of which are crucial for reproduction and fertility. Additionally, it protects against free radical damage that may impair sperm. Deficiency of zinc may lead to gonadal dysfunction and has been observed to be associated with male infertility and impotence.[45]

Zinc levels are typically much lower in infertile men with low sperm counts, indicating that a low zinc status may be the contributing factor in the infertility.[45–47] It has also been shown that zinc status directly correlates with an increase in sperm count and improvements in morphology and motility.[48] Finally, zinc has been shown to exert an antimicrobial effect in the seminal plasma; this effect can be important if sperm antibodies or underlying genitourinary infection is present.[49]

Several studies have evaluated the effect of zinc supplementation on sperm counts and motility.[50–52] The results of all of the studies support the use of zinc supplementation in the treatment of low sperm count, especially in the presence of low testosterone levels. The effectiveness of zinc is best illustrated by a study of 37 men with infertility of more than 5 years' duration whose sperm counts were less than 25 million/ml.[53] Blood testosterone levels were also measured. The men received a supplement of zinc sulfate (60 mg elemental zinc per day) for 45 to 50 days. In the 22 patients with initially low testosterone levels, mean sperm count rose significantly from 8 milllion to 20 million/ml. Testosterone levels also increased, and 9 of the 22 wives became pregnant during the study. This result is quite impressive given the long-term nature of the infertility and the rapidity of the results. In contrast, in the 15 men who had had normal testosterone levels before the study, sperm count increased slightly, but there was no change in testosterone levels and no pregnancies occurred.

Selenium. Selenium is a potent antioxidant that is essential for male fertility owing to its role in testosterone synthesis, normal sperm maturation, and sperm motility. Clinical trials reveal it has the ability to increase sperm motility and assist in the production of healthy spermatozoa.[54,55] Selenium also helps protect the sperm against oxidation.[56,57]

The effects of selenium on sperm motility are highlighted in a study involving a group of men with poorly motile sperm.[58] Over a three-month period men who were given selenium (either on it its own or as a combination of antioxidants that also included vitamins A, C, and E) showed increased sperm motility when compared with the placebo group. Five men in the treatment group (11%) impregnated their wives, in contrast to none in the placebo group. Though this study was small, it suggests that selenium supplementation can increase the chance of successful conception. This outcome is even more significant when one considers the cost and convenience of supplementation in comparison with in vitro fertilization and other methods.

More recently, selenium (200 mcg per day) in combination with the antioxidant n-acetylcysteine (600 mg per day) was found to improve sperm count, sperm motility, and normal sperm morphology.[59] However, once supplementation stopped, the sperm reverted back to baseline. This study did not measure pregnancy rate.

Folic Acid and Vitamin B_{12}. Folic acid and vitamin B_{12} are concentrated within the head of the sperm and are responsible for safeguarding the DNA within.[52,60–62] Multiple studies have shown that low levels of folic acid in seminal fluid are associated with increased sperm DNA damage, while a B_{12} deficiency is strongly associated with reduced sperm motility and count.[61,62] As the human body has a high turnover of these nutrients and requires a continual supply, supplementation is advisable for all men experiencing infertility regardless of whether there is a proven deficiency, especially in men who have a sperm count of less than 20 million/ml or a motility rate of less than 50%. In one study, 27% of men with a sperm count less than 20 million/ml who were given 1,000 mg per day of vitamin B_{12} were able to achieve a total sperm count in excess of 100 million/ml.[63] In another study, 57% of men with a low sperm count who took 6,000 mg per day demonstrated improvements.[64] As would be expected, men with elevated homocysteine levels—typically due to inadequate intake of B-complex vitamins—have greatly decreased fertility.

Alpha-Lipoic Acid. Alpha-lipoic acid is an antioxidant that is both fat- and water-soluble and assists in the chelation of heavy metals. It is especially useful because of its ability to regenerate other antioxidants, including vitamins C and E, CoQ_{10}, and glutathione.[65] In animal studies, alpha-lipoic acid has been shown to protect sperm.[66–68] It appears to act as a sort of shield, forming a protective barrier around and inside the midpiece of the sperm. This protection is crucial, as the midpiece has been identified as one of the first places free radicals attack.

Carnitine. Carnitine is a naturally produced compound in the body. It is derived from the amino acids lysine and/or methionine and plays a vital role in fatty acid metabolism. It works synergistically with coenzyme Q_{10}. Carnitine exerts protective antioxidant effects and provides energy to the testicles and sperm. Several studies comparing fertile men with infertile men found that fertile men had a statistically significant larger amount of carnitine in their seminal sample than the infertile men, and that low levels of L-carnitine in the seminal plasma may be a potent marker for infertility.[69]

Carnitine concentrations are extremely high in the epididymis and sperm, suggesting a role in male reproductive function. The epididymis derives the majority of its energy requirements from fatty acids, as do the sperm during transport through the epididymis. After ejaculation, the motility of sperm correlates directly with carnitine content—the higher the carnitine content, the more motile the sperm. Conversely, when carnitine levels are low, sperm development, function, and motility are drastically reduced.

Several clinical studies have shown that carnitine supplementation can produce dramatic improvements in sperm counts and sperm motility.[69] In the Italian Study Group on Carnitine and Male Infertility, 100 subjects were given 3,000 mg L-carnitine per day for four months.[70] Carnitine was able to increase sperm counts and sperm motility:

- The number of ejaculated sperm per ml increased from 142 billion to 163 billion.

- The proportion of motile sperm increased from 26.9 to 37.7%.

- The proportion of sperm that are able to swim in a straight line increased from 10.8 to 18%.

- The mean sperm velocity (how fast the sperm are able to swim) increased from 28.4 to 32.5%.

The results are even more impressive if results for only the patients with the poorest sperm motility are examined. This subgroup saw even more significant gains on all variables. For example, the proportion of motile sperm increased from 19.3 to 40.9%, and the proportion of sperm that are able to swim in

a straight line increased from 3.1 to 20.3%. These results have been confirmed in several double-blind studies.[71–75]

Coenzyme Q_{10} (CoQ_{10}). CoQ_{10} is concentrated in the head and midpiece (neck) of the sperm, and is also found in seminal fluid. It is considered to be the most crucial and powerful antioxidant in sperm structure owing to its role in mitochondrial energy release. It is believed to promote motility, foster sperm survival, and provide energy to assist the sperm's travel on its journey to the egg.

As a fat-soluble antioxidant and free radical scavenger, CoQ_{10} is required for the maintenance of healthy cell membrane integrity and cell functioning, specifically for new cells such as sperm. Decreased levels have been found in the seminal fluid and sperm of men with idiopathic and varicocele-associated asthenospermia.[76–78]

Arginine. The amino acid arginine is required for the replication of cells, so it is essential in sperm formation. A number of studies have shown that arginine can improve sperm count and motility. Stress in particular has been found to decrease the levels of arginine in the sperm production pathways. Arginine supplementation is often, but not always, an effective treatment for male infertility. The critical determinant appears to be the sperm count: if it is under 20 million/ml, arginine supplementation is less likely to be of benefit. In order to be effective, the dosage of arginine must be at least 4 g per day for three months. In perhaps the most favorable study, 74% of 178 men with low sperm count had significant improvements in sperm count and motility after arginine therapy.[79]

In one double-blind, randomized, placebo-controlled, crossover clinical trial, an improvement in semen variables was observed after administration of Prelox, a combination of

80 mg Pycnogenol and 3 g L-arginine.[80] Over a treatment period of four weeks, fifty men with idiopathic infertility experienced significant increase in ejaculate volume, concentration and number of sperm, and percentage of vital spermatozoa compared with the placebo group. The percentage of sperm with good motility also increased significantly, while the percentage of immotile sperm decreased. This effect appears to be due to a combination of the antioxidant activity of Pycnogenol and/or the ability of arginine to stimulate production of nitric oxide. Pycnogenol alone (200 mg per day for 90 days) was shown to improve sperm morphology by 38% and viability by 19% in a small pilot study.[81]

Botanical Medicines

Chinese Ginseng

Current scientific investigation suggests that Chinese ginseng (*Panax ginseng*) can be useful in supporting male fertility. It has a long history of use as a male tonic. In animal studies, Chinese ginseng has been shown to promote the growth of the testes, raise sperm formation and testosterone levels, and increase sexual activity and mating behavior. The active constituents (ginsenosides) have been shown to enhance nitric oxide production, thus improving fertilization ability and sperm motility.[82,83] Additionally, they have been shown to improve the functioning of parts of the endocrine system, which can assist in modulating stress-induced infertility or lowered testosterone from insufficient DHEA synthesis.[84] In clinical trials *Panax ginseng* has been shown to increase testosterone levels in men with low levels, improving erectile function and libido; it also improved sperm count and motility (including in some patients with varicoceles).[84–85] Note that ginseng does not increase testosterone in men with normal levels.

Pygeum

Pygeum (*Pygeum africanum*) has been shown to increase prostatic secretions and improve the composition of seminal fluid.[86–88] Specifically, pygeum administration to men with decreased prostatic secretion led to an increased total amount of seminal fluid plus increases in alkaline phosphatase and protein content. Pygeum appears to be most effective in men in whom the level of alkaline phosphatase activity is reduced (i.e., less than 400 IU/cm^3) and there is no evidence of inflammation or infection (i.e., absence of white blood cells and immunoglobulin A [IgA]). The absence of IgA in the semen is a good indicator of clinical success. In one study, patients with no IgA in the semen demonstrated an alkaline phosphatase increase from 265 to 485 IU/cm^3.[88] In contrast, patients with IgA showed only a modest increase from 213 to 281 IU/cm^3.

Pygeum extract has also shown an ability to improve the capacity to achieve an erection in patients with benign prostatic hypertrophy or prostatitis, as determined by nocturnal penile tumescence in a double-blind clinical trial.[89]

Tribulus

Tribulus (*Tribulus terrestris*) has been used traditionally in ayurvedic medicine as a tonic and aphrodisiac and in European folk medicine to increase sexual potency. A steroidal saponin, protodioscin, is considered the chief constituent responsible for the herb's effects on libido and sexual functioning. Of prime importance is the source of the extract. All of the clinical studies showing positive effects have used a leaf extract from Bulgaria, as it has been shown to be highest in protodioscin. A tribulus product made from the root or fruit of the plant or sourced from anywhere besides eastern Europe will probably contain low levels of protodioscin.

In animal studies tribulus has been shown to increase certain sex hormones (including testosterone) as well as nitric oxide synthesis;[90] however, these results have not been observed in some human studies.[91] One possible reason is differences in the extract used; another is that many of the studies have used healthy men with normal testosterone levels rather than men with testosterone abnormalities.

Tribulus appears to enhance male fertility owing to its ability to increase sperm count, viability, and libido; however, published studies are poorly designed and have produced conflicting results.[92]

QUICK REVIEW

- **The average sperm count has declined by 40% since 1940.**
- **A high sperm count means nothing if the percentage of healthy sperm is not also high.**
- **Reducing scrotal temperature in infertile men will often make them fertile.**
- **Infertile men should wear boxer-type underwear and periodically take a cold shower or apply ice to the scrotum.**
- **The presence of antisperm antibodies or of high levels of debris in a semen sample is considered a good indicator of a chronic infection.**
- **Increased exposure to environmental estrogens and other environmental pollutants during fetal development is suggested as a major cause of the tremendous rise in disorders that affect the development and function of the male sexual system.**
- **In one study cell phone use decreased sperm count, motility, viability, and normal morphology.**
- **Obese men are known to have lower sperm counts, reduced motility, reduced production of sperm, increased DNA fragmentation in sperm, and increased levels of erectile dysfunction.**
- **Free radical damage to sperm is thought to be responsible for many cases of male infertility.**
- **Antioxidants such as vitamin C, beta-carotene, selenium, and vitamin E have been shown to be very important in protecting the sperm against damage and improving male fertility.**
- **Zinc supplementation can be very helpful in achieving fertility, especially in men with low testosterone levels.**
- **Multiple studies have shown low levels of folic acid in seminal fluid to be associated with increased sperm DNA damage, while a vitamin B$_{12}$ deficiency is strongly associated with reduced sperm motility and count.**
- **Carnitine supplementation can lead to improvements in sperm counts and sperm motility.**
- **Pygeum has been shown to increase prostatic secretions and improve the composition of the seminal fluid.**
- **Ashwagandha inhibited lipid peroxidation, improved sperm count and motility, and had a positive effect on hormone levels.**

Velvet Bean

Velvet bean (*Mucuna pruriens*) has been used in ayurvedic medicine to improve stress endurance, increase general resistance against infection, retard the aging process, and improve male sexual function. It has been shown to help alleviate disorders including psychogenic impotence and unexplained infertility.[93] One paper showed that *Mucuna pruriens* seed powder produced dramatic improvements in 70% of study participants, helping to fight stress-mediated poor semen quality and acting as a restorative and invigorator in infertile subjects.[94] The effect appears to be due to significant improvements in levels of testosterone, luteinizing hormone, dopamine, adrenaline, and noradrenaline, plus reduction in levels of follicle-stimulating hormone and prolactin.[95] Sperm count and motility were also significantly improved in infertile men after treatment.

Ashwagandha

Ashwagandha (*Withania somnifera*) has shown considerable anti-stress and adaptogenic effects. In a three-month clinical trial, 75 normal healthy fertile men (control subjects) were compared with 75 men undergoing infertility screening who received 5 g powdered root per day. Results showed that ashwagandha inhibited lipid peroxidation and improved sperm count and motility. Treatment also significantly increased serum testosterone and luteinizing hormone and reduced levels of follicle-stimulating hormone and prolactin—all beneficial effects in infertile men.[96]

TREATMENT SUMMARY

There are many factors involved in male infertility, and a comprehensive treatment plan is essential to success. We recommend consulting a urologist or fertility specialist for a complete evaluation. It is advisable to go on a detoxification program at the start of treatment; see the chapter "Detoxification and Internal Cleansing."

Because elevated scrotal temperature is a common cause of infertility, we recommend scrotal cooling through the use of loose underwear, avoidance of activities that raise testicular temperature (e.g., hot tubs), and application of cold water or ice to the testes.

Optimize nutritional status and eliminate any unhealthy lifestyle practices; add fertility-enhancing nutritional supplements and botanicals as needed. Avoid pollutants and toxic substances such as cigarette smoke.

General Recommendations

- Maintain scrotal temperatures between 94° and 96.8°F
- Avoid exposure to free radicals
- Identify and eliminate environmental pollutants
- Talk to your doctor about stopping or reducing drugs such as antihypertensives, antineoplastics (e.g., cyclophosphamide), and anti-inflammatories (e.g., sulfasalazine)
- Utilize effective stress reduction techniques; employ psychological counseling if needed

- Avoid cigarette smoking and recreational drugs

Diet

- Follow the guidelines in the chapter "A Health-Promoting Diet"
- Avoid dietary sources of free radicals, saturated fats, and trans-fats; also avoid cottonseed oil
- Increase consumption of legumes (especially soy); good dietary sources of antioxidant vitamins, carotenes, and flavonoids (many dark- or bright-colored vegetables and fruits); and essential fatty acids and zinc (from nuts and seeds)
- Eat 8 to 12 servings of vegetables and 1 to 2 servings of fresh fruits per day
- Optimize protein intake from both vegetarian and organic animal sources
- Drink 6 to 8 glasses of water per day
- Eliminate caffeine, alcohol, sugar, and food additives (such as preservatives and colorings)

Nutritional Supplements

- A high-potency multiple vitamin and mineral formula as described in the chapter "Supplementary Measures"
- Key individual nutrients:
  - Vitamin B_6: 25 to 50 mg per day
  - Folic acid: 800 mcg to 2 mg per day
  - Vitamin B_{12}: 800 mcg per day
  - Vitamin C: 500 to 1,000 mg per day
  - Vitamin E (mixed tocopherols): 200 to 400 IU per day
  - Beta-carotene: 15,000 to 30,000 IU per day (preferably as mixed carotenoids)
  - Magnesium (bound to aspartate, citrate, fumarate, malate, or succinate): 200 to 300 mg three times per day
  - Selenium: 100 to 200 mcg per day
  - Zinc: 30 to 45 mg per day
  - Vitamin D_3: 2,000 to 4,000 IU per day (ideally, measure blood levels and adjust dosage accordingly)
  - Fish oils: 1,000 mg EPA + DHA per day
- One of the following:
  - Grape seed extract (>95% procyanidolic oligomers): 100 to 300 mg per day
  - Pine bark extract (>95% procyanidolic oligomers): 100 to 300 mg per day
  - Some other flavonoid-rich extract with a similar flavonoid content, super greens formula, or another plant-based antioxidant that can provide an oxygen radical absorption capacity (ORAC) of 3,000 to 6,000 units or more per day
- Specialty supplements:
  - Lycopene: 2 to 5 mg per day
  - CoQ_{10}: 200 to 400 mg per day
  - L-carnitine: 2,000 to 3,000 mg per day
  - L-arginine: 4,000 mg per day

Botanical Medicines

One or more of the following:

- Chinese ginseng (*Panax ginseng*):
  - High-quality crude ginseng root: 1.5 to 2 g per day
  - Fluid extract (containing a minimum of 10.5 mg/ml ginsenosides with Rg1:Rb1 greater than or equal to 0.5 by HPLC): 2 to 6 ml (½ to 1½ tsp) per day

- ○ Dried powdered extract standardized to contain 5% ginsenosides with an Rb1/Rg1 ratio of 2:1: 250 to 500 mg per day
- Pygeum *(Pygeum africanum)*, liposterolic extract standardized to contain 14% triterpenes: 100 to 200 mg per day in divided doses
- Tribulus *(Tribulus terrestris)*:
  - ○ Dried leaf with a protodioscin content of 12.22 mg/g: 9 to 18 g per day
  - ○ Dried powdered extract standardized to contain 45% steroidal saponins: 250 to 500 mg per day
  - ○ Fluid extract (2:1): 7 to 21 ml per day

- Velvet bean *(Mucuna pruriens)*: dosage equivalent to 5 g powdered dried seed per day
- Ashwagandha *(Withania somnifera)*:
  - ○ Powdered root: 5 g per day
  - ○ Dried powdered extract (root and leaves) standardized to contain 8% withanolide glycoside conjugates and 32% oligosaccharides: 125 to 250 mg per day
  - ○ Fluid extract (2:1), containing a minimum of 4 mg/ml withanosides: 2.5 to 5.0 ml per day

Insomnia

- Difficulty falling asleep (sleep-onset insomnia)
- Frequent or early awakening (sleep-maintenance insomnia)

Insomnia is one of the most common complaints seen by physicians. Within the course of a year, up to 30% of the population suffers from insomnia, and roughly 10% of the adult population has chronic insomnia.[1] Many people use over-the-counter medications to combat the problem, and others seek stronger sedatives. Approximately 12.5% of the adult population uses a prescribed anxiolytic or sedative hypnotic in the course of a year; about 2% of the population takes one on any given day. Nearly 100 million prescriptions are written each year for these drugs.[2]

Causes

Psychological factors such as depression and anxiety account for 50% of all cases of insomnia.[1] Psychological counseling with cognitive behavioral therapy can produce improvements in sleep quality.[3]

Eliminating factors that impair sleep quality is another important consideration. There are many recreational drugs, prescription and nonprescription drugs, and foods and beverages that can interfere with sleep, such as:

- Alcohol
- Beta-blockers
- Caffeine and related compounds:
  - Coffee
  - Tea
  - Chocolate
  - Caffeinated colas and energy drinks
- Marijuana
- Oral contraceptives
- Thyroid preparations

Sleep Apnea

It is important to rule out sleep apnea in anyone suffering from insomnia. First described in 1965, sleep apnea is a breathing disorder characterized by brief interruptions of breathing during sleep. These breathing pauses (as many as several hundred a night) are almost always accompanied by snoring between pauses, although not everyone who snores has this condition. Sleep apnea can also be characterized by a choking sensation. People with sleep apnea experience periods of anoxia (oxygen deprivation of the brain) with each episode; the anoxia arouses the sleeper enough to reinitiate breathing. Seldom does the sufferer awaken enough to be aware of the problem. But the frequent interruptions mean that people get less deep, restorative sleep, and this lack often leads to excessive daytime sleepiness, early morning headache, and other quality-of-life problems.[4] Approximately 18 million Americans are thought to suffer from sleep apnea.

Early recognition and treatment of sleep apnea are important because the disorder is also associated with irregular heartbeat, high blood pressure, heart attack, and stroke as well as a loss of memory function and of other intellectual capabilities. The patient usually does not know he or she has a problem. It is important that people see a doctor if they snore heavily or if their sleep partners have noticed periods of interrupted breathing during sleep. Sleep apnea should also be considered in anyone with significant daytime drowsiness or changes in intellectual function. Sleep apnea can be properly diagnosed only through the services of a sleep disorder specialist and usually in a sleep laboratory.

Sleep apnea is most often caused by narrowing of the airway from an accumulation of fatty tissue. This is called *obstructive sleep apnea*. With a narrowed airway, air cannot easily flow into or out of the nose or mouth. This results in heavy snoring, periods of no breathing, and frequent arousals (abrupt changes from deep sleep to light sleep). Alcohol and sleeping pills increase the frequency and duration of breathing pauses in people with sleep apnea. In some cases sleep apnea occurs even if no airway obstruction or snoring is present. This form, called *central sleep apnea*, is caused by a loss of brain control over breathing. In both obstructive and central sleep apneas, obesity is the major risk factor, and weight loss is the most important aspect of long-term management.

The most common treatment of sleep apnea is the use of nasal continuous positive airway pressure (CPAP). In this procedure, the patient wears a mask over the nose during sleep, and pressure from an air blower forces air through the nasal passages. The air pressure is adjusted so that it is just enough to prevent the throat from collapsing during sleep. Nasal CPAP prevents airway closure while in use, but apnea episodes return

Causes of Insomnia	
SLEEP-ONSET INSOMNIA*	SLEEP-MAINTENANCE INSOMNIA*
Anxiety or tension	Depression
Environmental change	Environmental change
Emotional arousal	Sleep apnea
Fear of insomnia	Nocturnal myoclonus
Phobia of sleep	Hypoglycemia
Disruptive environment	Parasomnias
Pain or discomfort	Pain or discomfort
Caffeine	Drugs
Alcohol	Alcohol

* The boundary between the categories is not entirely distinct.

when CPAP is stopped or is used improperly. Surgery to reduce soft tissue in the throat or soft palate should be used only as a last resort because it often does not work or can make the problem worse. Laser-assisted surgery (uvulopalatoplasty) is a highly promoted surgical option. In this procedure lasers are used to surgically remove excessive soft tissue from the back of the throat and from the palate. This procedure works well initially in about 90% of sleep apnea sufferers, but within one year many people are the same as or even worse than before because of the scar tissue that invariably forms.[4]

Therapeutic Considerations

Adequate sleep is absolutely necessary for long-term health and regeneration. Most people can tolerate a few days without sleep and fully recover. However, chronic sleep deprivation appears to accelerate aging of the brain, cause neuronal damage, and lead to nighttime elevations in cortisol.[5]

Avoidance of Stimulants, Especially Caffeine

As with all conditions, the best treatment is to first remove the causes. The average American consumes 150 to 225 mg caffeine per day, roughly the amount of caffeine in one to two cups of coffee. Although most people can handle this amount, there is a huge variation in the rate at which different people detoxify stimulants such as caffeine. Owing to the genetic variation in the liver enzyme that breaks down caffeine, some people can eliminate caffeine very quickly (for example, half of a dose of caffeine is eliminated within 30 minutes), while in others the breakdown process is much less effective (it can take as much as 12 hours to eliminate half of a dose of caffeine). Everyone who drinks more than one cup of coffee in the early morning and who has trouble sleeping should simply try caffeine avoidance for 7 to 10 days. All sources of caffeine—not just coffee but tea, chocolate, drugs with caffeine, and energy drinks—must be avoided.

Exercise

Regular physical exercise is known to improve general well-being and promote improvement in sleep quality.[3] Exercise should take place in the morning or early evening, not right before bedtime, and should be of moderate intensity. Usually 20 minutes of aerobic exercise at a heart rate between 60 and 75% of maximum (with the maximum rate calculated as 220 minus the patient's age in years) is sufficient.

Progressive Relaxation

Numerous techniques can promote relaxation and prepare the body and mind for sleep. One of the most popular and easy-to-use techniques is progressive relaxation, in which an individual is taught what it feels like to relax by comparing relaxation with muscle tension. Each muscle is contracted forcefully for a period of one to two seconds, then relaxed. The procedure begins with contraction and then relaxation of the muscles of the face and neck; next the upper arms and chest are contracted and then relaxed, followed by the lower arms and hands. The process is repeated progressively down the body—abdomen, buttocks, thighs, calves, and feet. Because the procedure goes progressively through all the muscles of the body, a deep state of relaxation eventually results. This whole procedure is repeated two or three times.

Nocturnal Glucose Levels

Dips in blood glucose levels during the night may be an important cause of sleep-maintenance insomnia, especially when the drops are rapid. The brain is highly dependent on glucose for energy, and a quick drop in blood glucose level stimulates the release of adrenaline and cortisol, which promote awakening. See the chapter "Hypoglycemia" for strategies to stabilize blood sugar levels.

Serotonin Precursor and Cofactor Therapy

Serotonin is an important initiator of sleep. The synthesis of serotonin in the central nervous system depends on availability of the amino acid tryptophan. Supplemental L-tryptophan has shown modest effects in the treatment of insomnia.[6–8] It is certainly not a panacea; however, excellent results have been reported even in severe cases. Although not every patient has shown response to tryptophan in clinical trials, those who do respond have experienced dramatic relief. The key advantage of tryptophan over prescription and over-the-counter pills is that, unlike these agents, tryptophan does not produce any significant distortions of normal sleep processes. Dosages of tryptophan smaller than 2,000 mg are generally ineffective.

Current knowledge about the sleep-inducing effects of tryptophan suggests that it is generally more effective in sleep-onset insomnia and less effective in sleep-maintenance insomnia.[6] The sleep-promoting effect is often thought to be the result of enhanced serotonin synthesis, but there is evidence to suggest that other mechanisms may play a role, including tryptophan-enhanced melatonin synthesis. For example, administration of large dosages of tryptophan causes a massive elevation of plasma melatonin concentration.[9] There may be other effects as well that do not involve either serotonin or melatonin.[10,11]

It appears that the insomnia-relieving and sleep-promoting actions of tryptophan are cumulative, in that it often takes a few nights for l-tryptophan to start working. In one double-blind study, the effects of 3 g tryptophan on sleep performance, arousal threshold, and brain electrical activity during sleep were assessed in 20 men with chronic sleep-onset insomnia.[12] After a sleep laboratory screening night, all subjects received a placebo for three consecutive nights; then 10 subjects received tryptophan and 10 received a placebo for six nights. All subjects received a placebo for the last two nights. L-tryptophan had no effect during the first three nights of administration. However, on nights four through six, the time it took to fall asleep was significantly reduced. Consistently with other studies, this study found that unlike sleeping pills (especially benzodiazepines), tryptophan did not alter sleep stages, impair daytime performance, or alter brain electrical activity during sleep. This study suggests that tryptophan should be used for a minimum of one week before its effects can be assessed in chronic insomnia. However,

single dosages of tryptophan can have good sleep-promoting effects in other situations, such as in people who regularly experience insomnia the first time they sleep in a new place, such as a hotel.

Administration of high-dose tryptophan (4 g) during the day can cause daytime sleepiness. This suggests that consumption of foods high in tryptophan during the day may contribute to daytime sleepiness. Conversely, an evening meal high in tryptophan relative to competing amino acids may promote sleep.

The important cofactors vitamin B_6, niacin, and magnesium should be administered along with the tryptophan to ensure its conversion to serotonin. Also, because other amino acids compete with tryptophan for transport into the central nervous system, avoid consuming protein at the same time as you take the tryptophan. But, because insulin increases tryptophan uptake, *do* take a carbohydrate source (such as fruit or fruit juice) with the tryptophan.

Niacin has been reported to have a sedative effect, probably owing to its ability to dilate peripheral blood vessels and shunt tryptophan metabolism toward serotonin synthesis.

5-Hydroxytryptophan (5-HTP)

Chemically speaking, 5-HTP is one step closer to serotonin than tryptophan is and does not depend on a transport system for entry into the brain. Several clinical studies have shown 5-HTP to produce dramatically better results than tryptophan in promoting and maintaining sleep, even though it is used at lower dosages.[13–16]

One of the key benefits of 5-HTP is its ability to increase REM sleep (typically by about 25%) while increasing deep sleep (stages 3 and 4) without lengthening total sleep time.[10,11] The sleep stages that are reduced to compensate for the increases are non-REM stages 1 and 2, the least important ones.

The dosage recommendation for 5-HTP is 100 to 300 mg taken 30 to 45 minutes before retiring. Start with the lower dose for at least three days before increasing it.

Melatonin

The most popular natural aid for sleep is melatonin. Supplementation with melatonin has been shown in several studies to be very effective in helping induce and maintain sleep in both children and adults and in both people with normal sleep patterns and those with insomnia. However, the sleep-promoting effects of melatonin are apparent only if melatonin levels are low.[17] When melatonin is taken just before going to bed by normal subjects or by patients with insomnia who have normal melatonin levels, it produces no sedative effect. This is because people normally have a rise in melatonin secretion before falling asleep. Melatonin supplementation appears to be most effective in treating insomnia in the elderly, in whom low melatonin levels are quite common.[18]

In one of the most interesting studies, 26 elderly insomniacs with lower than normal melatonin levels were given 1 to 2 mg melatonin two hours before the desired bedtime for one week. Although there was no discernible difference in sleep onset and sleep efficiency (time asleep as a percentage of total time in bed) between the two forms, the slow-release form yielded better effects on sleep maintenance.[19]

A dose of 3 mg at bedtime is more than enough (in fact, doses as low as 0.1 or 0.3 mg have been shown to produce a sedative effect when melatonin levels are low).[20] Although melatonin appears to have no serious side effects at recommended doses, melatonin supplementation could conceivably disrupt the normal circadian rhythm. In one study, a dosage of 8 mg per day for only four days resulted in significant alterations in hormone secretions.[21]

Restless Legs Syndrome and Nocturnal Myoclonus

Restless legs syndrome and nocturnal leg cramps (myoclonus) are significant causes of insomnia. Restless legs syndrome occurs when the patient is awake and is characterized by an irresistible urge to move the legs. Almost all patients with restless legs syndrome have nocturnal myoclonus.[1] Nocturnal myoclonus is a neuromuscular disorder characterized by repeated contractions of one or more muscle groups, typically of the leg, during sleep. Each jerk usually lasts less than 10 seconds. The patient is normally unaware of the myoclonus and complains only of either frequent nocturnal awakenings or excessive daytime sleepiness, but questioning of the sleep partner often reveals the myoclonus.

If there is a family history of restless legs syndrome (such a history is present in about one-third of all cases of the syndrome), high-dose folic acid, 35 to 60 mg per day, can be helpful.[22] Doses in this range require a prescription, because the U.S. Food and Drug Administration limits the amount available per capsule to 800 mcg. Restless legs syndrome is also a common finding in patients with malabsorption syndromes.[22]

If there is no family history, low iron levels may be the problem, so a blood test for serum ferritin should be done. The association between low iron levels and restless legs syndrome was documented in clinical studies more than 30 years ago. A later study reproduced these observations, finding serum ferritin levels to be lower in 18 patients with restless legs syndrome than in 18 control subjects.[23] Serum iron, vitamin B_{12}, folic acid, and hemoglobin levels did not differ in the two groups. However, serum ferritin levels were inversely correlated with the severity of symptoms. Fifteen of the patients with the syndrome were treated with iron (ferrous sulfate) at a dosage of 200 mg three times per day for two months. The severity of restless legs syndrome decreased by an average of 4 points in sixteen patients with an initial ferritin level lower than 18 mg/l, by 3 points in four patients with ferritin levels between 18 and 45 mg/l, and by 1 point in five patients with ferritin levels between 45 and 100 mg/l.

In addition to restless legs syndrome, low serum ferritin levels have been found in psychiatric patients experiencing a condition called akathisia, a drug-induced state of agitation (the name comes from the Greek and means "cannot sit down"). The drugs that most commonly produce akathisia are antidepressant drugs, such as fluoxetine (Paxil, Prozac) and sertraline (Zoloft). Level of iron depletion also correlates with the severity of akathisia. Anyone suffering from drug-induced akathisia should ask a physician to perform a serum ferritin assessment. If serum ferritin levels are below 35 mg/l, take 30 mg iron bound to either succinate or fumarate twice per day between meals. If this recommendation causes abdominal discomfort, try 30 mg with meals three times per day.

QUICK REVIEW

- **Psychological factors account for 50% of all insomnias evaluated in sleep laboratories.**
- **There are many recreational drugs, prescription and nonprescription drugs, and foods and beverages that can interfere with sleep.**
- **Early recognition and treatment of sleep apnea is important because it is associated with marked daytime fatigue, irregular heartbeat, high blood pressure, heart attack, and stroke as well as a loss of memory function and other intellectual capabilities.**
- **In both obstructive and central sleep apneas, obesity is the major risk factor, and weight loss is the most important aspect of long-term management.**
- **Chronic sleep deprivation appears to accelerate aging of the brain, causes neuronal damage, and leads to nighttime elevations in cortisol.**
- **Regular physical exercise promotes improvements in sleep quality.**
- **Rapid drops in blood glucose level can promote awakening during sleep.**
- **Several clinical studies have shown 5-HTP to be effective in promoting and maintaining sleep.**
- **Supplementation with melatonin has been shown in several studies to be very effective in helping induce and maintain sleep.**
- **More than 20 double-blind clinical studies have now substantiated valerian's ability to improve sleep quality and relieve insomnia.**

Botanicals with Sedative Properties

Numerous plants have sedative action. Plants commonly prescribed as aids in promoting sleep include:

Valerian (*Valeriana officinalis*)

Passionflower (*Passiflora incarnata*)

Hops (*Humulus lupulus*)

Skullcap (*Scutellaria lateriflora*)

Chamomile (*Matricaria chamomilla*)

Of the herbs listed, the one on which the most clinical research has been done is valerian. More than 20 double-blind clinical studies have now substantiated valerian's ability to improve sleep quality and relieve insomnia.[24,25] Additional research is warranted, but these studies show that extracts of valerian root improve sleep quality and reduce the time needed to fall asleep. The studies, which were usually performed under strict laboratory conditions, demonstrated quite clearly that valerian is as effective at bringing on sleep as small doses of barbiturates or benzodiazepines. However, although these latter compounds also increase morning sleepiness, valerian usually reduces morning sleepiness.

THE DARK SIDE OF SLEEPING PILLS

Most sleeping pills are technically "sedative hypnotics." This class of drugs is also widely used to treat anxiety and stress. Examples include:

Alprazolam (Alprazolam, Xanax)

Chlordiazepoxide (Librium)

Diazepam (Valium)

Eszopiclone (Lunesta)

Flurazepam (Dalmane)

Quazepam (Doral)

Ramelteon (Rozerem)

Temazepam (Restoril)

Triazolam (Halcion)

Zaleplon (Sonata)

Zolpidem (Ambien)

All of these drugs are associated with significant risks. Most of them are highly addictive and very poor candidates for long-term use. Common side effects include dizziness, drowsiness, and impaired coordination; it is important not to drive or engage in any potentially dangerous activities while on these drugs. Alcohol should never be consumed with these drugs, as it could be fatal.

The most serious side effects of the conventional antianxiety drugs relate to their effects on memory and behavior. Because these drugs have a powerful effect on brain chemistry, significant changes in brain function and behavior can occur. Severe memory impairment and amnesia, nervousness, confusion, hallucinations, bizarre behavior, and extreme irritability and aggressiveness may result. They have also been shown to increase feelings of depression, including suicidal thinking.

Daniel F. Kripke, M.D., professor of psychiatry emeritus at the University of California, San Diego, worked for over 30 years assessing the risk of sleeping pills. The most shocking of his findings was that people who take sleeping pills die sooner than people who do not use sleeping pills. Dr. Kripke examined data from a very large study known as the Cancer Prevention Study I. In this study, American Cancer Society volunteers gave questionnaires to more than 1 million Americans and then followed up six years later. Dr. Kripke and his colleagues found that 50% more of those who said that they often took sleeping pills had died, compared with participants of the same age, sex, and reported health status who never took sleeping pills.[26]

To reexamine these risks, the American Cancer Society agreed to ask new questions about sleeping pills to of 1.1 million new participants in another study, called the Cancer Prevention Study II, or CPSII. In the CPSII, it was again found that people who said that they used sleeping pills had significantly higher mortality. Those who reported taking sleeping pills 30 or more times per month had 25% higher mortality than those who said that they took no sleeping pills. Those that who took sleeping pills just a few times per month showed a 10% to 15% increase in mortality, compared with those who took no sleeping pills. Deaths from common causes such as heart disease, cancer, and stroke were all increased among sleeping pill users. Sleeping pills appeared unsafe in any amount.[27]

All told, there are now 18 population-based studies that show a clear link between the use of sleeping pills and increased mortality risk. Four of these studies specifically found that use of sleeping pills predicted increased risk of death from cancer.[27–29]

In a more recent study, Dr. Kripke's team obtained medical records for 10,529 people who were prescribed hypnotic sleeping pills and for 23,676 matched patients who were never prescribed sleeping pills. Over an average of 2.5 years, the death rate for those who did not use sleeping pills was 1.2%. It was 6.1% for people with sleeping pill prescriptions. They also had a 35% higher risk of cancer. Based on these findings, Kripke and colleagues estimate that sleeping pills are linked to 320,000 to 507,000 U.S. deaths each year.[29]

So what do all of these data really mean? They may mean that the use of sleeping pills is just an indicator of stress, anxiety, insomnia, and depression. In other words, maybe these people were taking sleeping pills because they were really stressed out or depressed, and it was actually the stress or depression that did them in. Or it could be that the drugs produce complications. For example, it is possible that the drugs interfere with normal sleep repair mechanisms as well as promote depression. The bottom line is that it is clear that the risks of taking the drugs far outweigh any benefits.

TREATMENT SUMMARY

The aim of treatment with natural measures is to improve sleep quality without any of the side effects of over-the-counter and prescription sleeping pills. In addition to psychological support if needed, the foremost component of treatment is the control of any factors known to disrupt normal sleep patterns, such as the following:

- Stimulants (e.g., coffee, tea, chocolate, energy drinks, coffee ice cream)
- Alcohol
- Hypoglycemia
- Stimulant-containing herbs (e.g., ephedra, guarana)
- Marijuana and other recreational drugs
- Numerous OTC medications
- Prescription drugs

If this approach produces no response, try natural sleep aids. Once a normal sleep pattern has been established, the recommended supplements and botanicals should be slowly decreased.

If there is a family history of restless legs syndrome, high-dose folic acid, 35 to 60 mg per day, can be helpful but requires a prescription. It is not known if lower dosages might work just as well. If there is no family history, ask for a serum ferritin test to rule out iron deficiency.

Exercise

Engage in a regular exercise program that elevates heart rate to 60 to 75% of maximum for at least 20 minutes a day (but do not exercise right before going to bed).

Diet

The guidelines given in the chapter "A Health-Promoting Diet" can be helpful. Especially important to preventing sleep maintenance insomnia is eating a low-glycemic-load diet to reduce blood sugar volatility. For additional information on how to stabilize blood sugar levels, see the chapter "Hypoglycemia."

Nutritional Supplements

The following supplements can be taken 45 minutes before bedtime:

- Niacin: 30 to 50 mg
- Vitamin B$_6$: 25 to 50 mg
- Magnesium: 150 to 200 mg
- 5-HTP: 25 to 50 mg
- Melatonin: 1 to 3 mg
- L-theanine: 200 to 600 mg

Botanical Medicines

- Valerian (*Valeriana officinalis*), 45 minutes before bedtime:
  - Dried root (or as tea): 2 to 3 g
  - Tincture (1:5): 4 to 6 ml (1 to 1½ tsp)
  - Fluid extract (1:1): 2 to 4 ml (½ to 1 tsp)
  - Dry powdered extract (0.8% valerenic acid): 150 to 300 mg

Irritable Bowel Syndrome

Characterized by some combination of:

- Abdominal pain or distension
- Altered bowel function, constipation, or diarrhea
- Hypersecretion of colonic mucus
- Dyspeptic symptoms (flatulence, nausea, anorexia)
- Varying degrees of anxiety or depression

Irritable bowel syndrome (IBS) is the most common gastrointestinal disorder and represents 30 to 50% of all referrals to gastroenterologists. Determining the true frequency is virtually impossible, as many sufferers never seek medical attention. It has, however, been estimated that approximately 15% of the population complains of IBS, with women predominating two to one (it is likely that an equal number of men have IBS but that they do not report symptoms as often). IBS has been attributed to physiological, psychological, and dietary factors.

Causes

IBS is a functional disorder of digestion that is the result of an interplay of digestive secretions, bacterial flora, and dietary factors. The diagnosis of IBS is often made by exclusion, as a result of ruling out other conditions that can mimic IBS (see the list opposite). We recommend that you consult a physician if you have symptoms suggestive of IBS. The physician will decide just how extensive the diagnostic process will be. A detailed medical history and physical examination are critical in diagnosing IBS. Abdominal distension, relief of pain with bowel movements, and the onset of loose or more frequent bowel movements with pain seem to correlate best with the diagnosis of IBS.

CONDITIONS THAT MIMIC IRRITABLE BOWEL SYNDROME

- Cancer
- Diarrhea caused by infections such as amebiasis or giardiasis
- Disturbed bacterial microflora as a result of antibiotic or antacid usage
- Diverticular disease
- Inflammatory bowel disease
- Intestinal candidiasis
- Lactose intolerance
- Laxative abuse
- Malabsorption diseases, such as pancreatic insufficiency and celiac disease
- Mechanical causes, such as fecal impaction
- Metabolic disorders, such as adrenal insufficiency, diabetes, or hyperthyroidism
- Response to dietary factors that interfere with digestion, such as excessive consumption of tea, coffee, carbonated beverages, and simple sugars

Therapeutic Considerations

Once other conditions have been ruled out, there appear to be several treatments to consider in the successful resolution of IBS:

- Increasing dietary fiber
- Eliminating allergic/intolerant foods
- Eliminating refined sugars
- Reducing dietary FODMAPs (fermentable oligo-, di-, and monosaccharides and polyols)
- Taking probiotics
- Taking enteric-coated peppermint oil
- Controlling psychological components, especially stress

Unfortunately, instead of addressing underlying factors, the medical treatment of IBS focuses on drugs that primarily suppress symptoms.[1,2] As a general measure, we recommend that you read the chapter "Digestion and Elimination." In our experience, improving digestion sometimes resolves the symptoms of IBS.

Dietary Fiber

The treatment of irritable bowel syndrome through an increase in dietary fiber has a long history of success. Patients with constipation are much more likely to show response to dietary fiber than those with diarrhea. One problem that has not been addressed in studies on the therapeutic use of dietary fiber is the role of food allergy. The type of fiber often used in both research and clinical practice is wheat bran.[3] Wheat and other grains are among the foods most commonly implicated in malabsorptive and allergic conditions, and food allergy is a significant etiological factor in IBS, so the use of wheat bran is usually contraindicated.

Increasing dietary fiber from fruit and vegetable sources rather than grain sources may offer more benefit to some individuals, although in one uncontrolled clinical study there was no significant difference in improvement when a diet including 30 g fruit and vegetable fiber and 10 g cereal fiber was compared with a diet consisting of the opposite ratio.[4] Although the two diets resulted in similar significant improvement in abdominal pain, bowel habits, and state of well-being, the presence of large quantities of potentially allergic cereal fiber in both diets probably would have obscured any differences.

Psyllium seed husks are a popular bulk-forming laxative (they are, for example, the primary ingredient in commercial products such as Metamucil) and can be very helpful in improving IBS symptoms.[5] Another type of soluble fiber that may be useful and that is without the allergenic component of a wheat-based fiber is partially hydrolyzed guar gum (PHGG). The guar plant, *Cyamopsis tetragonoloba*, has been grown in India and Pakistan since ancient times. PHGG is a natural, soluble dietary fiber derived from the guar plant and has been shown to decrease the frequency of IBS symptoms such as abdominal spasms, flatulence, and abdominal tension.[6] The researchers concluded that PHGG works well in cases of altered intestinal motility and is easy to use because of its nongelling properties, unlike unhydrolyzed gum, which is much higher in viscosity and more difficult to incorporate into the diet.

Put simply, for most cases of irritable bowel syndrome, nonwheat sources of fiber—fiber-rich vegetables and fruits, or bulk-forming soluble fiber, such as psyllium or guar gum—may be the best choice to help reduce symptoms associated with IBS.

Food Allergies

The importance of food allergies in IBS has been recognized since the early 1900s.[7,8] Later studies have further documented the association between food allergy and IBS.[9–12] According to double-blind challenge methods, approximately two-thirds of patients with IBS have at least one food intolerance, and some have multiple intolerances.[9] Foods rich in carbohydrates, as well as fatty food, coffee, alcohol, and hot spices, are most frequently reported to cause symptoms.[1,2] The most common allergens are dairy products (40 to 44%) and grains (40 to 60%).[11] Many patients have noted marked clinical improvement with the use of elimination diets.[9–13]

In one of the most recent studies, 20 patients with IBS who had had no success with standard medical therapy were evaluated for food allergies by means of IgG blood tests and treated with an elimination diet followed by an allergy rotation diet and probiotic supplementation. The results were impressive: 100% of the study subjects reported improvement in symptoms. There was a trend toward an increase in beneficial flora after treatment but no change in the number and type of abnormal flora.

For more information on elimination and allergy rotation diets, see the chapter "Food Allergy."

Sugar

Meals high in refined sugar can contribute to IBS as well as to small intestinal bacterial overgrowth by decreasing intestinal motility.[14] When blood glucose levels rise too rapidly, gastrointestinal tract peristalsis slows down. Because glucose is absorbed primarily in the first parts of the small intestine (the duodenum and jejunum), the message affects this portion of the gastrointestinal tract most

strongly. Basically, the duodenum and jejunum become paralyzed by high sugar intake. A diet high in refined sugar may be the most important reason that IBS is such a common condition in the United States.

Dietary FODMAPs (Fermentable Oligo-, Di-, and Monosaccharides and Polyols)

There is a group of short-chain carbohydrates that are poorly absorbed in the small intestine and thus are likely to be fermented by intestinal bacteria, producing large amount of gases (such as hydrogen and carbon dioxide) that cause abdominal bloating. These carbohydrates include fermentable oligosaccharides, disaccharides, monosaccharides, and polyols (FODMAPs for short). Recent work has identified these short-chain carbohydrates as important triggers of functional gut symptoms.

One particular type of FODMAP is the oligosaccharides called fructans, which are chains of fructose with one glucose molecule on the end. Fructans-rich foods include wheat and foods made from wheat flour (bread, pasta, pastries, cookies, etc.); onions; and artichokes. Fructans with more than 10 molecules of fructose in a chain are known as inulins, and those with fewer than 10 fructose molecules are referred to as fructooligosaccharides (FOS) or oligofructoses. These compounds are now commonly added to many foods and dietary supplements as a source of prebiotic fiber to promote the growth of "friendly" gut bacteria.

Similar to fructans are galactans (such as stachyose and raffinose), which are composed of chains of fructose with one galactose molecule on the end. Galactans-rich foods include legumes (soy, chickpeas, lentils, and other dried beans), cabbage, and brussels sprouts.

The major disaccharide that is an issue in IBS is lactose (milk sugar). Lactose is in dairy products, but it may be also found in chocolate and other sweets, beer, prepared soups and sauces, and so on. Lactose is poorly absorbed in individuals with lactose intolerance, an overgrowth of bacteria in the small intestine, Crohn's disease, and celiac disease.

Even fructose (fruit sugar), a monosaccharide, can be an issue for some people. Fructose-rich foods include honey, dried fruits (prunes, figs, dates, or raisins), apples, pears, sweet cherries, peaches, agave syrup, watermelon, and papaya. Fructose is often added to commercial foods and drinks as high-fructose corn syrup.

Polyols, also known as sugar alcohols (often used as artificial sweeteners in commercially produced foods and drinks), include mannitol, sorbitol, erythritol, arabitol, glycol, glycerol, lactitol, and ribitol. These may also be a problem, especially if consumed in large quantities.

Open studies have suggested that three out of four patients with IBS will see a decrease in symptoms when they restrict intake of FODMAPs.[15] A randomized placebo-controlled rechallenge trial confirmed that the benefit was likely to be due to reduction of FODMAP intake.[16]

Nutritional Supplements

Probiotics are dietary supplements containing beneficial live microorganisms. Among the most commonly utilized and studied are *Lactobacillus* (several species), *Bifidobacterium* (several species), and *Saccharomyces boulardii*. Randomized, controlled clinical trials using probiotics to treat IBS symptoms have shown some benefits, but probiotics are not likely to resolve all symptoms.[17] In two studies, *Bifidobacterium infantis* produced improvement in all IBS symptoms except stool frequency and consistency.[18,19] Other studies have also shown positive results with *Lactobacillus rhamnosus* GG and *Lacto-*

bacillus plantaris alone and in combination with other probiotic species.[20-22] One study used a probiotic mixture containing *Lactobacillus rhamnosus* GG, *L. rhamnosus*, *Bifidobacterium breve*, and *Propionibacterium freudenreichii* in IBS patients for a period of six months. There was improvement in total symptom scores (reflecting abdominal pain, distension, flatulence, and bowel rumbling) in the treatment group compared with the placebo group.[21] Other studies using combinations of species have also shown benefit.[19-25]

While probiotics appear to be a key component in a comprehensive approach to treating IBS, they should be used in combination with diet therapy. In general, we prefer probiotic formulations that include multiple species rather than a single one, as these are more similar to what is found in nature.

Botanical Medicines

Peppermint oil (and presumably other similar volatile oils) inhibits gastrointestinal smooth muscle action in both laboratory animal preparations and humans. Clinically, peppermint oil has been used to reduce colonic spasm during endoscopy,[26] and an enteric-coated peppermint oil (ECPO) capsule has been used in the treatment of IBS.[27] Enteric coating is believed to be necessary because menthol (the major constituent of peppermint oil) and other plant monoterpenes in peppermint oil are rapidly absorbed.[28] This rapid absorption tends to limit its effects to the upper intestine, resulting in relaxation of the cardioesophageal sphincter and common side effects, such as esophageal reflux and heartburn, after administration. A transient hot burning sensation in the rectum during defecation, due to unabsorbed menthol, has been noted in some patients taking ECPO.

A detailed analysis of five studies supported the efficacy of peppermint oil, with most of the studies using ECPO at a dosage of 0.2 ml twice per day between meals.[28,29] One well-designed study involved 110 patients with symptoms of IBS.[30] The patients took one capsule of either ECPO (0.2 ml) or a placebo three to four times per day, 15 to 30 minutes before meals, for one month. The results (listed below) are quite impressive, especially given the safety of ECPO. Only two cases of side effects were reported; one patient experienced heartburn (because of chewing the capsule), and one patient had a transient rash.

ECPO is thought to work by improving the rhythmic contractions of the intestinal tract and relieving intestinal spasm. An additional benefit of these volatile oils is their efficacy against *Candida albicans*.[31] This is because an overgrowth of *C. albicans* may be an underlying factor in IBS, especially in patients who do not respond to dietary advice and those who consume large amounts of sugar. Administration of the antifungal drug nystatin (600,000 IU per day for 10 days) to patients whose IBS did not respond to an elimination diet produced dramatic clinical improvement.[10]

ECPO is especially helpful for children with IBS as long as they can swallow the capsules. In one randomized, double-blind, controlled trial of 42 children with moderate levels of pain from IBS, peppermint oil was considered a safe and effective treatment.[32]

Psychological Factors

Mental and emotional problems—anxiety, fatigue, hostile feelings, depression, and sleep disturbances—are reported by almost all patients with IBS. Severity and frequency of symptoms tend to correlate with these psychological factors. Anxiety is associated with a high degree of food-related symptoms in IBS.[1] Especially significant is sleep quality; poor sleep quality results in a rise in symptom severity.[33] See the chapter "Insomnia" for recommendations to improve sleep quality if it is relevant.

Several theories link psychological factors to the symptoms of IBS. The "learning model" holds that when exposed to stressful situations, some children learn to develop gastrointestinal symptoms to cope with the stress. Another theory holds that IBS is a manifestation of depression, chronic anxiety, or both.

Stress is certainly an important factor to consider. Greater intestinal motility during exposure to stressful situations has been shown to occur in both normal subjects and people suffering from IBS.[34] This finding ap-

Percentage of Patients Showing Improvements with ECPO or Placebo on Major Symptoms of IBS		
PARAMETER	% SHOWING IMPROVEMENT WITH ECPO	% SHOWING IMPROVEMENT WITH PLACEBO
Abdominal pain	79	43
Abdominal distension	83	29
Stool frequency	83	33
Stomach rumbling	73	31
Flatulence	79	22

parently accounts for the increase in abdominal pain and irregular bowel function seen in both patients with IBS and normal subjects during periods of emotional stress.

Psychotherapy, in the form of relaxation therapy, biofeedback, hypnosis, counseling, or stress management training, has been shown to reduce symptom frequency and severity of IBS.[35–38]

QUICK REVIEW

- Irritable bowel syndrome is a functional disorder of the large intestine.
- Because IBS is caused by many inter-related factors, the best approach is to address each of the major ones.
- Rather than addressing underlying factors, conventional medical treatment of IBS focuses primarily on drugs that suppress symptoms.
- Increasing consumption of fiber can be a successful treatment for irritable bowel syndrome.
- The majority of patients with IBS have at least one food intolerance, and some have multiple intolerances.
- Meals high in refined sugar can contribute to irritable bowel syndrome.
- Open studies have suggested that three out of four patients with IBS respond well to restriction of FODMAP intake.
- Probiotics appear to be a key component in the comprehensive approach to treating IBS but should be used in combination with diet therapy.
- Enteric-coated peppermint oil is quite beneficial in relieving the symptoms of irritable bowel syndrome.

TREATMENT SUMMARY

Because IBS represents a health condition caused by many interrelated factors, the best approach is to address each of the following major factors:

- Increasing dietary fiber
- Eliminating foods to which there is an allergy or intolerance
- Eliminating refined sugars
- Reducing dietary FODMAPs
- Taking probiotics
- Taking enteric-coated peppermint oil
- Controlling psychological components, especially stress

Diet

The guidelines given in the chapter "A Health-Promoting Diet" are appropriate for improving IBS. Particularly important is increasing dietary fiber intake. It is also important to identify and eliminate food allergies. It may also help to eliminate or reduce FODMAPs.

Nutritional Supplements

- Follow the general recommendations in the chapter "Supplementary Measures."
- Probiotic supplement (multistrain, in- cluding species of lactobacillus and bi- fidobacteria): 5 billion to 20 billion live organisms per day

Botanical Medicines

- Enteric-coated peppermint oil: 0.2 to 0.4 ml twice per day between meals

Kidney Stones

- Usually without symptoms until stone becomes lodged in a ureter
- Excruciating intermittent radiating pain originating in the flank or kidney
- Nausea, vomiting, and abdominal distension
- Chills, fever, and urinary frequency if infection is present
- Diagnosed by ultrasound

Stone formation in the urinary tract has been recognized for thousands of years, but during the last few decades we have seen changes in the pattern and frequency of the disease. In the past, stone formation occurred almost exclusively in the bladder, whereas today most stones form in the kidneys. The frequency of stones has increased dramatically as well. It is now estimated that 10% of all American men will experience a kidney stone during their lifetime, with 0.1 to 6.0% of the general population having one in any given year. In the United States, 1 out of every 1,000 hospital admissions is for kidney stones. This increase in frequency parallels the rise in other diseases associated with the typical Western diet, including heart disease, high blood pressure, and diabetes.

In the United States, most kidney stones (75 to 85%) are composed of calcium salts, while 5 to 8% are uric acid stones and another 10 to 15% are magnesium ammonium phosphate stones. The prevalence of different types of stones varies geographically, reflecting differences in environmental factors, diet, and drinking water. Men are affected more than women, and most patients are over 30 years of age.

Components in human urine normally remain in solution due to pH control and the secretion of substances that inhibit crystal growth. However, where there is an increase in the substances that make up stones or a decrease in protective factors, these substances can form a tiny crystal, which can then grow in size to what we call a kidney stone. There are a number of metabolic diseases that can lead to kidney stones, so it is important to have your doctor rule out such conditions as hyperparathyroidism, cystinuria, Cushing's syndrome, and sarcoidosis.

Diagnostic Considerations

Diagnosing the type of stone is critical to determining the appropriate therapy. Careful evaluation of a number of criteria (diet; underlying metabolic or disease factors; urinalysis; urine culture; and blood levels of calcium, uric acid, creatinine, and electrolytes) will usually allow a physician to determine the composition of the stone if one is not available for chemical analysis.

Conditions favoring stone formation can be divided into two groups: factors increasing the concentration of the substances that make up stones, and factors favoring stone formation at normal urinary concentrations.

Chemical and Physical Characteristics of Urinary Stones					
COMPOSITION	**CRYSTAL NAME**	**FREQUENCY**	**X-RAY APPEARANCE**	**URINE CHARACTERISTICS**	**CRYSTAL CHARACTERISTICS**
Calcium oxalate	Whewellite	30–35%	Opaque	Nonspecific	Small; hemp seed or mulberry shape; brown or black color
Calcium oxalate + calcium phosphate		30–35	Opaque	pH > 5.5	Small; hemp seed or mulberry shape; brown or black color
Calcium phosphate	Apatite	6–8	Opaque	pH > 5.5	Staghorn configuration; light color
Magnesium ammonium phosphate	Struvite, triple phosphate	15–20	Opaque	pH > 6.2, infection	Staghorn configuration; light color
Uric acid		6–10	Translucent	pH < 6.0	Ellipsoid shape; tan or red-brown color
Cystine		2–3	Opaque	pH < 7.2	Multiple stones; faceted shape; maple sugar color

The first group includes reduction in urine volume (dehydration) and an increased rate of excretion of stone constituents. The second group of factors is related to stagnation of urine flow (urinary stasis), pH changes, foreign bodies, and reduction in levels of substances that normally keep stone constituents from forming crystals.

Therapeutic Considerations

The high frequency of calcium-containing stones in affluent societies is directly associated with the following dietary patterns:

- Low fiber intake[1]
- High consumption of refined carbohydrates[2,3]
- High alcohol consumption[4]
- Consumption of large amounts of animal protein[4,5]
- High fat consumption[6]
- High consumption of soft drinks[7]
- Excessively acid-forming diet

Today conventional medicine classifies most stones as having an "unknown cause" (idiopathic), but this ignores the dietary factors that lead to stone formation. The cumulative effect of these dietary factors is undoubtedly the reason for the rising incidence of kidney stones.

As a group, vegetarians have a decreased risk of developing stones.[5,8] Studies have shown that even among meat eaters, those who ate higher amounts of fresh fruits and vegetables had a lower incidence of stones.[8] Adding bran to the diet and changing from white bread to whole wheat bread are two

Causes of Excessive Excretion of Relatively Insoluble Urinary Constituents		
CONSTITUENT	**CAUSE OF EXCESS EXCRETION**	**LAB FINDINGS OR CAUSE**
Calcium (>250 mg excreted per day)	Absorptive hypercalciuria	Low serum PO_4
	Renal hypercalciuria (renal tubular acidosis)	High serum PTH, high urinary cAMP
	Primary hyperparathyroidism	High serum calcium, high calcitriol
	Hyperthyroidism	
	High vitamin D intake	High serum calcium
	Excess intake of milk and alkali	
	Aluminum salt intake	Low serum phosphate, high calcitriol
	Destructive bone disease	
	Sarcoidosis	
	Prolonged immobility	
	Consumption of an excessively acid-forming diet	
Oxalate	Familial oxaluria (rare)	
	Ileal disease, resection, or bypass	
	Steatorrhea	
	High oxalate intake	
	Ethylene glycol poisoning	
	Vitamin C excess (extremely unlikely)	Vitamin B_6 deficiency or abnormal oxalate metabolism
	Methoxyflurane anesthesia	
Uric acid (>750 mg excreted per day)	Gout	
	Idiopathic hyperuricosuria	
	Excess purine intake	
	Anticancer drugs	Rapid cell destruction
	Myeloproliferative disease	
Cystine	Hereditary cystinuria	

measures that have been shown to lower urinary calcium.[9]

Dietary factors may also play a role in acidifying or alkalinizing urine. Depending on the type of stone, this ability to alter urinary pH may help prevent and treat stones.[10]

In one study, 12 healthy men were given a standardized diet plus either cranberry, blackcurrant, or plum juice, then had their urine tested.[11] The researchers found that cranberry juice decreased urinary pH (made the urine more acidic) and significantly increased the excretion of oxalic acid, leading to a higher concentration of uric acid. Blackcurrant juice increased urinary pH (made the urine more alkaline), leading to excretion of citric acid and loss of oxalic acid. Plum juice demonstrated no effects. These results indicate that blackcurrant juice could support the prevention and treatment of uric acid and oxalate stones, while cranberry juice could be useful in the treatment of oxalate stones as well as magnesium ammonium phosphate stones.

Another study showed that cranberry juice reduced the amount of calcium in the urine by over 50% in patients with recurrent kidney stones.[12] Since high urinary calcium levels greatly increase the risk of developing a kidney stone, it appears that cranberry juice may offer significant benefit. Because most cranberry juice products on the market are loaded with sugar, it might be better to take a cranberry extract. For prevention of kidney stones in those at high risk, take the equivalent of 16 fl oz cranberry juice or follow dosage recommendations given on the product's label.

Drinking more water has long been recognized as one of the main approaches to preventing kidney stones. Increasing the urine volume results in a decrease in stone prevalence. Numerous clinical trials have found that consumption of more than about 48 fl oz of water per day lowers the long-term risk of kidney stone recurrence by approximately 60%.[13]

Another dietary recommendation is to decrease salt consumption. Urinary calcium excretion increases approximately 40 mg for each 2,300 mg increase in dietary sodium in normal adults; those who form kidney stones have an even greater increase in urinary calcium with an increase in salt intake. The best approach is to combine increased water intake with decreased sodium intake.[14]

Weight Control and Sugar Intake

Weight control and correction of carbohydrate metabolism are important, since excess weight and insulin insensitivity lead to increased urinary excretion of calcium and are high risk factors for stone formation.[15,16] A meal high in sugar is particularly detrimental, since urinary calcium levels rise following sugar intake, an effect that is exaggerated in most people (approximately 70%) with recurrent kidney stones.[17] Obviously people with recurrent kidney stones should avoid sugar; sports drinks are especially problematic, because they combine sugars and salt.

Magnesium and Vitamin B_6

A magnesium-deficient diet is one of the quickest ways to cause kidney stones in rats.[18] Adequate levels of magnesium have been shown to increase the solubility of calcium oxalate and inhibit the formation of both calcium phosphate and calcium oxalate stones.[18–20] A low urinary magnesium-to-calcium ratio is an independent risk factor in stone formation, and supplemental magnesium alone has been shown to be effective in preventing recurrences of kidney stones.[20–22] However, when it is used in conjunction with vitamin B_6, an even greater effect is noted.[23,24]

Many patients with recurrent oxalate stones show laboratory signs of vitamin B_6 deficiency. As with magnesium, vitamin B_6 deficiency also results in kidney stones. Supplemental vitamin B_6 is known to reduce the production and urinary excretion of oxalates.[25,26] Supplementing the diet with additional vitamin B$_6$ is very important in preventing recurrent kidney stones.

Calcium

Most conventional doctors tell their patients with kidney stones to avoid calcium supplements; the thinking is that because calcium-containing stones are so common, restricting the amount of calcium in the diet will help reduce the formation of stones. However, studies show that calcium supplementation (300 mg per day of calcium, given as calcium carbonate, citrate, or malate) actually reduced oxalate absorption and excretion, and thus would help to prevent stone formation. Taking 300 to 1,000 mg calcium per day may be a useful preventive strategy.[27]

Citrate

Citric acid (citrate) has the ability to reduce the concentration of calcium oxalate and calcium phosphate in the urine, thus retarding the formation and growth of stones. Potassium or sodium citrate has been shown to be quite effective in the treatment of patients with recurrent calcium oxalate stones, with nearly 90% of patients showing improvement.[28–31] For example, in one study, potassium citrate supplementation in recurrent stone formers resulted in a drop of stone formation from 0.7 to 0.13 per year.[30] In another study, which tracked 57 people with a history of calcium stones and low urinary citrate levels, those given potassium citrate developed fewer kidney stones over a period of three years than they had previously.[31] In comparison, the group given a placebo had no change in their rate of stone formation. However, it appears that magnesium citrate (rather than potassium or sodium citrate) offers the greatest benefit.

Another reason citrates decrease calcium oxalate stones is that they help reverse the acidification effects of the typical Western diet. One of the key ways the body works to neutralize excessive acid in the blood is by taking calcium from bone. Alkalinizing the diet decreases the excretion of calcium in the urine, suggesting that less calcium is being taken from the bones. For more information, see Appendix C, "Acid-Base Values of Selected Foods."

Vitamin K

Vitamin K is necessary in the manufacture of a molecule that is a powerful inhibitor of kidney stone formation.[32] The presence of vitamin K in green leafy vegetables may be one reason vegetarians have a lower incidence of kidney stones.[33]

Uric Acid Metabolism

The level of dietary purine consumption is directly related to the rate of urinary uric acid excretion.[34] This fact is important, since elevations in the uric acid content of urine are a causative factor in recurrent uric acid stones. People with uric acid stones should entirely avoid foods high in purine, including organ meats, other red meats, shellfish, yeast (brewer's and baker's), herring, sardines, mackerel, and anchovies. They should also watch their consumption of foods with moderate levels of purine, including dried legumes, spinach, asparagus, other types of fish, poultry, and mushrooms.

Low-Oxalate Diet

Dietary oxalate may be responsible for as much as 80% of the urine oxalate in some people with recurrent kidney stones, indicating that restricting dietary oxalate intake may have a protective action.[35–37] In one clinical trial, men with recurrent calcium oxalate stones who ate a diet that had normal amounts of calcium (1,200 mg per day), low amounts of animal protein, and low amounts of salt showed a significant reduction in oxalate excretion and a lower incidence of recurrent stones compared with men on a low-calcium diet (400 mg per day).[37] It appears that people with recurrent kidney stones have a tendency to absorb higher levels of dietary oxalates compared with normal subjects not prone to kidney stones. A low-oxalate diet is usually defined as one containing less than 50 mg oxalate per day, so foods that have high or moderate levels of oxalate should be avoided.

Oxalate Content of Selected Foods
Very high oxalate, >50 mg per serving

- Vegetables
  - Beets (greens or root)
  - Okra
  - Spinach
  - Swiss chard
- Fruits
  - Figs, dried
  - Rhubarb
- Grains
  - Buckwheat
- Nuts and seeds
  - Almonds
  - Peanuts
  - Peanut butter
  - Sesame seeds

High oxalate, >10 mg per serving

- Vegetables
  - Celery
  - Collards
  - Dandelion greens
  - Eggplant
  - Escarole
  - Green beans
  - Kale
  - Leeks
  - Parsley
  - Parsnips
  - Peppers, green
  - Potatoes
  - Pumpkin
  - Squash, yellow summer
  - Sweet potatoes
  - Tomato sauce, canned
  - Turnip greens
  - Watercress
- Fruits
  - Concord grapes
  - Kiwi
  - Lemon peel
  - Lime peel
  - Orange peel
- Grains
  - Bread, whole wheat
  - Oatmeal
  - Popcorn
  - Spelt
  - Wheat bran
  - Wheat germ
  - Whole wheat flour
- Legumes
  - Garbanzo beans
  - Lentils
  - Soybeans and all soy products
- Nuts and seeds
  - Brazil nuts

- ○ Hazelnuts
- ○ Pecans
- ○ Sunflower seeds
- Miscellaneous
  - ○ Beer
  - ○ Chocolate
  - ○ Cocoa
  - ○ Soy sauce (1 tbsp)
  - ○ Tea, black or green

Moderate oxalate, 6 to 10 mg per serving

- Vegetables
  - ○ Asparagus
  - ○ Artichokes
  - ○ Broccoli
  - ○ Brussels sprouts
  - ○ Carrots
  - ○ Cucumber
  - ○ Garlic
  - ○ Lettuce
  - ○ Mushrooms
  - ○ Mustard greens
  - ○ Onions
  - ○ Pumpkin
  - ○ Radishes
  - ○ Snow peas
  - ○ Tomato, fresh
  - ○ Tomato sauce, canned (¼ cup)
- Fruits
  - ○ Apples
  - ○ Apricots
  - ○ Blackberries
  - ○ Blueberries
  - ○ Cherries, sour
  - ○ Cranberries, dried

- ○ Currants, black
- ○ Oranges
- ○ Peaches
- ○ Pears
- ○ Pineapple
- ○ Plums
- ○ Prunes
- ○ Red raspberries
- ○ Tangerines
- Grains
  - ○ Bagel (1 medium)
  - ○ Barley, cooked
  - ○ Bread, white (2 slices)
  - ○ Corn
  - ○ Corn tortilla (1 medium)
  - ○ Cornbread
  - ○ Cornmeal, yellow (1 cup dry)
  - ○ Cornstarch (¼ cup)
  - ○ Pasta
  - ○ Rice, brown
  - ○ Spaghetti
  - ○ White flour
- Legumes
  - ○ Lima beans
  - ○ Split peas
- Nuts and seeds
  - ○ Cashews
  - ○ Flaxseed
  - ○ Walnuts
- Herbs
  - ○ Basil, fresh (1 tbsp)
  - ○ Dill (1 tbsp)
  - ○ Ginger, raw, sliced (1 tsp)
  - ○ Malt powder (1 tbsp)
  - ○ Nutmeg (1 tbsp)
  - ○ Pepper (1 tsp)

- Miscellaneous
  - Coffee
  - Red wine
  - Sardines
  - Tea, rose hip

Low oxalate, 2 to 5 mg per serving

- Vegetables
  - Acorn squash
  - Arugula
  - Ketchup (1 tbsp)
  - Onions
  - Peppers, red
  - Zucchini
- Fruits
  - Avocado
  - Cantaloupe
  - Cherries, sweet
  - Cranberries
  - Grapes
  - Lemons
  - Limes
  - Raisins
- Grains
  - Rice, white
  - Rice, wild
  - Rye bread
- Legumes
  - Peas, green
- Nuts and seeds
  - Coconut
- Herbs
  - Cinnamon, ground (1½ tsp)
  - Ginger, powdered (1 tbsp)

- Mustard, Dijon (¼ cup)
- Thyme, dried (1 tsp)
- Miscellaneous
  - Beef
  - Chicken
  - Corned beef
  - Eggs
  - Fish (haddock, plaice, and flounder)
  - Ham
  - Lamb
  - Pork
  - Turkey
  - Venison

Nutritional Supplements

Vitamin C

Vitamin C is often cited in the medical literature as a potential factor in the development of calcium oxalate kidney stones. However, numerous studies have now clearly demonstrated that high doses of vitamin C do not cause kidney stones. Studies have shown that vitamin C ingestion of up to 10 g per day does not have any effect on urinary oxalate levels.[38,39] While some studies showed that taking high dosages of vitamin C increased oxalate excretion;[40,41] it looks as if the vitamin C was converted to oxalates during the analytical process.[39]

Inositol Hexaphosphate

Inositol hexaphosphate is a naturally occurring compound found in whole grains, cereals, legumes, seeds, and nuts. One trial showed that 120 mg inositol hexaphosphate significantly reduced the formation of calcium oxalate crystals in the urine of people with a history of kidney stone formation, in only 15 days.[42]

Botanical Medicines

Compounds known as anthraquinones, isolated from herbs such as senna and aloe vera, bind calcium and significantly reduce the growth rate of urinary crystals when used in oral doses lower than the doses that cause a laxative effect.[43,44] Our recommendation is to use aloe vera or senna at levels that produce no laxative effect.

QUICK REVIEW

- **Up to 10% of all American men will develop a kidney stone during their lifetime.**
- **Kidney stones have been linked to the typical Western diet.**
- **Magnesium and vitamin B$_6$ supplementation can help prevent calcium oxalate kidney stones.**
- **Citrate supplementation stops calcium oxalate stone formation in nearly 90% of patients.**
- **Cranberry juice has been shown to reduce the amount of calcium in the urine by over 50% in patients with recurrent kidney stones.**
- **People who have uric acid stones should avoid foods high in purines.**
- **Drink at least 48 fl oz water per day.**

TREATMENT SUMMARY

Prevention of recurrence is the therapeutic goal in the treatment of kidney stones. Since dietary management is effective, relatively inexpensive, and free of side effects, it is the treatment of choice. The specific treatment is determined by the type of stone and may include reducing urinary calcium, reducing purine intake, avoiding high-oxalate foods, increasing foods high in magnesium-, and increasing foods rich in vitamin K.

For all types of stones, increasing urine flow to dilute the urine is vital. Drink at least 48 fl oz of water per day.

Note: In acute cases, surgical removal or breaking up the stone with sound waves (lithotripsy) may be necessary.

For Calcium Stones
Diet

Follow the general recommendations given in the chapter "A Health-Promoting Diet." In particular, increase fiber, complex carbohydrates, and green leafy vegetables, and decrease simple carbohydrates and foods high in purines (meat, fish, poultry, yeast). Increase consumption of magnesium-rich foods (barley, bran, corn, buckwheat, rye, soy, oats, brown rice, avocados, bananas, cashews, coconut, peanuts, sesame seeds, lima beans, potatoes). If you have calcium oxalate stones, reduce foods high in oxalate.

Nutritional Supplements

- Key individual nutrients:
  - ○ Vitamin B_6: 25 to 50 mg per day
  - ○ Vitamin K: 1 to 2 mg per day
  - ○ Magnesium (bound to aspartate, citrate, fumarate, malate, or succinate): 150 to 200 mg three times per day
  - ○ Vitamin D_3: 2,000 to 4,000 IU per day (ideally, measure blood levels and adjust dosage accordingly)
- Fish oils: 1,000 mg EPA + DHA per day
- One of the following:
  - ○ Cranberry extract: equivalent of 16 fl oz cranberry juice per day or follow label instructions
  - ○ Grape seed extract (>95% procyanidolic oligomers): 100 to 300 mg per day
  - ○ Pine bark extract (>95% procyanidolic oligomers): 100 to 300 mg per day
  - ○ Inositol hexaphosphate: 120 mg per day

Botanical Medicines

- Aloe vera or senna at a dosage just below the level that produces a laxative effect (this level will vary from one person to the next)

Other Considerations

- Avoid aluminum compounds and antacids

For Uric Acid Stones

Diet

- Decrease intake of purines

Nutritional Supplements

- See the chapter "Gout"

Other Considerations

- Alkalinize urine with citrate (see Appendix C)

For Magnesium Ammonium Phosphate Stones

- Eradicate any infections; see the chapter "Cystitis and Interstitial Cystitis/Painful Bladder"
- Acidify urine: ammonium chloride (100 to 200 mg three times per day).

For Cystine Stones

- Avoid methionine-rich foods (soy, wheat, dairy products, fish, meat, lima beans, garbanzo beans, mushrooms, and all nuts and seeds except coconut, hazelnuts, and sunflower seeds)
- Alkalinize the urine by eating an alkaline-rich diet and taking magnesium citrate (250 mg elemental magnesium three times daily): optimal pH is 7.5 to 8.0

Macular Degeneration

- Progressive visual loss due to degeneration of the macula
- Eye exam may reveal spots of pigment near the macula and blurring of the macular borders

The *macula* is the area of the retina where images are focused. It is the portion of the eye responsible for fine vision. Degeneration of the macula is the leading cause of severe visual loss in the United States and Europe in people 55 or older, and is second to cataracts as the leading cause of decreased vision in people over 65. It is estimated that more than 150,000 Americans are legally blind from age-related macular degeneration, with 20,000 new cases occurring each year.[1,2]

The major risk factors for macular degeneration are smoking, aging, atherosclerosis (hardening of the arteries), and high blood pressure.[1–4] The degeneration appears to be a result of free radical damage, similar to the type of damage that induces cataracts (see the chapter "Cataracts"). However, decreased blood and oxygen supply to the retina is the key factor leading to macular degeneration.

Types of Macular Degeneration

The two most common types of age-related macular degeneration (ARMD) are the *atrophic* ("dry") form, by far the more frequent, and the *neovascular* ("wet") form.[2,3] In either

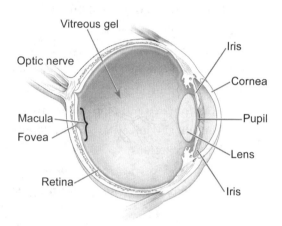

Anatomy of the Eye

form, patients may experience blurred vision. The patient may note that straight objects appear distorted or bent, that there is a dark spot near or around the center of the visual field, and that, while he or she is reading, parts of words are missing.

Dry ARMD

Between 80 and 85% of people with ARMD have the dry form of the disease. The primary lesions are atrophic changes in the *retinal pigmented epithelium* (RPE), which composes the innermost layer of the retina. Beginning in early life and continuing throughout life, cells of the RPE gradually accumulate sacs of cellular debris known as *lipofuscin*. The lipofuscin sacs are either remnants of incompletely degraded abnormal molecules from damaged RPE cells or derivatives of damaged membranes of nearby cells. Progressive engorgement of the RPE cells with lipofuscin is associated with the leakage (extrusion) of other cell components.[1–3] The hallmark feature of macular degeneration is the appearance of this extrusion beneath the RPE. This extrusion, which can be seen with the aid of an ophthalmoscope, is referred to as *drusen*.

The disease progresses slowly, and only central vision is lost; peripheral vision remains intact. It is rare for anyone to become totally blind from dry ARMD. Currently there is no standard medical treatment for this common form of ARMD, though the use of nutritional supplements designed to address the underlying oxidative damage is becoming the "unofficial" standard of care.

Wet Age-Related Macular Degeneration

Wet ARMD is also known as the neovascular form or advanced ARMD. It affects 5% to 20% of people with ARMD. Wet ARMD is characterized by the growth of abnormal blood vessels. Because the disease can rapidly progress to a point at which laser surgery cannot be used, treatment should be performed as soon as possible. A common early symptom of wet ARMD is that straight lines appear wavy.

Wet ARMD can be treated quite effectively in the early stages with laser surgery and other medical treatments such as lower-powered laser or low-dose radiation therapy. Drugs known as antiangiogenics or anti-VEGF (anti–vascular endothelial growth factor) agents are also used. These drugs can shrink the abnormal blood vessels and improve vision when injected directly into the vitreous humor of the eye. The injections have to be repeated on a monthly or bimonthly basis. Examples of these agents include ranibizumab (Lucentis), bevacizumab (Avastin), and pegaptanib (Macugen).[1,2]

Therapeutic Considerations

Treatment of the dry form and prevention of the wet form of ARMD involve the use of antioxidants and natural substances that correct the underlying free radical damage to the macula. Reduce the risk of ARMD by focusing on preventive factors against atherosclerosis, increasing dietary intake of fresh fruits and vegetables, supplementing with nutritional and botanical antioxidants, and not smoking.

In particular, smoking tobacco greatly increases the risk of ARMD.[3] Someone who smokes a pack of cigarettes a day for any significant length of time increases the risk of ARMD by two to three times that of someone who has never smoked.[3] The risk does not return to the normal level until after someone has stopped smoking for 15 years.

There is also a strong genetic component to consider. While a number of genetic markers have been identified, a family history may be the easiest screening method. The lifetime risk of developing late-stage macular degeneration is 50% for people who have a relative with macular degeneration, vs. 12% for people who do not.[5]

Interestingly, higher birth weight and a lower ratio of head circumference to birth weight are associated with significantly higher risk for ARMD.[6]

Diet

Not surprisingly, the dietary factors important in the prevention and treatment of ARMD are the same as those that prevent other chronic degenerative diseases including atherosclerosis. A diet rich in fruits and vegetables is associated with a lower risk for ARMD. Presumably this protection is

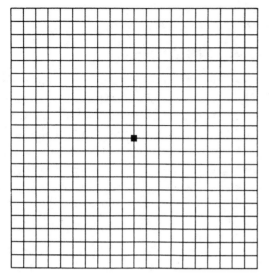

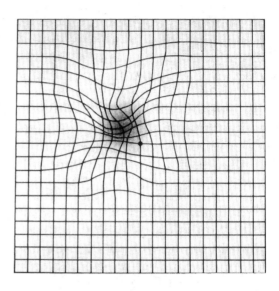

Normal Appearance of Amsler Grid

Appearance of Amsler Grid in Macular Degeneration

the result of greater intake of antioxidant vitamins and minerals.[7–10] However, various nonessential food components such as flavonoids and the carotenes lutein, zeaxanthin, and lycopene are proving to be even more significant in protecting against ARMD than traditional nutritional antioxidants such as vitamin C and E, zinc, and selenium. The macula, especially its central portion, the fovea, owes its yellow color to its high concentration of lutein and zeaxanthin. These yellow carotenoids function in preventing oxidative damage to the area of the retina responsible for fine vision and have a central role in protecting against the development of macular degeneration.[9,10]

The carotene lycopene, a component of tomatoes and other red fruit and vegetables, is also protective. In one study, individuals with the lowest levels of lycopene content were twice as likely to have ARMD.[11]

Moderate wine consumption is also associated with decreased risk of ARMD.[12] Red wine contains anthocyanins, powerful antioxidants that are probably responsible for

its protective effect. It is important to note that beer consumption increases drusen accumulation and the risk of exudative macular disease and therefore should be avoided.[13]

Just as in atherosclerosis, types of dietary fat appear to play a role in ARMD. A cohort study of 261 individuals with early or intermediate stages of ARMD revealed a twofold increased risk of progression with a diet high in animal fat and commercial baked goods (sources of sugar and trans-fatty acids). In contrast, higher intakes of fish and nuts are associated with a lower risk of ARMD progression.[14] A higher intake of long-chain omega-3 fatty acids was shown to be inversely associated with progression to ARMD over a period of 12 years.[15–17]

Nutritional Supplements

In addition to a diet high in antioxidants, supplementation with nutritional antioxidants such as vitamin C, selenium, beta-carotene, and vitamin E is certainly important in the treatment and prevention of macular de-

Food Sources of Carotenes Important for the Eyes	
CAROTENOID	**FOOD SOURCE**
Lycopene	Tomatoes, carrots, green peppers, apricots, pink grapefruit
Zeaxanthin	Spinach; paprika; corn; richly colored fruit, especially kiwi fruit and grapes
Lutein	Corn, potatoes, spinach and other greens, carrots, tomatoes, mangoes

generation. Studies conducted by the Age-Related Eye Disease Study Research Group (AREDS) confirm that a combination of these nutrients will be likely to produce better results than any single nutrient alone, because other studies have demonstrated that none of these antioxidants alone accounts for the impaired antioxidant status in ARMD.[18] Instead, the lower antioxidant status reflects decreases in a combination of nutrients. The specific amounts of antioxidants and zinc used in the study were 500 mg vitamin C, 400 IU vitamin E, 15 mg beta-carotene (often labeled as equivalent to 25,000 IU vitamin A), 80 mg zinc (as zinc oxide), and 2 mg copper (as cupric oxide).

Several other studies utilizing various commercially available broad-based antioxidant formulas have shown promising results. For example, a 1½-year study demonstrated that the progression of dry ARMD could be halted (but not reversed) with a broad-spectrum, 14-component antioxidant capsule (Ocuguard).[19,20] A retrospective study of a nutritional supplement called ICAPS Plus (which contains beta-carotene, vitamins C and E, zinc, copper, manganese, selenium, and riboflavin) compared 38 patients who used the preparation regularly with 37 patients who used only one bottle and who

served as controls. Fifteen of the treated patients showed improvement in their vision by one line or more on a vision acuity chart, compared with only 6 of the control group. In addition, only 3 of the 38 in the treatment group lost one line or more of vision, compared with 13 in the control group.[21] In a second blinded clinical trial reported in the same review, after six months, visual acuity was the same or better in 36 of 61 controls compared with 168 of 192 treated patients.

B vitamins are also important. In a randomized, double-blind, placebo-controlled trial, 5,442 female health care professionals 40 years or older with preexisting cardiovascular disease or three or more cardiovascular disease risk factors randomly received a combination of folic acid (2.5 mg per day), vitamin B_6 (50 mg per day), and vitamin B_{12} (1 mg per day) or a placebo. After an average of 7.3 years of treatment and follow-up, there were 55 cases of ARMD in the combination treatment group and 82 in the placebo group. There were 26 cases of more severe ARMD in the combination treatment group and 44 in the placebo group. These results indicate a 34% and 41% reduced relative risk, respectively.[22]

Lutein

In addition to a high-lutein diet, supplementation with additional lutein is of benefit. One 12-month double-blind study, the Lutein Antioxidant Supplementation Trial (LAST),[23] sought to determine whether nutritional supplementation with lutein or lutein together with antioxidants, vitamins, and minerals improves visual function and symptoms in ARMD. Patients receiving lutein (10 mg) alone or in combination with other vitamins and minerals in a broad-spectrum supplementation formula showed improvements in visual function.

In another study, 27 patients with ARMD

were randomly divided into two groups: 15 patients took vitamin C (180 mg), vitamin E (30 mg), zinc (22.5 mg), copper (1 mg), lutein (10 mg), zeaxanthin (1 mg), and astaxanthin (4 mg) every day for 12 months, while 12 patients served as controls. Visual acuity assessments indicated quite clearly that early-stage ARMD can respond positively to supplementation with carotenoids and antioxidants.[24]

Zinc

Zinc plays an essential role in the metabolism of the retina, and the elderly are at high risk for zinc deficiency. In addition to the studies with a combination of nutrients, a two-year, prospective, randomized, double-blind, placebo-controlled trial involving 151 subjects with dry ARMD demonstrated that the group taking 200 mg per day of zinc sulfate (approximately 80 mg elemental zinc) had significantly less visual loss than the placebo group.[25]

In another study, using a zinc-monocysteine (ZMC) supplement, 40 subjects with ARMD were randomly assigned to either ZMC 25 mg or a placebo twice per day for six months. The ZMC group showed improved visual acuity, contrast sensitivity, and macular light flash recovery time. No improvement occurred in the placebo group. ZMC was well tolerated, with a gastrointestinal irritation rate of under 2%.[26]

Flavonoid-Rich Extracts

Flavonoid-rich extracts of bilberry (*Vaccinium myrtillus*), ginkgo biloba, grape seed, or pine bark (e.g., Pycnogenol) offer significant benefits in the prevention and treatment of ARMD. In addition to exerting excellent antioxidant activity, all of these extracts have been shown to have positive effects on retinal blood flow and function. Clinical studies of humans have demonstrated that all three are also capable of halting the progressive visual loss of dry ARMD and possibly even improving visual function.[27–30] Of the three, bilberry extracts standardized to contain 25% anthocyanidins appear to be the most useful. The anthocyanosides of bilberry have a very strong affinity for the retinal pigmented epithelium, reinforcing the collagen structures of the retina and preventing free radical

. . . .

QUICK REVIEW

- **Degeneration of the macula is the leading cause of severe visual loss in the United States.**
- **The major risk factors for macular degeneration are smoking, aging, atherosclerosis (hardening of the arteries), and high blood pressure.**
- **The treatment goals in the dry form and prevention of the wet form involve the use of antioxidants and natural substances that protect against free radical damage and improve blood and oxygen supply to the macula.**
- **A diet rich in fruits and vegetables is associated with a greatly lowered risk for macular degeneration.**
- **In addition to a high-lutein diet, supplementation with additional lutein is of benefit.**
- **Antioxidant formulas have been shown to halt and even reverse macular degeneration.**

damage. Because the RPE is the portion of the eye affected in ARMD, bilberry anthocyanosides appear to be ideal therapeutic agents for the disorder. However, ginkgo biloba extract (24% ginkgo flavonglycoside content) is perhaps a better choice if a person is also showing signs of decreased blood flow to the brain.

TREATMENT SUMMARY

As with most diseases, prevention or treatment of ARMD at an early stage is most effective. The treatment of the wet form is clearly laser therapy, used as soon as possible. Because free radical damage and lack of blood and oxygen supply to the macula appear to be the primary causes of macular degeneration, consumption of antioxidant supplements and promotion of retinal blood flow are the keys to effective treatment.

The use of nutritional supplementation in ARMD has undergone extensive cost-benefit analysis. Compared with no therapy, antioxidant therapy yielded a cost-effective improvement in quality of life and lowered the percentage of patients with ARMD who ever developed visual impairment in the better-seeing eye from 7.0 to 5.6%.[31]

Diet

Follow the guidelines given in the chapter "A Health-Promoting Diet." Foods to avoid in cases of ARMD are:

- Fried and grilled foods, and other sources of free radicals
- Animal fat
- Processed baked goods
- Beer

Important foods to emphasize are:

- Yellow vegetables, green vegetables, tomato products
- Flavonoid-rich berries (blueberries, blackberries, cherries, etc.)
- Other fresh fruits and vegetables, nuts, and fish
- Moderate amounts of red wine

Nutritional Supplements

- A high-potency multiple vitamin and mineral formula as described in the chapter "Supplementary Measures"
- Key individual nutrients:
  ○ Vitamin B_6: 25 to 50 mg per day
  ○ Folic acid: 800 to 2,000 mg per day
  ○ Vitamin B_{12}: 800 mcg per day
  ○ Vitamin C: 500 to 1,000 mg per day
  ○ Vitamin E (mixed tocopherols): 100 to 200 IU per day
  ○ Magnesium (bound to aspartate, citrate, fumarate, malate, glycinate, or succinate): 200 to 300 mg three times per day
  ○ Selenium: 100 to 200 mcg per day
  ○ Zinc: 30 to 45 mg per day
  ○ Vitamin D_3: 2,000 to 4,000 IU per day (ideally, measure blood levels and adjust dosage accordingly)
- Fish oils: 1,000 mg EPA + DHA per day

- Lutein: 10 to 20 mg per day
- Zeaxanthin: 1 to 2 mg per day
- Astaxanthin: 4 to 6 mg per day

Botanical Medicines

One of the following:

- Ginkgo biloba extract (24% ginkgo fla-vonglycosides): 120 to 240 mg per day

- Bilberry extract (25% anthocyanidin content): 120 to 240 mg per day
- Grape seed or pine bark extract (95% procyanidolic content): 150 to 300 mg per day

Menopause

- Permanent cessation of menstruation in older women
- Average age of onset: 51
- Common complaints of menopause: hot flashes, headaches, atrophic vaginitis, frequent urinary tract infections, cold hands and feet, forgetfulness, inability to concentrate

Menopause is the permanent cessation of menstruation in women, which occurs on average around age 51 but may occur as early as 40 and as late as 55 years of age or even later. Six to 12 months without a menstrual period is the commonly accepted rule for diagnosing menopause. The time prior to menopause is referred to as *perimenopause*, and the time after menopause is referred to as *postmenopause*. During perimenopause, many women ovulate irregularly, owing to either decreased secretion of estrogen or resistance of the remaining follicles to ovulatory stimulus.

Many conventional doctors still see menopause as a disease rather than a normal physiological process. This view is in stark contrast to the perspective of many cultures, where menopause is viewed as a natural part of the life process and a positive event in a woman's life. In fact, in many parts of the world, most women do not experience the symptoms Americans tend to associate with menopause. This observation raises some interesting questions about menopause as a sociocultural event. However, there are certainly important dietary and environmental factors to consider as well.

Despite considerable research questioning its value, the current medical treatment of menopause primarily involves the use of hormone replacement therapy (HRT), utilizing a combination of estrogen and progesterone. The obvious question is whether hormone replacement therapy is necessary. The goal of this chapter is to answer that question and provide a natural approach to menopause and the postmenopausal period.

Causes

Menopause is thought to occur when there are no longer any viable eggs left in the ovaries. At birth, a woman has about 1 million eggs. This number drops to around 300,000 or 400,000 at puberty, but only about 400 of these ova will actually mature during the reproductive years. By the time a woman reaches the age of 50, few eggs remain.

With age, the absence of active *follicles* (the cellular housing of the egg) results in reduced production of estrogen and progesterone. In response to this drop in estrogen, the pituitary gland increases secretion of *follicle-stimulating hormone* (FSH) and *luteinizing hormone* (LH). After menopause, FSH and LH are secreted continuously in large quantities, even though there are no longer any follicles to stimulate. These two hormones cause the ovaries and the adrenal glands to secrete increased amounts of androgens (male sex hormones), which can be converted to estrogens by the fat cells of the hips and thighs. Converted androgens account for most of the circulating estrogen in the postmenopausal woman, but total estrogen levels are still far below the levels in women still in their reproductive years.

Major Symptoms

Many of the symptoms of menopause, especially hot flashes, appear to be a result of altered function of the hypothalamus, a mass of tissue at the center of the brain that serves as the bridge between the nervous system and the hormonal (endocrine) system. The hypothalamus is responsible for the control of many body functions, including body temperature, metabolic rate, sleep patterns, reactions to stress, libido, mood, and the release of pituitary hormones. Critical to proper functioning of the hypothalamus are the endorphins, the body's own mood-elevating and pain-relieving compounds. Endorphins are also thought to play a role in hot flashes. Several natural measures are thought to exert some of their beneficial effects against hot flashes by enhancing endorphin output. Two of the most effective measures are exercise and acupuncture.

Hot Flashes

Hot flashes are the most common symptom of menopause. The term *hot flash* refers to dilation of the peripheral blood vessels, which leads to a rise in skin temperature and flushing of the skin. In the typical hot flash, the skin, especially of the head and neck, becomes red and warm for a few seconds to a few minutes, with cold chills coming thereafter. Hot flashes can be accompanied by other symptoms, in-

cluding increased heart rate, headaches, dizziness, weight gain, fatigue, and insomnia.

In the United States, 65 to 80% of women around menopause experience hot flashes to some degree. Hot flashes are often the first sign that menopause is approaching, as they may begin prior to the cessation of menses. In most cases, hot flashes are at their most uncomfortable in the first and second years after menopause. As the body adapts to decreased estrogen levels, hot flashes typically subside.

Headaches

Headaches, especially migraines, often accompany menopause owing to increased instability of the blood vessels. Headaches often accompany hot flashes.

Atrophic Vaginitis

After menopause, the vaginal lining may become thin and dry owing to the lack of estrogen. As a result, menopausal and postmenopausal women may experience painful intercourse, an increased susceptibility to infection, and vaginal itching or burning.

Women with atrophic vaginitis should try to avoid substances that tend to dry the mucous membranes, including antihistamines, alcohol, caffeine, and diuretics. In addition, it is critical that the body stay well hydrated. Drink at least 32 to 48 fl oz water per day.

Underwear made from natural fibers, particularly cotton, is often recommended, as it allows the skin to breathe, thus decreasing the incidence of vaginal infections.

Regular sexual intercourse is also beneficial, as it increases blood flow to vaginal tissues; this blood flow helps improve tone and lubrication. However, good lubrication must be maintained; there are many oil- and water-based lubricants available, such as K-Y jelly.

Bladder Infections

About 15% of menopausal women experience frequent bladder infections. Apparently there is a breakdown in the natural defense mechanisms that protect against bacterial growth in the urinary tract. The primary goal in the natural approach to treating bladder infections is to enhance a woman's normal resistance to urinary tract infection. Specifically, increase the flow of urine through proper hydration, promote a pH that will inhibit the growth of microorganisms, and prevent bacteria from adhering to the endothelial cells of the bladder. In addition, there are several botanical medicines that can be employed. See the chapter "Cystitis and Interstitial Cystitis/Painful Bladder" for further information.

Cold Hands and Feet

Cold hands and feet are common among women in general, not just menopausal women. During the menopausal period they become even more common. In most instances, there are three major causes of cold hands and feet: hypothyroidism, low iron levels in the body, and poor circulation. It is important to rule out hypothyroidism by measuring blood levels of thyroid hormones. Along with a CBC (complete blood count) and chemistry panel that includes LDL/HDL cholesterol levels, there should also be a test for serum ferritin levels, the best indicator of body iron stores. A complete physical exam is also required, with particular attention to any other signs of decreased blood flow. Once the cause is identified, the treatment is straightforward.

Forgetfulness and Inability to Concentrate

Forgetfulness and an inability to concentrate are common symptoms of menopause. Often these symptoms are simply a result of decreased oxygen and nutrient supply to the brain, due not to menopause per se but rather to atherosclerosis (hardening of the arteries) of the blood vessels supplying oxygen and nutrition to the brain.

The brain is highly dependent on a constant supply of oxygen and nutrients. Although it weighs only 3 pounds, the brain utilizes about 20% of the oxygen supply of the entire body. To deal with symptoms of forgetfulness and inability to concentrate, the goal is to improve the supply of blood, oxygen, and nutrients to the brain.

Menopause as a Social Construct

While there is undeniably a physiological process involved in menopause, menopause is much more than simply a biological event. Social and cultural factors contribute greatly to how women react to menopause. Modern society has placed great value on the allure of youth, resulting in a deeply entrenched cultural devaluation of older people, particularly women. Advocates of a social and cultural explanation of menopause often point to this cultural devaluing of older women as the root of the negativity associated with achieving menopause.

In contrast, in many cultures of the world, women look forward to menopause because it brings with it greater respect.[1] Achieving an advanced age is viewed as a sign of divine blessing and great wisdom. Studies of menopausal women in many traditional cultures demonstrate that most will pass through menopause without hot flashes, vaginitis, and other symptoms common to menopausal women in developed countries. Even osteoporosis is extremely rare, despite the fact that the average woman in many traditional cultures lives longer than the average woman in the United States.

Cross-cultural research clearly demonstrates that the cultural view of menopause is directly related to the symptoms of menopause.[2] If the cultural view of menopause is largely negative, as in the United States, symptoms are quite common. In contrast, if menopause is associated with little negativity or viewed in a positive light, symptoms are far less frequent.

One of the most detailed studies of the effects of culture on menopause involved rural Mayans.[2] Detailed medical histories and examinations, including a physical examination, hormone-level measurement, and bone-density studies, were performed on 52 postmenopausal women. None of these women experienced hot flashes or any other menopausal symptom, and not one woman showed evidence of osteoporosis, despite the fact that their hormonal patterns (levels of the various female sex hormones) were identical to those of postmenopausal women living in the United States.

The researchers felt that the Mayan women's attitude toward menopause was responsible for their symptomless passage. The Mayan women saw menopause as a positive event that would provide them acceptance as respected elders, as well as relief from childbearing. This attitude is much different from the dominant attitude toward menopause that is common in industrialized societies. If our society adopted a different cultural view of older women, it is likely that the symptoms of menopause would cease to exist.

In 1966, Robert A. Wilson, M.D., released his landmark book *Feminine Forever*, which introduced the theory that menopause is an estrogen-deficiency disease that needs to be treated with estrogen to compensate for the normal decline of estrogen levels with aging. According to Wilson, without estrogen replacement therapy women were destined to become sexless "caricatures of their former selves . . . the equivalent of a eunuch."

Wilson's theory of menopause as a disease is still the dominant medical view of menopause, even within many alternative medical circles touting "bioidentical" hormones as a way for women to remain "forever feminine." These views place women who are entering menopause in a difficult situation: should they pass through this period of time naturally, or should they use hormonal therapy? Before this question can be answered, the benefits and risks of estrogen replacement therapy must be considered, as well as the natural alternatives.

Therapeutic Considerations

As we've noted, the current conventional medical treatment of menopause remains the short-term use (one to four years) of hormone replacement therapy for menopausal symptoms.

The use of HRT was widely accepted until 2002, when the National Institutes of Health (NIH) halted a major clinical trial designed to prove that HRT benefited postmenopausal women. This study, the Women's Health Initiative (WHI), found just the opposite and concluded that the risks of taking combined estrogen and progestin outweighed the benefits, increasing the risk of stroke, coronary heart disease, and breast cancer.[3]

HRT was shown to produce a:

- 26% increase in invasive breast cancer
- 41% increase in strokes
- 29% increase in heart attacks
- Doubling of the rate of blood clots in legs and lungs

- Two- to threefold increase in gallstone formation and liver disease

Once this study made the headlines, many doctors and the public became aware of other studies reporting similar alarming statistics. For example, HRT not only stimulates the growth of invasive breast cancers but also makes it harder to spot the potentially deadly tumors on mammograms, as the breast tissue remains denser on HRT; it doubled the risk of developing Alzheimer's and increased the risk of life-threatening blood clot formation.

While the WHI was viewed as a major revelation on the safety and efficacy of HRT, the reality is that this study and others only confirmed was what already known about the dangers of synthetic hormones.[4–8]

DECREASE IN BREAST CANCER RATES RELATED TO REDUCTION IN USE OF HRT

The immediate effect of the impact of the WHI was a sudden drop in the number of women using HRT. Not surprisingly, there was a parallel sharp decline in the rate of new breast cancer cases.[9] Keep in mind that prior to 2002, breast cancer rates in the United States had been climbing steadily.

Prescriptions for the two most commonly prescribed forms of HRT in the United States, Premarin and Prempro, dropped from 61 million in 2001 to 21 million in 2004. This drop produced a reduction in the annual rate of breast cancer in the United States of 8.4%. The decrease occurred only in women over the age of 50 and was more evident in women with cancers that were estrogen-receptor-positive. These tumors need estrogen in order to grow and multiply. The speed at which breast cancer rates declined after the WHI announcements may indicate that extremely small estrogen-receptor-positive breast cancers may have stopped progressing, or even regressed, after HRT was halted. Clearly, this dramatic drop in the breast cancer rate further strengthens the link between breast cancer and use of HRT.

Despite the results of the Women's Health Initiative and other studies showing the long-term problems associated with HRT, it is a sad fact that approximately 30 million prescriptions for HRT were still filled each year after 2002. Why on earth would doctors continue to prescribe HRT? Unfortunately, they are just not aware of effective natural strategies to deal with menopausal symptoms or reduce the risk of osteoporosis.

While there is no question that HRT is effective at relieving the symptoms of menopause, many health experts believe that long-term HRT is rarely justified in most women due to its risks. The only possible exception is women who are at high risk of developing osteoporosis (in the Women's Health Initiative study, women taking HRT had a 34% lower risk of hip fracture), but even then there are natural approaches that can dramatically reduce the risk of this bone disease. To determine your risk for osteoporosis and for more information on natural approaches, see the chapter "Osteoporosis."

Most women on HRT have no idea they are taking unnatural forms of estrogen and progesterone. Premarin, for example, contains forms of estrogen isolated from the urine of pregnant mares and includes more than 200 substances mostly foreign to humans. Animal rights activists also have long claimed that the methods used in Premarin's production cause suffering to the mares involved. The major health problem for women taking Premarin and other common forms of conjugated estrogens is that they are metabolized in the body to 17-beta-estradiol, the form of estrogen most strongly associated with cancer. The synthetic versions of progesterone used in HRT, such as megestrol, norethindrone, and norgestrel, are likely to be even more problematic than the conjugated estrogens.

Natural Hormone Replacement Therapy

Most naturopathic physicians prefer to use a type of HRT known as bioidentical hormone therapy. The bioidentical hormones most commonly used in menopause include estradiol, estrone, estriol, progesterone, and to a lesser extent, testosterone and dehydroepiandrosterone (DHEA). Bioidentical hormones are made from either beta-sitosterol extracted from soybeans or from diosgenin extracted from wild yam (*Dioscorea villosa*). These compounds are then processed to create hormones that are biochemically identical to human hormones. Bioidentical hormones require a prescription and are available from regular pharmacies or from compounding pharmacies. Using compounded forms of hormones offers a greater array of dosing and delivery options—customized doses of a particular hormone are available that pharmaceutical companies do not make; the hormones can be provided as capsules, sublingual lozenges or pellets, creams, gels, vaginal creams/gels or tablets, nasal sprays, injections, and pellets implanted under the skin; and any combination of estradiol, estriol, estrone, progesterone, testosterone, and DHEA can be formulated in a prescription optimized to the specific needs of each woman.

The basic concept behind bioidentical hormone therapy is that some of the detrimental effects of HRT may be related to the inherent problem in the synthetic forms of hormones being used. In addition, the dosage of hormones used with bioidentical hormone therapy is generally considerably less than that used in conventional HRT. However, even though there is a lot of circumstantial evidence of a better safety profile with bioidentical hormones, at this time there are no definitive studies proving that bioidentical hormone therapy is better than or safer

TAPERING OFF HRT

If you elect to discontinue HRT in favor of a natural, non-hormone approach, follow the dietary and supplementation strategies in the Treatment Summary (below) for one month and then reduce the dosage of HRT by half. Continue at this half dosage for one month, then cut the dosage in half again by taking it every other day for another month before discontinuing it entirely. Of course, before changing the dosage of any drug, always first consult your doctor.

than HRT. Because bioidentical hormones are natural, they are not patentable—hence, there are no big drug companies promoting them. Without the promise of a financial windfall it is highly unlikely that the large trials necessary to conclusively show the advantages of bioidentical hormones will ever be conducted. Nonetheless, it makes more sense to use bioidentical hormones if hormonal support is required. Because we suggest prescription forms, we recommend consulting with your physician or seeking the counsel of a naturopathic physician.

A critical factor in hormone replacement—whether natural or conventional—is to not only measure hormone levels but also determine the makeup of their metabolites after detoxification. These can be tested in the saliva, blood, and urine.

Natural Approaches to Menopausal Symptoms

Exercise

The health benefits of exercise for menopausal and postmenopausal women are extensive. In addition, regular physical exercise definitely reduces the frequency and severity of hot flashes. In one study, women who spent an average of 3½ hours per week exercising had no hot flashes whatsoever, whereas women who exercised less were more likely to have hot flashes.[10] Women can also achieve substantial reductions in cardiovascular disease, decrease their breast cancer risk, increase their bone density, and lower body fat and body mass index, as well as experience an improved sense of well-being.[11–13]

Health Benefits of Regular Exercise in Menopause

Relief from hot flashes

Decreased bone loss

Improved heart function

Improved circulation

Reduced blood pressure

Decreased blood cholesterol levels

Improved ability to deal with stress

Improved oxygen and nutrient utilization in all tissues

Increased self-esteem, mood, and frame of mind

Increased endurance and energy levels

Diet

The dietary guidelines discussed in the chapter "A Health-Promoting Diet" are very much indicated in helping improve menopausal symptoms. Perhaps the most important dietary recommendation may be to increase consumption of plant foods, especially those high in phytoestrogens, while reducing the consumption of animal foods. Phytoestrogens are plant-derived substances that are able to weakly bind to the estrogen receptors in mammals and have a very weak estrogen-like effect in some tissues and a weak antiestrogenic effect in other tissues. Soybeans and flaxseeds contain high amounts of phytoestrogens. Many other foods, such as apples, carrots, fennel, celery, parsley, and other legumes, contain smaller amounts of phytoestrogens. A high dietary intake of phytoestrogens is thought to explain why hot flashes and other menopausal symptoms appear to occur less frequently in cultures where the diet is predominantly plant-based. In addition, such a diet is promising for disease prevention, with some research showing a lower incidence of breast and prostate cancer in those consuming high-phytoestrogen diets.

Soy Products. Soy foods may be useful in menopause primarily for their potential benefits for hot flashes, but they may also slow bone loss, lower cholesterol and blood pressure levels, and reduce the risk of breast cancer. Some but not all clinical studies have shown eating soy foods (the equivalent of ⅔ cup soybeans per day) or taking a soy supplement to be effective in relieving hot flashes and vaginal atrophy.[14–19] Those studies that do show a benefit indicate that increased soy intake can help reduce hot flashes and/or night sweats by 30 to 55%.

One study explains why results with soy are so inconsistent.[20] In this six-month double-blind study, 66 women were given 135 mg soy isoflavones and 30 women were given a placebo. After one week, the women in the soy group were tested and further divided into two subgroups based upon their ability to metabolize the isoflavones into the phytoestrogen compound equol. Both of these subgroups were then given 135 mg isoflavones per day for six months. Compared with the results in the placebo group, symptoms of hot flashes and excessive sweating were significantly reduced after three months and total symptoms were significantly decreased after six months, but only in the group that broke down the isoflavones into equol. At six months, symptom scores had decreased by 84% in the equol-producing group, 58% in the non-equol-producing group, and 66% in the placebo group. Studies that had a higher percentage of women who were equol producers would show positive effects with soy supplementation, but if the study contained a lot of women who did not produce equol the results would have no effect.

So what determines the conversion of soy isoflavones into equol? It is the gut flora. It is thought that a higher level of health-promoting bacteria such as lactobacilli and bifidobacteria ensures proper conversion. Hence, we recommend that women using soy isoflavones to improve menopausal symptoms also take a probiotic supplement providing 5 billion to 20 billion live *Lactobacillus* and *Bifidobacterium* organisms.

Currently, a host of soy products can be found in most grocery stores, and even more in natural foods stores. They include dried soybeans, soy oil, soy milk, soy flour, roasted soy nuts, tofu, tofu paté, tempeh, miso, soy sauce, natto, edamame, soy ice cream, soy cheese, soy candy bars, soy burgers and hot dogs, and even soy marshmallows. For the greatest benefit, we recommend focusing on dietary sources vs. taking a supplement. Nonetheless, supplements containing soy iso-

flavones can also be used to deal with menopausal symptoms as well as possibly promote bone and cardiovascular health. The dosage should be in the same range as the dietary level of isoflavones in the traditional Asian diet: 45 to 90 mg per day of isoflavones.

Flaxseeds. Another significant dietary source of phytoestrogens is flaxseed. Flaxseed contains the lignans matairesinol and secoisolariciresinol, which are known to have estrogenic activity. In addition, these lignans are modified by intestinal bacteria to form other lignans that are absorbed in the circulation and have both estrogenic and antiestrogenic activity.[21,22] Although there is a lot of research on the protective effect of flax lignans against breast cancer, only a small amount of research has been done in the area of flaxseed and hot flashes. One study showed that women who consumed 2 tbsp of flaxseed twice per day halved their number of hot flashes within six weeks and reduced the intensity of the hot flashes by 57%.[23]

Nutritional Supplements

Fish Oils. In a study of fish oil supplementation in women between 40 and 55 years old with hot flashes and moderate to severe psychological distress, 120 women were randomly assigned to receive either a fish oil supplement providing 1,200 mg EPA + DHA or a placebo. The baseline level of hot flashes was an average of 2.8 per day. After eight weeks, the hot flash frequency decreased by an average of 1.58 per day (a 55% drop) in the fish oil group but by only 0.50 per day in the placebo group (25%). There was also a greater responder rate in the EPA + DHA group (58.5%) compared with the placebo group (34.4%).[24]

Vitamin C and Flavonoids. Combined with vitamin C, hesperidin and other citrus fla-

Isoflavone Content of Soy Foods		
SOY FOOD	**AMOUNT**	**ISOFLAVONES (MG)**
Roasted soy nuts	¼ cup	60
Tofu, low-fat and regular	½ cup	35
Tempeh	½ cup	35
Soy beverage powders	1–2 scoops	25–90
Regular soy milk	1 cup	30
Low fat soy milk	1 cup	20
Roasted soy butter	2 tbsp	17
Cooked soybeans	½ cup	150

vonoids may be effective in relieving hot flashes. In one clinical study, 94 women suffering from hot flashes were given a formula containing 900 mg hesperidin, 300 mg hesperidin methyl chalcone (another citrus flavonoid), and 1,200 mg vitamin C per day.[25] At the end of one month, hot flashes were significantly reduced in 53% of the patients and reduced in 34%. Improvements in nocturnal leg cramps, nosebleeds, and easy bruising were also noted. The only side effect was a slightly offensive body odor with a tendency for the perspiration to discolor the clothing.

Perhaps more useful than hesperidin are preparations containing procyanidolic oligomers (PCOs) such as extracts from grape seeds or pine bark. In a double-blind study, 230 perimenopausal Taiwanese women ages 45 to 55 were given either a placebo or 100 mg PCOs from pine bark (Pycnogenol) twice per day for six months.[26] Compared with the placebo, PCOs significantly improved both the severity and the frequency of problems relating to depression, vasomotor symptoms, memory, anxiety, sexual function, and sleep as soon as one month after the treatment was started.

Gamma-Oryzanol. Gamma-oryzanol (ferulic acid) is a growth-promoting substance found in grains and isolated from rice bran oil. In the treatment of hot flashes, its primary action is to enhance pituitary function and promote endorphin release by the hypothalamus. Gamma-oryzanol was first shown to be effective in menopausal symptoms, including hot flashes, in the early 1960s.[27] Subsequent studies have further documented its effectiveness.[28]

In one of the earlier studies, 8 menopausal women and 13 women whose ovaries had been surgically removed were given 300 mg per day of gamma-oryzanol. At the end of the 38-day trial, more than 67% of the women had a 50% or greater reduction in menopausal symptoms.[27] In a later study, the benefit of a 300 mg dose of gamma-oryzanol was even more effective, in that 85% of the subjects reported improvement in menopausal symptoms.[28]

Gamma-oryzanol is an extremely safe natural substance. No significant side effects have been produced in experimental and clinical studies. In addition to being helpful in improving the symptoms of menopause, gamma-oryzanol has also been shown to be quite effective in lowering blood cholesterol and triglyceride levels.[29]

Vitamin E. In the late 1940s, several clinical studies found vitamin E to be effective in relieving hot flashes and menopausal vaginal complaints compared with a placebo.[30–32] Unfortunately, there have been no further clinical investigations. In one study, vitamin E supplementation was shown to improve not only those symptoms but also the blood supply to the vaginal wall when taken for at least four weeks.[30] A follow-up study published in 1949 demonstrated that vitamin E (400 IU per day) was effective in about 50% of postmenopausal women with atrophic vaginitis.[31] Vitamin E oil, creams, ointments, or suppositories can be used topically to provide symptomatic relief of atrophic vaginitis. Vitamin E may be effective in relieving the dryness and irritation of atrophic vaginitis as well as other forms of vaginitis.[32]

Botanical Medicines

There are a number of botanicals with a long history of use in menopausal women. Rather than exerting a drug-like effect, these substances are thought to nourish and tone the female hormonal system and reproductive organs. Much of their effect is thought to be a result of phytoestrogens in the plants as well as the plants' ability to improve blood flow to the reproductive organs. This nonspecific mode of action makes many of these botanicals useful in a broad range of conditions.

Phytoestrogen-containing herbs offer significant advantages over the use of estrogens in the treatment of menopausal symptoms. Although both synthetic and natural estrogens may pose significant health risks, phytoestrogens have not been associated with these side effects. In fact, epidemiological data and experimental studies have demonstrated that phytoestrogens are extremely effective in inhibiting breast tumors, not only because they occupy estrogen receptors but also through other, unrelated anticancer mechanisms (see the chapter "Breast Cancer [Prevention]").

Black Cohosh. In the last 30 years, black cohosh (*Cimicifuga racemosa*) has emerged as the most frequently studied of the herbal alternatives to hormone replacement therapy for menopausal symptoms. The collective findings of studies involving black cohosh and long-term clinical anecdotal evidence indicate that it is most effective for hot flashes (both during the day and at night), mood swings, sleep disorders and body aches.[33]

In one of the largest studies, 629 women with menopausal complaints were treated with black cohosh.[34] As early as four weeks after the therapy began, a clear improvement in the menopausal ailments was seen in approximately 80% of the women. After six to eight weeks, symptoms completely disappeared in approximately 50%.

In perhaps the most detailed double-blind study to date, black cohosh extract was evaluated for its effect on menopausal symptoms, bone metabolism, and the lining of the uterus (endometrium).[35] The 62 postmenopausal women were treated either with black cohosh extract (40 mg per day), 0.6 mg conjugated estrogens, or a placebo for three months. Results indicated that the black cohosh extract was equal to the conjugated estrogens and superior to the placebo in reducing menopausal complaints. Both black cohosh extract and the conjugated estrogens produced beneficial effects on bone metabolism, but the black cohosh extract had no effect on endometrial thickness, which was significantly increased

Black Cohosh in the Treatment of Menopausal Symptoms: Results of a Large Clinical Trial			
SYMPTOM	% OF PATIENTS REPORTING SYMPTOM ELIMINATION	% OF PATIENTS REPORTING SYMPTOM IMPROVEMENT	TOTAL % REPORTING SYMPTOM IMPROVEMENT OR ELIMINATION
Ringing in the ears	54.8	38.1	92.9
Heart palpitation	54.6	35.2	90.4
Profuse perspiration	49.9	38.6	88.5
Vertigo	51.6	35.2	86.8
Hot flashes	43.3	43.3	86.6
Nervousness/irritability	42.4	43.2	85.6
Headache	45.7	36.2	81.9
Sleep disturbances	46.1	30.7	76.8
Depressive moods	46.0	36.5	82.5

by the conjugated estrogens (increased endometrial thickness is associated with a higher rate of uterine cancer). Vaginal superficial cells were increased with both black cohosh and conjugated estrogens. These results seem to confirm that black cohosh extracts contain substances with selective estrogen-receptor-modifying activity—that is, it shows positive effects in the brain/hypothalamus, bone, and vagina, but has no cancer-causing effects on the uterus.

Some recent studies have used black cohosh extract in combination with other botanical extracts. For example, healthy perimenopausal women who had typical symptoms and had not been on HRT for at least the previous three months were given black cohosh extract equivalent to 1 mg terpene glycosides and Saint-John's-wort extract equivalent to 0.25 mg hypericin.[36] Hot flash symptom scores at 4 and 12 weeks were significantly lower in the treatment group compared with the placebo group, though vaginal dryness and low libido did not improve.

A clinical trial involving 125 menopausal women showed that a combination of 40 mg black cohosh extract, 12 mg isoflavones from red clover, 60 mg isoflavones from soy, 30 mg chasteberry extract, 250 mg valerian extract, and 121 mg vitamin E resulted in a significant lowering of menopausal symptoms after four and six months.[37] These results suggest that it may take considerable time before women experience relief from black cohosh and other herbal approaches to menopausal symptoms.

Maca. Maca (*Lepidium meyenii*) is an herbal remedy from Peru most often thought of as enhancing male sexuality, but it also has effects on women. Research on menopausal women indicates that unlike HRT and phytoestrogenic botanicals, maca can increase the body's production of estrogen—vs. simply adding estrogen replacement to the body—and reduce levels of cortisol.[38] What makes this especially interesting is that the herb appears not to contain plant estrogens or hormones.[39,40] It has been suggested that maca's therapeutic actions rely on plant sterols stimulating the hypothalamus, pituitary, adrenal glands, and ovaries, and therefore also affecting the thyroid and pineal gland. Thus maca tends to work on all of a woman's menopausal symptoms instead of on any one specific symptom alone, such as hot flashes.

In one double-blind, randomized, four-month study of women in early a postmenopause, patients were given either a placebo or two 500-mg capsules of Maca-GO twice per day for a total of 2g per day.[38] After two months, estrogen (specifically estradiol) production had increased and FSH and cortisol had decreased. The maca also had a small effect on increasing bone density and alleviated numerous menopausal symptoms including hot flashes, insomnia, depression, nervousness, and diminished concentration.

Another double-blind trial of 14 postmenopausal women was completed using 3.5 g of powdered maca for 6 weeks or a placebo for 6 weeks.[41] Measurements of estradiol, FSH, LH, and sex-hormone-binding globulin were taken at baseline and weeks 6 and 12. There were no changes in hormone levels, but there was a significant reduction in anxiety, depression, and sexual dysfunction with maca consumption compared with the baseline and the placebo.

Red Clover. Red clover (*Trifolium praetense*), a member of the legume family, has been used worldwide as a source of hay for cattle, horses, and sheep and by humans as a source of protein (leaves and young sprouts). Historically, it has also been recognized as a medicinal plant for humans and, more recently, as a menopausal herb. The principal effective substances in red clover are isoflavones and coumestans.

At least six clinical trials have been conducted on the effect of red clover isoflavones on vasomotor symptoms; about half show benefit and the others do not.[42] To have an effect, red clover isoflavones probably require the same sort of healthful gut flora discussed above under "Soy Products." In fact, the inconsistent results with red clover are very similar to those seen with soy. The first two published studies on red clover and hot flashes showed no statistically significant difference between the red clover standardized extract and a placebo during a three-month period, although both groups did improve.[43,44] Two other studies using 40 mg standardized extract of red clover showed good effects. In the first study red clover extract produced a 75% reduction in hot flashes after 16 weeks in 30 women.[45] In the second study the red clover group had a 54% reduction in hot flashes after two months vs. a 30% reduction in the placebo group.[46] Two more recent studies continue the contradictions. In the first study, 80 mg isoflavones per day resulted in a significant reduction in hot flashes as compared with baseline.[47] Another recent study compared two different doses of red clover isoflavones (82 mg and 57 mg per day) with a placebo for 12 weeks, and no difference was observed between the groups.[48]

Dong Quai. Dong quai (*Angelica sinensis*) is one of the most famous herbal remedies in China, where it is often referred to as "female ginseng." By far the most popular use of dong quai is in the treatment of menopausal complaints. Although a double-blind, placebo-controlled study in women showed no significant benefit, the preparation used (a dried aqueous extract) was clearly lacking some of the important volatile compounds,

though it was standardized for ferulic acid content.[49] In addition, traditionally angelica has been used in combination with other plants. A study conducted in China showed that a combination of *A. sinensis*, along with other herbs (*Paeonia lactiflora, Ligusticum monnieri, Atractylodes chinensis, Sclerotium poriae,* and *Alisma orientalis*) was effective in roughly 70% of women experiencing menopausal symptoms.[50] Though not double-blind, this study shows promise for using angelica in combination with other compounds in the management of menopausal symptoms. Also, in a double-blind study, the combination of 100 mg dong quai extract, 60 mg soy isoflavones, and 50 mg black cohosh extract significantly reduced menstrual migraines.[51]

Saint-John's-Wort. Saint-John's-wort (*Hypericum perforatum*) extract research has focused on the area of mild to moderate depression. Several studies of menopausal symptoms have also been conducted. A recent randomized, double-blind, placebo-controlled clinical trial studied Saint-John's-wort in perimenopausal/menopausal hot flashes.[52] Fifty women (average age 50) received 20 drops three times per day of Saint-John's-wort extract (hypericin 0.2 mg/ml) and 50 women received a placebo. Clinical exams and interviews were performed at baseline, four weeks, and eight weeks. In women taking Saint-John's-wort, the frequency of hot flashes began to decline during the first month and showed more improvement during the second month. The decline in duration and severity of hot flashes was statistically significant at week eight and the decline was much more evident in the Saint-John's-wort group.

Another double-blind randomized clinical trial studied the effect of Saint-John's-wort extract on the symptoms and quality of life of 47 symptomatic perimenopausal women age 40 to 65 with three or more hot flashes per day.[53] Women were randomly assigned to receive a Saint-John's-wort extract (900 mg three times per day) or a placebo. After 12 weeks of treatment, a nonsignificant difference in favor of the Saint-John's-wort group was observed in daily hot flash frequency and hot flash score. After three months of treatment, women in the Saint-John's-wort group reported significantly better quality-of-life scores and significantly fewer sleep problems compared with the placebo group.

One study of women with menopause symptoms using 900 mg Saint-John's-wort extract for 12 weeks found that about three-quarters of the women experienced improvement in both psychological and psychosomatic menopausal symptoms as well as a feeling of sexual well-being.[54] And several double-blind studies (described above) have used a combination of Saint-John's-wort and black cohosh extract.

For information on possible drug interactions with Saint-John's-wort, see the chapter "Depression."

QUICK REVIEW

- In many parts of the world, most women do not experience the symptoms associated with menopause in the United States.

- Social and cultural factors contribute greatly to how women react to menopause.

- In the United States, 65 to 80% of menopausal women experience hot flashes to some degree.

- Women with atrophic vaginitis (vaginal drying and irritation due to lack of estrogen) should avoid substances that tend to dry the mucous membranes, including antihistamines, alcohol, caffeine, and diuretics.

- Rather than use estrogens to artificially counteract the symptoms of menopause, the natural approach focuses on improving physiology through diet, exercise, nutritional supplementation, and the use of botanical medicines.

- Regular exercise may reduce hot flashes.

- An especially important dietary recommendation in the relief of hot flashes and atrophic vaginitis, as well as the prevention of breast cancer, is to increase consumption of foods rich in phytoestrogens.

- Several nutrients have been shown to be effective in relieving hot flashes and atrophic vaginitis in clinical studies, including fish oils; hesperidin (a flavonoid) in combination with vitamin C; pine bark extract; gamma-oryzanol; and vitamin E.

- Black cohosh extract is the most widely used and thoroughly studied herbal alternative to hormone replacement therapy in menopause.

- Saint-John's-wort extract improves mood and sleep quality and reduces anxiety in menopause.

EstroG. EstroG is an herbal product containing a mixture of standardized extracts of *Cynanchum wilfordii*, *Phlomis umbrosa*, and *Angelica gigas* that has shown favorable results in clinical studies. In the most detailed double-blind study, 64 pre-, peri-, and postmenopausal women were randomly assigned to take either EstroG (517 mg per day) or a placebo for 12 weeks.[55] Menopausal symptoms were evaluated with the Kupperman menopause index (KMI) that includes 11 symptoms. After 12 weeks the mean KMI score was significantly reduced in the EstroG group, from 29.5 at baseline to 11.3, while there was no significant change in the placebo group. Statistically significant improvement in vaginal dryness in the EstroG group was also observed.

TREATMENT SUMMARY

Menopause is a normal and natural part of aging and each woman experiences it in her own unique way. However, premature menopause, surgical menopause, or medication-induced menopause is not normal, and the benefits and risks should be addressed individually under the guidance of a physician.

Many natural measures can help alleviate the most common symptoms of menopause. In most cases, HRT is not necessary to address these symptoms. However, for women at high risk for osteoporosis and women who have already experienced significant bone loss and also have menopause symptoms or do not tolerate osteoporosis medications, hormonal therapy may be indicated. In those circumstances, we definitely favor the use of biodentical hormones over conventional HRT, and we recommend that their metabolites be measured and optimized to maximize estrogens that work against cancer rather than promote it.

Exercise

Engage in a regular exercise program according to the recommendations in the chapter "A Health-Promoting Lifestyle."

Diet

The guidelines discussed in the chapter "A Health-Promoting Diet" are very much indicated in helping improve menopausal symptoms. Perhaps the most important dietary recommendation may be to increase consumption of plant foods, especially those high in phytoestrogens, while reducing the consumption of animal foods.

Nutritional Supplements

- A high-potency multiple vitamin and mineral formula as described in the chapter "Supplementary Measures"
- Key individual nutrients:
  - Vitamin C: 500 to 1,000 mg per day
  - Vitamin E (mixed tocopherols): 800 IU per day until symptoms have improved, then 200 to 400 IU per day

- Fish oils: 1,000 mg EPA + DHA
- One of the following:
  - Grape seed extract (>95% procyanidolic oligomers): 200 to 300 mg per day
  - Pine bark extract (>95% procyanidolic oligomers): 200 to 300 mg per day
  - Some other flavonoid-rich extract with a similar flavonoid content, super greens formula, or another plant-based antioxidant that can provide an oxygen radical absorption capacity (ORAC) of 3,000 to 6,000 units or higher per day
  - Gamma-oryzanol: 300 mg per day

Botanical Medicines

For general symptom relief, one or more of the following:

- Black cohosh extract: equivalent of 2 mg 27-deoxyacteine twice per day
- Maca: 1,000 mg gelatinized maca extract twice per day, or dosage equivalent to 3,500 mg dried powdered maca root per day

- Red clover extract: 40 to 80 mg per day
- Estro-G: 517 mg per day

If symptoms of anxiety or depression are significant, add:

- Saint-John's-wort extract standardized to 0.3% hypericin 900 to 1,800 mg per day

If symptoms of vaginal atrophy do not respond after two months of treatment with other botanicals, or if you are experiencing menopausal migraines:

- Black cohosh extract (if not previously used): see the dosage levels above
- Soy isoflavones (if no soy in the diet): 45 to 90 mg
- Dong quai (*Angelica sinensis*)
  - Powdered root or as tea: 1 to 2 g two or three times daily
- Tincture (1: 5): 4 ml (1 tsp) two or three times daily
- Fluid extract: 1 ml (¼ tsp) two or three times daily
- Dry powdered extract: 250 mg two or three times per day

Menstrual Blood Loss, Excessive (Menorrhagia)

- Blood loss greater than 80 ml occurring during regular menstrual cycles (cycles are usually of normal length)

Excessive menstrual bleeding, or menorrhagia, is a common female complaint that may be entirely prevented in many cases by taking proper nutritional measures. As with any disease, proper determination of the cause is essential for effective treatment. Physicians often believe they can assess menstrual blood loss by asking the patient to estimate the number of pads or tampons used during each period and the duration of the period. However, studies have demonstrated that there is no correlation between measured blood loss and these assessments.[1,2] A woman's assessment of her blood loss is extremely subjective, as demonstrated by one study finding that 40% of women with a menstrual blood loss exceeding 80 ml considered their periods only moderately heavy or scanty, whereas 14% of those with a measured loss of less than 20 ml judged their periods to be heavy.[2]

So how is excessive menstrual blood loss determined? Excessive blood loss should be a concern if a woman is bleeding longer than 7 straight days or more frequently than every 21 days, and is changing a pad or tampon every hour for more than half a day. Women who are changing a pad and/or tampon every half hour or at even shorter intervals often require urgent, perhaps emergency, attention. Symptoms such as lightheadedness, dizziness, and fainting are cause for immediate concern. Any amount of bleeding in a postmenopausal woman not taking hormone replacement therapy is considered abnormal.

Causes

The cause of functional menorrhagia (i.e., menorrhagia not caused by the presence of uterine fibroids or endometriosis) involves abnormalities in the biochemical processes of the endometrium (the lining of the uterus). Factors that may contribute to menorrhagia are iron deficiency, hypothyroidism, vitamin A deficiency, intrauterine devices (IUDs), and various local factors (e.g., endometrial polyps, thickening of the uterine lining, and infections).

Another cause of functional menorrhagia is abnormalities in arachidonic acid metabolism.[3,4] This fatty acid is converted to hormone-like compounds known as prostaglandins. The endometrium of women who have menorrhagia concentrates arachidonic acid to a much greater extent than normal, resulting in increased production of series 2 prostaglandins, which are thought to be the major factor both in the excessive bleeding and in the accompanying menstrual cramps. Arachidonic acid is found only in animal foods such as meats and dairy products.

As noted above, a common cause of functional menorrhagia is hypothyroidism. Even minimal thyroid dysfunction may be responsible for menorrhagia and other menstrual disturbances.[5] These patients often show dramatic response to thyroid hormone replacement. For more information, see the chapter "Hypothyroidism."

Therapeutic Considerations

The first issue to address is iron deficiency, as a menstrual blood loss exceeding 60 ml per period is associated with negative iron balance in most women.[6] A negative iron balance means that more iron is being lost than taken in. Although menstrual blood loss is well recognized as a major cause of iron deficiency anemia in fertile women, it is not as well known that chronic iron deficiency can be a cause of menorrhagia. This assertion is based on several observations:[7]

- Response to iron supplementation alone in 74 of 83 patients (in whom organic disease had been excluded)
- A significant double-blind placebo-controlled study displaying improvement in 75% of those given iron supplementation, compared with 32.5% of those given the placebo
- High rate of organic disease (fibroids, polyps, adenomyosis, etc.) in the patients with no response to iron supplementation
- Associated rise in serum iron levels in 44 of 57 patients
- Decreased response to iron therapy when initial serum iron levels were high

- Correlation of menorrhagia with depleted tissue iron stores (bone marrow) irrespective of serum iron level

In any woman suspected of having menorrhagia, it is important to rule out low iron stores by getting a blood test for serum ferritin (the first variable to indicate decreased iron levels). In one study, women who were menorrhagic had significantly lower serum ferritin levels than controls, but other iron indicators such as hemoglobin concentration, mean corpuscular volume, and mean corpuscular hemoglobin were not significantly different between the two groups.[8] Yet the investigators in this study erroneously stated that such women do not require prophylactic iron supplementation, since no hematological abnormalities appeared despite significantly reduced iron stores. In fact, a decreased serum ferritin level is a good indication of the need for iron supplementation.[9]

Nutritional Supplements

Vitamin C and Bioflavonoids

Capillary fragility is believed to play a role in some cases of menorrhagia. In a study from 1960, supplementation with vitamin C (200 mg three times per day) and bioflavonoids was shown to reduce menorrhagia in 14 out of 16 patients.[10] As vitamin C is known to significantly increase iron absorption, its therapeutic effect could be also due to enhanced iron absorption.

Vitamin K and Chlorophyll

Although bleeding time and clotting factors in women with menorrhagia are typically normal, vitamin K (usually in the form of crude chlorophyll preparations) has a long history of use and some clinical research support.[11,12]

Omega-3 Fatty Acids

As menorrhagia is associated with increased arachidonic acid availability in the uterus,[3,4] it makes sense to decrease the intake of animal products and increase the intake of omega-3 fatty acids and other beneficial oils. Consuming higher amounts of fish, nuts, and seeds and supplementing with fish oils may yield beneficial effects by reducing tissue levels of arachidonic acid.

Vitamin B Complex

There may be a correlation between a nutritional deficiency of B vitamins and menorrhagia. It has been shown that in vitamin B complex deficiency, the liver loses its ability to inactivate estrogen. Some cases of menorrhagia are due to the effect of excessive estrogen on the endometrium. Therefore, supplementing with a complex of B vitamins may normalize estrogen metabolism. A study conducted in the 1940s showed that a B-complex preparation (thiamine 3 to 9 mg, riboflavin 4.5 to 9 mg, and niacin up to 60 mg) was effective in improving menorrhagia.[13]

Botanical Medicines

Chasteberry

Chasteberry (*Vitex agnus-castus*) is probably the best-known botanical medicine for treatment of hormonal imbalances and abnormal bleeding in women. Since at least the time of the ancient Greeks, it has been used for the full scope of menstrual disorders, including heavy menses. Clinical studies have shown chasteberry extracts to be helpful in many types of menstrual abnormalities including menorrhagia. In a study observing 126 women with menstrual disorders who were given 15 drops of liquid extract, the duration between periods lengthened from an average of 20.1 days to 26.3 days in the 33 women with polymenorrhea, and the number of heavy bleeding days was shortened in the 58 patients with menorrhagia.[14] While chasteberry extract is the most important botanical medicine for normalizing menstrual flow, it may take three or four months to show effects.

. . . .

QUICK REVIEW

- **Nutritional factors are often responsible for excessive menstrual blood loss.**
- **Iron therapy is a key consideration in treating menorrhagia.**
- **A decreased serum ferritin level is a good indication of the need for iron supplementation.**
- **Even mild hypothyroidism can lead to excessive menstrual blood loss.**
- **Consuming higher amounts of fish, nuts, and seeds and supplementing with fish oils may yield beneficial effects.**
- **Clinical studies have shown chasteberry extracts to be helpful in many types of menstrual abnormalities including menorrhagia.**

TREATMENT SUMMARY

The first step in treating menorrhagia is to attempt to identify the cause. This step will usually require the help of a physician.

Diet

Follow the general recommendations given in the chapter "A Health-Promoting Diet." The diet should be relatively low in meat and dairy products, to reduce the intake of arachidonic acid. It should be higher in the beneficial oils from fish, nuts, and seeds. Green leafy vegetables, green tea, and other sources of vitamin K should be consumed freely.

Nutritional Supplements

- A high-potency multiple vitamin and mineral formula as described in the chapter "Supplementary Measures"
- Key individual nutrients:
  - Vitamin C: 500 to 1,000 mg three times per day
  - Vitamin D_3: 2,000 to 4,000 IU per day (ideally, measure blood levels and adjust dosage accordingly)
- Fish oils: 1,000 mg EPA + DHA per day
- One of the following:
  - Grape seed extract (>95% procyanidolic oligomers): 100 to 300 mg per day

- Pine bark extract (>95% procyanidolic oligomers): 100 to 300 mg per day
- Some other flavonoid-rich extract with a similar flavonoid content, super greens formula, or another plant-based antioxidant that can provide an oxygen radical absorption capacity (ORAC) of 3,000 to 6,000 units or more per day
- One of the following:
  - Chlorophyll: 25 mg per day (use a crude form)
  - 1 mg vitamin K_1

If low serum ferritin is confirmed:

- Iron (bound to either pyrophosphate, succinate, glycinate, or fumarate): 30 mg twice per day between meals (if this recommendation results in abdominal discomfort, take 30 mg with meals three times per day)

Botanical Medicines

- Chasteberry extract:
  - Tablets or capsules (often standardized to 0.5% agnuside): 175 to 225 mg per day
  - Liquid extract: 2 to 4 ml (½ to 1 tsp) per day

Migraine Headache

· ·

- Headache, typically pounding and on one side
- Attacks often preceded by psychological or visual disturbances: blurring or bright spots of vision, anxiety, fatigue, disturbed thinking, numbness or tingling of a hand or foot

Migraine headaches are caused by excessive dilation of blood vessels in the head. Vascular headaches, such as migraines, are characterized by a sharp throbbing or pounding pain. In nonvascular headaches, such as tension headache (usually caused by tightening in the muscles of the face, neck, or scalp as a result of stress or poor posture; see the chapter "Headache, Nonmigraine Tension Type"), the pain is steady, constant, and dull; it starts at the base of the skull or in the forehead and spreads over the entire head, giving the sensation of pressure, as if a vise has been applied to the skull.

Headache pain arises from the lining of the brain (the meninges), blood vessels, or muscles when stretched or tensed. Brain tissue itself has no sensory nerve endings.

Causes

Blood Vessel Instability

Considerable evidence supports an association between migraine headaches and instability of blood vessels.[1] The sequence of events causes excessive constriction of a blood vessel followed by rebound dilation. Most studies measuring brain blood flow have confirmed a reduction of blood flow, sometimes to very low and critical levels, during the period prior to a migraine attack. This decrease is followed by a stage of increased blood flow that can persist for more than 48 hours. The abnormal blood flow appears confined to the outer portion of the brain (cerebral cortex), while deeper structures have a normal blood supply.

There is some evidence that migraine patients have an inherited abnormality in their control of blood vessel constriction and dilation. Migraine patients suffer more often than normal people from dizziness upon standing suddenly, and they seem to be abnormally sensitive to the effects of physical and chemical factors that cause changes in blood vessels.

Platelet Disorder

Platelets are small blood cells involved in the formation of blood clots. The platelets of many migraine sufferers are very different from normal platelets, both during and between headaches. The differences include a significant increase in spontaneous clumping together (aggregation), highly significant differences in the manner of serotonin release, and significant differences in the structural composition of the platelets.

The biggest factor may be the differences in serotonin metabolism. Serotonin is a neurotransmitter, a compound used in the chemical transfer of information from one cell to another. Serotonin also plays a role in the state of relaxation or constriction of blood vessels. All of the serotonin normally in the blood is stored in the platelets and released by platelet aggregation. There is no difference in total serotonin content between normal platelets and the platelets of migraine patients. However, the quantity of serotonin released by the platelets of the migraine patient in response to serotonin stimulation (such as a food allergy), while initially normal, becomes progressively higher until a migraine is produced.

The platelet hypothesis is strengthened by the observation that patients with classic migraines have a twofold increase in incidence of mitral valve prolapse (that is, a leaky heart valve). This leaky valve can cause damage to blood platelets as they surge through the valve with each beat of the heart. Researchers have found that 16% of migraine patients have definite mitral valve prolapse, and another 15% have possible prolapse—a rate at least two times higher than normal. Interestingly, mitral valve prolapse is also found three times more frequently in individuals with deficient magnesium, a mineral that is especially effective in migraines.

Nerve Disorder

A third major hypothesis is that in migraines, the nervous system plays a role in initiating the vascular events. It has been suggested that nerve cells in the blood vessels of patients with migraines release a compound known as substance P. (You can probably guess what the *P* stands for: pain.) In addition to triggering pain, the release of substance P into the arteries is associated with the dilation of blood vessels and the release

of histamine and other allergic compounds by specialized white blood cells known as mast cells. Chronic stress is thought to be an important factor in this model. Some research has suggested that in as many as 40% of migraine sufferers the nerve mitochondria do not produce as much energy as in those without migraines. As a result, the nerves are overly reactive to the environment.

Serotonin Deficiency Syndrome

The final hypothesis is that migraine headache represents a serotonin deficiency state. The story of serotonin and headaches began in the 1960s, when researchers noted an increase in the serotonin breakdown product 5-hydroxyindoleacetic acid (5-HIAA) in the urine during a migraine. Initially it was thought that serotonin excess was the culprit. However, newer information indicates that the factor responsible for the increase in 5-HIAA is probably increased breakdown of serotonin as a result of increased activity of monoamine oxidase (MAO). Because migraine sufferers have low levels of serotonin in their tissues, researchers referred to migraines as "low-serotonin syndrome."[2]

Low serotonin levels are thought to lead to a decrease in the pain threshold in patients with chronic headaches. This contention is strongly supported by more than 35 years of research, including positive clinical results in double-blind studies with the serotonin precursor 5-hydroxytryptophan (5-HTP).

The link between low serotonin levels and headaches is the basis of many prescription drugs for the treatment and prevention of migraine headaches. For example, the serotonin agonist drug sumatriptan (Imitrex) is now among the most popular migraine prescriptions. In addition to sumatriptan, monoamine oxidase inhibitors (which increase serotonin levels) have also been shown to prevent headaches. The bottom line is there is considerable evidence that increasing serotonin levels leads to relief from chronic migraine headaches.

The effects of 5-HTP, sumatriptan, and other drugs on the serotonin system are extremely complex because of the multiple types of serotonin receptors. Many substances produce their effects on cells by first binding to receptor sites on the cell membrane. Some serotonin receptors are involved in triggering migraines and others prevent them. This situation is quite clear when we look at the different effects that various drugs exert in binding to these different serotonin receptors. Drugs that bind to serotonin receptors designated as 5-HT1c trigger migraines, while drugs such as methysergide, which inhibit 5-HT1c, are used to prevent migraines. In addition, the serotonin receptor 5-HT1d may play a role in migraine prevention, since drugs such as sumatriptan that bind to these receptors and mimic the effects of serotonin are quite effective in the acute treatment of migraine.

Because some serotonin receptors appear to undergo desensitization when exposed to higher levels of serotonin, these different receptors come into play with 5-HTP supplementation. It is thought that as 5-HTP increases serotonin levels, 5-HT1c receptors lose their ability or affinity to bind serotonin, resulting in more serotonin binding to the 5-HT1d receptor. The result is a lowered tendency to experience headache. One of the key pieces of evidence to support this concept is the fact that 5-HTP is more effective over time (better results are seen after 60 days of use than at 30 days).

Unified Hypothesis

The mechanism of migraine can be described as a three-stage process: initiation, prodrome (time between initiation and appearance of headache), and headache. Although a particular stressor may be associated with the onset of a specific attack, it appears that initiation is dependent on the accumulation of several stressors over time. These stressors ultimately affect serotonin metabolism. Once a critical point of susceptibility (or threshold) is reached, a "cascade event" or domino-like effect is set into motion, ultimately producing a headache. This susceptibility is probably a combination of decreased tissue serotonin levels, changes in the platelets, increased sensitivity to compounds such as substance P, and the buildup of histamine and other mediators of inflammation.

Factors That Trigger Migraine Headaches

- Low serotonin levels
  - Genetics
  - Shunting of tryptophan into other pathways
- Food allergies
  - Histamine-releasing foods
  - Histamine-containing foods
- Alcohol, especially red wine
- Food additives
  - Nitrates
  - MSG (monosodium glutamate)
- Nitroglycerin
- Withdrawal from caffeine or other drugs that constrict blood vessels
- Stress
- Emotional changes (especially letdown after stress) and intense emotions (such as anger)
- Hormonal changes, e.g., menstruation, ovulation, birth control pills
- Too little or too much sleep

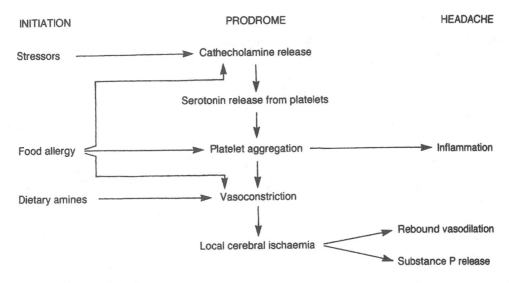

INITIATION   PRODROME   HEADACHE

Triggers of Migraine Headaches

- Exhaustion
- Poor posture
- Muscle tension
- Weather changes (barometric pressure changes, exposure to sun)
- Glare or eyestrain

Therapeutic Considerations

Modern drug treatment of headache tends to be inadequate because it fails to address the underlying cause in most cases. The first step in treating migraine headache is to identify the precipitating factor or factors. Although food intolerance/allergy is the most important, many other factors must be considered as either primary causes or contributors to the migraine process. Particularly important is to assess the role that headache medications may be playing, especially in chronic headaches.

Drug Reaction and Rebound Headaches

In the early 1980s it became apparent that headache medications could actually increase the tendency to experience chronic headache. Early reports identified increased frequency and intensity of headaches in heavy analgesic users. In one study migraine sufferers who took more than 30 analgesic tablets per month had twice as many headache days per month as those who took fewer than 30 tablets.[3] This finding led to the recommendation that analgesic use should be restricted in patients with chronic headaches. In another study 70 patients with daily headaches who were consuming 14 or more analgesic tablets weekly were advised to discontinue their use.[4] One month later, 66% of the patients were improved, and at the end of the second month, this percentage had grown to 81%.

Analgesic-rebound headaches should be suspected in anyone with chronic, predictable migraines who is taking large quantities of analgesics. The critical dosage that can lead to analgesic-rebound migraines is estimated to be 1,000 mg of either acetaminophen or aspirin. Analgesic medications used for migraines typically contain substances in addition to the analgesic such as caffeine or a sedative (e.g., butabarbital). These substances further contribute to the problem and may lead to withdrawal headache and related symptoms such as nausea, abdominal cramps, diarrhea, restlessness, sleeplessness, and anxiety. Withdrawal symptoms typically start 24 to 48 hours after the last dosage and in most cases subside in five or so days.

Food Allergies/Intolerance

There is little doubt that food allergies and intolerances play a role in many cases of migraine headache. Clinical studies have demonstrated that the detection and removal of allergenic or intolerable foods can eliminate or greatly reduce migraine symptoms in the majority of patients. Success rates range from 30 to 93%, with the majority of studies showing a remarkably high degree of success.[5–11] Several methods may be used to detect food allergies and are described in the chapter "Food Allergy."

Foods That Most Commonly Induce Migraine Headaches Listed in Descending Order of Frequency
Cow's milk and other dairy products
Wheat
Chocolate
Egg
Orange
Benzoic acid
Tomato
Tartrazine
Peanuts
Monosodium glutamate

Dietary Amines

Foods such as chocolate, cheese, beer, and wine may precipitate migraine attacks because they contain histamine or other compounds that have a vasodilation effect.[12–14] Red wine is more likely than white wine to trigger a headache because it contains up to twice as much histamine and tyramine, which stimulate the release of vasoactive compounds by platelets.[12,13,15] Red wine is additionally much higher in phenolic compounds, including flavonoids—the antioxidant components shown to help prevent heart disease. These compounds can also inhibit the enzyme phenolsulfotransferase, which normally breaks down serotonin and other vasoactive amines in platelets. Many migraine sufferers have been found to have significantly lower levels of this enzyme. Because red wine contains substances that are potent inhibitors of this enzyme, it often triggers migraines in these individuals, especially if consumed along with foods high in vasoactive amines such as cheese or chocolate. A standard treatment for histamine-induced headaches is a histamine-free diet, along with vitamin B_6 supplementation.[13,14]

The activity of the enzyme diamine oxidase, which breaks down histamine in the lining of the small intestine before it is absorbed into the circulation, appears to play a key role in determining reactivity to dietary histamine. Individuals sensitive to dietary histamine have lower levels (about 50%) of this enzyme in their tissues compared with control subjects.[13] Diamine oxidase is a vitamin B_6–dependent enzyme. Not surprisingly, compounds that antagonize vitamin B_6 also inhibit diamine oxidase.[13] These inhibitory factors include food coloring agents (specifically hydrazine dyes such as tartrazine, also known as yellow no. 5); some drugs (isoniazid, hydralazine, dopamine, and penicillamine); oral contraceptives; alcohol; and excessive protein intake.

Vitamin B_6 supplementation (usually 1 mg/kg) has been shown to improve histamine tolerance, presumably by increasing diamine oxidase activity.[13,16] Women have lower levels of diamine oxidase, which may explain their higher incidence of histamine-induced headaches. Women are also much more frequently unable to tolerate red wine. Interestingly, the level of diamine oxidase in a woman increases by more than 500 times during pregnancy.[17,18] Women with histamine-induced headaches commonly experience complete remission of their headaches during pregnancy.

Miscellaneous Diet-Related Triggers

Hypoglycemia can be a trigger for migraine headaches.[19,20] Blood sugar volatility is most often due to a diet of high-glycemic-index carbohydrates. For more information, see the chapter "Hypoglycemia." Excessive sodium intake, lactose intolerance, and aspartame, a common artificial sweetener, may also trigger migraines.[21–24]

Just as in other allergic or inflammatory disorders, it is important to reduce the consumption of animal fats (saturated fats and arachidonic acid) and increase consumption of the long-chain omega-3 fatty acids EPA and DHA from fish and fish oil supplements. Making such a dietary change can reduce platelet aggregation and the formation of inflammatory mediators and may play a role in preventing migraine headaches.[25–27] Several double-blind studies have shown a modest benefit with fish oil supplementation.[28–30] For example, a small double-blind study of adolescents with migraines revealed marked improvement in migraine headache frequency, duration, and severity with fish oil. However, the adolescents responded equally well to olive oil supplements, the placebo chosen

for this study.[30] Its possible that the olive oil also led to significant improvement in platelet function.

Treatment Considerations

Nutritional Supplements

5-Hydroxytryptophan (5-HTP)
The role of 5-HTP in preventing migraine headaches by increasing serotonin levels was discussed earlier. In addition to this mechanism, 5-HTP may also increase endorphin levels. The use of 5-HTP in migraine prevention offers considerable advantages over drug therapy. Although a number of drugs have been shown to be useful in the prevention of migraine headache, all of the currently used drugs carry with them a risk of significant adverse effects. 5-HTP is at least as effective as other pharmacological agents used in the prevention of migraine headaches and is safer and better tolerated. Although some studies have employed a dosage of 600 mg per day, equally impressive results have been achieved at a dosage as low as 200 mg per day.

Several studies have compared 5-HTP with methysergide in the prevention of migraine headaches. In one of the largest double-blind studies, 124 patients received either 5-HTP (600 mg per day) or methysergide (3 mg per day) for six months.[31] Treatment was determined to be successful if there was a greater than 50% reduction in the frequency of attacks or in the number of severe attacks. Although 75% of the patients taking methysergide demonstrated significant improvement, compared with 71% of the patients taking 5-HTP, this difference was not viewed as being statistically significant. The advantage of 5-HTP over methysergide was demonstrated when researchers looked at side effects. Side effects were more frequent

5-HTP vs. Methysergide, Clinical Effects of Treatment in 124 Patients		
	METHYSERGIDE (%)	**5-HTP (%)**
No attacks (100% reduction)	35	25
Improvement (>50% reduction)	40	46
No improvement	12.5	29
Withdrawal due to side effects	12.5	0

in the group receiving methysergide than in the 5-HTP group. In fact, five patients in the methysergide group had to withdraw during the trial because of side effects.

Two other studies comparing 5-HTP with drugs used in the prevention of migraine headaches (pizotifen and propranolol) demonstrated that 5-HTP compared quite favorably in terms of effectiveness.[32,33] Although these drugs have significant side effects, 5-HTP is extremely well tolerated even at dosages as high as 600 mg per day. One of the other key differences noted in these studies between 5-HTP and the drugs was 5-HTP's ability to improve mood and relieve feelings of depression.

Riboflavin (Vitamin B₂)

Migraine headaches may be the result of a deficit in the production of energy by the mitochondria, the energy-producing compartments of the cell.[34] Riboflavin (vitamin B₂) is required for the activity of key enzymes within the mitochondria. A double-blind study demonstrated that a dose of 400 mg riboflavin per day was superior to a placebo in preventing migraine attacks. The effect began at one month, with maximal effect after three months.[35] The ability of riboflavin to increase mitochondrial energy metabolism has been verified.[36,37] Riboflavin is well tolerated and is less expensive than typical migraine medications, so it is an excellent therapeutic option.[38] Other B vitamins including folic acid may also be instrumental in preventing or treating

migraine headache.[39] Diarrhea and increased urinary frequency may be associated with high doses of riboflavin.

Magnesium

The high frequency of magnesium deficiency seen in migraine sufferers is well established in research. Magnesium levels are depleted by a multitude of common factors, including stress, excessive alcohol intake, high estrogen levels, low progesterone, certain drugs, hyperthyroidism, and hyperparathyroidism. Inadequate dietary intake of magnesium is likely in 75% of the U.S. population,[40] and magnesium deficiency is thought to be the most common mineral deficiency, manifested in a diverse range of associated pathologies.[41] Physiological and psychological stress result in magnesium depletion, and both acute and chronic stress are associated with increased episodes of migraines.

Substantial documentation linking low magnesium levels to both migraine and tension headaches exists in the medical literature. Low brain and tissue magnesium concentrations have been found in patients with migraines, indicating a need for supplementation.[42–44] Among magnesium's central functions are maintaining vascular tone and preventing neuronal hyperexcitation. Positive results with magnesium supplementation have been shown in preventing migraines, specifically in people with low levels of magnesium.[45–47]

Low tissue levels of magnesium are common in patients with migraine, but most cases go unnoticed because physicians generally rely on serum magnesium levels to assess magnesium status. Because most of the body's magnesium is intracellular, serum levels are unreliable indicators. A low magnesium level in the serum reflects late-stage deficiency. More sensitive tests of magnesium status include red blood cell magnesium levels and ionized magnesium, the most physiologically active form.

The hypothesis that patients with an acute migraine episode and low serum levels (less than 0.54 mmol/l) of ionized magnesium are more likely to respond to an intravenous infusion of magnesium sulfate ($MgSO_4$) than patients with higher serum ionized magnesium levels has been tested.[48,49] Serum ionized magnesium levels were determined immediately before infusion of 1 g magnesium sulfate in 40 patients with an acute migraine. Pain reduction of 50% or more, as measured on a headache intensity verbal scale of 1 to 10, occurred within 15 minutes of infusion in 35 patients. In 21 patients, at least this degree of improvement or complete relief persisted for 24 hours or more. Pain relief lasted at least 24 hours in 18 of 21 patients (86%) with serum ionized magnesium levels below 0.54 mmol/l and in 3 of 19 patients (16%) with ionized magnesium levels at or above 0.54 mmol/l. The average ionized magnesium level in patients who had relief lasting for at least 24 hours was significantly lower than that in patients who experienced no relief or only fleeting relief.

Another possible benefit of magnesium supplementation in preventing migraines may be its ability to prevent mitral valve prolapse. Mitral valve prolapse is linked to migraines because it leads to damage to blood platelets, causing them to release vasoactive substances such as histamine, platelet-activating factor, and serotonin. Since research has shown that 85% of patients with mitral valve prolapse have chronic magnesium deficiency, magnesium supplementation is indicated.[50] This recommendation is further supported by several studies showing that oral magnesium supplementation improves mitral valve prolapse.

Magnesium bound to citrate, malate, or aspartate is better absorbed and better tolerated than inorganic forms such as magnesium sulfate, hydroxide, or oxide, which tend to produce a laxative effect.[51] If magnesium supplementation produces a loose stool or diarrhea, cut back to a level that is tolerable. Also, it is a good idea to take at least 50 mg vitamin B_6 per day, as this B vitamin has been shown to increase the intracellular accumulation of magnesium.[52]

Botanical Medicines

Feverfew

Perhaps the most popular herbal preventive treatment of migraine headaches is feverfew (*Tanacetum parthenium*). Scientific interest in feverfew began when a 1983 survey found that 70% of 270 migraine sufferers who had taken feverfew daily for prolonged periods reported that the herb decreased the frequency or intensity of their attacks.[53] Many of these patients had been unresponsive to routine medications. This survey prompted several clinical investigations that support the therapeutic and preventive effects of feverfew in the treatment of migraine frequency and intensity.[53–56]

The first double-blind study was done at the London Migraine Clinic, using patients who reported being helped by feverfew.[53] Those patients who received the placebo (and as a result stopped using feverfew) had a significant increase in the frequency and severity of headache, nausea, and vomiting during the six months of the study, while patients who continued taking feverfew showed no change in the frequency or severity of their symptoms. Two patients in the placebo group, who had been in complete remission during self-treatment with feverfew, developed recurrence of incapacitating migraine and had to withdraw from the study; when those two patients resumed self-treatment with feverfew, their symptoms abated. The second double-blind study, performed at the University of Nottingham, demonstrated that feverfew was effective in reducing the number and severity of migraine attacks.[54]

Follow-up studies have shown that feverfew works in the treatment and prevention of migraine headaches by inhibiting the release of blood-vessel-dilating substances from platelets, inhibiting the production of inflammatory substances, and reestablishing proper blood vessel tone.[55] The effectiveness of feverfew is dependent upon adequate levels of parthenolide.[56] However, at least three crossover, randomized, controlled trials found no benefit with feverfew, though each study had limitations.[57]

Key to understanding the inconsistency of the results with feverfew, as well as other natural agents, is recognizing that not everyone who suffers from migraines has the same disease. Rather, migraines are the end result of a diverse range of physiological dysfunctions. While conventional drugs often focus on relief of symptoms, most natural therapies address the cause—which for migraines can be quite diverse. If the natural therapy does

. . . .

QUICK REVIEW

- **The first step in treating migraine headache is identifying the precipitating factor.**
- **Several clinical studies have estimated that approximately 80% of patients with chronic headaches suffer from drug-induced headaches.**
- **Many double-blind, placebo-controlled studies have demonstrated that cutting out allergenic or intolerable foods will eliminate or greatly reduce migraine symptoms in the majority of patients.**
- **Foods such as chocolate, cheese, beer, and wine precipitate migraine attacks in many people because they contain histamines and/or other compounds that can trigger migraines in sensitive individuals by causing blood vessels to expand.**

- **5-HTP is at least as effective as other pharmacological agents used in the prevention of migraine headaches and is certainly much safer and better tolerated.**
- **Riboflavin has been shown to increase energy production in the brain and to effectively prevent migraines.**
- **Low magnesium levels may play a significant role in many cases of headaches.**
- **Feverfew, butterbur, and ginger extracts can help prevent migraine attacks.**
- **Biofeedback and relaxation training have been judged as effective as the drug approach but are without any side effects.**

not match the physiological dysfunction, then it is not going to work. The reason the early feverfew studies were so uniformly successful is that the patients had through trial and error preselected themselves: they had a physiological dysfunction that matched up well with the effects of feverfew.

Butterbur

There is significant documentation of the efficacy of butterbur (*Petasides hybridus*) in preventing migraines, and its recorded use for this purpose and others dates back at least 900 years. Butterbur has been shown to reduce the spasm of blood vessels as well as the formation of inflammatory compounds. Petadolex is a standardized extract from the butterbur plant that has been shown in several double-blind studies to produce excellent results in preventing migraine headaches without side effects. In one study, 60 patients suffering from headaches randomly received 50 mg Petadolex twice per day for 12 weeks. Compared with the beginning of the trial, Petadolex reduced the frequency of attacks by 46% after 4 weeks, 60% after 8 weeks, and 50% after 12 weeks of treatment (the figures for the placebo group were 24%, 17%, and 10%, respectively).[58] Petadolex is generally well tolerated, but diarrhea has been reported in some individuals. If this side effect occurs, discontinue use. It is important to use Petadolex or similarly prepared products that have had the liver-damaging and cancer-causing substances in butterbur (pyrrolizidine alkaloids) removed. No drug interactions have been identified, but its safety during pregnancy or lactation has not been determined, so it should not be used in these instances.[59]

Ginger

Gingerroot (*Zingiber officinalis*) has been shown to exert significant effects in sup-pressing inflammation and platelet aggregation.[60–62] With respect to migraine headache, there is much anecdotal information and speculation about its usefulness based on its known properties. Ginger may be commonly used in clinical practice for migraine treatment, but little clinical investigation has been performed to date. The most active anti-inflammatory components of ginger are found in fresh preparations and the oil.

Acupuncture

Sufficient evidence exists to support the use of acupuncture to relieve migraine pain.[63–67] The mechanism of action may involve normalization of serotonin levels.

Biofeedback and Relaxation Therapy

The most widely used nondrug therapies for migraine headaches are thermal biofeedback and relaxation training. Thermal biofeedback uses a feedback gauge to monitor the temperature of the hands. The patient is then taught how to raise (or lower) the temperature of the hands, while the device provides feedback regarding temperature measurements. Relaxation training involves teaching patients techniques designed to produce the relaxation response—a physiological state that opposes the stress response (see the chapter "A Positive Mental Attitude" for more information).

Biofeedback/Relaxation Compared with Propranolol	
THERAPY	**AVERAGE IMPROVEMENT PER PATIENT (%)**
Biofeedback/relaxation	56.4
Propranolol	55.2
Placebo	14.3
Untreated	3.2

The effectiveness in reducing the frequency and severity of recurrent migraine headaches with biofeedback and relaxation training has been the subject of more than 35 clinical studies.[66] When the results from these studies were compared with studies using the beta-blocking drug propranolol (Inderal), it was apparent that this nondrug approach was as effective as the drug approach but was without adverse effects.

TREATMENT SUMMARY

Migraine headaches are often debilitating, frequently interfering significantly with an individual's quality of life. Owing to the many contributing factors, a comprehensive approach is necessary for an effective outcome. Specifically, identification and avoidance of precipitating factors are important in reducing the frequency of headaches. Owing to the high frequency (80 to 90%) of food allergy/intolerance in patients with migraine headache, we recommend beginning treatment by identifying and eliminating food allergies. This can be accomplished through blood analysis or by the use of an elemental diet (see the chapter "Food Allergy").

Diet

All food allergens must be eliminated and a four-day rotation diet utilized. Foods that contain vasoactive amines should initially be eliminated; after symptoms have been controlled, such foods can be carefully reintroduced. The primary foods to eliminate are alcoholic beverages (especially red wine), cheese, chocolate, citrus fruits, and shellfish. The diet should be low in sources of arachidonic acid (animal fats) and high in foods that inhibit platelet aggregation (olive oil, fish oils, flavonoid-rich berries, garlic, and onion).

Nutritional Supplements

- A high-potency multiple vitamin and mineral formula as described in the chapter "Supplementary Measures"
- Key individual nutrients:
  - Magnesium (citrate, malate, succinate, aspartate, or glycinate is preferred): 150 to 250 mg three to four times per day
  - Vitamin B_6: 50 to 75 mg per day
  - Vitamin B_2 (riboflavin): 400 mg once per day
- Fish oils: 1,000 mg EPA + DHA per day
- One of the following:
  - Grape seed extract (>95% procyanidolic oligomers): 100 to 300 mg per day
  - Pine bark extract (>95% procyanidolic oligomers): 100 to 300 mg per day
  - Some other flavonoid-rich extract with a similar flavonoid content, super greens formula, or another plant-based antioxidant that can pro-

vide an oxygen radical absorption capacity (ORAC) of 3,000 to 6,000 units or higher per day

- 5-HTP: 50 to 100 mg three times per day

Botanical Medicines

One of the following:

- Feverfew: extract providing a dosage of 0.25 to 0.5 mg parthenolide twice per day.
- Butterbur: extract equivalent to Petadolex, 50 to 100 mg twice per day with meals

- Ginger:
  ○ Fresh: approximately 10 g per day (¼-inch slice)
  ○ Powdered: 500 mg four times per day
  ○ Extract standardized to contain 20% of gingerol and shogaol: 100 to 200 mg three times per day for prevention and 200 mg every two hours (up to six times per day) in the treatment of an acute migraine

Physical Medicine and Relaxation Therapies

- Acupuncture
- Biofeedback

Multiple Sclerosis

- Sudden transient motor and sensory disturbances, including blurred vision, dizziness, muscle weakness, and tingling sensations
- Evidence of demyelination visible on MRI

Multiple sclerosis (MS) is a syndrome of progressive nerve disturbances that usually occurs early in adult life. It is caused by gradual loss of the myelin sheath that surrounds the nerve cell. This process is called demyelination. One of the key functions of this myelin sheath is to facilitate the transmission of the nerve impulse. Without the myelin sheath, nerve function is lost. Symptoms correspond to the nerves that have lost their myelin sheath.

In about two-thirds of the cases, onset is between ages 20 and 40 (rarely is the onset after age 50), and women are affected more often than men (60% female to 40% male). MS affects about 1 of 1,000 people in the United States, Canada, and northern Europe.[1]

Clinically, MS can cause various neurological problems depending on the location and severity of MS plaques (see the table opposite). In about 85% of cases, MS starts with a relapsing-remitting course.[2] Patients experience relapses or attacks of MS during which they confront a new neurological problem, the return of an old problem that had resolved, or worsening of preexisting symptoms. Relapses develop over a few days or weeks, and then a period of improvement and stability ensues. In between relapses, patients are clinically stable, although they may have residual permanent neurological symptoms from previous relapses of MS; and they can continue to have demyelination without additional symptoms.[3]

Causes

The cause of MS remains to be identified conclusively. One of the more interesting features of MS is the geographic and racial distribution of the disease. First, MS is most common among Caucasians, particularly those of northern European descent.[4,5] Typical MS is rare among Asians and black Africans but is relatively common among African-Americans, suggesting a dietary link. The racial predilection of MS is one piece of evidence indicating the strong influence of genetics on the risk of developing MS.

In regard to the geographic distribution of the disease, areas with the highest prevalence are located in higher latitudes in both the northern and southern hemispheres.[6,7] These high-risk areas include the northern United States, Canada, Great Britain, Scandinavia, northern Europe, New Zealand, and Tasmania. It appears that the initial event in the development of MS may occur in early life. This statement is based on the observation that people who move from a low-risk area to a high-risk area before age 15 have a higher risk of developing MS, whereas those who make the same move after age 15 retain their

Symptoms of Multiple Sclerosis and Their Neurological Causes	
SYMPTOMS	**CAUSES**
Weakness, numbness, and tingling in legs and arms; stiffness in legs	Spinal cord lesions
Urinary urgency, retention, incontinence, and recurrent bladder infections	Spinal cord lesions
Constipation	Spinal cord lesions; diet
Sexual dysfunction	Spinal cord lesions
Blurred vision and blindness	Optic nerve lesions
Double vision	Brain stem lesions
Imbalance	Spinal cord and cerebellar lesions
Tremor of arms	Brain lesions
Impaired memory and concentration	Brain lesions; effects of inflammatory cytokines
Fatigue	Effects of inflammatory cytokines; nerve fiber fatigability resulting from demyelination
Heat sensitivity and elevations in body temperature	Sensitivity of demyelinations to elevations in body temperature
Depression and other mood disorders	Associated with elevations in inflammatory cytokines

low risk. There are many possible reasons for the geographic distribution of MS, such as genetics, vitamin D, diet, and other environmental factors. These factors are discussed more fully below.

Genetics

Substantial evidence indicates that genetic background influences the risk of developing MS.[8,9] Having a parent or sibling with MS increases your risk of developing MS by five-fold to tenfold. Perhaps the most compelling evidence of the genetic influence on the risk of developing MS comes from studies of twins in which at least one twin has the disease.[10] Among fraternal twins, the chance of the second twin's having MS is 1 to 2%, which is similar to that of non-twin sibling pairs. Among identical twins, the chance of the second twin's having MS is 25%, indicating a strong genetic influence. An estimated 10 to 15 different genes may affect the risk of developing MS, and major research efforts are under way to identify these genes. However, the fact that only 25% of identical twins develop MS if their twin develops it clearly shows that dietary, environmental, and lifestyle factors are required for the disease to manifest itself in most cases. In other words, genetics alone does not inevitably lead to MS.[11]

Viruses

Viruses and other microbes have been suggested as possible factors in developing MS. Viruses can cause several demyelinating diseases in humans and animals that are quite similar to MS. A number of viruses have been isolated from cultures of material in patients with multiple sclerosis, including herpes simplex virus, scrapie virus, parainfluenza virus, subacute myelo-opticoneuropathy virus, measles virus, Epstein-Barr virus, and coronavirus. The most suspicious viruses now are the measles and Epstein-Barr viruses. However, all of these viruses may simply be bystanders, rather than the cause of MS.[12,13]

The *cerebrospinal fluid* (the fluid that surrounds the brain and spinal cord) of most MS patients contains an elevated level of antibodies (protein molecules made by white blood cells that bind to foreign molecules such as bacteria, viruses, and cancer cells) in a pattern that is characteristic of an infectious process. According to one theory, this pattern is, in fact, due to an unrecognized infectious agent that causes MS. This theory has been termed the "sense antibody" theory. An alternative theory states that MS is not an infectious disease and that the antibodies in the cerebrospinal fluid are nonspecific or "nonsense" antibodies. At present, the available data do not appear to support a common virus as the cause for the increased antibody levels, which are more likely the result of an autoimmune reaction. However, it is possible that the trigger is a virus or another organism.

Geographic and Seasonal Influences

As we have noted, MS is more common in populations that live farther from the equator. People who move from a low-risk area to a high-risk area before age 15 acquire a higher risk of developing MS, whereas those who make the same move after adolescence retain a lower risk. These observations suggest that environmental exposure,[14] and in particular early sunlight exposure (which is correlated to serum vitamin D levels), in the first two decades of life influences the risk of developing MS.

Although not consistently seen in all geographic areas, an association between season of birth and risk of developing MS has been shown in several European population studies.[15] These studies observe that there is a lower risk of MS for births occurring after October and a higher risk for MS for births occurring after May. The authors reporting these findings suggest that maternal levels of vitamin D levels during the third trimester of pregnancy may influence risk of MS: there is a lower risk when maternal vitamin D levels are high (summer months) and a higher risk when maternal vitamin D levels are low (winter months).

The research is now very clear: low levels of vitamin D, as measured by serum 25-hydroxyvitamin D, are strongly correlated with an increased risk of MS. Early trials of supplementation with vitamin D in MS are showing encouraging results.

Of particular interest is a recent study showing that the MS protection afforded by being closer to the equator may not be due simply to increased vitamin D production.[16] Apparently sun exposure itself is protective against MS, independent of increasing vitamin D levels.

Diet

Diet may play a role as an additional risk factor in acquiring MS. The first investigations into diet and MS led by Roy Swank, M.D., centered on trying to explain why inland farming communities in Norway had a higher incidence than areas near the coastline. It was discovered that the diets of the farmers were much higher in animal and dairy products than the diets of the coastal dwellers, whose diet featured more cold-water fish.[17] Additional studies have since correlated MS with consumption of meat and animal fat.[18]

However, a large prospective cohort study using data from the Nurses Health Study and Nurses Health Study II found no evidence linking risk of MS with intake of saturated fats. The authors did note, however, that intake of alpha-linolenic acid, an omega-3 fatty acid, but not fish oils, was associated with a trend toward a lower risk for MS.[19] Data from this study also showed no relationship between intake of fruits and vegetables and risk of MS.[20] A study in Canada found a positive association between animal fat intake and risk of MS.[21] Taken together, these studies suggest that diet has a modest influence on the risk of developing MS.

Therapeutic Considerations

From a natural medicine standpoint, the primary approach is to utilize dietary therapy and nutritional supplements shown to be helpful in arresting the disease process, along with exercise and effective stress management.

The conventional medical approach to treating MS includes the use of medications to control disease activity and additional medications plus rehabilitation interventions designed to alleviate symptoms resulting from damage to the central nervous system. Medications that help decrease disease activity (also called disease-modifying agents) in relapsing-remitting MS include human recombinant interferon beta (Avonex, Betaseron, and Rebif), glatiramer acetate (Copaxone), a monoclonal antibody against alpha-4 integrin (Tysabri), and the immunosuppressant mitoxantrone (Novantrone). Compared with a placebo, these medications decrease the relapse rate by about one-third, decrease new lesion formation in the brain as detected by MRI, and decrease the risk of developing permanent neurological disability.[22–27] The immunosuppressant mitoxantrone has also been shown to decrease disease activity in pa-

tients with rapidly progressive forms of MS.[28] Tysabri, which prevents inflammatory cells from entering the central nervous system, has been shown to decrease the rate of MS exacerbations and reduce the disease activity (new lesions) when compared with a placebo.[22] Corticosteroids, such as methylprednisolone, given in high doses can decrease the duration of relapses of MS but do not affect the degree of eventual recovery from those relapses. A number of different medications are useful for treating various symptoms of MS such as fatigue, bladder dysfunction, and spasticity, but these medications do not reverse damage that has already occurred or decrease disease activity.

Although conventional medications are able to reduce disease activity in relapsing-remitting MS, they have limitations: they have only a modest effect on prolonging time to disability; they are available in an injectable form only; the average cost is $20,000 to $30,000 per year; and they have a high incidence of side effects (e.g., injection site reactions, neutralizing antibodies). Given these consideration, identifying natural therapies that have benefit for people with MS is warranted.

The Swank Diet

Roy Swank, M.D., former professor of neurology at the University of Oregon Medical School, provided strong evidence over a lifetime of research that a diet low in saturated fats, maintained over a long period of time, tends to retard the disease process, reduce the number of attacks, and decrease mortality.[29–31] Swank began treating patients with his low-fat diet in 1948. The idea of using a low-fat diet supplemented with cod liver oil was based on population studies that found a decreased incidence of MS in populations with a low consumption of animal fats and a high consumption of cold-water fish (such as mackerel, salmon, and herring).

On the basis of our current knowledge of the disease process of MS, the rationale for using the Swank Diet or other diets low in saturated fats in patients with MS relates to the general health benefits of such a diet and the anti-inflammatory and perhaps nerve-cell-membrane-stabilizing effects of a diet rich in the long-chain omega-3 fatty acids EPA and DHA. Although red meat consumption is significantly restricted on the Swank Diet, fish is highly recommended because of its excellent protein content and, perhaps more important, its high omega-3 fatty acid content. In addition, because optimal neuronal functioning depends on cell membrane fluidity, which in turn depends on lipid composition, optimal essential fatty acid levels may have an important neuroprotective effect.[32]

Since Dr. Swank's observational studies suggesting that this diet is beneficial for patients with MS, two pilot studies evaluating diet in MS have been conducted. An open-label study looked at the effects of a diet low in saturated fats combined with fish oil supplementation, vitamin B complex, and vitamin C in newly diagnosed relapsing-remitting MS.[33] Besides dietary modifications, subjects were advised to reduce their sugar, coffee, tea, and alcohol consumption and to stop smoking. Diet was monitored over two years by dietary record, and plasma fatty acid levels were noted at baseline, year one, and year two. Patients on the diet showed a significant increase in plasma levels of omega-3 fatty acids and a significant decrease in plasma omega-6 fatty acids. They also had a significant reduction in both relapse rates and disability.

One study evaluated the effect of low-fat dietary intervention with omega-3 fatty acid supplementation in 31 MS patients.[34] Subjects were randomized into one of two groups: those on a low-fat diet (no more than 15% of calories from fat) plus fish oil (EPA 1.98 g and DHA 1.32 g per day), and those on a moderate-fat diet (no more than 30% of calories from fat) plus olive oil capsules (1 g per day). The group on the low-fat diet plus fish oil had better quality-of-life scores (as measured on a questionnaire) for physical well-being than the group taking olive oil supplementation, although the result was not statistically significant. The mental health scores were similar in the two intervention groups. The olive oil group reported an improvement in fatigue as compared with the fish oil group. For both intervention groups, relapse rates were reduced as compared with the year prior to their entering the study. This study thus suggested that a diet low in fat (especially saturated fat) with fish oil supplementation might promote better physical and mental health for people with MS.

Nutritional Supplements

Fish Oil Supplements and Other Beneficial Fats

As we have seen, there is a good rationale for supplementation with fish oil in the treatment of MS. For example, one published study documented the effects of fish oil supplementation on the production of inflammatory compounds known as cytokines in MS patients.[35] Twenty subjects with MS and 15 age-matched healthy controls were given 6 g per day of fish oil containing 3 g EPA and 1.8 g DHA for six months. All MS subjects had had a stable course of MS for at least three months before enrollment, had not modified their diet as a consequence of developing MS, and were not on any disease-modifying therapies. After three and six months of fish oil supplementation, a significant decrease in the levels of inflammatory cytokines was noted. Cytokine levels returned to baseline values when fish oil supplementation was discontinued for three months.

Another large double-blind study in which 312 MS patients were given 3.1 g EPA + DHA daily for two years reported a trend in improvement in the omega-3 group compared with controls. Although the results did not achieve statistical significance, both groups in the study were advised to follow a diet low in animal fat, and this may have affected the results.[36]

While linoleic acid—an essential omega-6 fatty acid—has shown some benefit in some (but not all) clinical trials in MS,[37] nonetheless we recommend restricting omega-6 fatty acid intake by eliminating common vegetable oils such as corn, safflower, sunflower, and soy from the diet and instead focusing on using monounsaturated oils such as olive oil and macadamia nut oil for cooking and flaxseed oil (which is high in alpha-linolenic acid, a shorter-chain omega-3 fatty acid) in salad dressing. Though evening primrose oil, which is rich in the omega-6 fatty acid gamma-linoleic acid, is commonly used by MS patients, we do not recommend it, because it is an omega-6 oil and clinical research has shown it to be of little if any benefit in MS.[38]

Vitamin D

As we have noted, population-based and clinical studies have found that low vitamin D intake and low serum vitamin D levels may increase the risk of MS.[39–41] A recent study looked at the serum vitamin D levels in 199 people with MS and found 84% of them to be deficient.[42] In addition to this circumstantial evidence, studies involving the animal model of MS have shown that vitamin D has the ability to decrease immune-cell-mediated

inflammation and prevent MS-like lesions.[43,44] The vitamin D may affect the ability of inflammatory white blood cells from entering the central nervous system.[45]

In human studies, higher levels of vitamin D are associated not only with a lower incidence of MS (in women) but also with lower levels of the inflammatory cytokines linked to MS.[46,47] Given the extremely high frequency of vitamin D deficiency in MS patients, it makes sense to evaluate serum vitamin D levels.

Alpha-Lipoic Acid

Alpha-lipoic acid (ALA) is a unique antioxidant with multiple modes of action. ALA can regenerate other antioxidants such as glutathione, vitamin C, and vitamin E; serve as a reactive oxygen species scavenger; repair oxidative damage; and chelate metallic ions involved in oxidative injury.[48–50] ALA is present in both lipid (fat) and aqueous (water) compartments of cells and exerts antioxidant effects in both locations.[51]

In studies using an animal model of MS, ALA has been shown to suppress the development of disease by preventing inflammatory immune cells from entering the central nervous system (this is similar to the way vitamin D acts).[52,53] ALA has also been shown to modulate the immune system in a manner very beneficial in MS.[54]

One double-blind study evaluated ALA in 37 MS patients. The patients were randomly assigned to one of four groups: placebo; ALA, 600 mg twice a day; ALA, 1,200 mg once a day; or ALA, 1,200 mg twice a day. The study found that ALA given at 600 mg twice a day was barely measurable in serum, while ALA given at dose of 1,200 mg showed significantly higher serum levels. The study also found an association between higher ALA serum levels and lower inflammatory mediator levels.[55]

Proteolytic Enzymes

Proteolytic enzymes (proteases) digest protein by breaking it down into smaller units. These enzymes include chymotrypsin and trypsin from pancreatin (from hog pancreas), bromelain (pineapple enzyme), papain (papaya enzyme), and fungal and bacterial proteases. Like other autoimmune diseases, MS is associated with an increased level of circulating immune complexes. Experimental and clinical studies have shown that proteolytic enzyme preparations are effective in reducing levels of circulating immune complexes in several autoimmune diseases, including MS. In the treatment of multiple sclerosis, pancreatic enzyme preparations have been shown to reduce the severity and frequency of symptom flare-ups. Especially good results were noted in cases of visual disturbance, bladder and intestinal malfunction, and sensory dis-

. . . .

QUICK REVIEW

- **Multiple sclerosis appears to be an autoimmune disease, but what triggers the autoimmune process has not been determined conclusively.**
- **Although genetics plays a role, it is clear that dietary, environmental, and lifestyle factors are required for the disease to manifest itself in most cases.**
- **Areas with the highest prevalence of MS are located in higher latitudes, in both the northern and the southern hemispheres.**
- **There is a lower risk of MS for births occurring after the summer and a higher risk of MS for births occurring after the winter, suggesting that maternal vitamin D levels during the third trimester of pregnancy may influence the risk of MS.**
- **Population-based and clinical studies have found that low vitamin D intake and low serum vitamin D levels increase the risk of MS.**
- **A high intake of saturated fats and animal fats is linked to MS.**
- **The conventional medical approach to treating MS includes the use of medications to control disease activity plus other medications and rehabilitation interventions designed to alleviate symptoms resulting from damage to the central nervous system.**
- **There is evidence that the Swank Diet (low in saturated fats), maintained over a long period of time, tends to retard the disease process, reduce the number of attacks, and decrease mortality.**
- **Alpha-lipoic acid is a unique antioxidant that may be of benefit in MS.**
- **Ginkgo biloba extract has shown a number of beneficial effects that might be helpful in MS, including an ability to improve mental function.**
- **Regular exercise is beneficial for people with MS.**
- **Hyperbaric oxygen does not seem to be warranted for treatment of MS.**

turbances. However, little effect on spasticity, dizziness, or tremor was reported.[56]

Botanical Medicines

Cognitive impairment affects up to 40 to 50% of people with MS, and ginkgo biloba extract has shown a number of beneficial effects that might be helpful in MS, including an ability to improve mental function.[57] It has also been evaluated for its effect on cognitive impairment in Alzheimer's disease, with mixed findings (see the chapter "Alzheimer's Disease"). In the only study to look at the effects of ginkgo biloba on cognitive performance in MS, 43 patients were randomly assigned to receive either 120 mg ginkgo biloba extract twice a day or a placebo for 12 weeks. Ginkgo biloba was shown to significantly improve performance on several tests that measured attention and executive function.[58]

Other Considerations

Exercise

In the past MS patients were often advised not to exercise because increased body temperature and nerve fiber fatigue resulting from exercise were thought to induce transient symptomatic worsening and provide no long-term benefit. However, research has since shown that regular exercise is beneficial for people with MS, as it leads to an improvement in feelings of fatigue, quality of life, well-being, and walking ability.[59–62] The exercise need not be strenuous: yoga, tai chi, swimming, and light exercise have shown significant benefit.[63–66]

Stress

MS patients often report that stress worsens their MS symptoms. A review of the scientific literature concluded that perceived stress is definitely associated with flare-ups of MS.[67,68] For natural ways to manage stress, see the chapter "Stress Management."

Hyperbaric Oxygen

Early reports described promising results from the use of hyperbaric (higher-pressure) oxygen in the treatment of MS. However, these reports were largely anecdotal or from uncontrolled clinical trials. The first double-blind, placebo-controlled trial of hyperbaric oxygen indicated an apparently beneficial effect in the treatment of MS.[69] Objective improvement was noted in 12 of 17 patients in the study group, compared with only 1 of 20 in the placebo group. Although the improvements were mild and transient in most of the patients, it appeared that patients with milder forms of MS and a shorter duration of disease derived a more pronounced and longer-lasting benefit. This encouraging preliminary study led to further trials on a larger number of subjects, with longer periods of follow-up. The results showed no significant improvement, apart from a subjective improvement in bowel and bladder function in one of the studies. The results from these larger, well-designed studies cast substantial doubt on the efficacy of hyperbaric oxygen in MS. Detailed reviews and analysis of the 14 controlled trials of hyperbaric oxygen treatment showed that only one of the trials produced a significant positive effect. At this time, we do not feel the evidence warrants use of hyperbaric oxygen therapy in MS.[70,71]

TREATMENT SUMMARY

Treatment of MS with diet, nutritional supplementation, exercise, and stress reduction should be the basis for the natural medicine approach to MS. Although this approach (combined therapies) has not so far been proven to be beneficial for MS in randomized, controlled trials, its individual components have shown considerable benefit, indicating that a combination of these benefits could be quite profound. (One of our major frustrations with medical research is that it studies individual therapies rather than comprehensive approaches, which are much more likely to be effective.) The natural medicine approach can be used in conjunction with conventional therapies that have been proven in controlled trials to be beneficial for MS.

Diet

Follow the general recommendations given in the chapter "A Health-Promoting Diet," while also incorporating the following features of the Swank Diet:

- Saturated fat intake: 15 g per day or less
- Unsaturated fat intake: minimum 20 g per day, maximum 50 g per day
- No red meat consumption for the first year (this includes dark meat of turkey and chicken); following the first year, only 3 oz red meat weekly
- White-meat poultry, fish, and shellfish are permissible in any amounts as long as they are low in saturated fat

- Elimination of dairy products containing 1% fat or more

Nutritional Supplements

- A high-potency multiple vitamin and mineral formula as described in the chapter "Supplementary Measures"
- Fish oils: 3,000 mg EPA + DHA per day
- Vitamin C: 500 to 1,000 mg per day
- Vitamin D_3: 2,000 to 4,000 IU per day (we strongly recommend relying on blood levels in the treatment of MS, with an ideal range of 50 to 80 ng/ml 25-hydroxyvitamin D)
- One of the following:
  - Grape seed extract (>95% procyanidolic oligomers): 150 to 300 mg per day
  - Pine bark extract (>95% procyanidolic oligomers): 150 to 300 mg per day
- Specialty supplements:
  - Alpha-lipoic acid: 600 to 1,200 mg once per day with meals
  - Proteolytic enzymes: pancreatin (10X USP) 350 to 750 mg between meals three times per day, or bromelain 250 to 750 mg (1,800 to 2,000 MCU) between meals three times per day

Botanical Medicines

- Ginkgo biloba extract (24% ginkgo flavonglycosides): 120 to 160 mg twice a day is recommended for patients with cognitive impairment

Exercise

Mild to moderate exercise for at least 30 minutes three times per week is recommended. Types of exercises recommended for MS include walking, stretching, bicycling, low-impact aerobics, stationary bicycling, swimming or water aerobics, yoga, and tai chi.

Stress Reduction

Stress reduction therapies recommended for MS include meditation, deep breathing or breathing exercises, and prayer.

Nonalcoholic Fatty Liver Disease (NAFLD)/ Nonalcoholic Steatohepatitis (NASH)

- Most patients with NAFLD have few or no symptoms.
- Patients may complain of fatigue, malaise, and dull right-upper-quadrant abdominal discomfort.
- Liver enzymes may be elevated.
- On ultrasound exam of the liver, the presence of fatty accumulations can be seen.

Non-alcoholic fatty liver disease (NAFLD) is one cause of a fatty liver, occurring when fat is deposited in the liver (steatosis), though not because of excessive alcohol use. It ranges in severity from a rather benign impairment of liver function to an inflammation of the liver referred to as nonalcoholic steatohepatitis (NASH), which may advance to cirrhosis and end-stage liver disease.

Simple steatosis is associated with obesity, occurring in 70% of patients who are 10% above ideal body weight and nearly 100% of those who are obese. In addition to obesity, NASH is also associated with other factors that impair liver function, including nutritional abnormalities, drugs, and occupational exposure to toxins.

NAFLD is thought to affect more than 20% of Americans, making it the most common liver disease in the United States. NASH affects roughly 2 to 3% of those with NAFLD, making it a major cause of cirrhosis of the liver. Almost 20% of patients with NASH progress to cirrhosis over a decade.

Causes

NAFLD is associated with insulin resistance, which may be evident as obesity, type 2 diabetes, and elevations in blood triglycerides.[1-3] When the liver is exposed to damaging compounds, such as the pro-oxidants that are seen with the inflammation accompanying insulin resistance, the first reaction is the infiltration of fat into the liver. NAFLD can also be caused by some medications:

- Amiodarone
- Antiviral drugs (nucleoside analogues)
- Aspirin (rarely, as part of Reye's syndrome in children)
- Corticosteroids

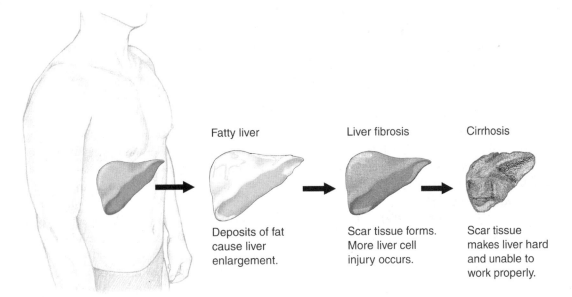

Fatty liver	Liver fibrosis	Cirrhosis
Deposits of fat cause liver enlargement.	Scar tissue forms. More liver cell injury occurs.	Scar tissue makes liver hard and unable to work properly.

Progression of NAFLD/NASH

- Diltiazem
- Methotrexate
- Nifedipine
- Tamoxifen
- Tetracycline

Therapeutic Considerations

The primary goal in most cases is improving insulin sensitivity through diet and supplementation. Weight loss is the most effective treatment for NAFLD in overweight individuals[4] (see the chapter "Obesity and Weight Management"). NAFLD patients with diabetes will need to follow the recommendations in the chapter "Diabetes."

Treatment in lean individuals with NAFLD, and a secondary treatment in overweight individuals, involves the use of liver-protecting compounds and herbal compounds that promote the flow of bile and fat to and from the liver (choleretics).

All individuals with NASH should follow the recommendations below as well as those given in the chapter "Hepatitis."

Diet

Elimination of high-glycemic-index foods is a critical step in both the prevention and the treatment of NAFLD. It is interesting to note that in one study 80% of NAFLD patients drank enough soft drinks and juices to add the equivalent of 12 tsp sugar or more to their diet.[5] The recommendations in the chapter "A Health-Promoting Diet" should be followed. In addition, special foods rich in factors that help protect the liver from damage and improve liver function include high-sulfur foods such as garlic, legumes, onions, and eggs; good sources of soluble fiber such as pears, oat bran, apples, and legumes; vegetables in the brassica family, especially broccoli, brussels sprouts, and cabbage; artichokes, beets, carrots, and dandelion; many herbs and spices such as turmeric, cinnamon, and cilantro; and green leafy vegetables that enhance detoxification processes in the liver.

Considerable research indicates an increase in iron concentration in the liver in people with NAFLD.[6–8] Given its ability to generate pro-oxidants, iron should be avoided unless there is a medical reason for iron supplementation (e.g., iron-deficiency anemia). Follow a low-iron diet and avoid iron supplements.

Nutritional Supplements

Betaine and Other Lipotropic Factors

Betaine, choline, methionine, vitamin B_6, folic acid, and vitamin B_{12} are important lipotropic agents, compounds that promote the flow of fat and bile to and from the liver. Lipotropic agents have a long history of use in naturopathic medicine; in essence, they produce a "decongesting" effect on the liver and promote improved liver function and fat metabolism. Lipotropic formulas appear to increase the levels of two important liver substances: SAM-e and glutathione.

Betaine as a single agent has been shown to be quite helpful in NAFLD when given at dosages up to 10 g twice a day.[9] However, we feel that taking a lower dosage in conjunction with other lipotropic agents is a more rational approach. Most major manufacturers of nutritional supplements offer lipotropic formulas. The important thing in taking a lipotropic formula is to take enough to provide a daily dose of 1,000 mg betaine, 1,000 mg choline, and 1,000 mg methionine and/or cysteine. Alternatively, SAM-e can be used at a dosage of 200 to 400 mg per day.

Carnitine

Our bodies can make carnitine, but sometimes we may not manufacture sufficient quantities—NAFLD may be an example. Carnitine plays an extremely important role

. . . .

QUICK REVIEW

- **Insulin resistance is the primary risk factor for NAFLD.**
- **Weight loss is the most effective treatment for NAFLD in overweight individuals.**
- **Elimination of high-glycemic foods is a critical step in both prevention and treatment of NAFLD.**
- **A diet low in iron and avoidance of iron supplements is indicated in NAFLD.**
- **Betaine, choline, methionine, vitamin B_6, folic acid, and vitamin B_{12} are important lipotropic agents.**

- **Carnitine supplementation has been shown to significantly inhibit and even reverse alcohol-induced fatty liver disease.**
- **Prescription bile acid therapy with ursodeoxycholic acid is a very important consideration, especially in NASH.**
- **Milk thistle extract protects the liver from damage, enhances detoxification processes, and increases the liver's content of glutathione—a key compound in liver function that is low in patients with NAFLD.**

in the utilization and metabolism of fatty acids in the liver as well as in the function of mitochondria, the energy-producing part of cells. Low levels of carnitine in the liver can increase susceptibility to NAFLD. Carnitine supplementation has been shown to significantly inhibit and even reverse alcohol-induced fatty liver disease.[10]

Since carnitine normally facilitates fatty acid transport and oxidation in the mitochondria, a high carnitine level may be needed to handle the increased fatty acid load produced by alcohol consumption or other liver injury. In addition to studies in NAFLD, supplemental carnitine has been shown to reduce free fatty acid levels in patients with cirrhosis and to reduce serum triglycerides and liver enzyme levels while elevating HDL cholesterol in patients with alcohol-induced fatty liver disease.[10,11]

In a recent study, 45 NAFLD patients were given either carnitine (600 mg per day) or placebo. Results demonstrated significant improvements in the carnitine group, including improvement in liver function and evidence of improved mitochondrial function.[12]

Carnitine's use in liver disorders associated with fatty infiltration, including NAFLD, is very important, especially when these changes are due to the ingestion of alcohol or exposure to toxins such as pesticides and herbicides.

Bile Acids

Bile acids are naturally occurring compounds such as ursodeoxycholic acid and taurourso-deoxycholic acid that, like the liptropic agents described above, are effective in promoting the flow of bile and fat to and from the liver. Bile acid preparations are available by prescription, but mixtures of bile acids from ox bile are available in health food stores and may prove to be suitable alternatives. Bile acids appear to be a very useful treatment for NASH. Normally, the daily dosage of ursodeoxycholic acid is 13 to 15 mg/kg.[9] However, a recent study assessed the efficacy and safety of high-dose ursodeoxycholic acid in patients with NASH.[13] This 12-month double-blind study used a daily dosage of 28 to 35 mg/kg in 126 patients with biopsy-proven NASH and elevated liver enzymes (alanine aminotransferase, ALT). The results showed that treatment with high-dose ursodeoxycholic acid was safe and improved ALT levels and other markers of liver function.

Botanical Medicines

There is a long list of plants that have beneficial effects on liver function. However, the most impressive research is with the extract of milk thistle (*Silybum marianum*) known as silymarin. The flavonoids in silymarin effectively protect the liver from damage and enhance detoxification processes, including increasing the liver's content of glutathione—a key compound in liver function that is low in patients with NAFLD. For more information on silymarin, see the chapter "Detoxification and Internal Cleansing."

TREATMENT SUMMARY

Diet

Follow the guidelines in the chapter "A Health-Promoting Diet." In addition, the recommendations in the chapter "Obesity and Weight Management" are very important.

Certain foods are particularly helpful because they contain the nutrients the liver needs to produce and activate the dozens of enzymes involved in the various phases of detoxification or aid in the effective elimination of toxins. Such foods include:

- Garlic, legumes, onions, eggs, and other foods with a high sulfur content.
- Good sources of soluble fiber, such as pears, oat bran, apples, and legumes or soluble fiber supplements such as PGX (PolyGlycopleX)
- Vegetables in the brassica family, especially broccoli, brussels sprouts, and cabbage because they aid in detoxification reactions
- Artichokes, beets, carrots, dandelion greens, and many herbs and spices such as turmeric, cinnamon, and cilantro
- Green leafy vegetables as well as green foods such as wheatgrass, barley grass, chlorella, and spirulina

Nutritional Supplements

- A high-potency multiple vitamin and mineral formula as described in the chapter "Supplementary Measures"

- Fish oils: 1,000 mg EPA + DHA
- One of the following:
  - Grape seed extract (>95% procyanidolic oligomers): 100 to 300 mg per day
  - Pine bark extract (>95% procyanidolic oligomers): 100 to 300 mg per day
  - Some other flavonoid-rich extract with a similar flavonoid content, super greens formula, or another plant-based antioxidant that can provide an oxygen radical absorption capacity (ORAC) of 3,000 to 6,000 units or higher per day
- One of the following:
  - Lipotropic formula providing 1,000 mg betaine, 1,000 mg choline, and 1,000 mg cysteine and/or methionine
  - SAM-e: 200 to 400 mg per day
  - Bile acids (mixed, from ox bile): 500 mg with meals
- PGX (PolyGlycopleX): 1,500 to 5,000 mg before meals

Botanical Medicines

- Milk thistle (*Silybum marianum*): Dosage is based on silymarin content (standardized extracts are preferred) and the best results are achieved at higher dosages, i.e., 140 mg to 210 mg silymarin three times per day; dosage for silymarin phytosome is 120 mg two to three times per day between meals.

Osteoarthritis

- Mild early-morning stiffness, stiffness following periods of rest, pain that worsens on joint use, loss of joint function
- Local tenderness, soft tissue swelling, joint crepitus (crackling sound), bony swelling, and restricted mobility
- X-ray findings (narrowed joint spaces, cartilage erosion, bone spurs, etc.)

Arthritis is inflammation of the joints. The most common form of arthritis is osteoarthritis, which is also known as degenerative joint disease because it is characterized by joint degeneration and loss of cartilage, the shock-absorbing gel-like material between joints.

The percentage of people who have osteoarthritis increases dramatically with age. Surveys have indicated that more than 40 million Americans have osteoarthritis, including 80% of those over the age of 50. Under age 45, osteoarthritis is much more common in men; after 45, it is a little more common in women.[1,2] The hands and the weight-bearing joints—knees, hips, and spine—are most often affected by the degenerative changes of osteoarthritis. These joints are under greater stress because of weight and use.

Osteoarthritis is divided into two categories: primary and secondary. In primary osteoarthritis, the degenerative wear-and-tear process occurs after the fifth or sixth decade of life, with no apparent predisposing abnormalities. The cumulative effects of decades of use leads to the degenerative changes by stressing the collagen matrix, the support structure of the cartilage. Damage to the cartilage results in the release of enzymes that destroy cartilage components. With aging, the ability to restore and synthesize normal cartilage structures decreases. The incidence of osteoarthritis increases dramatically with age and body mass index for weight-bearing joints.[1–3]

Secondary osteoarthritis is associated with some predisposing factor that is responsible for the degenerative changes.[4] Predisposing factors for secondary osteoarthritis include inherited abnormalities in joint structure or function, trauma (fractures along joint surfaces, surgery, etc.), presence of abnormal cartilage, and previous inflammatory disease of joints (rheumatoid arthritis, gout, septic arthritis, etc.).

Contributors to Osteoarthritis

Age-related changes in collagen-matrix repair mechanisms

Altered biochemistry

Fractures and mechanical damage

Genetic predisposition

Hormonal and sex factors

Hypermobility/joint instability

Inflammation

Inflammatory joint disease

Other factors

One of the most interesting clinical features of osteoarthritis is the lack of correlation between its severity as determined by X-rays and the degree of pain. In some cases the joint appears essentially normal, with little if any joint space narrowing, yet the pain can be excruciating. On the other hand, there are cases where there is tremendous deformity, yet little if any pain. In fact, about 40% of individuals with the worst X-ray classification for osteoarthritis are pain free.[5] Depression and anxiety appear to increase the perception of pain from osteoarthritis.

Therapeutic Considerations

Normally the body deals with damage to cartilage by attempting to repair itself. This damage can be halted and sometimes reversed. The major therapeutic goal should be to decrease the rate of damage and enhance the repair and regeneration of the collagen matrix.[6,7]

One group of researchers studied people with osteoarthritis of the hip over a 10-year period without treatment. All subjects had X-ray changes suggestive of advanced osteoarthritis, yet the researchers reported marked clinical improvement and X-ray evidence of repair in 14 of 31 hips over time.[8]

Conventional Drug Treatment

Nonsteroidal anti-inflammatory drugs (NSAIDs) have become the main treatment of osteoarthritis in conventional medicine. Although these drugs provide short-term symptomatic relief, they do not address the cause of the problem and may actually increase the rate of degeneration of the joint cartilage. Experimental studies have shown that aspirin and other NSAIDs inhibit collagen matrix synthesis and accelerate cartilage destruction.[9] Some retrospective clinical studies have shown that NSAID use is associated with acceleration of osteoarthritis and increased joint destruction.[10–13]

A patient is unlikely to die from osteoarthritis, but NSAID use is associated with significant risk for mortality. With older NSAIDs the risk is primarily related to gastrointestinal bleeding, while newer cyclooxygenase-2 (COX-2) inhibitors such as celecoxib (Celebrex) are associated with an increase in deaths due to heart disease.

Diet and Exercise

The key dietary focus in the prevention and treatment of osteoarthritis is the achievement of normal body weight and improvement in insulin sensitivity. Excess weight means increased stress on weight-bearing joints, and there is also considerable evidence linking osteoarthritis to insulin resistance (see the chapter "Obesity and Weight Management"). Insulin resistance not only increases inflammation but also impairs cartilage regeneration.[14] Proper sensitivity to insulin is required to signal cartilage cells to increase the synthesis and assembly of structural molecules known as proteoglycans, and the most prominent early change seen in the articular cartilage in osteoarthritis is a decrease in both proteoglycan content and structure.

Weight reduction, possibly due to a combination of mechanical and physiological factors, reduces the risk for osteoarthritis and has also been shown to reduce pain and improve cartilage function in existing osteoarthritis, especially when combined with exercise.[3,15,16] Lack of exercise decreases the hydration of the joint cartilage and retards diffusion of nutrients into the affected area. When arthritis pain develops, sufferers often tend to reduce activity, and inactivity in turn decreases muscle strength. Muscle weakness increases joint wear, and the inactivity can lead to weight gain, which can worsen osteoarthritis, causing this cycle to repeat itself. In addition, patients with diabetes and cardiovascular concerns who limit their exercise may also increase their risk related to these illnesses. Weight loss and exercise independently decrease the causative factors of osteoarthritis and produce clinical improvement, but the best results are achieved by a combined approach. One study involved 252 obese elderly patients with a body mass index greater than 28 and X-ray-confirmed osteoarthritis who were randomized into healthful-lifestyle (control), diet-only, exercise-only, and diet-plus-exercise groups.[16] The exercise program involved hour-long sessions that focused on aerobics and resistance training three times a week. The dietary interventions were intended to produce an average weight loss of 5% during the 18-month period. The most benefit was demonstrated in the diet-plus-exercise group. Compared with control patients and the diet-only group, subjects in the diet-plus-exercise group gained a significant improvement in self-reported physical function, six-minute walking distance, stair-climb times, and knee pain scores. Improvements in the exercise-only group were limited to the six-minute walking distance.

In general, the principles detailed in the chapter "A Health-Promoting Diet" are appropriate for osteoarthritis. As with other degenerative health conditions, the Mediterranean diet may show positive effects in arthritis. The Mediterranean diet includes abundant plant foods (fruits, vegetables, whole grains, beans, nuts and seeds); minimally processed, seasonal, locally grown foods; fish and poultry; olive oil as the main source of fat; and dairy products, red meat, and wine in low to moderate amounts. Thus the diet is rich in monounsaturated fatty acids, long-chain polyunsaturated fatty acids, antioxidants, and unrefined carbohydrates.

The Mediterranean diet has shown significant effects in rheumatoid arthritis in two recent studies and may show similar benefit in osteoarthritis.[17,18]

One popular dietary practice in the treatment of osteoarthritis is eliminating foods from the family Solanaceae (nightshade family). A horticulturist, Norman Childers, arrived at this method after finding that this simple dietary elimination cured his own arthritis.[19] His theory is that genetically susceptible individuals might develop arthritis and other complaints from long-term, low-level consumption of the alkaloids found in tomatoes, potatoes, eggplant, peppers, and pimento. Presumably these alkaloids inhibit normal collagen repair in the joints or promote inflammatory degeneration of the joint. Although as yet unproved, this diet has been of benefit to some individuals.

Nutritional Supplements

Glucosamine

Glucosamine sulfate has emerged as the most popular nutritional approach to osteoarthritis. It is a simple molecule composed of glucose and an amine. Its main physiological function in joints is to stimulate the manufacture of glycosaminoglycans (GAGs)—molecules that provide the structural framework of cartilage and attract water to provide the gel-like nature of cartilage. Glucosamine also promotes the incorporation of sulfur into cartilage. It appears that as some people age, they lose the ability to manufacture sufficient levels of glucosamine. The result is that cartilage loses its gel-like nature and consequently its ability to act as a shock absorber. Extensive preclinical and clinical research, including long-term double-blind studies, supports a potential role for glucosamine as a primary treatment for arthritis.

Numerous double-blind studies have

shown glucosamine to produce much better results compared with NSAIDs, placebos, or acetaminophen in relieving the pain and inflammation of osteoarthritis. While some of the studies comparing glucosamine with NSAIDs or acetaminophen show similar reductions in pain and symptom scores, only glucosamine improves indicators of joint function and markers showing improvement in cartilage structure. Typically the advantages of glucosamine over these other treatments are seen after two to four weeks of use, but there is some evidence that the longer glucosamine is used, the greater the therapeutic benefit.[20-37]

Not all studies have shown clear positive results; a few have shown no greater benefit for glucosamine over a placebo in improving symptom scores.[38-41] However, it must be kept in mind that the placebo response in osteoarthritis is quite high and may confound the true benefit of glucosamine and other approaches to osteoarthritis. Fortunately, there have been several studies showing objective improvements. The results from the two longest placebo-controlled trials show quite convincingly that glucosamine slows down the progression of osteoarthritis and in many cases produces regression of the disease, as noted by X-ray improvements, and significantly reduces the incidence of total joint replacement even as much as five years after glucosamine treatment is discontinued.[26-30]

In the first long-term study, 212 patients with knee osteoarthritis were randomly assigned 1,500 mg oral glucosamine or a placebo once per day for three years. X-rays were taken of weight-bearing joints at enrollment and after one and three years. Average joint-space width was assessed along with symptoms of pain, stiffness, and functionality.[26] The 106 patients on the placebo had progressive joint-space narrowing, with a mean joint-space loss after three years of 0.31 mm.

In the glucosamine group, no significant joint-space loss occurred. Furthermore, among patients with a greater joint-space width (over 6.2 mm), those in the placebo group demonstrated a 14.9% narrowing of joint space, while patients from the glucosamine group experienced a narrowing of only 6%.[28]

In the second long-term study, 202 patients with knee osteoarthritis were randomly assigned to receive glucosamine (1,500 mg once per day) or a placebo.[27] Changes in CAT scan and symptom scores were used to judge efficacy. Symptoms improved more significantly in the glucosamine group, but the most telling result was the fact that joint space narrowed 0.19 mm with placebo use, while there was as actually an 0.04-mm increase in joint space with glucosamine use.

Of 414 participants in the two long-term studies, 319 were postmenopausal women. After three years, postmenopausal participants in the glucosamine group showed no joint space narrowing, whereas participants in the placebo group experienced a narrowing of 0.33 mm.[29] After three years, the glucosamine group showed a 14.1% improvement in symptom scores, while the placebo group actually worsened by 5.4%. These results may indicate that postmenopausal women may be especially responsive to glucosamine.[28]

Several head-to-head, double-blind studies have shown glucosamine to produce much better results compared with NSAIDs and analgesics in relieving the pain and inflammation of osteoarthritis, despite the fact that glucosamine exhibits little direct anti-inflammatory effect and no direct analgesic or pain-relieving effects.[31-37] As we have noted, NSAIDs and analgesics such as acetaminophen offer purely symptomatic relief, and NSAIDs may actually promote the disease process; by contrast, glucosamine appears to address the cause of osteoarthritis by promoting joint repair, thus relieving symptoms. The clinical effect is impressive, especially when glucosamine's safety and lack of side effects are considered.

In one of the earlier comparative studies in which glucosamine (1,500 mg per day) was compared with ibuprofen (1,200 mg per day), pain scores decreased faster in the first two weeks in the ibuprofen group. However, by week four the group receiving glucosamine experienced a significantly better improvement than the ibuprofen group.[31] Physicians rated the overall response as good in 44% of the glucosamine-treated patients as compared with only 15% of the ibuprofen group.

Additional studies designed to further evaluate the comparative effectiveness of glucosamine and NSAIDs provide even better evidence.[32–37] One study consisted of 200 subjects with osteoarthritis of the knee who were given either glucosamine (500 mg three times per day) or ibuprofen (400 mg three times per day) for four weeks.[32] Consistently with previous studies, the ibuprofen group experienced quicker pain relief. However, by the end of the second week, the group taking glucosamine experienced results as good as those of the ibuprofen group. In addition, although the side effects of glucosamine were mild and affected only 6% of the group, ibuprofen produced more significant side effects much more frequently, with 35% of the group experiencing them.

Glucosamine was shown to offer significant benefit in an open trial involving 1,506 patients in Portugal.[42] The patients received 500 mg glucosamine three times per day over a mean period of 50 days. Symptoms of pain at rest, on standing, and during exercise, as well as in limited active and passive movements, all improved steadily throughout the treatment period. Objective therapeutic efficacy was rated by doctors as "good" in 59% of the patients and "sufficient" in a further 36%.

Although this was not a controlled study, a 95% response rate is impressive. The results with glucosamine were rated by both doctors and patients as being significantly better than those obtained with previous treatment including NSAIDs, vitamin therapy, and cartilage extracts. Glucosamine produced good benefit in a significant portion of patients who had not responded to any other medical treatment. The improvement with glucosamine lasted for 6 to 12 weeks after the end of treatment. Obesity was associated with a significant shift from a "good" to a "sufficient" outcome. This finding may indicate that higher dosages may be required for obese individuals or that glucosamine is not enough to counteract the added stress of obesity on the joints. Patients with peptic ulcers and patients taking diuretics were also associated with a shift from "good" to "sufficient" in efficacy as well as tolerance. Individuals with current peptic ulcers should take glucosamine with foods. People taking diuretics may need to increase the dosage to compensate for the reduced effectiveness.

Glucosamine may also have a role as a preventive measure against the development of osteoarthritis, especially in athletes subjected to joint strain. One study to investigate the cartilage-protective action of glucosamine in athletes compared biomarkers for cartilage breakdown and manufacture in soccer players and nonathlete controls before and after they took glucosamine or a placebo. Based on the ratio of cartilage breakdown to manufacture, it was concluded that glucosamine exerts a cartilage-protective effect in athletes by preventing cartilage degradation but maintaining cartilage synthesis.[43]

Glucosamine only mildly affects the speed of recovery from an injury. In a study of 106 male athletes after acute knee injury who were given either glucosamine (1,500 mg per day) or a placebo for 28 days, no significant dif-

Results of a Double-Blind Study of Glucosamine vs. Ibuprofen[34]			
TIME	**GLUCOSAMINE**		**IBUPROFEN**
Knee Pain (Average Score)			
Before treatment	8.42		8.46
Week 2	5.54		5.63
Week 4	3.60		4.18
2 weeks after treatment	3.26		3.84
Knee Swelling (Average Score)			
Before treatment	1.43		1.48
Week 2	0.77		0.89
Week 4	0.47		0.48
2 weeks after treatment	0.36		0.54
Clinical Improvement			
	Glucosamine		Ibuprofen	
Effectiveness	After 4 Weeks (%)	After 6 Weeks (%)	After 4 Weeks (%)	After 6 Weeks (%)
Symptom free	45	55	32	36
Improved	39	32	45	41
Unchanged	11	7	15	14
Worsened	5	6	8	9
Side Effects			
	Glucosamine Sulfate		Ibuprofen	
Side effects	6%		16%	
Dropouts	0%		10%	

ference was found between the glucosamine group and the placebo group in pain intensity scores for resting and walking, or in degree of knee swelling, at the 7-day, 14-day, 21-day, and 28-day assessments. The only finding that placed glucosamine over the placebo was in knee flexibility after 28 days of treatment.[44] For more information on natural approaches for acute sports injuries, see the chapter "Sports Injuries, Tendinitis, and Bursitis."

The standard dosage for glucosamine is 1,500 mg per day. It may be administered as a single dose or divided doses with equal effectiveness. Obese individuals may need higher dosages, based on their body weight (e.g., 20 mg/kg per day). Also, individuals taking diuretics may need to take higher dosages. Athletes or individuals who subject their joints to greater wear and tear may need to increase the dosage to 3,000 mg to maintain positive cartilage synthesis.

Glucosamine sulfate appears to be more effective than glucosamine hydrochloride. Unfortunately several large, well-publicized studies have utilized the hydrochloride form. For example, the Glucosamine/Chondroitin Arthritis Intervention Trial involved 1,583 patients with symptomatic knee osteoarthritis.[45,46] Patients were randomly assigned to receive 1,500 mg glucosamine hydrochloride per day, 1,200 mg chondroitin sulfate per day, both glucosamine hydrochloride and chondroitin sulfate, 200 mg celecoxib per day, or a placebo. Overall, glucosamine hydrochloride and chondroitin sulfate were not significantly better than the placebo in reducing knee pain by 20%.

Glucosamine sulfate has an excellent safety record in animal and human studies. On the basis of these studies, many experts have recommended that glucosamine be considered as a preferred treatment for osteoarthritis. Side effects, when they do appear, are generally limited to light to moderate gastrointestinal symptoms, including stomach upset, heartburn, diarrhea, nausea, and indigestion. If these symptoms occur, glucosamine should be taken with meals.

Some people are sulfur-sensitive and may worry about taking glucosamine sulfate. However, an important distinction needs to be made. When patients report that they are allergic to sulfur, what they usually mean is that they are allergic to sulfa drugs or sulfite-containing food additives. It is impossible to be allergic to sulfur, as sulfur is an essential mineral. The sulfate form of sulfur is present in human blood. In short, glucosamine is extremely well tolerated, and only a few allergic reactions have been reported, although millions of people take glucosamine.

Concern has been expressed that glucosamine may influence insulin secretion or action, or both. This concern is based primarily on in vitro studies with high concentrations of glucosamine that are impossible to achieve with oral supplementation at recommended dosages. Detailed human studies show glucosamine has no impact on insulin secretion or action in healthy subjects, those with type 2 diabetes, or those with insulin resistance.[47–50] In fact, in long-term studies, glu-

cosamine actually produced a nonsignificant lowering of fasting blood glucose concentrations in all groups of subjects.[50]

Glucosamine may potentiate the effect of warfarin (Coumadin). The World Health Organization adverse drug reactions database documented 21 spontaneous case reports in which glucosamine interfered with warfarin; 17 of these resolved when glucosamine was stopped. Given the widespread use of glucosamine, this potentiation does not appear to be a significant concern. Nonetheless, patients using both warfarin and glucosamine should be monitored by a physician.[51]

Chondroitin

Chondroitin sulfate (as well as shark cartilage, bovine cartilage extracts, and sea cucumber) contains a mixture of intact or partially hydrolyzed GAGs. Chondroitin sulfate is composed of repeating units of derivatives of glucosamine sulfate with attached sugar molecules. Although the absorption rate of glucosamine sulfate is 90% to 98%, the absorption of intact chondroitin sulfate is estimated to be much lower, anywhere from 0% to 13%.[52–54] The difference in absorption is largely due to the difference in size. A molecule of chondroitin sulfate is at least 50 to 300 times larger than a molecule of glucosamine sulfate—too large to pass through the normal intact intestinal barrier or into cartilage cells. These absorption problems suggest that any direct effect of these compounds in osteoarthritis is highly unlikely. Furthermore, chondroitin sulfate levels are typically elevated in the synovial tissues in patients with osteoarthritis.[55] Any clinical benefit from chondroitin sulfate is most likely due to the absorption of sulfur or smaller GAG molecules broken down by the digestive tract. However, even this is controversial, as in one human study, 1 g chondroitin sulfate failed to increase serum GAG concentration at all. These results prompted the researchers to conclude that oral chondroitin has no effect on cartilage.[56,57]

Despite the fact that direct action by the chondroitin molecule is unlikely, one study using 800 mg chondroitin sulfate for two separate periods of three months over the course of one year showed decreased pain and improved knee function, as well as a decrease in the progression of joint space reduction.[58] This study reveals that even intermittent use of chondroitin may be effective.

The clinical studies that have been done with orally administered chondroitin sulfate demonstrate that it is less effective than glucosamine sulfate.[59–64] Furthermore, there is no evidence that using glucosamine and chondroitin together is more effective than using either alone. In general, the more impressive results have been achieved with glucosamine sulfate. Nevertheless, given the safety record of chondroitin and evidence that it may modify joint space pathology, chondroitin is a reasonable addition to an osteoarthritis patient's glucosamine regimen. Although it has no apparent direct action, chondroitin may provide a modest benefit by exerting some indirect effect on improving joint health (see next section).

Hyaluronic Acid

Hyaluronic acid is an important GAG in joints, where it provides a structural framework and affects the ability of the cartilage to hold water. By the time most people reach the age of 70, the hyaluronic acid content in their body has dropped by 80% from when they were 40, predisposing them to a decrease in connective tissue integrity, particularly in the skin and joints. Weekly injections of hyaluronic acid (Synvisc, Hyalgan, Supartz, etc.) into joints affected by osteoarthritis have been shown to be an effective treatment, with improvement noted in pain, function, and patients' self-assessment at different postinjection periods, but especially at 5 to 13 weeks postinjection.[65]

Oral supplementation with hyaluronic acid has been shown to be a practical method of increasing body hyaluronic acid stores. Supplements feature hyaluronic acid derived either from animal sources or from bacterial fermentation.

Two double-blind, placebo-controlled studies have been done on the effects of hyaluronic acid in osteoarthritis. In the first, 20 patients with knee osteoarthritis were given either hyaluronic acid (80 mg per day) or a placebo for eight weeks.[66] Compared with the placebo group, pain scores were significantly improved in the hyaluronic acid group. In the second study, 60 patients with osteoarthritis were randomized to receive either 200 mg hyaluronic acid, 100 mg hyaluronic acid, or a placebo for eight weeks.[67] Significant reductions in pain scores and total symptom scores were seen with the 200-mg dosage but not with the 100-mg dosage.

Niacinamide

In the 1940s and 1950s Dr. William Kaufman, and later Dr. Abram Hoffer, reported good clinical results in the treatment of hundreds of patients with rheumatoid arthritis and osteoarthritis using high-dose niacinamide (900 to 4,000 mg per day in divided doses).[68,69] Dr. Kaufman documented improvements in joint function, range of motion, muscle strength and endurance, and sedimentation rate. Most patients achieved noticeable benefits within one to three months of use, with peak benefits noted between one and three years of continuous use.

These clinical results were more rigorously evaluated in the 1990s in a well-designed, double-blind, placebo-controlled trial.[70]

Seventy-two patients with osteoarthritis were randomized for treatment with niacinamide (3,000 mg per day in divided dosages) or a placebo for 12 weeks. Outcome measures included global arthritis impact and pain, joint range of motion and flexibility, erythrocyte sedimentation rate, complete blood count, liver function tests, serum cholesterol, serum uric acid, and fasting blood sugar. The researchers found that niacinamide produced a 29% improvement in global arthritis impact, compared with a 10% worsening in the placebo group. Pain levels did not change, but those on niacinamide reduced their NSAID use. Niacinamide supplementation reduced the sedimentation rate by 22% and increased joint mobility by 4.5 degrees over controls (8 degrees vs. 3.5 degrees). There were no other changes in blood chemistry. Side effects, primarily mild gastrointestinal complaints, were more common in the niacinamide group but could be effectively managed by taking the pills with food or fluids.

Niacinamide at this high dose can result in significant side effects (e.g., glucose intolerance, liver damage) and therefore requires strict medical supervision—at the very least regular blood tests to assess liver damage.

S-adenosyl-methionine (SAM-e)

S-adenosyl-methionine (SAM-e) is an important substance that the body forms by combining the essential amino acid methionine with adenosine triphosphate. A deficiency of SAM-e in the joint tissue, just like a deficiency of glucosamine, leads to loss of the gel-like nature and shock-absorbing qualities of cartilage. A detailed analysis of 11 studies reports that SAM-e reduces pain and functional limitations in patients with osteoarthritis.[71]

SAM-e has been shown to be important in the manufacture of cartilage components.[72] In one double-blind study, supplemental SAM-e increased cartilage formation, as determined by MRI, in 14 patients with arthritis of the hands.[73] In addition to this effect, SAM-e has also demonstrated some mild pain-relieving and anti-inflammatory effects in animal studies.

In double-blind trials, SAM-e has produced reductions in pain scores and in clinical symptoms similar to the reductions seen with NSAIDs such as ibuprofen, indomethacin, naproxen, and piroxicam.[71–82] All of these studies indicate that SAM-e offers significant advantages over NSAIDs. The drugs are associated with a significant risk of toxicity, side effects, and actual promotion of the disease process in osteoarthritis, while SAM-e offers similar benefits with minimal risk and minimal side effects. Side effects are uncommon but can include occasional gastrointestinal disturbances, mainly diarrhea. As with glucosamine sulfate, its major benefit is enhancing cartilage regeneration rather than simply relieving symptoms.

Vitamin C

Results from the Framingham Osteoarthritis Cohort Study indicate that a high intake of antioxidant nutrients, especially vitamin C, may reduce the risk of cartilage loss and disease progression in people with osteoarthritis.[83] A threefold reduction in the risk of osteoarthritis progression was found with higher vitamin C intake. These results highlight the importance of a diet rich in plant-based antioxidant nutrients for protection against chronic degenerative diseases, including arthritis.

Low intake of vitamin C is common in the elderly, resulting in altered collagen synthesis and compromised connective tissue repair.[84,85] Several test tube studies have demonstrated that vitamin C has an anabolic effect on cartilage.[86,87] Research has confirmed the importance of—indeed, necessity for—vitamin C in human cartilage cell protein synthesis.[87] A study showed that people who reported a history of vitamin C supplementation saw a halt in the progression of their osteoarthritis.[88] Vitamins C and E appear to possess synergistic effects in osteoarthritis.[84]

Vitamin D

Several studies have shown that low serum levels of vitamin D appear to be associated with an increased risk for progression of osteoarthritis, especially in people under 60 years of age.[89–91] In one study of people undergoing hip replacement, patients with vitamin D deficiency had lower hip function scores before surgery and were significantly less likely to see an excellent outcome after surgery.[91] Low serum levels of vitamin D also predict loss of cartilage, as assessed by loss of joint space and increase in bony growths. It seems reasonable to consider that exposure to adequate amounts of sunlight, as well as sufficient intake of vitamin D in childhood and young adulthood, may help decrease the risk of osteoarthritis. It is not known, however, whether increasing vitamin D intake will help decrease or reverse already established arthritis.

Vitamins A and E, Pyridoxine, Zinc, Copper, and Boron

These nutrients are required for the synthesis of collagen and maintenance of normal cartilage structures. A deficiency of any one of these would allow accelerated joint degeneration. In addition, supplementation at appropriate levels may promote cartilage repair and synthesis.

For example, boron supplementation has been used in the treatment of osteoarthritis in Germany since the mid-1970s. This use was recently evaluated in a small, double-blind clinical study and an open trial. In the double-blind study, of the patients given 6 mg boron, 71% improved, compared with only 10% in the placebo group.[92] In the open trial, boron supplementation (6 to 9 mg per day) produced effective relief in 90% of arthritis patients, including patients with osteoarthritis, juvenile arthritis, and rheumatoid arthritis.[93] The preliminary indication is that boron supplements are of value in arthritis, with many osteoarthritis patients experiencing complete resolution of symptoms.

Vitamin K

Studies have shown that low vitamin K status is associated with knee osteoarthritis,[94,95] so vitamin K may offer some protection against arthritis. Foods rich in vitamin K include green tea, kale, turnip greens, spinach, and other green leafy vegetables.

Botanical Medicines

Historically, many herbs have been used in the treatment of osteoarthritis.

Curcumin

Curcumin is the yellow pigment of turmeric (*Curcuma longa*). It may be helpful in osteoarthritis due to a variety of anti-inflammatory effects.[96] One concern regarding curcumin has been absorption, but there now exist a number of methods and products that enhance absorption. One of those methods involves complexing the curcumin with soy phospholipids to produce a product sold as Meriva. Absorption studies in animals indicate that peak plasma levels of curcumin after administration of Meriva were five times higher than those after administration of regular curcumin.[97] Studies with another advanced form of curcumin, Theracurmin, show even better absorption (27 times greater than regular curcumin).[98]

Meriva has been used in two studies of patients with osteoarthritis. In the first study, 50 patients were given 1,000 mg Meriva (providing 200 mg curcumin) for three months, after which symptom scores decreased by 58%, walking distance in the treadmill test was prolonged from 76 meters to 332 meters, and the level of an inflammatory marker (CRP) in the blood decreased from 168 to 11.3 mg/l in the subgroup of patients with high CRP.[99] In the second study, 100 patients with osteoarthritis were given 1,000 mg Meriva for eight months. Just as in the previous study, symptom scores, walking distance, and blood measurements of inflammation were significantly improved.[100]

Boswellia

Boswellia (*Boswellia serrata*), a large branching tree native to India, yields a gum resin known as salai guggul that has been used for centuries for arthritic and other conditions. Newer preparations concentrated for the active components (boswellic acids) are showing significant clinical results. Initially, boswellic acid extracts demonstrated antiarthritic effects in various animal models. Among several mechanisms of action are inhibition of inflammatory mediators, prevention of decreased GAG synthesis, and improved blood supply to joint tissues.[101,102] Clinical studies using herbal formulas with boswellia have yielded good results in osteoarthritis of the knee, with patients experiencing decreased knee pain, decreased swelling, and increased knee flexion and walking distance.[103–106] Corroborating the improvements in pain scores and joint function were significant reductions in cartilage breakdown products, indicating

improved collagen matrix stability. No side effects due to boswellic acids have been reported.

Procyanidolic Oligomers

Procyanidolic oligomers are among the most useful plant flavonoids. Grape seed and pine bark extract (e.g., Pycnogenol) are two popular commercial sources, but these compounds are also found in many foods, especially berries. Two double-blind studies have been conducted using Pycnogenol for osteoarthritis and showing very good effects. In the first study, Pycnogenol (100 mg per day) or a placebo was given for three months to 156 patients with osteoarthritis.[107] Overall signs and symptoms of osteoarthritis decreased by 56% in the treatment group vs. 9.6% in the placebo group. Walking distance in the treadmill test was prolonged from 68 meters at the start to 198 meters in the Pycnogenol group, compared with an increase from 65 meters to 88 meters in the placebo group. The use of drugs decreased by 58% in the Pycnogenol group vs. 1% in the placebo group. Foot swelling decreased in 79% of the Pycnogenol patients vs. 1% of the controls. Similar results were seen in a second study when Pycnogenol was given at the same dosage.[108]

Ginger

Ginger (*Zingiber officinalis*) exerts some anti-inflammatory effects. In a six-week study of 261 patients with knee osteoarthritis given ginger extract or a placebo, a moderate effect on symptoms was seen: 63% of the ginger group found relief vs. 50% of the placebo group.[109] Those in the ginger group resorted to acetaminophen less frequently and had a reduction in knee pain on standing and after walking. Patients receiving ginger extract did experience more gastrointestinal adverse events than did the placebo group (59 patients vs. 21 patients), though the problems were mild. One double-blind crossover trial found ginger (170 mg three times per day) to be effective before the crossover, but by the end of the study, there was no benefit of ginger over the placebo.[110] Clearly, more studies are necessary to assess ginger's effectiveness for osteoarthritis.

Devil's Claw

Devil's claw (*Harpagophytum procumbens*) is a South African plant that grows in regions bordering the Kalahari Desert. Extracts of the root are usually standardized for harpagosides, the principal active compound. A systematic review of the clinical efficacy of devil's claw concluded that products providing less than 30 mg harpagosides per day were of little benefit in the treatment of knee and hip osteoarthritis, while dosages providing 60 mg harpagoside per day showed moderate evidence of efficacy in the treatment of spine, hip, and knee osteoarthritis.[111] Some of the individual studies showed significant benefit. For example, in a two-month double-blind study of spine and knee osteoarthritis, 670 mg devil's claw powder three times a day was more effective than a placebo in reducing pain scores.[112] In a four-month double-blind study of hip and knee osteoarthritis, 2.6 g devil's claw powder per day was equal in efficacy to 200 mg diacerhein per day in improving pain scores but was better tolerated than the drug.[113] In a review of 28 clinical trials of devil's claw extract, adverse events occurred at a rate of about 3% and did not exceed the rate of side effects experienced with placebos.[114] Long-term use appears to be safe.

Topical Analgesics

The mainstays of natural topical preparations for osteoarthritis are those containing menthol-related compounds, One popular combination contains 4% camphor, 10% menthol, and 30% methyl salicylate and/or capsaicin (typically creams contain 0.075% capsaicin). These time-tested and clinically proved topical analgesics can often provide significant relief in arthritis. An alternative are products containing Celadrin, a mixture of cetylated fatty acids. Celadrin has been shown to affect several key factors that contribute to inflammation. Its main action appears to be its ability to enhance cell membrane health and integrity. As a result, it halts the production of inflammatory compounds known as prostaglandins. It also reduces the production of negative immune factors such as IL-6 that play a central role in inflammation. Studies have assessed both the oral and the topical use of Celadrin. In a study with oral Celadrin, 64 patients with chronic osteoarthritis of the knee were evaluated at baseline and at 30 and 68 days. Results indicated that compared with a placebo, Celadrin improves knee range of motion.[115]

The effect of Celadrin cream was studied in osteoarthritis of the knees. Forty patients were randomly assigned to receive either the Celadrin cream or a placebo. Patients were tested on three occasions: baseline, 30 minutes after initial treatment, and after 30 days of treatment in which the cream was applied twice per day. Assessments included knee range of motion, timed "up-and-go" from a chair, timed stair climbing, and two other functional tests. For stair climbing ability and the up-and-go test, significant decreases in time were observed 30 minutes after the first administration and after one month of use only in the Celadrin group. Likewise, range of motion of the knees increased with Celadrin, both 30 minutes after the initial application and after one month's use. In contrast, no difference was observed in the placebo group. The other functional tests also clearly demonstrated improvements with

Celadrin, while the placebo failed to produce results.[116]

In another study involving patients with knee osteoarthritis, patients were assessed by having them stand on a special platform for 20 and 40 seconds to measure their ability to stand comfortably in one place for a period of time. Again, only those subjects using the Celadrin cream demonstrated improvements.[117]

One of the significant features of Celadrin is that, unlike many other natural approaches, it produces almost immediate results.

Physical Therapy

Joint misalignment stresses joints and increases the risk for osteoarthritis. Although this concept is relatively simple, it is only recently that it has been investigated scientifically. An 18-month study of 230 patients with osteoarthritis of the knee and at least some difficulty with activity requiring movement of the knee revealed conclusively that bowlegged patients had a fourfold increased risk of osteoarthritis progression on the inner side of the knee.[118] Similarly, knock-kneed patients showed almost five times the risk of osteoarthritis progression on the outer side of the knee. Not surprisingly, the greater the misalignment, the more severe the arthritis. Individuals with misalignments may need to consider chiropractic or osteopathic treatment, as well as orthotics.

Various physical therapy modalities (e.g., exercise, heat, cold, diathermy, ultrasound) are often beneficial in improving joint mobility and reducing pain in osteoarthritis, especially when administered regularly. Much of the benefit of physical therapy is thought to be a result of achieving proper hydration within the joint capsule.

Clinical and experimental studies seem to indicate that short-wave diathermy may be of the greatest benefit.[119–121] Combining short-wave diathermy therapy with periodic ice massage, rest, and appropriate exercises appears to be the most effective approach. Ultrasound and laser therapy have also been shown to be helpful.[122,123]

The best exercises are isometrics and swimming. These types of exercises increase circulation to the joint and strengthen surrounding muscles without placing excessive strain on joints. Increasing quadriceps strength has been shown to improve the clinical features and reduce pain in osteoarthritis of the knee.[124] Walking programs help to improve functional status and relieve pain in patients with arthritis of the knee.[125] Patient-specific physical therapies may also be useful. For example, four older adults with hand osteoarthritis benefited from keyboard playing for 20 minutes a day, four days a week.[126]

Effective Nonpharmacological Approaches to Pain in Osteoarthritis

Acupuncture

Diathermy

Exercise

Laser therapy

Magnetic therapy

Massage

Physical therapy

Psychological aids

Thermal baths

Transcutaneous nerve stimulation (TENS)

Ultrasound

Weight loss

Acupuncture and Electroacupuncture

Acupuncture has been shown to be safe and effective in reducing pain from osteoarthritis.[127,128] Other studies have shown very good results with either electroacupuncture or transcutaneous electrical nerve stimulation (TENS) in relieving pain due to arthritis, but only electroacupuncture improved joint function.[129] Electroacupuncture has also been tested against the NSAID diclofenac in a head-to-head, 186-patient controlled trial.[130] For these knee patients, improvement of osteoarthritis symptoms was greatest in the electroacupuncture group. Unlike the diclofenac and placebo groups, most of the patients receiving electroacupuncture rated their results

as "much better," and substantially better pain management and functionality were obtained in the electroacupuncture group as well.

Magnetic Therapy

Magnetic therapy has been used in the treatment of a wide variety of chronic pain syndromes.[131] A number of studies clearly support magnetic therapy used for knee osteoarthritis.[132–135] One double-blind trial enrolled 75 patients with osteoarthritis of

· ·

QUICK REVIEW

- **Osteoarthritis is the most common cause of arthritis.**
- **NSAIDs appear to suppress the symptoms of osteoarthritis but accelerate its progression.**
- **The key dietary focus in the prevention and treatment of osteoarthritis is the achievement of normal body weight and improvement in insulin sensitivity.**
- **The Mediterranean diet may show positive effects in osteoarthritis.**
- **One popular dietary practice in the treatment of osteoarthritis is eliminating foods from the family Solanaceae (nightshade family).**
- **Numerous double-blind studies have shown that glucosamine produces much better results compared with NSAIDs, placebos, or acetaminophen in relieving the pain and inflammation of osteoarthritis.**
- **Clinical studies suggest that orally administered chondroitin is less effective than glucosamine.**

- **A high intake of antioxidant nutrients, especially vitamin C, may reduce the risk of cartilage loss and disease progression in people with osteoarthritis.**
- **Meriva, a special form of curcumin bound to phosphatidylcholine to improve absorption, has been shown in two double-blind studies to produce benefits in osteoarthritis.**
- **Two double-blind studies have been conducted with Pycnogenol, showing very good effects in osteoarthritis.**
- **Natural topical preparations for osteoarthritis (menthol, capsaicin, or Celadrin) can reduce inflammation.**
- **Joint misalignment stresses joints and increases the risk for osteoarthritis.**
- **Physical therapy (e.g., exercise, heat, cold, diathermy, ultrasound, acupuncture, TENS, and electroacupuncture) can improve joint mobility and reduce pain in osteoarthritis.**

the knee who had previously been unable to obtain acceptable results using conventional treatments.[134] Low-frequency pulsed magnetic fields produced notable improvements in pain, functionality, and physician evaluation of patients' condition. Mean morning stiffness also decreased by 20 minutes in the group using magnetic therapy, while increasing by 2 minutes in the placebo group. A second double-blind study of 176 patients with knee osteoarthritis also showed significant results from using low-amplitude and low-frequency fields.[135] Reduction in pain after a treatment session was significantly greater in the magnet-on group (46%) compared with the magnet-off group (8%). A smaller, 29-subject study of knee osteoarthritis used either high-strength magnetic or a placebo knee-sleeve treatment for four hours in a monitored setting and self-treatment six hours per day for six weeks.[135] This study demonstrated a significant decrease in pain scores in the treatment group and only a minimal improvement in the placebo group after four hours of treatment, but no sig-nificant differences after six weeks of self-treatment—indicating either that monitored treatment is more effective or that the benefits subside with time. Nonetheless, there is evidence that magnetic therapies may be a useful treatment for arthritis.

Relaxation Techniques

Relaxation techniques such as meditation, deep breathing, and guided imagery have been used for many types of pain conditions. A study of 66 elderly people suffering from chronic osteoarthritis pain evaluated the effect of daily music listening on pain levels.[136] Differences in perceptions of pain were measured over 14 days in experimental subjects who listened to Mozart selections for 20 minutes per day and control subjects who sat quietly for 20 minutes per day. Those who listened to music had less pain when compared with those who sat quietly and did not listen to music. The amount of pain perceived by the Mozart group also decreased incrementally over the 14-day study period.

TREATMENT SUMMARY

The natural approach to osteoarthritis is a rational program based on reducing joint stress and trauma, promoting collagen repair mechanisms, and eliminating foods and other factors that may inhibit normal collagen repair. NSAIDs should be avoided as much as possible. If you must take NSAIDs, also take deglycyrrhizinated *Glycyrrhiza glabra* (DGL) to help protect the gastrointestinal tract, and discontinue use of the NSAIDs as soon as possible.

Diet

Achieving ideal body weight is the primary dietary goal; see the chapter "Obesity and Weight Management." The general recommendations in the chapter "A Health-Promoting Diet" are appropriate here as well. In addition, some people have reported benefits by eliminating plants of the Solanaceae family (tomatoes, potatoes, eggplant, peppers, etc.). Regular consumption of flavonoid-rich berries and naturally occurring vitamin C sources such as broccoli, dark leafy greens (kale, mustard greens, spinach, etc.), and citrus fruit is important, as is consuming a Mediterranean-type diet.

Nutritional Supplements

- A high-potency multiple vitamin and mineral formula as described in the chapter "Supplementary Measures"
- Key individual nutrients:
  - Vitamin B_6: 50 mg per day
  - Vitamin K: 100 mcg per day
  - Zinc: 30 to 45 mg per day
  - Copper: 0.5 to 1 mg per day
  - Boron: 6 mg per day
  - Vitamin C: 500 to 1,000 mg per day
  - Selenium: 100 to 200 mcg per day
  - Vitamin E (mixed tocopherols): 100 to 200 IU per day
  - Vitamin D_3: 2,000 to 4,000 IU per day
- Fish oils: 1,000 mg EPA + DHA per day
- One of the following:
  - Grape seed extract (>95% procyanidolic oligomers): 100 to 300 mg per day
  - Pine bark extract (>95% procyanidolic oligomers): 100 to 300 mg per day
  - Some other flavonoid-rich extract with a similar flavonoid content, super greens formula, or another plant-based antioxidant that can provide an oxygen radical absorption capacity (ORAC) of 3,000 to 6,000 units or higher per day

- Specialty supplements (begin with glucosamine; if no benefit is seen after four to six weeks, add SAM-e, followed by hyaluronic acid, and then niacinamide):
  - Glucosamine sulfate: 1,500 mg per day (dosages up to 3,000 mg per day may be necessary in obese individuals, those on diuretics, and athletes or individuals who are subjecting their joints to greater wear and tear)
  - SAM-e: 200 to 400 mg three times per day
  - Hyaluronic acid: 100 to 200 mg per day
  - Niacinamide: 1,000 mg three times per day (under medical supervision; liver enzymes must be regularly checked)

Botanical Medicines

One or more of the following:

- Curcumin:
  - Meriva: 500 to 1,000 mg twice daily
  - BCM95 Complex: 750 to 1,500 mg twice daily
  - Theracurmin: 300 mg one to three times daily
- Boswellia extract: equivalent of 400 mg boswellic acids three times per day
- Ginger: 8 to 10 g dried powdered ginger or ginger extracts standardized to contain 20% gingerol and shogaol at a dosage of 100 to 200 mg three times per day
- Devil's claw:
  - Dried root powder (tablet or capsule): 2,000 mg three times per day
  - Fluid extract (1:1): 2 ml three times per day

○ Dry powdered extract (standardized to contain 2.5% harpagosides): 750 to 1,000 mg three times per day

Topical Treatments

One of the following, applied to affected areas twice per day:

- Menthol preparations
- Capsaicin preparations
- Cetylated fatty acid cream (Celadrin)

Exercise

Physical activity that causes too much strain on affected joints should be avoided. Make sure you maintain good posture, and if you have any structural abnormalities (e.g., bowlegs, knock-knees), see an orthopedist; these measures will help limit joint strain. The best exercises are isometrics, walking, and swimming.

Physical Therapy and Acupuncture

Various physical therapy modalities such as exercise, heat, cold, diathermy, ultrasound, acupuncture, TENS, and electro-acupuncture often improve joint mobility and reduce pain in osteoarthritis.

Osteoporosis

- Usually without symptoms until severe backache or hip fracture occurs
- Most common in postmenopausal white women
- Spontaneous fractures of the hip and vertebrae
- Decrease in height
- Demineralization of spine and pelvis, as confirmed by bone mineral density test

Osteoporosis literally means "porous bone." It is the most common bone disease in humans and poses a serious health threat for many postmenopausal women. It is characterized by diminished bone strength, which leads to an increased risk of fracture. Osteoporosis is now determined primarily by bone mineral density (BMD) testing and is defined by BMD scores less than or equal to a standard deviation of –2.5 at the total hip, femoral neck, or lumbar spine.[1,2]

Osteoporosis most commonly occurs in postmenopausal women, and the risk increases with age. Although the prevalence is 4% in women between 50 and 59 years of age, it rises to 52% in women age 80 and above.[3] Osteoporosis of the hip occurs in 13% to 18% of white American women, and another 37% to 50% have low bone mass (often called osteopenia) of the hip.[4]

The big consequence of osteoporosis is fractures. It is estimated that osteoporosis causes approximately 1.5 million fractures every year. Of these, 250,000 are fractures of the hip.[5,6] Even with considerable advances in medical care, up to 20% of women with hip fractures still die within a year of the fracture, and an additional 25% require long-term nursing care. Approximately half the women who suffer from a hip fracture are permanently unable to walk without the assistance of a cane or walker. The hip is not the only site where fractures result in serious consequences. Fractures of the bones in the spine (the vertebrae) begin to be seen more commonly in women in their mid-70s and cause significant pain as well as loss of height and exaggerated kyphosis (hunchback). In addition to pain, restricted range of motion, changes in posture, restricted lung function, and digestive problems can all be caused by vertebral fractures. Once a vertebral fracture has occurred, there is at least a five- to sevenfold increase in the risk of additional vertebral fractures.[7,8]

Men are not immune to osteoporosis, though their risk is only about 25% of women's risk. Nonetheless, hip fractures in men account for one-third of all hip fractures and have a higher mortality rate than those in women.[9] In addition, men who break a hip suffer worse outcomes.

Causes

Bone is dynamic living tissue that is constantly remodeling. The breaking down and rebuilding of bone are the result of the actions of two types of bone cells, osteoclasts and osteoblasts. Osteoclasts stimulate the production of acids and enzymes that dissolve minerals and protein in bone and thus promote bone breakdown (resorption). Osteoblasts create a protein matrix, primarily of collagen, that provides the structural framework upon which mineralization can occur. Bone remodeling is normally a balance of bone resorption and bone formation. An imbalance between bone removal and bone replacement results in bone loss and the development of osteoporosis.

In childhood, bone mass rapidly increases and then slows in the late teens (around age 17 for women), but it continues to increase during the 20s. After achieving a peak bone mass around age 28, women slowly lose an average of 0.4% of bone mass in the femoral neck each year. After menopause, the rate of loss is faster, with an average 2% loss annually during the first 5 to 10 years. Bone loss continues in older women (past age 70) but at a much slower rate.

Diagnostic Considerations

Risk Factors

Major risk factors for osteoporosis in postmenopausal women are advanced age, genetics, lifestyle issues (low calcium, low vitamin D intake, and smoking), thinness, and menopausal status. The most common risk factors are as follows:

- Age (50–90 years)
- Female
- Thinness
- Small stature
- Prior fragility fracture
- Parental history of hip fracture

- Current tobacco smoker
- Long-term use of glucocorticoids
- Rheumatoid arthritis
- Other causes of secondary osteoporosis (e.g., primary hyperparathyroidism, renal calcium leak)
- More than two alcoholic drinks per day
- Low level of vitamin D
- Genetic variations of vitamin D receptors

Genetic Factors

The level of peak bone mass is greatly influenced by genetic factors.[10–12] Young daughters of women with osteoporotic fractures have lower bone mass compared with other children their age.[13] The risk of hip fractures is almost 50% higher if there is a family history of fractures and 127% higher if a hip fracture has occurred in a parent.[14] One key genetic factor now being recognized is differences (polymorphisms) of the vitamin D receptor site. Some of these differences significantly increase the need for vitamin D.

Vitamin D Deficiency

The importance of vitamin D sufficiency in bone health has been underappreciated in the past. Emerging research is showing a direct correlation between both bone density and blood levels of vitamin D_3. Higher blood levels of vitamin D are associated with a lower rate of fractures of virtually all types; lower blood levels of vitamin D_3 are associated with a higher rate of fractures of all types.[15]

It is well known that vitamin D stimulates the absorption of calcium. Since vitamin D can be produced in our bodies by the action of sunlight on 7-dehydrocholesterol (a compound the body can manufacture from cholesterol) in the skin, many experts consider it more of a hormone than a vitamin. Strictly defined, a

Relative Activities of Vitamin D₃ Forms	
FORM	**RELATIVE ACTIVITY LEVEL**
Vitamin D₃ (cholecalciferol)	1
25-(OH) vitamin D (calcidiol)	2 to 5
1,25-(OH) vitamin D (calcitriol)	10

vitamin is an essential compound the human body cannot manufacture, while a hormone is a compound that the human body manufactures and that serves to control a particular function. In the case of vitamin D, the compound serves to control calcium absorption.

The process of vitamin D manufacture begins when sunlight changes the 7-dehydrocholesterol in the skin into vitamin D_3 (cholecalciferol). This form of vitamin D is also the most popular supplement form, so taking it in supplement form bypasses the need to manufacture it in the skin. From the bloodstream vitamin D_3 is then transported to the liver and converted by an enzyme into 25-(OH) vitamin D, which is two to five times more potent than vitamin D_3. The 25-(OH) vitamin D is then converted by an enzyme in the kidneys to 1,25-(OH) vitamin D, which is 10 times more potent than vitamin D_3.

Disorders of the liver or kidneys result in impaired conversion of cholecalciferol to more potent vitamin D compounds. In some patients who have osteoporosis, there are high levels of calcidiol, while the level of calcitriol is quite low, signifying a problem with the kidneys. So, it may not be enough to supplement with vitamin D_3, as many people with osteoporosis may not be converting it fully to calcitriol. Many theories have been proposed to account for this decreased conversion seen in some patients with osteoporosis, including lack of parathyroid hormone,

lack of estrogen, magnesium deficiency, and deficiency of the trace mineral boron.

Diet and Lifestyle

As significant as genetic factors are in osteoporosis risk, there is no question that the major determinants of bone health are diet and lifestyle. Factors that influence bone health include physical activity; protein intake; acid-base homeostasis; smoking; alcohol consumption; and intake of calcium, vitamin K, and vitamin D. To achieve peak bone mass, a young woman requires adequate calories, protein, and calcium.[16]

Dietary Protein

Both too much protein (especially animal protein) and too little protein lead to an increased risk for osteoporosis.[17] Too much animal protein promotes osteoporosis, as diets high in red meat are acid-producing, and calcium from bone may be mobilized to offset the acid and maintain the acid-base balance the body requires. (Diets high in fruits, vegetables, and plant proteins are alkaline-forming.) Too little protein leads to osteoporosis because it leads to impaired formation of the collagen matrix of bone.

Smoking

Women smokers tend to lose bone more rapidly and have a lower bone mass than those who do not smoke.[18,19] Some studies show that smokers also have a higher fracture rate.[20,21] In addition, smokers reach menopause up to two years earlier than nonsmokers. It may be that smoking interferes with estrogen metabolism, although the mechanism is not clearly known.

Alcohol

Consumption of seven alcoholic drinks or more per day, which is considered heavy, has

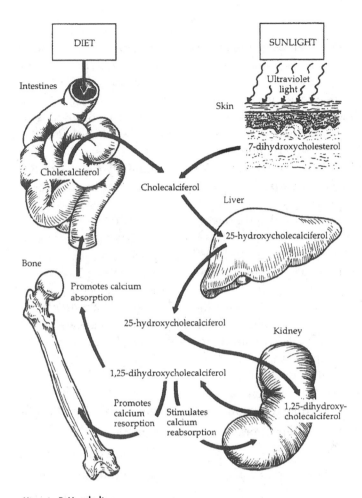

Vitamin D Metabolism

been shown to increase the risk of falls and hip fractures. However, moderate alcohol consumption seems to lower the risk of hip fractures in older women. It is thought that moderate amounts of alcohol inhibit bone resorption by increasing estradiol concentrations.[22,23]

Physical Activity

The benefits of physical activity for reducing the risk of osteoporosis cannot be overemphasized. The evidence is overwhelming that highly active individuals have higher bone mass[24] and those who are sedentary have a lower bone mass. Individuals who require bed rest[25] or who are confined to a wheelchair experience a rapid and dramatic loss of bone. Exercise functions primarily to reduce osteoporosis risk by stimulating the activity of osteoblasts, the bone-building cells.

Hormonal Factors

A woman's hormonal status clearly influences bone mass and the rate of bone resorption. After menopause, all women lose bone, and this loss is especially accelerated in the first five years. The drop in estrogen production that comes with menopause, no matter at what age, increases the rate of bone resorption. The earlier menopause occurs before the average age of onset (51 years), the sooner the bones lose the protective effect of endogenous estrogen.

Women who have premature menopause (before age 40), who began menstruating late in adolescence (e.g., after age 15 years), who have undergone surgical menopause, and/or who have experienced periods of no menstruation due to low estrogen levels in their reproductive years are at greater risk of osteoporosis. Women who missed up to half of their expected menstrual periods because of low estrogen had 12% less vertebral bone mass than did those with normal menstrual cycles; those who missed more than half had 31% less bone mass than healthy controls.[26]

The concentration of calcium in the blood is strictly maintained within narrow limits. If levels start to decrease, there is an increase in the secretion of parathyroid hormone by the parathyroid glands and a decrease in the secretion of calcitonin by the thyroid and parathyroids. If calcium levels in the blood start to increase, there is a decrease in the secretion of parathyroid hormone and an increase in the secretion of calcitonin.

Parathyroid hormone increases serum calcium levels primarily by increasing the activity of the osteoclasts, although it also decreases the excretion of calcium by the kidneys and increases the absorption of calcium in the intestines. In the kidneys, parathyroid hormone increases the conversion of calcidiol to calcitriol.

Assessing Risk

The more risk factors are present, the greater the potential for lower bone mass and the higher the risk of fracture. Risk factors alone cannot adequately determine whether an individual has low bone mass; rather, they are important guides in determining osteoporosis and fracture risks, and an understanding of these risks contributes to optimal prevention strategies. In addition, various medical conditions and medications can interrupt normal bone physiology and lead to osteoporosis.

Secondary Causes of Bone Loss

- Genetic disorders
  - Hemochromatosis
  - Hypophosphatasia
  - Osteogenesis imperfecta
  - Thalassemia
- Hormonal disorders
  - Cortisol excess
  - Cushing's syndrome
  - Gonadal insufficiency
  - Hyperthyroidism
  - Primary hyperparathyroidism
  - Type 1 diabetes
  - Hypothalamic amenorrhea
  - Premature ovarian failure
- Gastrointestinal diseases
  - Primary biliary cirrhosis
  - Celiac disease
  - Crohn's disease
  - Total astrectomy
  - Gastric bypass
- Other conditions
  - Ankylosing spondylitis
  - Chronic renal disease
  - Lymphoma and leukemia
  - Multiple myeloma
  - Anorexia nervosa
  - Bulimia
  - Rheumatoid arthritis

- Medications
  - Aromatase inhibitors
  - Cytotoxic agents
  - Excessive thyroid dosing
  - Gonadotropin-releasing hormone agonists or analogs
  - Some long-term anticonvulsants (e.g., phenytoin)
  - Glucocorticoid use for more than three months

Bone Mineral Density Testing

While bone mineral density (BMD) testing alone may not be a good predictor of fracture risk (see the box on page 852), it is a great way to increase the awareness of and establish a diagnosis of osteoporosis. There are several techniques to measure BMD, but the gold standard is dual energy X-ray absorptiometry (DEXA). Other methods of assessing bone mass include computerized tomography (CT) scans, ultrasounds of the heel, and standard X-rays, none of which is as optimal for diagnosis and follow-up as the DEXA scan.[27]

In addition to providing the most reliable measurement of bone density, the DEXA test requires less radiation exposure than a conventional X-ray or CT scan. Usually the DEXA scan is used to measure both the hip and the lumbar spine densities. The hip is the preferred site for BMD testing, especially in women older than 60, because the spinal measurements can be unreliable. Although peripheral DEXA sites are accurate, they may be less useful because they may not correlate as well with fracture risk and BMD at the hip and spine. The guidelines for indications for BMD testing established by many reputable and independent organizations are as follows:

- Individuals with secondary causes of bone loss (e.g., steroid use, hyperparathyroidism)
- Individuals in whom there is X-ray evidence of osteopenia (insufficient bone mineral density)
- All women 65 years and older (not only for a diagnosis, but also as a historical reference point for comparisons in the future)
- Younger postmenopausal women with fractures due to fragile bones since menopause, low body weight, or family history of spine or hip fracture

Results of BMD tests are reported as standard deviations—either a Z-score or a T-score. A Z-score is based on the standard deviation (SD) from the mean BMD of women in the same age group. A T-score is based on standard deviation from mean peak BMD of a normal young woman. The World Health Organization's criteria for the diagnosis of osteoporosis uses T-scores. A T-score below –2.5 is associated with osteoporosis. People with a BMD in between that of normal bone and osteoporosis are classified as having osteopenia. Keep in mind that using the T-score instead of a Z-score increases the likelihood that you will be classified as having

Bone Mineral Density Score Interpretation		
STATUS	**T-SCORE**	**INTERPRETATION**
Normal	Above –1	BMD is within 1 SD of a young normal adult
Osteopenia	Between –1 and –2.5	BMD is between 1 and 2.5 SD below a young normal adult
Osteoporosis	Below –2.5	BMD is 2.5 SD or more below a young normal adult

Osteoporosis Risk Assessment and Recommendations

Choose the item in each category that best describes you, and fill in the point value for that item in the space to the right.

	POINTS	SCORE

Frame Size (choose one)

	POINTS	SCORE
Small or petite frame	10	_____
Medium frame, very lean	5	_____
Medium frame, average or heavy build	0	_____
Large frame, very lean	5	_____
Large frame, heavy build	0	_____

Ethnic Background (choose one)

	POINTS	SCORE
Caucasian	10	_____
Asian	10	_____
Other	0	_____

Activity Level (how often you walk briskly, jog, engage in aerobics/sports, or perform hard physical labor for at least 30 continuous minutes; choose one)

	POINTS	SCORE
Seldom	30	_____
1–2 times per week	20	_____
3–4 times per week	5	_____
5 or more times per week	0	_____

Smoking (choose one)

	POINTS	SCORE
Smoke 10 or more cigarettes a day	20	_____
Smoke fewer than 10 cigarettes a day	10	_____
Quit smoking	5	_____
Never smoked	0	_____

Personal Health Factors (choose all that apply)

	POINTS	SCORE
Family history of osteoporosis	20	_____
Long-term corticosteroid use	20	_____
Long-term anticonvulsant use	20	_____
Drink more than three glasses of alcohol each week	20	_____
Drink more than one cup of coffee per day	10	_____
Seldom get outside in the sunlight	10	_____

(continues)

Osteoporosis Risk Assessment and Recommendations		
	POINTS	**SCORE**
Personal Health: Women Only (choose only one)		
Had ovaries removed	10	_____
Premature menopause	10	_____
Had no children	10	_____
Dietary Factors (choose all that apply)		
Consume more than 4 oz meat on a daily basis	20	_____
Drink soft drinks regularly	20	_____
Consume the equivalent of 3–5 servings of vegetables each day	–10	_____
Consume at least 1 cup of green leafy vegetables each day	–10	_____
Take 1,000 mg supplemental calcium and 1,000 IU of Vitamin D	–10	_____
Consume a vegetarian diet	–10	_____
Total Score		_____

If your score is greater than 50, you are at significant risk for osteoporosis. However, you can reduce your score significantly by taking steps to reduce or eliminate risk factors as described in this chapter. For women who are at risk of osteoporosis or who have already experienced significant bone loss, the benefits of natural hormone therapy (described below) outweigh the risks. The exception is women at high risk for breast cancer or women with a disease aggravated by estrogen, such as active liver diseases or certain cardiovascular diseases.

osteopenia, even though it is normal to lose some bone mass with aging.

Laboratory Tests of Bone Metabolism

Tests for biochemical markers of bone turnover include a urine test that measures the breakdown products of bone, such as cross-linked N-telopeptide of type I collagen or deoxypyridium. These tests can be correlated with the rate of bone loss, but they are not intended to be used for the diagnosis of osteoporosis or monitoring of bone loss. Such tests may be used to monitor the success (or failure) of therapy, as they provide quicker feedback compared with DEXA, with which it can take up to two years to detect a thera-peutic response. The reduction of urinary levels of these markers of bone breakdown over a 2-year period has been correlated with increases in bone density measurements.[28]

Therapeutic Considerations

Osteoporosis is a complex condition involving genetic, hormonal, lifestyle, nutritional, and environmental factors. A comprehensive plan that addresses all of these factors offers the greatest protection. Fortunately, osteoporosis in most cases is entirely preventable through diet, lifestyle, and proper supplementation. Rarely should medical therapy (i.e., hormones

DOES BONE MINERAL DENSITY PREDICT FRACTURE RISK?

While BMD testing provides useful information on bone strength, a careful review of the literature and the results of a very large study suggest that there is no correlation between bone mineral density testing alone and ability to predict future fractures.[29] It turns out that bone density is not the only risk factor that contributes to future fractures. In fact, osteoporosis accounts for only about 15 to 30% of all hip fractures in postmenopausal women; one-third of all women who experience a hip fracture have normal bone density, with the rest somewhere in between normality and osteoporosis. An important risk factor for hip fracture is an increased risk of falling due to poor balance and lack of muscle strength.[30] For many people, efforts to prevent falls by changing diet and lifestyle as well as improving balance and increasing muscle strength are more important in preventing fractures than increasing bone strength.[31]

In addition, while current drug therapy increases BMD, it does not improve bone quality or "toughness." As an illustration, chalk is denser than bamboo, but bamboo is tougher and less likely to break. Factors that promote improved bone quality and a healthy collagen matrix are likely to be just as critical, or perhaps even more critical, to bone quality and toughness compared with the mineral content of bone.

and drugs) be required if proper steps are taken. However, since drug therapy is such a major focus in the conventional prevention and treatment of osteoporosis, it is important for us to discuss it. Drug treatment focuses on the use of estrogen and progesterone, bisphosphonates, Evista (a selective estrogen receptor modulator), parathyroid hormone, and calcitonin. There are currently no prospective studies comparing the efficacy of these therapies.

Hormone Replacement Therapy

As women approach menopause and immediately after, estrogen levels decline and bone resorption outpaces bone formation. Both estrogen replacement therapy (ERT) and hormone replacement therapy (HRT, using a combination of estrogen and progesterone) reduce the rate of bone turnover and resorption, leading to reduced fracture rates in postmenopausal women. In two-year trials, the average increase in BMD after ERT or HRT was 6.8% at the lumbar spine and 4.1% at the femoral neck.[32,33] However, there are significant risks with HRT (see the chapter "Menopause"). For women at high risk for osteoporosis, those who underwent surgical menopause or early menopause, and other special cases, we definitely recommend consideration of bioidentical hormone therapy (see the chapter "Menopause").

Bisphosphonates

The most widely prescribed drugs for prevention and treatment of osteoporosis are the bisphosphonates:

- Alendronate (Fosamax, Fosamax Plus D)
- Etidronate (Didronel)
- Ibandronate (Boniva)
- Pamidronate (Aredia)
- Risedronate (Actonel, Actonel with Calcium)
- Tiludronate (Skelid)
- Zoledronic acid (Reclast, Zometa)

These drugs are a $7 billion business, yet they are of marginal benefit at best and carry significant risks.

The first bisphosphonate was Fosamax,

produced by the drug company Merck. Its launch coincided with the publishing of a Merck-funded study called the Fracture Intervention Trial.[34] At first glance the claims made in Merck's advertisements for Fosamax were quite impressive. Merck claimed that Fosamax reduced the rate of hip fracture, compared with a placebo, by 50%, but at a closer look the numbers do not seem so rosy. First of all, the women in the study were high-risk women who had a history of a fracture due to osteoporosis. Next, only 2 out of 100 women in the placebo group had a hip fracture during the trial, compared with 1 out of 100 in the Fosamax group. In other words, 98 women out of 100 in the Fosamax group would have fared just the same if they had been on a placebo. While in severely high-risk individuals bisphosphonate therapy may offer some benefits, we believe that in time nondrug measures will be shown to be even more effective. In fact, clinical studies examining the effect of diet, lifestyle measures, and proper supplementation (discussed below) suggest that the natural approach may be far superior.

An important consideration is that in the Fracture Intervention Trial and many others, the women studied were at extremely high risk for a fracture. Such women are a small group. In fact, bisphosphonates are prescribed just as often for women with osteopenia (bone mineral density that is lower than normal but not low enough to be classified as osteoporosis) as they are for women with osteoporosis, even though there is no correlation between osteopenia and hip fracture risk. Neither bisphosphonates nor other drugs have shown effectiveness or are indicated in the treatment of osteopenia, despite considerable efforts by drug companies to convince doctors otherwise.[35] Instead of relying on a drug to reduce the risk of osteoporosis and hip fracture, the more rational approach would be to focus on diet, lifestyle, and supplement strategies.

Most of the side effects of bisphosphonates are mild, such as minor digestive disturbances (heartburn, diarrhea, flatulence), muscle and joint pain, headaches, and allergic reactions. However, these drugs can cause severe damage to the esophagus. It is very important that anyone taking an oral bisphosphonate remain standing or seated upright for 45 to 60 minutes after taking the medication.

Bisphosphonates have also been associated with severe bone destruction (osteonecrosis) of the jaw. This side effect is most often seen in cancer patients or those undergoing dental work to eliminate potential sites of infection.

One consequence of bisphosphonate use is the development of "brittle bones" and severe fractures of the thighbone (femur). Risk for brittle bones may be associated with long-term use and is one reason the use of bisphosphonates should be limited to five years at most.

Selective Estrogen-Receptor Modulators

Selective estrogen-receptor modulators (SERMs) are compounds that modulate the effects of estrogen receptors without producing the cancer-causing effects of estrogen. Currently the only SERM approved for the treatment of osteoporosis is Evista (raloxifene). In a 20-year study, raloxifene at 60 mg per day significantly improved BMD at the lumbar spine by 1.6% and at the femoral neck by 1.2%.[36] In the Multiple Outcomes of Raloxifene Evaluation trial, three years of raloxifene therapy at 60 mg per day in postmenopausal women increased BMD by 2.6% at the spine and 2.1% at the femoral neck.[37] Yet these benefits are not achieved without risk.

The most serious side effect for Evista is the formation of clots that can block veins or lodge in the lungs or heart. Though these side effects occur in only about 1 out of 100 patients treated with Evista, women treated with Evista were more than twice as likely to develop clot-related disease than women taking a placebo. More common side effects of Evista include difficult, burning, or painful urination; fever; increased rate of infections; leg cramps; skin rash; swelling of hands, ankles, or feet; and vaginal itching. Less common side effects include body aches and pains, congestion in the lungs, decreased vision or other changes in vision, diarrhea, difficulty breathing, hoarseness, loss of appetite, nausea, trouble swallowing, and weakness.

Parathyroid Hormone

Parathyroid hormone is given by injection under the skin once per day. Parathyroid hormone stimulates osteoblastic bone formation and increases bone density in women with osteoporosis.[38–40] One parathyroid hormone medication in particular, teriparatide (Forteo), is approved for the treatment of osteoporosis in postmenopausal women. Nineteen months of teriparatide treatment (20 mcg per day) increased bone density in the spine by 8.6% and in the femoral neck by 3.5% compared with a placebo.[40] In addition, the incidence of new vertebral fractures was reduced by 65% and that of nonvertebral fractures by 53%. It is interesting to note that the process of injecting a placebo increased bone density by 3.5%, a degree of improvement greater than that seen with bisphosphonates or Evista.

Calcitonin

Calcitonin is approved for postmenopausal osteoporosis treatment but not for prevention. It is available as a nasal spray and a subcutaneous injection. In the Prevent Recurrence of Osteoporotic Fractures trial,[41] an intranasal spray containing calcitonin (delivering 200 IU per day) was used for five years by postmenopausal women with osteoporosis; this was found to reduce the risk of new vertebral fractures by 33% compared with a placebo. No effect was seen on hip or nonvertebral fractures. Calcitonin spray may also be helpful in women with osteoporosis in that it can reduce bone pain from vertebral compression fractures.

Lifestyle

Smoking

Smoking tends to cause more rapid bone loss and lower bone mass. Women who smoke also tend to experience menopause two years earlier than nonsmokers.[42–44] Postmenopausal smokers have higher fracture rates,[45] and meta-analyses have suggested that hip fracture risk may be increased in current smokers.[46] Such fractures may be a particular risk for women over age 60. The World Health Organization reports that a history of smoking causes a substantial risk for future fracture independent of BMD.[47]

Alcohol

Alcohol consumption affects bone in a dose-dependent manner. While moderate alcohol consumption is associated with an increased BMD in postmenopausal women,[48,49] heavy alcohol consumption—more than seven drinks a day—is associated with an increased risk of falls and fractures.[50] One drink is equal to 12 fl oz beer, 4 fl oz wine, or 1 fl oz hard liquor.[51]

Exercise

Exercise is the major determinant of bone density. One hour of moderate physical activity three times a week has been shown to prevent bone loss and actually increase bone mass in postmenopausal women.[52–57] Both weight-bearing and strength-training exercises are beneficial to the development of bone and maintenance of bone health and function.[58–60] In a meta-analysis of postmenopausal women, those who exercised increased their spine BMD by approximately 2%.[61] That equals the benefits noted with bisphosphonate drugs. In addition to increasing BMD, muscle-strengthening and balance-enhancing exercises have been shown to reduce the risk of falls and fall-related injuries by 75% in women 75 years of age and older.[62] Weight-bearing exercises can be simple, such as walking or tai chi. Strength-training exercises can also be simple, with hand weights or resistance bands that can be used at home.

Diet

Many dietary factors play a role in bone health:[63–65]

- Low intake of calcium and/or high intake of phosphorus
- High-protein diet

PREVENTING SARCOPENIA

Sarcopenia is the loss of skeletal muscle mass and strength as we age. Sarcopenia is to our muscle mass what osteoporosis is to our bones. The degree of sarcopenia as we age is a predictor of mortality and disability. Sarcopenia is linked not just to a significantly shorter life expectancy but also to decreased vitality, poor balance and gait speed, and increased falls and fractures. Just as we want to build bone while we are young to help us preserve it longer through the aging process, the same is true for muscle: we want to reach peak muscle mass while we are young. And just as it is important to engage in dietary, lifestyle, and exercise strategies to fight osteoporosis in our later years, we must do the same to fight sarcopenia. For more information on sarcopenia and what you can do about it, see the discussion in the chapter "Longevity and Life Extension."

- Low-protein diet
- A diet high in acid ash (high in meat and dairy products, low in fruits and vegetables)
- High salt intake
- High sugar intake
- Trace mineral deficiencies

A vegetarian diet (either a vegan diet or one that includes milk and eggs) is associated with a lower risk of osteoporosis.[66,67] Although bone mass in vegetarians does not differ significantly from that in omnivores in the third, fourth, and fifth decades, there are significant differences in the later decades. These findings indicate that the decreased incidence of osteoporosis in vegetarians is due not to increased initial bone mass but rather to decreased bone loss.

Several factors are probably responsible for the decrease in bone loss observed in vegetarians. The most important of these is probably a lowered intake of protein coupled with an alkaline-ash diet. A high-protein diet or a diet high in phosphates is associated with increased excretion of calcium in the urine, as the calcium is used to buffer the extra acid this type of diet generates in the body. Raising daily protein intake from 47 to 142 g doubles the excretion of calcium in the urine.[68] A diet this high in protein is common in the United States and may be a significant factor in the increasing number of people suffering from osteoporosis in this country.[69] But perhaps more important than reducing protein intake is increasing the dietary intake of fruits and vegetables for their alkalinizing effect. When the diet induces acidosis—which is typical of a diet high in protein and salt—the body maintains pH by buffering with calcium, which is taken from the bones.[70] For some additional guidance on an alkaline diet, see Appendix C, "Acid-Base Values of Selected Foods."

Gastric Acid

It has long been believed that the absorption of calcium depends on its becoming ionized in the intestines, largely on the basis of the secretion of gastric acid, and that poor ionization of calcium is a major problem with calcium carbonate—the most widely used form of calcium for nutritional supplementation. There is still some validity to these beliefs, but the situation is a bit more complicated. The biggest detriment to calcium absorption in regard to stomach acid production may be the use of acid-blocking drugs.

Although decreased gastric acidity is seen in as many as 40% of postmenopausal women,[71] a critical review of available studies indicates that the effects of increased gastric pH are apparent only when poorly soluble calcium salts (such as calcium carbonate) are taken on an empty stomach.[72] In a fasting state, patients with insufficient stomach acid output can absorb only about 4% of an oral dose of calcium as calcium carbonate, whereas a person with normal stomach acid can typically absorb about 22%.[72] Patients with low stomach acid secretion need a form of calcium that is already in a soluble and ionized state, such as calcium citrate, calcium lactate, or calcium gluconate, if they are going to take it on an empty stomach. About 45% of the calcium is absorbed from calcium citrate in patients with reduced stomach acid.[73] However, when any form of calcium is taken with meals, there is little difference in its absorption even in elderly subjects who secrete little stomach acid or those taking acid-blocking drugs. That said, there is an association between increased risk of hip fractures and long-term use of proton-pump-inhibiting acid-blocking drugs such as these:[74,75]

- Omeprazole (Losec, Prilosec, Zegerid, Ocid, Lomac, Omepral, Omez)
- Lansoprazole (Prevacid, Zoton, Monolitum, Inhibitol, Levant, Lupizole)
- Dexlansoprazole (Kapidex, Dexilant)
- Esomeprazole (Nexium, Esotrex)
- Pantoprazole (Protonix, Somac, Pantoloc, Pantozol, Zurcal, Zentro, Pan, Controloc)
- Rabeprazole (Zechin, Rabecid, Nzole-D, AcipHex, Pariet, Rabeloc.
- Revaprazan (Revanex)

Sugar

Refined sugar is another dietary factor that increases the loss of calcium from the body. Following sugar intake, there is an increase in the urinary excretion of calcium.[76] Considering that the average American consumes 125 g sucrose, 50 g corn syrup, and other refined simple sugars every day, it is little wonder that so many suffer from osteoporosis.

Soft Drinks

Soft drinks are a major contributor to osteoporosis for those who drink them, as they are high in phosphates (phosphoric acid) and sugar. This leads to lower calcium and higher phosphate levels in the blood. The United States ranks first among countries for soft drink consumption, with an average per capita consumption of approximately 15 oz per day.

The link between soft drink consumption and bone loss is going to be even more significant as children practically weaned on soft drinks reach adulthood. Soft drink consumption among children poses a significant risk factor for impaired calcification of growing bones. Because there is such a strong correlation between maximum BMD and the risk of osteoporosis, the rate of osteoporosis may eventually reach even greater epidemic proportions.

The severely negative effect that soft drinks have on bone formation in children was clearly demonstrated in a study that compared 57 children with low blood calcium, age 18 months to 14 years, with 171 matched controls with normal calcium levels.[77] The goal of the study was to assess whether the intake of at least 1.5 quarts per week of soft drinks containing phosphates is a risk for the development of low blood calcium levels. Of the 57 children with low blood calcium levels, 38 (66.7%) drank more than four bottles (12 to 16 fl oz each) per week, but only 48 (28%) of the 171 children with normal serum calcium levels drank that many soft drinks. For all 228 children, a significant inverse correlation between serum calcium level and the amount of soft drinks consumed each week was found.[78]

Green Leafy Vegetables

Green leafy vegetables (kale, collard greens, parsley, lettuce, etc.) offer significant protection against osteoporosis. These foods are a rich source of a broad range of vitamins and minerals that are important to maintaining healthy bones, including calcium, vitamin K_1, and boron.

Vitamin K_1 (phylloquinone or phytoquinone) is the form of vitamin K that is found in plants. A function of vitamin K that is often overlooked is its role in converting inactive osteocalcin (the major noncollagen protein in bone) to its active form. Osteocalcin's role is to anchor calcium molecules and hold them in place within the bone.[79] A deficiency of vitamin K leads to impaired bone health due to inadequate osteocalcin levels. In one study, very low blood levels of vitamin K_1 were found in patients who had fractures due to osteoporosis.[80] The severity of fractures was strongly correlated with the level of circulating vitamin K: the lower the level of vitamin K, the greater the severity of the fracture. In the Nurses Health Study a low dietary intake of vitamin K was linked

to increased hip fractures.[81] Despite some studies showing that the lower the level of circulating vitamin K, the lower the bone density,[82] more recent studies indicate that while low dietary vitamin K levels are linked to fractures due to osteoporosis, they do not appear to be correlated with low BMD.[83]

This evidence clearly indicates the importance of vitamin K in preventing fractures; it probably increases the tensile strength of bone without affecting BMD. Since vitamin K is found in green leafy vegetables, it may be one of the key protective factors against osteoporosis in a vegetarian diet. The richest sources of vitamin K_1 are dark green leafy vegetables (such as broccoli, lettuce, cabbage, and spinach) and green tea. Other good sources are asparagus, oats, whole wheat, and fresh green peas.

In addition to vitamin K_1, the high levels of many minerals in green leafy vegetables, such as calcium and boron, may also be responsible for this protective effect.

Boron

Boron is a trace mineral that is a protective factor against osteoporosis. In one study, supplementing the diet of postmenopausal women with 3 mg boron per day reduced urinary calcium excretion by 44% and dramatically increased levels of 17-beta-estradiol, the most biologically active estrogen.[84] It appears that boron is required to activate certain hormones, including estrogen and vitamin D.[85] It was mentioned previously that vitamin D is converted to its most active form (1,25-[OH] vitamin D, or calcitriol) within the kidney, and that this conversion is impaired in postmenopausal osteoporosis. Boron is apparently required for this conversion to occur. A boron deficiency may contribute greatly to osteoporosis and to menopausal symptoms.

Because fruits and vegetables are the main dietary sources of boron, diets low in these

PRUNES TO BUILD BONES

Prunes (dried plums) are well known for their ability to prevent and relieve constipation. Prunes may also be able to help offset women's significantly increased risk for accelerated bone loss during the first three to five years after menopause. When 58 postmenopausal women ate about 12 prunes each day for three months, they were found to have higher blood levels of enzymes and growth factors that indicate bone formation than women who did not consume prunes. Also, none of the women suffered any adverse gastrointestinal side effects. Prunes' beneficial effects on bone formation may be due to their high concentration of phenolic compounds that act as antioxidants and help curb bone loss. Prunes also provide a good supply of boron, a trace mineral integral to bone metabolism that is thought to play an important role in the prevention of osteoporosis. A single serving (3.5 oz) of prunes provides 2 to 3 mg boron.[86]

foods may be deficient in boron. The standard American diet is severely deficient in these foods. In order to guarantee adequate boron levels, supplement with 3 to 5 mg boron per day.

Soy Isoflavones

Soy products contain a class of compounds called isoflavones, including genistein, daidzein, and glycitein, all of which are considered to be phytoestrogens because they share a structure similar to that of 17-beta-estradiol, the main form of estrogen produced in the body. The binding of soy isoflavones to estrogen receptors is preferential for the estrogen receptor beta and thus indicates that soy isoflavones act as selective estrogen modulators similar to Evista, but seemingly without the side effects.[87] The daidzein molecule is similar in shape to the molecule of a drug called ipriflavone, which is used in Europe and Japan to treat osteoporosis (as discussed below). In the United States, ipriflavone is available as a nutritional supplement.

Soy foods or soy isoflavone supplements have the potential to favorably affect bone metabolism, yet they remain a bit controversial in the medical literature due to the inconsistencies in the studies that have been done to date.[88] These variations include differences in the dosage and form of soy products studied (soy protein isolate, whole soy foods, or extracted soy isoflavones), differences in the menopausal status of the women studied (perimenopausal, early postmenopausal, or late postmenopausal), differences in the duration of the various trials, and differences in the tests used to assess bone density and bone metabolism. Nonetheless, there is considerable evidence that soy has a bone-building effect, as many studies have shown that soy or soy isoflavones can slow bone turnover and increase bone density in women. Menopausal women taking 55 to 90 mg soy isoflavones for six months had an increase in mineral levels and density in the lumbar spine.[89–91]

Several detailed analyses of the clinical trials of soy and soy isoflavones concluded that a dose of 90 mg per day of soy isoflavones is required to achieve benefits for bone health.[92,93] Studies that have used lower levels of soy isoflavones have consistently failed to show any real benefit to bone health. In addition, the benefits of soy in bone health may be more apparent in postmenopausal women than in premenopausal women.[94,95]

A nutritional influence of soy foods that may be overlooked is the amount of calcium in some of these foods or in diets that contain soy foods. A diet that includes greater amounts of soy products can account for a meaningful amount of calcium, and some soy foods can offer at least as much calcium as a serving of dairy products.

Calcium Content of Selected Soy Products		
SOY PRODUCT	**SERVING SIZE**	**CALCIUM (MG)**
Tofu, firm	¼ block	553
Tofu, regular	¼ block	406
Soy milk, calcium-fortified	1 cup	80–300
Soy milk	1 cup	7
Soybeans, roasted	¼ cup	119
Soybeans, boiled	¼ cup	88
Tempeh	¼ cup	77

Nutritional Supplements

Calcium

Adequate calcium intake has an established role in maintaining bone health, primarily in very young women and the elderly. However, calcium alone provides very little benefit in protecting against osteoporosis; vitamin D, vitamin K, and other nutrients are required as well).[96] In a detailed analysis of all controlled trials with calcium supplementation evaluating bone health up to 2002, supplementation with 500 to 2,000 mg per day of calcium had only a modest benefit for bone density in postmenopausal women: the difference in the amount of bone loss between calcium and placebos was 2.05% for the total body, 1.66% for the lumbar spine, and 1.64% for the hip.[97] Closer examination of the largest study, the Women's Health Initiative, which enrolled more than 36,000 postmenopausal women, showed a surprising result: while overall data showed that supplementation with 1,000 mg per day of calcium and 400 IU per day of vitamin D decreased the risk of hip fractures by 12% when compared with a placebo, when the analysis was restricted to women who actually took the tablets at least 80% of the time, calcium plus vitamin D decreased hip fractures by 29% compared with the placebo.[98] That is significant, especially because in the study vitamin D was supplemented at levels now known to be less than ideal.

In postmenopausal women, calcium supplementation has been shown to decrease bone loss by as much as 50% at nonvertebral sites. The effects were greatest in women whose baseline calcium intake was low, in older women, and in women with established osteoporosis.[99] There are other studies that have shown some effects in preventing vertebral bone loss as well.[100]

Here are our recommendations for calcium supplementation. First, there is no reason to take more than 1,000 mg per day as a supplement. Studies are clear that the benefits seen at 2,000 mg per day are not greater than those seen with 1,000 mg. Taking large doses of calcium can impair the absorption of magnesium and other minerals. Avoid oyster-shell calcium, dolomite, and bonemeal products because these forms tend to have higher lead levels. We prefer easily ionized forms of calcium such as calcium citrate, but the reality is that if taken with meals even calcium carbonate is effectively absorbed in most people. We also like tricalcium phosphate, for the following reasons: [101,102]

- Tricalcium phosphate provides three molecules of calcium for every molecule of phosphorus, so it is a highly efficient source of both calcium and phosphorus.

- Clinical studies indicate that consuming calcium with phosphorus in the form of tricalcium phosphate is more effective at building strong bones than consuming calcium alone.

- Calcium cannot be utilized in the absence of phosphorus.

- Approximately 50% of North American women are deficient in phosphorus.

DOES MILK CONSUMPTION PREVENT OR CAUSE OSTEOPOROSIS?

While numerous clinical studies have demonstrated that calcium and vitamin D supplementation can help prevent bone loss, the data are inconclusive in regard to any link between a high dietary calcium intake from milk and prevention of osteoporosis and bone fractures. In fact, the current available data indicate that frequent milk consumption actually increases the risk for osteoporosis. When reviewing the data from the Nurses' Health Study, a study involving 77,761 women, researchers found that women who drank two or more glasses of milk per day had a 45% increased risk for hip fracture compared with women consuming 1 glass or less per week.[103] In other words, the more milk a woman consumed, the more likely she was to experience a hip fracture. This negative effect may turn out to be due to the vitamin A added to milk (at higher levels, vitamin A, but not beta-carotene, may interfere with bone formation). Interestingly, the rate of osteoporosis is considerably higher in countries where milk intake is highest.

- Phosphorus is an essential component of bone, with 85% of the phosphorus in your body found in your bones.

- Clinical research indicates that calcium supplements without phosphorus may actually decrease the phosphorus available to the body for bone health, thus contributing to osteoporosis.

While too much phosphorus is not a good thing, especially when it is not accompanied by calcium (as in soft drinks and animal meats), so too is not enough, especially in regard to the absorption of calcium.

Vitamin D

As discussed above under "Diagnostic Considerations," vitamin D plays a major role in bone health. Given its importance in bone health as well for general health, vitamin D supplementation seems critical. While the results from large randomized, controlled trials have found that the combination of calcium and vitamin D produces some benefits in reducing fracture risk, virtually all of these studies used vitamin D dosages that were inadequate to raise blood levels of vitamin D_3 into the effective range (45 to 90 ng/ml).[104,105] Nonetheless, a detailed analysis of randomized controlled trials in elderly postmenopausal women found that even at a low dose of 700 to 800 IU per day vitamin D was associated with significant reductions in the risk of hip and nonvertebral fractures.[106] Vitamin D in combination with calcium supplementation definitely reduces the rate of postmenopausal bone loss, especially in older women.[107] Vitamin D has also been shown to improve muscle strength[108] and balance,[109] thereby reducing the risk of falling.[110]

So, how much vitamin D do you need? As detailed in the chapter "Supplementary Measures," the only way to accurately know your vitamin D status is to measure it in the blood. Studies indicate that for proper health, serum vitamin D levels should be between 50 and 80 ng/ml (125 to 200 nmol/l). We definitely recommend testing to ensure that optimal levels of vitamin D levels are being achieved. While some people can achieve an optimal level with just 600 IU a day (or 20 minutes of sunlight exposure per day) others have a genetic requirement for as much 10,000 IU a day. The only way to determine your optimal dosage is by testing.

For general health we recommend a dosage of 2,000 IU per day, but for women or men with reduced bone density or osteoporosis we recommend a dosage of 5,000 IU per day. Pregnant and lactating women are likely to need more vitamin D as well. In the past, breastfeeding longer than six months was considered a cause of vitamin D deficiency in children. We now know that the problem is not breastfeeding, but rather that almost all women are deficient in vitamin D.

Magnesium

Magnesium is just as important in bone mineralization as calcium, but it does not receive nearly the same level of attention. Low magnesium status is common in women with osteoporosis, and magnesium deficiency is associated with abnormal bone mineral crystals.[111] Some women with reduced BMD do not have an increased fracture rate, possibly because their bone mineral crystals are of high quality, owing in part to high levels of magnesium. In a group of postmenopausal women, supplementation with 250 to 750 mg per day of magnesium for 6 months followed by 250 mg per day for 6 to 18 months resulted in an increase in bone density in 71% of the women. This increase was noteworthy because it occurred without calcium supplementation.[112]

Zinc

Zinc is essential for the proper formation and function of osteoblasts and osteoclasts, and it enhances the biochemical action of vitamin D. Zinc is also is necessary for the synthesis of various proteins found in bone. Low zinc levels have been found in the serum and bone in people with osteoporosis.[113]

Copper

A deficiency of copper is known to produce abnormal bone development in growing children and may be a contributing cause of osteoporosis. In vitro studies have shown that copper supplementation inhibits bone resorption.[114,115] In a double-blind trial, supplementation with 3 mg per day of copper for two years significantly decreased bone loss in postmenopausal women.[116]

Manganese

A deficiency of manganese may be one of the lesser-known but more important nutritional factors related to osteoporosis. Manganese deficiency causes a reduction in calcium deposition in bone. Manganese also stimulates the production of important compounds in the collagen matrix that provides a framework for the mineralization process.[117]

Combinations of Minerals

In a double-blind study of postmenopausal women, the combination of zinc, copper, manganese, and calcium appeared to be more effective than calcium alone for preventing bone loss in postmenopausal women.[117]

Silicon

During bone growth and the early phases of bone calcification, silicon has an essential role in the formation of cross-links between collagen and proteoglycans. In animals, silicon-deficient diets have produced abnormal skull development and growth retardation,[118] and supplemental silicon partially prevented bone loss in female rats that had their ovaries removed.[119]

A highly bioavailable form of silica (choline stabilized orthosilicic acid, sold as BioSil) showed impressive clinical results in improving bone health in a double-blind study in postmenopausal women with low bone density.[120] Compared with a control treatment consisting of calcium and vitamin D alone, the addition of BioSil (6 mg per day) was able to increase the collagen content of the bone by 22% and increase BMD by 2% within the first year of use. The ability to improve the collagen matrix as well as BMD indicates that BioSil produced greater bone tensile strength and flexibility, thereby greatly increasing the resistance to fractures. The recommended dosage is 6–10 mg per day.

Folic Acid, Vitamin B$_6$, and Vitamin B$_{12}$

Accelerated bone loss in menopausal women may in part be due to increased levels of homocysteine, a breakdown product of methionine that will be elevated if folic acid, vitamin B$_6$, or vitamin B$_{12}$ levels are insufficient. Homocysteine has the potential to promote osteoporosis if it is not eliminated adequately. In a prospective study, women with high homocysteine levels had almost twice as high a risk of nonvertebral osteoporotic fractures as women with low homocysteine levels.[121] Since a deficiency of any of the B vitamins involved in homocysteine metabolism may be the factor in the elevated homocysteine levels, it is important to supplement all three at recommended levels. Restoration of the proper status of these B vitamins will bring elevated homocysteine levels down. Deficiencies of at least one of these nutrients are common in postmenopausal women.

Vitamin C

Vitamin C promotes the formation and cross-linking of some of the structural proteins in bone. Animal studies have shown that vitamin C deficiency can cause osteoporosis,[122] and it has been known for decades that scurvy, a disease caused by vitamin C deficiency, is also associated with abnormalities of bone.

Vitamin K

Vitamin K, as discussed above, is required for the production of the bone protein osteocalcin, a key component in the matrix of bone. Various forms of vitamin K supplements have been used in human trials: vitamin K$_1$ (phylloquinone or phytoquinone), menaquinone-4 (MK4, a form of vitamin K$_2$), and menaquinone-7 (MK7, another form of vitamin K$_2$).

Studies of the effects of vitamin K supplementation on bone health have produced mixed results. We feel it is because the variable used to assess effectiveness, BMD, is probably not the right measure. Most of the double-blind studies with vitamin K$_1$ have shown only a modest effect or no effect on bone density, and while studies with MK4 have shown positive results in reducing bone loss and fracture rates, the dosage used (45 mg per day) was extremely high, suggesting that the positive results are probably due to a drug-like effect rather than a nutritional effect.[106,123–129] One double-blind study with vitamin K$_1$ showed that taking 5 mg a day for two to four years did not protect against an age-related decline in BMD in postmenopausal women with osteopenia but did result in significantly fewer fractures.[124] Because vitamin K affects osteocalcin, it is entirely possible that it has an effect on improving bone health without improving BMD.

MK7 (a longer-chain form of vitamin K$_2$) is found in high concentrations in natto (a fermented soy food popular in Japan) and is produced by gut bacteria in small amounts from dietary vitamin K$_1$.[128] MK7 has been found in animal studies to be more potent and more bioavailable as well as to have a longer half-life than MK4. When taken as a supplement (0.22 mmol per day), MK7 is more effective than K$_1$ in activating osteocalcin and stays in the blood circulation much longer (half-life of 8 hours for K$_1$ and MK4 vs. 96 hours for MK7).[129–130] In a study of postmenopausal Japanese women, a significant inverse association was found between natto consumption and the incidence of hip fractures.[131] In a study of osteoporosis after organ transplantation, one year of MK7 supplementation (180 mcg per day) resulted in increased bone mineralization compared with a placebo.[132] However, a study of early menopausal women given one year of supplementation of 360 mcg per day of MK7 did not show a significant improvement in BMD despite a reduction in inactive osteocalcin.[133] Again, there is no question that vitamin K is performing a vital function in bone health and appears to reduce fractures, but it is unlikely to produce a significant improvement in BMD on its own.

Strontium

Strontium is a nonradioactive earth element physically and chemically similar to calcium. Strontium ranelate is the specific strontium salt used in clinical trials for osteoporosis, but this form of strontium is not available in the United States. Strontium in large doses stimulates bone formation and reduces bone resorption. In one double-blind study, 2 g per day of oral strontium ranelate (containing 680 mg per day of elemental strontium) for three years was shown to reduce the risk of vertebral fractures and to increase BMD in 1,649 postmenopausal women with osteoporosis.[134] In the first year, there was a 49% reduction in the incidence of vertebral fractures in the strontium ranelate group; and there was a 41% reduction at the end of three years. A 6.8% increase in BMD was seen at the lumbar spine after three years of strontium supplementation. There was also an 8.3% increase at the femoral neck.

In a two-year trial, 353 postmenopausal women with osteoporosis and a history of at least one vertebral fracture received a placebo or one of three different doses of strontium: 170 mg per day, 340 mg per day, or 680 mg per day.[135] A small increase in lumbar BMD was seen with each dose of strontium, but the difference compared with a placebo was statistically significant only for the highest dose. The incidence of new vertebral fractures was lowest (38.8%) with the lowest dose of strontium (170 mg), vs. 54.7%, 56.7%, and 42.0% in the placebo, 340 mg, and 680 mg

groups, respectively. The fact that the highest dosage increased BMD the most while the lowest dosage had the greatest effect on preventing vertebral fractures indicates that the goal with strontium supplementation may not be trying to increase BMD to the highest possible degree. In addition, since there are potential adverse effects with strontium, including rickets, bone mineralization defects, and interference with vitamin D metabolism, it makes sense to use the lowest dosage possible.

There are many questions to be answered about strontium, including whether strontium chloride (the most common form of strontium used in U.S. supplements) is equal to strontium ranelate. Strontium chloride has not been the subject of published research. Other questions relate to safety and long-term benefits. Until these questions are answered, our advice is to consider supplementation with any strontium salt only as a last resort for elderly women who are at extremely high risk for fractures or who have a significant history of fractures.

Ipriflavone

Ipriflavone is a semisynthetic isoflavonoid, similar in structure to soy isoflavones, that has been approved in Japan, Hungary, and Italy for the treatment and prevention of osteoporosis. The compound, ipriflavone, has shown impressive results in a number of clinical studies. For example, in one study, ipriflavone (200 mg three times per day) increased bone density measurements by 2% and 5.8% after 6 and 12 months, respectively, in 100 women with osteoporosis.[136] In another study of women with osteoporosis, ipriflavone (600 mg per day) produced a 6% increase in bone mineral density after 12 months, while the bone density of the placebo group dropped by 0.3%.[137] Longer-term studies showed equally promising results given the safety and apparent efficacy of ipriflavone.[138,139] The effectiveness of ipriflavone suggests that naturally occurring soy isoflavones such as genistein and diadzein may offer similar benefits. Given the protective effect of soy isoflavones against breast cancer, the regular consumption of soy foods is encouraged. The mechanism of action appears to involve the enhancement of the effect of calcitonin on calcium metabolism (see above), as ipriflavone exerts no estrogen-like effects.[140]

In one study of ipriflavone published in 2001, the results were not nearly so positive.[141] In this double-blind, placebo-controlled four-year study, 474 postmenopausal Caucasian women with osteoporosis were randomly assigned to receive 200 mg ipriflavone three times a day plus 500 mg calcium or a placebo plus 500 mg calcium. Bone density was measured in the spine, hip, and forearm, as were biochemical markers of bone resorption. After 36 months of treatment, the annual percentage change in bone mineral density did not differ significantly between the two groups. The biochemical markers were also similar between the groups. The number of women with new spinal fractures was the same in the two groups at all points in the 36 months. Unexpected results included decreased lymphocytes (a type of white blood cell) in the blood in 31 women treated with ipriflavone.

So why did earlier studies of early and later postmenopausal women and of women with osteoporosis show positive results with ipriflavone and not this study? The most likely explanation is that the study population could have been too osteoporotic to show any benefit. Or it could be that this ipriflavone study, the largest and best-designed to date,

reveals that ipriflavone just does not have a significant role in the treatment of osteoporosis. It may be more appropriate for women with osteopenia or in the prevention of osteoporosis, but not for women whose BMD has dropped to osteoporosis. And why did ipriflavone cause a decrease in lymphocytes in this study but not in others? Subsequent studies done with ipriflavone since 2001 have demonstrated very positive results with no significant side effects.[142–144]

Our feeling is that until the issue of the decreased lymphocyte concentrations is cleared up, we recommend using soy isoflavones instead of ipriflavone. If you choose to use ipriflavone, monitor blood lymphocyte levels on a quarterly basis to detect any adverse effect.

Botanical Medicines

Green Tea

Population-based studies as well as experimental studies have demonstrated that consumption of green tea (*Camellia sinensis*) may offer significant protection against osteoporosis.[145] Green tea is rich not only in health-promoting polyphenols but also in vitamin K_1. In order to take advantage of this protection you need to drink three to five cups per day, providing a minimum of 250 mg per day of polyphenols (also referred to as catechins); alternatively, take a green tea extract providing the same level of polyphenols. In the experimental studies, the basic mechanism of green tea polyphenols was to impair bone resorption while at the same time stimulating osteoblast activity.[146–148] This effect would have tremendous significance if confirmed in human clinical trials.

QUICK REVIEW

- Osteoporosis is now determined primarily by bone mineral density testing.

- The big consequence of osteoporosis is fractures, especially in older women and men.

- Men are not immune to osteoporosis, though their risk is only about 25% that of women.

- Bone is dynamic living tissue that is constantly remodeling.

- Emerging research is showing a direct correlation between bone density and blood levels of vitamin D_3.

- As significant as genetic factors are in osteoporosis risk, there is no question that the major determinants of bone health are diet and lifestyle.

- The benefits of physical activity in reducing the risk of osteoporosis cannot be overemphasized.

- Women who have experienced premature menopause (before age 40), late onset of menstruation in adolescence, surgical menopause, or periods of no menstruation due to low estrogen levels in their reproductive years are at greater risk of osteoporosis.

- While BMD testing alone may not be a good predictor of fracture risk, it is a great way to increase the awareness of osteoporosis.

- Osteoporosis in most cases is entirely preventable through diet, lifestyle, and proper supplementation.

- Bisphosphonates are a $7 billion business, yet they are of marginal benefit at best and carry significant risks.

- Smoking, alcohol consumption, and physical activity are key lifestyle factors that affect bone health.

- When any form of calcium is taken with meals, there is little difference in its absorption, even in elderly subjects who secrete little stomach acid or in those taking acid-blocking drugs.

- There is an association between long-term use of proton-pump acid-blocking drugs and an increased risk of hip fracture.

- The link between soft drink consumption and bone loss is significant.

- A deficiency of vitamin K leads to impaired bone health due to inadequate osteocalcin levels.

- Boron is a trace mineral that is also a protective factor against osteoporosis.

- Soy consumption is associated with greater bone density.

- Calcium alone has very little benefit in protecting against osteoporosis; it requires vitamin D (and possibly other nutrients as well).

- There is no reason to take more than 1,000 mg calcium per day as a supplement.

- Vitamin D in combination with calcium supplementation definitely reduces the rate of postmenopausal bone loss, especially in older women.

- Vitamin D has also been shown to improve muscle strength and balance, thereby reducing the risk of falling.

- Low magnesium status is common in women with osteoporosis, and magnesium deficiency is associated with abnormal bone mineral crystals.

- A highly bioavailable from of silica (Bio-Sil) showed impressive clinical results in improving bone health in postmenopausal women with low bone density.

- Strontium in large doses stimulates bone formation and reduces bone resorption, but there are still many questions about its use as a dietary supplement.

- Population-based studies as well as experimental studies have demonstrated that green tea consumption may offer significant protection against osteoporosis.

. . . .

TREATMENT SUMMARY

As with most chronic health conditions, the most effective approach to osteoporosis is prevention. The risk of developing osteoporosis may be reduced by optimizing peak bone mass in the younger years and minimizing subsequent bone loss with aging. In order to maximize peak bone mass (even in the context of hereditary and other nonmodifiable risk factors), a healthful lifestyle, proper nutrition, and moderate exercise should begin during childhood and adolescence and continue into adulthood. Avoid smoking and excessive alcohol consumption.

For women (and men) who have already been diagnosed with osteoporosis, drug therapies can serve as a short-term adjunct to the recommendations in this chapter if required. But there is no question that the nutritional and lifestyle factors recommended here should serve as the primary approach to slow bone loss and decrease the risk of fractures.

Lifestyle

- Weight-bearing exercise four times a week plus strength training two or more times a week
- Fewer than seven alcoholic drinks per week; no more than two per day
- Avoidance of smoking and secondhand smoke

Diet

The guidelines discussed in the chapter "A Health-Promoting Diet" are very much indicated in helping to build strong healthy bones. A key area of attention is getting adequate protein, soy isoflavones, and green leafy vegetables each day while limiting the intake of factors that promote calcium excretion, such as salt, sugar, excessive protein, and soft drinks.

Nutritional Supplements

- A high-potency multiple vitamin and mineral formula as described in the chapter "Supplementary Measures"
- Key individual nutrients:
  - Calcium: 1,000 mg per day
  - Magnesium: 350 to 500 mg per day
  - Vitamin B_6: 25 to 50 mg per day
  - Folic acid: 800 mcg per day
  - Vitamin B_{12}: 800 mcg per day
  - Vitamin K_2 (MK7): 100 mcg per day
  - Vitamin D_3: 5,000 IU per day (ideally, measure blood levels and adjust dosage accordingly)
- Fish oils: 1,000 mg EPA + DHA per day
- One of the following:
  - Grape seed extract (>95% procyanidolic oligomers): 100 to 300 mg per day
  - Pine bark extract (>95% procyanidolic oligomers): 100 to 300 mg per day
  - Some other flavonoid-rich extract with a similar flavonoid content, super greens formula, or another plant-based antioxidant that can provide an oxygen radical absorption capacity (ORAC) of 3,000 to 6,000 units or more per day
- Specialty supplements:
  - Soy isoflavones: 90 mg per day
  - Strontium: 170 to 680 mg per day (but read the discussion above)
  - Ipriflavone: 600 mg per day (but read the discussion above)
  - Choline-orthosilicic acid (BioSil): 6 to 10 mg per day

Botanical Medicines

- Green tea: three to five cups per day, or a green tea extract that provides 250 to 300 mg polyphenols (also referred to as catechins) per day

Parkinson's Disease

A progressive neurological disorder of movement and mental function characterized by the following:

- "Pill rolling" motion of the thumb and forefinger

- Tremor (worst when the limb is at rest; diminishes with voluntary movement and sleep)

- Slow movement or inability to move; difficulties not only with execution of movement but also with planning and initiation of movement

- Postural instability; impaired balance leading to frequent falls

- Stooped posture

- Abnormal gait

- Reduced or fixed facial expressions ("masked face"), low-volume or monotone voice, or both

- Gastrointestinal symptoms: constipation (often one of the earliest symptoms), difficulty swallowing (later in the disease)

- Cognitive disturbances, including an inability to make decisions and adapt to new environments, poor problem solving, fluctuations in attention, and memory problems

- Behavior and mood alterations, including depression, apathy, and anxiety

Parkinson's disease was first described by James Parkinson in 1817. Parkinson's disease affects more than 7 million people worldwide and at least 1 million in the United States, where about 50,000 new cases are reported annually. These figures are expected to increase as the average age of the population rises. The average age of onset is approximately 60 and the prevalence increases with age.[1]

Parkinson's disease is the result of damage to the nerves in the area of the brain that is responsible for controlling muscle tension and movement—the substantia nigra of the basal ganglia. The damaged cells are the ones needed to produce the neurotransmitter called dopamine.

The disease usually begins as a slight tremor of one hand, arm, or leg. In the early stages the tremors are more apparent while the person is at rest, such as while sitting or standing, and are less noticeable when the hand or limb is being used. A typical early symptom of Parkinson's disease is "pill rolling," in which the person appears to be rolling a pill back and forth between the fingers. As the disease progresses, symptoms often get worse. The tremors and weakness affect the limbs on both sides of the body. The hands and the head may shake continuously. The person may walk with stiff, shuffling steps. In many cases, the disease causes a permanent rigid, stooped posture and an unblinking, fixed expression.[1]

Causes

Parkinson's disease is classified as a neurodegenerative disease, like Alzheimer's disease, and shares with Alzheimer's some underlying causes, such as oxidative damage, inflammation, and dysfunction of the mitochondria, the energy-producing parts of cells. Many of the underlying issues in Parkinson's disease are discussed in the chapter "A Cellular Approach to Health," and that chapter also provides a deeper understanding of the preventive and therapeutic strategies that are important in Parkinson's disease.

The first biochemical abnormality in Parkinson's disease is a decrease in the level of glutathione, the brain cell's primary antioxidant. Low glutathione makes the cells more susceptible to oxidative damage, such as that caused by environmental toxins. This sets the stage for the destruction of the neuron.

The first hint that Parkinson's disease may be related to an environmental toxin came from a report based on a series of patients who developed Parkinson's disease after exposure to MPTP, a contaminant found in synthetic heroin.[2] MPTP can freely cross the blood-brain barrier, is selectively taken up by the dopamine system cells of the substantia nigra, and inhibits mitochondrial energy production; this inhibition results in cell death. As of 2012, MPTP is the only environmental agent that has been directly linked to development of Parkinson's disease, but there are many more suspects. Population-based studies and animal experimental models have identified an association between Parkinson's disease and a number of environmental factors, including living in a rural area, farming, drinking well water, exposure to pesticides, and long-term occupational exposure to copper, iron, lead, and manganese.[3-16] Additionally, it is possible that pesticides and metals act synergistically with other neurotoxins to increase the risk of Parkinson's disease. In other words, it may be the total load of neurotoxins—instead of any single agent—that matters in the development of Parkinson's.

What all of these environmental toxins have in common is that they cause depletion of glutathione and disruption of the mitochondrial function.[17] That is a one-two punch that ultimately destroys the brain cell. By the time Parkinson's disease is typically diagnosed, more than 50% of the substantia nigra has been destroyed.

Therapeutic Considerations

At this point in time, Parkinson's disease is best treated with drug therapy along with key dietary, nutritional, and herbal recommendations to address the underlying disease process and/or enhance the effectiveness of drug therapy.

The most popular drug used in Parkinson's disease is Sinemet, which contains two key ingredients: levodopa and carbidopa. Levodopa, or L-dopa, is the "middle step" in the conversion of the amino acid tyrosine into dopamine. L-dopa, but not dopamine, crosses the blood-brain barrier. Carbidopa is a drug that works by ensuring that more L-dopa is converted to dopamine within the brain, where it is needed, and not within the other tissues of the body. Other drugs used include Eldepryl (selegiline or deprenyl), bromocriptine, and amantadine.

Unfortunately, although effective in the early stages of the disease in providing relief of symptoms, drug therapy does alter the disease progression and loses efficacy over time. Also, L-dopa and other drugs for Parkinson's disease are associated with common side effects such as motor complications, nausea, vomiting, sedation, hallucinations, and delusions. The primary focus with naturopathic care is to reduce these side effects while protecting the neurons from further damage.[1,18]

There are preliminary studies of gene therapy, which involves the use of a noninfectious virus to shuttle a gene into a specific part of the brain. The goal is to set in motion a series of biochemical processes that will increase the amount of GABA, which helps to manage Parkinson's disease symptoms. A more controversial therapy involves transplanting stem cells into the substantia nigra. Another therapy that is regaining traction is deep brain stimulation, which involves implanting a brain stimulator (a device similar to a heart pacemaker) in certain areas of the brain. All of these treatments are promising but still considered experimental.

Low-Protein Diet

A low-protein diet can enhance the action of L-dopa therapy. This simple dietary recommendation has been demonstrated to be extremely helpful in several clinical studies and is now a well-accepted supportive therapy. The usual recommendation is to eliminate as much protein as possible from breakfast and lunch while eating a typical dinner, so that total daily protein intake is less than 50 g per day for men and 40 g per day for women. This simple dietary practice can be effective in reducing tremors and other symptoms of Parkinson's disease during waking hours.[19]

Since L-dopa absorption is delayed or diminished by the amino acids in protein, patients on L-dopa should take their medication with a high-carbohydrate meal.

Nutritional Supplements

Antioxidants
Given the abundance of data suggesting that an excessive free radical burden contributes to Parkinson's disease, it is logical to consider that increasing antioxidant intake through dietary supplementation may offer some therapeutic benefit. Unfortunately, the research that exists on this line of therapy has focused on a rather limited number of antioxidant nutrients and the results have been rather disappointing. High supplemental dosages of vitamin E and C do not seem to affect Parkinson's disease. However, population-based studies have mostly indicated that high dietary intakes of antioxidant nutrients, especially vitamin E, may prevent Parkinson's disease.[20,21] The results from these preliminary studies led to a trial of high-dose vitamins C and E in early Parkinson's disease as well as a large study of high-dose vitamin E and the drug selegiline.[22]

In the double-blind study in patients with early Parkinson's disease given 3,000 mg vitamin C and 3,200 IU of vitamin E each day for a period of seven years, the supplement group fared better than the placebo group.[23] Although all patients eventually required drug treatment, the patients receiving the vitamins were able to delay the need for medication for up to two to three years longer. These results were quite promising, but a 10-year study of vitamin E only, at 2,000 IU per day, failed to show any real benefit in slowing or improving the disease.[24] It is likely that a combination of nutrients and a very broad antioxidant supplement program may be required in order to see any significant benefit in preventing the progression of Parkinson's disease.[25]

Coenzyme Q_{10} (CoQ_{10})
Given that CoQ_{10} is a powerful antioxidant and is also essential for the specific mitochondrial function that is damaged in Parkinson's disease, it seems that CoQ_{10} should be helpful, but the research is not clear. Reduced levels of CoQ_{10} have been demonstrated in

the platelets of individuals with Parkinson's disease, and CoQ_{10} levels were strongly correlated with activity in mitochondrial energy production.[26]

Results of clinical trials have been inconsistent. In one trial of CoQ_{10} supplementation, progression of Parkinson's disease was reduced by 44%.[27] All of the patients had the three primary features of Parkinson's disease—tremor, stiffness, and slowed movements—and had been diagnosed with the disease no more than five years before enrolling in the study. After an initial screening and baseline blood tests, the patients were randomly divided into four groups. Three of the groups received CoQ_{10} at different doses (300, 600, or 1,200 mg per day) while a fourth group received a placebo, for 16 months. The subjects who received the largest dose of CoQ_{10} displayed significant improvement in mental function, motor function, and ability to carry out activities of daily living, such as feeding or dressing themselves; the greatest effect was in activities of daily living. The subjects who received 300 mg per day and 600 mg per day developed slightly less disability than the placebo group, but the effects were less than those in the group that received the highest dosage of CoQ_{10}. Average plasma levels of CoQ_{10} were approximately 1.8, 2.1, and 4.5 mcg/ml, respectively, for the 300-, 600-, and 1,200-mg dosages. These results indicate that the beneficial effects of CoQ_{10} in Parkinson's disease may require adequate blood levels. It is important to point out that in this study CoQ_{10} was administered along with vitamin E at a dosage of 1,200 IU day, which may have prevented the achievement of higher levels of CoQ_{10}. If vitamin E is not used, target CoQ_{10} levels may be reached at lower dosages. The researchers were aware of this issue but chose to include the vitamin E given its apparent protective role against Parkinson's disease.

Two recent studies have cast doubt on the therapeutic efficacy of CoQ_{10} in Parkinson's disease, however. In a German study, a highly absorbable form of CoQ_{10} at a dosage of 100 mg three times per day or a placebo was given to 131 patients with Parkinson's disease for three months. Plasma levels of CoQ_{10} reached 4.6 mcg/ml in the treatment group, yet no effect on symptoms was seen. These results indicate that other factors may be responsible for determining the efficacy of CoQ_{10} in Parkinson's disease beyond achieving effective plasma levels.

On May 27, 2011, the National Institute of Neurological Diseases and Strokes stopped a phase III study of coenzyme Q_{10} for treatment of early stage Parkinson's disease.[28] The study enrolled 600 patients with early Parkinson's disease and randomly assigned them to receive 1,200 or 2,400 mg per day of active CoQ_{10} or a placebo. All subjects also received vitamin E at a dosage of 1,200 IU per day. While CoQ_{10} was shown to be extremely safe, results of an interim analysis showed that longer patient follow-up was not likely to demonstrate any statistically significant difference between active treatment and the placebo.

Despite this result, we recommend making CoQ_{10} a part of a comprehensive protocol for dealing with Parkinson's disease because of its safety and the rationale for its use.

Reduced Nicotinamide Adenine Dinucleotide (NADH)

NADH is the active form of vitamin B_3 that is required by the brain to make various neurotransmitters as well as chemical energy. Human studies indicate that NADH is effective in raising the level of dopamine within the brain. In two studies NADH has been shown to significantly increase brain dopamine levels in patients with Parkinson's disease, reducing symptoms and improving brain function.[29–31]

Phosphatidylserine (PS)

Phosphatidylserine is the major phospholipid in the brain, where it plays a key role in determining the integrity and fluidity of cell membranes. Normally the brain can manufacture sufficient levels of phosphatidylserine, but there is evidence that insufficient production can lead to depression and/or impaired mental function, especially in people over the age of 50. In numerous double-blind studies phosphatidylserine supplementation has been shown to improve mental function, mood, and behavior in elderly subjects, including those with Parkinson's disease.[32]

5-Hydroxytryptophan (5-HTP)

When used in combination with Sinemet, 5-HTP can alleviate the depression often associated with Parkinson's disease.[33] While it may be helpful as a supplement to Sinemet, 5-HTP should never be used alone in Parkinson's disease.[34–36] It is converted to serotonin in the brain, and increasing serotonin without increasing dopamine can worsen symptoms, especially rigidity. People taking Eldepryl should also not take 5-HTP unless under a physician's care, since there is a significant risk that this combination can raise serotonin to excessively high levels.[37]

N-acetylcysteine

N-acetylcysteine (NAC) has shown promising results in animal models of Parkinson's disease.[38] It may work by increasing brain glutathione levels. Early research on intravenous glutathione showed some benefit, which lasted for several weeks even after treatment was stopped.[39] Some nutritionally oriented doctors are reporting good results with both intravenous and intranasal glutathione. It is

QUICK REVIEW

- Parkinson's disease is the result of damage to the nerves in the area of the brain that is responsible for controlling muscle tension and movement
- The first biochemical abnormality in Parkinson's disease is a decrease in the level of glutathione, the brain cell's primary antioxidant
- Parkinson's disease may be related to exposure to environmental toxins
- Parkinson's disease is best treated with drug therapy along with key dietary, nutritional, and herbal recommendations to address the underlying disease process and/or enhance the effectiveness of drug therapy
- A low-protein diet can enhance the action of L-dopa therapy
- Results of clinical trials with supplemental dietary antioxidants have been inconsistent
- Phostphatidylserine has been shown in numerous double-blind studies to improve mental function, mood, and behavior in elderly subjects, including those with Parkinson's disease
- Population-based studies consistently demonstrate that consumption of green tea offers protection against the development of Parkinson's disease
- Velvet bean and fava bean are natural sources of L-dopamine

too early to make specific recommendations, but we hope these encouraging results will soon be followed up with rigorous research.

Botanical Medicines

Green Tea

Population-based studies consistently demonstrate that consumption of green tea (*Camellia sinensis*) offers protection against the development of Parkinson's disease. Specifically, green tea polyphenols may play a role in preventing and treating the oxidative stress underlying Parkinson's disease. In cell cultures and animal models, green tea polyphenols have demonstrated an ability to protect brain cells against neurotoxins.[40,41]

Ginkgo Biloba Extract

Ginkgo biloba extract has a number of beneficial effects that may help in Parkinson's disease. In a one-year open trial of 25 patients with Parkinson's disease who had signs of impaired mental function, it produced significant improvements in brain wave tracings, signifying improved brain metabolism.[42] Ginkgo has also been shown to be useful in animal models of Parkinson's disease and has demonstrated the ability to protect the substantia nigra from damage induced by the neurotoxin MPTP.[43]

Velvet Bean

The powdered seed of the velvet bean (*Mucuna pruriens*) has long been used in traditional ayurvedic medicine for Parkinson's disease and other conditions. It is a rich natural source of L-dopamine, but other components also contribute to its medicinal actions. An extract of velvet bean (7.5 g of velvet bean extract dissolved in water, given three to six times per day) was studied in 60 patients with Parkinson's disease (26 patients were taking Sinemet before treatment with the extract, and the remaining 34 were not taking any medication).[44] Statistically significant reductions in symptom scores were seen from the beginning to the end of the 12-week study. In another study, eight Parkinson's disease patients were given single doses of 200/50 mg L-dopa/carbidopa (LD/CD) and 15 and 30 g velvet bean preparation in randomized order at weekly intervals.[45] Compared with standard LD/CD, the 30 g velvet bean preparation led to a considerably faster onset of effect (34.6 vs. 68.5 minutes), reflected in shorter times to peak L-dopa concentrations in the blood, and fewer side effects. The researchers felt that the velvet bean might possess advantages over conventional L-dopa preparations. This conclusion has been confirmed in various animal models.[46,47] Individuals on medications such as Sinemet and L-dopa should be aware that velvet bean consumption may increase L-dopa levels too much.

Fava Bean

L-dopamine was also found in the fava or broad bean (*Vicia faba*) in 1913. Since then, anecdotal cases of symptomatic improvement after broad bean consumption have been described in patients with Parkinson's disease. In one small clinical study, 250 g cooked broad beans produced a substantial increase in L-dopamine blood levels, which correlated with a significant improvement in motor performance.[48] Individuals on medications such as Sinemet and L-dopamine should be aware that consumption of fava beans may increase L-dopamine levels too much.

TREATMENT SUMMARY

Treatment of Parkinson's disease from a naturopathic perspective involves trying to address the underlying disease process by employing strategies to protect the neurons in the substantia nigra as well as support current drug therapy.

Dietary Recommendations

Follow the guidelines in the chapter "A Health-Promoting Diet," along with the following recommendations:

- Eat a diet that is high in fiber, specifically from legumes and vegetables, and low in animal products.
- Eat antioxidant-rich foods: nuts and seeds, green leafy vegetables (bok choy, chard, etc.), beans, spices (turmeric, clove, cinnamon), coffee, and chocolate.
- Avoid pesticides by using organic produce when possible.
- To maintain bowel health and facilitate the liver's detoxification processes, eat high-sulfur foods such as garlic, onions, and eggs, as well as soluble fiber such as guar gum, oat bran, pectin, and psyllium seed.
- For patients taking L-dopa, a lower protein intake is recommended (50 g per day for men and 40 g per day for women). They should take their medication with a high-carbohydrate meal and delay protein intake until the final meal of the day in an effort to optimize the medication's therapeutic efficacy.

Nutritional Supplements

- A high-potency multiple vitamin and mineral formula as described in the chapter "Supplementary Measures" (without iron)
- Vitamin D_3: 2,000 to 4,000 IU per day (ideally, measure blood levels and adjust dosage accordingly)
- Fish oils: 1,000 to 3,000 mg EPA + DHA per day
- Specialty supplements:
  - N-acetylcysteine: 400 to 600 mg per day
  - NADH (Enada): 10 to 20 mg per day
  - CoQ_{10}:
    - Ubiquinone powder in hard gelatin capsule: 400 mg three times daily with meals
    - Ubiquinone suspended in rice bran oil in soft gelatin capsule: 200 mg three times daily with meals
    - Ubiquinone ==solubilized (e.g., Q-gel) in soft gelatin capsule: 100 mg three times daily with meals
    - Ubiquinone nanonized in soft or hard gelatin capsule: 100 mg three times daily with meals
    - Ubiquinone emulsified with soy peptide (BioQ10 SA) in soft or hard gelatin capsule: 100 mg twice daily with meals
    - Ubiquinol in soft gelatin capsule: 100 mg twice daily with meals

Botanical Medicines

- One of the following:
  - ○ Green tea extract (90% polyphenol content): 150 to 300 mg per day
  - ○ Grape seed extract (>95% procyanidolic oligomers): 150 to 300 mg per day
  - ○ Pine bark extract (>95% procyanidolic oligomers): 150 to 300 mg per day
  - ○ Ginkgo biloba extract (24% ginkgo flavonglycosides): 240 to 320 mg per day
- Velvet bean (*Mucuna puriens*): dosage equivalent to 30 g dried powdered seed

Peptic Ulcer

- Abdominal distress 45 to 60 minutes after meals or during the night; both relieved by food, antacids, or vomiting
- Abdominal tenderness
- Chronic but periodic symptoms
- Ulcer crater or deformity in the stomach or upper small intestine visible on X-ray or endoscopic exam
- Positive test for blood in the stool

A peptic ulcer is an erosion of the tissue, producing a crater-like lesion. When it occurs in the stomach it is called a gastric ulcer; when it occurs in the first portion of the small intestine, it is called a duodenal ulcer. Duodenal ulcers are more common, occurring in an estimated 6 to 12% of the adult population in the United States. Duodenal ulcers are four times more common in men than in women, and four to five times more common than gastric ulcers.

Although symptoms of a peptic ulcer may be absent or quite vague, most peptic ulcers are associated with abdominal discomfort noted 45 to 60 minutes after meals or during the night. In the typical case, the pain is described as gnawing, burning, cramp-like, or aching, or as "heartburn." Eating or taking antacids usually results in great relief.

Causes

Even though duodenal and gastric ulcers occur at different locations, they appear to be the result of similar mechanisms: damage to the protective factors that line the stomach and duodenum.

Gastric acid is extremely corrosive (pH 1 to 3), and though it is very effective at digesting food, it would eat right through the skin or mucous membrane. To protect against ulcers, the lining of the stomach and small intestine has a layer of slippery mucus called *mucin*. Other protective factors include the constant renewal of intestinal cells and the secretion of factors that neutralize the acid when it comes into contact with the lining of the stomach and intestine.

Contrary to popular opinion, excessive secretion of gastric acid output is rarely a factor in the development of gastric ulcers. In fact, patients who have gastric ulcers tend to secrete normal or even reduced levels of gastric acid. In duodenal ulcer patients, however, almost half have increased gastric acid output. This increase may be due to an increased number of acid-producing cells, known as *parietal cells*. As a group, patients with duodenal ulcers have twice as many parietal cells in their stomach as people without ulcers.

Even with an increase in gastric acid output, under normal circumstances there are enough protective factors to prevent either gastric or duodenal ulcer formation. However, when the integrity of these protective factors is impaired, an ulcer can form. A loss of integrity can be a result of infection by the bacterium *Helicobacter pylori*, use of aspirin and other nonsteroidal anti-inflammatory drugs (NSAIDs), excessive use of alcohol, nutrient deficiency, stress, and many other factors. Of these factors, *H. pylori* and NSAIDs are by far the most significant.

Helicobacter pylori

The role of the bacterium *H. pylori* in peptic ulcer disease has been extensively investigated. It has been shown that 90 to 100% of patients with duodenal ulcers, 70% with gastric ulcers, and about 50% of people over the age of 50 test positive for this bacterium.[1] Physicians can determine if it is present by measuring the level of antibodies to *H. pylori* in the blood or saliva, or by culturing material collected during an endoscopy.

Predisposing factors for *H. pylori* infection are low gastric acid output and low antioxidant content in the gastrointestinal lining. *Helicobacter pylori* infection increases gastric pH, thereby setting up a positive-feedback scenario.[2] In other words, *H. pylori* infection leads to ulcer formation, and ulcer formation leads to *H. pylori* infection—a vicious circle.

Aspirin and Other Nonsteroidal Anti-inflammatory Drugs

Use of aspirin and other nonsteroidal anti-inflammatory drugs is associated with a significant risk of peptic ulcer. In addition, the combination of NSAID use and smoking is particularly harmful to the ulcer patient. Although most studies documenting the relative frequency of peptic ulcers as a consequence of aspirin and NSAIDs have focused on their use in the treatment of arthritis and headaches, in one study the risk of gastrointestinal bleeding due to peptic ulcers was evaluated for aspirin at daily dosages of 300, 150, and 75 mg—dosages commonly recommended to prevent heart attacks and strokes.[3] The study was conducted at five test hospitals in England and found an increased risk of gastrointestinal bleeding due to peptic ulcer at all dosage levels. However, the dosage of 75 mg per day was associated with 40% less bleeding than 300 mg per day and 30% less bleeding than 150 mg per day. The researchers concluded: "No conventionally used prophylactic aspirin regimen seems free of the risk of peptic ulcer complications."

Stress and Emotions

Stress is universally believed to be an important causative factor in peptic ulcers. However, this link is not well established in the medical literature. One of the big problems is that studies attempting to examine this assumption about stress and ulcers have been poorly designed. Several studies have shown that the number of stressful life events is not significantly different in peptic ulcer patients compared with carefully selected, ulcer-free controls.[4] The data suggest that the significant factor is not simply the amount of stress but rather an individual's response to it.[5] Psychological factors are probably important in some people with peptic ulcer disease, but not in others. As a group, ulcer patients have been characterized as tending to repress emotions. At the very least, we encourage our patients with ulcers to discover enjoyable outlets of self-expression as well as to develop effective stress management in their lives.

Smoking

Smoking is a significant factor in the occurrence and severity of peptic ulcers. Increased frequency of occurrence, decreased response to peptic ulcer therapy, and an increased mortality due to peptic ulcers are all related to smoking. Smoking causes ulcers by at least three mechanisms. First of all, smoking increases the backflow (reflux) of bile salts into the stomach. Bile salts are extremely irritating to the stomach and initial portions of the duodenum. Bile salt reflux induced by smoking appears to be the primary reason for the increased peptic ulcer rate in smokers. Smoking also decreases the secretion of bicarbonate (an important neutralizer of gastric acid) by the pancreas and accelerates the passage of food from the stomach into the duodenum, thus not allowing the acid enough time to interact with food.[6]

The psychological aspects of smoking are also important, since the chronic anxiety and psychological stress associated with smoking appear to worsen ulcer activity.

Food Allergies

Clinical and experimental evidence points to food allergy as a primary factor in many cases of peptic ulcer.[7–10] In one study, 98% of patients who had X-ray evidence of peptic ulcer had coexisting lower- and upper-respiratory-tract allergic disease.[9] In another study, 25 of 43 allergic children had peptic ulcers as diagnosed by X-rays.[10] A diet that eliminates food allergens has been used with great success in treating and preventing recurrent ulcers.[8,9] It is ironic that many people with peptic ulcers soothe their stomachs by consuming milk, a highly allergenic food. Milk should be avoided on this basis alone. However, population studies offer additional evidence that increased milk consumption leads to a greater likelihood of ulcer. The reason is probably that milk significantly increases stomach acid production.[11]

Therapeutic Considerations

Individuals experiencing any symptoms of a peptic ulcer need competent medical care.

Complications such as hemorrhage, perforation, and obstruction represent medical emergencies that require immediate hospitalization.

Obviously, the best treatment of a peptic ulcer involves identification of the causative factor and its appropriate elimination.

Diet

Fiber

A diet rich in fiber and low in refined sugar is associated with a reduced rate of duodenal ulcers as compared with a low-fiber diet. The therapeutic use of a high-fiber diet or soluble fiber supplement in patients with recently healed duodenal ulcers reduces the recurrence rate by half.[12] This is probably a result of fiber's ability to delay the emptying of the stomach, counteracting the rapid movement of food into the duodenum that is normally seen in ulcer patients. In addition to a high-fiber diet, several fiber supplements (e.g., pectin, guar gum, and psyllium) have been shown to produce beneficial effects.[13,14]

Cabbage

Raw cabbage juice was first documented as having remarkable success in treating peptic ulcers in 1949.[15,16] One liter per day of the fresh juice, taken in divided doses, resulted in total ulcer healing in an average of only 10 days. Further research has shown that the high glutamine content of the juice is probably responsible for its efficacy in treating ulcers. In a double-blind clinical study of 57 patients, 24 using 1.6 g per day of glutamine and the rest using conventional therapy (antacids, antispasmodics, milk, and a bland diet), glutamine proved to be the more effective treatment. Half of the patients using glutamine showed complete healing (according to radiographic analysis) within two weeks, and 22 of the 24 showed complete relief and healing within four weeks.[17] Although the mechanism for these results is not known, the authors postulate that it is related to the role of glutamine in the biosynthesis of certain mucoproteins. This could stimulate mucin synthesis, which would benefit peptic ulcer patients.

In addition, isothiocyanates such as sulforaphane, from vegetables in the brassica family, have shown considerable activity against *H. pylori*. In one double-blind study, 48 *H. pylori*–infected patients were randomly assigned to consume broccoli sprouts (70 g per day for eight weeks), which contain sulforaphane, or to consume an equal amount of alfalfa sprouts, which do not contain sulforaphane, as a placebo. Broccoli sprouts decreased markers for both *H. pylori* and gastric inflammation. Values returned to their original levels two months after treatment was discontinued.[18]

Bismuth Subcitrate

Bismuth is a naturally occurring mineral that can both act as an antacid and exert activity against *H. pylori*. The best-known and most widely used bismuth preparation is bismuth subsalicylate (Pepto-Bismol). However, bismuth subcitrate has produced the best results against *H. pylori* in the treatment of peptic ulcers.[19,20] In the United States, bismuth subcitrate preparations are available through compounding pharmacies. To find a compounding pharmacist in your area, call the International Academy of Compounding Pharmacists at (800) 927–4227.

An advantage of bismuth preparations over standard antibiotic approaches to eradicating *H. pylori* is that although the bacterium may develop resistance to various antibiotics, it is unlikely to develop resistance to bismuth.[21,22]

The usual dosage for bismuth subcitrate is 240 mg twice per day before meals. For bismuth subsalicylate, the dosage is 500 mg four times per day. Bismuth preparations are extremely safe when taken at prescribed dosages. Bismuth subcitrate may cause a temporary and harmless darkening of the tongue, the stool, or both. Bismuth subsalicylate should not be taken by children recovering from the flu, chicken pox, or other viral infection, as it may mask the nausea and vomiting associated with Reye's syndrome, a rare but serious illness.

Nutritional Supplements

Vitamins A and E

Vitamins A and E have been shown to inhibit the development of stress ulcers in rats and are important factors in maintaining the integrity of the mucosal barrier.[23,24] High-dose vitamin A therapy was shown to be useful in the treatment of chronic gastric ulcers in one clinical trial, but we recommend using it only at smaller dosages, for nutritional support.[25]

Zinc

Zinc increases mucin production in vitro and has been shown to have a protective effect against peptic ulcers in animal studies and a curative effect in humans.[26] Zinc bound to carnosine is perhaps the most beneficial. Carnosine is a small protein composed of the amino acids histidine and alanine. It is found in relatively high concentrations in several body tissues, most notably skeletal muscle, heart muscle, and the brain. The exact biological role of carnosine is still under investigation, but numerous animal studies have demonstrated that it possesses strong and specific antioxidant properties, protects against radiation damage, improves heart function, and promotes wound healing. Zinc bound to carnosine exerts significant protection against ulcer formation and has ulcer-healing properties. Clinical studies with humans demonstrate the same effects, including an ability to antagonize *H. pylori*, which is linked to indigestion and stomach cancer as well as to peptic ulcer. When 60 patients with *H. pylori* infection who were suffering from indigestion were given either antibiotics alone or antibiotics plus zinc carnosine for seven days, better results were seen with the group getting zinc carnosine (94% success rate vs. 77%).[27]

Botanical Medicines

Licorice

Licorice root (*Glycyrrhiza glabra*) has historically been regarded as an excellent medicine for peptic ulcer. However, one of the substances in licorice, glycyrrhizinic acid, has known side effects that include salt and water retention, leading to hypertension. A procedure was developed to remove glycyrrhizinic acid from licorice, forming deglycyrrhizinated licorice (DGL). The result is a very successful antiulcer agent without any known side effects.[28–31] Researchers think that DGL works by stimulating the secretion of the protective substance mucin that lines the stomach and intestines. Clinical studies have demonstrated that DGL is as effective as cimetidine in preventing recurrence of ulcers.[28]

DGL contains several flavonoids that have been shown to inhibit *H. pylori*.[32] In addition, unlike antibiotics, the flavonoids were also shown to augment natural defense fac-

- -

QUICK REVIEW

- **Individuals with peptic ulcer must be monitored by a physician, because complications can be serious if not effectively treated.**
- **Ulcers are usually the result of a breakdown in protective factors that line the stomach or small intestine.**
- **The bacterium *Helicobacter pylori* has been linked to both duodenal and gastric ulcers.**
- **Use of aspirin and other nonsteroidal anti-inflammatory drugs (NSAIDs) is associated with a significant risk of developing an ulcer.**
- **Smoking contributes to the occurrence and severity of peptic ulcers.**
- **An allergy to milk may be a causative factor in many cases of ulcers.**

- **A diet rich in fiber is associated with a reduced rate of duodenal ulcers.**
- **Raw cabbage juice is well documented as having remarkable success in treating peptic ulcers.**
- **Bismuth is a naturally occurring mineral that can act as an antacid and exert activity against *H. pylori*.**
- **Zinc carnosine has been shown to heal ulcers and help control *H. pylori*.**
- **DGL, a special form of licorice, has been shown to be as effective as ulcer medications like Tagamet and Zantac in head-to-head comparison studies.**
- **Rhubarb or aloe vera preparations can be used to stop the bleeding of an ulcer.**

tors that prevent ulcer formation. The activity of the most potent flavonoid was shown to be similar to that of bismuth subcitrate.

It appears that in order to be effective in healing peptic ulcers, DGL must mix with saliva. DGL may promote the release of salivary compounds that stimulate the growth and regeneration of stomach and intestinal cells. DGL in capsule form has not been shown to be effective.

The standard dosage for DGL is two to four 380-mg chewable tablets between meals or 20 minutes before meals. Taking DGL after meals is associated with poor results. DGL therapy should be continued for at least 8 to 16 weeks after symptoms disappear.

Mastic

Mastic is a resin obtained from the mastic tree (*Pistacia lentiscus*). Originally liquid, the resin is sun-dried into brittle, translucent drops. When chewed, the resin softens and becomes a bright white and opaque gum. The flavor is bitter at first, but after being chewed the drops release a refreshing, slightly piney or cedary flavor.

People in the Mediterranean region have used mastic as a medicine for gastrointestinal ailments for several thousand years. Recent studies indicate that it may be of benefit in healing peptic ulcers. In a double-blind clinical trial carried out on 38 patients with symptomatic and endoscopically proved duodenal ulcer, the patients were given either mastic gum (1 g per day) or a placebo for two weeks. Symptomatic relief was obtained in 16 patients on mastic (80%) and in 9 patients on the placebo (50%), while endoscopically proved healing occurred in 14 patients on mastic (70%) and only 4 patients on the placebo (22%).[33]

In another study, mastic gum showed some bactericidal activity on *H. pylori*, but it was not sufficient to eradicate the bacteria, compared with conventional drug therapy.[34]

Rhubarb and Aloe Vera

In cases of active intestinal bleeding, rhubarb (*Rheum* species) and aloe vera preparations can be extremely effective. In one double-blind study, rhubarb extract stopped bleeding from gastric or duodenal ulcers in more than 90% of 312 patients, and accomplished this in less than 60 hours.[35]

The beneficial actions of rhubarb are due to the presence of anthraquinones and flavonoids, which stop the bleeding by acting as astringents (basically, drying agents). Aloe vera contains similar compounds. In cases of active gastrointestinal bleeding, we recommend rhubarb or aloe vera preparations. The most accessible treatment may be drinking aloe vera juice, about 4 cups per day, during these times.

· ·

TREATMENT SUMMARY

Peptic ulcer disease has a number of causes, all of which lead to an ulcerative lesion in either the stomach or the duodenum. Patients must be carefully evaluated to determine which of the factors discussed earlier in this chapter are most relevant to their situation. This can be difficult, however, so a more general approach may be necessary.

The first step is to identify and eliminate or reduce all factors implicated in peptic ulcers: *H. pylori*, food allergy,

cigarette smoking, stress, and drugs (especially aspirin and other NSAIDs). Once the causative factors have been controlled, attention should be directed at healing the ulcers, inhibiting exacerbating factors (e.g., reducing excess acid secretion if present), and promoting tissue resistance. Finally, make diet and lifestyle changes in order to prevent further recurrence.

WARNING: Peptic ulcer complications—hemorrhage, perforation, and obstruction—are medical emergencies that require immediate hospitalization.

Diet

Eliminate common food allergens, especially milk. Eat a diet high in dietary fiber, and consume fresh cabbage juice and other vegetable juices on a regular basis.

Nutritional Supplements

- A high-potency multiple vitamin and mineral formula as described in the chapter "Supplementary Measures"
- Key individual nutrients:
  - Vitamin C: 500 mg three times per day
  - Vitamin E (mixed tocopherols): 100 IU per day
  - Zinc: 20 to 30 mg per day (but do not supplement with extra zinc if using zinc carnosine)
  - Vitamin D_3: 2,000 to 4,000 IU per day (ideally, measure blood levels and adjust dosage accordingly)
- Fish oils: 1,000 mg EPA + DHA per day
- One of the following:
  - Grape seed extract (>95% procyanidolic oligomers): 100 to 300 mg per day
  - Pine bark extract (>95% procyanidolic oligomers): 100 to 300 mg per day
  - Some other flavonoid-rich extract with a similar flavonoid content, super greens formula, or another plant-based antioxidant that can provide an oxygen radical absorption capacity (ORAC) of 3,000 to 6,000 units or higher per day
- Specialty supplements:
  - Glutamine: 1,000 mg three times per day
  - Zinc carnosine: 75 mg once or twice per day

Botanical Medicines

- One of the following:
  - DGL (deglycyrrhizinated licorice): 380 to 760 mg taken 20 minutes before meals three times per day
  - Mastic gum: 350 to 1,000 mg three times per day
  - Aloe vera juice: 2 to 4 cups per day

Periodontal Disease

- Gingivitis: inflammation of the gums, characterized by redness, contour changes, and bleeding

- Periodontitis: localized pain, loose teeth, presence of dental pockets, redness, swelling, or pus; X-ray may reveal bone destruction

Periodontal disease is an inflammatory condition of the gums (gingivitis) and/or support structures (periodontitis). Periodontal disease typically progresses from gingivitis to periodontitis. It may be a manifestation of a more systemic condition, such as diabetes, anemia, vitamin deficiency states, leukemia, or other disorders of white blood cell function.[1] An association with hardening of the arteries has also been reported, as periodontal disease is associated with an elevation in C-reactive protein—an important marker for systemic inflammation and an independent risk factor for heart disease.[2]

Since there can be significant loss of the bone that supports the teeth (alveolar bone) without much inflammation, the definition of periodontal disease used in this chapter excludes the processes that cause only tooth loss (the majority of which is due to osteoporosis).[1] These noninflammatory conditions reflect systemic disease, with local factors playing only a minor role. Therefore, the focus in such cases should be on treating the underlying condition rather than the "periodontal disease." For a discussion of the factors involved in noninflammatory alveolar bone loss, see the chapter "Osteoporosis."

The focus of this chapter is on the use of nutrition and lifestyle factors to aid in prevention and control of inflammatory periodontal disease. This disease is a good example of a condition that is probably best treated with the combined expertise of a dentist or periodontist and a nutritionally minded physician. Although oral hygiene is of great importance in treating and preventing periodontal disease, it is not sufficient in many cases. The patient's immune system and other defense mechanisms must be normalized if development and progression of the disease are to be controlled.[1,3] To a large extent, a person's nutritional status determines the status of his or her defense mechanisms.

The frequency of periodontal disease increases directly with age. The rate of periodontal disease is approximately 15% at age 10, 38% at age 20, 46% at age 35, and 54% at age 50. As a group, men have a higher prevalence and severity of periodontal disease than women. The occurrence of periodontal disease is inversely related to increasing levels of education and income; rural dwellers have a higher level of severity and prevalence than city dwellers.[1]

Causes

Understanding the underlying process of any disease leads to a more effective treatment plan. In periodontal disease, this means understanding the normal protective factors in the gums and supporting structures (periodontium). Many experts agree that the presence of bacteria is not sufficient to cause disease; a person's immune status and other defense mechanisms must be involved.[3] These are discussed below.

The Environment of the Gingival Sulcus

The gingival sulcus is the V-shaped crevice that surrounds each tooth. The anatomy of the gingival sulcus is ideal for growth of bacteria, as it is resistant to the cleansing action of saliva. Furthermore, the gingival fluid (the fluid found in the sulcus) provides a rich nutrient source for microorganisms. The clinical determination of the depth of the gingival sulcus is an important part of the diagnosis. Individuals who have periodontal disease should see their dentist no less than once every six months for proper evaluation and cleaning.

Bacterial Factors

Bacterial plaque has long been considered the causative agent in most forms of periodontal disease.[1] However, immune system factors are now known to be involved as well.[1,3] Bacteria secrete numerous compounds that weaken a person's immune system, including endotoxins and exotoxins, free radicals and collagen-destroying enzymes, and waste products.[1]

Neutrophil Function

White blood cells known as *neutrophils* constitute a first line of defense against microbial overgrowth. When neutrophils function inadequately, the periodontium can be damaged.[1,3] Neutrophil function is lower in older people generally, as well as in patients with diabetes, Crohn's disease, and Down syndrome.[1,3] These patients are at extremely high risk for developing rapidly progressing periodontal disease, as are people with temporarily low levels of neutrophils.

Neutrophils can also play a role in tissue destruction. As they defend the body against microbes, neutrophils release numerous free radicals (which break down collagen), inflammatory compounds, and a compound that stimulates alveolar bone destruction.[1,3]

Complement Activation

The complement system is composed of at least 22 proteins that circulate in the blood. Upon activation, complement components act in a cascade fashion. The complement system plays a critical role in the resistance to infection, but it also plays a big role in the tissue injury of periodontal disease, because complement activation increases gingival permeability, allowing bacteria and bacterial by-products to penetrate gum tissue.[1,3] In periodontal disease, activation of complement within the periodontal pocket is possibly the major factor in tissue destruction.

IgE and Mast Cell Function

Mast cells are white blood cells that reside in tissues. They contain histamine and other inflammatory compounds in packets known as *granules*. The release of the contents of these packets (in response to allergy antibodies, complement activation, trauma, endotoxins, and free radicals) is a major factor in periodontal disease.[1] The finding of increased allergy antibody (IgE) concentrations in the gingiva of patients with periodontal disease suggests that allergic reactions may be a factor in the progression of the disease in some patients.[4]

Amalgam Restorations

Faulty dental work is a common cause of gingival inflammation and periodontal destruction.[1] Overhanging margins from a poorly done filling or crown provide an ideal location for the accumulation of plaque and the multiplication of bacteria. If the restoration is a silver amalgam filling, there may be even more involvement because over time the mercury in those fillings is released into the body, where it decreases the activity of antioxidant enzymes, including glutathione peroxidase, superoxide dismutase, and catalase.[5] The support structures of the teeth are particularly sensitive to free radical damage.[6]

The Collagen Matrix

The collagen matrix of the periodontal membrane serves to anchor the tooth to the alveolar bone and allows the dissipation of the tremendous amount of pressure exerted during chewing. The health of this collagen matrix affects its ability to resist inflammatory mediators, bacteria and their by-products, and destructive enzymes. Because periodontal collagen is constantly being renewed, it is extremely vulnerable when the necessary cofactors for collagen synthesis (protein, zinc, copper, vitamins C, B_6, and A, etc.) are absent or deficient.

Miscellaneous Factors

Numerous local factors favor the progression of periodontal disease. These include food residue, unreplaced missing teeth, malocclusion, tongue thrusting, bruxism (grinding of the teeth), toothbrush trauma, mouth breathing, and tobacco smoking.

Tobacco smoking is associated with increased susceptibility to severe periodontal disease and tooth loss.[1,7,8] Many of the harmful effects of smoking are a result of free radical damage. Furthermore, smoking greatly reduces vitamin C levels, thereby intensifying its damaging effects.[9]

Therapeutic Considerations

From a nutritional perspective, therapeutic goals in treating periodontal disease are:

- Decrease wound healing time (the time needed for wound healing is longer in patients who are more susceptible to periodontal disease)[10]
- Improve membrane and collagen integrity
- Decrease inflammation and free radical damage (inflammation can promote periodontal disease)
- Enhance immune status

Diet and Nutritional Supplements

Vitamin C

Vitamin C plays a major role in preventing periodontal disease, as is evident from many experimental studies.[1,11–14] The classical symptom of gingivitis seen in scurvy (severe vitamin C deficiency) illustrates the vital function vitamin C plays in maintaining the integrity of the periodontal membrane and collagen matrix.[1] The effects of deficiency on the bone include osteoporosis and retardation or cessation of bone formation. Subclinical vitamin C deficiency plays a significant role in periodontal disease through these effects and through its role in delaying wound healing.

Decreased vitamin C levels are also associated with increased susceptibility of the oral tissues to endotoxins and bacterial by-products, as well as impaired function of white blood cells (particularly neutrophils).

Sugar

Sugar is known to significantly increase plaque accumulation while decreasing white blood cell function.[15,16] The inhibition of neutrophil function is due to competition with vitamin C. Vitamin C and glucose are known to compete for intracellular transport sites, with this intracellular transport being largely insulin-dependent. (See the chapter "Immune System Support" for further information on nutrient factors and immune function.)

If we consider the fact that the average American consumes in excess of 150 g sucrose and other refined carbohydrates per day, it is safe to say that most Americans have a chronically depressed immune status, which puts them at increased risk for periodontal disease.

Vitamin A

Vitamin A deficiency predisposes a person to periodontal disease. Deficiency of vitamin A is associated with abnormal cell structures in the periodontium, inflammatory infiltration and degeneration, periodontal pocket formation, plaque formation, increased susceptibility to infection, and abnormal alveolar bone formation.[1] Vitamin A is necessary for collagen synthesis, wound healing, and enhancing numerous immune functions.

Zinc

Zinc's importance in treating periodontal disease cannot be overstated. Zinc functions synergistically with vitamin A in many body processes.[17] The severity of periodontal disease is directly associated with decreased zinc levels.[18] In the United States, marginal zinc deficiency is widespread, particularly among the elderly. This is clearly a factor in the increasing prevalence of periodontal disease with age, although the geriatric population as a whole is at higher risk for developing numerous nutrient deficiencies.

The functions of zinc in the gingiva and periodontium include stabilization of membranes, antioxidant activity, collagen synthesis, inhibition of plaque growth, inhibition of mast-cell degranulation, and numerous immune-enhancing activities.[17–20] Zinc is also known to significantly reduce wound healing time.

Plaque growth can be inhibited by the use twice per day of a mouthwash that contains 5% zinc.[19] However, lower concentrations of zinc or less frequent mouthwash use is not particularly successful.

Vitamin E and Selenium

These two nutrients function synergistically in antioxidant mechanisms and seem to potentiate each other's effect. Vitamin E alone has been demonstrated to be of considerable value in treating patients with severe periodontal disease.[1,21] This can largely be attributed to the decreased wound healing time associated with vitamin E.

The antioxidant effects of vitamin E are particularly needed if amalgam fillings are present. Mercury depletes the tissues of the antioxidant enzymes superoxide dismutase, glutathione peroxidase, and catalase. In animal studies, this effect is prevented by supplementation with vitamin E.[5] Another reason supplemental selenium is beneficial is that it is displaced by mercury from several enzyme systems. Higher levels allow it to better compete with mercury for inclusion in the enzymes.

The antioxidant activities of selenium and vitamin E also deter periodontal disease because the effects of free radicals are extremely damaging to gums.

Coenzyme Q$_{10}$

Coenzyme Q$_{10}$ is involved in energy production, and it is also an effective antioxidant. Coenzyme Q$_{10}$ is widely used in Japan to treat many conditions, including periodontal disease. A review of seven studies found that 70% of the 332 patients involved responded favorably to CoQ_{10} supplementation.[22] A double-blind study comprising 56 subjects found that the supplemented group responded significantly, while the placebo group displayed very little change in periodontal pocket depth and tooth mobility.[23]

Flavonoids

As a group, these compounds are an essential nutritional component of any periodontal disease treatment program. Flavonoids are extremely effective in reducing inflammation and stabilizing collagen structures. Flavonoids affect collagen structure by decreasing membrane permeability, thereby decreasing the load of inflammatory mediators and bacterial products; preventing free radical damage; inhibiting destruction of collagen; inhibiting mast cell degranulation; and cross-linking with collagen fibers directly to increase their stability and strength.[24-26]

Perhaps the most useful source of flavonoids is either grape seed or pine bark extract, as the proanthocyanidins in both have been shown to possess a wide range of actions useful against periodontal disease.[27,28]

The flavonoid components of green tea (*Camellia sinensis*) are also useful, as they have demonstrated activity against gingival

. . . .

QUICK REVIEW

- **Periodontal disease is best treated with the combined expertise of a dentist or periodontist and a nutritionally minded physician.**
- **Although oral hygiene is of great importance in treating and preventing periodontal disease, it is not sufficient in many cases.**
- **The immune system and other defense mechanisms are essential in preventing and controlling periodontal disease.**
- **Faulty dental work is a common cause of gingival inflammation and periodontal destruction.**
- **Tobacco smoking is associated with increased susceptibility to severe periodontal disease and tooth loss.**
- **Vitamin C plays a major role in preventing periodontal disease.**
- **Sugar is known to significantly increase plaque accumulation while decreasing white blood cell function.**
- **Vitamin E has been demonstrated to be of considerable value in treating patients with severe periodontal disease.**
- **Coenzyme Q_{10} is useful in periodontal disease.**
- **Flavonoids, particularly those found in grape seed, pine bark, and green tea extract, are extremely effective in reducing inflammation and stabilizing collagen structures of the gums.**
- **Folic acid has produced significant reductions of gingival inflammation in double-blind studies.**
- **Sanguinarine, an alkaloid derived from bloodroot, is useful in preventing dental plaque.**

bacteria and direct anti-inflammatory effects as well. Population-based studies have shown that green tea intake protects against periodontal disease and tooth loss.[29] Clinical studies have focused on direct, local effects with either chewable candy alone or dissolvable strips impregnated with green tea catechins. In the study with the strips, pocket depth and proportion of disease-causing bacteria were markedly decreased.[30] The study using the chewable candy was double-blind and indicated that the green tea chews significantly reduced plaque and the inflammatory degree of the gingiva.[31] A double-blind study showed that chewing gum containing procyanidolic oligomers also minimizes gingival bleeding and plaque accumulation.[32]

Folic Acid

The use of folic acid in double-blind studies, either as a mouthwash or as a pill, has produced significant reductions of gingival inflammation, as determined by reduction in redness, bleeding tendency, and plaque scores.[33–37] Folic acid mouthwash (0.1% folic acid) is significantly more effective than oral supplementation consisting of either 2 or 5 mg folic acid per day, suggesting a local mechanism of action.[35–37] Folic acid has also been demonstrated to bind plaque-derived toxins.

The use of folic acid mouthwash is particularly indicated for pregnant women and women using birth control pills, in whom hormonal changes appear to reduce the amount of folic acid in the cells of the oral cavity.[38–40] People taking drugs that interfere with folic acid (e.g., chemotherapy agents, epilepsy drugs, and drugs used in Crohn's disease and ulcerative colitis) also benefit from folic acid mouthwash.

Botanical Medicines

A number of botanical compounds have shown an ability to inhibit plaque formation, including green tea polyphenols and glycyrrhetinic acid from licorice, but the most extensively studied compound is an alcoholic extract of bloodroot.

Bloodroot

Bloodroot (*Sanguinaria canadensis*) contains a mixture of alkaloids, but chiefly sanguinarine, which is available in commercial toothpastes and mouth rinses. Sanguinarine demonstrates properties that are useful in preventing dental plaque formation. It has broad antimicrobial activity and anti-inflammatory properties. In vitro studies indicate that the antiplaque action of sanguinarine is due to its ability to prevent bacteria from adhering to tissue. Electron microscope studies demonstrate that bacteria exposed to sanguinarine aggregate and become morphologically irregular.[41]

Sanguinarine appears to be less effective than chlorhexidine mouthwash, but it is effective in many cases and does have the advantage of being a natural compound as opposed to a synthetic one.[41,42]

Gotu Kola

An extract containing the triterpenoids of gotu kola (*Centella asiatica*) has demonstrated impressive wound-healing properties. These properties can be put to good use in treating severe periodontal disease or if surgery is required. One study demonstrated that gotu kola extract was quite helpful in speeding recovery after laser surgery for severe periodontal disease.[43]

TREATMENT SUMMARY

Since many factors are involved in the initiation and promotion of periodontal disease, effective therapy requires that all relevant factors be controlled. Since there are as yet no clear guidelines for determining which factors are most important for any given person, a general approach is recommended here. If you are a smoker, we strongly encourage you to stop, as continued smoking greatly decreases the success of any therapy for periodontal disease.

Oral Hygiene

Visit a dentist periodically to have plaque and tartar removed. Brushing after meals and daily flossing are necessary.

Diet

A diet high in fiber may have a protective effect by increasing salivary secretion. Avoiding sugar and refined carbohydrates is extremely important. Follow the general guidelines detailed in the chapter "A Health-Promoting Diet."

Nutritional Supplements

- A high-potency multiple vitamin and mineral formula as described in the chapter "Supplementary Measures"
- Key individual nutrients:
  - Vitamin B_6: 25 to 50 mg per day
  - Folic acid: 800 mcg to 2 mg per day, or wash mouth with ½ fl oz of a 0.1% solution of folic acid twice a day
  - Vitamin B_{12}: 800 mcg per day
  - Vitamin C: 500 to 1,000 mg three times per day
  - Vitamin E (mixed tocopherols): 100 to 200 IU per day
  - Selenium: 100 to 200 mcg per day
  - Zinc: 30 mg zinc picolinate per day (45 mg per day if another form), or wash mouth with ½ fl oz of a 5% zinc solution twice per day
  - Vitamin D_3: 2,000 to 4,000 IU per day (ideally, measure blood levels and adjust dosage accordingly)
- Fish oils: 1,000 mg EPA + DHA per day
- One of the following:
  - Grape seed extract (>95% procyanidolic oligomers): 100 to 300 mg per day
  - Pine bark extract (>95% procyanidolic oligomers): 100 to 300 mg per day
  - Green tea extract (>80% polyphenol content): 150 to 300 mg per day
- Coenzyme Q_{10}: 50 to 100 mg three times per day

Botanical Medicines

- Bloodroot: use toothpaste containing the extract sanguinarine
- Gotu kola: Dosage is based upon the triterpenic acid content. Recommended dosage is 30 mg of triterpenoids twice daily. For example, for an extract containing 6% triterpenoids, the dosage would be 500 mg twice daily.

Premenstrual Syndrome

· ·

- Recurrent signs and symptoms that develop during the 7 to 14 days prior to menstruation
- Typical symptoms include decreased energy level, tension, irritability, depression, headache, altered sex drive, breast pain, backache, abdominal bloating, and swelling of the fingers and ankles

Premenstrual syndrome (PMS) is estimated to affect between 30 and 40% of menstruating women, with peak occurrences among women in their 30s and 40s. In most cases, symptoms are relatively mild. However, in about 10% of all women, symptoms can be quite severe. Severe PMS, with depression, irritability, and extreme mood swings, is referred to as premenstrual dysphoric disorder (PMDD).

**Signs and Symptoms of
Premenstrual Syndrome**
Psychological

- Nervousness, anxiety, and irritability
- Mood swings and mild to severe personality change
- Fatigue, lethargy, and depression

Gastrointestinal

- Abdominal bloating
- Diarrhea and/or constipation
- Change in appetite (usually cravings for sugar)

Breasts and reproductive system

- Tender and enlarged breasts
- Uterine cramping
- Altered libido

General

- Headache
- Backache
- Acne
- Swelling of fingers and ankles

Causes

The Normal Menstrual Cycle

In order to appreciate the hormonal abnormalities that have been found in some women with PMS, it is important to briefly review the normal menstrual cycle. The menstrual cycle reflects the monthly rhythmic changes in the secretion rates of the female hormones and corresponding changes in the lining of the uterus and other female organs.

The menstrual cycle is controlled by the complex interactions of the hypothalamus, pituitary, and ovaries. Each month during the reproductive years, the secretion of various hormones is designed to accomplish two primary goals: (1) ensure that only a single egg is released by the ovaries each month, and (2) prepare the lining of the uterus (the endometrium) for implantation of the fertilized egg. To accomplish these goals, the concentrations of the primary female sexual hormones, estrogen and progesterone, fluctuate during the menstrual cycle.

The control center for the female hormonal system is the hypothalamus, a region of the brain roughly the size of a cherry, situated above the pituitary gland and below another area of the brain called the thalamus. The hypothalamus and pituitary gland are housed in the middle of the head just behind the eyes. The hypothalamus controls the female hormonal system by releasing hormones, such as gonadotropin-releasing hormone (GnRH) and follicle-stimulating hormone–releasing hormone (FSH-RH), which stimulate the release of pituitary hormones.

In response to the hypothalamus, the pituitary gland releases follicle-stimulating hormone (FSH) and luteinizing hormone (LH). FSH is the hormone primarily responsible for the maturation of the egg during the first phase of the menstrual cycle. It is called follicle-stimulating hormone because each egg within the ovary is housed inside an individual follicle. LH is responsible for initiating ovulation, the release of the fully developed egg.

The release of LH is triggered by increasing estrogen levels as a result of the growing follicle. After ovulation, the eggless follicle is transformed into the corpus luteum, which functions primarily to secrete progesterone and estrogen to help a fertilized egg become well established in the uterine lining. If fertilization does not occur, the corpus luteum recedes, hormone production decreases, menstruation occurs approximately two weeks later, and the entire menstrual cycle begins anew.

The usual menstrual cycle is completed in about a month. It is divided into three phases, in order of occurrence: follicular, ovulatory, and luteal. The follicular phase lasts for 10 to 14 days, the ovulatory phase lasts for about 36 hours and involves the release of the egg, and the luteal phase lasts for 14 days.

Other Hormones

Because of the complex interrelationships among the components of the endocrine system, disorder of any of the individual parts of the system (pituitary, ovaries, adrenals, thyroid, parathyroids, and pancreas) can lead to menstrual abnormalities and/or PMS. For example, low thyroid function (hypothyroidism) and elevated levels of cortisol (an adrenal hormone) are common in women with PMS.

Prolactin, another hormone produced by the pituitary, also plays an important role in PMS and female infertility. Prolactin's chief function is to promote the development of the mammary glands and milk secretion during pregnancy and nursing. Increased production of prolactin in lactating women can inhibit the maturation of the follicles in the ovaries, thus delaying the return of fertility after childbirth. In nonlactating women, elevated levels of prolactin are often linked to cases of PMS, menstrual abnormalities, ovarian cysts, breast tenderness, and absence of ovulation.

Hormonal Patterns in Women with PMS

There is no consistent alteration in hormonal patterns among PMS patients compared with women who have no symptoms of PMS. For many years it was commonly believed that women with PMS experienced elevated estrogen levels and reduced progesterone levels 5 to 10 days before the menses, increasing the ratio of estrogen to progesterone. While this association is no longer accepted in the medical literature as a causative factor in most cases of PMS, it may be a factor for some women. Other factors in some cases of

PMS may include hypothyroidism, elevated prolactin levels, elevated FSH levels six to nine days prior to the onset of menses, and excessive amounts of aldosterone (a hormone produced by the adrenal glands that leads to sodium and water retention).

The dominant belief now is that PMS is the result of alterations in brain chemistry that affects the brain's sensitivity to hormones. Lower levels of the neurotransmitter serotonin are most often suggested as the underlying issue in PMS. The influence of serotonin on mood and behavior is fully discussed in the chapter "Depression." It is thus not surprising that recent research and therapy have focused on the use of antidepressant drugs for PMS, particularly the selective serotonin reuptake inhibitor drugs such as fluoxetine (Prozac), sertraline (Zoloft), and paroxetine (Paxil). Interestingly, many of the natural antidepressant agents also show benefits in PMS.

Therapeutic Considerations

Even though it is now understood that there is no significant disturbance in serum estrogen or progesterone levels in most cases of PMS, it is possible that a relative excess or insufficiency of either hormone may have an effect on the central nervous system. Owing to the lack of scientific understanding in this area and to clinical experience with improving estrogen metabolism in women with PMS, it is still something to be considered. The bottom line is that there is no single cause of PMS; rather, each woman needs to understand her unique imbalances, which then need to be addressed.

Estrogen Metabolism

In the early 1940s, Morton Biskind, M.D., observed an apparent relationship between B vitamin deficiency and PMS.[1,2] He postulated that PMS, as well as fibrocystic breast disease, was due to an elevation in estrogen levels caused by decreased detoxification and elimination of estrogen in the liver as a result of B vitamin deficiency.

There appears to be support for Biskind's theory. Estrogen excess is known to produce cholestasis (diminished bile flow or "sluggish liver"). Cholestasis reflects minimal impairment of liver function because normal indicators of liver status (such as concentrations of the liver enzymes in the blood) are not elevated. These enzyme measurements, the conventional means of assessing liver status, are not very useful, however, as they serve only to indicate liver damage, being elevated only when the liver cells are leaking enzymes. Because of the liver's important role in numerous metabolic processes, even a minor impairment of liver function can have profound effects.

Cholestasis can be caused by a large number of factors besides excess estrogen, chief among them being obesity and/or insulin resistance (see the chapter "Non-Alcoholic Fatty Liver Disease (NAFLD)/Non-Alcoholic Steatohepatitis (NASH)"). The presence of cholestasis may be a predisposing factor in PMS, because with cholestasis there is reduced estrogen detoxification and clearance, producing a positive feedback cycle. The high incidence of gallstones and nonalcoholic fatty liver disease is a clear indication that many American women suffer from cholestasis.

One study found a direct correlation between the estrogen/progesterone ratio and endorphin activity in the brain.[3] In essence, when the estrogen/progesterone ratio increased, there was a decline in endorphin levels. This reduction is significant considering the known ability of endorphins to normalize or improve mood. Other studies have shown that low endorphin levels during the luteal phase are common in women with PMS.[4] Endorphins are lowered by stress and raised by exercise. The role of endorphins is discussed further later.

The way in which estrogen levels during the luteal phase negatively affect neurotransmitter and endorphin levels may be connected to the way in which estrogen impairs the action of vitamin B_6. Vitamin B_6 levels are typically quite low in depressed patients, especially women taking estrogens (birth control pills or conjugated estrogens such as Premarin).[5,6] Vitamin B_6 supplementation has been shown to have positive effects on all PMS symptoms, particularly depression, in many women (discussed in greater detail later). Historically, this improvement was thought to be the result of a combination of a reduction in estrogen levels and an increase in progesterone levels in the mid-luteal phase. Now, however, the possible explanation centers on the influence of B_6 on brain chemistry. Vitamin B_6 has the ability to increase the synthesis of several neurotransmitters in the brain, including serotonin, dopamine, norepinephrine, epinephrine, taurine, and histamine.

Diet

Women suffering from PMS typically eat a diet that is even worse than the standard American diet. Compared with the diets of symptom-free women, the diets of PMS patients are more likely to feature the following:[7]

- 62% more refined carbohydrates
- 275% more refined sugar
- 79% more dairy products
- 78% more sodium
- 53% less iron
- 77% less manganese
- 52% less zinc

A diet that is high in dairy products may also contribute to some PMS symptoms. A survey of 39 women with PMS and 14 women without reported that the women with PMS consumed five times more dairy products and three time more refined sugar than the women without PMS.[8] Another study observed that women with PMS tend to have an increased intake of dietary fat, carbohydrates, and simple sugars and a decreased protein intake.[9]

Food cravings are also more often present in women with PMS; this may in part be due to a decrease in serotonin during the luteal phase in PMS sufferers. Serotonin-enhancing treatments (e.g., 5-HTP) may be helpful in controlling such food cravings.[10]

Another nutritional factor in PMS is the effect of refined sugars. These produce a rapid increase in insulin, which then causes the retention of sodium and subsequent water retention, resulting in swelling in the hands and feet, abdominal bloating, and breast engorgement. Sugar, especially combined with caffeine, has a detrimental effect on mood (discussed later).[11] A high intake of sugar also impairs estrogen metabolism. The evidence is based on the higher frequency of PMS symptoms in women consuming a high-sugar diet and the fact that a high sugar intake is also associated with higher estrogen levels.[12] One study found that a low-fat, high-complex-carbohydrate diet alleviated premenstrual breast tenderness.[13] Of course, eating sugar and other refined carbohydrates results in increased cravings for more when blood sugar levels drop, creating a vicious circle. (See the chapter "Hypoglycemia" for a more complete discussion.)

C-reactive protein, a marker of inflammation, has been correlated with the severity of both physical and psychological symptoms of PMS.[14] A diet that includes large amounts of sugar, poultry, eggs, cheese, milk, white flour, white rice, and partially hydrogenated oils stimulates inflammatory pathways. Foods that can reduce inflammation include fresh fruits (especially berries), green leafy vegetables, fish, nuts, seeds, turmeric, garlic, and onions.

Vegetarian women have been shown to excrete two to three times more estrogen in their feces and to have 50% lower levels of free estrogen in their blood than omnivores.[15,16] These differences are thought to be due to vegetarians' lower fat consumption and higher fiber intake. These dietary differences may also explain the lower incidence of breast cancer, endometriosis, and uterine cancer in vegetarian women, and perhaps play a role in PMS.

At the very least, women suffering from PMS should lower saturated fat and cholesterol intake by reducing consumption of animal foods and increasing consumption of fiber-rich plant foods (fruits, vegetables, whole grains, and legumes).

Decreasing the percentage of calories as fat, in particular saturated fat, has dramatic effects on the reduction of circulating estrogen.[17,18] In one study, when 17 women switched from the standard American diet (40% of calories from fat and only 12 g fiber per day) to a low-fat, high-fiber diet (25% of calories from fat and 40 g fiber per day), there was a 36% reduction in blood estrogen levels, with 16 out of the 17 women demonstrating significant reductions in only 8 to 10 weeks.[19]

It should be noted that not all nutrition research shows a clear-cut association with PMS. In the Study of Women's Health Across the Nation, a cross-sectional analysis was conducted of PMS symptoms in a multiethnic sample of 3,302 midlife women.[20] The researchers sought to determine if the frequency of physical or emotional premenstrual symptoms was associated with dietary intake of phytoestrogens, fiber, fat, or calcium; consumption of alcohol or caffeine; exposure to cigarette smoke; lack of physical exercise; and race/ethnicity or socioeconomic status. In this study, most dietary factors did not appear to be related to PMS. A lower fat intake was associated with food cravings and bloating. A higher fiber intake was associated with a reduction in breast pain. Alcohol intake was negatively associated with anxiety, mood changes, and headaches. Exposure to cigarette smoke, whether passive or active, was associated with cramps and back pain. Ethnic differences in the reporting of symptoms and in associations with other medical conditions were observed as well.

Thyroid Function

Low thyroid function (hypothyroidism) has been shown to affect a large proportion of women with PMS.[21,22] For example, in one study, 51 of 54 subjects with PMS demonstrated low thyroid status compared with 0 of 12 in the control group.[23] In another study, 7 of 10 subjects in the PMS group had low thyroid status compared with 0 of 9 in the control group.[22] Other studies have shown hypothyroidism to be only slightly more common in women with PMS than in controls.[23,24] Many women with PMS and confirmed hypothyroidism who are given thyroid hormone experience complete relief of symptoms.[21] For more information, see the chapter "Hypothyroidism."

Stress

Study of the interaction of stress/serotonin and PMS has shown that serotonin levels in women with PMS fall after ovulation. Those without PMS had much higher levels of serotonin during the last half of the menstrual cycle.[25] A key factor may be how women with PMS handle stress, as many women with PMS tend to employ negative coping styles, including:[26]

- Overeating
- Watching too much television
- Emotional outbursts
- Overspending
- Excessive behavior
- Dependence on chemicals
  - Drugs, legal or illicit
  - Alcohol
  - Smoking

There are also some important relationships between PMS and depression. Depression is a common feature in many cases of PMS, and PMS symptoms are typically more severe in depressed women. The reason appears to be a decrease in the brain level of various neurotransmitters, with serotonin and GABA being the most significant.[27,28] The standard medical approach to both PMS and depression involves antidepressant drugs. However, various psychotherapy methods have been equally if not more successful in improving the psychological aspects of PMS. In particular, biofeedback and short-term individual counseling (especially cognitive therapy) have documented clinical efficacy.[29,30] One of the advantages of these therapies over antidepressant drug therapy in the treatment of PMS is that learning better coping skills can produce excellent results that are maintained over time.

Exercise

Several studies have shown that women who engage in regular exercise do not suffer from PMS nearly as often as sedentary women.[31–33] In one of the more thorough studies, mood and physical symptoms at various points during the menstrual cycle were assessed in 97 women who exercised regularly and in a second group of 159 women who did not exercise.[31] Mood scores and physical symptoms showed that exercise significantly decreased negative mood states and physical symptoms. The regular exercisers had significantly lower scores for impaired concentration, negative mood, unwanted behavior changes, and pain.

In another study, 143 women were monitored for 5 days in each of the three phases of their cycles.[32] The group included 35 competitive athletes, two groups of exercisers (33 high-frequency exercisers and 36 low-frequency exercisers), and 39 sedentary women. The high-frequency exercisers experienced the greatest positive mood scores and sedentary women the least. The high-frequency exercisers also reported the least depression and anxiety. The differences were most apparent during the premenstrual and menstrual phases. These results are consistent with the belief that women who exercise frequently (but not competitive athletes) are protected from PMS symptoms. In particular, regular exercise protects against the deterioration of mood before and during menstruation.

These studies provide convincing evidence that women with PMS should engage in regular exercise. Exercise may reduce PMS symptoms by a number of different mechanisms, including elevating endorphin levels.[34]

Nutritional Supplements

Vitamin B$_6$

The first use of vitamin B$_6$ in the management of cyclic conditions in women was in the successful treatment of depression caused by birth control pills, as noted in several studies in the early 1970s. These results led researchers to try to determine the effectiveness of vitamin B$_6$ in relieving PMS symptoms. Since 1975 at least a dozen double-blind clinical trials have been performed. Some of these studies have shown no effect, but most of the studies have demonstrated a significant effect on the whole range of PMS symptoms at dosage ranges from 50 to 500 mg per day.[35] For example, in one double-blind crossover trial, 84% of the subjects had a lower symptom score during the B$_6$ treatment period.[36] In another double-blind crossover trial, 50 mg per day of B$_6$ was effective in decreasing premenstrual depression, fatigue, and irritability.[37]

Although B$_6$ supplementation alone appears to benefit most patients, not all double-blind studies of vitamin B$_6$ have shown a positive effect.[35,38] Additional support may be required. For example, the negative results in some trials may have been caused by the inability of some women to convert B$_6$ to its active form, pyridoxal-5-phosphate (P5P), owing to a deficiency in another nutrient (e.g., vitamin B$_2$ or magnesium) that was not supplemented.

We do not feel that high dosages of B$_6$ are necessary or a good idea. For most indications, the therapeutic dosage of vitamin B$_6$ is 50 to 100 mg per day. A single dose of 100 mg pyridoxine did not lead to significantly higher pyridoxal-5-phosphate levels in the blood than a 50-mg dose, possibly indicating that a 50-mg oral dose of pyridoxine is about all the liver can handle at once.[39] We recommend a dosage of 25 to 50 mg twice per day. This dosage level is well below any reported toxicity. If you do not see enough improvement, then try 15 mg per day of the more expensive P5P.

Magnesium

Another mechanism by which vitamin B$_6$ may improve the symptoms of PMS is by increasing the accumulation of magnesium within body cells.[40] Without vitamin B$_6$, magnesium does not get inside the cell. Magnesium deficiency has been implicated as a causative factor in PMS.[41] Red blood cell (RBC) magnesium levels have been shown to be significantly lower in patients with PMS than in normal subjects.[42] Because magnesium plays such an integral part in normal cell function, magnesium deficiency may account for the wide range of symptoms attributed to PMS. Furthermore, magnesium deficiency and PMS have many common features, and magnesium supplementation has been shown to be an effective treatment for PMS. In one study involving 32 women with PMS, 360 mg magnesium three times per day was given from midcycle to the onset of menstrual flow.[43] Relief of premenstrual mood fluctuations and depression during magnesium treatment was significant.

The most recent study designed to improve understanding of the association between magnesium and the menstrual cycle measured plasma, RBC, and mononuclear blood cell (MBC) magnesium concentrations in 26 women with confirmed PMS and in a control group of 19 women during the follicular, ovulatory, early luteal, and late luteal phases of the menstrual cycle.[44] Although there were no significant differences in plasma magnesium levels between PMS patients and control subjects and there was no menstrual cycle effect on plasma magnesium, women with PMS had significantly lower RBC magnesium concentrations than those in the control group, and this finding was consistent throughout the menstrual cycle.

The observation of low RBC magnesium concentrations in patients with PMS has now been confirmed by four independent studies. In general, it is thought that women with PMS have a "vulnerability to luteal phase mood state destabilization"[44] and that chronic intracellular magnesium depletion serves as a major predisposing factor.

In addition to emotional instability, magnesium deficiency in PMS is characterized by excessive nervous sensitivity, with generalized aches and pains and a lower premenstrual pain threshold. One clinical trial of magnesium in PMS showed a remarkable reduction of nervousness in 89% of subjects, of breast tenderness in 96%, and of weight gain in 95%.[7] In another double-blind study, high-dose magnesium supplementation (360 mg three times per day) was shown to dramatically relieve PMS-related mood changes.[43]

Although magnesium has been shown to be effective on its own, even better results may be achieved by combining it with vitamin B_6 and other nutrients. Several studies have shown that when PMS patients are given a multivitamin/multimineral supplement containing high doses of magnesium and pyridoxine, they experience a substantial reduction in PMS symptoms.[45,46]

The optimal intake of magnesium should be based on body weight, 6 mg/kg. For a 110-lb woman, the recommendation would be 300 mg; for a 200-lb. woman, 540 mg. Because these dosages are difficult to achieve by diet alone, supplementation is recommended. In the treatment of PMS, a dosage of twice this amount, 12 mg/kg, may be needed.

Magnesium bound to aspartate, citrate, fumarate, malate, glycinate, or succinate is preferred to magnesium oxide, gluconate, sulfate, or chloride because of better absorption and less chance of a laxative effect.[47,48]

Calcium

Calcium has emerged as a common nutrient to supplement for PMS. Because calcium deficiency can actually mimic some PMS symptoms, supplemental calcium has been tested as a treatment. An important multicenter clinical trial was conducted with 479 women who were given either 1,200 mg calcium carbonate or a placebo for three menstrual cycles.[49] A significantly lower symptom score was observed in the calcium group during the luteal phase of the cycle for both the second and the third cycles. By the end of the third cycle, calcium resulted in a 48% reduction in total symptom scores from baseline compared with a 30% reduction in the placebo group. Other studies also show improvements in PMS symptoms with calcium supplementation (1,000 to 1,336 mg).[50,51] In one of the later studies, calcium and manganese supplementation (1,336 and 5.6 mg, respectively) improved mood, concentration, and behavior. In another study, 1,000 mg per day improved mood and water retention.[50]

Zinc

Zinc levels have been shown to be low in women with PMS.[52] Zinc is required for proper action of many body hormones, including the sex hormones, as well as in the control of the synthesis and secretion of hormones. In particular, zinc serves as one of the control factors for prolactin secretion.[53] When zinc levels are low, prolactin release increases; high zinc levels inhibit this release. Hence in high-prolactin states, zinc supplementation is very useful. An effective dosage range for zinc supplementation for elevated prolactin levels in women is 30 to 45 mg in the picolinate form.

Vitamin E

Although vitamin E research concerning PMS has focused primarily on breast tenderness, significant reduction of other PMS symptoms has also been demonstrated in double-blind studies.[7,54] Nervous tension, headache, fatigue, depression, and insomnia were all significantly reduced. In one double-blind study, patients receiving vitamin E (400 IU per day) demonstrated a 33% reduction in physical symptoms (such as weight gain and breast tenderness), a 38% reduction in anxiety, and a 27% reduction in depression after three months of use.[54] In contrast, the placebo group reported only a 14% reduction in physical symptoms. The group taking vitamin E also noted higher energy levels, fewer headaches, and fewer cravings for sweets.

Essential Fatty Acids

Women with PMS have been shown to exhibit essential fatty acid and prostaglandin abnormalities, the chief abnormality being a decrease in gamma-linolenic acid (GLA).[55] Evening primrose, blackcurrant, and borage oils contain GLA, typical levels being 9%, 12%, and 22%, respectively. Although these essential fatty acid sources are quite popular, the research on GLA supplements in the treatment of PMS shows no benefit over placebos. In the four double-blind, controlled crossover trials of evening primrose oil, this issue may be complicated by a very high response in the placebo group.[56,57] One of these studies used 3 g per day and the others used 4 g per day. A meta-analysis of the clinical trials of evening primrose oil concluded that it is of little value in the management of PMS.[56]

A better recommendation for PMS will probably turn out to be fish oils, given the benefits of the long-chain omega-3 fatty acids EPA and DHA in depression (see the chapter "Depression"). As of this writing, there are no clinical studies of fish oil supplementation for PMS despite considerable evidence of possible benefits.

Multivitamin and Multimineral Supplements

Given the numerous nutrients demonstrating benefit in PMS, it is clear that a high-quality multivitamin/multimineral supplement providing all of the known vitamins and minerals can serve as a foundation on which to build. Women with PMS have two very sound reasons for taking a high-potency multiple vitamin: nutritional deficiency is relatively common among women with PMS, and high-potency multivitamin/multimineral formulations have been shown to have significant benefits in PMS.

The frequency of nutritional supplementation and the calculated intake of selected nutrients have been shown to be much lower in patients with PMS than in normal women.[16] Several double-blind studies have shown that patients with PMS who were given a multivitamin/multimineral supplement containing high doses of magnesium and pyridoxine experienced reductions (typically of at least 70%) in symptoms.[45,46]

Tryptophan

As discussed earlier in this chapter, decreases in serotonin may be the cause of PMS or at least may exacerbate PMS. Tryptophan is a precursor to serotonin. Studies using tryptophan in doses of 6 g per day for 17 days from ovulation to day three of menses demonstrated significant reductions in mood swings, insomnia, carbohydrate cravings, tension, irritability, and dysphoria.[58,59] However, we feel that a stronger recommendation is the use of 5-HTP—the intermediate compound between tryptophan and serotonin—which can be used at much lower dosages and with greater efficacy. The benefits of 5-HTP in low-serotonin conditions is detailed in the chapter "Depression."

Botanical Medicines

Chasteberry

Chasteberry (*Vitex agnus-castus*) is native to the Mediterranean and has long been used for women's health. Chasteberry extract is probably the single most important herb in the treatment of PMS, not only because of its long tradition of use but also as a result of modern scientific research. In two surveys of gynecological practices in Germany, physicians graded chasteberry extract as good or very good in the treatment of PMS. More than 1,500 women participated in the studies.[60,61] One-third of the women experienced complete resolution of their symptoms, and another 57% reported significant improvement.

The beneficial effects of chasteberry in PMS and certain other conditions appear to be related to profound effects on the hypothalamus and pituitary function. As a result, it is able to normalize the secretion of various hormones—for instance, reducing the secretion of prolactin and reducing the estrogen-to-progesterone ratio.

In one of the more recent studies, a double-blind trial compared 20 mg of chasteberry extract standardized for casticin with a placebo in 170 women with PMS over three consecutive menstrual cycles.[62] Women were asked to rate changes in PMS symptoms, such as irritability, mood changes, anger, headache, breast tenderness, and bloating. At the end of the trial, women taking the chasteberry reported a 52% overall reduction in PMS symptoms, compared with only 24% for those taking the placebo. Women taking the chasteberry extract reported significantly greater reductions in irritability,

mood changes, anger, headache, and breast tenderness than the women taking the placebo; bloating was the only symptom that did not change significantly. Another study has looked at the effectiveness of chasteberry extract vs. fluoxetine (Prozac) in decreasing PMS symptoms and found the two treatments to have comparable results, with the main difference being that fluoxetine was more effective in treating psychological symptoms and chasteberry was more effective with physical symptoms.[63] Additional well-designed studies show a significant advantage of chasteberry extract in moderate to severe PMS.[64]

A combination of Saint-John's-wort extract and chasteberry extract was studied in the treatment of PMS-like symptoms in women approaching menopause.[65] This clinical trial was conducted over 16 weeks, and information rating PMS scores in perimenopausal women who were experiencing irregular menses was collected at 4-week intervals. Results for the active treatment group were statistically superior to those for the placebo group for total PMS symptoms as well as subgroups of PMS-related depression and food cravings.

Ginkgo Biloba

In the first randomized placebo-controlled clinical trial evaluating ginkgo biloba extract in PMS, 165 women of reproductive age who had fluid retention, breast tenderness, and vascular congestion were assigned to receive either ginkgo biloba at 80 mg twice per day or a placebo from day 16 of one cycle to day 5 of the next. Symptom diaries kept by patients and physician evaluation of symptoms demonstrated that ginkgo biloba extract was effective against the congestive symptoms of PMS, particularly breast pain and breast tenderness.[66]

In a subsequent study, 85 women were given ginkgo biloba extract (40 mg three times per day) or a placebo from day 16 of one cycle to day 5 of the next. Overall severity of symptoms in the ginkgo group was 34.80 before the treatment and fell to 11.11 after the treatment (comparable rates in the placebo group were 34.38 and 25.64).[67]

Saint-John's-Wort

Saint-John's-wort (*Hypericum perforatum*) is frequently used for depression because of its influence on raising serotonin, so it should not be surprising that this herb would be an important botanical in the treatment of PMS. In a double-blind trial of 36 women with regular menstrual cycles and mild PMS the women were randomly assigned to receive Saint-John's-wort extract (900 mg per day and standardized to 0.18% hypericin and 3.38% hyperforin) or a placebo for two menstrual cycles.[68] After a one-month washout period, the women were crossed over to the opposite group for two additional cycles. Saint-John's-wort was statistically more beneficial than the placebo in relieving food cravings, swelling, poor coordination, insomnia, confusion, headaches, crying, and fatigue. Saint-John's-wort was not statistically more beneficial for anxiety, irritability, depression, nervous tension, mood swing, feeling out of control, or pain-related symptoms during two cycles of treatment. However, these pain-related symptoms appeared to improve more than with the placebo toward the end of each treatment period.

In an observational study, 19 women who were diagnosed with PMS completed a daily symptom rating questionnaire for one menstrual cycle and underwent a screening interview with physicians. The participants then took Saint-John's-wort extract daily for two complete menstrual cycles.[69] The degree of improvement in overall PMS scores between the beginning of the study and the end was 51%, with more than two-thirds of the women having at least a 50% decrease in the severity of symptoms. The mood subscale showed the most improvement (57%); the specific symptoms with the greatest reductions in scores were crying (92%), depression (85%), confusion (75%), feeling out of control (72%), nervous tension (71%), anxiety (69%), and insomnia (69%).

Saffron

Saffron (*Crocus sativus L.*) has been shown to have an antidepressant effect in women with mild to moderate depression, so again it is not surprising that it would be beneficial in PMS. A double-blind placebo-controlled trial was done to study whether saffron could be used to relieve PMS symptoms. Fifty women of reproductive age with regular menstrual cycles and PMS symptoms for at least the last six months were randomly assigned to receive 15 mg saffron twice per day or a placebo twice per day for four full menstrual cycles.[70] According to daily symptom reports, 19 of the 25 women in the saffron group responded with at least a 50% reduction in severity of symptoms vs. only 2 of 25 in the placebo group. A significant difference between the saffron and the placebo groups occurred between the third and fourth cycles and was statistically significant by the end of the study. Based on a depression rating scale, 15 of 25 women in the saffron group responded to treatment vs. only 1 of 25 in the placebo group.

Saffron, which is the dried stigmas of the flowers, can be very expensive, so we recommend using extracts prepared from the petals of the saffron crocus. Please see the discussion on saffron in the chapter "Depression" for more information.

QUICK REVIEW

- Premenstrual syndrome (PMS) is estimated to affect between 30 and 40% of menstruating women.

- There is no consistent alteration in hormonal patterns among PMS patients compared with women who have no symptoms of PMS.

- The dominant thought now is that PMS is the result of alterations in brain chemistry that influence many factors, including the sensitivity of the brain to hormones.

- Impaired liver function could lead to reduced levels of serotonin in the brain, lower endorphin levels, impaired vitamin B_6 activity, and alterations in other hormone levels.

- The primary nutritional recommendations for PMS are to increase consumption of plant foods (vegetables, fruits, legumes, whole grains, nuts, and seeds), consume small to moderate quantities of meat and dairy products, reduce fat and sugar intake, eliminate caffeine intake, and keep salt intake low.

- Low thyroid function (hypothyroidism) has been shown to affect a large percentage of women who have PMS.

- Most women who have PMS tend to employ negative coping styles to deal with stress.

- Vitamin B_6 and magnesium are the two most important nutritional supplements for treating PMS.

- Exercise is extremely helpful in eliminating PMS.

- Chasteberry extract is probably the single most important herb in the treatment of PMS.

- Ginkgo biloba extract is well known for its effects in improving blood flow to the brain, and it has also been shown to be of great benefit in PMS in several clinical trials.

- Saint-John's-wort extract and saffron have also shown benefits in relieving PMS symptoms.

TREATMENT SUMMARY

Dealing with PMS usually requires a comprehensive plan involving many general health-improving strategies. Diet, lifestyle, attitude, and proper nutritional supplementation are all very important in reducing symptoms. PMS has many diverse causes and treatments, so each woman needs to learn which therapies work best for her unique needs.

Diet

The dietary recommendations in the chapter "A Health-Promoting Diet" are important in PMS. It is very important to avoid salt, eat a low-glycemic Mediterranean-style diet, increase consumption of fiber-rich plant foods (fruits, vegetables, grains, legumes, nuts, and seeds), and avoid caffeine and alcohol.

Lifestyle and Attitude

- Exercise at least 30 minutes at least three times a week.
- Spend 10 to 15 minutes per day on relaxation or stress reduction techniques.
- Follow the recommendations in the chapter "A Positive Mental Attitude."

Nutritional Supplements

- A high-potency multiple vitamin and mineral formula as described in the chapter "Supplementary Measures"
- Key individual nutrients:
  - Vitamin B_6: 100 mg per day
  - Magnesium (aspartate, citrate, malate, succinate, or glycinate: 250 mg two times per day
  - Zinc: 15 to 20 mg per day
  - Vitamin E (mixed tocopherols): 400 IU per day
  - Vitamin C: 500 to 1,000 mg per day
  - Vitamin D_3: 2,000 to 4,000 IU per day

- Fish oils: 1,000 mg EPA + DHA per day
- One of the following:
  - Grape seed extract (>95% procyanidolic oligomers): 100 to 300 mg per day
  - Pine bark extract (>95% procyanidolic oligomers): 100 to 300 mg per day
  - Some other flavonoid-rich extract with a similar flavonoid content, super greens formula, or another plant-based antioxidant that can provide an oxygen radical absorption capacity (ORAC) of 3,000 to 6,000 units or more per day
- 5-HTP: 50 to 100 mg three times per day

Botanical Medicines

- One or more of the following:
  - Chasteberry: tablets or capsules standardized for 0.5% agnuside, 175 to 225 mg per day; liquid extract, 2 to 4 ml (½ to 1 tsp) per day
  - Saint-John's-wort extract (0.3% hypericin content): 600 to 1,800 mg per day, or from day 17 of one menstrual cycle through day 3 of the next
  - Ginkgo biloba extract (24% ginkgo flavonglycosides): 240 to 320 mg per day
  - Saffron petal extract: 15 mg twice per day

Prostate Cancer (Prevention)

Prostate cancer can cause any of the following symptoms:

- A need to urinate frequently, especially at night
- Difficulty starting urination or holding back urine
- Inability to urinate
- Weak or interrupted flow of urine
- Painful or burning urination
- Difficulty in having an erection
- Painful ejaculation
- Blood in urine or semen
- Frequent pain or stiffness in the lower back, hips, or upper thighs

Prostate cancer is a form of cancer that develops in the prostate, a doughnut-shaped gland about the size of a walnut that lies below the bladder and surrounds the urethra (the tube that connects the bladder to the tip of the penis). Prostate cancer is the most-diagnosed form of cancer in American men. Each year roughly 200,000 men are diagnosed with prostate cancer and more than 30,000 will die from it. In many respects, prostate cancer is the mirror of breast cancer in women: it is a hormone-sensitive cancer that will affect at least one out of every six men now living in the United States.

Most prostate cancers are slow-growing; however, there are cases of aggressive prostate cancer. The cancer cells may metastasize (spread) from the prostate to other parts of the body, particularly the bones and lymph nodes. Next to lung cancer, in men prostate cancer is the second-leading cause of death due to cancer.

The symptoms listed above are not specific for prostate cancer, especially the first four, which are usually a sign of benign prostatic hyperplasia (BPH), a noncancerous enlargement of the prostate (see the chapter "Prostate Enlargement [BPH]"). The symptoms listed can also indicate a prostate infection. If you are experiencing any of these symptoms, it is important to see a doctor immediately.

Causes

Researchers are studying factors that may increase the risk of this disease. Studies have found that the following risk factors are associated with prostate cancer:

- **Family history of prostate (or breast) cancer.** A man's risk for developing prostate cancer is two times higher if his father has had the disease, five times higher if a brother has had it, and two times higher if his mother or sister has had breast cancer.

903

- **Age.** In the United States, prostate cancer is found mainly in men over age 55, and more than 8 out of 10 cases are in men over 65. The average age of patients at the time of diagnosis is 70.

- **Race.** Prostate cancer is roughly twice as common in African-American men as in white men. It is less common in Asian and Native American men.

- **Hormonal factors.** Testosterone is thought to stimulate hormone-dependent prostate cancer in much the same way that estrogen stimulates breast cancer. Other hormones implicated are estrogen and prolactin.

- **Diet and dietary factors.** Current research indicates that diets high in red meat, dairy, and saturated fat are associated with an increased risk of developing prostate cancer. Risks are also increased for those who have diets low in fruits, vegetables, phytoestrogens, selenium, vitamin E, lycopene, and other dietary antioxidants.

Diagnostic Considerations

The most important aspect of detecting prostate cancer for men over the age of 50 years is seeing a physician for an annual physical exam that includes:

- **Digital rectal exam.** The doctor inserts a lubricated, gloved finger into the rectum and feels the prostate through the rectal wall to check for hard or lumpy areas.

- **Blood test for prostate-specific antigen (PSA).** PSA is usually elevated in men with prostate cancer. A normal PSA level ranges from 0 to 4 ng/ml. A PSA level of 4 to 10 ng/ml is considered slightly elevated, levels between 10 and 20 ng/ml are con-

sidered moderately elevated, and anything above that is considered highly elevated. The higher the PSA level, the more likely it is that cancer is present. However, approximately 35% of men with diagnosed prostate cancer will have a PSA of less than 4 ng/ml. The level of PSA in the blood tends to rise with prostate cancer, but minor elevations may be due to less serious conditions such as prostatitis (inflammation of the prostate) and BPH. PSA levels alone do not give doctors enough information to distinguish between benign prostate conditions and cancer; the doctor will take the result of this test into account in deciding whether to check further for signs of prostate cancer. In addition to being used as a screening test, PSA is also used to monitor patients with a history of prostate cancer to see if the cancer has come back. Researchers are looking for ways to distinguish between cancerous and benign conditions, and between slow-growing cancers and fast-growing, potentially lethal cancers. Some of the methods being studied are:

- **PSA velocity.** PSA velocity is based on changes in PSA levels over time. A sharp rise in the PSA level raises the suspicion of cancer.

- **Age-adjusted PSA.** Age is an important factor in increasing PSA levels. For this reason, some doctors use age-adjusted PSA levels to determine when diagnostic tests are needed. When age-adjusted PSA levels are used, a different PSA level is defined as normal for each 10-year age group. Doctors who use this method suggest that men younger than age 50 should have a PSA level below 2.5 ng/ml, while a PSA level up to 6.5 ng/ml would be considered normal for men in their 70s.

○ **PSA density.** PSA density considers the relationship of the PSA level to the size and weight of the prostate. In other words, an elevated PSA might not arouse suspicion in a man with a very enlarged prostate. The use of PSA density to interpret PSA results is controversial because cancer might be overlooked in a man with an enlarged prostate.

○ **Free vs. attached PSA.** PSA circulates in the blood in two forms: free or attached to a protein molecule. With benign prostate conditions, there is more free PSA, while cancer produces more of the attached form. If the PSA is between 4 and 10 mg/ml, a free PSA of less than 10% suggests a high risk of cancer, while a free PSA of more than 25% suggests a low risk of cancer.

• **Biopsy.** A biopsy of the prostate involves taking tissue samples from the prostate via the rectum with the use of a biopsy gun that inserts and removes special hollow-core needles (usually three to six on each side of the prostate) in less than a second. Prostate biopsies are routinely done on an outpatient basis. The tissue samples are then examined under a microscope to determine whether cancer cells are present and to evaluate the microscopic features (or Gleason score) of any cancer found. In general, the higher the Gleason score, the more aggressive the cancer.

Therapeutic Considerations

The therapeutic goal is to reduce as many risk factors as possible while simultaneously implementing dietary and lifestyle factors associated with prostate cancer prevention. Most of the lifestyle factors linked to preventing cancer in general, such as avoiding

TO SCREEN OR NOT TO SCREEN?

The rationale for early detection of cancer is that it leads to more effective treatment. Unfortunately, the data on PSA screening for prostate cancer do not support this notion. Several reviews on the impact of PSA screening showed no statistically significant difference in death due to prostate cancer between men randomly assigned to screening and those who were not screened.[1,2] In fact, the Centers for Disease Control and Prevention and the U.S. Preventive Services Task Force believe that PSA screening produces more harm than good based upon very extensive analyses. Harms of screening included high rates of false-positive results for the PSA test and the adverse events associated with biopsies (such as infection, bleeding, and pain) and with the treatment of prostate cancer with chemotherapy and radiation. It is believed that in most cases the prostate cancer would not have seriously affected the patient's life expectancy if it had simply been left alone. Most prostate cancers are extremely slow-growing, meaning that men can live with prostate cancer, rather than die from it. In fact, autopsy studies report that more than 30% of all men over the age 50 have evidence of prostate cancer, but only 3% will die from it.

Our feeling is that the problem with early screening is not the screening but what happens after the screening. In the case of PSA screening, the approach should be "watchful waiting" vs. immediate biopsy unless accompanied by significant PSA velocity or family history or unless the patient is African-American. And if the biopsy is positive, even then a conservative approach should be taken with the majority of men. Now, that does not mean that we advocate idleness with watchful waiting. In fact, we recommend just the opposite: an aggressive focus on the measures detailed in this chapter, which can help prevent or even reverse the disease.

cigarette smoke or excessive intake of alcohol, also apply to prostate cancer. The same is true for dietary factors. Therefore, we recommend strengthening the "four cornerstones of good health" detailed in Section II of this book:

- A positive mental attitude
- A health-promoting lifestyle
- A health-promoting diet
- Supplementary measures

Focusing on these key foundations provides the strongest general protection against cancer of any type.

Diet

There is so much convincing evidence on the role of diet in prostate cancer that

---

MALE-PATTERN BALDNESS AND PROSTATE CANCER

Men with male-pattern baldness appear to have an increased risk for prostate cancer, according to a study of more than 4,000 men tracked since the 1970s by a research team from the National Institutes of Health. The results indicated that men with any degree of male-pattern baldness (characterized by gradual hair loss at the front and/or crown of the head) in their mid-twenties were 50% more likely to develop prostate cancer.[3]

It was hypothesized that there might be an association between male-pattern baldness and prostate cancer on the basis that both conditions are sensitive to testosterone levels. There are receptors for testosterone on the cells of both hair follicles and the prostate. Male-pattern baldness has also been linked to a higher risk for heart disease.

These findings mean not that balding men will definitely get prostate cancer, but only that they are at increased risk, meaning that they would be wise to be more aggressive with dietary and supplementation programs to reduce their risk of developing prostate cancer.

Dr. William Fair and colleagues from Memorial Sloan-Kettering Cancer Center went so far as to suggest that prostate cancer may be a nutritional disease.[4] Key causative dietary factors include diets rich in animal foods (particularly grilled and broiled meats, saturated fat, and dairy products) and low in protective nutrients such as lycopene, selenium, vitamin E, soy isoflavones and other dietary phytoestrogens, omega-3 fatty acids (particularly those from fish), and isothiocyanates from vegetables in the brassica (cabbage) family. As is also the case in breast cancer, these dietary factors are known to affect sex hormone levels, detoxification mechanisms, and antioxidant status.[5,6]

In fact, it would be worthwhile to read the chapter "Breast Cancer (Prevention)" to gain an even greater appreciation of how diet can affect hormone-sensitive tissues like the breast and prostate. One of the interesting dietary associations in breast cancer is the high risk that comes with eating well-done or charbroiled meat; frequent consumption of well-done meat, for example, was associated with a nearly 500% increase in breast cancer. With prostate cancer the risk is a little less but still very significant. Higher consumption of hamburgers, processed meats, grilled meats, and well-done meat was associated with an approximately 50 to 80% increase in aggressive forms of prostate cancer.[7]

Another food that has been strongly implicated in prostate cancer is milk. In a study conducted in Canada, researchers found a twofold increased risk of prostate cancer associated with an increased intake of milk. Interestingly, it was the only dairy product associated with an increased risk for prostate cancer.[8] Initially researchers thought the risk might be due to the calcium, but it now appears that it is due to milk's high phosphorus content.[9]

High intakes of certain foods are associated with a reduction in prostate cancer risk, while high intakes of other foods are associated with increased risk:[5–10]

- Fish: 44% reduced risk
- Tomatoes, tomato sauce, tomato juice: 35% reduced risk
- Green leafy vegetables: 34% reduced risk
- Soy: 30% reduced risk
- Vegetables high in carotenoids: 29% reduced risk
- High-glycemic-index foods: 64% increased risk
- Hamburgers: 79% increased risk
- Processed meat: 57% increased risk
- Grilled red meat: 63% increased risk
- Well-done red meat: 52% increased risk
- Milk: 111% increased risk

Without question the dietary recommendations in the chapter "A Health-Promoting Diet" are powerful in helping to protect against prostate cancer. It is also important to point out that the Mediterranean diet has been shown to help prevent prostate cancer. That would be expected given that it is high in vegetables, legumes, dried and fresh fruits, and fish; olive oil is its main fat source; it is low in animal fats, processed red meat, milk and dairy products; and it includes regular but low alcohol intake (wine with meals).[11]

Soy Products

The isoflavones of soy—genistein and daidzein—exert significant protection against prostate cancer, according to population-based studies.[12] Test tube and animal studies have confirmed that soy isoflavones inhibit the growth of prostate cancer cells.[13] Since both testosterone-dependent and testosterone-independent prostate cancer cells are inhibited, it appears that soy isoflavones possess several types of anticancer action. The high intake of soy may be one of the key protective factors accounting for the low rate of prostate cancer in Japan and China compared with other parts of the world: blood and urine concentrations of soy isoflavones (an indicator of intake) were found to be 7 to 10 times higher in Japanese men consuming a traditional Japanese diet compared with Finnish men consuming a typical Western diet.[12] A study of 12,395 California Seventh-Day Adventist men found that men who drank soy milk had a 70% reduction in the risk of prostate cancer.[14] A study of 42 countries found soy to have a higher protective value against prostate cancer than any other dietary factor.[12] Higher blood levels of genistein are associated with a significantly reduced risk of developing prostate cancer.[15] A daily dietary intake of 45 to 90 mg soy isoflavones is recommended for prevention of prostate cancer. Information on the isoflavone content of common soy foods can be found on page 788.

Omega-3 Fatty Acids

The risk of prostate cancer is reduced with a higher intake of fish rich in the omega-3 fatty acids eicosapentaenoic acid (EPA) and docosahexaenoic acid (DHA). In a population-based study, reduced prostate cancer risk was associated with a high red blood cell content of EPA and DHA.[16] This study provided further support to previous population-based studies as well as test tube and animal experiments showing that these omega-3 fatty acids inhibit prostate cancer cells.

Just as in breast cancer again, the benefits of these long-chain omega-3 fatty acids are magnified when the level of animal fat (saturated fat, and arachidonic acid in particular) is also reduced. A high ratio of dietary omega-6 to omega-3 fatty acids is major risk factor for prostate cancer.[17]

While the data are clear that increased consumption of long-chain omega-3 fatty acids from fish offers protection against prostate cancer, there has been some controversy about recommending flaxseed oil, which contains the omega-3 fatty acid alpha-linolenic acid (ALA), to men; we believe this is based upon the misunderstanding of some research results. While ALA shows benefit against breast cancer, some initial studies indicated that ALA may actually increase the risk of prostate cancer.[18-20] However, in some of these studies ALA intake was used simply as a marker for meat intake. In the absence of consuming vegetable sources of ALA, such as flaxseed or canola oil, the primary dietary source is from meat. It is also possible that deficiencies of zinc or other nutrients involved in the conversion of the shorter-chain ALA to the longer-chain EPA and DHA are ultimately responsible for the elevations in ALA noted in men with prostate cancer. About 50% of all men with prostate cancer are deficient in zinc. More recent analysis shows that there is no concern with ALA as a risk factor in prostate cancer.[21]

Nonetheless, studies also seem to indicate that if diets are high in ALA and low in antioxidants (especially lycopene, discussed below) it could be a problem. Unfortunately, no one has actually looked at the effect of flaxseed oil in prostate cancer. It is very likely that the lignan content overrides any problem with ALA. At this time it appears that men in general may be better off avoiding flaxseed oil supplements and focusing on ground flaxseed (for the lignans) and fish (for the omega-3 fatty acids).

Flaxseed

Ground flaxseed appears to be quite helpful not only in preventing prostate cancer but also in men with existing prostate cancer.

AFRICAN-AMERICAN MEN, FAT INTAKE, AND PROSTATE CANCER

African-American men develop prostate cancer twice as frequently as white men. Although genetics could play a role, a more likely explanation is dietary differences. In a study conducted by the National Cancer Institute of men who had been newly diagnosed with biopsy-proved prostate cancer and matched controls without prostate cancer, it was shown that increased consumption of foods high in animal fat was linked to prostate cancer (independent of intake of other calories) among black men compared with whites. The higher the intake of animal fat, the greater the risk for advanced prostate cancer. These results indicate that diet plays a major role in why black men have a higher rate of prostate cancer and show that a reduction of fat from animal sources in the diet could lead to decreased incidence and mortality rates for prostate cancer, particularly among African-Americans.[22]

In addition to its phytoestrogenic effect, flaxseed lignans also bind to male hormone receptors and promote the elimination of testosterone. In a study of men with prostate cancer, a low-fat diet (with fat providing 20% or less of total calories) supplemented with 30 g ground flaxseed (roughly 2 tbsp) reduced serum testosterone by 15%, slowed the growth rate of cancer cells, and increased the death rate of cancer cells after only 34 days.[23]

Vitamin E

Several population-based studies suggested that vitamin E supplementation prevents prostate cancer.[5,6] The same sort of protection has been demonstrated in some clinical studies as well. In one, a total of 29,133 male smokers ages 50 to 69 from southwestern Finland were randomly assigned to receive vitamin E (50 mg), beta-carotene (20 mg), both nutrients, or a placebo for 5 to 8 years (median 6.1 years). A 32% decrease in the incidence of prostate cancer was observed among the 14,564 subjects receiving vitamin E compared with the 14,569 not receiving it. Mortality from prostate cancer was 41% lower among men receiving vitamin E. However, in the 14,560 subjects receiving beta-carotene, prostate cancer incidence was actually 23% higher and mortality was 15% higher compared with the 14,573 not receiving it.[24] Once again these results emphasize the importance of broad-spectrum antioxidant support.

Another form of vitamin E, known as gamma-tocopherol, may prove to be more important against prostate cancer than the alpha-tocopherol form, which has been used in virtually all the vitamin E research. Eight different compounds—four tocopherols and four tocotrienols—make up the vitamin E family. They have some functions that are similar and other functions that are completely different. Alpha-tocopherol became synonymous with vitamin E for two main reasons: (1) of the eight, it is the most abundant in the human body, and (2) it is by far the most effective of the eight for what was originally thought of as vitamin E's main function—to support reproduction.

Our blood and tissue contain much more alpha-tocopherol than gamma-tocopherol despite the fact that in the typical American diet we consume twice as much gamma-tocopherol as alpha. The reason is that the liver is able to identify the alpha-tocopherol as it is absorbed from the gut and bind it to a special protein, called the alpha-tocopherol transfer protein. It recognizes the alpha-tocopherol and preferentially puts more of it in lipoproteins—proteins that carry fat and cholesterol (e.g., LDL, VLDL, and HDL).

So why is gamma-tocopherol important? It has some actions of its own, but more likely it is metabolized to a more active compound known as LLU-alpha-tocopherol. This compound and other metabolites may act to better protect the prostate from oxidative damage as well as promote apoptosis (programmed cell death), which helps prevent cells from becoming cancerous.

In one study, 117 men who developed prostate cancer and 233 matched control subjects had toenail and plasma samples assayed for selenium, alpha-tocopherol, and gamma-tocopherol.[25] The risk of prostate cancer declined (but not linearly) with increasing concentrations of alpha-tocopherol. For gamma-tocopherol, men with the highest levels had a fivefold reduction in the risk of developing prostate cancer compared with men with the lowest levels. The association between selenium and prostate cancer risk was in the protective direction. Statistically significant protective associations for high levels of selenium and alpha-tocopherol were observed only when gamma-tocopherol concentrations were high as well. These results indicate that in order to achieve the greatest degree of protection, natural mixed tocopherols that include both alpha- and gamma-tocopherol should be used, rather than only alpha-tocopherol.

Remember that vitamin E is available in many different forms. First of all, there is natural vs. synthetic. Natural forms of vitamin E are designated *d-*, as in d-alpha-tocopherol, while synthetic forms are *dl-*, as in dl-alpha-tocopherol. The prefixes *d-* and *l-* refer to two versions of the vitamin E molecule that are, in effect, mirror images of each other, the way your right hand is a mirror image of your left. In the human body, only the natural form is recognized. Although the synthetic form has antioxidant activity, it may actually inhibit the natural form from entering cell membranes. Therefore, natural vitamin E (d-alpha-tocopherol) has greater benefit than the synthetic form (dl-alpha-tocopherol). We strongly recommend avoiding synthetic vitamin E.

Selenium

Like vitamin E, selenium has also shown benefit in preventing prostate cancer in some studies. A 10-year cancer prevention trial found that selenium supplementation appears to significantly lower the incidence of not only prostate cancer but also lung and colon cancers in people with a history of skin cancer.[26] The primary purpose of the study was to see if dietary supplements of selenium could lower the incidence of basal cell or squamous cell skin cancers, but seven years into the study several secondary end points (including the incidence of three commonly

occurring cancers: lung, colorectal, and prostate) were added.

The results of the study were exciting to researchers because they showed the cancer prevention potential of simply adding a nutritional supplement to a normal diet. Participants in the randomized, double-blind study took either 200 mcg of selenium per day or a placebo for four and a half years and were followed for more than six additional years. Three-quarters of the participants were men. Total cancer incidence was significantly lower in the selenium group than in the placebo group (77 cases vs. 119), as was the incidence of some specific cancers: the selenium group had fewer lung cancers (17 vs. 31), fewer colorectal cancers (8 vs. 19), and fewer prostate cancers (13 vs. 35, a 63% reduction).

THE SELECT PROSTATE CANCER PREVENTION TRIAL

Because the evidence from preliminary studies with vitamin E and selenium was so convincing, the SELECT Prostate Cancer Prevention Trial, the largest prostate cancer prevention trial to date, sought to determine whether these two dietary supplements can protect against prostate cancer. The study randomly assigned 35,533 men to four groups: selenium (200 mcg per day) plus a placebo, vitamin E (400 IU per day) plus a placebo, selenium plus vitamin E, or placebo and placebo. Eligibility criteria were age 50 years or older for African-Americans, 55 years or older for Caucasians, a serum PSA level of 4 ng/ml or less, a digital rectal examination not suspicious for cancer, and normal blood pressure. While the study was planned to last 12 years, it was terminated after 7 years because no effect on the risk of prostate cancer in these relatively healthy men could be demonstrated by selenium, vitamin E, or the combination at the doses and formulations used in the study. Concerns of the SELECT trial were a modest increase in the risk of prostate cancer with vitamin E (6% increased risk) and in the risk of type 2 diabetes in the selenium group (7% increased risk).[27]

Reasons why selenium and vitamin E, alone or in combination, failed to prevent prostate cancer in the SELECT trial are not clear. However, our feeling is that the researchers may have been looking at the wrong form of tocopherol (see the discussion above about gamma-tocopherol). Also, other trials studying high-dose vitamin E for disease prevention have shown no benefit either. It may be that when taken at such high dosages, vitamin E loses its preventive effects. In the absence of companion antioxidants vitamin E may become a free radical itself or be unable to perform its function (see the discussion of lycopene below). The earlier positive studies used a dosage of 50 IU, not the 400 IU used in the SELECT Study. Next, several studies suggested that vitamin E is more protective against prostate cancer in smokers, and less than 60% of SELECT men were current or former smokers, whereas in some of the other studies with vitamin E all men were smokers. The fact that selenium was ineffective in preventing prostate cancer could be due to the subjects' having sufficient levels of selenium before the trial started.[28]

The results also showed that overall mortality was 17% less in the selenium group than in the control group (108 deaths vs. 129), with this difference largely due to a 50% reduction in cancer deaths (29 vs. 57).

Lycopene

One of the most important anticancer nutrients, especially for the prostate, is lycopene—a carotene that provides the red color in tomato products. Lycopene is one of the major carotenes in the diet of North Americans and Europeans. More than 80% of lycopene consumed in the United States is derived from tomato products, although apricots, papaya, pink grapefruit, guava, and watermelon also contribute to dietary intake. Lycopene content of tomatoes can vary significantly, depending on type of tomato and stage of ripening. In the reddest strains of tomatoes, lycopene concentration is close to 50 mg/kg, compared with only 5 mg/kg in the yellow strains. Lycopene appears to be relatively stable during cooking and food processing. In fact, the absorption and utilization of lycopene from tomato paste or juice are up to five times greater compared with the absorption from raw tomatoes because it has been better liberated from the plant cell. Eating a lycopene source with some oil (e.g., olive oil) can also improve its absorption.

Lycopene is a more potent scavenger of oxygen radicals than other major dietary carotenes, and it exerts additional anticancer effects. Lycopene's role as a protector against prostate cancer was highlighted in a finding by Harvard researchers that of all the different types of carotenes, only lycopene was clearly linked to protection against prostate cancer.[29] The men who had the greatest amounts of lycopene in their diet (6.5 mg per day) showed a 21% decreased risk of prostate cancer compared with those eating the least. When the researchers looked at only advanced prostate cancer, the high-lycopene group had an 86% decreased risk (although this did not reach statistical significance due to the small number of cases). In a study of patients with existing prostate cancer, lycopene supplementation (15 mg per day) was shown to slow tumor growth. In subjects consuming the lycopene supplement, prostate tumors shrank and produced reduced levels of prostate-specific antigen.[30]

Population-based studies also indicate that lycopene protects against cancers of the colon, cervix, lung, and breast. Researchers have also found a statistically significant association between high dietary lycopene and a lower risk of heart disease.[31]

Clearly, increasing the intake of lycopene is a key goal in preventing many cancers, including prostate cancer. Although lycopene supplements are available in pill form, there are excellent food sources of lycopene. For example, a 12-oz can of tomato paste contains 192 mg lycopene and costs around $1.59 (less than 1 cent per mg of lycopene). But a bottle of 30 lycopene capsules (15 mg each) totaling 450 mg costs $18.99 (nearly 6 cents per mg). While lycopene alone has clear benefit, it is important to point out that in a test tube study it was found that lycopene alone was not a potent inhibitor of prostate cancer cell proliferation. However, the simultaneous addition of lycopene together with alpha-tocopherol (vitamin E) resulted in a 90% decrease in cell proliferation.[32]

Vitamin D

Population-based studies suggest that vitamin D protects against prostate cancer, although evidence is limited and inconsistent. In the most recent study, it was shown that men deficient in vitamin D were twice as likely to suffer from more aggressive prostate cancers, but there was no evidence of an association with overall prostate cancer risk.[33]

Berries and Other Sources of Proanthocyanidins

Blackberries, raspberries, blueberries, black-currants, cranberries, acai berries, and strawberries, as well as other fruits rich in similar flavonoids, such as pomegranates, cherries, and plums, appear to be extremely helpful in preventing prostate cancer, as test tube studies have shown impressive anticancer actions.[34–37] In addition, a study showed that *any* use of grape seed extract was associated with a 41% reduced risk of prostate cancer.[38] Studies in Italy showed similar protection with procyandin intake and a variety of cancers.[39] It can be concluded that the same degree of protection would be found in other concentrated sources of procyanidolic oligomers (e.g., pine bark or extracts of cranberry, blueberry, pomegranate, or acai berry). Regular consumption of these foods and supplementation with a concentrated source of procyanidolic oligomers are recommended.

. . . .

QUICK REVIEW

- **Prostate cancer is the most-diagnosed form of cancer in American men.**
- **It is important to reduce as many risk factors as possible while simultaneously implementing dietary and lifestyle factors associated with prostate cancer prevention.**
- **There is so much convincing evidence on the role of diet in prostate cancer that some authorities have suggested that prostate cancer may be a nutritional disease.**
- **Higher consumption of hamburgers, processed meats, grilled meats, and well-done meat was associated with an approximately 50 to 80% increase in aggressive forms of prostate cancer.**
- **A Mediterranean-style diet has been shown to help prevent prostate cancer.**
- **Studies suggest that men who drink soy milk have a lower risk of prostate cancer.**
- **A high ratio of dietary omega-6 to omega-3 fatty acids is a major risk factor for prostate cancer.**
- **Diet plays a major role in why black men have a higher rate of prostate cancer.**
- **Selenium and vitamin E have not been proved to have any effect on the risk of prostate cancer.**
- **Gamma-tocopherol may prove to be more important against prostate cancer than alpha-tocopherol.**
- **Men who consume the greatest amounts of lycopene had a lower risk of prostate cancer.**
- **Use of grape seed extract was associated with a reduced risk of prostate cancer.**
- **Green tea polyphenols have shown considerable benefit in preventing prostate cancer.**

Green Tea

Population-based studies have demonstrated that consumption of green tea *(Camellia sinensis)* may offer significant protection against many forms of cancer, including prostate cancer.[40] In order to take advantage of this protection you would need to drink three to five cups per day, providing a minimum of 250 mg per day polyphenols (also referred to as catechins). However, emerging clinical data suggest that this dosage level may not be sufficient in high-risk individuals.

The best data on green tea's anticancer effects may actually be on prostate cancer. Test tube and animal studies have shown that epigallocatechin gallate (EGCG)—a major polyphenol in green tea—inhibits both hormone-sensitive and hormone-insensitive prostate cancer cells. In one study, men with clinically localized prostate cancer were divided into groups and consumed either six cups of green tea per day or water for three to six weeks before undergoing surgery to remove the prostate (radical prostatectomy).[41] With the use of highly sensitive lab analysis, metabolites of EGCG were detectable in both prostate tissue and urine in men consuming the green tea. This study also showed initial indications that EGCG metabolites in the prostate cancer cells helped induce apoptosis.

In another study, men who were about to undergo radical prostatectomy for prostate cancer were given either 1,300 mg per day of green tea polyphenols or a placebo until the time of the surgery. The results showed a significant reduction in serum levels of PSA in men with prostate cancer after brief treatment with green tea polyphenols.[42]

A proof-of-principle clinical trial was designed to assess the safety and efficacy of green tea polyphenols in preventing precancerous lesions from developing into prostate cancer within one year.[43] The 60 men in the study were given either a placebo or 600 mg green tea polyphenol extract per day. After one year, only one tumor was diagnosed among the 30 extract-treated men, whereas nine cancers were found among the 30 placebo-treated men. Total PSA levels were consistently lower in the green tea group than in the placebo group. Men who had benign prostate hyperplasia (BPH) also significantly improved on the green tea polyphenol extract.

Pygeum

Pygeum *(Pygeum africanum)* is an evergreen tree native to Africa. An extract made from its bark has been well studied in promotion of a healthy prostate (see the chapter "Prostate Enlargement [BPH]"). Current treatment of prostate cancer often involves the use of antiandrogens, synthetic compounds that block the action of testosterone by inhibiting androgen receptors. These compounds have numerous side effects and typically are effective for only about 16 to 24 months, after which the prostate cancer cells cease being androgen-dependent. By contrast, pygeum has a different mechanism of action and efficiently represses the growth of both androgen-dependent prostate cancer cells and some types of androgen-independent prostate cancer cells. We recommend the use of pygeum extract in men with a high risk for prostate cancer.[44,45]

TREATMENT SUMMARY

Focus on reducing risk factors for prostate cancer along with implementing dietary and lifestyle factors associated with prevention. In many cases, men with prostate cancer also have BPH, so if you have BPH, follow the recommendations in that chapter as well.

Diet and Lifestyle

- Follow the recommendations in the chapter "A Health-Promoting Lifestyle."
- Follow the recommendations in the chapter "A Health-Promoting Diet." In particular, employ the principles of the Mediterranean diet: eat more fish, whole grains, vegetables, and mono-unsaturated fats; consume soy foods and vegetables from the brassica (cabbage) family on a regular basis; add 1 tbsp ground flaxseed to the diet per day; avoid high-glycemic foods and unhealthful fats; and achieve and maintain ideal body weight.

Nutritional Supplements

- A high-potency multiple vitamin and mineral formula as described in the chapter "Supplementary Measures"

- Key individual nutrients:
  - Vitamin E (mixed tocopherols): 100 to 200 mg per day
  - Selenium: 100 to 200 mcg per day
  - Lycopene: 10 to 15 mg per day
  - Vitamin D_3: 2,000 IU per day
- Fish oils: 1,000 mg EPA + DHA
- One of the following:
  - Grape seed extract (>95% procyanidolic oligomers): 100 to 300 mg per day
  - Pine bark extract (>95% procyanidolic oligomers): 100 to 300 mg per day
  - Some other flavonoid-rich extract with a similar flavonoid content, super greens formula, or another plant-based antioxidant that can provide an oxygen radical absorption capacity (ORAC) of 3,000 to 6,000 units or more per day

Botanical Medicines

- Green tea extract (>80% total polyphenol content): 300 to 400 mg per day
- Pygeum extract (14% triterpene content): 50 to 100 mg per day for high-risk individuals

Prostate Enlargement (BPH)

- Symptoms of bladder outlet obstruction (increased urinary frequency, urgency, and need to urinate during the night; difficulty beginning to urinate; urine stream starts and stops; slow urine flow)

- Enlarged, nontender prostate

The prostate is a doughnut-shaped gland about the size of a walnut that lies below the bladder and surrounds the urethra. The prostate secretes a thin, milky, alkaline fluid that increases sperm motility, lubricates the urethra, and helps prevent infection. Prostate secretions are extremely important to successful fertilization of the egg as well as the male sexual experience.

Prostate enlargement refers to benign prostatic hyperplasia (BPH), a condition that affects more than 50% of men in their lifetime. The actual incidence increases with advancing age, from approximately 5 to 10% at age 30 to 50% at age 50 and more than 90% in men older than 85.[1]

Although BPH is usually more of a bothersome condition that can dramatically affect quality of life, it can also lead to serious consequence, as it can progress to urinary retention, with an accompanying risk of recurrent

---

WARNING: Prostate disorders can be diagnosed only by a physician. Do not self-diagnose. If you are experiencing any symptoms associated with BPH or prostate cancer, see your physician immediately for proper diagnosis.

---

urinary tract infections, bladder stones, and occasionally kidney failure.

Causes

Genetic predisposition plays a minor role in BPH, particularly when BPH occurs in a younger man.[1–3] Genetics can set the stage, but ultimately BPH is a condition caused by the influence of dietary, lifestyle, and environmental factors on the metabolism of male sex hormones (androgens). Levels of testosterone, particularly free testosterone, decrease with age after the fifth decade. By contrast, hormones such as prolactin, estradiol, sex-hormone-binding ligand, luteinizing hormone (LH), and follicle-stimulating hormone (FSH) are all increased. The ultimate effect of these changes is that within the prostate there is an increased concentration of dihydrotestosterone (DHT), the potent androgen derived from testosterone. This increase is largely due to a decreased rate of removal combined with an increase in the activity of the enzyme that converts testosterone to DHT.[4] Estrogens come into play because they inhibit the proper excretion of testosterone and DHT.

Diagnostic Considerations

It is often recommended that men over the age of 40 have yearly prostate exams. This exam is not high-tech. It simply involves a doctor inserting a gloved finger into the rectum and feeling the lower part of the prostate for any abnormality. However, in the case of BPH, often the prostate has not enlarged to a point that can be recognized by physical exam. And in the case of cancer, a digital exam is not reliable enough.

The classic enlarged prostate due to BPH will usually feel softer than normal and may be two to three times larger than normal. In BPH, the prostate is not tender; this differentiates it from prostatitis—an infection of the prostate. The classic finding in prostatic cancer is that the prostate feels much harder and its border is not as well-defined as that of a healthy prostate.

The definitive diagnosis of BPH can be made with the aid of ultrasound measurements. However, because the symptoms of BPH and prostate cancer can be similar, a simple blood test is used to differentiate BPH from the more serious prostate cancer. The blood test measures the levels of prostate-specific antigen (PSA), a protein that is produced in the prostate. The PSA test is regarded as a highly significant and sensitive marker for prostate cancer. The normal value for PSA is less than 4 ng/ml. A level above 10 ng/ml is highly indicative of prostate cancer.

There has been concern that the use of PSA as a screening test for prostate cancer is not reliable enough and leads to many unnecessary biopsies in the attempt to rule out prostate cancer. Making matter worse, many forms of prostate cancer are very slow-growing, so that the treatment is often more serious than the disease. Although an elevated level of prostate-specific antigen indicates prostate cancer about 90% of the time, it must be kept in mind that midrange elevations in PSA can be caused by BPH, and that in some instances there may be prostate cancer yet PSA levels are not elevated. De-

spite the fact that this test is not perfect, it is a simple, relatively noninvasive test that can provide valuable information.

If you are a man over the age of 50 and if any of your immediate relatives—father, brother, or uncle—has had prostate cancer, an annual prostate exam and PSA test are a very good idea. See the chapter "Prostate Cancer (Prevention)" for more information.

Therapeutic Considerations

If left untreated, BPH can eventually obstruct the bladder outlet, resulting in the retention of urine and eventually kidney damage. As this situation is potentially life-threatening, proper treatment is crucial. Surgery may be indicated in patients for whom medical therapy has not worked, who have recurrent infection, or who display signs of kidney failure. In the past, medical treatment involved a procedure known as transurethral resection of the prostate. Because this surgery is associated with a high rate of morbidity (sexual dysfunction, incontinence, and bleeding) and often makes matters worse, it should be avoided unless absolutely necessary. Surgical procedures that use microwaves or lasers are also available. Generally, these newer procedures are less expensive than transurethral resection of the prostate and have fewer complications, although subsequent therapies are often required.[5]

Exercise

There is an association between greater physical activity and lower rates of BPH, and there is also an association between abdominal obesity and BPH.[6,7] Higher caloric intake not also encourages abdominal obesity but also increases sympathetic nervous system activity (the fight-or-flight response); this may cause the smooth muscle of the prostate to contract, resulting in a worsening of urinary symptoms. Interestingly, higher caloric intake does not seem to increase BPH risk when accompanied by increased physical activity.[7]

It seems possible that physical activity may serve a threefold purpose: (1) it may increase blood flow to the area, allowing the body to remove wastes efficiently; (2) it can decrease sympathetic stress responses, thus relaxing prostatic tissue; and (3) it can reduce excess abdominal weight, decreasing sympathetic nervous system activity and thus relaxing the prostate/rectal region and improving blood flow into and out of the area.

Diet

Diet appears to play a critical role in the health of the prostate. Diets high in overall fat, particularly saturated fat, are associated with an increased risk of BPH, as are diets high in red meat.[7] A study of Chinese farmers revealed a correlation between diets higher in animal products and the frequency of BPH (91.1% of those those eating diets high in animal products had BPH vs. 11.8% in those not eating animal protein).[8]

The recommendations in the chapter "A Health-Promoting Diet" are appropriate for BPH. It is particularly important to avoid pesticide residues on fruits and vegetables, increase consumption of fruits and vegetables,[9,10] increase the intake of zinc and essential fatty acids, decrease coffee consumption,[11] decrease butter consumption, and avoid margarine and other sources of trans fats.[9–11] It is also important to keep blood cholesterol levels below 200 mg/dl.

Zinc

Paramount in an effective BPH treatment plan is adequate zinc intake and absorption.

Studies done in the 1970s showed that zinc supplementation reduces the size of the prostate and decreases symptoms in the majority of patients.[12,13] The clinical efficacy of zinc is probably due to its critical involvement in many aspects of androgen metabolism. Intestinal absorption of zinc is impaired by estrogens but enhanced by androgens. Because estrogen levels are increased in men with BPH, zinc uptake may be low.

Studies have demonstrated that zinc inhibits the activity of the enzyme that converts testosterone to DHT.[14–18] Zinc also inhibits the binding of androgens to androgen receptors in the cell.[14]

Zinc has been shown to inhibit prolactin secretion by the pituitary gland.[19,20] Prolactin increases the uptake of testosterone by the prostate, thereby leading to increased levels of DHT.[20] Drugs that block prolactin have been shown to reduce many of the symptoms of prostatic hyperplasia. However, these drugs have severe side effects and are of limited value.[21] Beer (but not pure alcohol), tryptophan, and stress all increase prolactin secretion and may therefore be aggravating factors.[22,23]

The authors of one study of 184 patients and 356 controls reported a positive association between zinc and BPH. A possible reason for this result is that in this study higher zinc may have been associated with intake of meat, a known risk factor for increased BPH.[24] It appears that a high meat intake can cancel out the positive effects of zinc against BPH.

Alcohol

Although only beer raises prolactin levels, higher alcohol intake may be associated with BPH. In a 17-year study of 6,581 men in Hawaii, it was noted that an alcohol intake of at least 25 fl oz a month was directly correlated with the diagnosis of BPH.[25] The association was most significant for beer, wine, and sake and less for distilled spirits. A smaller study of 889 men described an inverse association between alcohol intake and men treated surgically for BPH or in "watchful waiting" for surgical intervention. In other words, the higher the alcohol intake, the more likely it was that men experienced more severe BPH.

Amino Acids

The combination of glycine, alanine, and glutamic acid has been shown in several studies to relieve many BPH symptoms. In a controlled study of 45 men, increased nighttime urinary frequency was relieved or reduced in 95%, urgency reduced in 81%, daytime urinary frequency reduced in 73%, and delayed urination alleviated in 70%.[26] These results have also been reported in other controlled studies.[27] The mechanism of action is unknown but is probably related to the amino acids acting as inhibitory neurotransmitters and reducing the feelings of a full bladder. In other words, amino acid therapy is effective only at reducing symptoms.

Cholesterol

Toxic cholesterol metabolites are irritating to the bladder. They have been shown to accumulate in an enlarged prostate or in one with cancer. Cholesterol that has been damaged by free radicals can in turn damage prostate cells, leading to the increased cell growth seen in BPH. Every effort should be made to decrease cholesterol levels by using the principles outlined in the chapter "High Cholesterol and/or Triglycerides," as well as to prevent the formation of toxic forms by maintaining a high intake of dietary antioxidants.

Soy Products

Soybeans are especially rich in phytosterols, especially beta-sitosterol. The cholesterol-lowering effects of phytosterols are well docu-

mented.[28] Phytosterols have also been shown to improve BPH. A recent double-blind study consisted of 200 men receiving beta-sitosterol (20 mg) or placebo three times per day.[29] The beta-sitosterol produced an increase in urine flow rate and a decrease in the urine left behind in the bladder after voiding. No changes were observed in the placebo group. A 3.5-oz serving of soybeans, tofu, or other soy food provides approximately 90 mg beta-sitosterol. Increased consumption of soy and soy foods is also associated with a decrease in the risk of prostate cancer (see the chapter "Prostate Cancer [Prevention]").

Botanical Medicines

Plant-based medicines are much more popular prescriptions in Europe for BPH than their synthetic counterparts. Specifically, in Germany and Austria botanical medicines are considered first-line treatments for BPH and account for more than 90% of all drugs in the medical management of BPH. In Italy plant extracts account for roughly 50% of all medications prescribed for BPH, while alpha-blockers and 5-alpha-reductase inhibitors account for only 5.1% and 4.8%, respectively.[30]

About 30 plant-based compounds are currently available in Europe for the treatment of BPH. At least 15 of them contain saw palmetto (*Serenoa repens*) extract. Other popular botanical medicines include pygeum (*Pygeum africanum*), stinging nettle (*Urtica dioica*), and Cernilton, a special flower pollen extract. On the basis of careful examination of the published literature, we rate saw palmetto as the most effective, followed by Cernilton, pygeum, and stinging nettle. However, each plant has a slightly different mechanism of action, and one herb may work better for a particular person than another herb. Combinations may also prove to be more effective than any single agent.

The chance of clinical success with any of the botanical treatments of BPH appears to be determined by the degree of obstruction, as indicated by residual urine content (urine left in the bladder after urination). For levels less than 50 ml, the results are usually excellent. For levels between 50 and 100 ml, the results are usually quite good. Residual urine levels between 100 and 150 ml will make it tougher to see significant improvements. If the residual urine content is greater than 150 ml, saw palmetto extract and other botanical medicines are unlikely to produce any significant improvement on their own.

Saw Palmetto

The fat-soluble extract of the fruit of the saw palmetto tree (*Serenoa repens*), native to Florida, has been shown to significantly diminish the signs and symptoms of BPH. The mechanism of action is related to inhibition of DHT binding to cellular receptors, inhibition of the enzyme 5-alpha-reductase, and interfering with prostate estrogen receptors. Excellent results have been produced in numerous clinical studies, with roughly 90% of men who have mild to moderate BPH experiencing some improvement in symptoms during the first four to six weeks of therapy with saw palmetto extract.[31–34] As a matter of fact, men treated with saw palmetto had results comparable to those seen by men taking finasteride (Proscar). Adverse effects from the saw palmetto extract were mild and infrequent, with erectile dysfunction appearing more frequently with finasteride (4.9%) than with saw palmetto (1.1%).[31] In general, saw palmetto is well tolerated, and it has

---

Over the years many of us in the natural health field have seen the media disseminate questionable results from research studies in major medical journals, holding them up as "proof" that the public is being duped into spending money on worthless natural products. Of course, those knowledgeable about the merits of these same natural products try to mobilize the resources that we have available to counteract these negative statements, but this is often difficult when we are up against an article published in a respected journal such as the *New England Journal of Medicine, Lancet, British Medical Journal,* or *Journal of the American Medical Association.* Such journals are seemingly more credible than even the natural product industry's most reputable organizations, companies, and experts.

To illustrate this point, let's take a quick look at a double-blind study that the media presented as evidence that saw palmetto extract does not work in relieving the symptoms of benign prostatic hyperplasia (BPH). The study was published in the *New England Journal of Medicine.*[35] The news releases that ensued included the Associated Press reporting that a "popular herbal pill used by millions of men doesn't reduce the frequent urge to go to the bathroom or other annoying symptoms of an enlarged prostate." That is not true at all. We have been writing about the benefits of saw palmetto extract in the treatment of BPH for over 20 years. We have always pointed out that the success of saw palmetto extract is most obvious in the early stages of BPH. The problem is that the study that got a lot of publicity was done in men with severe, advanced disease, in which saw palmetto is already known not to work. The media did not make this distinction, simply asserting that saw palmetto does not work.

What the media should have reported is that the study reinforced the importance of taking saw palmetto extract early in the disease process, as soon as symptoms of BPH appear (e.g., increased urinary frequency, urgency, increased nighttime urination, difficulty beginning to urinate, urine stream starts and stops, and slow urine flow). If a man waits until his prostate has enlarged so severely that it results in significant obstruction of the bladder, saw palmetto is simply not likely to work. But if he starts it early enough, it is as effective as or more effective than popular prescriptionı drugs without the side effects.

no known drug interactions.[34] One possible side effect is gastrointestinal distress, which is mild and is easily remedied by taking saw palmetto with food. Future studies will hopefully include head-to-head trials comparing saw palmetto with alpha-blockers such as tamsulosin (Flomax), doxazosin (Cardura), and prazosin (Minipress).

Cernilton

Cernilton, an extract of rye-grass flower pollen, has been used to treat prostatitis and BPH in Europe for more than 40 years.[36] It has been shown to be quite effective in several double-blind clinical studies in the treatment of BPH.[37,38] The overall success rate in patients with BPH is about 70%.[37] Patients who respond typically have reductions of around 70% in both nighttime and daytime urinary frequency, as well as significant reductions in urine that is left behind in the bladder after urination.[38] The extract has been shown to exert some anti-inflammatory action and produce a contractile effect on the bladder while simultaneously relaxing the urethra. In addition, Cernilton contains a substance that inhibits the growth of prostate cells.[39]

In one study, the efficacy of Cernilton in the treatment of symptomatic BPH was examined over a one-year period.[36] Seventy-nine men averaging 68 years of age (range 62 to 89) were given 63 mg Cernilton twice per day for 12 weeks. They saw improvements in average urine maximum flow rate, average flow rate, and residual urine volume. Overall, 85% of the test subjects experienced benefit: 11% reporting "excellent," 39% reporting

QUICK REVIEW

- **More than 50% of men will develop an enlarged prostate in their lifetime.**
- **BPH is largely the result of hormonal changes associated with aging.**
- **Obesity is a major risk factor for BPH.**
- **Paramount to an effective BPH treatment plan is adequate zinc intake and absorption.**
- **Cholesterol damaged by free radicals is particularly toxic and carcinogenic to the prostate.**
- **Increased consumption of soy and soy foods is associated with a decrease in the risk of getting prostate cancer and may help in treating BPH.**
- **In Europe, plant-based medicines are the most popular prescriptions for BPH.**

- **Saw palmetto extract and other herbal approaches to BPH are most effective in mild to moderate cases. Saw palmetto is not likely to be effective in severe cases.**
- **Roughly 90% of men with mild to moderate BPH experience some improvement in symptoms during the first four to six weeks after beginning to take saw palmetto extract.**
- **Pygeum, a flower pollen extract (Cernilton), and stinging nettle root extract all have shown excellent results in improving BPH symptoms in double-blind studies.**

"good," 35% reporting "satisfactory," and 15% reporting "poor" as a description of their outcome.

A summary review of two placebo-controlled studies, two comparative trials (both lasting 12 to 24 weeks), and three double-blind studies of 444 men showed that although Cernilton did not improve urinary flow rates, residual volume, or prostate size, it did improve self-rated urinary symptom scores and reduced nighttime urinary frequency compared with a placebo and an amino acid mixture.[40] Clearly, more long-term studies of Cernilton need to be conducted in order to elucidate the terms of its usefulness as an alternative or adjunct to saw palmetto.

Pygeum

The bark of *Pygeum africanum*, an evergreen tree native to Africa, has historically been used in the treatment of urinary tract disorders. The major active components of the bark are fat-soluble sterols and fatty acids. Virtually all of the research on pygeum has featured an extract standardized to contain 14% triterpenes, including beta-sitosterol and 0.5% n-docosanol. This extract has been extensively studied in both experimental animal studies and clinical trials with humans. A study on rat prostatic cells suggests that the therapeutic effect of pygeum may be due in part to the inhibition of growth factors (e.g., EGF, bFGF, and IGF-I) that are responsible for the prostatic overgrowth.[41]

Numerous clinical trials with more than 600 patients have demonstrated pygeum extract to be effective in reducing the symptoms and clinical signs of BPH, especially in early cases.[41] However, in a double-blind study that compared pygeum extract with the extract of saw palmetto, the saw palmetto produced a greater reduction of symptoms and was better tolerated.[42] In addition, the effects on urine flow rate and residual urine content are better in the clinical studies with saw palmetto. However, there may be circumstances where pygeum is more effective than saw palmetto. For example, saw palmetto has not been shown to produce some of the effects on prostate secretion that pygeum has. Of course, as the two extracts have somewhat overlapping mechanisms of actions, they can be used in combination.

Stinging Nettle

Extracts of the root of stinging nettle (*Urtica dioica*) have also been shown to be effective in the treatment of BPH. Fewer studies have been done with stinging nettle root extract than with the other botanical medicines discussed. Two double-blind studies have shown it to be more effective than a placebo.[43,44] However, like pygeum, the results with stinging nettle are less impressive than those with saw palmetto extract or Cernilton. A randomized, multicenter, double-blind study of 431 patients using both the extracts of saw palmetto and stinging nettle found clinical benefit equal to that of finasteride.[45] Like the extract of saw palmetto, stinging nettle extract appears to interact with binding of DHT to cellular and nuclear receptors.[46] Test tube studies show that stinging nettle root extract may also modulate hormonal effects.[47]

TREATMENT SUMMARY

Therapeutic goals for BPH are to normalize prostate nutrient levels, inhibit excessive conversion of testosterone to DHT, inhibit DHT receptor binding, and limit prolactin, which promotes prostate cell growth.

Severe BPH, resulting in significant acute urinary retention, may require catheterization for relief; a sufficiently advanced case may not respond rapidly enough to therapy and may require the short-term use of an alpha-1 antagonist drug (e.g., Flomax, Cardura, Hytrin, Uroxatral) or surgical intervention.

Exercise

Exercise is protective against BPH. Follow the recommendations in the chapter "A Health-Promoting Lifestyle."

Diet

The recommendations in the chapter "A Health-Promoting Diet" are appropriate in BPH. It is important to limit the consumption of meat and other animal products; alcohol and coffee; drug-, pesticide-, and hormone-contaminated foods; and cholesterol-rich foods. Soy foods should be consumed regularly.

Nutritional Supplements

- A high-potency multiple vitamin and mineral formula as described in the chapter "Supplementary Measures"

- Zinc: 30 to 45 mg per day (picolinate form preferred)
- Fish oils: 1,000 mg EPA + DHA
- One of the following:
  - Grape seed extract (>95% procyanidolic oligomers): 150 to 300 mg per day
  - Pine bark extract (>90% procyanidolic oligomers): 150 to 300 mg per day
  - Some other flavonoid-rich extract with a similar flavonoid content, super greens formula, or another plant-based antioxidant that can provide an oxygen radical absorption capacity (ORAC) of 3,000 to 6,000 units or more per day
- Specialty supplements:
  - Glycine: 200 mg per day
  - Glutamic acid: 200 mg per day
  - Alanine: 200 mg per day
  - Beta-sitosterol: 60 to 100 mg per day

Botanical Medicines

- One or more of the following:
  - Saw palmetto extract (standardized at 85% to 95% fatty acids and sterols): 320 to 640 mg per day
  - Flower pollen extract (e.g., Cernilton): 63 mg two to three times per day
  - Pygeum extract (14% triterpene content): 50 to 100 mg per day
  - Stinging nettle root extract: 120 to 150 mg twice per day

Psoriasis

- Sharply bordered reddened rash or plaques covered with overlapping silvery scales
- Characteristic locations: scalp; back of the wrists, elbows, knees, buttocks, and ankles; and sites of repeated trauma
- Family history in 50% of cases
- Nail involvement results in characteristic "oil drop" stippling (thimble-like appearance)
- Possible arthritis

Psoriasis is an extremely common skin disorder. In the United States, it occurs in 2 to 4% of the population. Psoriasis affects mainly Caucasians. It affects few blacks in tropical zones but is more common among blacks in temperate zones. It appears commonly among Japanese but is rare in American Indians and is entirely absent in natives of the Andean region of South America. Psoriasis affects men and women equally, and the mean onset is 27.8 years of age, although 2% show onset by two years of age.[1]

In addition to affecting the skin, psoriasis can cause an inflammatory form of arthritis and affect the nails. The nails take on a characteristic thimble-like appearance referred to as "oil drop" stippling.

Causes

Psoriasis is caused by a pileup of skin cells that have replicated too rapidly. The rate at which skin cells divide in psoriasis is roughly one thousand times greater than in normal skin. This high rate of replication is simply too fast for the cells to be shed, so they accumulate, resulting in the characteristic silvery scale of psoriasis.

Psoriasis is the result of a basic defect that lies within the skin cells. The frequency of psoriasis is increased in people with certain genetic markers, reflecting a possible genetic error in the control over how skin cells divide. The genetic link is also confirmed by the observation that 36% of psoriasis patients have one or more family members with psoriasis. There are also multiple defects noted in the skin and immune cells of psoriatic patients, indicating a complex interplay of genetic factors.[2-4] The primary defect in psoriasis appears to be an increase in cell signaling through compounds known as chemokines and cytokines, secreted by white blood cells, which cause skin cells to replicate excessively. It appears that rather than being a disorder of the skin cells, psoriasis is primarily a condition that affects the immune system.[5-7]

Perhaps the strongest evidence of a link to the immune system is that psoriasis has been shown to develop in those who have received bone marrow transplants from donors with psoriasis and to clear up in bone marrow recipients with psoriasis when they receive a transplant from donors without psoriasis. Drugs that suppress the immune system are effective in reducing psoriasis.[8,9]

While psoriasis has a very strong genetic component, how those genes are expressed can be modified. There is a clear relationship between psoriasis and conditions associated with altered gastrointestinal permeability, such as celiac disease[10] and Crohn's disease,[11] and in conditions associated with impaired liver function.[12] Furthermore, the gastrointestinal lining of psoriatic patients has shown microscopic lesions and greater intestinal permeability.[13] Factors leading to poor intestinal function and increased gut permeability ultimately allow food and microbial antigens and endotoxins to be absorbed from the gastrointestinal tract, travel through the bloodstream, and initiate activated immune activity that ultimately leads to skin cell replication. These data provide a clear focus of therapy.

Therapeutic Considerations

Although psoriasis has a significant genetic component, addressing the factors that can activate the immune system or skin cells can result in significant clinical improvement.

Incomplete Protein Digestion

Incomplete protein digestion or poor intestinal absorption of protein breakdown products can result in elevations of amino acids and polypeptides in the bowel. These are metabolized by bowel bacteria into several toxic compounds. In particular, toxic metabolites of the amino acids arginine and ornithine, known as polyamines (e.g., putrescine, spermidine, and cadaverine), have been shown to be higher in the blood in individuals with psoriasis. These polyamines have been shown to contribute to the excessive rate of cell proliferation in psoriasis.[14–16] Lowered skin and urinary levels of polyamines are associated with clinical improvement in psoriasis.[14]

A number of natural compounds can inhibit the formation of polyamines and may be of benefit in the treatment of psoriasis. For example, vitamin A and the alkaloids of goldenseal (*Hydrastis canadensis*) such as berberine inhibit bacterial decarboxylase, the enzyme that converts amino acids into polyamines.[17,18] However, the best way to prevent the excessive formation of polyamines is to ensure adequate hydrochloric acid and pancreatic enzyme secretion in the gastrointestinal system. See the chapter "Digestion and Elimination" for more information, as ensuring proper digestion is a key step in dealing with psoriasis.

Bowel Toxemia

A number of gut-derived toxins are also implicated in the development of psoriasis, including endotoxins (cell-wall components of gram-negative bacteria), *Candida albicans*, and yeast compounds.[19–21] Endotoxins have been found in high levels in the blood of psoriatic patients,[22] and these compounds lead to dramatic increases in the rate of skin cell proliferation. Overgrowth of *C. albicans* in the intestines (chronic candidiasis) may play a role in some patients with psoriasis.

A diet low in dietary fiber is associated with increased levels of gut-derived toxins.[19] Dietary fiber is critical to maintaining a healthy colon. Many fiber components bind bowel toxins and promote their excretion in the feces. It is therefore essential that the diet of an individual with psoriasis be rich in beans, fruits, and vegetables. Natural compounds that bind endotoxins and promote their excretion may also be used. For example, an aqueous extract of the herb sarsaparilla (*Smilax sarsaparilla*) was found in a 1942 study to be effective in psoriasis, particularly the more chronic, large-plaque-forming variety.[23] In this controlled study of 92 patients, sarsaparilla greatly improved psoriasis in 62% of the patients and resulted in complete clearance in another 18% (i.e., 80% of the subjects experienced significant benefits). This benefit is apparently due to the components of sarsaparilla binding to bacterial endotoxins and promoting their excretion.

Because the severity of psoriasis as well as therapeutic response have been shown to correlate well with the level of circulating endotoxins, control of gut-derived toxins is important in the treatment of psoriasis.

Liver Function

The correction of abnormal liver function may be of benefit in the treatment of psoriasis.[12,24] The connection between the liver and psoriasis relates to one of the liver's basic tasks—filtering and detoxifying the blood returning through the portal circulation from the bowels. Altered liver function is common in psoriatic patients.[25] As mentioned previously, psoriasis has been linked to the presence of several microbial by-products in the blood. If hepatic function is compromised by excessive levels of these toxins from the bowel or if there is a decrease in the liver's detoxification ability, the systemic toxin level rises and the psoriasis worsens.

Alcohol consumption is known to significantly worsen psoriasis.[26] Alcohol has this effect because it both increases the absorption of toxins from the gut (by damaging the gut mucosa) and impairs liver function. Alcohol intake must be restricted in individuals with psoriasis.

Silymarin, the flavonoid component of milk thistle (*Silybum marianum*), has been reported to be of value in the treatment of psoriasis.[27] Presumably this is a result of its ability to improve liver function, inhibit inflammation, and reduce excessive cellular proliferation.[27,28]

Bile Acid Deficiency

In the psoriatic patient, endotoxins are absorbed from the intestine into the bloodstream.[22] Bile acids normally present in the intestines act to detoxify bacterial endotoxins. In the absence of sufficient amounts of bile acids, endotoxins can move into the bloodstream and produce a variety of problems, including the release of inflammatory cytokines known to play a role in psoriasis.

A study of 800 psoriatic patients was conducted in which 551 were treated with oral bile acid (dehydrocholic acid) supplementation for one to six weeks for acute cases and three to eight weeks for chronic cases. Conventional therapies were administered to 249 patients as a comparison group. Both groups were encouraged to eat a diet high in vegetables and fruits and were instructed to avoid hot spices, alcohol, raw onion, garlic, and carbonated soft drinks. Of the 551 patients receiving the bile acid, 434 (78.8%) experienced complete resolution of their psoriasis, whereas only 62 (24.9%) of the 249 patients receiving conventional therapies demonstrated clinical recovery during this treatment period. Additionally, the curative effect of bile acid supplementation was more pronounced in the acute form of psoriasis: 95.1% of the patients in this group became asymptomatic. In follow-up assessments two years later, 319 of the 551 patients with acute and chronic psoriasis who had been treated with bile acid (57.9%) were asymptomatic, compared with only 15 of the 249 patients (6%) who had received the conventional treatment.[22] The dosage of dehydrocholic acid used in the studies was 250 mg per day given in two to three doses. Dehydrocholic acid is available by prescription, but mixtures of bile acids from ox bile are available in health food stores and may prove to be suitable alternatives.

Diet and Nutrition

Omega-3 Fatty Acids

Just as in other inflammatory conditions (e.g., rheumatoid arthritis), it is important to reduce the consumption of meat and dairy products to reduce the intake of arachidonic acid—a fatty acid that is known to increase the inflammatory response and is found in high levels in psoriatic skin—while increasing the intake of the long-chain omega-3 fatty acids eicosapentaenoic acid (EPA) and docosahexaenoic acid (DHA). Several double-blind clinical studies have demonstrated that supplementing the diet with 3,000 mg EPA and DHA results in significant improvement in psoriasis.[29–32] Detailed studies support a number of beneficial effects of EPA and DHA in psoriasis, including a reduction in the production of inflammatory compounds that stimulate skin cell proliferation. In addition, EPA and DHA tamp down some of the immune mechanisms that also trigger skin cell replication. While increasing the intake of EPA and DHA is important in improving psoriasis, it is imperative to reduce the intake of arachidonic acid as well.

Fasting, Vegetarian Diet, and Food Allergy Control

Dietary treatment of psoriasis is very similar to that for rheumatoid arthritis (see that chapter). Research studying the effects of fasting and vegetarian regimens on chronic inflammatory disease found that a therapeutic fast followed by a vegetarian diet with careful attention to any food allergy is very therapeutic in both conditions. The fast con-

sisted of herbal teas, garlic, vegetable broth, a decoction of potatoes and parsley, and the juice of carrots, beets, and celery. The fast was followed by a systematic reintroduction of a single food item every two days with elimination of foods that aggravated symptoms.[33] The improvement was probably due to decreased intestinal permeability, leading to reduced levels of gut-derived toxins and polyamines entering the bloodstream. Other studies have also shown considerable benefits from elimination diets as well as gluten-free diets (see the chapter "Celiac Disease").[34,35]

A vegetarian diet often includes the herbs and spices turmeric, red pepper, cloves, ginger, cumin, anise, fennel, basil, rosemary, garlic, and pomegranate, all of which can block the activation of the inflammatory cytokines linked to psoriasis, providing another possible route of benefit with such a diet.[36] Liberal use of these herbs and spices is recommended.

Individual Nutrients

Decreased levels of vitamin A and zinc are common in patients with psoriasis.[37–39] Given the critical roles of these nutrients in the health of the skin, supplementation might be warranted even without this association.

Chromium supplementation may be indicated to increase the sensitivity of insulin receptors, since psoriatic patients typically have evidence of insulin resistance (increased serum levels of both insulin and glucose) and carry an increased risk for type 2 diabetes and metabolic syndrome.[40]

Substantial evidence indicates that psoriasis is an independent risk factor for cardiovascular disease.[41] Inflammatory factors such as C-reactive protein (CRP) and other risk factors for atherosclerosis are found significantly more often in psoriasis patients.[42] This association alone stresses the importance of omega-3 fatty acids, folic acid, vitamin B$_6$, and vitamin B_{12}.[43] High homocysteine (a metabolite of the amino acid methionine that is linked to atherosclerosis; levels will be elevated if a person is low in folic acid, vitamin B_6, and vitamin B_{12}) and decreased folic acid levels are linked to an increase in the severity of psoriasis. The rapid skin cell turnover rate in psoriasis may result in increased folic acid utilization and subsequent deficiency.[44] The authors of one study concluded that "dietary supplementation of folic acid, B_6, and B_{12} appears reasonable in psoriasis patients, particularly those with elevated homocysteine, low folate and additional cardiovascular risk factors."[45]

Levels of the selenium-containing antioxidant enzyme glutathione peroxidase are low in psoriatic patients, possibly because of such factors as alcohol abuse, malnutrition, and the excessive replication and loss of skin cells. Depressed levels of glutathione peroxidase normalize with oral selenium and vitamin E therapy.[46] Several investigations have found that patients with longer-term psoriasis (three years or more) demonstrated low plasma selenium status.[47,48]

Vitamin D status is low in patients with psoriasis and appears to be a contributing factor.[49] Skin cells convert naturally produced 7-dehydrocholesterol to vitamin D_3 in the presence of ultraviolet B light. Not surprisingly, sunlight, UVB phototherapy, oral vitamin D analogues, and topical vitamin D_3 all improve psoriasis, validating vitamin D's ability to control the excessive skin cell replication seen in psoriasis.[50] Vitamin D also favorably affects the immune system and the expression of genes by skin cells in a way that could also explain the improvements seen in psoriasis.[51–54]

Given the importance of vitamin D in psoriasis as well for general health, supplementation seems critical. And while sunlight can be helpful in psoriasis, it may not help increase vitamin D levels. Studies conducted in Honolulu, Miami, and southern Arizona showed that abundant sun exposure did not necessary ensure vitamin D adequacy; this finding points to the need for vitamin D supplementation to achieve optimal blood levels.[55] In psoriasis, we recommend the upper limit of vitamin D: doses of up to 5,000 IU per day.[56]

Fumaric Acid

Over the past three decades, fumaric acid therapy has become increasingly popular in western Europe for psoriasis. Therapy consists of the oral intake of dimethylfumaric acid (240 mg per day) or monoethylfumaric acid (720 mg per day) and the topical application of 1% to 3% monoethylfumaric acid. Clinical studies have shown that it is useful in many patients with psoriasis,[57] but side effects such as flushing of the skin, nausea, diarrhea, general malaise, gastric pain, and mild liver and kidney disturbances can occur.[58] We recommend using fumaric acid therapy only after other natural therapies have proved ineffective.

Psychological Aspects

Stress is often a precipitating factor in psoriasis flare-ups. Hence stress management, psychotherapy, and biofeedback training can be of benefit.[59] For more information, see the chapter "Stress Management."

Sunlight and Ultraviolet Light

Exposure to sunlight is extremely beneficial for individuals with psoriasis.[60,61] In one study, an outdoor four-week sunbathing therapy was shown to promote significant clearance of psoriatic symptoms in 84% of 373 subjects.[62] Studies employing commercial tanning beds have shown that a majority of patients find them helpful;[63] they also facilitate improvements in quality of life.[64]

Sunlight and ultraviolet light exposure may also be of benefit owing to its induction of vitamin D synthesis in the skin. The standard ultraviolet medical treatment of psoriasis typically involves the use of the drug psoralen and ultraviolet A (PUVA therapy). Ultraviolet B (UVB) exposure alone also leads to inhibition of cell proliferation; in certain studies, it has been shown to be as effective as PUVA therapy, with fewer side effects.[65,66] At the Dead Sea, where 80% to 85% of psoriatic conditions clear in four weeks, UVB wavelengths are known to be dominant.[67,68] All together, what these studies indicate is that the drug psoralen may not be necessary and the key factor may be sunlight or UVB exposure; both need to be used carefully, especially by those at risk for skin cancer.

Topical Treatments

A number of natural proprietary formulas as well as over-the-counter preparations can be used to provide symptomatic relief in mild to moderate psoriasis.

Topical Vitamin D

Topical corticosteroids are the most common treatment for psoriasis; however, their long-term use is associated with a potential risk for side effects. Topical vitamin D modulators have been developed as an option for use in place of or in addition to topical corticosteroids. Topically, vitamin D inhibits skin cell proliferation and modulates immune cell activity in a positive manner in psoriasis.[69] Calcipotriene (Dovonex), an analogue of vitamin D, is the most widely used topical vitamin D. Although evidence suggests that in the long term it is approximately as effective as low- to medium-potency corticosteroids (response is not obtained as quickly as with

corticosteroids), it is associated with skin irritation, especially when used on sensitive skin. Calcitriol ointment was recently approved; it contains the naturally occurring active form of vitamin D_3 and is associated with a low rate of cutaneous and systemic adverse effects.

Aloe Vera

One double-blind study found that topical application of an aloe extract in a cream was highly effective in psoriasis vulgaris.[70] Sixty patients with slight to moderate chronic plaque-type psoriasis applied either the aloe or a placebo cream three times a day. By the end of the study (4 to 12 months of treatment), the aloe extract cream had improved the psoriasis in 25 of 30 patients (83.3%) compared with the placebo improvement rate of only 2 of 30 (6.6%), resulting in significant clearing of psoriatic plaques (82.8% with the aloe vs. 7.7 % with the placebo). In another double-blind study, 80 patients with psoriasis applied either aloe vera or a popular prescription corticosteroid cream (0.1% triamcinolone acetonide).[71] After eight weeks of treatment, the mean psoriasis clinical score decreased from 11.6 to 3.9 in the aloe group and from 10.9 to 4.3 in the corticosteroid group. These results indicate aloe's effects may be on a par with conventional corticosteroid cream, but without the side effects.

Capsaicin

Capsaicin, from cayenne pepper *(Capsicum frutescens)*, is known to stimulate and then block small-diameter pain fibers by depleting them of the neurotransmitter substance P, which is thought to be the principal chemical mediator of pain impulses. In addition, substance P has been shown to activate inflammatory mediators in psoriasis. Several clinical studies have found that the topical application of 0.025 or 0.075% capsaicin is effective in relieving psoriasis.[72,73]

For example, in one study 98 patients applied 0.025% capsaicin cream four times per day for six weeks, while 99 patients applied a placebo cream.[72] Efficacy was evaluated based on a physician's global evaluation and a combined psoriasis severity score including scaling, thickness, redness, and itching. Capsaicin-treated patients demonstrated significantly greater improvement in global evaluation and in relief of itching, as well as a significantly greater reduction in combined psoriasis severity scores.

Curcumin

Curcumin, from turmeric (*Curcuma longa*), is a well-known anti-inflammatory agent. In one study, topical application of curcumin in a gel yielded 90% resolution of plaques in 50% of patients within two to six weeks;

the remainder of the study subjects showed 50% to 85% improvement.[74] Curcumin was found to be twice as effective as calcipotriene cream, which generally takes three months to exert its full effect.

Emollients

The scaliness and hardness of psoriasis skin benefits from the use of emollients (skin softening agents) such as ceramides. These compounds can help improve the skin's water-holding capacity, and it has been shown that ceramides are decreased in psoriatic skin. Newer ceramide-containing emollients (e.g., CeraVe, MimyX, Aveeno Eczema Therapy, etc.) have shown benefit in psoriasis and may improve skin barrier function and decrease water loss.[75]

. . . .

QUICK REVIEW

- **Psoriasis is caused by a pileup of skin cells that have replicated too rapidly.**
- **There are multiple abnormalities noted in the skin and immune cells of psoriatic patients, indicating a complex interplay of genetic factors.**
- **Although psoriasis has a significant genetic component, addressing the factors that can activate the immune system or skin cells can result in significant clinical improvement**
- **Incomplete protein digestion, bowel toxemia, impaired liver function, and bile acid deficiency are linked to psoriasis.**
- **Reducing the intake of arachidonic acid, a fat found exclusively in animal foods, while increasing the intake of** omega-3 fatty acids is a primary nutritional recommendation.
- **A therapeutic fast followed by a vegetarian diet with careful attention to any food allergy is very therapeutic in psoriasis.**
- **Sunlight, UVB phototherapy, oral vitamin D analogues, and topical vitamin D$_3$ all improve psoriasis, validating vitamin D's effect on controlling the excessive skin cell replication seen in psoriasis.**
- **Outdoor sunbathing therapy was shown to promote significant clearance of psoriatic symptoms.**
- **Topical treatments with preparations containing vitamin D, aloe vera, curcumin, or capsaicin can be helpful.**

TREATMENT SUMMARY

Despite the complexity of this disease, the therapeutic approach is fairly straightforward: decrease bowel toxemia, rebalance fatty acid levels and inflammatory processes systemically and in the skin, reduce the abnormal proliferation of skin cells, and apply topical agents to provide quicker symptom relief and aid the healing process. The protocol given below accomplishes all of these goals. In the case of psoriatic arthritis, we recommend following the treatment summary for rheumatoid arthritis (see that chapter).

Diet

The first step is a therapeutic fast or elimination diet, followed by careful reintroduction of individual foods to detect those that trigger symptoms. Although any food can cause a reaction, the most common are wheat, corn, dairy products, beef, foods in the nightshade family (tomatoes, potatoes, eggplant, peppers), pork, citrus, oats, rye, egg, coffee, peanuts, cane sugar, lamb, and soy.

After all allergens have been isolated and eliminated, a vegetarian or Mediterranean-style diet rich in organic whole foods, vegetables, cold-water fish (anchovies, mackerel, herring, sardines, and salmon), olive oil, and berries and low in sugar, meat, refined carbohydrates, and animal fats is indicated. The recommendations in the chapter "A Health-Promoting Diet" are appropriate for long-term support.

Nutritional Supplements

- A high-potency multiple vitamin and mineral formula as described in the chapter "Supplementary Measures"
- Key individual nutrients:
  - Vitamin C: 500 to 1,000 mg per day
  - Vitamin E (mixed tocopherols): 200 to 400 IU per day
  - Vitamin D_3: 5,000 IU per day (ideally, measure blood levels and adjust dosage accordingly)
  - Vitamin B_6: 25 to 50 mg per day
  - Folic acid: 800 mcg per day
  - Vitamin B_{12}: 800 mcg per day
  - Selenium: 100 to 200 mcg per day
  - Chromium: 200 to 400 mcg per day
- Fish oils: 3,000 mg EPA + DHA per day
- One of the following:
  - Grape seed extract (>95% procyanidolic oligomers): 100 to 300 mg per day
  - Pine bark extract (>95% procyanidolic oligomers): 100 to 300 mg per day
  - Some other flavonoid-rich extract with a similar flavonoid content, super greens formula, or another plant-based antioxidant that can provide an oxygen radical absorption capacity (ORAC) of 3,000 to 6,000 units or higher per day
- Specialty supplements:
  - Soluble fiber (psyllium, pectin, guar gum, etc.): 5 g at bedtime

- Bile acids (mixed, from ox bile): 500 mg with meals
- Pancreatin (10X USP): 350 to 750 mg with meals three times per day; or equivalent multiple enzyme formula with meals
- Probiotic (*Lactobacillus* species and *Bifidobacterium* species): a minimum of 5 billion to 10 billion colony-forming units
- Fumaric acid: dimethylfumaric acid (240 mg per day) or monoethylfumaric acid (720 mg per day) and topical application of 1% to 3% of monoethylfumaric acid (to be used only when other approaches fail)

Botanical Medicines

- Milk thistle *(Silybum marianum)*: Dosage is based on silymarin content (standardized extracts are preferred) and the best results are achieved at higher dosages, i.e., 140 mg to 210 mg silymarin three times per day; dosage for silymarin phytosome is 120 mg two to three times per day between meals.

  Consider the following if suffering from impaired digestion:

- Goldenseal (standardized extracts preferred):
  - Dried root or as tea: 2 to 4 g three times per day

- Fluid extract (1:1): 2 to 4 ml (0.5 to 1 tsp) three times per day
- Solid (powdered dry) extract (4:1 or 8 to 12% alkaloid content): 250 to 500 mg three times per day
- Sarsaparilla:
  - Dried root or as decoction: 1 to 4 g three times per day
  - Liquid extract (1: 1): 4 to 8 ml (1 to 2 tsp) three times per day
  - Solid extract (4: 1): 250 to 500 mg three times per day

Psychological Measures

Utilize stress management strategies.

Physical Medicines

- Sunbathing (taking precautions not to become sunburned): as much as possible.
- UVB: 295 to 305 nm, 2 mW/cm^2, three minutes three times weekly

Topical Treatments

- Vitamin D, aloe vera, capsaicin, or curcumin creams: apply to affected areas of the skin two to three times per day (try different ones to see which works best)
- Ceramide-containing emollient: apply to affected areas of the skin two to three times per day

Rheumatoid Arthritis

- Fatigue, low-grade fever, weakness, weight loss, joint stiffness, and vague joint pain may precede the appearance of painful, swollen joints by several weeks
- Severe joint pain with considerable inflammation that usually begins in the small joints and progresses to eventually affect all joints
- X-ray findings usually show soft tissue swelling, erosion of cartilage, and joint space narrowing
- Rheumatoid factor is present in the blood

Rheumatoid arthritis (RA) is a chronic inflammatory condition that affects the entire body, but especially the joints. The joints typically involved are the hands, feet, wrists, ankles, and knees. Between 1% and 3% of the population is affected, and the number of women with RA exceeds the number of males by almost three to one. The usual age of onset is 20 to 40, although rheumatoid arthritis may begin at any age.

The onset of RA is usually gradual but occasionally is quite abrupt. Several joints are usually involved in the onset, typically in a symmetrical fashion (i.e., both hands, wrists, or ankles). In about one-third of people with RA, initial involvement is confined to one or a few joints.

Involved joints will characteristically be quite warm, tender, and swollen, with prolonged morning stiffness. The skin over the joint will take on a ruddy purplish hue. As the disease progresses, deformities develop in the joints of the hands and feet. The common terms used to describe these deformities include *swan neck*, *boutonniere*, and *cock-up toes*.

Diagnostic Considerations

The diagnosis of RA is based upon the presence of pain and inflammation in at least one joint, with no alternative explanation, and (see table below) a score of 6 or greater in a four-tier rubric.[1]

Joint involvement (select the one with highest point value):	
1 medium-large joint	0 points
2–10 medium-large joints	1 point
1–3 small joints	2 points
4–10 small joints	3 points
10+ small joints	5 points
Serology:	
Seronegative for RF and anti-CCP	0 points
Low-titer of RF and/or anti-CCP	2 points
High-titer of RF and/or anti-CCP (>3 times upper normal limit)	3 points
Duration of synovitis:	
Less than 6 weeks	0 points
6+ weeks	1 point
Acute phase reactants:	
Normal ESR and CRP	0 points
Elevated CRP or ESR	1 point

Anti-CCP = anti-cyclic citrullinated peptide antibodies
CRP = C-reactive protein.
ESR = erythrocyte sedimentation rate
RF = rheumatoid factor

Causes

There is abundant evidence that RA is an autoimmune reaction, in which antibodies develop against components of joint tissues. Yet what triggers this autoimmune reaction remains largely unknown. Speculation and investigation have centered on genetic factors, abnormal bowel permeability, lifestyle and nutritional factors, food allergies, and microorganisms. RA is a classic example of a multifactorial disease, wherein assorted genetic, dietary, and environmental factors contribute to the disease process.

Diagnostic Considerations

Other Autoimmune Diseases Affecting Connective Tissue

In addition to RA, there are several other autoimmune diseases that affect connective tissue (collagen structures that support internal organs as well as cartilage, tendons, muscles, and bone). These diseases include systemic lupus erythematosus (SLE or lupus; see that chapter), ankylosing spondylitis, scleroderma, polymyalgia rheumatica, and mixed connective tissue disease. There is tremendous overlap among these diseases in terms of underlying causes, symptoms, and treatment. They share many features with RA, but the autoimmune and inflammatory process is a bit different in each of these diseases. From a natural medicine perspective the treatment of any of these other autoimmune diseases should focus on the same treatment recommendations given here in this chapter for RA.

Genetic Susceptibility

A positive family history is a risk factor for developing RA. Evidence of a genetic factor was first noted in studies of twins, yet in identical twins the chance that one twin will develop the disease if the other already has it is only 15%. If RA were purely a genetic disease, both twins would be affected every time. These results have led geneticists to focus on epigenetic factors—factors that can turn off or turn on the expression of the genetic code.[2] The biggest determinants of epigenetic influence on the expression of DNA are nutrition and environmental toxins. Epigenetic factors are thought to be associated with more aggressive disease by affecting immune function, antioxidant pathways, detoxification mechanisms, and other processes. Interestingly, patients with RA also have changes in fecal flora that are thought to contribute to the disease process (see discussion below), and studies have shown that the flora of identical twins is more similar than that of fraternal twins, independent of other contributing factors, indicating that genetic factors influence the type of bacterial flora a person has.[3]

Environmental Factors

Genetic studies indicate that dietary and environmental factors are required for RA to be manifested. For example, toxins in cigarette smoke interact with epigenetic factors to enhance the inflammatory process and increase the risk of RA.[4] The risk for smokers of developing RA is nearly 8-fold in genetically susceptible individuals and nearly 16-fold for identical twins. Smoking also increases RA risk in the general population, and quitting smoking results in decreased risk of RA.[5] Other factors such as poor diet, drinking more than three cups of coffee per day, silicate exposure, and psychological factors may also play a role in the development of the disease and affect the levels of pain and physical disability experienced by RA patients,[6] while oral contraceptives (birth control pills), tea (black or green) intake, and increased vitamin D consumption have been found to be protective. Other environmental factors such as low temperature, high atmospheric pressure, and high humidity have been correlated with increased RA pain.[7]

Oxidative Stress

Several studies have shown that the risk of RA is highest in people with the lowest levels of nutrient antioxidants. Low antioxidant levels may be exacerbated by genetic factors.[8] The resulting increase in oxidative stress could produce free radical damage to DNA and mutations that may contribute to the development of RA.[9] Once disease is established, synovial concentrations of free radicals are elevated and concentrations of antioxidants are diminished, accelerating inflammation and joint destruction.

Autoantibody Production

The serum of most individuals with RA contains an antibody called rheumatoid factor (RF) and cyclic citrullinated peptide autoantibodies (anti-CCP). The blood levels of these antibodies often reflect the severity of arthritis symptoms and prognosis, but not in every case, and the antibodies are not directly responsible for joint destruction. Autoantibodies have been detected as much as 10 years prior to the onset of clinical disease, and other inflammatory markers have been elevated for up to 12 years prior to diagnosis.[10,11] This suggests a "multiple hit" model in which the disease progresses in distinct stages, perhaps explaining why autoantibodies are present for years before clinical symptoms.

Microbial Influences: Infection and Cross-Reactivity

Microorganisms may play a role in the disease process of RA. The onset of RA is preceded by a specific inciting event, such as an infection, in 8 to 15% of cases, and antimicrobials such as metronidazole, clotrimazole, acyclovir, roxithromycin, tetracycline, sulfasalazine, and minocycline have been associated with improvement in symptoms and, in some cases, complete remission.[12–18] Many disease-causing organisms, such as Epstein-Barr virus, cytomegalovirus, parvovirus, rubella virus, mycoplasma, amebic organisms, *E. coli*, *Proteus* species, and influenza virus AH2N2, have been associated with RA. Yet no single microbial agent has been consistently isolated in patients with the disease, indicating that a multitude of organisms may directly or indirectly contribute to the disease process by the formation of cross-reacting antibodies that attack body cells instead of the infectious organism. It is well established that over a dozen different organisms can produce arthritis similar to RA after a gastrointestinal, urinary tract, or respiratory infection in genetically susceptible individuals and that the condition can become chronic in 15 to 60% of cases.

Dysbiosis and Small Intestinal Bacterial Overgrowth

Perhaps more important than specific disease-causing organisms is the subtler influence of the intestinal microflora on our internal gut environment. There are more microflora in our digestive tract than human cells in our bodies, and the composition of the hundreds of species of microorganisms is known to be affected by genetics, medical treatment, diet, and stress.[19] The bacterial flora of our intestinal tract has a profound influence on immune function, nutritional status, and stress response and can contribute to many diseases.[20,21] Many of these intestinal functions are thought to be involved in the disease process of RA.

It is well established that the fecal flora is significantly altered in RA, including significantly less bifidobacteria and bacteria of the *Bacteroides*, *Porphyromonas*, and *Prevotella* genera.[22] This condition is called *dysbiosis*. Clinical studies have demonstrated improvement with changes in microbial flora.[23,24] Likewise, many RA patients have small-intestine bacterial overgrowth (SIBO), 51% in one study, and the degree of SIBO was associated with the severity of symptoms and disease activity.[25] Even bacteria from the periodontal tissue in the mouth may play a role. One study found identical periodontal bacterial DNA in 100% of joint fluid samples and 83.5% of blood samples of RA patients,[26] and another study found a correlation between the severity of periodontitis and the severity of RA symptoms.[27] Antibodies to periodontal bacteria are associated with elevated anti-CCP antibodies and promoting the autoimmune response in RA.[28]

Adverse Food Reactions

As much as 10% of the population has food allergies and, for patients who have tested positive for food allergies, consumption of those allergenic foods is associated with increases in inflammatory markers in the blood.[29,30] Outcomes of food allergy studies in RA have been conflicting. It is also important to point out that adverse food reactions such as food intolerance and sensitivity are not antibody-mediated and, therefore, not apparent with antibody testing.[31] Yet these reactions may be contributory.

One group analyzed the studies that considered the quantitative exposure to allergenic foods and found that studies utilizing larger doses of food antigens tend to show a positive correlation between RA and food allergies in 20 to 40% of patients.[32] These same authors examined jejunal and serum antibody secretions of RA patients and compared them with controls. While serum food antibodies were not correlated with RA, jejunal IgA, IgG, and especially IgM were significantly elevated against nearly all food antigens in RA patients compared with controls, and the antibodies were substantially cross-reactive with normal body proteins. These researchers conclude that RA patients may have multiple modest hypersensitivity reactions and that the additive effect could lead to widespread antibody-mediated tissue destruction.

Toxins and Autoantibody Production

Pesticides, herbicides, and other synthetic toxins are particularly problematic to both RA patients and people at risk for RA, owing to impaired detoxification processes.[33] Slow detoxification also predicts the severity of RA.[34]

Other toxins also appear to induce similar autoimmune responses in genetically susceptible patients. Bacterial toxins can bind to the lining of the intestines and stimulate antibody production against peptides and normal tissue proteins.[35] This same response was stimulated by gliadin peptides (from grains, especially wheat, rye, and barley), casein (a milk protein), and ethyl mercury (the vaccine adjuvant Thimerosal).[36]

Abnormal Gut Permeability

Individuals with RA have excessive intestinal permeability to dietary and bacterial antigens as well as alterations in the bacterial flora.[37–39] Chronic inflammation in the gut can cause increased intestinal permeability and is associated with joint inflammation. Adverse food reactions and bacterial endotoxins[40] may contribute greatly to chronic gut inflammation, and nonsteroidal anti-inflammatory drugs (NSAIDs) that are commonly prescribed for RA can worsen this situation as well.[41] However, increased gut inflammation and permeability also occur in RA independent of NSAID use.[42] This "leaky gut" facilitates the migration of dietary and gut-derived antigens and bacterial gut flora to blood, mesenteric lymph nodes, spleen, and kidneys.[43] In conjunction with dysbiosis and bacterial overgrowth, increased gut permeability to bacterial endotoxins and food antigens can produce immune activation and circulating immune complexes, many of which have been recovered in synovial fluid and could contribute to joint inflammation and degeneration.

Decreased Androgen Levels

Low levels of androgens (male sex hormones) are linked to RA. Specifically, chronically low levels of testosterone and dehydroepiandrosterone (DHEA) have been found in early-stage and established RA.[44–46] A small study showed that testosterone replacement therapy had positive effects in male RA patients, decreasing RF levels, the number of affected joints, and NSAID use.[47]

Abnormal Estrogen Levels

Unlike androgens, estrogens (female sex hormones) may be involved in sustaining the inflammatory activity of activated immune cells.[48] Estradiol levels have been found to be higher in RA patients than controls and strongly and positively associated with markers of inflammation. A five-year study of 689 patients with similar disease duration and severity found that gender was a major predictor of remission in early RA. Women had a lower androgen-to-estrogen ratio and, at two and five years, had more severe disease and 16 to 22% fewer remissions than men. This effect could not be explained by any other differences between the groups, including disease duration, age, or treatments used.[49]

Therapeutic Considerations

Standard medical therapy is limited by its overreliance on drugs designed to suppress the disease process and its symptoms, while failing to address the complex underlying causes of this disease.[50] The effects and side effects of these drugs actually worsen many factors contributing to the disease process, and the drugs have significant morbidity and mortality risks of their own. Drug therapies generally fall into three categories: nonsteroidal anti-inflammatory drugs (NSAIDs), disease-modifying antirheumatic drugs (DMARDs), and biological therapies.

Nonsteroidal Anti-inflammatory Drugs and Cyclooxygenase Inhibitors

NSAIDs suppress of symptoms while accelerating factors that promote the disease process. While relieving symptoms by decreasing inflammation, NSAIDs can inhibit cartilage formation and actually promote joint destruction.[51,52] Furthermore, they promote several factors thought to contribute to the disease process of RA by increasing gastrointestinal tract hyperpermeability, dysbiosis (alteration in normal gut flora), free radicals in joint synovial fluid, and bacterial overgrowth.[53,54] NSAIDs also cause serious gastrointestinal tract side effects, including ulcers, hemorrhage, and perforation, which according to one study led to 107,000 hospitalizations and 16,500 deaths in one year among arthritis patients alone.[55]

To mitigate GI toxicity, NSAIDs are sometimes given along with acid-blocking medications. These acid-blocking drugs help alleviate the upper GI damage but end up causing additional issues, including lower levels of hydrochloric acid in the stomach (resulting in impaired food digestion and hence more food allergies) and overgrowth of bacteria in the small intestine (still another factor contributing to the disease process of RA).[56]

Newer NSAIDs such as Celebrex, a cyclooxygenase inhibitor, are easier on the stomach, but they do not completely protect the lower GI tract from injury and are associated with adverse cardiovascular events.[57,58] Because RA patients are already at increased risk for cardiovascular disease, these drugs may not be appropriate for general use with RA patients.[59] Finally, all drugs in this class also have been connected to kidney toxicity, and chronic use of high doses in arthritis patients increases risk for kidney failure.[60]

Corticosteroids

Corticosteroid medications such as prednisone are generally reserved for patients who do not respond to NSAID therapy. By more completely blocking the inflammatory response, including the production and secretion of inflammatory mediators such as histamine, prostaglandins, and leukotrienes, they suppress not only inflammation but the normal immune response as well. These medications may be of great benefit in acute symptom management, but they become problematic with long-term use. Corticosteroids are associated with more frequent serious infections (those requiring hospitalization) and increased mortality. Even small doses (up to 7.5 mg prednisone or the equivalent) carry increased risk for infection and death when used over the long term. One study found the risk of mortality increased 14% after one year and 49% after more than 10 years of use when the subjects were compared with RA patients who had not been treated with low-dose corticosteroids.[61]

Common side effects of long-term use that negatively affect RA include severe cartilage damage, osteoporosis, increased intestinal permeability, and cardiovascular disease.[61-65] Furthermore, the risk of peptic ulcers and GI bleeding in patients already using NSAIDs is greatly increased with simultaneous use of corticosteroids. Insomnia is also a side effect, and patients with RA are more susceptible to insomnia than the general population.[66] In fact, one study concluded that the fatigue experienced by RA patients may be more a product of sleep fragmentation than a constitutional symptom of the disease itself.[67] Finally, depression is a common side effect of prednisone and is also common among patients experiencing chronic pain from diseases such as RA. Patients with RA who experience depression have worse outcomes than those who are not depressed, further contraindicating the use of corticosteroids.[68]

Synthetic Disease-Modifying Antirheumatic Drugs

Once reserved for severe cases, disease-modifying antirheumatic drugs (DMARDs) are now used as first-line therapies in conventional treatment guidelines. Methotrexate is the most common drug used, with the best balance of efficacy and toxicity.[69] Originally used as a chemotherapeutic agent, it exerts an immunosuppressive effect by decreasing white blood cell production. The more severe side effects of methotrexate include gastrointestinal ulceration, severe bone marrow suppression, frequent infections, elevated risk of cancer, and damage to lungs, liver, or kidneys. Other drugs in this class include hydroxychloroquine (Plaquenil), azathioprine, cyclophosphamide, and leflunomide and have similar and sometimes more severe side effects. Many patients may not actually continue long-term therapy with any DMARDs beyond the first few years owing to adverse effects or lack of efficacy. However, there is evidence that beginning a DMARD within the first three months of diagnosis is associated with decreased risk of joint erosion. Therefore, patients presenting with a diagnosis of RA will now most often be on DMARDs, individually or increasingly in combination, and perhaps additional drugs to manage their side effects.

Biological Disease-Modifying Antirheumatic Drugs

Newer biological agents include infliximab, etanercept, and adalimumab. Other members of this class include tocilizumab and abatacept. These medications are no more effective than methotrexate when used as a sole therapy. However, in an analysis of comparative trials, a combination of these drugs with methotrexate was more effective than methotrexate alone, especially in initially severe RA.[70] Unfortunately, drug-free remission is still very rarely achieved and most patients experience higher disease activity upon discontinuation of therapy. Biological agents also carry significant health risks, including infections, anemia, and perhaps acceleration of atherosclerosis.[71,72]

Diet

Population studies have demonstrated that RA is found at higher rates in societies consuming a Western-style diet.[73] A diet of organic whole foods, rich in vegetables and fiber and low in sugar, meat, refined carbohydrates, saturated fat, and additives, appears to offer some protection against the development of RA, as well as promise in its treatment.[74–79]

Adverse Food Reactions

Elimination of food allergens or reactive foods has been shown to offer significant benefit to some individuals with RA.[79–82] The most common triggers in one study included corn (56%), wheat (54%), bacon/pork (39%), oranges (39%), milk or oats (37%), rye (34%), egg, beef, and coffee (32%), malt (27%), cheese or grapefruit (24%), tomato (22%), peanuts or cane sugar, (20%), and butter, lamb, soy, or lemon (17%). Of those participants who continued to avoid their reactive foods, 19% remained well without medications for follow-up periods of up to 5 years.[83]

Dietary elimination and challenge are methods of identifying triggering foods, which can be different for each patient. Some studies that fail to show benefit of dietary intervention provide the entire experimental group with the same hypoallergenic diet, not one customized to each participant's particular sensitivity or sensitivities.

Therapeutic Fasting

Patients with RA have historically benefited from fasting. Short-term fasts of three to five days' duration are recommended during acute flare-ups to induce a substantial reduction of joint pain, swelling, morning stiffness, and other symptoms of RA.[84] It is an obvious method for eliminating reactive foods but has effects that extend beyond allergen avoidance. Fasting increases serum DHEA, decreases serum inflammatory mediators,[85] and favorably affects intestinal permeability.[86] Juice, broth, and water fasts of longer duration, up to 10 days, have been shown to be effective as well.[87] For more information on nutritional cleansing, see the chapter "Detoxification and Internal Cleansing."

Vegetarian Diet

A predominantly vegetarian diet has considerable support in the medical literature in the treatment of RA. One 13-month controlled study began with a 7-to-10-day fast before transitioning to a vegetarian diet.[88] The fast consisted of herbal teas, garlic, vegetable broth, decoction of potatoes and parsley, and the juice of carrots, beets, and celery. The diet was followed by a systematic reintroduction of a single food item every two days with elimination of foods that aggravated RA symptoms. The treatment group showed significant improvements compared with controls, and these improvements were maintained at one-year follow-ups in those patients still sticking to the diet. This study supported the positive results noted in prior studies of short-term fasting followed by a vegetarian diet, and the pooling of these data in a systematic review showed a statistically and clinically significant beneficial long-term effects.[89–91] Beyond allergy elimination, vegetarian diets are also associated with higher fiber intake and improved gut flora, including decreased antibodies to suspected organisms linked to RA, less SIBO, and improvement in RA symptoms.[92] Other changes include increased potassium intake (which may lead to improved biosynthesis and release of cortisol) and favorable fatty acid and antioxidant intake.

Mediterranean Diet

Patients with established RA in one study experienced a reduction in inflammatory activity, an increase in physical function, and improved vitality in 12 weeks on a Mediterranean-style diet.[93,94] Rich in seasonally fresh plant-derived foods, the Mediterranean diet is similar to a vegetarian diet with the addition of fish and poultry, low to moderate amounts red meat, consumption of moderate amounts of dairy foods and red wine, and olive oil as the main source of lipids. Different types of dietary fats can either alleviate or aggravate RA by influencing eicosanoid metabolism.[93,95] Both vegetarian and Mediterranean diets are inherently low in saturated fats and arachidonic acid, the precursor to the inflammatory series-2 prostaglandins and leukotrienes; and rich in gamma-linolenic and alpha-linolenic acids, the precursors to anti-inflammatory series-1 and series-3 prostaglandins. The consumption of cold-water fish such as anchovies, mackerel, herring, sardines, and salmon, which are rich in eicosapentaenoic acid (EPA) and docosahexaenoic acid (DHA), further promotes anti-inflammatory prostaglandins.

A population-based case-control study of women living in the Seattle area compared fish consumption in 324 cases of RA with 1,245 control cases.[96] Consumption of broiled or baked fish was associated with a dose-dependent decreased risk of RA. This may explain some of the anti-inflammatory effects of the Mediterranean diet, which includes fish but relatively little meat. Excluding meats removes not only pro-inflammatory arachidonic acid from the diet but also a potential food allergen: several studies have found that RA patients are commonly allergic to meats, especially beef and pork.[97,98] Furthermore, the inclusion of olive oil produces additional benefits in RA, including antioxidant and anti-inflammatory effects, competitive inhibition of omega-6 fatty acids, pain reduction, reduced morning stiffness, and improved patient evaluation of overall health.[99] Additionally, these effects seem to be synergistic with fish oils.

Antioxidants

The continuous production of free radicals within arthritic joints promotes joint degeneration, exhausts antioxidant systems, and may cause the low antioxidant levels commonly seen in RA patients.[100] The importance of consuming a diet rich in fresh fruits and vegetables in the dietary treatment of RA cannot be overstated. These are the best sources of antioxidants such as vitamin C, carotenoids, vitamin E, selenium, and bioflavonoids, which promote healthy joints by neutralizing inflammation and supporting collagen structures. Antioxidants work synergistically in systems—for example, vitamin C is needed to regenerate vitamin E—and this may explain why systematic reviews have not found single antioxidant supplements to be effective, but have documented the benefit of antioxidant-rich diets. The antioxidant content of vegetarian and Mediterranean diets almost certainly contributes to their effectiveness in treating RA.

Nutritional Supplements

Blood and tissue samples from RA patients have been shown to be deficient in many nutrients, including magnesium, folate, vitamin B_{12}, vitamin B_6, zinc, and selenium.[101–106] Many factors may contribute to this, including decreased dietary nutrient intake among RA patients, decreased absorption due to impaired gut function, increased utilization of antioxidant nutrients due to elevated oxidative stress, and increased excretion of nutrients due to stress and medications. Studies are few in number and have produced conflicting results, and systematic reviews have failed to demonstrate benefit from sup-

plementation of individual nutrients, but it is almost certainly the case that a multifactorial condition such as RA requires a multifaceted approach to treatment rather than a nutrient monotherapy. It appears reasonable, safe, and at least hypothetically efficacious to address deficiencies of multiple nutrients simultaneously.

This is a key conceptual difference from conventional medicine, where typically a single drug is used to inhibit or poison an enzyme system to impair the production of inflammatory mediators or some other mechanism in the disease process. With natural medicine we are working to normalize the many dysfunctions that together result in the disease. Single natural therapies are rarely able to address all of a person's physiological needs. A comprehensive approach that addresses all, or at least most, of the causes is always far more effective. Unfortunately, virtually all the research on nutrition is on single agents. Drawing on our decades of clinical experience, we can confidently tell you that the comprehensive natural medicine approach—combining diet, lifestyle, and supplementation—is far more effective than single agents. Nonetheless, since most of the research that is available addresses only single agents, we cover here specific nutrients that have been found to be deficient and/or beneficial in some clinical trials with RA.

Selenium and Vitamin E

These nutrients work together in reducing the production of inflammatory compounds and controlling free radical tissue damage. Clinical studies have not demonstrated improvement from selenium supplementation in RA; however, one clinical study did indicate that selenium combined with vitamin E had a positive effect.[107,108] In another randomized, controlled trial, patients already diagnosed with RA who received 600 mg vitamin E twice a day showed significant pain reduction but no changes in clinical and biochemical indicators of inflammation.[109] However, a review of five studies found no conclusive evidence of benefit from vitamin E or selenium supplementation alone.[107] In order to be of benefit, both nutrients must be provided.

Zinc

Zinc deficiency is common in RA patients, and it may predispose them to increased inflammation. Lower plasma zinc levels are associated with higher blood levels of inflammatory compounds.[110] Zinc also has antioxidant effects and is a cofactor for the enzyme superoxide dismutase (SOD). Patients using corticosteroids may be at increased risk for zinc deficiency because these medications have been shown to decrease plasma zinc and increase loss of zinc in the urine.[111] Several studies have demonstrated a slight therapeutic effect from zinc supplementation in RA patients.[112–114]

Manganese and Superoxide Dismutase

Manganese functions in the antioxidant enzyme superoxide dismutase (SOD), which prevents the damage caused by the toxic oxygen molecule known as superoxide. Manganese-containing SOD is deficient in patients with RA.[115] The injectable form of this enzyme has been shown to be effective in the treatment of RA;[116] however, it has not been demonstrated that oral supplementation with SOD affects tissue SOD levels.[117] What has been established is that oral manganese supplementation increases SOD activity.[118] Although no clinical studies have been conducted to determine the effectiveness of manganese in the treatment of RA, it appears to be indicated on the basis of the low levels seen in patients with RA as well as its biochemical functions.

Vitamin C

Vitamin C is an important antioxidant, but vitamin C concentrations in white blood cell and plasma are significantly decreased in patients with RA.[119] Supplementation with vitamin C increases SOD activity, reduces histamine levels, and provides anti-inflammatory action.[120,121] One intervention study with a Mediterranean diet showed a negative correlation between plasma vitamin C levels and RA disease activity,[122] which was corroborated by another study that found higher vitamin C levels associated with lower markers of inflammation, such as CRP.[123]

Pantothenic Acid

Blood pantothenic acid levels have been reported to be lower in patients with RA than in normal controls and inversely correlated with disease activity.[124] Correction of low pantothenic acid levels brings about some alleviation of RA symptoms. In one double-blind study, subjective improvement of RA symptoms was noted in patients receiving 2 g per day of calcium pantothenate.[125] Patients noted improvements in duration of morning stiffness, degree of disability, and severity of pain.

Pyridoxine (Vitamin B$_6$)

There is a clear relationship between low blood levels of vitamin B$_6$ and inflammatory indicators of RA and more disability, pain, fatigue, and swollen joints.[126] The low pyridoxine levels were attributed not to deficiency of intake but rather to ongoing chronic inflammatory processes using it up more quickly. Higher levels of homocysteine—a risk factor for heart disease—were also noted and correlated with low vitamin B$_6$ status in RA patients.[127]

Copper

The wearing of copper bracelets has been a longtime folk remedy that appears to have some scientific support, as found in a double-blind study performed in Australia. Presumably, copper is absorbed through the skin and is chelated to another compound that is able to exert anti-inflammatory action.[128] Copper is also utilized in SOD. Deficiency may result in significant susceptibility to free radical damage as a result of decreased SOD levels. However, an excessive intake of copper may be detrimental.[129]

Vitamin D

Population-based studies indicate a significant association between vitamin D deficiency and an increased incidence of several autoimmune diseases, including RA.[130] One study identified lower vitamin D levels and higher incidence of RA in northern European countries compared with southern European countries. In both northern and southern Europe, however, low 25(OH)-vitamin D levels were significantly correlated with worse RA symptoms.[131]

Pancreatic Enzymes and Hydrochloric Acid

Impaired digestion from inadequate secretion of pancreatic enzymes and/or of hydrochloric acid, which is common in RA patients, can be a major contributor to the disease process.[132,133] In addition to poor assimilation of ingested nutrients, incompletely digested food molecules can be inappropriately absorbed, stimulating an immune response (i.e., food allergy). In one study, 80% of untreated RA patients had reduced gastric acid output.[134] Gastric acid also plays a role in protecting against infection, and so individuals who produce insufficient hydrochloric acid may be predisposed to small-intestine bacterial overgrowth (SIBO). Half of RA patients who have inadequate hydrochloric acid secretion also have SIBO, and restoration of gastric pH can help resolve the overgrowth.

For information on hydrochloric acid supplementation, see the chapter "Digestion and Elimination."

Beyond their role in aiding digestion, pancreatic enzymes may offer additional benefits when taken between meals. Specifically, the protein-digesting enzymes (proteases) have been shown to reduce circulating levels of immune complexes in RA and other autoimmune diseases.[135,136] Because clinical improvements usually correspond with decreases in immune complex levels, proteolytic enzyme supplementation is very important.

Probiotics

Probiotic supplementation can modulate the immune system in a positive manner, reduce inflammation, and reduce the growth of organisms linked to RA.[137] One small-scale human trial of *Lactobacillus rhamnosus* GG did not show a clinical benefit; however, a recent study of *Bacillus coagulans* GBI-30, 6080 produced statistically significant improvement in pain scale compared with a placebo.[138] Treatment also resulted in greater improvement in patient global assessment, self-assessed disability, CRP, ability to walk two miles, and participation in daily activities.[139]

Omega-3 Fatty Acids

Many published studies have documented the efficacy of fish oil supplementation in RA.[140-147] Supplementation has been shown to be effective in decreasing long-term utilization of NSAIDs in these trials. A recent very detailed review concluded that there is convincing evidence of benefit in RA, including reduction of duration of morning stiffness, number of tender or swollen joints, joint pain, length of fatigue, and serum markers of inflammation.[147] Supplements may need to be consumed for at least 12 weeks at a minimum dose of 3 g per day combined

EPA and DHA before effects are apparent. Furthermore, fish oil may further benefit RA patients by decreasing cardiovascular risk. It is important to select a product that has been rigorously tested for contaminants such as heavy metals, polychlorinated biphenyls (PCBs), dioxins, and lipid peroxides. Also, the benefits of omega-3 fatty acid supplementation are substantially enhanced when sources of arachidonic acid, including red meat and dairy products, are also significantly reduced.

Botanical Medicines

Many botanicals possess significant anti-inflammatory action and are useful in the treatment of RA. The suggestions made here represent some of those with long historical use and stronger research support.

Curcumin

Curcumin, the yellow pigment of turmeric (*Curcuma longa*), exerts excellent anti-inflammatory and antioxidant effects and has been found to be as effective as cortisone or phenylbutazone in models of acute inflammation.[148] In RA, one double-blind clinical trial compared curcumin (1,200 mg per day) with phenylbutazone (300 mg per day).[149] The improvements in the duration of morning stiffness, walking time, and joint swelling were comparable in both groups. Furthermore, while phenylbutazone is associated with significant adverse effects, curcumin has not been shown to produce any side effects. It is noteworthy that curcumin has no direct pain-relieving effects, so the ability to reduce pain is the result of reducing the inflammatory factors that cause pain.

One concern regarding curcumin has been absorption, but there now exist a number of methods and products that enhance the absorption of curcumin. One of the first methods was using piperine, a compound found in black pepper.[150] A more recent improved method is complexing the curcumin with soy phospholipids to produce a product sold under the name Meriva.[151] Absorption studies of animals indicate that peak plasma levels of curcumin after administration of Meriva were five times higher than those after administration of regular curcumin. Studies with another advanced form of curcumin, Theracurmin, show even greater absorption (27 times greater than regular curcumin).[152]

Bromelain

Bromelain refers to a mixture of enzymes found in pineapple. Since 1957, more than 200 scientific papers have appeared in the research literature documenting a wide variety of beneficial effects, including reducing inflammation in RA.[153,154] Much of its effect is due to activation of compounds that break down the inflammation-induced matrix of fibrin (a kind of internal scarring protein) that leads to inadequate tissue drainage and swelling. Bromelain also blocks the production of kinins, compounds produced during inflammation that increase swelling and cause pain. A protein-digesting enzyme product containing bromelain, papain (an enzyme from papaya), and trypsin and chymotrypsin (pancreatic enzymes from pigs) was shown to decrease excessive level of transforming growth factor (TGF),[155] an inflammatory marker linked to the progression of joint destruction in RA.[156]

Ginger

Ginger (*Zingiber officinalis*) contains antioxidants and exerts anti-inflammatory effects by inhibiting formation of a number of different inflammatory mediators. A preliminary clinical study was conducted with seven RA patients for whom conventional drugs had provided only temporary or partial relief.[157]

All patients were treated with ginger. One patient took 50 g per day of lightly cooked ginger, and the other six took either 5 g per day of fresh ginger or 0.1 to 1 g per day of powdered ginger. Despite the difference in dosage, all patients reported a substantial improvement, including pain relief, joint mobility, and a decrease in swelling and morning stiffness.

In the follow-up to this study, 28 patients with RA, 18 with osteoarthritis, and 10 with muscular discomfort who had been taking 500 to 4,000 mg powdered ginger for periods ranging from 3 to 30 months were evaluated.[158] On the basis of clinical observations, it was reported that 75% of the patients with arthritis (either RA or osteoarthritis) and 100% of those with muscular discomfort experienced relief in pain or swelling and that the effects were dose-dependent.

Fresh ginger contains higher levels of gingerols and a protease that may have anti-inflammatory action similar to that of bromelain, and therefore may be more effective in the treatment of RA than dried preparations.[159] Most studies have utilized 1 g powdered gingerroot, which is a relatively small dose compared with the average of 8 to 10 g consumed per day in India. A dose of 2 to 4 g powdered ginger per day is safe and may be effective in RA. This amount is roughly equivalent to 20 g fresh gingerroot,

QUICK REVIEW

- **Rheumatoid arthritis is an autoimmune reaction in which antibodies develop against components of joint tissues.**
- **RA is a classic example of a multifactorial disease, wherein an assortment of genetic, nutritional, and environmental factors contribute to the disease process.**
- **Standard medical therapy is of limited value in treating most cases of RA, as it fails to address the complex underlying causes of this disease.**
- **Diet has been strongly implicated in rheumatoid arthritis for many years, in regard to both cause and cure.**
- **Elimination of allergenic foods has been shown to offer significant benefit to some individuals with rheumatoid arthritis.**
- **Altered gastrointestinal tract flora have been linked to RA and other autoimmune diseases.**
- **A vegetarian diet has been shown to produce significant benefits in treating RA.**
- **In the dietary treatment of RA, the importance of consuming a diet rich in fresh fruits and vegetables cannot be overstated.**
- **Several natural anti-inflammatory compounds (e.g., curcumin, bromelain, and ginger) have shown positive effects in treating RA.**
- **Physical therapy (i.e., exercise, heat, cold, massage, diathermy, lasers, and paraffin baths) has a major role in the management of RA.**

or a ½-inch slice. These amounts of ginger can easily be incorporated into the diet in fresh fruit and vegetable juices.

Exercise

Exercise can improve strength and performance while maintaining range of motion in RA patients. Furthermore, it decreases cardiovascular risk, RA disease activity, and systemic inflammation.[160] Patients with well-developed disease should begin with progressive, passive range-of-motion and isometric exercises, gradually introducing active range-of-motion and isotonic exercises as appropriate. One randomized, controlled trial studied the effects of high-intensity exercise in more than 300 patients with RA. Participants were given either standard physical therapy or a high-intensity exercise program for two years. While there was no X-ray evidence of increased damage to the large joints, except possibly in those patients who had considerable baseline damage, high-intensity exercise improved functionality and mood and provided a sense of well-being.[161]

Hydrotherapy

Heat is typically used to help relieve stiffness and pain, relax muscles, and increase range of motion. Moist heat (e.g., moist packs, hot baths) is more effective than dry heat (e.g., a heating pad), and paraffin baths are used if skin irritation from regular water immersion develops. Cold packs are of value during acute inflammatory flare-ups or following hot applications.

Psychological Considerations

Optimistic patients with RA report better psychosocial and physical functioning than pessimistic patients who adopt passive coping strategies such as staying in bed for many hours a day. Patients who believe they have a high ability to control and decrease pain by utilizing spiritual or religious coping methods tend to have less joint pain and fewer negative moods and are much more likely to have higher levels of general social support.[162] Positive support from a spouse or family is inversely related to depression and can significantly enhance quality of life.[163]

- -

TREATMENT SUMMARY

Rheumatoid arthritis is often an aggressive disease that needs aggressive treatment. In mild to moderate RA, the measures below are extremely effective. Foremost is the use of diet to reduce the causes and ameliorate the symptoms of RA. Symptom relief can also be attained through the use of nutritional supplements, botanical medicines, and physical medicine techniques. In severe cases, drug therapy may be necessary, at least in the acute phase. However, do not abandon natural measures, because they will actually enhance the effectiveness of the drugs, allowing for lower dosages when drugs are necessary, while providing a foundation for healing by addressing the underlying causative factors and utilizing modalities that are both safe and beneficial in long-term use.

Diet

The first step is a therapeutic fast or elimination diet, followed by careful reintroduction of individual foods to detect those that trigger symptoms. Although any food can cause a reaction, the most common are wheat, corn, dairy products, beef, foods in the nightshade family (tomatoes, potatoes, eggplant, peppers), pork, citrus, oats, rye, egg, coffee, peanuts, cane sugar, lamb, and soy.

After all allergens have been isolated and eliminated, a vegetarian or Mediterranean-style diet rich in organic whole foods, vegetables, cold-water fish (mackerel, herring, sardines, and salmon), olive oil, and berries and low in sugar, meat, refined carbohydrates, and animal fats is indicated. The recommendations in the chapter "A Health-Promoting Diet" are appropriate in the long-term support of RA.

Nutritional Supplements

- A high-potency multiple vitamin and mineral formula as described in the chapter "Supplementary Measures"
- Key individual nutrients:
  - Vitamin B_6: 25 to 50 mg per day
  - Vitamin C: 500 to 1,000 mg per day
  - Vitamin E (mixed tocopherols): 200 to 400 IU per day
  - Vitamin D_3: 2,000 to 4,000 IU per day
  - Selenium: 100 to 200 mcg per day
  - Zinc: 15 to 30 mg per day
  - Manganese: 1.5 to 2 mg per day

- Fish oils: 3,000 mg EPA + DHA per day
- One of the following:
  - Grape seed extract (>95% procyanidolic oligomers): 100 to 300 mg per day
  - Pine bark extract (>95% procyanidolic oligomers): 100 to 300 mg per day
  - Some other flavonoid-rich extract with a similar flavonoid content, super greens formula, or another plant-based antioxidant that can provide an oxygen radical absorption capacity (ORAC) of 3,000 to 6,000 units or more per day
- Probiotic (*Lactobacillus* species and *Bifidobacterium* species): a minimum of 5 billion to 10 billion colony-forming units
- One of the following:
  - Pancreatin (10X USP): 350 to 750 mg between meals three times per day or
  - Bromelain: 250 to 750 mg (1,800 to 2,000 MCU) between meals three times per day

Botanical Medicines

- One of the following:
  - Meriva: 500 to 1,000 mg twice daily
  - BCM95 Complex: 750 to 1,500 mg twice daily
  - Theracurmin: 300 mg one to three times daily
- Ginger: 8 to 10 g dried powdered ginger daily; or ginger extract (standardized to contain 20% gingerol and shogaol) 100 to 200 mg three times per day

Physical Medicine

Physical therapy (i.e., exercise, heat, cold, massage, diathermy, lasers, and paraffin baths) has a major role in the management of RA.

- Heat (moist packs, hot baths, etc.): 20 to 30 minutes one to three times per day
- Cold packs for acute flare-ups or following heat

Other Considerations

Improving digestion with hydrochloric acid supplementation may be useful. Positive results from other tests may indicate that DHEA, testosterone, and treatment for intestinal permeability, dysbiosis, and environmental toxicity are advisable.

Rosacea

- Chronic acne-like eruption on the face of middle-aged and older adults, associated with facial flushing
- Primary involvement occurs over the flushed areas of the cheeks and nose
- More common in women but more severe in men

Rosacea is a common, chronic, progressive inflammatory skin disorder in which the nose and cheeks are abnormally red and may be covered with pimples similar to those seen in acne (see that chapter). Rosacea was originally called "acne rosacea" because its inflammatory papules and pustules so closely mimic those of acne. However, acne is based on the interaction of abnormal keratinization, increased sebum production, and bacterially induced inflammation, whereas the inflammation in rosacea is vascular in nature. Rosacea generally occurs in patients between the ages of 25 and 70 years, and it is much more common in people with fair complexions. Women are three times more likely than men to have rosacea, although the disease is generally more severe in men. At least 13 million Americans are known to be affected.[1]

Rosacea is divided into the following three stages, but since progression does not necessarily occur, rosacea is also often divided into four specific subtypes (erythematotelangiectatic, papulopustular, phymatous, and ocular): [1,2]

- **Stage I:** In stage I, or erythematotelangiectatic rosacea, redness and flushing of the skin are triggered by hot beverages, spicy foods, and alcohol and may persist for hours; spider veins (telangiectasias) are noticeable on the central third of the face; and burning, stinging, and itching after the application of cosmetics, fragrances, and sunscreens become a major complaint.
- **Stage II:** Inflammatory whiteheads and pimples are the hallmarks of stage II, or papulopustular rosacea. Flushing, telangiectasia, increased skin oiliness (seborrhea), and minimal facial pore enlargement become obvious.
- **Stage III:** A small number of patients progress to stage III, or phymatous rosacea, which is characterized by deep inflammatory nodules, large spider veins, markedly dilated facial pores, sebaceous gland enlargement, and enlargement of the nose (rhinophyma).

Ocular rosacea is the spectrum of eye findings associated with the skin involvement. Ocular rosacea can cause the eyes to have a watery or bloodshot appearance, the sensation of a foreign body, burning or stinging, dryness, itching, light sensitivity, and a host of other signs and symptoms. Sties are a common sign of rosacea-related ocular disease, and some individuals may have decreased visual acuity owing to corneal complications.

It is important to point out that what differentiates the flushing that rosacea patients experience from the flushing that accompanies embarrassment, exercise, or hot environments is the prolonged nature and intensity of rosacea flushing. While normal flushing episodes last from several seconds to a few minutes, the flushing that the typical rosacea patient describes lasts longer than 10 minutes and is more red than pink, with an accompanying burning or stinging sensation. The stimuli that bring on such flushing in rosacea patients may be acutely felt emotional stress, hot drinks, alcohol, spicy foods, exercise, cold or hot weather, and hot baths or showers. However, many times the episodes are without known stimuli.

Causes

The cause of rosacea is poorly understood, although numerous theories have been offered. Included in the factors that have been suspected of causing acne rosacea are the following:

- The mite *Demodex folliculorum*
- *Helicobacter pylori*
- Alcoholism
- Lack of stomach acid
- Menopausal flushing
- Local infection
- Food allergies
- B vitamin deficiencies
- Gastrointestinal disorders

Most cases of rosacea are associated with moderate to severe seborrhea (oiliness), although sebum production is not increased in many. Vasomotor lability is prevalent, and migraine headaches are three times more common in persons with rosacea than in age- and sex-matched controls.

There is also emerging evidence for a role for *Helicobacter pylori* in rosacea. It is known that *H. pylori* infection increases the production of several vasoactive substances such as histamines, prostaglandins, and leukotrienes. However, these vascular mediators are found only with *H. pylori* strains that also produce a specific cytotoxin, CagA. The presence of *H. pylori* capable of producing this cytotoxin may be more important in rosacea than that of other strains. When the presence of CagA was assessed in 60 rosacea patients and compared with control subjects indigestion researchers found that when infected with *H pylori*, 67% of rosacea patients, vs. only 32% of controls, had positive findings for CagA. After eradication of *H. pylori* infection in the rosacea patients, symptoms disappeared in almost all patients (51 of 53).[3]

The bottom line is that since many of the implicated triggers of rosacea are experienced by healthy people who never go on to develop the symptoms or signs of rosacea, rosacea-prone individuals very likely have an inherent sensitivity to these triggers.

Therapeutic Considerations

One of the first recommendations is to avoid those stimuli that tend to exacerbate the disease—exposure to extremes of heat and cold, excessive sunlight, and ingestion of hot liquids, alcohol, and spicy foods. The conventional medical treatment of rosacea is usually oral tetracycline, especially for the papular or pustular lesions, although this treatment usually only controls rather than eradicates the disease. Topical therapy for rosacea using antibiotics or synthetic retinoids is generally less successful than systemic antibiotic treatment. Also, although topical corticosteroids may initially improve signs and symptoms, long-term corticosteroid therapy is not advisable because it may actually lead to rosacea. The treatment of chronic skin changes and severe rhinophyma may require laser treatments and surgical intervention, respectively.

The natural approach to rosacea is to try to identify and eliminate contributing factors if possible. Key factors to address are hypochlorhydria (lack of stomach acid), eradication of *Helicobacter pylori*, elimination of food allergies, and optimal intake of B vitamins.

Hypochlorhydria

Gastric analysis of patients with rosacea has led to the belief that it is the result of hypochlorhydria.[4] Psychological factors, such as worry, depression, and stress, often reduce gastric acidity. Hydrochloric acid supplementation results in marked improvement in those patients with rosacea who have achlorhydria or hypochlorhydria.[4,5] Patients with rosacea have also been shown to have diminished secretion of lipase (a fat-digesting enzyme secreted by the pancreas) and to benefit from pancreatic supplementation.[6] For more information, see the chapter "Digestion and Elimination."

Helicobacter pylori

Given the high incidence of hypochlorhydria, it is perhaps not surprising that a high incidence of *H. pylori* infection in the stomach has also been found in patients with rosacea.[7,8] In a pilot study, *H. pylori* was found in 46 of 94 patients with rosacea, 38 of 88 patients with other inflammatory diseases, and 5 of 14 patients without an inflammatory disease. The researchers believed that

the flushing reaction in rosacea is caused by gastrin or vasoactive intestinal peptides. They also quoted an Irish study that found that 19 of 20 patients with acne rosacea tested positive for *H. pylori*.

Another study that evaluated biopsies of sections of the stomach lining found that 84% of 31 patients were *H. pylori* positive.[9] Interestingly, 20% of the patients who tested positive on biopsy tested negative by blood test for the organism. The antibiotic metronidazole is effective in rosacea, and the elimination of *H. pylori* is also associated with clinical improvement. These factors further incriminate *H. pylori*. It is interesting to note that patients with rosacea complain significantly more frequently of "indigestion" and use more antacids than the general population.[10]

Nutritional Supplements

B Vitamins

The administration of large doses of B vitamins has been shown to be quite effective,[11] with riboflavin appearing to be the key factor. It is interesting to note that researchers were able to infect the skin of riboflavin-deficient rats with the mite *D. folliculorum*, but not the skin of normal rats.[12] This mite was once considered a causative factor in rosacea and may still be a factor in some patients, especially those with more granulomatous lesions. Evidence suggests that a delayed hypersensitivity reaction in follicles is triggered by *D. folliculorum* antigens and stimulates the progression of the affection to the papulopustular stage.[13]

Although B vitamins are important for patients with rosacea, care must be exercised because some patients' rosacea may be aggravated by large dosages of these common nutrients. There is a case report of a 53-year-old female who presented to a dermatology clinic with a nine-month history of a facial eruption resembling acne rosacea. Treatment with oral hydroxychloroquine, ibuprofen, terfenadine, prednisone, erythromycin, and tetracycline had been tried during the nine months without success. Topical corticosteroids (desoximetasone, hydrocortisone) and cosmetic elimination also yielded no benefit. Patch test showed a positive reaction to nickel. The eruption began at the time of a personal stress when the patient went through a marital separation. To help with her stress, the patient began taking 100 mg per day of pyridoxine and 100 mcg per day of vitamin B_{12}. Discontinuation of the vitamins resulted in dramatic improvement, and with rechallenge, the condition reappeared. The investigators noted that inflammation and exacerbations of acne related to vitamins B_2, B_6, and B_{12} have been reported in the European literature.[14]

Zinc

Zinc supplementation has been shown to be helpful in acne vulgaris and may also be effective in acne rosacea. To test this hypothesis, 25 patients with rosacea were assessed with a clinical score, then randomly allocated to receive either zinc (23 mg from zinc sulfate) or identical placebo capsules three times per day. Following three months of treatment, the patients crossed over. Nineteen patients completed the study. In the group started on zinc, the score before therapy ranged from 5 to 11. The mean started to decrease directly after the first month of therapy with zinc sulfate to a significantly lower level. After the subjects shifted to the placebo treatment, the mean started to rise gradually in the fifth month but remained significantly lower than the levels before therapy. In the group started on the placebo,

QUICK REVIEW

- **Rosacea was originally called acne rosacea because its inflammatory papules and pustules so closely mimic those of acne.**
- **Most cases of rosacea are associated with moderate to severe seborrhea (oiliness).**
- **One of the first recommendations is to avoid those stimuli that tend to exacerbate the disease—exposure to extremes of heat and cold, excessive sunlight, and ingestion of hot liquids, alcohol, and spicy foods.**
- **Hydrochloric acid supplementation results in marked improvement in those patients with rosacea who have achlorhydria or hypochlorhydria.**

- **A high incidence of *H. pylori* infection in the stomach has also been found in patients with rosacea.**
- **Although B vitamins are important for patients with rosacea, care must be exercised because some patients' rosacea may be aggravated by large dosages of these common nutrients.**
- **Zinc supplementation has been shown to be helpful in acne vulgaris and may also be effective in rosacea.**
- **Topical applications of azelaic acid (AzA) appear to be extremely effective in papulopustular rosacea.**

the score before therapy ranged from 5 to 9. The mean remained high in the first three months of therapy while the patients were on the placebo. After they shifted to zinc sulfate, the mean started to decrease after the fourth month to significantly low levels. No important side effects were reported apart from mild gastric upset in three (12%) of the patients on zinc sulfate. The authors concluded that zinc is a good option in the treatment of rosacea, as it was safe, effective, and without significant side effects.[15]

Topical Treatments

Topical applications of azelaic acid (AzA) appear to be extremely effective in papulo-pustular rosacea. Initially AzA was released in a 20% cream formulation and was shown in this vehicle to be effective in the treatment of mild to moderate rosacea. A 15% gel formulation of AzA vastly improved the delivery of AzA and has been proved in head-to-head studies to be superior to the 20% AzA cream and as effective as metronidazole cream or gel.[16–18] In a meta-analysis of five double-blind trials involving topical AzA (cream or gel) for the treatment of rosacea compared with a placebo or other topical treatments, four of the five studies demonstrated significant decreases in the average number of inflammatory lesions and redness after treatment with azelaic acid compared with the placebo and effects equal to those of metronidazole in papulopustular rosacea. However, no significant decrease in telangiectasia severity occurred with any treatment group.[16]

. . . .

TREATMENT SUMMARY

Eradication of *H. pylori* infection (when present) and control of hypochlorhydria and food intolerance form the basis of therapy. This approach is supported with B-complex supplementation and the avoidance of vasodilating foods.

General Recommendations

See the chapter "Acne" for general recommendations for acne.

Diet

Avoid coffee, alcohol, hot beverages, spicy foods, and any other food or drink that causes a flush. Eliminate from the diet all refined and/or concentrated sugars; foods containing trans-fatty acids such as milk, milk products, margarine, shortening, and other synthetically hydrogenated vegetable oils; and fried foods.

Nutritional Supplements

- A high-potency multiple vitamin and mineral formula as described in the chapter "Supplementary Measures" (but note that the B vitamins may aggravate rosacea in some cases)
- Key individual nutrients:
  - ○ Zinc: 45 to 60 mg per day for three months, followed by 20 to 30 mg per day thereafter
- Fish oils: 3,000 mg EPA + DHA per day

- One of the following:
  - Grape seed extract (>95% procyanidolic oligomers): 100 to 300 mg per day
  - Pine bark extract (>95% procyanidolic oligomers): 100 to 300 mg per day
  - Some other flavonoid-rich extract with a similar flavonoid content, super greens formula, or another plant-based antioxidant that can provide an oxygen radical absorption capacity (ORAC) of 3,000 to 6,000 units or more per day

- Probiotic (*Lactobacillus* species and *Bifidobacterium* species): a minimum of 5 billion to 10 billion colony-forming units per day
- Pancreatin (8 to 10X USP): 350 to 500 mg before meals
- Hydrochloric acid: follow guide on page 136

Topical Treatments

- Topical application of 15% azelaic acid gel

Seborrheic Dermatitis

- Superficial reddened small bumps and scaly eruptions occurring on the scalp, cheeks, and skin folds (armpit, groin, and neck)
- Usually does not itch
- Seasonal; worse in winter

Seborrheic dermatitis is a common skin condition with an appearance similar to eczema. It may be associated with excessive oiliness (seborrhea) and dandruff. The scales may be yellowish and either dry or greasy. The reddened, scaly bumps may coalesce to form large plaques or patches.

Seborrheic dermatitis often occurs in infancy as "cradle cap" (usually between 2 and 12 weeks of age) and has a prognosis of lifelong recurrence, tending to be worse with advancing age.

Causes

The cause of seborrheic dermatitis is unknown. Genetic predisposition, emotional stress, diet, hormones, and infection with yeast-like organisms have all been implicated. Seborrheic dermatitis is now recognized as one of the most common manifestations of AIDS, affecting as many as 83% of AIDS patients. This recent observation has given increased credence to the infection theory of seborrheic dermatitis.

Food Allergies

Seborrheic dermatitis, although not primarily an allergic disease, has been associated with food allergies—67% of people with seborrheic dermatitis develop some form of allergy by 10 years of age.[1]

Therapeutic Considerations

A deficiency of one or more B vitamins may be involved in seborrheic dermatitis. For example, the underlying factor in infants appears to be a biotin deficiency.[2] A syndrome clinically similar to seborrheic dermatitis has been produced by feeding rats a diet high in raw egg white, which is high in avidin, a protein that binds biotin and makes it unavailable for absorption. Since a large portion of the human biotin supply is provided by intestinal bacteria and since newborns have a sterile gastrointestinal tract, it has been postulated that the absence of normal intestinal flora may be responsible for biotin deficiency in infants.[2] A number of studies have demonstrated successful treatment of seborrheic dermatitis with biotin in both the nursing mother and the infant.[3]

In adults, treatment with biotin alone is usually of no value. It must be used in combination with other B vitamins (pyridoxine, pantothenic acid, niacin, thiamine, etc.) that are vital for proper skin metabolism.

Nutritional Supplements

Vitamin B$_6$

Taking a drug that causes vitamin B$_6$ deficiency (4-deoxypyridoxine) and placing rats on a vitamin B$_6$–deficient diet cause skin lesions indistinguishable from seborrheic dermatitis.[4] Vitamin B$_6$ has been shown to be effective in a form of seborrhea (seborrhea sicca) that involves only the scalp (dandruff), brow, nasolabial folds, and beard area, with varying degrees of greasy adherent scales on a reddened base.

Folic Acid and Vitamin B$_{12}$

Oral treatment with folic acid has been only moderately successful; the best results are obtained with a special form, tetrahydrofolate.[5] It should also be used in combination with vitamin B$_{12}$. Injections of vitamin B$_{12}$ have been shown to be very effective in many cases.[6] This may be due to vitamin B$_{12}$'s role as a cofactor in converting folic acid into its active form, tetrahydrofolate.

Botanical Medicines

Aloe Vera Gel

Aloe vera gel can be quite helpful when applied topically. In one double-blind trial involving people with seborrheic dermatitis, the application of a 30% crude aloe emulsion cream twice a day for four to six weeks produced improvements in scaling and itching in 62% of subjects, compared with improvements in only 25% of the placebo group.[7]

Tea Tree Oil

Tea tree (*Melaleuca alternifolia*) oil may be of benefit in the treatment of seborrheic dermatitis owing to its antifungal effects.[8] It seems to be especially helpful when there is involvement of the scalp. In a study of 126 patients, treatment with 5% tea tree oil shampoo produced a 41% improvement in severity vs. 11% in the placebo group.[9] Tea tree oil shampoos are available, or you may add the oil to your favorite shampoo (1 tbsp tea tree oil for every 8 oz shampoo).

. . . .

QUICK REVIEW

- **Seborrhea may be due to a B vitamin deficiency.**
- **A biotin deficiency is the most frequent cause of cradle cap.**

- **Aloe vera gel applied topically can help.**

. . . .

TREATMENT SUMMARY

For infants, biotin supplementation (3 mg twice per day) and control of food allergies are the keys. For adults, supplementing with large doses of vitamin B complex within a high-potency multiple vitamin is the key therapy. We also recommend op- **timal intake of essential fatty acids, using both flaxseed oil and fish oils.**

Diet

Rule out food allergies. For nursing infants, the food allergies of the mother

should be considered. Otherwise, the recommendations in the chapter "A Health-Promoting Diet" should be followed.

Nutritional Supplements

- A high-potency multiple vitamin and mineral formula as described in the chapter "Supplementary Measures"
- Fish oils: 1,000 mg EPA + DHA per day
- Flaxseed oil: 1 tbsp per day
- One of the following:
  - Grape seed extract (>95% procyanidolic oligomers): 100 to 300 mg per day
  - Pine bark extract (>95% procyanidolic oligomers): 100 to 300 mg per day
  - Some other flavonoid-rich extract with a similar flavonoid content, super greens formula, or another plant-based antioxidant that can provide an oxygen radical absorption capacity (ORAC) of 3,000 to 6,000 units or more per day
- Probiotic (*Lactobacillus* species and *Bifidobacterium* species): a minimum of 5 billion to 10 billion colony-forming units

Topical Applications

- Aloe vera gel: apply twice per day to affected areas
- Tea tree oil shampoo: wash hair and scalp daily

Sinus Infections

· ·

- History of acute viral respiratory infection, dental infection, or nasal allergy

  - Nasal congestion and thick mucus discharge

  - Fever, chills, and frontal headache

  - Pain, tenderness, redness, and swelling over the involved sinus

  - In chronic infection, often no symptoms other than mild postnasal discharge, a musty odor, or a nonproductive cough

Sinus infection, or sinusitis, is a bacterial infection of the sinus passages—it may be either acute or chronic. The most common predisposing factor in acute bacterial sinusitis is viral upper respiratory infection (the common cold). Nasal allergies and other factors that interfere with normal protective mechanisms may precede the viral infection and therefore are the more likely predisposing factors. The key point is that any factor that induces swelling or inflammation of the mucous membranes that line the nasal and sinus passages will predispose a person to bacterial sinusitis, as the environment that is produced serves as a suitable medium for bacterial overgrowth, with streptococci, pneumococci, staphylococci, and *Haemophilus influenzae* being the most commonly cultured bacteria.

In chronic bacterial sinusitis an allergy is the most common cause; in 25% of cases there is an underlying dental infection.

Therapeutic Considerations

Although antibiotic therapy is the dominant treatment of acute and chronic bacterial sinusitis, it is of limited value.[1] A detailed analysis of clinical trials with adults concluded that there was insufficient evidence to say that antibiotic treatment was effective in acute sinusitis.[2] Nonetheless, in severe or unresponsive cases, antibiotics may be appropriate. In a Cochrane review it was shown that although 80% of participants treated without antibiotics improve within two weeks, antibiotics have a small effect in patients with uncomplicated acute sinusitis who have symptoms for more than seven days. Newer, more potent antibiotics (e.g., cephalosporins) appear to be more effective than penicillin, amoxicillin, and other less potent antibiotics.[3]

In children, there is even less evidence that antimicrobial therapy is of significant benefit.[4] Overuse of antibiotics for children with sinusitis or otitis media is a growing concern, as it is leading to antibiotic-resistant strains of bacteria.

In chronic sinusitis, antibiotics are also usually of little or no benefit.[5] Clearly the most rational approach seems to be to address the underlying cause of chronic sinusitis (respiratory or food allergens) along with providing supportive therapy (saline nasal rinse, immune-enhancing herbs, natural decongestants).

Studies indicate that among most patients with chronic sinusitis, perhaps as many as 84%, have allergies.[6,7] Environmental control requires the elimination of dust mites (washing at a temperature of at least 136°F), use of air-filtering vacuum cleaners, installation of an air cleaner with a high-efficiency particulate air filter, and whatever methods are necessary to maintain the humidity under 50%. Some particularly sensitive patients may need to have all pets removed, along with carpeting and featherbedding.[8] Other recommendations are in the chapter "Hay Fever."

Mucolytics

The ability to clear particulate matter and microorganisms from the sinuses depends on the properties and volume of secreted mucus and the hairlike appendages (cilia) of the cells that line the sinuses. In chronic sinusitis, the mucus is usually thicker and sticker. Guaifenesin (also known as glycerol guiacolate) is a derivative of a compound originally isolated from beech wood that has expectorant and mucolytic properties and is available in many over-the-counter preparations. The goal with a mucolytic is to reduce the thickness and stickiness of the mucus to help promote effective clearance.[9]

Alternative mucolytics include N-acetylcysteine (NAC) and proteolytic enzymes. NAC is very effective in this role, interacting with the protein bonds of mucus to break it down into less viscous strands. NAC has been shown to be effective for chronic bronchitis.[10] These same properties make it useful for sinusitis. Proteolytic (protein-digesting) enzymes may break down complex proteins at the site of inflammation, exert some antimicrobial effects, or act directly on mucus proteins. Trypsin, chymotrypsin, *Serratia* peptidase, and bromelain are the proteolytic enzymes that can break down mucus proteins

and other proteins when they are administered topically. Of these enzymes, *Serratia* peptidase may be the most effective, while bromelain is probably the most popular and readily available. *Serratia* peptidase is an enzyme derived from bacteria that reside in the intestines of silkworms. It is also called "silkworm enzyme," as it is the enzyme used to break down the cocoon of the silkworm. It is more powerful and has broader pH stability than the pancreatic enzymes chymotrypsin and trypsin. It has been used in Europe and Japan for over 25 years as a mucolytic and natural anti-inflammatory. When *Serratia* peptidase was given at a dose of 30 mg per day for four weeks to patients with chronic sinusitis, it significantly reduced the thickness of nasal mucus.[11] When *Serratia* peptidase was administered at the same dose to patients with chronic bronchitis, it significantly increased mucus clearance.[12] In a double-blind, placebo-controlled study of 193 subjects suffering from various acute or chronic ear, nose, or throat disorders, including sinusitis, *Serratia* peptidase demonstrated greater efficacy and more rapid action against all the symptoms examined.[13] Orally administered bromelain has also shown benefit in the treatment of chronic sinusitis.[14]

Botanical Medicines

Many herbs have been shown to have antibacterial, antiviral, and immune-enhancing effects that would be appropriate for bacterial sinusitis. The most popular herbal medicines historically used in the United States for sinusitis are goldenseal (*Hydrastis canadensis*) and echinacea (*Echinacea* species); see the information on echinacea in the chapter "Common Cold," as it may be more useful than goldenseal in viral infections. The discussion below includes goldenseal and other berberine-containing plants as well as South African geranium (*Pelargonium sidoides*). Extracts from the rhizomes and tubers of South African geranium have been shown to exert a number of effects beneficial in upper respiratory tract infections, particularly acute bronchitis, for which it is an approved drug in Germany (see the chapter "Bronchitis and Pneumonia").

Goldenseal and Other Berberine-Containing Plants

Goldenseal (*Hydrastis canadensis*), barberry (*Berberis vulgaris*), Oregon grape (*Berberis aquifolium*), and coptis or goldthread (*Coptis chinensis*) are valued for their high content of alkaloids, of which berberine has been the most widely studied. Berberine has demonstrated significant antibiotic and immune-enhancing effects in both experimental and clinical settings. Berberine has also been shown to inhibit the adherence of bacteria to human cells, so they cannot infect the cells.

The primary immune-enhancing action of berberine is the activation of white blood cells known as macrophages. These cells are responsible for engulfing and destroying bacteria, viruses, tumor cells, and other particulate matter. Historically, berberine-containing plants have also been used to bring down fevers. In animal studies, berberine has produced a fever-lowering effect three times as potent as that of aspirin. However, while aspirin suppresses fever through its action on hormone-like compounds known as prostaglandins, berberine appears to lower fever by enhancing the immune system's ability to handle fever-producing compounds produced by bacteria and other microorganisms.

South African Geranium

South African geranium (*Pelargonium sidoides*) has demonstrated immune-enhancing effects as well as antibacterial and antiviral effects and the ability to prevent adhesion of bacteria to epithelial cells.[15] In one double-blind, placebo-controlled trial, 103 patients with acute sinusitis of presumably bacterial origin were given an extract of *P. sidoides* (EPs 7630, sold under the name Umcka) for a maximum of 22 days.[16] The average decrease in symptom severity score was 5.5 points in the EPs 7630 group compared with 2.5 points in the placebo group. Patients in the EPs 7630 group also had a faster rate of recovery.

Nasal Irrigation

Use of a neti pot to deliver a saline wash is also recommended. A neti pot is a ceramic pot that looks like a cross between a small teapot and Aladdin's magic lamp. The neti pot originally comes from the ayurvedic/

QUICK REVIEW

- **Any factor that causes swelling of the lining of the sinuses may result in obstruction of drainage and subsequent infection.**
- **Antibiotic therapy is of limited value.**
- **Addressing the underlying cause of**

- **chronic sinusitis along with supportive therapy appears to be the most rational approach.**
- **A daily nasal rinse with a saline wash is recommended during active infection.**

yoga medical tradition but has been used worldwide for centuries. Typically, to use the neti pot or another nasal irrigation device you would mix about 16 fl oz lukewarm water with 1 tsp salt. Once you've filled the neti pot, tilt your head over the sink at about a 45-degree angle. Put the spout into your top nostril and gently pour the saline solution into that nostril. The fluid will flow through your nasal cavity and out the other nostril. It may also run into your throat. If this occurs, just spit it out. Blow your nose to get rid of any remaining liquid, then refill the neti pot and repeat the process on the other side. Use the neti pot once per day when symptoms are present. A more convenient way of doing nasal rinsing is with a plastic squeeze bottle filled with the lukewarm saline solution. It is available commercially as NeilMed Sinus Rinse.

TREATMENT SUMMARY

In acute sinusitis, the immediate therapeutic goals are to reestablish drainage and clear the acute infection. Various measures can be used: local application of saline through the use of a neti pot, botanicals with antibacterial and immune-enhancing properties, and basic immune system support (see the chapter "Immune System Support").

Because chronic bacterial sinusitis is often secondary to allergy, long-term control depends on isolation and elimination of the food or airborne allergens and correction of the underlying problem that allowed the allergy to develop. During the acute phase, elimination of common food allergens (milk, wheat, eggs, citrus, corn, and peanuts) is indicated until a more definitive diagnosis can be made.

Nutritional Supplements

- A high-potency multiple vitamin and mineral formula as described in the chapter "Supplementary Measures"
- Key individual nutrients:
  - Vitamin A: 5,000 international units per day
  - Vitamin C: 500 to 1,000 mg every two hours
- One of the following:
  - Bioflavonoids (mixed citrus): 1,000 mg per day
  - Grape seed extract (>95% procyanidolic oligomers): 150 to 300 mg per day
  - Pine bark extract (>95% procyanidolic oligomers): 150 to 300 mg per day.
- Zinc: 20 to 30 mg per day
- N-acetylcysteine: 200 mg three times per day
- One of the following:
  - Bromelain (1,200 to 1,800 MCU): 250 to 500 mg three times per day between meals
  - *Serratia* peptidase (enteric-coated): 30 to 50 mg three times per day between meals

Botanical Medicines

- Goldenseal *(Hydrastis canadensis)* or another berberine-containing plant (standardized extracts recommended):
  - Dried root or as infusion (tea): 2 to 4 g three times per day
  - Tincture (1: 5): 6 to 12 ml (1.5 to 3 tsp) three times per day
  - Fluid extract (1: 1): 2 to 4 ml (0.5 to 1 tsp) three times per day
  - Solid (powdered dry) extract (4:1 or 8 to 12% alkaloid content): 250 to 500 mg three times per day
- *Echinacea* species:
  - Fluid extract of the fresh aerial portion of *E. purpurea* (1:1): 2 to 4 ml (½ to 1 tsp) three times per day (preferred form)
  - Juice of aerial portion of *E. purpurea* stabilized in 22% ethanol: 2 to 4 ml (½ to 1 tsp) three times per day (preferred form)
  - Dried root (or as tea): 1 to 2 g three times per day
  - Freeze-dried plant: 325 to 650 mg three times per day
  - Tincture (1:5): 2 to 4 ml (½ to 1 tsp) three times per day
  - Fluid extract (1:1): 2 to 4 ml (½ to 1 tsp) three times per day
  - Solid (dry powdered) extract (6.5:1 or 3.5% echinacoside): 150 to 300 mg three times per day
- South African geranium (*Pelargonium sidoides*, EPs 7630 or equivalent preparation): adults, 3 ml three times per day or two 20-mg tablets three times per day for up to 14 days; children ages 7 through 12, 30 drops (1.5 ml) three times per day; age 6 years or less, 10 drops (0.5 ml) three times per day

Physical Medicine

- Nasal rinse with warm saline solution once per day, increasing to several times a day during acute attacks

Sports Injuries, Tendinitis, and Bursitis

· ·

- Tendinitis:
  - Acute or chronic pain localized in a tendon
  - Limited range of motion
- Bursitis
  - Severe pain in the affected joint, particularly on movement
  - Limited range of motion

This chapter deals with sports injuries (e.g., sprains, strains, and bruises), tendinitis, and bursitis. *Tendinitis* is an inflammatory condition of a tendon—the tissue that connects muscles to bones. Tendinitis usually results from a strain. Although acute tendinitis usually heals within a few days to two weeks, it may become chronic, in which case calcium salts will typically deposit along the tendon fibers. The tendons most commonly affected are the Achilles tendon (back of ankle), the biceps (front of shoulder), the pollicis brevis and longus (thumb), the upper patellar tendon (knee), the posterior tibial tendon (inside of foot), and the rotator cuff (shoulder).

Bursitis is inflammation of the bursa, the sac-like membrane that contains fluid which lubricates the joints. Bursitis may result from trauma, strain, infection, or arthritic conditions. The most common locations are shoulder, elbow, hip, and lower knee. Occasionally the bursa can develop calcified deposits and become a chronic problem.

Causes

The most common cause of sports injury is sudden excessive tension on a tendon or bursa, producing a strain or sprain. Repeated muscle contraction, leading to exhaustion of the muscle, can result in similar injury. Sometimes tendinitis develops when the grooves in which the tendons move develop bone spurs or other mechanical abnormalities. Proper stretching and warm-up before exercise are important preventive measures.

Therapeutic Considerations

After an injury or sprain, immediate first aid is very important. The acronym RICE summarizes the approach:

- Rest the injured part as soon as it is hurt, to avoid further injury.
- Ice the area of pain to decrease swelling and bleeding.
- Compress the area with an elastic bandage to limit swelling and bleeding.

- Elevate the injured part above the level of the heart to increase drainage of fluids out of the injured area.

Proper application of these procedures is important for optimal results. When icing, first cover the injured area with a towel, then place an ice pack on it. It is important not to wrap the injured part so tightly that circulation is impaired. The ice and compress should be applied for 30 minutes, followed by 15 minutes without the ice to allow recirculation. You want to get the affected area cold, but not so cold that it freezes or damages the tissues.

Of course, for any serious injury, a physician should be consulted immediately. Conditions that indicate the need to see a physician include severe pain, injury to a joint, loss of function, and bruising around or below or pain that persists for more than two weeks.

After the acute inflammatory stage (24 to 48 hours), gradually increase range-of-motion and stretching exercises, to maintain and improve mobility and prevent adhesions (abnormal scar formation). Alternating hot and cold packs are also useful to improve circulation, thus bringing in nutrients and more rapidly clearing the debris from the injured tissues.

Nutritional Considerations

Several nutrients are important for the promotion of healing. For example, vitamin C supplementation is important, since vitamin C plays a major role in the prevention and repair of injuries. Deficiency of vitamin C is associated with defective formation and maintenance of tendon and bursal tissues. In addition to vitamin C, vitamin A, zinc, vitamin E, and selenium are important not only for their wound-healing properties but also for their antioxidant effects.

Flavonoids

Flavonoids, a group of plant pigments responsible for the colors of many fruits and flowers, are extremely effective in reducing inflammation and strengthening collagen structures. Collagen is the major protein in tendons and other connective tissues. Flavonoids help maintain a healthy collagen structure by (1) decreasing blood vessel permeability, thereby decreasing the influx of inflammatory mediators into areas of damage; (2) preventing free radical damage by means of their potent antioxidant properties; (3) inhibiting damage to collagen tissue caused by enzymes that break down collagen; (4) inhibiting the release of inflammatory chemicals; and (5) reinforcing the natural cross-linking of collagen fibers to make them stronger.

Double-blind, placebo-controlled studies have shown that supplemental citrus flavonoids cut in half the time needed to recover from sports injuries.[1,2] But, given the greater biological activity of the procyanidolic oligomers found in pine bark or grape seed extract, we prefer these sources over citrus flavonoids.

Bromelain and Other Proteolytic Enzymes

Bromelain (the protein-digesting enzyme complex of pineapple) was introduced as a medicinal agent in 1957, and since that time more than 400 scientific papers on its therapeutic applications have appeared in medical literature. In these studies, bromelain has been reported to exert a wide variety of beneficial effects, including reducing inflammation in cases of sports injury or trauma and preventing swelling after trauma or surgery.[3]

One of the most interesting studies that used bromelain to treat sports-related injuries involved 146 boxers.[4] Seventy-four received bromelain; in 58, all signs of bruising cleared completely within 4 days. In the remainder, complete clearance took 8 to 10 days. Among the 72 boxers who did not take bromelain, at the end of 4 days only 10 had completely cleared bruises; the remainder took 7 to 14 days. These results indicate that bromelain goes a long way in reducing bruising, inflammation, and swelling due to trauma.

It is important to recognize that while bromelain has been shown to effectively reduce pain, this probably is the result of a reduction in tissue inflammation and swelling, rather than a direct analgesic effect.

A couple of studies have used a commercial preparation (Phlogenzym) containing bromelain (90 mg), trypsin (48 mg), and rutin (100 mg per tablet). In a study of ankle sprain, Phlogenzym was not found to be effective.[5] However, in another study, conducted at the Canadian College of Naturopathic Medicine, postal workers with shoulder (rotator cuff) tendinitis for a duration of more than 6 weeks were randomly assigned to receive naturopathic care or standardized physical exercises over 12 weeks. Participants in the naturopathic care group received dietary counseling, acupuncture, and Phlogenzym (two tablets three times a day). The physical exercise group received passive, active-assisted, and active range-of-motion exercises and a matched placebo. Final total shoulder pain and disability scores decreased by 54.5% in the naturopathic care group and by 18% in the physical exercise group.[6]

Botanical Medicines

Curcumin

Curcumin—the yellow pigment of turmeric, *Curcuma longa*—exerts excellent anti-inflammatory and antioxidant effects. Curcumin is as effective as cortisone or the potent anti-inflammatory drug phenylbutazone in animal studies. However, while phenylbutazone and cortisone are associated with significant toxicity, curcumin is without side effects. In human studies, curcumin has also demonstrated beneficial effects comparable to those of standard drugs.[7]

QUICK REVIEW

- **Proper stretching and warm-up before exercise are important preventive measures.**
- **After an injury or sprain, immediate first aid to the injured area (RICE: rest, ice, compression, and elevation) is very important.**
- **Deficiency of vitamin C is associated with defective formation and maintenance of tendon and bursal tissues.**
- **Vitamin A, zinc, vitamin E, and selenium, as well as vitamin C, are important not only for their wound-healing properties but also for their antioxidant effects.**
- **Bromelain has been reported in scientific studies to exert a wide variety of beneficial effects, including reducing inflammation in cases of sports injury or trauma.**
- **Curcumin exerts excellent anti-inflammatory and antioxidant effects.**
- **Physical therapy can aid in pain relief and recovery from injury.**

One concern regarding curcumin has been absorption, but there now exist a number of methods and products that enhance the absorption of curcumin. One of those methods is complexing the curcumin with soy phospholipids to produce a product called Meriva. Absorption studies in animals indicate that peak plasma levels of curcumin after administration of Meriva were five times higher than those after administration of regular curcumin.[8] Studies with another advanced form of curcumin, Theracurmin, shows even greater absorption (e.g., 27 times greater than regular curcumin).[9]

Physical Therapy

There are a number of physical therapy techniques that can be quite helpful in speeding recovery and relieving pain. Perhaps the two most popular techniques are transcutaneous electrical nerve stimulation (TENS) and ultrasound. TENS involves the use of electricity to stimulate muscular contractions. The use of TENS to control pain has been well documented. Individuals with tendinitis have been found to respond well to TENS. TENS therapy may be applied by a physical therapist or physician. In addition, home units are now available.

Ultrasound is a form of high-frequency sound vibration used to heat an area and increase its blood supply and lymphatic drainage. While it is useful during the acute stage (the first 24 to 48 hours) of an injury, it offers the greatest benefit in the recovery phase. It is particularly useful when the bursitis or tendinitis forms calcium deposits, or when adhesions (scar tissue) have formed inappropriately, thus limiting function and increasing the risk of future injury.

- -

TREATMENT SUMMARY

Treatment of the muscle, joint, tendon, or bursal damage caused by acute and chronic injuries involves two phases: inflammation inhibition and protection of the injured tissues, followed by promotion of healing after the acute phase has resolved. For any serious injury (involving severe pain, injuries to the joints, loss of function, or pain that persists for more than two weeks), consult a physician immediately. Utilize RICE therapy for 24 to 48 hours, after which increasing range-of-motion and stretching exercises should be used to maintain and improve mobility and prevent abnormal scar formation.

Nutritional Supplements

- A high-potency multiple vitamin and mineral formula as described in the chapter "Supplementary Measures"
- Key individual nutrients:
  - Vitamin C: 500 to 1,000 mg one to three times per day
  - Vitamin D_3: 2,000 to 4,000 IU per day (ideally, measure blood levels and adjust dosage accordingly)

- Fish oils: 3,000 mg EPA + DHA per day until symptoms resolve, then 1,000 mg EPA + DHA per day thereafter
- One of the following:
  - Grape seed extract (>95% procyanidolic oligomers): 150 to 300 mg per day
  - Pine bark extract (>95% procyanidolic oligomers): 150 to 300 mg per day
  - Some other flavonoid-rich extract with a similar flavonoid content, "super greens formula," or another plant-based antioxidant that can provide an oxygen radical absorption capacity (ORAC) of 3,000 to 6,000 units or more per day

Botanical Medicines

- Bromelain (1,800 to 2,000 MCU): 250 to 750 mg three times per day between meals
- One of the following:
  - Meriva: 500 to 1,000 mg twice daily
  - BCM95 Complex: 750 to 1,500 mg twice daily
  - Theracurmin: 300 mg one to three times daily

Physical Medicine

- TENS if needed for pain control
- Ultrasound: three times per week during the recovery phase and if adhesions or contractures develop

Strep Throat
(Streptococcal Pharyngitis)

- Abrupt onset of sore throat, fever, malaise, nausea, and headache
- Throat red and swollen, with or without exudation
- Tender lymph nodes along the neck
- Positive rapid detection of streptococcal antigen
- Group A streptococci on throat culture

Over 90% of sore throats are caused by viruses. Nonetheless, if you have a sore throat, we recommend consulting a physician to rule out strep throat (group A beta-hemolytic streptococci pharyngotonsillitis or GABHS). You simply cannot tell the difference between the two just by looking at the throat and tonsils. Strep throat is more common in children, with about 15% to 36% of children with sore throats seeking medical care turning out to be positive for strep. Slightly lower percentages occur in adults. However, it must be kept in mind that 10% to 25% of the general population are carriers for group A streptococci; therefore, the true number of cases of sore throat due to strep is probably less than reported. In other words, some people have strep present all of the time in their throat and do not have an active infection.

Diagnostic Considerations

There are now tests available in doctors' offices that provide an immediate or rapid screening for strep. These tests detect the presence of group A streptococcal antigens and are a major clinical advancement that helps to prevent unnecessary prescribing of antibiotics. Prior to these tests doctors had to rely on throat cultures that usually took two days to show results. Often antibiotics were started before the results were known, leading to unnecessary exposure to antibiotics and a greater likelihood of development of antibiotic-resistant organisms. Rapid strep screening will someday soon replace throat culture as the diagnostic gold standard. That said, these tests remain underutilized, as one analysis found they were performed on only 53% of patients with acute sore throat for whom an antibiotic was prescribed.[1]

Therapeutic Considerations

From a natural medicine perspective, the primary therapeutic consideration is improving the status of the immune system. If the person's immune system is functioning well, the illness will be short-lived. Enhancing general immune function, as described in the chapter

"Immune System Support," may shorten the course of the sore throat. In cases of poor immune function, every effort should be made to strengthen the immune system by following the recommendations in that chapter.

While many physicians continue to rely on antibiotics in the treatment of strep throat, in most cases antibiotics are not necessary. Strep throat is usually a self-limiting disease—meaning that it will resolve on its own with time—and most research has shown that clinical recovery is similar in cases in which antibiotics are prescribed and those in which they are not.[2–4]

The primary concern about not using antibiotics is the development of what is called *nonsuppurative poststreptococcal syndromes* (rheumatic fever, poststreptococcal glomerulonephritis, etc.). However, antibiotic administration does not significantly reduce the incidence of these complications. The issue seems to be related to a combination of host defense factors and the particular strength (virulence) of some group A strep bacteria that are more likely to cause rheumatic fever and glomerulonephritis.[5] It is also important to point out that although many physicians believe that acute rheumatic fever can be caused only by group A strep infection of the upper respiratory tract, population-based studies indicate that strep infections of the skin are the major cause in high-incidence communities. In contrast, in settings in which rheumatic fever has become rare, the group A streptococcal strains causing pharyngitis are of relatively lower virulence in terms of causing rheumatic fever.[5]

At this time, it appears that the use of antibiotics should be reserved for those who are suffering from severe infection, those whose sore throat is unresponsive to therapy (i.e., no response after one week of immune-supportive therapy), and those with a prior history of rheumatic fever or glomerulonephritis.

If antibiotics are used or have been used, it is important to use a probiotic supplement containing *Lactobacillus* and *Bifidobacterium* species. Probiotic supplementation is very important for preventing and treating antibiotic-induced diarrhea, candida overgrowth, and urinary tract infections. Although it is commonly believed that acidophilus supplements are not effective if taken during antibiotic therapy, research actually supports the use of *L. acidophilus* during antibiotic administration.[6,7] Reductions of friendly bacteria and/or superinfection with antibiotic-resistant flora may be prevented by administering *L. acidophilus* products during antibiotic therapy. A dosage of at least 15 billion to 20 billion organisms is required during antibiotic usage. We recommend taking the probiotic supplement as far between antibiotic doses as possible. After the antibiotic course is finished, a dosage of 2 billion to 5 billion live organisms is usually sufficient.

Nutritional Supplements

Vitamin C

During the 1930s there was considerable interest in the relationship between malnutrition and the development of the complications of strep throat. Both experimental animal work and population-based surveys demonstrated a correlation between vitamin C deficiency and the development of these complications. Rheumatic fever is virtually nonexistent in the tropics, where vitamin C intake is higher; and 18% of children in high-risk groups have subnormal serum vitamin C levels.[8,9]

Vitamin C supplementation of strep-infected, vitamin-C-deficient, rheumatic-fever-susceptible guinea pigs totally prevents the development of rheumatic fever.[8,9] Uncontrolled clinical studies demonstrated very positive results when children were given orange juice supplementation. Unfortunately, this promising line of research appears to have been dropped, probably owing to the advent of supposedly effective antibiotics.

Botanical Medicines

The guidelines for enhancing the immune system, as presented in the chapter "Immune System Support," are particularly well indicated for streptococcal pharyngitis. In addition, the botanicals goldenseal (*Hydrastis canadensis*) and *Echinacea* species are well respected in the support of the immune system during strep infections. The berberine alkaloid of goldenseal exerts antibiotic activity against streptococci and, perhaps more important, has been shown to inhibit the attachment of group A streptococci to pharyngeal epithelial cells. Echinacea also exerts action against streptococci infection. To promote the spread of colonies, streptococci secrete large amounts of hyaluronidase. This enzyme is inhibited by echinacea as well as by many bioflavonoids. Echinacea also inactivates group A streptococci and reduces the pro-inflammatory response to strep infection[10] as well as promoting greater ability of white blood cells to identify and destroy bacteria.

South African Geranium

Extracts of this African plant (*Pelargonium sidoides*) have been shown to exert a number of effects beneficial in upper respiratory tract infections, particularly acute bronchitis, an indication for which it is an approved drug in Germany (see the chapter "Bronchitis and Pneumonia"). A special extract of *P. sidoides* known as EPs 7630 or Umcka has demonstrated immune-enhancing effects as well as antibacterial effects and the ability to prevent adhesion of bacteria to epithelial cells.[11] In a double-blind study, 143 children ages six to ten with non-GABHS sore throat were given either EPs 7630 or a placebo for six days. Treatment with EPs 7630 reduced the severity of symptoms (the decrease in the severity score from day 0 to day 4 was 7.1 points with EPs 7630 and 2.5 points in the placebo group) and shortened the duration of illness by at least two days, consistent with the results seen in acute bronchitis.[12] Although this study addressed non-GABHS sore throat, it does raise the possibility that *P. sidoides* may have benefit for GABHS.

QUICK REVIEW

- **More than 90% of all sore throats are caused by viruses.**
- **If you have a sore throat, see a physician to rule out strep throat as the cause.**
- **Before antibiotics are used, an in-office rapid strep screening test should be performed.**
- **If antibiotics are used or have been used, it is important to use a probiotic supplement containing *Lactobacillus acidophilus* and *Bifidobacterium bifidus*.**
- **Vitamin C is very important in the prevention of rheumatic fever.**
- **Goldenseal prevents the adherence of strep bacteria to the lining of the throat.**
- **Echinacea inactivates group A strep and reduces the pro-inflammatory response to strep infection.**

TREATMENT SUMMARY

For further information, consult the chapter "Immune System Support." If antibiotics are used, follow the recommendations for *Lactobacillus acidophilus* supplementation in the chapter "Diarrhea."

Nutritional Supplements

- A high-potency multiple vitamin and mineral formula as described in the chapter "Supplementary Measures"
- Key individual nutrients:
  - Vitamin C: 500 to 1,000 mg every two waking hours
  - Vitamin A: 5,000 IU per day (women who are pregnant or who may become pregnant should take no more than 3,000 IU per day)
  - Zinc: 30 mg per day
- One of the following:
  - Grape seed extract (>95% procyanidolic oligomers): 100 to 300 mg per day
  - Pine bark extract (>95% procyanidolic oligomers): 100 to 300 mg per day
  - Mixed citrus bioflavonoids: 1,000 mg per day

Botanical Medicines

One or more of the following can be used:

- *Echinacea* species:
  - Fluid extract of the fresh aerial portion of *E. purpurea* (1:1): 2 to 4 ml (½ to 1 tsp) three times a day (preferred form)
  - Juice of aerial portion of *Echinacea purpurea* stabilized in 22% ethanol: 2 to 4 ml (½ to 1 tsp) three times a day (preferred form)
  - Dried root (or as tea): 1 to 2 g three times a day
  - Freeze-dried plant: 325 to 650 mg three times a day
  - Tincture (1:5): 2 to 4 ml (½ to 1 tsp) three times a day
  - Fluid extract (1:1): 2 to 4 ml (½ to 1 tsp) three times a day
  - Solid (dry powdered) extract (6.5:1 or 3.5% echinacoside): 150 to 300 mg three times a day
- Goldenseal (*Hydrastis canadensis*), standardized extracts recommended:
  - Dried root or as infusion (tea): 2 to 4 g three times a day
  - Tincture (1:5): 6 to 12 ml (1.5 to 3 tsp) three times a day
  - Fluid extract (1:1): 2 to 4 ml (0.5 to 1 tsp) three times a day
  - Solid (powdered dry) extract (4:1 or 8% to 12% alkaloid content): 250 to 500 mg three times a day
- South African geranium (*Pelargonium sidoides*, EPs 7630 or equivalent preparation): adults, 3 ml three times per day or two 20-mg tablets three times per day for up to 14 days; children ages 7 through 12, 30 drops (1.5 ml) three times per day; age 6 years or less, 10 drops (0.5 ml) three times per day

Stroke (Recovery From)

Signs of stroke include:

- Sudden, unexplained dizziness, trouble with walking, loss of balance, or unsteadiness

- Confusion, trouble speaking or understanding communication

- Unexplained weakness or numbness of the face, arms, or legs, or on one side of the body

- Loss of vision in one or both eyes

- Sudden, unexplained severe headache

A stroke is the loss of nerve function for at least 24 hours due to lack of oxygen. The time limit is specified to distinguish it from a transient ischemic attack (TIA), which does not cause permanent disability. A stroke can be the result of a lack of blood flow (ischemia) caused by blockage from a blood clot (embolism) or a hemorrhage (leakage of blood). Without oxygen, the nerve cells become damaged or die, and the affected area of the brain becomes unable to function. A stroke may result in an inability to move one or both limbs on one side of the body, inability to understand or formulate speech, or an inability to see on one side of the visual field. If the stroke is severe enough or occurs in a certain location, such as parts of the brainstem, it can result in coma or death.

Stroke is the leading cause of adult disability in the United States and the third-leading cause of death. Risk factors for stroke include old age, hypertension (high blood pressure), previous stroke or transient ischemic attack (TIA), diabetes, high cholesterol, cigarette smoking, and atrial fibrillation. High blood pressure is the most important risk factor for a stroke.

A stroke is diagnosed through a neurological examination and is usually confirmed with a CT or MRI scan.

Risk Factors for a Stroke	
RISK FACTOR	**SIGNIFICANCE**
High blood pressure	Accounts for 35–50% of stroke risk
Atrial fibrillation	Risk of 5% each year to develop stroke
Diabetes	At least two to three times more likely to develop stroke
Surgery	Particularly carotid endarterectomy (see the chapter "Cerebral Vascular Insufficiency")
Dietary factors	High saturated fat intake; low consumption of fruit, vegetables, and omega-3 fatty acids
Smoking	Increases the risk of developing atherosclerosis
High cholesterol	Increases the risk of developing atherosclerosis

One of the key factors in limiting the damage to the brain caused by a stroke is how quickly a person receives the drug form of the naturally occurring compound tissue plasminogen activator (rtPA). It must be administered within a few hours of a stroke to produce significant benefit. Unfortunately, only 1 to 3% of stroke patients receive rtPA treatment.

The results of stroke can affect patients physically, mentally, or emotionally, or in any combination of the three ways, and can vary widely depending on size and location of the lesion. Disability corresponds to areas in the brain that have been damaged.

The physical disabilities that can result from stroke include muscle weakness, numbness, pressure sores, pneumonia, incontinence, apraxia (inability to perform learned movements), difficulties carrying out daily activities, appetite loss, speech loss, vision loss, and pain.

Emotional problems after a stroke can result from direct damage to emotional centers in the brain or from frustration and difficulty adapting to new limitations. Poststroke emotional difficulties include anxiety, panic attacks, flat affect (failure to express emotions), mania, apathy, and psychosis.

Almost half of stroke survivors suffer poststroke depression, which is characterized by lethargy, irritability, sleep disturbances, lowered self-esteem, and withdrawal. Emotional lability, another consequence of stroke, causes the patient to switch quickly between emotional highs and lows and to express emotions inappropriately, for instance with an excess of laughing or crying with little or no provocation. While these expressions of emotion usually correspond to the patient's actual emotions, a more severe form of emotional lability causes patients to laugh and cry pathologically, without regard to context or emotion. Some patients show the opposite of what they feel, such as crying when they are happy. Emotional lability occurs in about 20% of stroke patients.

Cognitive deficits resulting from stroke include perceptual disorders, speech problems, dementia, and problems with attention and memory. A stroke sufferer may be unaware of his or her own disabilities, a condition called anosognosia. In a condition called hemispatial neglect, a patient is unable to attend to anything on the side of space opposite to the damaged hemisphere.

Up to 10% of all stroke patients develop seizures, most commonly in the week subsequent to the event; the severity of the stroke increases the likelihood of seizures.

Therapeutic Considerations

For most stroke patients who suffer from poststroke disability, recovery is a concerted effort that involves physical therapy, occupational therapy, and speech-language therapy. We recommend taking advantage of these services, as they can greatly aid the rehabilitation process.

Medical care is often focused on preventing another stroke and most often utilizes anticoagulant therapy with warfarin (Coumadin) or antiplatelet therapy with aspirin or clopidogrel (Plavix), ticlopidine (Ticlid), and so on. These drugs are designed to prevent blood clots from forming and lodging in the brain, where they can produce another stroke. These drugs are not, of course, used when the stroke is from a hemorrhage.

From a natural medicine perspective the goals are similar, but more focused on maximizing blood flow and nutrition to the damaged areas. In addition, acupuncture has shown significant benefits in aiding stroke recovery.

The general guidelines offered in the chapter "Cerebral Vascular Insufficiency" are valid here. In particular, ginkgo biloba extract is very important in stroke recovery. Ginkgo biloba extract increases blood flow to the brain, improves the production of energy within nerve cells, and favorably affects blood viscosity (thickness), resulting in improved blood flow characteristics within the brain.[1] We also recommend coenzyme Q_{10}, as it may help improve energy production within the recovering brain cells.

Natural Antiplatelet and Fibrinolytic Therapy

There are a number of dietary and supplements to reduce the aggregation of platelets as well as reduce the formation of fibrin and thereby prevent blood clots from forming. The general dietary factors that reduce platelet aggregation and promote fibrin breakdown (fibrinolysis) are discussed in the chapter "Heart and Cardiovascular Health." These factors include omega-3 fatty acids, antioxidant nutrients, flavonoids, flavonoid-rich extracts (e.g., grape seed and pine bark extract), nattokinase, and garlic preparations standardized for alliin content. Fish oil supplementation can definitely be used in combination with aspirin and other platelet inhibitors,[2] but if several natural antiplatelet agents are used at the same time or if nattokinase is used, it is important to avoid the use of antiplatelet drugs (including aspirin). There are case reports of hemorrhagic strokes that occurred when a natural agent (e.g., nattokinase) was combined with an antiplatelet drug.[3] However, aspirin alone is also associated with similar case reports, so it is hard to gauge the significance of an interaction. Nonetheless, the caution not to mix antiplatelet therapies applies.

Precautions with Coumadin

The drug Coumadin works by blocking the action of vitamin K. Since green leafy vegetables and green tea contain high levels of vitamin K, you should avoid increasing your intake of these foods while taking Coumadin. You can usually eat the same levels you're accustomed to—just don't increase your consumption. Your physician will monitor your blood clotting ability and will change your dose up or down as needed. In addition to foods high in vitamin K, other natural remedies may interact with Coumadin. For example:

- Coenzyme Q_{10} and Saint-John's-wort (*Hypericum perforatum*) may reduce Coumadin's efficacy

- Proteolytic enzymes, such as nattokinase and bromelain, and several herbs, including Chinese ginseng (*Panax ginseng*), devil's claw (*Harpagophytum procumbens*), and dong quai (*Angelica sinensis*), can increase Coumadin's effects.

- It's likely that you can continue using these products, but don't change the dosage from what your body is accustomed to. Clotting values must be monitored appropriately.

- Garlic (*Allium sativum*) and ginkgo biloba extracts may reduce the ability of platelets to stick together, increasing the likelihood of bleeding. However, neither appears to interact directly with Coumadin. We generally tell people taking Coumadin to avoid these products at higher dosages (more than the equivalent of one clove of garlic per day for garlic or more than 240 mg per day of ginkgo extract) but not to worry if they are just on the typical support dose of garlic or ginkgo.

- Iron, magnesium, and zinc may bind with Coumadin, potentially decreasing its absorption and activity. Take Coumadin and products that contain iron, magnesium, or zinc products at least two hours apart.

To reduce the likelihood of bleeding and easy bruising with Coumadin, we recommend taking 150 to 300 mg of either grape seed or pine bark extract per day.

Citicoline and Gylcerophosphocholine

Citicoline (CDP-choline) and glycerophosphocholine (GPC) are well absorbed and highly bioavailable sources of choline. In double-blind studies both have been shown to be useful in promoting recovery from a stroke.[4]

A 2002 analysis looked at four double-blind studies with oral citicoline for acute ischemic stroke.[5] All were performed in the United States and used various doses of oral citicoline (500, 1,000, or 2,000 mg per day) or placebos. In all cases, citicoline was begun within 24 hours after stroke onset and continued for six weeks. At the three-month check-up, results indicated that citicoline improved by 29% the probability that the patient would recover the ability to participate in activities of daily living and by 42% the probability of recovering functional capacity. However, it did not increase neurological recovery to any significant degree. Nonetheless, these results are very encouraging, as any improvement over a placebo can have profound real-life benefits.[6]

GPC is even better studied, as it has been administered in six clinical trials to almost 3,000 patients suffering from a stroke.[7-13] In all of these trials, the patients were started within 10 days after having a stroke. The trials consisted of two phases: during the first phase of 28 days, generally in a hospital, GPC was given intramuscularly at 1,000 mg per day. During the second phase, from day 29 to day 180, GPC was given orally at 1,200 mg per day (400 mg three times per day). The single largest trial was conducted at 176 centers in Italy and included 2,044 patients.[8] At the end of the six-month trial, the investigators found that GPC significantly helped

QUICK REVIEW

- **Stroke is the leading cause of adult disability in the United States and the third-leading cause of death.**
- **High blood pressure is the most important risk factor of stroke.**
- **Ginkgo biloba extract increases blood flow to the brain, improves the production of energy within nerve cells, and favorably affects blood viscosity (thickness), resulting in improved blood flow characteristics within the brain.**
- **It is important to use natural products with caution when taking drugs that inhibit platelets or blood clotting.**
- **Citicoline and glycerophosphocholine are well absorbed and highly bioavailable sources of choline shown to be useful in promoting recovery from a stroke.**
- **Acupuncture can often help stroke patients perform self-care better, can mean that patients require less nursing care and less rehabilitation therapy, and can possibly cut health care costs.**

more than 95% of patients and was without side effects. Overall, GPC was judged by 78% of investigators as "very good" or "good," by 17% as "moderate," and by just 5% as having "poor" or "no" efficacy.

Acupuncture

There is some clinical research showing that acupuncture can facilitate recovery from a stroke. Specifically, acupuncture can often help stroke patients perform self-care better, can mean that patients require less nursing and less rehabilitation therapy, and can possibly cut health care costs. Possible mechanisms of its effects include stimulation of nerve cell regrowth, facilitation of improved nerve cell function, reduction of poststroke inflammatory reactions, and prevention of nerve cell death. Given its safety and possible benefits, acupuncture is very much worth the effort.[14,15]

TREATMENT SUMMARY

In most cases, a stroke is a consequence of atherosclerosis. That being the case, appropriate prevention of further strokes involves following the recommendations in the chapter "Heart and Cardiovascular Health." It may also be appropriate to consult the chapter "High Cholesterol and/or Triglycerides" and the chapter "High Blood Pressure," especially as hypertension is a major cause of stroke. The primary therapeutic goal in the recovery from a stroke is to enhance the blood and oxygen supply to the brain as well as improve nerve cell function.

Nutritional Supplements

- A high-potency multiple vitamin and mineral formula as described in the chapter "Supplementary Measures"
- Vitamin D$_3$: 2,000 to 4,000 IU per day (ideally, measure blood levels and adjust dosage accordingly)
- Fish oils: 1,000 to 3,000 mg EPA + DHA per day

- One of the following:
  - Grape seed extract (>95% procyanidolic oligomers): 100 to 300 mg per day
  - Pine bark extract (>95% procyanidolic oligomers): 100 to 300 mg per day
  - Some other flavonoid-rich extract with a similar flavonoid content, super greens formula, or another plant-based antioxidant that can provide an oxygen radical absorption capacity (ORAC) of 3,000 to 6,000 units or more per day
- One of the following:
  - Citicoline: 1,000 to 2,000 mg per day
  - Glycerophosphocholine: 400 mg three times per day
  - CoQ$_{10}$: 50 to 100 mg three times per day

Botanical Medicines

- Ginkgo biloba extract (24% ginkgo flavonglycosides): 240 to 320 mg per day
- Garlic: the equivalent of 4,000 mg per day of fresh garlic

Systemic Lupus Erythematosus

Systemic lupus erythematosus (SLE) is a systemic autoimmune disease that can affect any part of the body. In autoimmune diseases the immune system attacks the body's cells and tissue, resulting in inflammation and tissue damage. In SLE, the tissues most often damaged are the heart, joints, skin, lungs, blood vessels, liver, kidneys, and nervous system.

SLE can vary in severity and clinical course. There are often times of remission interrupted by periods of illness (called flares). SLE occurs nine times more often in women than in men. It most often affects women in their childbearing years (ages 15 to 35) and is also more common in women of non-European descent.

Causes

There is abundant evidence that SLE is an autoimmune reaction in which antibodies formed by the immune system attack components of joint tissues. Yet what triggers this autoimmune reaction remains largely unknown. Speculation and investigation have centered on genetic factors, abnormal bowel permeability, lifestyle, nutritional factors, food allergies, and microorganisms.

As with other autoimmune diseases, there is definitely a genetic predisposition for SLE. However, research indicates that this predis-

position requires an environmental trigger. Since 90% of patients with SLE are female, there appears to be a hormonal aspect or some protective factor on the X chromosome. Defective manufacture of male sex hormones (androgens) has been proposed as a potential predisposing factor for SLE.[1]

Researchers have also sought to find a connection between certain infectious agents (viruses and bacteria), but no organism can be consistently linked to the disease.

Drug-induced lupus erythematosus (DILE) is an autoimmune disorder similar to SLE and caused by chronic use of certain drugs. There is a long list of medications known to cause DILE, but the three associated with the highest number of cases are hydralazine, procainamide, and isoniazid. Generally, the symptoms recede after the drugs are discontinued.

Therapeutic Considerations

The general approach to SLE from a naturopathic perspective is nearly identical to the approach to rheumatoid arthritis (RA); see that chapter. Just as in RA, the major focus in dietary therapy for SLE is to eliminate food allergies, increase the intake of antioxidant-rich food and nutrients, follow a vegetarian diet, and alter the intake of dietary fats and oils. Vegetarian diets are often beneficial in the treatment of inflammatory conditions such as SLE, presumably as a result of decreasing the availability of arachidonic acid (found in animal products) for conversion to inflammatory compounds. Another important way in which a vegetarian diet may be helpful is that is has a higher alkalinity than a meat-based diet. And, just as in RA, fish oils have shown considerable benefit in improving symptoms and disease activity scores in SLE.[2–4]

DHEA

As stated above under "Causes," a defect in male sex hormone production is common in SLE. Supplemental DHEA has shown therapeutic benefits in patients with SLE in several studies. Clinical research began with a small preliminary study in which DHEA use was associated with improved SLE disease activity index scores and decreased prednisone use.[5] Each patient received 200

> **WARNING:** For SLE treatment, given the high dosages of DHEA required to show benefit, we strongly recommend against self-medication. Because of substantial risk of side effects, working with a physician to monitor the proper dosage and benefit of DHEA is necessary.

mg per day of DHEA for three to six months. Eight of the 10 patients reported improvements in overall well-being, fatigue, energy, and/or other symptoms. For the group as a whole, there was a significant improvement in the physician's overall assessment of disease activity. After three months, the average prednisone requirement had decreased from 14.5 to 9.4 mg per day.

This study has been followed up with several higher-quality studies. In a double-blind study, 28 female patients with mild to moderate SLE were given DHEA (200 mg per day) or a placebo for three months.[6] In the patients receiving DHEA, the average dosage of corticosteroids dropped by 30% while

- -

QUICK REVIEW

- **Systemic lupus erythematosus (SLE) is a systemic autoimmune disease that can affect any part of the body.**
- **Like other autoimmune diseases, there is definitely a genetic predisposition for SLE. However, research indicates that this predisposition requires an environmental trigger.**
- **The general approach to SLE from a naturopathic perspective is nearly identical to the approach to rheumatoid arthritis.**
- **Vegetarian diets are often beneficial in the treatment of inflammatory conditions such as SLE, presumably as a result of decreasing the availability of arachidonic acid for conversion to inflammatory compounds.**
- **Fish oils have shown considerable benefit in improving symptoms and disease activity scores in SLE.**
- **A defect in male sex hormone production is common in SLE. Supplemental DHEA (under physician supervision) has shown therapeutic benefits in patients with SLE in several studies.**

the dosage rose by 40% in the placebo group. There were three lupus flare-ups in the DHEA group, compared with eight in the placebo group. A larger double-blind trial involving 191 patients with SLE confirmed that DHEA supplementation could be associated with a modest stabilization of disease and reduction in steroid dose.[7] Other studies have also showed that DHEA improved quality-of-life scores in SLE patients.[8,9] In all of these studies, mild acne was a common side effect of DHEA at these dosages.

Botanical Medicines

Please consult the chapter "Rheumatoid Arthritis" for more information. Dosages are given below for our recommendations.

- -

TREATMENT SUMMARY

SLE is often an aggressive disease that needs aggressive treatment. In mild to moderate cases, the measures below are extremely effective. Foremost is the use of diet to reduce the causes and ameliorate the symptoms. Symptom relief can also be attained through the use of nutritional supplements, botanical medicines, and physical medicine techniques. In severe cases, drug therapy may be necessary, at least in the acute phase. However, do not abandon natural measures, because they will actually enhance the effectiveness of the drugs, allowing for lower dosages when drugs are necessary, while providing a foundation for healing by addressing the underlying causative factors and utilizing modalities that are both safe and beneficial in long-term use. Please see the chapter "Rheumatoid Arthritis" for a more complete discussion of our recommended treatments.

Diet

The first step is a therapeutic fast or elimination diet, followed by careful reintroduction of individual foods to detect those that trigger symptoms. Although any food can cause a reaction, the most common are wheat, corn, dairy products, beef, foods in the nightshade family (tomatoes, potatoes, eggplant, peppers), pork, citrus, oats, rye, egg, coffee, peanuts, cane sugar, lamb, and soy.

After all allergens have been isolated and eliminated, a vegetarian or Mediterranean-style diet rich in organic whole foods, vegetables, cold-water fish (mackerel, herring, sardines, and salmon), olive oil, and berries and low in sugar, meat, refined carbohydrates, and animal fats is indicated. The recommendations in the chapter "A Health-Promoting Diet" are appropriate in the long-term support of SLE.

Nutritional Supplements

- A high-potency multiple vitamin and mineral formula as described in the chapter "Supplementary Measures"
- Key individual nutrients:
  ○ Vitamin C: 500 to 1,000 mg per day
  ○ Selenium: 200 to 400 mcg per day

- ○ Vitamin E (mixed tocopherols): 200 to 400 IU per day
- ○ Vitamin D$_3$: 2,000 to 4,000 IU per day (ideally, measure blood levels and adjust dosage accordingly)
- Fish oils: 3,000 mg EPA + DHA per day for seven days; 1,000 mg per day thereafter
- One of the following:
  - ○ Grape seed extract (>95% procyanidolic oligomers): 150 to 300 mg per day
  - ○ Pine bark extract (>90% procyanidolic oligomers): 150 to 300 mg per day
- Probiotic (*Lactobacillus* species and *Bifidobacterium* species): a minimum of 5 billion to 10 billion colony-forming units
- One of the following:
  - ○ Pancreatin (10X USP): 350 to 750 mg between meals three times per day
  - ○ Bromelain: 250 to 750 mg (1,800 to 2,000 MCU) between meals three times per day

Botanical Medicines

- One of the following:
  - ○ Meriva: 500 to 1,000 mg twice daily
  - ○ BCM95 Complex: 750 to 1,500 mg twice daily
  - ○ Theracurmin: 300 mg one to three times daily
- Ginger:
  - ○ 8 to 10 g dried ginger
  - ○ Ginger extracts standardized to contain 20% gingerol and shogaol: 100 to 200 mg three times per day

Physical Medicine

- Heat (moist packs, hot baths, etc.): 20 to 30 minutes, one to three times per day
- Cold packs for acute flare-ups or following heat

Other Considerations

- Improving digestion with hydrochloric acid supplementation may be useful. Positive results from other tests may indicate that treatment for intestinal permeability, dysbiosis, and environmental toxicity is advisable.
- DHEA may be taken under the supervision of a physician.

Uterine Fibroids

- The majority are without symptoms but may be associated with vague feelings of discomfort, pressure, congestion, bloating, and heaviness; can include pain with vaginal sexual activity, urinary frequency, backache, abdominal enlargement, and abnormal bleeding
- Abnormal bleeding in 30% of women with fibroids

Uterine fibroids are bundles of smooth muscle and connective tissue that can be as small as a pea or as large as a grapefruit. Although they are sometimes called tumors, fibroids are not cancerous. However, because they disrupt the blood vessels and glands in the uterus, they can cause bleeding and loss of other fluids. Around 30% of women over age 30 have at least one fibroid. Hysterectomies due to fibroids are the most common major surgery in women. Uterine fibroids are classified according to their location, as follows:

- Submucosal (just under the lining of the uterus)
- Intramural (within the uterine muscle wall)
- Subserosal (just inside the outer wall of the uterus)
- Interligamentous (in the cervix between the two layers of the broad ligament)
- Pedunculated (on a stalk, either submucosal or subserous)

Causes

Increases in local estrogen (specifically estradiol) concentration within the fibroid itself are thought to play a role in the development and growth of fibroids. Concentrations of estrogen receptors are higher in fibroid tissue than in the surrounding tissue. In addition to an excess of estrogen production within the body, a strong case can be made for the role of the most significant environmental factor assaulting female hormonal health—compounds known as xenoestrogens. These compounds are also known as endocrine or hormone disrupters, environmental estrogens, hormonally active agents, estrogenic substances, estrogenic xenobiotics, and bioactive chemicals. Examples of xenoestrogens include phthalates (used in plastics), pesticides, tobacco smoke by-products, and various solvents. Xenoestrogens enhance or block the effects of estrogen in the body by binding to estrogen receptors. They also promote a shift from healthy estrogen breakdown products to cancer-causing estrogen metabolites.

Therapeutic Considerations

Reducing the size as well as the symptoms of uterine fibroids with natural medicines is easily accomplished in most cases. Unfortunately, this statement is supported more by the clinical experiences of naturopathic physicians than by scientific evidence, though the approach is scientifically rational—that is, if uterine fibroids are caused by an excess of estrogen produced in the body as well as the effects of xenoestrogens, it makes sense that reducing estrogenic influences should shrink uterine fibroids. Keep in mind that as women pass through menopause there is less estrogen and so there will also be a tendency for the fibroid to shrink on its own.

Diet

The most important dietary recommendations are to eat a high-fiber diet rich in phytoestrogens (plant estrogens) and to avoid saturated fat, sugar, and caffeine. These simple changes can dramatically reduce circulating estrogen levels and reduce estrogen's influence on the fibroid. One study looked at what happened when women switched from the standard American diet (40% of calories from fat; only 12 g fiber per day) to a healthier diet (25% of calories from fat; 40 g fiber). Results showed a 36% reduction in blood estrogen levels within 8 to 10 weeks.[1]

Phytoestrogens are able to bind to the same cell receptors as the estrogen your body produces. That's a good thing, because when phytoestrogens occupy the receptors, estrogen can't affect cells. By competing with estrogen, phytoestrogens cause a drop in estrogen effects, and are thus sometimes called antiestrogens. Great sources of phytoestrogens include soy and soy foods, ground flaxseed, and nuts and seeds. In particular, we recommend eating 1 to 2 tbsp of ground flaxseed per day.

These dietary recommendations have extreme significance not only in treating uterine fibroids but also in reducing endometrial cancer. Women with uterine fibroids have a fourfold increase in the risk of endometrial cancer. In a case-control study of a multi-

ethnic population (Japanese, white, Native Hawaiian, Filipino, and Chinese) examining the role of dietary soy, fiber, and related foods and nutrients in the risk of endometrial cancer, 332 women with endometrial cancer were compared with women in the general multiethnic population, and all women were interviewed by means of a dietary questionnaire.[2] The researchers found the following associations: a higher fat intake increased the risk of endometrial cancer, a higher fiber intake reduced the risk for endometrial cancer, and a high consumption of soy products and other legumes decreased the risk of endometrial cancer. Similar reductions in risk were found for greater consumption of other sources of phytoestrogens, such as whole grains, vegetables, fruits, and seaweed. The researchers concluded that plant-based diets low in calories from fat, high in fiber, and rich in legumes (especially soybeans), whole grain foods, vegetables, and fruits reduce the risk of endometrial cancer. These dietary associations may explain at least in part the lower rates of uterine cancer in Asian countries than in the United States. Vegetarians also have lower circulating estrogen levels than omnivorous women.[3]

Some have suggested that since soy foods are high in phytoestrogens (specifically isoflavones), which have a weak estrogenic effect, women with uterine fibroids or endometrial cancer should avoid phytoestrogens. This recommendation does not have merit. Soy isoflavones appear to be selective in terms of the tissues in which they have an estrogenic effect and the tissues in which their effect is antiestrogenic. Soy phytoestrogens do not appear to have an estrogenic effect on the human uterus and may in fact help shrink uterine fibroids due to an antiestrogenic effect. We recommend moderate but not excessive soy consumption in the range of 45 to 90 mg soy isoflavones per day. See the chapter "Menopause" for more information on the isoflavone content of soy foods.

Nutritional Supplements

Historically, naturopaths have used lipotropic factors such as inositol and choline to support the healthy detoxification of estrogen. Lipotropic factors promote the removal of fat from the liver. Lipotropic supplements usually are a combination of vitamins and herbs designed to support the liver's function in removing fat, detoxifying the body's wastes, detoxifying external harmful substances (pesticides, flame retardants, plastics, etc.), and metabolizing and excreting estrogens. These lipotropic products vary in their formulations depending on the manufacturer, but they are all similar and are meant for the same uses.

Many now contain anticancer phytonutrients found in vegetables from the brassica family, such as indole-3-carbinol, di-indoylmethane, and sulforaphane. Research has shown that these compounds help to break down cancer-causing forms of estrogens to nontoxic forms, making them especially important for women with uterine fibroids.[4–6]

Botanical Medicines

Many plants have been used in traditional herbal medicines in the treatment of women with uterine fibroids. Most of these plants contain phytoestrogens. However, their activity is certainly less than the effects of dietary phytoestrogens such as soy and flax. So we recommend focusing on dietary phytoestrogens rather than botanical sources.

QUICK REVIEW

- **Increases in local estrogen (specifically estradiol) concentration within the uterine fibroid itself are thought to play a role in cause and growth.**
- **Xenoestrogens are thought to also play a role in uterine fibroids.**
- **The most important dietary recommendations are to eat a high-fiber diet rich in phytoestrogens while avoiding saturated fat, sugar, and caffeine.**
- **Research has shown that compounds from vegetables in the brassica family help to break down cancer-causing forms of estrogens to nontoxic forms, making them especially important in women with uterine fibroids.**

TREATMENT SUMMARY

When uterine fibroids cause heavy bleeding, medical management is definitely necessary. Sometimes surgery is required. Newer, nonsurgical techniques such as high-intensity focused ultrasound are also now available.

Diet

Follow the guidelines in the chapter "A Health-Promoting Diet." Consume a diet low in fat and high in fiber, whole grains, and soy foods and avoid saturated fats, sugar, caffeine, and alcohol. Soy isoflavone intake should be between 45 and 90 mg per day. Ground flaxseed at a dosage of 1 to 2 tbsp per day is also recommended.

Nutritional Supplements

- A high-potency multiple vitamin and mineral formula as described in the chapter "Supplementary Measures"
- Vitamin D_3: 2,000 to 4,000 IU per day (ideally, measure blood levels and adjust dosage accordingly)
- Fish oils: 1,000 mg EPA + DHA per day
- Flaxseed oil: 1 tbsp per day
- One of the following:
  - Grape seed extract (>95% procyanidolic oligomers): 100 to 300 mg per day
  - Pine bark extract (>95% procyanidolic oligomers): 100 to 300 mg per day
  - Some other flavonoid-rich extract with a similar flavonoid content, super greens formula, or another plant-based antioxidant that can provide an oxygen radical absorption capacity (ORAC) of 3,000 to 6,000 units or more per day
- Specialty supplements, one of the following:
  - Lipotropic formula providing 1,000 mg betaine, 1,000 mg choline, and 1,000 mg cysteine or methionine
  - SAM-e: 200 to 400 mg per day
- One or a combination of the following:
  - Indole-3-carbinol (I3C): 300 to 600 mg per day
  - Di-indoylmethane (DIM): 100 to 200 mg per day

Vaginitis

· ·

- Increased volume of vaginal secretions
- Abnormal color, consistency, or odor of vaginal secretions
- Vulvovaginal itching, burning, or irritation
- Painful urination or intercourse

Vaginitis is an infection of the vaginal tract. It is one of the most common reasons for women to seek medical attention. In addition to causing physical discomfort and embarrassment, vaginitis is medically important for several reasons: (1) it may be a symptom of a more serious underlying problem, such as chronic inflammation of the cervix (cervicitis) or a sexually transmitted disease; (2) the infection may travel into the uterus and lead to pelvic inflammatory disease, a serious situation that can result in infertility due to scarring of the fallopian tubes; and (3) chronic vaginal infections are often the underlying cause of recurrent urinary tract infections because they serve as a reservoir of the infectious bacteria.

Causes

Vaginitis may be sexually transmitted or may arise from a disturbance to the delicate ecology of the healthy vagina. In many instances, vaginal infections involve an overgrowth of common organisms normally found in the vagina of many healthy women. In normal situations these microbes do not cause any problems, but when there is a disturbance in the vaginal environment a normally present microbe can overgrow and produce an infection.

Factors influencing the vaginal environment include pH, tissue sugar (glycogen) content, blood sugar (glucose) level, presence of "friendly" organisms (particularly *Lactobacillus acidophilus*), natural flushing action of vaginal secretions, presence of blood (menstruation), spermicides and lubricants, and presence of antibodies and other compounds in the vaginal secretions. These factors are, in turn, affected by such things as low immune function as a result of nutritional deficiencies, medications (e.g., steroids, birth control pills), pregnancy, serious illness, diabetes, and the wearing of panty hose (which tend to prevent drying of the area). In fact, vaginal yeast infections are three times more prevalent in women wearing panty hose than those wearing cotton underwear.[1]

Risk factors for sexually transmitted infections include increased numbers of sexual partners, unusual sexual practices, and the type of birth control used (barrier methods reduce risk of infection, while birth control pills increase risk of infection).

Approximately 90% of cases of vulvovaginitis will be associated with one of three organisms, *Trichomonas vaginalis*, *Candida albicans*, or *Gardnerella vaginalis*. The relative frequency of each form varies with the population studied, as well as with sexual activity levels. Less frequent causes of vaginitis include *Neisseria gonorrhea*, herpesvirus,

Diagnostic Differentiation of Common Causes of Infectious Vaginitis	CANDIDA	NSV/BV	TRICHOMONAS	GONORRHEA	HERPES	CHLAMYDIA
Key symptoms	Itching	Odor	Odor and itching	No symptoms, or painful cervicitis	Vesicles (small blisters) or ulcers	Usually without symptoms
Discharge pH	<4.5	>4.5	>5.0	<4.5	<4.5	<4.5
Odor	None	Fishy/amines	May be fishy	None	None	None
Appearance	Curdy, adherent, scant to thick	Gray, even consistency	Greenish yellow, frothy	Bloody and pus-filled	None	None
Pelvic exam	Adherent white patches with a reddened border	Unremarkable	May show reddened bumps on cervix—a "strawberry" cervix—or vaginal lining	Cervical discharge, may have pelvic tenderness	Small, multiple vesicles or ulcers on cervix or labia	May show signs of pelvic inflammatory disease

and *Chlamydia trachomatis*. Each is described more fully below.

The preceding table summarizes the diagnostic differentiation of the most common causes of infectious vaginitis.

Candida albicans

The relative frequency and the total incidence of vaginal yeast infections (candidal vaginitis) have increased dramatically in the past 40 years. Several factors have contributed to this increased incidence, chief among them being the increased use of antibiotics. The problem with vaginal yeast infections as a result of antibiotic use is well known by virtually every woman.

Most cases of recurrent candidal vaginitis are due either to transmission of candida from the gastrointestinal tract or to failure to recognize and treat the presence of one or more predisposing factors.[2] In extremely persistent cases, sexual partners may be a source of reinfection. Allergies have also been reported to cause recurrent candidiasis, which resolves when the allergies are treated.[3]

Predisposing Factors in Candidal Vaginitis

Allergies

Antibiotics

Diabetes

Elevated vaginal pH

Gastrointestinal candidiasis

Oral contraceptives

Panty hose

Pregnancy

Steroids

The primary symptom of a vaginal yeast infection is vulvar itching, which can be quite severe. Candida vaginitis is often associated with the presence of a thick, curdy, or "cottage cheese" discharge, which may reveal pinpoint bleeding when removed. The presence of such a discharge is strong evidence of a yeast infection, but its absence does not rule out candida.

Nonspecific Vaginitis or Bacterial Vaginosis

This category is defined as vaginitis not due to trichomonas, gonorrhea, or candida. Whereas itching is the predominant symptom of candidal vaginitis, the presence of a discharge and odor are the keynotes of nonspecific vaginitis (NSV) or bacterial vaginosis (BV). Both terms are used to describe a shift in vaginal flora from a predominance of lactobacilli to a predominance of a type of bacteria that degrade the mucins forming a natural barrier on the vaginal lining. This destruction of the mucin layer causes a vaginal discharge characteristic of NSV/BV. The odor is variously described as fishy, foul, or rotten, and reflects the production of the breakdown of proteins by bacteria. The discharge is nonirritating, gray, and usually of even consistency, though it may occasionally be frothy or even thick and pasty.

One of the most common causes of NSV/BV is routine douching. This practice is associated with a loss of vaginal lactobacilli. The organism most frequently cited as responsible for NSV/BV is *Gardnerella vaginalis* (formerly called *Haemophilus vaginalis*). However, although this bacterium is found in 95% of women with NSV/BV, it is also found in 40% of women who do not have vaginitis. It is very likely that *Gardnerella vaginalis* prospers in the conditions of NSV/BV but that the responsible organism may be another type of bacteria or simply the loss of proper balance in the vagina.

Trichomonas vaginalis

Trichomonas vaginalis is a single-celled organism that is transmitted by sexual intercourse. Trichomonas does not invade tissues and rarely causes serious complications. The most frequent symptom is vaginal discharge with itching and burning. The discharge is frequently smelly, greenish yellow, and frothy. This organism grows optimally at a pH of 5.5 to 5.8. Thus, a vaginal pH outside this range in a woman with vaginitis is suggestive of an agent other than trichomonas. Looking at vaginal fluid under a microscope will confirm the diagnosis in 80 to 90% of cases.

Gonorrhea

Neisseria gonorrhea is an uncommon cause of vaginitis, responsible for less than 4% of cases. Gonococcal vaginitis is more common in young girls because the vaginal epithelium is thinner before puberty. During the reproductive years, severe infection of the cervix is the primary symptom (painful, bloody, pus-filled discharge). Gonorrhea, either alone or in combination with other organisms, is cultured in 40 to 60% of cases of pelvic inflammatory disease, a major cause of infertility. Because of the potential for serious consequences, sexually active women experiencing any symptoms suggestive of gonorrhea must consult a physician immediately.

Herpes simplex

Herpes simplex (herpesvirus infection) is the most common cause of genital ulcers in the United States. For a more thorough discussion see the chapter "Herpes."

Chlamydia trachomatis

Chlamydia trachomatis is a parasite that lives within human cells. It rarely causes vaginitis on its own but is frequently found in association with other common causes such as *Candida albicans*. Chlamydia is another sexually transmitted disease that is now recognized as a major health problem in the United States. Chlamydia infects 5 to 10% of sexually active women and is usually without symptoms until the development of complications, such as infections of the cervix, fallopian tubes, or urethra. Chlamydia is the organism most frequently recovered in cultures of women with pelvic inflammatory disease, a severe infection of the female genital tract. Chlamydia infections are the major cause of infertility due to scarring of the fallopian tubes.

Chlamydial infection during pregnancy increases the risk of prematurity and infant death. If a healthy baby is born to an infected woman, there is a 50% chance it will develop chlamydial infection of the eyes and a 10% chance of pneumonia. Because of the considerable risks of untreated chlamydia, we again recommend consulting a physician immediately if you are suffering from any suspicious symptoms.

Therapeutic Considerations

Although vaginitis is usually due to *Candida albicans* and is almost always self-treated with over-the-counter preparations, there is the possibility of a more serious cause of vaginitis, and so we strongly recommend consulting a physician for a definitive diagnosis. The natural treatments given below are recommended only after consultation with a health care provider. The focus is on the treatment of candida vaginitis, but the same principles also apply to trichomonas, NSV, and BV. For chlamydial and gonorrheal vaginitis we recommend conventional antibiotic therapy given the serious risk of tubal scarring and other complications.

The goals of therapy are to identify and eliminate or reduce contributing factors, to improve immune function and defense mechanisms, and to reestablish proper bacterial flora.

Diet

The recommendations in the chapter "Candidiasis, Chronic," are appropriate here, especially in dealing with candida vaginitis. Do not eat refined carbohydrates and simple sugars. Do not eat foods with a high content of yeast or mold, including alcoholic beverages, cheeses, dried fruits, melons, and peanuts. Avoid all known or suspected food allergies.

Nutritional Supplements

Lactobacillus acidophilus

The normal microflora of the vagina is dominated by lactobacilli capable of inhibiting the adhesion and growth of infectious organisms. Lactobacilli produce this effect through at least three mechanisms: (1) they help to produce lactic acid and other acids to provide a normal vaginal acidic environment of 3.5 to 4.5, which inhibits the growth of many disease-causing organisms; (2) lactobacilli

produce hydrogen peroxide, which inhibits microbial growth; and (3) lactobacilli are competitive with other microorganisms for adherence to the vaginal lining.[4-6]

Due to the importance of lactobacilli, one of the primary goals in successfully treating and preventing recurrent vaginal infections is reestablishing the normal vaginal flora. In particular, *Lactobacillus acidophilus* is an integral component of the normal vaginal flora and helps to prevent the overgrowth of *Candida albicans* and less desirable bacterial species.

Reestablishment of normal vaginal lactobacilli can be accomplished by douching twice a day with an acidophilus-containing solution. The solution can be prepared by using a high-quality acidophilus supplement or an active-culture yogurt (careful reading of labels is important, since most commercially available yogurts do not use live lactobacilli). Dissolve enough of either choice in 10 ml water to provide 10 billion organisms. Use a syringe to douche the material into the vagina. Since lactobacilli are normal inhabitants of the vaginal flora, the douche can be retained in the vagina as long as desired. We suggest also taking lactobacilli orally, as women with vaginal yeast overgrowth will often have an overgrowth in the gut as well. Several clinical studies have confirmed that the use of lactobacillus in the vagina as well as oral supplementation is effective in eliminating candidal vaginitis and improving the vaginal flora.[7-11]

Topical Treatments

Vitamin C

Vaginal vitamin C therapy has been used to treat BV. A randomized, double-blind, placebo-controlled study used one 250-mg tablet of vitamin C inserted vaginally once a day for six days. Fifty subjects were given the active treatment and 50 were given a placebo. Significantly more patients still had BV in the placebo group (35.7%) compared with the vitamin C group (14%). Anaerobic bacteria disappeared in 77% of the vitamin C group vs. 54% of the placebo group, and lactobacilli reappeared in 79.1% of vitamin C group vs. 53.3% in the placebo group.[12]

Local Antiseptics

There are a number of natural antiseptic compounds that can be used during the infectious stage to get rid of the offending organisms. The discussion below will focus on iodine, boric acid, and tea tree oil, as these appear to be the most effective. In fact, their effectiveness has been shown to be as good as or better than that of standard antibiotic therapy for the common causes of vaginitis (*Trichomonas vaginalis*, *Candida albicans*, and *Gardnerella vaginalis*). Be sure to always follow these antimicrobial douches with lactobacilli douches.

Iodine. Iodine used topically as a douche is effective against a wide range of infectious agents linked to vaginal infections, including those due to trichomonas, candida, chlamydia, and nonspecific vaginitis. This is the strongest of the douches, so we recommend it be used only if the gentler approaches are inadequate. Povidone-iodine solution (Betadine) has all the advantages of iodine without the disadvantages of stinging and staining. Betadine is available at any pharmacy. A douching solution diluted to 1 tsp povidone-iodine solution in 2 cups water used twice per day for 14 days is effective against most organisms.[13–19] A study published in 1962 found povidone-iodine to be effective in treating 100% of cases of candidal vaginitis, 80% of cases of trichomonas, and 93% of cases of combination infections.[18] However, excessive use must be avoided, since some iodine will be absorbed into the system and can cause suppression of thyroid function. In addition, recognize that iodine is indiscriminate in the bacteria it kills, so following up with a lactobacilli douche is critical.

Boric Acid. Capsules of boric acid inserted into the vagina have been used to treat candidiasis with success rates equal to or better than those of nystatin and creams containing miconazole, clotrimazole, or butoconazole.[20–23] Boric acid treatment offers an inexpensive, easily accessible therapy for vaginal yeast infections. In a study of 92 women with chronic vaginal yeast infections, boric acid treatment was shown to be significantly more effective.[23] The dosage was 600 mg boric acid in a vaginal suppository twice per day for two weeks. As well as being more effective in relieving symptoms, boric acid also demonstrated a more significant improvement with microscopic examination of a vaginal swab. In fact, no patient receiving antifungal drugs had a normal microscopic exam. All exams in these patients demonstrated continued presence of yeast, damaged

Outcome of Therapy with Conventional Antifungal Agents and Boric Acid		
AGENT	**RESOLUTION OF SYMPTOMS (% OF PATIENTS)**	**ABNORMAL MICROSCOPIC FINDINGS (% OF PATIENTS)**
Antifungals	52%	100%
Boric acid	98%	2%

cells lining the vagina, or some other abnormality.

In chronic cases of vaginal yeast infections standard antifungal agents are often ineffective. In these cases, it is definitely recommended that boric acid (600 mg) be used twice a day for four months. After this time further use may not be necessary except during menstruation.

Side effects with boric acid are quite rare. The most common side effect is burning of the labia due to boric acid leaking out of the vagina. If this occurs, reduce the amount of boric acid or discontinue use.

Tea Tree Oil. Tea tree (*Melaleuca alternifolia*) oil diluted to 1% in water exerts a strong antibacterial and antifungal action. It was shown in one study to be effective in treatment of trichomoniasis, candidiasis, and cervicitis. Treatment consists of a daily douche combined with saturated tampons used weekly. No adverse reactions were reported, and patients commented favorably on its soothing effect.[24]

QUICK REVIEW

- **Consult a physician for immediate and accurate diagnosis of vaginal infections.**
- **Infectious vaginitis may be sexually transmitted or may arise from a disturbance to the ecology of the healthy vagina.**
- **Approximately 90% of vulvovaginitis will be associated with one of three organisms: *Trichomonas vaginalis, Candida albicans,* or *Gardnerella vaginalis.***
- **The goals of therapy are to identify and eliminate or reduce contributing factors, improve immune function and defense mechanisms, and reestablish proper bacterial flora with *Lactobacillus acidophilus.***
- **Iodine, boric acid, and tea tree oil can be used as vaginal antiseptics.**

TREATMENT SUMMARY

Since approximately 90% of all vaginitis is due to candida, trichomonas, or *Gardnerella* infections, the following recommendations are primarily directed toward treatment of these organisms. Immune support (through proper diet, nutritional supplementation, and botanical medicines) is an important aspect of the therapy. For recurrent infections, please follow the recommendations in the chapter "Immune System Support."

General Recommendations

- Consult a physician for accurate diagnosis.
- Treatment failures may be due to incor-

rect diagnosis, reinfection, failure to treat predisposing factors, or resistance to the treatment used.

- In all cases of vaginitis, it is important to use live lactobacillus preparations to reestablish in the vagina a healthy colony of these desirable organisms.

- Sexual activity should be avoided during treatment to avoid reinfection and to reduce trauma to inflamed tissues. If this is not possible, at least ensure that condoms are used.

- In recurrent cases consider treating sexual partners.

- Wear cotton underwear.

Diet

The recommendations in the chapter "Candidiasis, Chronic," are appropriate here, especially in dealing with candida vaginitis. Do not eat refined carbohydrates and simple sugars. Do not eat foods with a high content of yeast or mold, including alcoholic beverages, cheeses, dried fruits, melons, and peanuts. Avoid all known or suspected food allergies.

Nutritional Supplements

- A high-potency multiple vitamin and mineral formula as described in the chapter "Supplementary Measures"

- Vitamin D_3: 2,000 to 4,000 IU per day (ideally, measure blood levels and adjust dosage accordingly)

- Fish oils: 1,000 mg EPA + DHA per day

- One of the following:
  - Grape seed extract (>95% procyanidolic oligomers): 100 to 300 mg per day

  - Pine bark extract (>95% procyanidolic oligomers): 100 to 300 mg per day

  - Or some other flavonoid-rich extract with a similar flavonoid content, super greens formula, or another plant-based antioxidant that can provide an oxygen radical absorption capacity (ORAC) of 3,000 to 6,000 units or more per day

- Probiotic (*Lactobacillus* species and *Bifidobacterium* species): a minimum of 5 billion to 20 billion colony-forming units per day

Topical Treatments

- One or more of the following agents (do not try to include all at once, as the variety provides alternatives for use in resistant cases):
  - Betadine (povidone-iodine solution): 1:100 dilution used as a douche twice per day for 14 days

  - Boric acid capsules: 600-mg capsule placed in vagina twice per day for 14 days (*Caution:* Repeated use of povidone-iodine solution or boric acid may cause irritation, and use for more than seven days may result in problems from systemic absorption.)

  - *Lactobacillus* species: Dissolve enough in 10 ml water to provide 10 billion organisms and use as a douche once per day for 14 days.

Varicose Veins

- Dilated, twisted veins in the legs
- May have no symptoms, or may be associated with fatigue, aching discomfort, a feeling of heaviness, or pain
- Possible swelling, darkening, and ulceration of the skin of the leg below the knee
- Women are affected four times as frequently as men

Veins are fairly frail structures. Defects in the wall of a vein and excessive pressure lead to dilation of the vein and damage to the valves. When the valves become damaged, the higher static pressure (which results when the valves no longer break up the gravitational pressure) results in the bulging veins known as *varicose veins*.

Varicose veins affect nearly 50% of middle-aged adults. The subcutaneous veins of the legs are the veins most commonly affected, owing to the gravitational pressure that standing exerts on them. When an individual stands for long periods, the pressure in the vein can increase by up to 10 times. Hence, individuals with occupations that require long periods of standing are at greatest risk for development of varicose veins.

Women are affected about four times as frequently as men; obese individuals have a much greater risk; and the risk rises with age owing to loss of tissue tone, loss of muscle mass, and weakening of the walls of the veins. Pregnancy, which increases venous pressure in the legs, may also lead to the development of varicose veins.

In general, varicose veins pose little harm if the involved vein is near the surface. These types of varicose veins are, however, cosmetically unappealing. Although significant symptoms are not common, the legs may feel heavy, tight, and tired. If the varicose veins are associated with significant chronic venous insufficiency, leg ulcers may form that are often difficult to resolve.

A more serious form of varicose vein involves obstruction and valve defects of the deeper veins of the leg. This type of varicose vein can lead to problems such as thrombophlebitis, pulmonary embolism, myocardial infarction, and stroke. Diagnosis is made by clinical signs and symptoms and diagnostic ultrasound.

Causes

The following are theories as to the causes of varicose veins:

- Genetic or functional weakness of the veins or venous valves.
- Excessive venous pressure due to a low dietary fiber–induced increase in straining during defecation.
- Long periods of standing and/or heavy lifting.
- Damage to the veins or venous valves secondary to thrombophlebitis.

The major cause of varicose veins is weakness of the vascular walls due to either abnor-

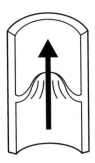 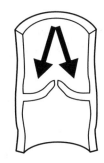

Healthy venous valves

Venous blood flows upward against gravity and any backflow is prevented by valves that shut against the flow.

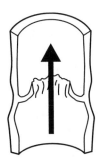 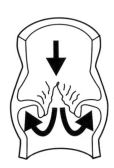

Varicose veins

The valves become damaged and do not function properly. Backflow of blood is not prevented and "pooling" of blood stretches and balloons the vein walls.

Vein Function in Normal and Varicose Veins

malities in the support structures of the vein or excessive expression, activity, or release of enzymes that degrade structural compounds. Damage to the lining of the vein also triggers infiltration of white blood cells, which can cause inflammation and lead to further vein wall damage, thus leading to chronic and progressive varicose vein formation.[1,2]

Therapeutic Considerations

The treatment of varicose veins ranges from conservative measures to surgical interventions. Conservative therapy involves the following:

- Elevating the legs periodically
- Wearing graduated compression stockings with variable pressure gradients, especially if standing for long periods of time is unavoidable
- Exercise, especially walking, riding a bike, or jogging, as contraction of the leg muscles pushes pooled blood back into circulation
- Achieving or maintaining ideal body weight.
- Maintaining adequate intake of dietary fiber to avoid straining during a bowel movement, which increases venous pressure
- Using nutritional and botanical agents to assist in improving the function and structural integrity of the veins

For severely affected veins, more aggressive treatment may be necessary. The traditional surgical treatment has been vein stripping to remove the affected veins. Newer, less invasive treatments seal the main leaking vein on the highest point of valvular dysfunction on the thigh. Because most of the blood in the legs is returned by the deep veins, the superficial veins, which return only about 10% of the total blood of the legs, can usually be removed or blocked off without serious harm.

Diet

A low-fiber diet that is high in refined foods contributes to the development of varicose veins.[3,4] Individuals consuming a low-fiber diet tend to strain more during bowel movements, because their smaller and harder stools are more difficult to pass. This straining raises the pressure in the abdomen, obstructing the flow of blood up the legs. The increased pressure, over time, may significantly weaken the vein walls, leading to the formation of varicose veins or hemorrhoids, or may weaken the wall of the large intestine and produce diverticuli.[5]

A diet rich in vegetables, fruits, legumes, and grains promotes peristalsis, and many fiber components attract water and form a gelatinous mass, which keeps the feces soft, bulky, and easy to pass. The net effect of a high-fiber diet is significantly less straining during defecation. Natural bulking compounds can also be used. These substances, particularly psyllium seed, pectin, and guar gum, possess mild laxative action owing to their ability to attract water and form a gelatinous mass. Soluble fiber is generally less irritating than wheat bran and other cellulose fiber products.

Flavonoids

Berries, such as hawthorn berries, cherries, blueberries, blackcurrants, and blackberries, appear to be beneficial in the prevention and treatment of varicose veins. These berries are very rich sources of proanthocyanidins and anthocyanidins.[6-8] These flavonoids are noted for their ability to improve the function and integrity of the vascular system. Extracts of several of these berries are used widely in Europe for various circulatory conditions.

Another rich source of flavonoids is buckwheat (*Fagopyrum esculentum*), which is high in rutin. In one double-blind, placebo-controlled study, 77 patients with chronic venous insufficiency were given placebo tea or buckwheat tea for 12 weeks. The tea was standardized to contain 5% total flavonoids, yielding a daily dosage of 270 mg rutin. A statistically significant reduction in the total volume of fluid in the leg was seen in the treated group, along with statistically insignificant improvements in capillary permeability and symptoms. No adverse effects were noted.[9]

Consumption of these berries, their extracts, or other flavonoid-rich extracts such as grape seed or pine bark (Pycnogenol) is indicated for individuals with varicose veins as well as for those who wish to prevent them. These extracts' efficacy is related to their ability to accomplish the following:

- Reduce capillary fragility
- Increase the integrity of the venous wall
- Improve the muscular tone of the vein.

Numerous double-blind studies with Pycnogenol have validated the effectiveness of procyanidolic oligomers in chronic venous insufficiency. Pycnogenol has an ability to decrease venous ulcer size,[10,11] reduce the swelling and blood clots associated with airline travel, reduce nighttime claudication (muscle pain), and reduce other signs and symptoms of chronic venous insufficiency.[12-16]

The most useful single flavonoid for varicose veins may be micronized diosmin. Micronization involves a high-technology grinding process with a jet of air at supersonic velocities, reducing the size of standard particles from more than 20 μm to less than 2 μm. As a result, there is better and faster absorption, and thus increased bioavailability, which lends greater clinical efficacy. Micronized diosmin has shown considerable benefits in promoting the healing of varicose veins, venous ulcers, and hemorrhoids.[17-20]

Botanical Medicines

Horse Chestnut

The horse chestnut (*Aesculus hippocastanum*) tree is native to western Asia but is now widely distributed all over the world. The seeds of the horse chestnut tree have been valued for centuries for their ability to improve hemorrhoids and varicose veins. This historical use ultimately has led to the development of topical and oral preparations with confirmed clinical benefits for these conditions.[21,22]

Horse chestnut compounds (escin, proanthocyanidin, and esculin) have shown a number of effects beneficial in the treatment of varicose veins. All three active components have been shown to exert significant protective and venotonic effects, such as antioxidant effects, combined with an ability to inhibit enzymes that destroy venous structures, such as collagenase, hyaluronidase, beta-glucuronidase, and elastase, thus improving the integrity and function of critical venous structures. In addition, horse chestnut seed extract prevents the accumulation of white blood cells in varicose veins. It appears that the ultimate effect of horse chestnut seed extract is the prevention of vascular leakage along with increase in the tone of the vein itself.[23]

The therapeutic benefits of horse chestnut seed extract have been confirmed in more than 16 double-blind clinical trials that demonstrate a positive effect in the treatment of varicose veins and thrombophlebitis.[21] In fact, extracts of horse chestnut seed extract standardized for escin appear to be as effective as compression stockings without the nuisance. In one well-designed study, the effectiveness of horse chestnut seed extract vs. compression stockings was examined in 240 patients with varicose veins.[24] Patients received either horse chestnut seed extract (50 mg escin per day), compression stockings, or a placebo for 12 weeks. Effectiveness was evaluated by a phlethysmograph, a machine that measures the volume of fluid in the leg. After the 12-week trial, fluid volume in the more severely affected leg decreased an average of 56.5 ml with compression therapy and 53.6 ml with horse chestnut seed extract, whereas it rose by 9.8 ml with the placebo.

In the treatment of varicose veins, escin can be given orally as well as topically. The topical formula is also of benefit in the treatment of bruises, owing to escin's ability to reduce capillary fragility and swelling.

Gotu Kola

When given orally, an extract of gotu kola (*Centella asiatica*) containing 70% triterpenic acids (asiatic acid, madecassic acid, and asiatoside) has demonstrated impressive clinical results in the treatment of cellulite, venous insufficiency of the lower limbs, and varicose veins.[25–28] The effect of centella in

QUICK REVIEW

- **A diet high in fiber helps prevent varicose veins.**
- **Veins can be strengthened with flavonoid-rich extracts.**
- **Several herbal extracts have been** shown to act as venotonics—agents that enhance the structure, function, and tone of veins—and produce excellent clinical results.

venous insufficiency and varicose veins appears to be related to its ability to enhance connective tissue structure, reduce hardening of the vein, and improve blood flow.

Butcher's Broom

The shrub butcher's broom (*Ruscus aculeatus*) is a member of the lily family that grows in the Mediterranean region. The rhizome from butcher's broom has a long history of use in treating venous disorders such as hemorrhoids and varicose veins. The active ingredients in butcher's broom are ruscogenins. These compounds have demonstrated a wide range of pharmacological actions, including anti-inflammatory and tonic effects on blood vessels. In Europe, butcher's broom extracts are used extensively, both internally and externally, in the treatment of varicose veins and hemorrhoids. Double-blind clinical studies have shown that these preparations offer benefits in both symptom relief and improved venous blood flow.[29–31]

Bromelain and Other Fibrinolytic Compounds

Individuals with varicose veins have a decreased ability to break down fibrin.[32] This fact is extremely important because fibrin is deposited in the tissue near the varicose veins. The skin then becomes hard and "lumpy" owing to the presence of the fibrin and fat (lipodermatosclerosis). In addition, decreased fibrinolytic activity raises the risk of clot formation, which may result in thrombophlebitis, myocardial infarction, pulmonary embolism, or stroke.

Herbs and spices that increase the fibrinolytic activity of the blood are therefore indicated. Capsicum (cayenne),[32] garlic,[33] onion,[34] and ginger[35] all promote fibrin breakdown. Liberal consumption of these spices in foods is recommended for individuals with varicose veins and other disorders of the cardiovascular system.

The proteolytic enzymes from pineapple, bromelain, also appears to be indicated in the treatment of varicose veins. Vein walls are an important source of plasminogen activator, which promotes the breakdown of fibrin. Veins that have become varicose have decreased levels of plasminogen activator. Bromelain acts in a manner similar to plasminogen activator to cause fibrin breakdown.[36]

Another useful substance is nattokinase from natto, a traditional Japanese food prepared from fermented soybeans using *Bacillus subtilis*. Nattokinase is a protein-digesting enzyme that has potent fibrinolytic and thrombolytic (clot-busting) activity and has shown significant potential in improving cardiovascular conditions associated with clot formation and excessive fibrin deposits.[37]

Bromelain and nattokinase may help prevent the development of the hard and lumpy skin found around varicosed veins.

- -

TREATMENT SUMMARY

Conservative therapy, as described above, should be employed as early as possible for patients with varicose veins. It may halt the progression and prevent the need for more aggressive therapy. Note that patience is needed, as improving the structure and function of the veins takes time.

Diet

Follow the recommendations in the chapter "A Health-Promoting Diet." A diet rich in dietary fiber is definitely indicated. The diet should also contain liberal amounts of proanthocyanidin- and anthocyanidin-rich foods, such as blackberries, cherries, and blueberries. Garlic, onions, ginger, and cayenne should also be consumed liberally.

Nutritional Supplements

- A high-potency multiple vitamin and mineral formula as described in the chapter "Supplementary Measures"
- Vitamin D_3: 2,000 to 4,000 IU per day (ideally, measure blood levels and adjust dosage accordingly)
- Fish oils: 1,000 mg EPA + DHA per day
- The following may be useful as an adjunct:
  - Bromelain (minimum 1,500 MCU): 500 to 750 mg three times per day between meals
  - Nattokinase: 100 mg (2,000 FU) per day

Botanical Medicines

- One or more of the following:
  - Micronized diosmin: 500 to 1,000 mg per day
  - Grape seed extract (>95% procyanidolic oligomers): 150 to 300 mg per day
  - Pine bark extract (>95% procyanidolic oligomers): 150 to 300 mg per day
  - Horse chestnut:
    - Bark of root: 500 mg three times per day
    - Escin: 50 mg two to three times per day (alternatively, escin preparations may be applied topically in a 1% concentration)
  - Gotu kola (*Centella asiatica*) extract (70% triterpenic acid content): 30 mg three times per day
  - Butcher's broom extract (9% to 11% ruscogenin content): 100 mg three times per day

Abortifacient: A substance that induces abortion.

Abscess: A localized collection of pus and liquefied tissue in a cavity.

Acetylcholine: One of the chemicals that transmit impulses between nerves and between nerves and muscle cells.

Acrid: Pungent and biting, causing irritation.

Acute: Having a rapid onset, severe symptoms, and a short course; not chronic.

Adaptogen: A substance that is safe, increases resistance to stress, and has a balancing effect on body functions.

Adjuvant: A substance that enhances the effect of a medicinal agent or increases the antigenicity of a cancer cell.

Adrenaline: A hormone secreted by the adrenal gland that produces the "fight-or-flight" response. Also called epinephrine.

Aldosterone: A hormone secreted by the adrenal gland that causes the retention of sodium and water.

Alkaloids: Naturally occurring amines (nitrogen-containing compounds) arising from heterocyclic and often complex structures that display pharmacological activity. The names of alkaloids usually end in -ine.

Allopathy: The conventional method of medicine that combats disease by using substances and techniques specifically targeting the disease.

Alterative: A substance that produces a balancing effect on a particular body function.

Amebiasis: An intestinal infection characterized by severe diarrhea caused by the parasite *Entamoeba histolytica*.

Amino acids: A group of nitrogen-containing chemical compounds that form the basic structural units of proteins.

Analgesic: A substance that reduces the sensation of pain.

Androgen: A hormone that stimulates male charateristics.

Anthelminthic: A substance that causes the elimination of intestinal worms.

Anthocyanidin: A particular class of flavonoids that gives plants, fruits, and flowers colors ranging from red to blue.

Antibody: A protein manufactured by the body that binds to antigens to neutralize, inhibit, or destroy it.

Antidote: A substance that neutralizes or counteracts the effects of a poison.

Antigen: A substance that when introduced into the body causes the formation of antibodies against it.

Antihypertensive: Having a blood-pressure-lowering effect.

Antioxidant: A compound that prevents free-radical or oxidative damage.

Aphrodisiac: A substance that increases sexual desire.

Artery: A blood vessel that carries oxygen-rich blood away from the heart.

Astringent: An agent that causes the contraction of tissue.

Atherosclerosis: A process in which fatty substances (cholesterol and triglycerides) are deposited in the walls of medium to large arteries, eventually leading to their blockage.

Atopy: A predisposition to various allergic conditions, including eczema and asthma.

Autoimmunity: A process in which antibodies develop against the body's own tissues.

Balm: A soothing or healing medicine applied to the skin.

Basal metabolic rate: The rate of metabolism when the body is at rest.

Basophil: A type of white blood cell involved in allergic reactions.

Benign: Term describing a mild disorder that is usually not fatal.

Beta-carotene: Provitamin A; a plant carotene that can be converted to two vitamin A molecules.

Beta cells: The cells in the pancreas that manufacture insulin.

Bilirubin: The breakdown product of the hemoglobin molecule of red blood cells.

Biopsy: A diagnostic test in which tissue or cells are removed from the body for examination under a microscope.

Bleeding time: The time required for the cessation of bleeding from a small skin puncture as a result of platelet disintegration and blood vessel constriction. Ranges from 1 to 4 minutes.

Blood-brain barrier: A barrier that prevents the passage of materials from the blood to the brain.

Blood pressure: The force exerted by blood as it presses against and attempts to stretch blood vessels.

Bromelain: The protein-digesting enzyme found in pineapple.

Bursa: A sac or pouch containing a special fluid that lubricates joints.

Bursitis: Inflammation of a bursa.

Calorie: A unit of heat. A nutritional calorie is the amount of heat necessary to raise 1 kilogram of water 1°C.

Candida albicans: A yeast common to the intestinal tract.

Candidiasis: A complex medical syndrome produced by a chronic overgrowth of the yeast *Candida albicans.*

Carbohydrates: Sugars and starches.

Carcinogen: Any agent or substance capable of causing cancer.

Carcinogenesis: The development of cancer caused by the actions of certain chemicals, viruses, and unknown factors on primarily normal cells.

Cardiac output: The volume of blood pumped from the heart in one minute.

Cardiopulmonary: Pertaining to the heart and lungs.

Cardiotonic: A compound that tones and strengthens the heart.

Carminative: A substance that promotes the elimination of intestinal gas.

Carotene: A fat-soluble plant pigment, some of which can be converted into vitamin A by the body.

Cartilage: A type of connective tissue that acts as a shock absorber at a joint interface.

Cathartic: A substance that stimulates the movement of the bowels; more powerful than a laxative.

Cholagogue: A compound that stimulates the contraction of the gallbladder.

Cholecystitis: Inflammation of the gallbladder.

Cholelithiasis: Gallstones.

Choleretic: A compound that promotes the flow of bile.

Cholestasis: The stagnation of bile within the liver.

Cholinergic: Pertaining to the parasympathetic portion of the autonomic nervous system and the release of acetylcholine as a transmitter substance.

Chronic: Long-term or frequently recurring.

Cirrhosis: A severe disease of the liver characterized by the replacement of liver cells with scar tissue.

Coenzyme: A necessary nonprotein component of an enzyme, usually a vitamin or mineral.

Cold sore: A small skin blister anywhere around the mouth caused by the herpesvirus.

Colic: Severe, spasmodic pain that occurs in waves of increasing intensity, reaches a peak, then abates for a short time before returning.

Colitis: Inflammation of the colon that is usually associated with diarrhea containing blood and mucus.

Collagen: The protein that is the main component of connective tissue.

Compress: A linen or cotton pad applied under pressure to an area of skin and held in place.

Congestive heart failure: A chronic disease that results when the heart is not capable of supplying the oxygen demands of the body.

Connective tissue: The type of tissue that performs the function of providing support, structure, and cellular cement to the body.

Contagious: Transferable from one person to another by social contact, such as sharing the home or workplace.

Coronary artery disease: A condition in which the heart receives an inadequate blood and oxygen supply, owing to atherosclerosis.

Corticosteroid drugs: A group of drugs similar to the natural corticosteroid hormones that are used predominantly in the treatment of inflammation and to suppress the immune system.

Corticosteroid hormones: A group of hormones produced by the adrenal glands that control the body's use of nutrients and the excretion of salt and water in the urine.

Cushing's syndrome: A condition caused by a hypersecretion of cortisone and characterized by spindly legs, "moon face," "buffalo hump," abdominal obesity, flushed facial skin, and poor wound healing.

Cyst: An abnormal lump or swelling filled with fluid or semisolid material in any body organ or tissue.

Cystitis: Inflammation of the inner lining of the bladder. It is is usually caused by a bacterial infection.

Decoction: A tea prepared by boiling a botanical in water for a specified period of time, followed by straining or filtering.

Dehydration: Excessive loss of water from the body.

Dementia: Senility; loss of mental function.

Demineralization: Loss of minerals from bones.

Demulcent: A substance soothing to irritated mucous membranes.

Dermatitis: Inflammation of the skin, sometimes due to allergy.

Diastolic: The lower number in a blood pressure reading; the measure of the pressure in the arteries during the relaxation phase of the heartbeat.

Disaccharide: A sugar composed of two monosaccharide units.

Diuretic: A substance that increases urination.

Diverticuli: Saclike outpouchings of the wall of the colon.

Double-blind study: A way of controlling against experimental bias by ensuring that neither the researcher nor the subject knows when an active agent or a placebo is being used.

Douche: Introduction of water and/or a cleansing agent into the vagina with the aid of a bag with a tube and nozzle attached.

Dysfunction: Abnormal function.

Dysplasia: An abnormality of growth.

Edema: Accumulation of fluid in tissues (swelling).

Eicosapentaenoic acid (EPA): A fatty acid found primarily in cold-water fish.

Electroencephalogram: A machine that measures and records brain waves.

Elimination diet: A diet that eliminates allergenic foods.

Emulsify: To disperse large fat globules into smaller, uniformly distributed particles.

Encephalitis: Inflammation of the brain, usually due to viral infection.

Endometrium: The mucous membrane lining of the uterus.

Enteric-coated: A tablet or capsule that is coated to ensure that it does not dissolve in the stomach so it can reach the intestinal tract.

Enzyme: An organic catalyst that speeds chemical reactions.

Epidemiology: The study of the occurrence and distribution of diseases in human populations.

Epinephrine: See **Adrenaline.**

Epithelium: The cells that cover the entire surface of the body and that line most of the internal organs.

Epstein-Barr virus: The virus that causes infectious mononucleosis and is associated with Burkitt's lymphoma and nasopharyngeal cancer.

Essential fatty acid: A fatty acid that the body cannot manufacture; examples are linoleic acid and linolenic acid.

Essential oil: Also known as volatile oil, ethereal oil, or essence. Usually a complex mixture of a wide variety of organic compounds (alcohols, ketones, phenols, acids, ethers, esters, aldehydes, oxides, etc.) that evaporate when exposed to air. Generally represents the odoriferous principles of plants.

Estrogen: A hormone that stimulates female characteristics.

Excretion: The process of elimination of waste products from a cell, a tissue, or the entire body.

Extracellular space: The space outside the cell, composed of fluid.

Extract: A concentrated form of a natural product that is obtained by treating a crude material containing a certain substance with a solvent and then removing the solvent completely or partially from the preparation. The most common are fluid extracts, solid extracts, powdered extracts, tinctures, and native extracts.

Exudate: Escaping fluid or semifluid material that oozes from a space that may contain serum, pus, and cellular debris.

Faruncle: Another name for a boil that involves a hair follicle.

Fibrin: A white insoluble protein formed by the clotting of blood that is the starting point for wound repair and scar formation.

Fibrinolysis: The dissolution of fibrin or a blood clot by the action of enzymes that convert insoluble fibrin into soluble particles.

Flavonoid: A generic term for a group of flavone-containing compounds that are found widely in nature. They include many of the compounds that account for plant pigments (anthocyanins, anthoxanthins, apigenins, flavones, flavonols, bioflavonols, etc.). They exert a wide variety of physiological effects in the human body.

Fluid extract: Typically a hydroalcoholic solution with a strength of 1 part solvent to 1 part herb. The alcohol content varies with each product. In essence, a concentrated tincture.

Free radical: A highly reactive molecule characterized by an unpaired electron that can bind to and destroy cellular compounds.

Gerontology: The study of aging.

Giardiasis: An infection of the small intestine caused by the protozoan (single-celled organism) *Giardia lamblia.*

Gingivitis: Inflammation of the gums.

Glaucoma: A condition in which the pressure of the fluid in the eye is so high that it causes damage.

Glucose: A monosaccharide found in the blood that is one of the body's primary energy sources.

Gluten: One of the proteins in wheat and certain other grains that gives dough its tough, elastic character.

Glycoside: A sugar-containing compound composed of a glycone (sugar component) and an aglycone (non-sugar-containing component) that can be cleaved on hydrolysis. The glycone portion may be glucose, rhamnose, xylose, fructose, arabinose, or any other sugar. The aglycone portion can be any kind of compound, e.g., a sterol, triterpene, anthraquinone, hydroquinone, tannin, carotenoid, or anthocyanidin.

Goblet cell: A goblet-shaped cell that secretes mucus.

Ground substance: The thick, gel-like material in which the cells, fibers, and blood capillaries of cartilage, bone, and connective tissue are embedded.

Helper T cell: A lymphocytes that helps the immune response.

Hematocrit: The expression of the percentage of blood occupied by blood cells.

Hemorrhoid: A distended vein in the lining of the anus.

Hepatic: Pertaining to the liver

Hepatomegaly: Enlargement of the liver.

Holistic medicine: A form of therapy aimed at treating the whole person, not just the part or parts in which symptoms occur.

Hormone: A secretion of an endocrine gland that controls and regulates body functions.

Hyperglycemia: High blood sugar.

Hyperlipidemia: High levels of of cholesterol and triglycerides in the blood.

Hypersecretion: Excessive secretion.

Hypertension: High blood pressure.

Hypochlorhydria: Insufficient gastric acid output.

Hypoglycemia: Low blood sugar.

Hypolipidemia: Low levels of cholesterol and triglycerides in the blood.

Hypotension: Low blood pressure.

Hypoxia: An inadequate suppy of oxygen.

Iatrogenic: Literally "physician produced," the term can be applied to any medical condition, disease, or other adverse occurrence that results from medical treatment.

Idiopathic: Of unknown cause.

Immunoglobulin: Antibody.

Incidence: The number of new cases of a disease occurring during a given period (usually years) in a defined population.

Incontinence: The inability to control urination or defecation.

Infarction: Death of a localized area of tissue due to lack of oxygen supply.

Infusion: A tea produced by steeping a botanical in hot water.

Insulin: A hormone secreted by the pancreas that lowers blood sugar levels.

Interferon: A potent immune-enhancing substance that is produced by the body's cells to fight off viral infection and cancer.

In vitro: Outside a living body and in an artificial environment.

In vivo: In a living body of an animal or plant.

Jaundice: A condition caused by elevation of bilirubin in the body and characterized by yellowing of the skin.

Keratin: An insoluble protein found in hair, skin, and nails.

Lactase: An enzyme that breaks down lactose into the monosaccharides glucose and galactose.

Lactose: One of the sugars present in milk. It is a disaccharide.

Laxative: A substance that promotes the evacuation of the bowels.

LD^{50}: The dosage that will kill 50 percent of the animals taking a substance.

Lesion: Any localized, abnormal change in tissue formation.

Lethargy: A feeling of tiredness, drowsiness, or lack of energy.

Leukocyte: White blood cell.

Leukotriene: An inflammatory compound produced when oxygen interacts with polyunsaturated fatty acids.

Lipids: Fats, phospholipids, steroids, and prostaglandins.

Lipotropic: Promoting the flow of lipids to and from the liver.

Lymph: Fluid contained in lymphatic vessels that flows through the lymphatic system to be returned to the blood.

Lymphocyte: A type of white blood cell found primarily in lymph nodes.

Malabsorption: Impaired absorption of nutrients, most often due to diarrhea.

Malaise: A vague feeling of being sick or of physical discomfort.

Malignant: A term used to describe a condition that tends to worsen and eventually causes death.

Manipulation: As a therapy, the skillful use of the hands to move a part of the body or a specific joint or muscle.

Mast cell: A cell found in many tissues of the body that contributes greatly to allergic and inflammatory processes by secreting histamine and other inflammatory particles.

Menorrhagia: Excessive loss of blood during menstrual periods.

Menstrum: A solvent used for extraction, e.g., water, alcohol, acetone.

Metabolism: A collective term for all the chemical processes that take place in the body.

Metabolite: A product of a chemical reaction.

Metalloenzyme: An enzyme that contains a metal at its active site.

Microbe: A popular term for microorganism.

Microflora: The microbial inhabitants of a particular region, e.g., the colon.

Mites: Eight-legged animals less than $\frac{1}{20}$ inch (1.2 mm) long that are similar to tiny spiders.

Molecule: The smallest complete unit of a substance that can exist independently and still retain the characteristic properties of the substance.

Monoclonal antibody: A genetically engineered antibody specific to one particular antigen.

Monosaccharide: A simple, one-unit sugar such as fructose or glucose.

Mortality rate: The number of deaths per 100,000 population per year.

Mucosa: Another term for mucous membrane.

Mucous membrane: The soft pink tissue that lines most of the body's cavities and tubes, including the respiratory tract, gastrointestinal tract, genitourinary tract, and eyelids. The mucous membranes secrete mucus.

Mucus: The slick, slimy fluid secreted by the mucous membranes that acts as a lubricant and mechanical protector of the mucous membranes.

Mycotoxin: A toxin produced by yeast or a fungus.

Myelin sheath: A white fatty substance that surrounds nerve cells to aid in nerve impulse transmission.

Neoplasia: A tumor formation characterized by a progressive, abnormal replication of cells.

Neurofibrillary tangle: A cluster of degenerated nerves.

Neurotransmitter: A substance that modifies or transmits nerve impulses.

Night blindness: The inability to see well in dim light or at night.

Nocturia: Disturbance of a person's sleep at night by the need to pass urine.

Oleoresin: Generally, a mixture of resins and volatile oils either occuring naturally or made by extracting the oily and resinous materials from botanicals with organic solvents (e.g., hexane, acetone, ether, alcohol). The solvent is then removed under vacuum, leaving behind a viscous, semisolid extract that is the oleoresin. Examples of prepared oleoresins are paprika, ginger, and capsicum.

Oligoantigenic diet: See **Elimination diet.**

Otitis media: Acute infection of the middle ear.

Pancreatin: An extract of pork pancreas.

Papain: The protein-digesting enzyme in papaya.

Parkinson's disease: A slowly progressive, degenerative nervous system disease characterized by resting tremor, "pill rolling" by the fingers, a masklike facial expression, a shuffling gait, and muscle rigidity and weakness.

Pathogen: Any agent, particularly a microorganism, that causes disease.

Pathogenesis: The process by which a disease originates and develops, particularly cellular and physiological processes.

Peristalsis: Successive muscular contractions of the intestines that move food through the intestinal tract.

Physiology: The study of the functioning of the body, including the physical and chemical processes of its cells, tissues, organs, and systems.

Physostigmine: A drug that blocks the breakdown of acetylcholine.

Phytoestrogen: A plant compound that exerts an estrogenic effect.

Placebo: An inert or inactive substance used to test the efficacy of another substance.

Polysaccharide: A molecule composed of many sugar molecules linked together.

Powdered extract: A solid extract that has been dried as a powder.

Prostaglandin: A hormonelike compound manufactured from essential fatty acids.

Psychosomatic: Pertaining to the relationship between the mind and body. Commonly used to refer to physiological disorders thought to be caused entirely or partly by psychological factors.

Putrefaction: The process of breaking down protein compounds by rotting.

RDA: Recommended Dietary Allowance.

Resin: A complex oxidative product of a terpene that occurs naturally as a plant exudate or is prepared by alcohol extraction of a botanical that contains a resinous principle.

Saccharide: A sugar molecule.

Saponin: A nonnitrogenous glycoside, typically with sterol or triterpene as the aglycone, that possesses the property of foaming, or making suds, when strongly agitated in aqueous solution.

Satiety: A feeling of fullness or gratification.

Saturated fat: A fat whose carbon atoms are bonded to the maximum number of hydrogen atoms; found in animal products such as meat, milk, milk products, and eggs.

Sclerosis: The process of hardening or scarring.

Senile dementia: Mental deterioration associated with aging.

Slow-reacting substance of anaphylaxis (SRSA): A potent allergic mediator produced and released by mast cells.

Solid extract: An extract from which all of the residual solvent or liquid has been removed.

Submucosa: The tissue just below the mucous membrane.

Suppressor T cell: A lymphocyte controlled by the thymus gland that suppresses the immune response.

Syndrome: A group of signs and symptoms that occur together in a pattern characteristic of a particular disease or abnormal condition.

T cell: A lymphocyte that is under the control of the thymus gland.

Tincture: An alcoholic or hydroalcoholic solutions that usually contains the active principles of a botanical in a low concentration. It is usu-ally prepared by maceration, percolation, or dilution of its corresponding fluid or native extracts. The strength of a tincture is typically 1 to 10 or 1 to 5; the alcohol content varies.

Tonic: A substance that exerts a gentle strengthening effect on the body.

Trans-fatty acid: A detrimental type of fat found in margarine, dairy products, and many processed foods.

Uremia: The retention of urine by the body and the presence of high levels of urine components in the blood.

Urinalysis: The analysis of urine.

Urticaria: Hives.

Vasoconstriction: The constriction of blood vessels.

Vasodilation: The dilation of blood vessels.

Vitamin: An essential compound necessary to act as a catalyst in normal processes of the body.

Western diet: A diet characteristic of Western societies, i.e., a diet high in fat, refined carbohydrates, and processed foods and low in dietary fiber.

Wheal: The characteristic lesion in hives; a small welt.

ARE YOU AN OPTIMIST?

What distinguishes an optimist from a pessimist is the way in which they explain both good and bad events. Dr. Martin Seligman has developed a simple test to determine your level of optimism (see *Learned Optimism*, Knopf, 1981). Take as much time as you need. There are no right or wrong answers. It is important that you take the test before you read the interpretation. Read the description of each situation and vividly imagine it happening to you. Choose the response that most applies to you by circling either A or B. Ignore the letter and number codes for now; they will be explained later.

1. The project you are in charge of is a great success. **PsG**

   A. *I kept a close watch over everyone's work.* 1

   B. *Everyone devoted a lot of time and energy to it.* 0

2. You and your spouse (boyfriend/girlfriend) make up after a fight. **PmG**

   A. *I forgave him/her.* 0

   B. *I'm usually forgiving.* 1

3. You get lost driving to a friend's house. **PsB**

   A. *I missed a turn.* 1

   B. *My friend gave me bad directions.* 0

4. Your spouse (boyfriend/girlfriend) surprises you with a gift. **PsG**

   A. *He/she just got a raise at work.* 0

   B. *I took him/her out to a special dinner the night before.* 1

5. You forget your spouse's (boyfriend's/girlfriend's) birthday. **PmB**

   A. *I'm not good at remembering birthdays.* 1

   B. *I was preoccupied with other things.* 0

6. You get a flower from a secret admirer. **PvG**

   A. *I am attractive to him/her.* 0

   B. *I am a popular person.* 1

7. You run for a community office position and you win. **PvG**

   A. *I devoted a lot of time and energy to campaigning.* 0

   B. *I work very hard at everything I do.* 1

8. You miss an important engagement. **PvB**

   A. *Sometimes my memory fails me.* 1

   B. *I sometimes forget to check my appointment book.* 0

9. You run for a community office position and you lose. **PsB**

   A. *I didn't campaign hard enough.* 1

   B. *The person who won knew more people.* 0

10. You host a successful dinner. **PmG**

    A. *I was particularly charming that night.* 0

    B. *I am a good host.* 1

11. You stop a crime by calling the police. **PsG**

    A. *A strange noise caught my attention.* 0

    B. *I was alert that day.* 1

12. You were extremely healthy all year. **PsG**

    A. *Few people around me were sick, so I wasn't exposed.* 0

    B. *I made sure I ate well and got enough rest.* 1

13. You owe the library ten dollars for an overdue book.   **PmB**

   A. *When I am really involved in what I am reading, I often forget when it's due.*   1

   B. *I was so involved in writing the report that I forgot to return the book.*   0

14. Your stocks make you a lot of money.   **PmG**

   A. *My broker decided to take on something new.*   0

   B. *My broker is a top-notch investor.*   1

15. You win an athletic contest.   **PmG**

   A. *I was feeling unbeatable.*   0

   B. *I train hard.*   1

16. You fail an important examination.   **PsB**

   A. *I wasn't as smart as the other people taking the exam.*   1

   B. *I didn't prepare for it well.*   0

17. You prepared a special meal for a friend and he/she barely touched the food.   **PvB**

   A. *I wasn't a good cook.*   1

   B. *I made the meal in a rush.*   0

18. You lose a sporting event for which you have been training for a long time.   **PvB**

   A. *I'm not very athletic.*   1

   B. *I'm not good at that sport.*   0

19. Your car runs out of gas on a dark street late at night.   **PsB**

   A. *I didn't check to see how much gas was in the tank.*   1

   B. *The gas gauge was broken.*   0

20. You lose your temper with a friend.   **PmB**

   A. *He/she is always nagging me.*   1

   B. *He/she was in a hostile mood.*   0

21. You are penalized for not returning your income tax forms on time.   **PmB**

   A. *I always put off doing my taxes.*   1

   B. *I was lazy about getting my taxes done this year.*   0

22. You ask a person out on a date and he/she says no.   **PvB**

   A. *I was a wreck that day.*   1

   B. *I got tongue-tied when I asked him/he on the date.*   0

23. A game-show host picks you out of the audience to participate in the show.   **PsG**

   A. *I was sitting in the right seat.*   0

   B. *I looked the most enthusiastic.*   1

24. You are frequently asked to dance at a party.   **PmG**

   A. *I am outgoing at parties.*   1

   B. *I was in perfect form that night.*   0

25. You buy your spouse (boyfriend/girlfriend) a gift he/she doesn't like.   **PsB**

   A. *I don't put enough thought into things like that.*   1

   B. *He/she has very picky tastes.*   0

26. You do exceptionally well in a job interview.   **PmG**

   A. *I felt extremely confident during the interview.*   0

   B. *I interview well.*   1

27. You tell a joke and everyone laughs.   **PsG**

   A. *The joke was funny.*   0

   B. *My timing was perfect.*   1

28. Your boss gives you too little time in which to finish a project, but you get it finished anyway.   **PvG**

   A. *I am good at my job.*   0

   B. *I am an efficient person.*   1

29. You've been feeling run-down lately.   **PmB**

   A. *I never get a chance to relax.*   1

   B. *I was exceptionally busy this week.*   0

30. You ask someone to dance and he/she says no.   **PsB**

   A. *I am not a good enough dancer.*   1

   B. *He/she doesn't like to dance.*   0

31. You save a person from choking to death.   **PvG**

   A. *I know a technique to stop someone from choking.*   0

   B. *I know what to do in crisis situations.*   1

32. Your romantic partner wants to cool things off for a while.   **PvB**

   A. *I'm too self-centered.*   1

   B. *I don't spend enough time with him/her.*   0

33. A friend says something that hurts your
feelings.   PmB

    A. *She always blurts things out without
thinking of others.*   1

    B. *My friend was in a bad mood and
took it out on me.*   0

34. Your employer comes to you for advice.   PvG

    A. *I am an expert in the area about
which I was asked.*   0

    B. *I'm good at giving useful advice.*   1

35. A friend thanks you for helping him/her
get through a bad time.   PvG

    A. *I enjoy helping him/her through
tough times.*   0

    B. *I care about people.*   1

36. You have a wonderful time at a party.   PsG

    A. *Everyone was friendly.*   0

    B. *I was friendly.*   1

37. Your doctor tells you that you are in
good physical shape.   PvG

    A. *I make sure I exercise frequently.*   0

    B. *I am very health-conscious.*   1

38. Your spouse (boyfriend/girlfriend) takes
you away for a romantic weekend.   PmG

    A. *He/she needed to get away for a
few days.*   0

    B. *He/she likes to explore new areas.*   1

39. Your doctor tells you that you eat too
much sugar.   PsB

    A. *I don't pay much attention to my diet.*   1

    B. *You can't avoid sugar, it's in everything.*   0

40. You are asked to head an important
project.   PmG

    A. *I just successfully completed a similar
project.*   0

    B. *I am a good supervisor.*   1

41. You and your spouse (boyfriend/
girlfriend) have been fighting a great deal.   PsB

    A. *I have been feeling cranky and
pressured lately.*   1

    B. *He/she has been hostile lately.*   0

42. You fall down a great deal while skiing.   PmB

    A. *Skiing is difficult.*   1

    B. *The trails were icy.*   0

43. You win a prestigious award.   PvG

    A. *I solved an important problem.*   0

    B. *I was the best employee.*   1

44. Your stocks are at an all-time low.   PvB

    A. *I didn't know much about the
business climate at the time.*   1

    B. *I made a poor choice of stocks.*   0

45. You win the lottery.   PsG

    A. *It was pure chance.*   0

    B. *I picked the right numbers.*   1

46. You gain weight over the holidays and
you can't lose it.   PmB

    A. *Diets don't work in the long run.*   1

    B. *The diet I tried didn't work.*   0

47. You are in the hospital and few people
come to visit.   PsB

    A. *I'm irritable when I am sick.*   1

    B. *My friends are negligent about things
like that.*   0

48. They won't honor your credit card at a
store.   PvB

    A. *I sometimes overestimate how much
money I have.*   1

    B. *I sometimes forget to pay my credit
card bill.*   0

Scoring Key

PmB _____		PmG _____
PvB _____		PvG _____
	HoB _____	
PsB _____		PsG _____
Total B _____		Total G _____
	G–B _____	

Interpreting Your Test Results

The test results will give you a clue as to your explanatory style. In other words, the results will tell you about the way in which you explain things to yourself. It tells you your habit of thought. Again, remember that there are no right or wrong answers.

There are three crucial dimensions to your explanatory style: permanence, pervasiveness, and personalization. Each dimension, plus a couple of others, will be scored from your test.

Permanence. When pessimists are faced with challenges or bad events, they view the events as being permanent. In contrast, people who are optimists tend to view the challenges or bad events as temporary. Here are some statements that reflect the subtle differences:

PERMANENT (PESSIMISTIC)	TEMPORARY (OPTIMISTIC)
"My boss is always a jerk."	"My boss is in a bad mood today."
"You never listen."	"You are not listening."
"This bad luck will never stop."	"My luck has got to turn."

To determine how you view bad events, look at the eight items coded PmB (for Permanent Bad): 5, 13, 20, 21, 29, 33, 42, and 46. Each one with a "0" after it is optimistic; each one followed by a "1" is pessimistic. Total the numbers at the right-hand margin of the questions coded PmB, and write the total on the PmB line on the scoring key.

If you totaled 0 or 1, you are very optimistic on this dimension; 2 or 3 is a moderately optimistic score; 4 is average; 5 or 6 is quite pessimistic; and 7 or 8 is extremely pessimistic.

Now let's take a look at the difference in explanatory style between pessimists and optimists when there is a positive event in their lives. It's just the opposite of what happened with a bad event. Pessimists view positive events as temporary, while optimists view them as permanent. Here again are some

subtle differences in how pessimists and optimists might communicate their good fortune:

TEMPORARY (PESSIMISTIC)	PERMANENT (OPTIMISTIC)
"It's my lucky day."	"I am always lucky."
"My opponent was off today."	"I am getting better every day."
"I tried hard today."	"I always give my best."

Now total all the questions coded PmG (for Permanent Good): 2, 10, 14, 15, 24, 26, 38, and 40. Write the total on the line in the scoring key marked PmG.

If you totaled 7 or 8, you are very optimistic on this dimension; 6 is a moderately optimistic score; 4 or 5 is average; 3 is pessimistic; and 0, 1, or 2 is extremely pessimistic.

Are you starting to see a pattern? If you are scoring as a pessimist, you may want to learn how to be more optimistic. Your anxiety may be due to your belief that bad things are always going to happen, while good things are only a fluke.

Pervasiveness. Pervasiveness refers to the tendency to describe things in universals (everyone, always, never, etc.) vs. specifics (a specific individual, a specific time, etc.). Pessimists tend to describe things in universals, while optimists describe things in specifics.

UNIVERSAL (PESSIMISTIC)	SPECIFIC (OPTIMISTIC)
"All lawyers are jerks."	"My attorney was a jerk."
"Instruction manuals are worthless."	"This instruction manual is worthless."
"He is repulsive."	"He is repulsive to me."

Total your score for the questions coded PvB (for Pervasive Bad): 8, 17, 18, 22, 32, 44, and 48. Write the total on the PvB line.

If you totaled 0 or 1, you are very optimistic on this dimension; 2 or 3 is a moderately optimistic score; 4 is average; 5 or 6 is quite pessimistic; and 7 or 8 is extremely pessimistic.

Now let's look at the level of pervasiveness of good events. Optimists tend to view good events as universal, while pessimists view them as specific. Again, it's just the opposite of how each views a bad event.

Total your score for the questions coded PvG (for Pervasive Good): 6, 7, 28, 31, 34, 35, 37, and 43. And write the total on the line labeled PvG.

If you totaled 7 or 8, you are very optimistic on this dimension; 6 is a moderately optimistic score; 4 or 5 is average; 3 is pessimistic; and 0, 1, or 2 is extremely pessimistic.

Hope. Our level of hope or hopelessness is determined by our combined level of permanence and pervasiveness. Your level of hope may be the most significant score for this test. Take your PvB and add it to your PmB score. This is your hope score.

If it is 0, 1, or 2, you are extraordinarily hopeful; 3, 4, 5, or 6 is a moderately hopeful score; 7 or 8 is average; 9, 10, or 11 is moderately hopeless; and 12, 13, 14, 15, or 16 is severely hopeless.

People who make permanent and universal explanations for their troubles tend to suffer from stress, anxiety, and depression; they tend to collapse when things go wrong. According to Dr. Seligman, no other score is as important as your hope score.

Personalization. The final aspect of explanatory style is personalization. When bad things happen, either we can blame ourselves (internalize) and lower our self-esteem as a consequence, or we can blame things beyond our control (externalize). Although it may not be right to deny personal responsibility, people who tend to externalize blame in relation to bad events have higher self-esteem and are more optimistic.

Total your score for the questions coded PsB (for Personalization Bad): 3, 9, 16, 19, 25, 30, 39, 41, and 47.

A score of 0 or 1 indicates very high self-esteem and optimism; 2 or 3 indicates moderate self-esteem; 4 is average; 5 or 6 indicates moderately low self-esteem; and 7 or 8 indicates very low self-esteem.

Now let's take a look at personalization and good events. Again, just the exact opposite occurs compared with bad events. When good things happen, the person with high self-esteem internalizes while the person with low self-esteem externalizes.

Total your score for those questions coded PsG (for Personalization Good): 1, 4, 11, 12, 23, 27, 36, and 45. Write your score on the line marked PsG on your scoring key.

If you totaled 7 or 8, you are very optimistic on this dimension; 6 is a moderately optimistic score; 4 or 5 is average; 3 is pessimistic; and 0, 1, or 2 is extremely pessimistic.

Your Overall Scores. To compute your overall scores, first add the three B's (PmB + PvB + PsB). This is your B (bad event) score. Do the same for all of the G's (PmG + PvG + PsG). This is your G score. Subtract B from G; this is your overall score.

If your B score is from 3 to 6, you are marvelously optimistic when bad events occur; 10 or 11 is average; 12 to 14 is pessimistic; anything above 14 is extremely pessimistic.

If your G score is 19 or above, you think about good events extremely optimistically; 14 to 16 is average; 11 to 13 indicates pessimism; and a score of 10 or less indicates great pessimism.

If your overall score (G minus B) is above 8, you are very optimistic across the board; if it's from 6 to 8, you are moderately optimistic; 3 to 5 is average; 1 or 2 is pessimistic; and a score of 0 or below is very pessimistic.

GLYCEMIC INDEX, CARBOHYDRATE CONTENT, AND GLYCEMIC LOAD OF SELECTED FOODS

A complete list of the glycemic index and glycemic load of all tested foods is beyond the scope of this book; it would be a book in itself. So we have selected the most common foods. This listing will give you a general sense of what are high-GL and low-GL foods. We have listed the items by food groups, from low to high glycemic loads. You may notice that certain food groups are not listed.

For example, you won't see nuts, seeds, fish, poultry, and meats listed, because these foods have little impact on blood sugar levels as they are low in carbohydrates.

If you would like to see an even more complete listing, visit www.mendosa.com, a free website operated by the medical writer Rick Mendosa. It is an excellent resource.

FOOD	GI	CARBOHYDRATES (G)	FIBER (G)	GL
BEANS (LEGUMES)				
Soybeans, cooked, ½ cup, 100 g	14	12	7.0	1.6
Peas, green, fresh, frozen, boiled, ½ cup, 80 g	48	5	2.0	2.0
Beans, navy,, white, boiled, ½ cup, 90 g	38	11	6.0	4.2
Beans, lima, boiled, ½ cup, 90 g	27	18	7.3	4.8
Peas, split, yellow, boiled, ½ cup, 90 g	32	16	4.7	5.1
Lentils, ½ cup, 100g	28	19	3.7	5.3
Beans, lima, baby, ½ cup cooked, 85 g	32	17	4.5	5.4
Beans, black, canned, ½ cup, 95 g	45	15	7.0	5.7
Beans, pinto, canned, ½ cup, 95 g	45	13	6.7	5.8
Chickpeas, canned, drained, ½ cup, 95 g	42	15	5.0	6.3
Beans, kidney, canned and drained, ½ cup, 95 g	52	13	7.3	6.7
Beans, broad, frozen, boiled, ½ cup, 80 g	79	9	6.0	7.1
Peas, dried, boiled, ½ cup, 70 g	22	4	4.7	8.0
Baked beans, canned in tomato sauce, ½ cup, 120 g	48	21	8.8	10.0
Black-eyed peas, soaked, boiled, ½ cup, 120 g	42	24	5.0	10.0

FOOD	GI	CARBOHYDRATES (G)	FIBER (G)	GL
BREAD				
Multigrain, unsweetened, 1 slice, 30 g	43	9	1.4	4.0
Oat bran and honey loaf, 1 slice, 40 g	31	14	1.5	4.5
Sourdough, rye, 1 slice, 30 g	48	12	0.4	6.0
Stone-ground whole wheat, 1 slice, 30 g	53	11	1.4	6.0
Wonder, enriched white, 1 slice, 20 g	73	10	0.4	7.0
Sourdough, wheat, 1 slice, 30 g	54	14	0.4	7.5
Pumpernickel, 1 slice, 60 g	41	21	0.5	8.6
Whole wheat, 1 slice, 35 g	69	14	1.4	9.6
Healthy Choice, hearty 7-grain, 1 slice, 38 g	56	18	1.4	10.0
White (wheat flour), 1 slice, 30 g	70	15	0.4	10.5
Healthy Choice, 100% whole grain, 1 slice, 38 g	62	18	1.4	11.0
Gluten-free multigrain, 1 slice, 35 g	79	15	1.8	12.0
French baguette, 30 g	95	15	0.4	14.0
Hamburger bun, 1, 50 g	61	24	0.5	15.0
Rye, 1 slice, 50 g	65	23	0.4	15.0
Light rye, 1 slice, 50 g	68	23	0.4	16.0
Dark rye, black, 1 slice, 50 g	76	21	0.4	16.0
Croissant, 1, 50 g	67	27	0.2	18.0
Kaiser roll, 1, 50 g	73	25	0.4	18.0
Pita, 1, 65 g	57	38	0.4	22.0
Bagel, 1, 70 g	72	35	0.4	25.0
BREAKFAST CEREALS				
Oat bran, raw, 1 tablespoon, 10 g	55	7	1.0	4.0
Bran with psyllium, ⅓ cup, 30 g	47	12	12.5	5.6
Bran, ⅓ cup, 30 g	58	14	14.0	8.0
All-Bran Soy 'n Fiber, ½ cup, 45 g	33	26	7.0	8.5
All-Bran, ½ cup, 40 g	42	22	6.5.	9.2
Oatmeal, cooked with water, 1 cup, 245 g	42	24	1.6	10.0
Shredded Wheat, ⅓ cup, 25 g	67	18	1.2	12.0
Kellogg's Frosted Mini-Wheats (whole wheat), 1 cup, 30 g	58	21	4.4	12.0
All-Bran Fruit 'n Oats, ½ cup, 45 g	39	33	6.0	13.0
Weetabix, 2, 30 g	69	19	2.0	13.0
Cheerios, ½ cup, 30 g	74	20	2.0	15.0

FOOD	GI	CARBOHYDRATES (G)	FIBER (G)	GL
Kellogg's Frosted Flakes, ¾ cup, 30 g	55	27	1.0	15.0
Corn Bran, ½ cup, 30 g	75	20	1.0	15.0
Kellogg's Honey Smacks, ¾ cup, 30 g	56	27	1.0	15.0
Total, 30 g	76	22	2.0	16.7
Healthwise for Heart Health, 45 g	48	35	2.0	16.8
Puffed wheat, 1 cup, 30 g	80	22	2.0	17.6
Bran flakes, ¾ cup, 30 g	74	24	2.0	18.0
Kellogg's Crunchy Nut, ¾ cup, 30 g	72	25	2.0	18.0
Froot Loops, 1 cup, 30 g	69	27	1.0	18.0
Cocoa Pops, ¾ cup, 30 g	77	26	1.0	20.0
Corn Chex, 1 cup, 30 g	83	25	1.0	20.8
Just Right, ¾ cup, 30 g	60	36	2.0	21.6
Cornflakes, 1 cup, 30 g	84	26	0.3	21.8
Rice Krispies, 1 cup, 30 g	82	27	0.3	22.0
Rice Chex, 1 cup, 30 g	89	25	1.0	22.0
Kellogg's Crispix, 1 cup, 30 g	87	26	1.0	22.6
Kellogg's Just Right Just Grains, 1 cup, 45 g	62	38	2.0	23.5
Oats'n Honey, 1 cup, 45 g	77	31	2.0	24.0
Raisin bran, 1 cup, 45 g	73	35	4.0	25.5
Grape Nuts, ½ cup, 58 g	71	47	2.0	33.3
CAKE				
Cake, angel food, 1 slice, 30 g	67	17	<1.0	11.5
Cake, sponge, 1 slice, 60 g	46	32	<1.0	14.7
Cake, cupcake, with icing and cream filling, 1, 38 g	73	26	<1.0	19.0
Cake, chocolate fudge (Betty Crocker), 73 g cake + 33 g frosting	38	54	<1.0	20.5
Cake, banana, 1 slice, 80 g	47	46	<1.0	21.6
Cake, pound, 1 slice, 80 g	54	42	<1.0	22.6
Cake, French vanilla (Betty Crocker), 73 g Cake + 33 g frosting	42	58	<1.0	24.4
Cake, Lamingtons, 1, 50 g	87	29	<1.0	25
Cake, flan, 1 slice, 80 g	65	55	<1.0	35.8
Scones, made from mix, 1, 40 g	92	90	<1.0	83.0

FOOD	GI	CARBOHYDRATES (G)	FIBER (G)	GL
CRACKERS				
Kavli, 4, 20 g	71	13	3.0	9.2
Breton wheat, 6, 25 g	67	14	2.0	9.4
Ryvita or Wasa (regular), 2, 20 g	69	16	3.0	11.0
Stoned Wheat Thins, 5, 25 g	67	17	1.0	11.4
Premium soda, 3, 25 g	74	17	0.0	12.5
Water, 5, 25 g	78	18	0.0	14.0
Graham, 1, 30 g	74	22	1.4	16.0
Rice cake, 2, 25 g	82	21	0.4	17.0
MILK, SOY MILK, AND JUICES				
Milk, full fat, 1 cup, 250 ml	27	12	0.0	3.0
Milk, soy, 1 cup, 250 ml	31	12	0.0	3.7
Milk, skim, 1 cup, 250 ml	32	13	0.0	4.0
Juice, grapefruit, unsweetened, 1 cup, 250 ml	48	16	1.0	7.7
Nesquik chocolate powder, 3 teaspoons in 1 cup (250 ml) milk	55	14	0.0	7.7
Milk, chocolate, low fat, 1 cup, 250 ml	34	23	0.0	7.8
Juice, orange, 1 cup, 250 ml	46	21	1.0	9.7
Gatorade, 1 cup, 250 ml	78	15	0.0	11.7
Juice, pineapple, unsweetened, canned, 1 cup, 250 ml	46	27	1.0	12.4
Juice, apple, unsweetened, 1 cup, 250 ml	40	33	1.0	13.2
Ocean Spray cranberry juice cocktail, 1 cup, 250 ml	68	34	0.0	23.0
Coca-Cola, 12 ounces; 375 ml	63	40	0.0	25.2
Other soft drinks sweetened with sugar or high-fructose corn syrup, 12 ounces; 375 ml	68	51	0.0	34.7
Milk, sweetened condensed, ½ cup, 125 ml	61	90	0.0	55.0
FRUIT				
Cherries, 20, 80 g	22	10	2.4	2.2
Plums, 3–4 small, 100 g	39	7	2.2	2.7
Peach, fresh, 1 large, 110 g	42	7	1.9	3.0
Apricots, fresh, 3 medium, 100 g	57	7	1.9	4.0
Apricots, dried, 5–6, 30 g	31	13	2.2	4.0
Kiwi, 1 raw, peeled, 80 g	52	8	2.4	4.0

FOOD	GI	CARBOHYDRATES (G)	FIBER (G)	GL
Orange, 1 medium, 130 g	44	10	2.6	4.4
Peach, canned, in natural juice, ½ cup, 125 g	38	12	1.5	4.5
Pear, canned, in natural juice, ½ cup, 125 g	43	13	1.5	5.5
Watermelon, 1 cup, 150 g	72	8	1.0	5.7
Pineapple, fresh, 2 slices, 125 g	66	10	2.8	6.6
Apple, 1 medium, 150 g	38	18	3.5	6.8
Grapes, green, 1 cup, 100 g	46	15	2.4	6.9
Apple, dried, 30g	29	24	3.0	6.9
Prunes, pitted (Sunsweet), 6, 40 g	29	25	3.0	7.3
Pear, fresh, 1 medium, 150 g	38	21	3.1	8.0
Fruit cocktail, canned, in natural juice, 1½ cup, 125 g	55	15	1.5	8.3
Apricots, canned, in light syrup, ½ cup, 125 g	64	13	1.5	8.3
Peach, canned, in light syrup, ½ cup, 125 g	52	18	1.5	9.4
Mango, 1 small, 150 g	55	19	2.0	10.4
Figs, dried, tenderized (water added), 50 g	61	22	3.0	13.4
Sultanas, ¼ cup, 40 g	56	30	3.1	16.8
Banana, raw, 1 medium, 150 g	55	32	2.4	17.6
Raisins, ¼ cup, 40 g	64	28	3.1	18.0
Dates, dried, 5, 40 g	103	27	3.0	27.8
GRAINS				
Rice bran, extruded, 1 tablespoon, 10 g	19	3	1.0	0.6
Barley, pearl, boiled, ½ cup, 80 g	25	17	6.0	4.3
Millet, cooked, ½ cup, 120 g	71	12	1.0	8.5
Bulgur, cooked, ⅔ cup, 120 g	48	22	3.5	10.6
Rice, brown, steamed, 1 cup, 150 g	50	32	1.0	16.0
Couscous, cooked, ⅔ cup, 120 g	65	28	1.0	18.0
Rice, white, boiled, 1 cup, 150 g	72	36	0.2	26.0
Rice, arborio, white, boiled, 100 g	69	35	0.2	29.0
Rice, basmati, white, boiled, 1 cup, 180 g	58	50	0.2	29.0
Buckwheat, cooked, ½ cup, 80 g	54	57	3.5	30.0
Rice, instant, cooked, 1 cup, 180 g	87	38	0.2	33.0
Tapioca, steamed 1 hour, 100 g	70	54	<1.0	38.0
Tapioca, boiled with milk, 1 cup, 265 g	81	51	<1.0	41.0
Rice, jasmine, white, long grain, steamed, 1 cup, 180 g	109	39	0.2	42.5

FOOD	GI	CARBOHYDRATES (G)	FIBER (G)	GL
ICE CREAM				
Ice cream, low-fat French vanilla, 2 scoops, 50 g	38	15	0.0	5.7
Ice cream, full fat, 2 scoops, 50 g	61	10	0.0	6.1
JAM				
Jam, no sugar, 1 tablespoon, 25 g	55	11	<1.0	6.0
Jam, sweetened, 1 tablespoon, 25 g	48	17	<1.0	8.0
MUFFINS AND PANCAKES				
Muffin, chocolate butterscotch, from mix, 50 g	53	28	1.0	15.0
Muffin, apple, oat, and sultana, from mix, 50 g	54	28	1.0	15.0
Muffin, apricot, coconut, and honey, from mix, 50 g	60	27	1.5	16.0
Muffin, banana, oat, and honey, from mix, 50 g	65	28	1.5	18.0
Muffin, apple, 1 muffin, 80 g	44	44	1.5	19.0
Muffin, bran, 1 muffin, 80 g	60	34	2.5	20.0
Muffin, blueberry, 1 muffin, 80 g	59	41	1.5	24.0
Pancake, buckwheat, from dry mix, 1 small, 40 g	102	30	2.0	30.0
Pancake, from dry mix, 1 large, 80 g	67	58	1.0	39.0
PASTA				
Tortellini, cheese, cooked, 1 cup, 180 g	50	21	2.0	10.5
Ravioli, meat filled, cooked, 1 cup, 220 g	39	30	2.0	11.7
Vermicelli, cooked, 1 cup, 180 g	35	45	2.0	15.7
Rice noodles, fresh, boiled, 1 cup, 176 g	40	44	0.4	17.6
Spaghetti, whole grain, cooked, 1 cup, 180 g	37	48	3.5	17.8
Fettucine, cooked, 1 cup, 180 g	32	57	2.0	18.2
Spaghetti, gluten-free, in tomato sauce, 1 small can, 220 g	68	27	2.0	18.5
Macaroni and cheese, packaged, cooked, 220 g	64	30	2.0	19.2
Star pastina, cooked, 1 cup, 180 g	38	56	2.0	21.0
Spaghetti, white, cooked, 1 cup, 180 g	41	56	2.0	23.0
Rice pasta, brown, cooked, 1 cup, 180 g	92	57	2.0	52.0
SUGARS				
Fructose, 1 teaspoon, 10 g	23	10	0.0	2.3
Honey, 1½ tablespoon, 10 g	58	16	0.0	4.6

FOOD	GI	CARBOHYDRATES (G)	FIBER (G)	GL
Lactose, 1 teaspoon, 10 g	46	10	0.0	4.6
Sucrose, 1 teaspoon, 10 g	65	10	0.0	6.5
Glucose, 1 teaspoon, 10 g	102	10	0.0	10.2
Maltose, 1 teaspoon, 10 g	105	10	0.0	10.5
SNACKS				
Corn chips, Doritos original, 50 g	42	33	<1.0	13.9
Snickers bar, 59 g	41	35	0.0	14.3
Tofu frozen dessert (nondairy), 100 g	115	13	<1.0	15.0
Real Fruit bar, strawberry, 20 g	90	17	<1.0	15.3
Twix bar (caramel), 59 g	44	37	<1.0	16.2
Pretzels, 50 g	83	22	<1.0	18.3
Mars bar, 60 g	65	41	0.0	26.6
SOUPS				
Tomatoes, canned, 7/8 cup, 220 ml	38	15	1.5	6.0
Black bean, 7/8 cup, 220 ml	64	9	3.4	6.0
Lentil, canned, 7/8 cup, 220 ml	44	14	3.0	6
Split pea, canned, 7/8 cup, 220 ml	60	13	3.0	8
VEGETABLES				
Carrots, raw, 1/2 cup, 80 g	16	6	1.5	1
Low-glycemic vegetables:	≈20	≈7	≈1.5	≈1.4
Asparagus, 1 cup cooked or raw				
Bell peppers, 1 cup cooked or raw				
Broccoli, 1 cup cooked or raw				
Brussels sprouts, 1 cup cooked or raw				
Cabbage, 1 cup cooked or raw				
Cauliflower, 1 cup cooked or raw				
Cucumber, 1 cup				
Celery, 1 cup cooked or raw				
Eggplant, 1 cup				
Green beans, 1 cup cooked or raw				
Kale, 1 cup cooked, 2 cups raw				
Lettuce, 2 cups raw				
Mushrooms, 1 cup				

FOOD	GI	CARBOHYDRATES (G)	FIBER (G)	GL
Spinach, 1 cup cooked or 2 cups raw				
Tomatoes, 1 cup				
Zucchini, 1 cup cooked or raw				
Carrots, peeled, boiled, ½ cup, 70 g	49	3	1.5	1.5
Beets, canned, drained, 2–3 slices, 60 g	64	5	1.0	3.0
Pumpkin, peeled, boiled, ½ cup, 85 g	75	6	3.4	4.5
Parsnips, boiled, ½ cup, 75 g	97	8	3.0	8.0
Corn on the cob, sweet, boiled 20 minutes, 80 g	48	14	2.9	8.0
Corn, canned and drained, ½ cup, 80 g	55	15	3.0	8.5
Sweet potato, peeled, boiled, 80 g	54	16	3.4	8.6
Sweet corn, ½ cup boiled, 80 g	55	18	3.0	10.0
Potato, peeled, boiled, 1 medium, 120 g	87	13	1.4	10.0
Potato, with skin on, boiled, 1 medium, 120 g	79	15	2.4	11.0
Yam, boiled, 80 g	51	26	3.4	13.0
Potato, baked in oven, 1 medium, 120 g	93	15	2.4	14.0
Potatoes, mashed, ½ cup, 120 g	91	16	1.0	14.0
Potatoes, instant mashed, prepared, ½ cup	83	18	1.0	15.0
Potatoes, new, unpeeled, boiled, 5 small, 175 g	78	25	2.0	20.0
Cornmeal (polenta), ⅓ cup, 40 g	68	30	2.0	20.0
French fries, fine cut, small serving, 120g	75	49	1.0	36.0
Gnocchi, cooked, 1 cup, 145 g	68	71	1.0	48.0
YOGURT				
Yogurt, low fat, artificially sweetened, 200 g	14	12	0.0	2.0
Yogurt, with fruit, 200 g	26	30	0.0	8.0
Yogurt, low fat, 200 g	33	26	0.0	8.5

ACID-BASE VALUES OF SELECTED FOODS

One of the goals of the body is to maintain the proper balance of acidity and alkalinity (pH) in the blood and other body fluids in order to function properly. The acid-alkaline theory of disease is an oversimplification, but it essentially states that many diseases are caused by excess acid accumulation in the body. There is accumulating evidence that certain disease states such as osteoporosis, rheumatoid arthritis, gout, and many others may be influenced by the dietary acid-alkaline balance. For example, osteoporosis may be the result of a chronic intake of acid-forming foods that consistently outweighs the intake of alkaline foods, with the result that the bones are constantly forced to give up their alkaline minerals (calcium and magnesium) in order to buffer the excess acid.

The dietary goal for good health is simple: make sure that you consume more alkaline-producing foods than acid-producing foods. Keep in mind that there is a difference between acidic foods and acid-forming foods. For example, although foods like lemons and citrus fruits are acidic, they actually have an alkalizing effect on the body. What determines the pH nature of a food in the body is the metabolic end product when it is digested. For example, the citric acid in citrus fruit is metabolized in the body to its alkaline form (citrate) and may even be converted to bicarbonate, another alkaline compound.

The following table was prepared by Professor Jürgen Vormann of the Institute for Prevention and Diet in Ismaning, Germany (used with permission; see http: //jn.nutrition .org/content/138/2/413S for original). Foods with a negative value exert a base (B) or alkaline effect, foods with a positive value an acid (A) effect. Neutral foodstuffs are labeled N. The calculation is based upon the potential acid load to the kidneys in milliequivalents per 100-g (3½-oz) serving.

FOOD	A, B, OR N	POTENTIAL ACIDIC LOAD
BEVERAGES		
Beer, draft	B	−0.2
Beer, pale	A	0.9
Beer, stout	B	−0.1
Coca-Cola	A	0.4
Cocoa, made with semi-skim milk	B	−0.4
Coffee, espresso	B	−2.3

FOOD	A, B, OR N	POTENTIAL ACIDIC LOAD
Coffee, brewed, 5 minutes	B	−1.4
Juice, apple, unsweetened	B	−2.2
Juice, beet	B	−3.9
Juice, carrot	B	−4.8
Juice, grape	B	−1.0
Juice, lemon	B	−2.5
Juice, mixed vegetable (tomato, beet, carrot)	B	-3.6
Juice, orange, unsweetened	B	−2.9
Juice, tomato	B	−2.8
Tea, fruit	B	−0.3
Tea, green	B	−0.3
Tea, herbal	B	−0.2
Tea, Indian	B	−0.3
Water, mineral (Apollinaris)	B	−1.8
Water, mineral (Volvic)	B	−0.1
Wine, red	B	−2.4
Wine, white, dry	B	−1.2
FATS, OILS, AND NUTS		
Almonds	A	4.3
Butter	A	0.6
Hazelnuts	B	−2.8
Margarine	B	−0.5
Oil, olive	N	0.0
Oil, sunflower seed	N	0.0
Peanuts, plain	A	8.3
Pistachios	A	8.5
Walnuts	A	6.8
FISH AND SEAFOOD		
Carp	A	7.9
Cod, fillets	A	7.1
Eel, smoked	A	11.0
Haddock	A	6.8
Halibut	A	7.8
Herring	A	7.0

FOOD	A, B, OR N	POTENTIAL ACIDIC LOAD
Matjes (herrings), salted	A	8.0
Mussels	A	15.3
Prawns, tiger	A	18.2
Rosefish	A	10.0
Salmon	A	9.4
Sardines, in oil	A	13.5
Shrimp	A	7.6
Sole	A	7.4
Trout, steamed	A	10.8
FRUITS		
Apples	B	−2.2
Apricots	B	−4.8
Bananas	B	−5.5
Currants, black	B	−6.5
Cherries	B	-3.6
Figs, dried	B	−18.1
Grapefruit	B	−3.5
Grapes	B	−3.9
Kiwifruit	B	−4.1
Lemon	B	−2.6
Mango	B	−3.3
Oranges	B	−2.7
Peaches	B	−2.4
Pears	B	−2.9
Pineapple	B	−2.7
Raisins	B	−21.0
Strawberries	B	−2.2
Watermelon	B	−1.9
GRAINS AND FLOUR		
Amaranth	A	7.5
Barley, whole grain	A	5.0
Buckwheat, whole grain	A	3.7
Corn, whole grain	A	3.8
Cornflakes	A	6.0

FOOD	A, B, OR N	POTENTIAL ACIDIC LOAD
Flour, rye	A	4.4
Flour, rye, whole grain	A	5.9
Flour, wheat, white	A	6.9
Flour, wheat, whole grain	A	8.2
Millet, whole grain	A	8.6
Oat flakes	A	10.7
Rice, brown	A	12.5
Rice, white	A	4.6
Spelt	A	8.8
PASTA		
Macaroni	A	6.1
Noodles	A	6.4
Spaetzle (German pasta)	A	9.4
Spaghetti, white	A	6.5
Spaghetti, whole wheat	A	7.3
BREAD		
Bread, pumpernickel	A	4.2
Bread, rye	A	4.1
Bread, rye, mixed	A	4.0
Bread, wheat, mixed	A	3.8
Bread, white	A	3.7
Bread, whole wheat	A	7.2
Bread, whole wheat, coarse	A	5.3
Crispbread, rye	A	3.3
LEGUMES		
Beans, green/French	B	−3.1
Lentils, green or brown, whole, dried	A	3.5
Peas	A	1.2
Soybeans	B	−3.4
Soy milk	B	−0.8
Tofu	B	−0.8

FOOD	A, B, OR N	POTENTIAL ACIDIC LOAD
MEAT AND SAUSAGES		
Beef, lean only	A	7.8
Beef, corned, canned	A	13.2
Beef, rump steak, lean and fat	A	8.8
Chicken, meat only	A	8.7
Duck	A	4.1
Duck, lean only	A	8.4
Frankfurters/ hot dogs	A	6.7
Goose, lean only	A	13.0
Lamb, lean only	A	7.6
Liver, beef	A	15.4
Liver, pork	A	15.7
Liver, veal	A	14.2
Liver sausage	A	10.6
Pork, lean only	A	7.9
Rabbit, lean only	A	19.0
Salami	A	11.6
Sausage, cervelat	A	8.9
Sausage, chasseur	A	7.2
Sausage containing ham	A	8.3
Sausage, pork	A	7.0
Turkey, meat only	A	9.9
Veal, filet	A	9.0
MILK, DAIRY PRODUCTS, AND EGGS		
Buttermilk	A	0.5
Cheese, Camembert	A	14.6
Cheese, cheddar-type, reduced fat	A	26.4
Cheese, cottage, plain	A	8.7
Cheese, Emmental, full fat	A	21.1
Cheese, Edam, full fat	A	19.4
Cheese, full-fat soft	A	4.3
Cheese, Gouda	A	18.6
Cheese, hard varieties	A	19.2
Cream, fresh, sour	A	1.2
Cheese, Parmesan	A	34.2

FOOD	A, B, OR N	POTENTIAL ACIDIC LOAD
Cheese, processed, plain	A	28.7
Cheese, rich creamy full fat	A	13.2
Egg, chicken, white	A	1.1
Egg, chicken, whole	A	8.2
Egg, chicken, yolk	A	23.4
Ice cream, fruit, mixed	B	−0.6
Ice cream, vanilla	A	0.6
Milk, skim	A	0.7
Milk, whole, evaporated	A	1.1
Milk, whole, pasteurised and sterilized	A	0.7
Whey	B	−1.6
Yogurt, whole milk, fruit	A	1.2
Yogurt, whole milk, plain	A	1.5
SWEETS		
Chocolate, bitter	A	0.4
Chocolate, milk	A	2.4
Honey	B	−0.3
Madeira cake	A	3.7
Marmalade	B	−1.5
Nougat hazelnut cream	B	−1.4
Sugar, brown	B	−1.2
Sugar, white	N	0.0
VEGETABLES		
Arugula	B	−7.5
Asparagus	B	−0.4
Broccoli, green	B	−1.2
Brussels sprouts	B	−4.5
Carrots	B	−4.9
Cauliflower	B	−4.0
Celery	B	−5.2
Chicory	B	−2.0
Cucumber	B	−0.8
Eggplant	B	−3.4
Fennel	B	−7.9

FOOD	A, B, OR N	POTENTIAL ACIDIC LOAD
Garlic	B	–1.7
Gherkin, pickeled	B	–1.6
Kale	B	–7.8
Kohlrabi	B	–5.5
Leeks	B	–1.8
Lettuce, iceberg	B	–1.6
Lettuce, romaine	B	–2.5
Mushrooms, white	B	–1.4
Onions	B	–1.5
Peppers, green bell	B	–1.4
Potatoes	B	–4.0
Radishes, red	B	–3.7
Sauerkraut	B	–3.0
Spinach	B	–14.0
Tomato	B	–3.1
Zucchini	B	–4.6
HERBS AND VINEGAR		
Basil	B	–7.3
Chives	B	–5.3
Parsley	B	–12.0
Vinegar, apple cider	B	–2.3
Vinegar, wine, balsamic	B	–1.6

The references provided are by no means intended to be a complete list for all of the studies reviewed or mentioned in this book. In fact, we have chosen to focus on key studies and comprehensive review articles that readers, especially medical professionals, may find helpful.

We encourage those interested to visit the website of the National Library of Medicine (NLM) at www.nlm.nih.gov for additional studies. The NLM Gateway (http://gateway .nlm.nih.gov) is a web-based system that lets users search simultaneously in multiple retrieval systems at the NLM. From this site you can access all of the NLM databases, including the PubMed database. The PubMed database was developed in conjunction with publishers of biomedical literature as a search tool for accessing literature citations and linking to full-text journal articles at websites of participating publishers. Publishers participating in PubMed electronically supply NLM with their citations prior to or at the time of publication. If the publisher has a website that offers full text of its journals, PubMed provides links to that site, as well as sites with other biological data, sequence centers, and so on. User registration, a subscription fee, or some other type of fee may be required to access the full text of articles in some journals.

PubMed provides access to bibliographic information, including MEDLINE, the NLM's premier bibliographic database covering the fields of medicine, nursing, dentistry, veterinary medicine, the health care system, and the preclinical sciences. MEDLINE contains bibliographic citations and author abstracts from more than 4,000 medical journals published in the United States and 70 other countries. The file contains more than 12 million citations dating back to the mid-1960s. Coverage is worldwide, but most records are from English-language sources or have English abstracts (summaries). Conducting a search is quite easy, and the site has a link to a tutorial that fully explains the search process.

What Is Natural Medicine?

1. Lust B. *Universal naturopathic directory and buyer's guide.* American Naturopathic Association, New York, 1918.
2. Campion F. *AMA and U.S. health policy since 1940.* Chicago: AMA Publications, 1984.
3. French GL. The continuing crisis in antibiotic resistance. *International Journal of Antimicrobial Agents* 2010 Nov;36 suppl 3:S3–S7.
4. Gootz TD. The global problem of antibiotic resistance. *Critical Reviews in Immunology* 2010; 30(1):79–93.
5. Wolfe MM, Lichtenstein DR, Singh G. Gastrointestinal toxicity of nonsteroidal anti-inflammatory drugs. *The New England Journal of Medicine* 1999;340: 1888–1899.
6. Vaithianathan R, Hockey PM, Moore TJ, Bates DW. Iatrogenic effects of COX-2 inhibitors in the US population: findings from the Medical Expenditure Panel Survey. *Drug Safety* 2009;32(4):335–343.
7. Dingle JT. The effect of NSAIDs on human articular cartilage glycosaminoglycan synthesis. *European Journal of Rheumatology and Inflammation* 2009;16:47–52.
8. Brandt KD. Effects of nonsteroidal anti-inflammatory drugs on chondrocyte metabolism in vitro and in vivo. *The American Journal of Medicine* 1987; 83 suppl 5A:29–34.
9. Shield MJ. Anti-inflammatory drugs and their effects on cartilage synthesis and renal function. *European Journal of Rheumatology and Inflammation* 1993;13:7–16.
10. Brooks PM, Potter SR, Buchanan WW. NSAID and osteoarthritis—help or hindrance? *The Journal of Rheumatology* 1982;9:3–5.
11. Newman NM, Ling RSM. Ace-

tabular bone destruction related to non-steroidal anti-inflammatory drugs. *The Lancet* 1985;2: 11–13.

12. Solomon L. Drug induced arthropathy and necrosis of the femoral head. *Journal of Bone and Joint Surgery* 1973;55B: 246–251.

13. Ronningen H, Langeland N. Indomethacin treatment in osteoarthritis of the hip joint. *Acta Orthopaedica* 1979;50:169–174.

14. Bruyere O, Honore A, Ethgen O, et al. Correlation between radiographic severity of knee osteoarthritis and future disease progression. Results from a 3-year prospective, placebo-controlled study evaluating the effect of glucosamine sulfate. *Osteoarthritis and Cartilage* 2003;1:1–5.

15. Christgau S, Henrotin Y, Tanko LB, et al. Osteoarthritic patients with high cartilage turnover show increased responsiveness to the cartilage protecting effects of glucosamine sulphate. *Clinical and Experimental Rheumatology* 2004;22:36–42.

16. Bruyere O, Pavelka K, Rovati LC, et al. Total joint replacement after glucosamine sulphate treatment in knee osteoarthritis: results of a mean 8-year observation of patients from two previous 3-year, randomised, placebo-controlled trials. *Osteoarthritis and Cartilage* 2008 Feb;16(2):254–60.

17. Muller-Fassbender H, Bach GL, Haase W, et al. Glucosamine sulfate compared to ibuprofen in osteoarthritis of the knee. *Osteoarthritis and Cartilage* 1994;2:61–69.

18. Rovati LC, Giacovelli G, Annefeld M, et al. A large, randomized, placebo controlled, double-blind study of glucosamine sulfate vs piroxicam and vs their association, on the kinetics of the symptomatic effect in knee osteoarthritis. *Osteoarthritis and Cartilage* 1994;2 suppl 1:56.

19. Qiu GX, Gao SN, Giacovelli G, et al. Efficacy and safety of glucosamine sulfate versus ibuprofen in patients with knee osteoarthritis. *Arzneimittelforschung* 1998;48:469–474.

20. Sawitzke AD, Shi H, Finco MF, et al. Clinical efficacy and safety of glucosamine, chondroitin sulphate, their combination, celecoxib or placebo taken to treat osteoarthritis of the knee: 2-year results from GAIT. *Annals of the Rheumatic Diseases* 2010 Aug;69(8):1459–1464.

21. Pelletier KR. A review and analysis of the health and cost-effective outcome of comprehensive health promotion and disease promotion at the worksite: 1991–1993 update. *American Journal of Health Promotion* 1993;8:50–61.

22. Wilper AP, Woolhandler S, Lasser KE, et al. A national study of chronic disease prevalence and access to care in uninsured U.S. adults. *Annals of Internal Medicine* 2008;149: 170–176.

23. Verbrugge LM, Patrick DL. Seven chronic conditions: their impact on U.S. adults' activity levels and use of medical services. *The American Journal of Public Health* 1995;85:173–182.

24. Oojendijk WTM, Mackenbach JP, Limberger HHB. What is better? An investigation into the use and satisfaction with complementary and official medicine in the Netherlands. Netherlands Institute of Preventive Medicine and the Technical Industrial Organization, London, UK, 1980.

25. Oakley GP. Folic acid–preventable spina bifida and anencephaly. *JAMA, The Journal of the American Medical Association* 1993;269:1292–1293.

The Healing Power Within

1. Klopfer B. Psychological variables in human cancer. *Journal of Projective Techniques* 1957; 21:331–340.

2. Benedetti F. Mechanisms of placebo and placebo-related effects across diseases and treatments. *Annual Review of Pharmacology and Toxicology* 2008;48:33–60.

3. Price DD, Finniss DG, Benedetti F. A comprehensive review of the placebo effect: recent advances and current thought. *Annual Review of Psychology* 2008;59:565–590.

4. Beecher HK. The powerful placebo. *JAMA, The Journal of the American Medical Association* 1955;159:1602–1606.

5. Benson H, Friedman R. Harnessing the power of the placebo effect and renaming it "remembered wellness." *Annual Review of Medicine* 1996;47: 193–199.

6. Benedetti F, Lanotte M, Lopiano L, Colloca L. When words are painful: unraveling the mechanisms of the nocebo effect. *Neuroscience* 2007;147(2): 260–271.

7. Olshansky B. Placebo and nocebo in cardiovascular health: implications for healthcare, research, and the doctor-patient relationship. *Journal of the American College of Cardiology* 2007;49(4):415–421.

8. O'Hara DP. Is there a role for prayer and spirituality in health care? *Medical Clinics of North America* 2002;86(1):33–46.

9. Pizzorno L. Spirituality and Healing. In *A Textbook of Natural Medicine*, ed. Pizzorno JE, Murray MT. London: Churchill-Livingston, 2005, 519–532.

10 McNichol T. The new faith in medicine. *USA Today*, April 7, 1996, 4.

11. Benson H. The relaxation response: therapeutic effect. *Science* 1997;278:1694–1651.

12. Levin J. Spiritual determinants of health and healing: an epidemiologic perspective on salutogenic mechanisms. *Alternative Therapies in Health and Medicine* 2003;9(6):48–57.

A Positive Mental Attitude

1. Maruta T, Colligan RC, Malinchoc M, Offord KP. Optimism-pessimism assessed in the 1960s and self-reported health status 30 years later. *Mayo Clinic Proceedings* 2002;77:748–753.
2. Taylor SE, Kemeny ME, Reed GM, et al. Psychological resources, positive illusions, and health. *American Psychologist* 2000;55:99–109.
3. Schweizer K, Beck-Seyffer A, Schneider R. Cognitive bias of optimism and its influence on psychological wellbeing. *Psychological Reports* 1999;84:627–636.
4. Segerstrom SC. Optimism, goal conflict, and stressor-related immune change. *Journal of Behavioral Medicine* 2001;24:441–467.
5. Maruta T, Colligan RC, Malinchoc M, Offord KP. Optimists vs pessimists: survival rate among medical patients over a 30-year period. *Mayo Clinic Proceedings* 2000;75:140–143.
6. Kubzansky LD, Sparrow D, Vokonas P, Kawachi I. Is the glass half empty or half full? A prospective study of optimism and coronary heart disease in the normative aging study. *Psychosomatic Medicine* 2001;63:910–916.
7. Peterson C, Seligman M, Valliant G. Pessimistic explanatory style as a risk factor for physical illness: a thirty-five year longitudinal study. *Journal of Personality and Social Psychology* 1988;55:23–27.
8. Wood AM, Joseph S. The absence of positive psychological (eudemonic) wellbeing as a risk factor for depression: a ten year cohort study. *Journal of Affective Disorders* 2010;122:213–217.
9. Brennan FX, Charnetski CJ. Explanatory style and immunoglobulin A (IgA). *Integrative Physiological and Behavioral Science* 2000;35:251–255.
10. Kamen-Siegel L, Rodin J, Seligman ME, Dwyer J. Explanatory style and cell-mediated immunity in elderly men and women. *Health Psychology* 1991;10:229–235.
11. Imai K, Nakachi K. Personality types, lifestyle, and sensitivity to mental stress in association with NK activity. *International Journal of Hygiene and Environmental Health* 2001;204:67–73.
12. Segerstrom SC. Personality and the immune system: models, methods, and mechanisms. *Annals of Behavioral Medicine* 2000;22:180–190.
13. Jung W, Irwin M. Reduction of natural killer cytotoxic activity in major depression: interaction between depression and cigarette smoking. *Psychosomatic Medicine* 1999;61:263–270.
14. Kiecolt-Glaser JK, McGuire L, Robles TF, Glaser R. Emotions, morbidity, and mortality: new perspectives from psychoneuroimmunology. *Annual Review of Psychology* 2002;53:83–107.
15. Kiecolt-Glaser JK, Glaser R. Psychoneuroimmunology and cancer: fact or fiction? *European Journal of Cancer* 1999;35:1603–1607.
16. Raikkonen K, Matthews KA, Flory JD, et al. Effects of optimism, pessimism, and trait anxiety on ambulatory blood pressure and mood during everyday life. *Journal of Personality and Social Psychology* 1999;76:104–113.
17. Maslow A. *The farther reaches of human nature.* New York: Viking, 1971.
18. Seligman M. *Learned optimism.* New York: Knopf, 1991.

A Health-Promoting Lifestyle

1. Chandler MA, Rennard SI. Smoking cessation. *Chest* 2010 Feb;137(2):428–435.
2. Law M, Tang JL. An analysis of the effectiveness of interventions intended to help people stop smoking. *Archives of Internal Medicine* 1995;155:1933–1941.
3. Nettle H, Sprogis E. Pediatric exercise: truth and/or consequences. *Sports Medicine and Arthroscopy Review* 2011 Mar;19(1):75–80.
4. Farmer ME, Locke BZ, Mosciki EK, et al. Physical activity and depressive symptomatology: the NHANES 1 epidemiologic follow-up study. *American Journal of Epidemiology* 1988;1328:1340–1351.
5. Carr DB, Bullen BA, Skrinar GS, et al. Physical conditioning facilitates the exercised-induced secretion of beta-endorphin and beta-lipoprotein in women. *The New England Journal of Medicine* 1981;305:560–565.
6. Lobstein D, Mosbacher BJ, Ismail AH. Depression as a powerful discriminator between physically active and sedentary middle-aged men. *Journal of Psychosomatic Research* 1983;27:69–76.
7. Blair SN. Changes in physical fitness and all-cause mortality: a prospective study of healthy and unhealthy men. *JAMA, The Journal of the American Medical Association* 1995;273:1093–1098.
8. Dement WC, Vaughan C. *The promise of sleep: a pioneer in sleep medicine explores the vital connection between health, happiness, and a good night's sleep.* New York: Dell, 2000.

A Health-Promoting Diet

1. Ryde D. What should humans eat? *Practitioner* 1985;232:415–418.
2. Milton K. Nutritional characteristics of wild primate food: do the diets of our closest living relatives have lessons for us? *Nutrition* 1999;15:488–498.
3. Cordain L, Eaton SB, Miller JB, et al. The paradoxical nature of hunter-gatherer diets: meat-based, yet non-atherogenic. *European Journal of Clinical Nutrition* 2002;56 suppl 1:S42–S52.
4. Eaton SB, Eaton SB 3rd.

Paleolithic vs. modern diets—selected pathophysiological implications. *European Journal of Nutrition* 2000;39:67–70.

5. Trowell H, Burkitt D. *Western diseases: their emergence and prevention.* Cambridge, Mass.: Harvard University Press, 1981.

6. Steinmetz KA, Potter JD. Vegetables, fruit, and cancer. II. Mechanisms. *Cancer Causes and Control* 1991;2:427–442.

7. Steinmetz KA, Potter JD. Vegetables, fruit, and cancer prevention: a review. *Journal of the American Dietetic Association* 1996;96:1027–1039.

8. La Vecchia C, Tavani A. Fruit and vegetables, and human cancer. *European Journal of Cancer Prevention* 1998;7:3–8.

9. Van Duyn MA, Pivonka E. Overview of the health benefits of fruit and vegetable consumption for the dietetics professional: selected literature. *Journal of the American Dietetic Association* 2000;100:1511–1521.

10. Baris D, Zahm SH. Epidemiology of lymphomas. *Current Opinion in Oncology* 2000;12:383–394.

11. Blair A, Zahm SH. Agricultural exposures and cancer. *Environmental Health Perspectives* 1995;103 suppl 8:205–208.

12. Mao Y, Hu J, Ugnat AM, White K. Non-Hodgkin's lymphoma and occupational exposure to chemicals in Canada. Canadian Cancer Registries Epidemiology Research Group. *Annals of Oncology* 2000;11 suppl 1:69–73.

13. Aronson KJ, Miller AB, Woolcott CG, et al. Breast adipose tissue concentrations of polychlorinated biphenyls and other organochlorines and breast cancer risk. *Cancer Epidemiology, Biomarkers & Prevention* 2000;9:55–63.

14. Jaga K, Brosius D. Pesticide exposure: human cancers on the horizon. *Reviews on Environmental Health* 1999;14:39–50.

15. Lu C, Knutson DE, Fisker-Andersen J, Fenske RA. Biological monitoring survey of organophosphorus pesticide exposure among preschool children in the Seattle metropolitan area. *Environmental Health Perspectives* 2001;109(3):299–303.

16. Consumers Union of United States. *Do you know what you're eating? An analysis of U.S. government of data of pesticide residues in foods.* Washington, D.C.: Consumers Union, 1999.

17. Jenkins DJ, Kendall CW, Augustin LS, et al. Glycemic index: overview of implications in health and disease. *The American Journal of Clinical Nutrition* 2002;76:266S–273S.

18. Willett W, Manson J, Liu S. Glycemic index, glycemic load, and risk of type 2 diabetes. *The American Journal of Clinical Nutrition* 2002;76:274S–280S.

19. Liu S, Willett WC, Stampfer MJ, et al. A prospective study of dietary glycemic load, carbohydrate intake, and risk of coronary heart disease in US women. *The American Journal of Clinical Nutrition* 2000;71:1455–1461.

20. Sinha R, Cross AJ, Graubard BI, et al. Meat intake and mortality: a prospective study of over half a million people. *Archives of Internal Medicine* 2009 Mar 23;169(6):562–571.

21. Bingham SA. High-meat diets and cancer risk. *Proceedings of the Nutrition Society* 1999;58:243–248.

22. Segasothy M, Phillips PA. Vegetarian diet: panacea for modern lifestyle diseases? *QJM* 1999;92:531–544.

23. Zheng W, Gustafson DR, Sinha R, et al. Well-done meat intake and the risk of breast cancer. *Journal of the National Cancer Institute* 1998;90:1724–1729.

24. Blot WJ, Henderson BE, Boice JD Jr. Childhood cancer in relation to cured meat intake: review of the epidemiological evidence. *Nutrition and Cancer* 1999;34:111–118.

25. Preston-Martin S, Pogoda JM, Mueller BA, et al. Maternal consumption of cured meats and vitamins in relation to pediatric brain tumors. *Cancer Epidemiology, Biomarkers & Prevention* 1996;5:599–605.

26. Bougnoux P. N-3 polyunsaturated fatty acids and cancer. *Current Opinion in Clinical Nutrition and Metabolic Care* 1999;2:121–126.

27. Bucher HC, Hengstler P, Schindler C, Meier G. N-3 polyunsaturated fatty acids in coronary heart disease: a meta-analysis of randomized controlled trials. *The American Journal of Medicine* 2002;112:298–304.

28. Fraser GE. Nut consumption, lipids, and risk of a coronary event. *Clinical Cardiology* 1999;22 suppl:11–15.

29. Jiang R, Manson JE, Stampfer MJ, et al. Nut and peanut butter consumption and risk of type 2 diabetes in women. *JAMA, The Journal of the American Medical Association* 2002;288:2554–2560.

30. Alarcon de la Lastra C, Barranco MD, Motilva V, Herrerias JM. Mediterranean diet and health: biological importance of olive oil. *Current Pharmaceutical Design* 2001;7:933–950.

31. Whelton PK, He J. Potassium in preventing and treating high blood pressure. *Seminars in Nephrology* 1999;19:494–499.

32. Sacks FM, Svetkey LP, Vollmer WM, et al. Effects on blood pressure of reduced dietary sodium and the Dietary Approaches to Stop Hypertension (DASH) diet. DASH–Sodium Collaborative Research Group. *The New England Journal of Medicine* 2001;344:3–10.

33. Jansson B. Potassium, sodium, and cancer: a review. *Journal of Environmental Pathology, Toxicology and Oncology* 1996;15:65–73.

34. Boris M, Mandel FS. Foods and additives are common causes of the attention deficit hyperactive disorder in children. *Annals of Allergy, Asthma & Immunology* 1994;72:462–468.

35. Lessof MH. Reactions to food additives. *Clinical & Experimental Allergy* 1995;25 suppl 1: 27–28.

36. Groten JP, Butler W, Feron VJ, et al. An analysis of the possibility for health implications of joint actions and interactions between food additives. *Regulatory Toxicology and Pharmacology* 2000;31:77–91.

37. Simon RA. Adverse reactions to food additives. *Current Allergy and Asthma Reports* 2003;3: 62–66.

38. Lasky T. Foodborne illness—old problem, new relevance. *Epidemiology* 2002;13:593–598.

39. Tauxe RV. Emerging foodborne pathogens. *International Journal of Food Microbiology* 2002; 78:31–41.

40. Kleiner SM. Water: an essential but overlooked nutrient. *Journal of the American Dietetic Association* 1999;99:200–206.

Supplementary Measures

1. Centers for Disease Control and Prevention. National Health and Nutrition Examination Survey. NHANES 2007–2008. www.cdc.gov/nchs/nhanes/nhanes2007–2008/nhanes07_08.htm.

2. Davis DR, Epp MD, Riordan HD. Changes in USDA food composition data for 43 garden crops, 1950 to 1999. *Journal of the American College of Nutrition* 2004;23:669–682.

3. Thomas D. A study on the mineral depletion of the foods available to US as a nation over the period 1940 to 1991. *Nutrition and Health* 2003;17:85–115.

4. Havsteen BH. The biochemistry and medical significance of the flavonoids. *Pharmacology & Therapeutics* 2002;96:67–202.

5. Calder PC, Yaqoob P. Understanding omega-3 polyunsaturated fatty acids. *Postgraduate Medicine* 2009 Nov;121(6):148–157.

6. Prentice A. Vitamin D deficiency: a global perspective. *Nutrition Reviews* 2008 Oct;66(10 suppl 2):S153–S164.

7. Goldstein D. The epidemic of vitamin D deficiency. *Journal of Pediatric Nursing* 2009 Aug; 24(4):345–346.

8. Holick MF, Chen TC. Vitamin D deficiency: a worldwide problem with health consequences. *The American Journal of Clinical Nutrition* 2008 Apr; 87(4):1080S–1086S.

9. Semba RD, Houston DK, Ferrucci L, et al. Low serum 25-hydroxyvitamin D concentrations are associated with greater all-cause mortality in older community-dwelling women. *Nutrition Research* 2009;29(8):525–523

10. Hollis BW, Johnson D, Hulsey TC, et al. Vitamin D supplementation during pregnancy: double-blind, randomized clinical trial of safety and effectiveness. *Journal of Bone and Mineral Research* 2011;26(10): 2341–2357.

A Cellular Approach to Health

1. Schmitz G, Ecker J. The opposing effects of n-3 and n-6 fatty acids. *Progress in Lipid Research* 2008 Mar;47(2):147–155.

2. Siscovick DS, Raghunathan TE, King I, et al. Dietary intake and cell membrane levels of long-chain n-3 polyunsaturated fatty acids and the risk of primary cardiac arrest. *JAMA, The Journal of the American Medical Association* 1995 Nov 1;274(17): 1363–1367.

3. Block RC, Harris WS, Reid KJ, et al. EPA and DHA in blood cell membranes from acute coronary syndrome patients and controls. *Atherosclerosis* 2008 Apr;197(2):821–828.

4. Lemaitre RN, King IB, Raghunathan TE, et al. Cell membrane trans-fatty acids and the risk of primary cardiac arrest. *Circulation* 2002 Feb 12;105(6): 697–701.

5. Salmeron J, Hu FB, Manson JE, et al. Dietary fat intake and risk of type 2 diabetes in women. *The American Journal of Clinical Nutrition* 2001;73:1019–1026.

6. Rivellese AA, De Natale C, Lilli S. Type of dietary fat and insulin resistance. *Annals of the New York Academy of Sciences* 2002;967:329–335.

7. Ramel A, Martinéz A, Kiely M, et al. Beneficial effects of long-chain n-3 fatty acids included in an energy-restricted diet on insulin resistance in overweight and obese European young adults. *Diabetologia* 2008 Jul; 51(7):1261–1268.

8. Abete I, Parra D, Crujeiras AB, et al. Specific insulin sensitivity and leptin responses to a nutritional treatment of obesity via a combination of energy restriction and fatty fish intake. *Journal of Human Nutrition and Dietetics* 2008 Dec;21(6): 591–600.

9. Mozaffarian D, Aro A, Willett WC. Health effects of trans-fatty acids: experimental and observational evidence. *European Journal of Clinical Nutrition* 2009 May;63 suppl 2: S5–S21.

10. Wilson JX. Regulation of vitamin C transport. *Annual Review of Nutrition* 2005;25: 105–125.

11. Biolo G, Williams BD, Fleming RY, Wolfe RR. Insulin action on muscle protein kinetics and amino acid transport during recovery after resistance exercise. *Diabetes* 1999 May;48(5): 949–957.

12. Christensen NJ, Hilsted J. Insulin facilitates transport of macromolecules and nutrients to muscles. *International Journal of Obesity and Related Metabolic Disorders* 1993 Dec;17 suppl 3:S83–S85.

13. Bonadonna RC, Saccomani MP, Cobelli C, et al. Effect of insulin

on system A amino acid transport in human skeletal muscle. *Journal of Clinical Investigation* 1993 Feb;91(2):514–521.

14. Duarte AI, Santos MS, Seiça R, de Oliveira CR. Insulin affects synaptosomal GABA and glutamate transport under oxidative stress conditions. *Brain Research* 2003 Jul 4;977(1):23–30.

15. Longo N. Insulin stimulates the Na+,K(+)-ATPase and the Na+/K+/Cl- cotransporter of human fibroblasts. *Biochimica et Biophysica Acta* 1996 May 22; 1281(1):38–44.

16. Tiwari S, Riazi S, Ecelbarger CA. Insulin's impact on renal sodium transport and blood pressure in health, obesity, and diabetes. *American Journal of Physiology—Renal Physiology* 2007 Oct;293(4):F974–F984.

17. Bhopal RS, Rafnsson SB. Could mitochondrial efficiency explain the susceptibility to adiposity, metabolic syndrome, diabetes and cardiovascular diseases in South Asian populations? *International Journal of Epidemiology* 2009 Aug;38(4):1072–1081.

18. Richter C, Park JW, Ames BN. Normal oxidative damage to mitochondrial and nuclear DNA is extensive. *Proceedings of the National Academy of Sciences of the United States of America* 1988 Sep;85(17):6465–6467.

19. Lee HC, Wei YH. Oxidative stress, mitochondrial DNA mutation, and apoptosis in aging. *Experimental Medicine and Biology (Maywood)* 2007 May; 232(5):592–606.

20. Aliev G, Palacios HH, Walrafen B, et al. Brain mitochondria as a primary target in the development of treatment strategies for Alzheimer disease. *The International Journal of Biochemistry & Cell Biology* 2009 Oct;41(10):1989–2004.

21. Palmieri L, Papaleo V, Porcelli V, et al. Altered calcium homeostasis in autism-spectrum disorders: evidence from biochemical and genetic studies of the mitochondrial aspartate/glutamate carrier AGC1. *Molecular Psychiatry* 2010;15:38–52.

22. Myhill S, Booth NE, McLaren-Howard J. Chronic fatigue syndrome and mitochondrial dysfunction. *International Journal of Clinical and Experimental Medicine* 2009;2(1):1–16.

23. Di Donato S. Multisystem manifestations of mitochondrial disorders. *Journal of Neurology* 2009 May;256(5):693–710.

24. Finsterer J. Central nervous system manifestations of mitochondrial disorders. *Acta Neurologica Scandinavica* 2006 OctZS114(4):217–238.

25. Monroe RK, Halvorsen SW. Environmental toxicants inhibit neuronal Jak tyrosine kinase by mitochondrial disruption. *Neurotoxicology* 2009 Jul;30(4): 589–598.

26. Lim S, Ahn SY, Song IC, Chung MH. Chronic exposure to the herbicide, atrazine, causes mitochondrial dysfunction and insulin resistance. *PLoS One* 2009; 4(4):e5186.

27. Lee HK, Cho YM, Kwak SH, et al. Mitochondrial dysfunction and metabolic syndrome—looking for environmental factors. *Biochimica et Biophysica Acta* 2010;1800(3):282–289.

28. Przedborski S, Jackson-Lewis V, Muthane U, et al. Chronic levodopa administration alters cerebral mitochondrial respiratory chain activity *Annals of Neurology* 1993;34:715–723.

29. Kupsch K, Hertel S, Kreutzmann P, et al. Impairment of mitochondrial function by minocycline. *FEBS Journal* 2009 Mar;276(6):1729–1738.

30. Golomb BA, Evans MA. Statin adverse effects: a review of the literature and evidence for a mitochondrial mechanism. *American Journal of Cardiovascular Drugs* 2008;8(6):373–418.

31. Quinzii CM, DiMauro S, Hirano M. Human coenzyme Q10 deficiency. *Neurochemical Research* 2007;32:723–727.

32. Quinzii CM, Hirano M. Coenzyme Q and mitochondrial disease. *Developmental Disabilities Research Reviews* 2010 Jun;16(2):183–188.

33. Miles MV, Horn PS, Tang PH, et al. Age-related changes in plasma coenzyme Q10 concentrations and redox state in apparently healthy children and adults. *Clinica Chimica Acta* 2004;34:139–144.

34. Rundek T, Naini A, Sacco R, et al. Atorvastatin decreases the coenzyme Q10 level in the blood of patients at risk for cardiovascular disease and stroke. *Archives of Neurology* 2004; 61(6):889–892.

35. Mortensen SA, Leth A, Agner A, Rohde M. Dose-related decrease of serum coenzyme Q_{10} during treatment with HMG-CoA reductase inhibitors. *Mol Aspects Med* 1997;18:S137–S144.

36. Bonakdar RA, Guarneri E. Coenzyme Q10. *American Family Physician* 2005;72:1065–1070.

37. Littarru GP, Tiano L. Bioenergetic and antioxidant properties of coenzyme Q10: recent developments. *Molecular Biotechnology* 2007;37:31–37.

38. Kumar A, Kaur H, Devi P, Mohan V. Role of coenzyme Q10 (CoQ10) in cardiac disease, hypertension and Ménière-like syndrome. *Pharmacology & Therapeutics* 2009;124:259–268.

39. Ochiai A, Itagaki S, Kurokawa T, et al. Improvement in intestinal coenzyme q10 absorption by food intake. *Yakugaku Zasshi* 2007 Aug;127(8):1251–1254.

40. Bhagavan HN, Chopra RK. Plasma coenzyme Q10 response to oral ingestion of coenzyme Q10 formulations. *Mitochondrion* 2007;7 suppl:S78–S88.

41. Hosoe K, Kitano M, Kishida H, et al. Study on safety and bioavailability of ubiquinol (Kaneka QH) after single and 4-week multiple oral administration to healthy volunteers. *Regulatory Toxicology and Pharmacology* 2007 Feb;47(1):19–28.

42. Beg S, Javed S, Kohli K. Bioavailability enhancement of coenzyme Q10: an extensive review of patents. *Recent Patents on Drug Delivery & Formulation* 2010 Nov;4(3):245–255.

43. Takeda R, Sawabe A, Nakano R, et al. Effect of various food additives and soy constituents on high CoQ10 absorption. *Japanese Journal of Medicine and Pharmaceutical Science* 2011; 64(4):614–620.

44. Vormann J, Worlitschek M, Goedecke T, Silver B. Supplementation with alkaline minerals reduces symptoms in patients with chronic low back pain. *Journal of Trace Elements in Medicine and Biology* 2001; 15(2–3):179–183.

Cancer Prevention

1. Greenlee RT, Murray T, Bolden S, Wingo PA. Cancer statistics, 2000. *CA: A The Cancer Journal for Clinicians* 2000; 50:7–33.

2. Hackshaw AK, Law MR, Wald NJ. The accumulated evidence on lung cancer and environmental tobacco smoke. *BMJ* 1997; 315:980–988.

3. Thune I, Furberg AS. Physical activity and cancer risk: dose-response and cancer, all sites and site-specific. *Medicine & Science in Sports & Exercise* 2001;33 suppl 6:S530–S550.

4. Hardman AE. Physical activity and cancer risk. *Proceedings of the Nutrition Society* 2001; 60(1):107–113.

5. Segerstrom SC. Personality and the immune system: models, methods, and mechanisms. *Annals of Behavioral Medicine* 2000;22:180–190.

6. Imai K, Nakachi K. Personality types, lifestyle, and sensitivity to mental stress in association with NK activity. *International Journal of Hygiene and Environmental Health* 2001;204:67–73.

7. Sturm R, Wells KB. Does obesity contribute as much to morbidity as poverty or smoking? *Public Health* 2001;115: 229–235.

8. Lash TL, Aschengrau A. Active and passive cigarette smoking and the occurrence of breast cancer. *American Journal of Epidemiology* 1999;149:5–12.

9. Caplan LS, Schoenfeld ER, O'Leary ES, Leske MC. Breast cancer and electromagnetic fields: a review. *Annals of Epidemiology* 2000;10(1):31–44.

10. Terry P, Lichtenstein P, Feychting M, et al. Fatty fish consumption and risk of prostate cancer. *The Lancet* 2001;357(9270): 1764–1766.

11. Singh PN, Fraser GE. Dietary risk factors for colon cancer in a low-risk population. *American Journal of Epidemiology* 1998; 148:761–774.

12. Zheng W, Gustafson DR, Sinha R, et al. Well-done meat intake and the risk of breast cancer. *Journal of the National Cancer Institute* 1998;90:1724–1729.

13. Terry P, Giovannucci E, Michels KB, et al. Fruit, vegetables, dietary fiber, and risk of colorectal cancer. *Journal of the National Cancer Institute* 2001;93:525–533.

14. Silverman DT, Swanson CA, Gridley G, et al. Dietary and nutritional factors and pancreatic cancer: a case-control study based on direct interviews. *Journal of the National Cancer Institute* 1998;90:1710–1719.

15. Zhang S, Folsom AR, Sellers TA, et al. Breast cancer survival for postmenopausal women who are less overweight and eat less fat. *Cancer* 1995;76:275–283.

16. Slattery ML, Benson J, Berry TD, et al. Dietary sugar and colon cancer. *Cancer Epidemiology, Biomarkers & Prevention* 1997;6(9):677–685.

17. Levi F, Pasche C, La Vecchia C, et al. Food groups and colorectal cancer risk. *British Journal of Cancer* 1999;79:1283–1287.

18. Franceschi S, Dal Maso L, Augustin L, et al. Dietary glycemic load and colorectal cancer risk. *Annals of Oncology* 2001;12: 173–178.

19. Penninx BW, Guralnik JM, Pahor M, et al. Chronically depressed mood and cancer risk in older persons. *Journal of the National Cancer Institute* 1998; 90:1888–1893.

20. Bruske-Hohlfeld I, Mohner M, Ahrens W, et al. Lung cancer risk in male workers occupationally exposed to diesel motor emissions in Germany. *American Journal of Industrial Medicine* 1999;36:405–414.

21. Johnson K. Dairy products linked to ovarian cancer risk. *Family Practice News* 2000 June 15:8.

22. Chan JM, Giovannucci EL. Dairy products, calcium, phosphorus, vitamin D, and risk of prostate cancer. *Cancer Causes and Control* 1998;9:559–566.

23. Levi F, Pasche C, La Vecchia C, et al. Food groups and colorectal cancer risk. *British Journal of Cancer* 1999;79:1283–1287.

24. La Vecchia C, Favero A, Franceschi S. Monounsaturated and other types of fat, and the risk of breast cancer. *European Journal of Cancer Prevention* 1998; 7(6):461–464.

25. Zhong L, Goldberg MS, Gao YT, Jin F. Lung cancer and indoor air pollution arising from Chinese-style cooking among nonsmoking women living in Shanghai, China. *Epidemiology* 1999;10:488–494.

26. Prescott E, Gronbaek M, Becker U, Sorensen TI. Alcohol intake and the risk of lung cancer: influence of type of alcoholic beverage. *American Journal of Epidemiology* 1999; 149:463–470.

27. Garland M, Hunter DJ, Colditz GA, et al. Alcohol consumption in relation to breast cancer risk in a cohort of United States women 25–42 years of age. *Cancer Epidemiology, Biomarkers & Prevention* 1999;8: 1017–1021.

28. Mannisto S, Virtanen M, Kataja V, et al. Lifetime alcohol consumption and breast cancer: a case-control study in Finland. *Public Health Nutrition* 2000;3: 11–18.

29. Garland CF, Garland FC. Do sunlight and vitamin D reduce the likelihood of colon cancer? *International Journal of Epidemiology* 1980 Sep;9(3):227–231.

30. Autier P, Gandini S. Vitamin D supplementation and total mortality: a meta-analysis of randomized controlled trials. *Archives of Internal Medicine* 2007;167:1730–1737.

31. Trump DL, Deeb KK, Johnson CS. Vitamin D: considerations in the continued development as an agent for cancer prevention and therapy. *The Cancer Journal* 2010 Jan–Feb;16(1):1–9.

32. Giovannucci E, Stampfer MJ, Colditz GA, et al. Multivitamin use, folate, and colon cancer in women in the Nurses' Health Study. *Annals of Internal Medicine* 1998;129(7):517–524.

33. Michaud DS, Spiegelman D, Clinton SK, et al. Fluid intake and the risk of bladder cancer in men. *The New England Journal of Medicine* 1999;340: 1390–1397.

34. Combs GF Jr, Clark LC, Turnbull BW. Reduction of cancer risk with an oral supplement of selenium. *Biomedical and Environmental Sciences* 1997;10: 227–234.

35. van Poppel G, Verhoeven DT, Verhagen H, Goldbohm RA. Brassica vegetables and cancer prevention. Epidemiology and mechanisms. *Advances in Experimental Medicine and Biology* 1999;472:159–168.

36. Michaud DS, Spiegelman D, Clinton SK, et al. Fruit and vegetable intake and incidence of bladder cancer in a male prospective cohort. *Journal of the National Cancer Institute* 1999; 91:605–613.

37. Jacobsen BK, Knutsen SF, Fraser GE. Does high soy milk intake reduce prostate cancer incidence? The Adventist Health Study (United States). *Cancer Causes and Control* 1998;9:553–557.

38. Messina MJ. Legumes and soybeans: overview of their nutritional profiles and health effects. *The American Journal of Clinical Nutrition* 1999;70 suppl 3:439S–450S.

39. Kristal AR, Stanford JL, Cohen JH, et al. Vitamin and mineral supplement use is associated with reduced risk of prostate cancer. *Cancer Epidemiology, Biomarkers & Prevention* 1999; 8:887–892.

40. Hardman AE. Physical activity and cancer risk. *Proceedings of the Nutrition Society* 2001; 60(1):107–113.

41. Cohen JH, Kristal AR, Stanford JL. Fruit and vegetable intakes and prostate cancer risk. *Journal of the National Cancer Institute* 2000;92(1):61–68.

42. Clinton SK. The dietary antioxidant network and prostate carcinoma. *Cancer* 1999;86:1629–31.

43. Michaud DS, Spiegelman D, Clinton SK, et al. Prospective study of dietary supplements, macronutrients, micronutrients, and risk of bladder cancer in US men. *American Journal of Epidemiology* 2000;152:1145–1153.

44. Inoue M, Tajima K, Mizutani M, et al. Regular consumption of green tea and the risk of breast cancer recurrence: follow-up study from the hospital-based Epidemiologic Research Program at Aichi Cancer Center (HERPACC), Japan. *Cancer Letters* 2001;167:175–182.

45. Setiawan VW, Zhang ZF, Yu GP, et al. Protective effect of green tea on the risks of chronic gastritis and stomach cancer. *International Journal of Cancer* 2001;92:600–604.

46. Nakachi K, Matsuyama S, Miyake S, et al. Preventive effects of drinking green tea on cancer and cardiovascular disease: epidemiological evidence for multiple targeting prevention. *Biofactors* 2000;13:49–54.

47. Fleischauer AT, Poole C, Arab L. Garlic consumption and cancer prevention: meta-analyses of colorectal and stomach cancers. *The American Journal of Clinical Nutrition* 2000;72: 1047–1052.

48. German JB, Walzem RL. The health benefits of wine. *Annual Review of Nutrition* 2000;20: 561–593.

49. Lappe JM, Travers-Gustafson D, Davies KM, et al. Vitamin D and calcium supplementation reduces cancer risk: results of a randomized trial. *The American Journal of Clinical Nutrition* 2007 Jun;85(6):1586–1591.

Detoxification and Internal Cleansing

1. Passwater RA, Cranton EM. *Trace elements, hair analysis and nutrition.* New Canaan, Conn.: Keats, 1983.

2. Rutter M, Russell-Jones R, eds. *Lead versus health: sources and effects of low level lead exposure.* New York: John Wiley, 1983.

3. Yost KJ. Cadmium, the environment and human health. An overview. *Experentia* 1984;40: 157–164.

4. Gerstner BG, Huff JE. Clinical toxicology of mercury. *Journal of Toxicology and Environmental Health* 1977;2:471–526.

5. Nation JR, Hare MF, Baker DM, et al. Dietary administration of nickel: effects on behavior and metallothionein levels. *Physiology & Behavior* 1985;34: 349–353.

6. Toxicologic consequences of oral aluminum (editorial). *Nutrition Reviews* 1987;45:72–74.

7. Marlowe M, Cossairt A, Welch K, Errara J. Hair mineral content as a predictor of learning disabilities. *Journal of Learning Disabilities* 1984;17:418–421.

8. Pihl R, Parkes M. Hair element content in learning disabled children. *Science* 1977; 198:204–206.

9. David O, Clark J, Voeller K. Lead and hyperactivity. *The Lancet* 1972;2:900–903.

10. David O, Hoffman S, Sverd J. Lead and hyperactivity. Behavioral response to chelation: a pilot study. *The American Journal of Psychiatry* 1976;133: 1155–1188.

11. Benignus VA, Otto DA, Muller KE, Seiple KJ. Effects of age and body lead burden on CNS function in young children: EEG spectra. *Electroencephalography and Clinical Neurophysiology* 1981;52:240–248.

12. Rimland B, Larson G. Hair mineral analysis and behavior: an analysis of 51 studies. *Journal of Learning Disabilities* 1983;16:279–285.

13. Hunter B. Some food additives as neuroexcitors and neurotoxins. *Clinical Ecology* 1984;2: 83–89.

14. Cullen MR, ed. *Workers with multiple chemical sensitivities.* Philadelphia: Hanley & Belfus, 1987.

15. Stayner LT, Elliott L, Blade L, et al. A retrospective cohort mortality study of workers exposed to formaldehyde in the garment industry. *American Journal of Industrial Medicine* 1988;13: 667–681.

16. Kilburn KH, Warshaw R, Boylen CT, et al. Pulmonary and neurobehavioral effects of formaldehyde exposure. *Archives of Environmental Health* 1985;40:254–260.

17. Sterling TD, Arundel AV. Health effects of phenoxy herbicides. *Scandinavian Journal of Work, Environment & Health* 1986;12:161–173.

18. Dickey L, ed. *Clinical ecology.* Springfield, Ill.: Charles C. Thomas, 1976.

19. Linstrom K, Riihimaki H, Hannininen K. Occupational solvent exposure and neuropsychiatric disorders. *Scandinavian Journal of Work, Environment & Health* 1984;10:321–323.

20. Talska G. Genetically based n-acetyltransferase metabolic polymorphism and low-level environmental exposure to carcinogens. *Nature* 1994;369: 154–156.

21. Gallagher JE, Everson RB, Lewtas J, et al. Comparison of DNA adduct levels in human placenta from polychlorinated biphenyl exposed women and smokers in which CYP 1A1 levels are similarly elevated. *Teratogenesis, Carcinogenesis, and Mutagenesis* 1994;14:183–192.

22. Campbell ME, Grant DM, Inaba T, Kalow W. Biotransformation of caffeine, paraxanthine, theophylline, and theobromine by polycyclic aromatic hydrocarbon-inducable cytochrome P-450 in human liver microsomes. *Drug Metabolism and Disposition* 1987;15:237–249.

23. Beecher CWW. Cancer preventive properties of varieties of *Brassica oleracea*. A review. *The American Journal of Clinical Nutrition* 1994;59 suppl:1166S–1170S.

24. Crowell PL, Gould MN. Chemoprevention and therapy of cancer by d-limonene. *Critical Reviews in Oncogenesis* 1994;5: 1–22.

25. Yee GC, Stanley DL, Pessa LJ, et al. Effect of grapefruit juice on blood cyclosporin concentration. *The Lancet* 1995;345: 955–956.

26. Nagabhushan M, Bhide SV. Curcumin as an inhibitor of cancer. *Journal of the American College of Nutrition* 1992;11: 192–198.

27. Polasa K, Raghuram TC, Krishna TP, Krishnaswamy K. Effect of turmeric on urinary mutagens in smokers. *Mutagenesis* 1992;7:107–109.

28. Hagen TM, Wierzbicka GT, Bowman BB, et al. Fate of dietary glutathione. Disposition in the gastrointestinal tract. *American Journal of Physiology—Gastrointestinal and Liver Physiology* 1990;259: G524–G529.

29. Witschi A, Reddy S, Stofer B, Lauterburg BH. The systemic availability of oral glutathione. *European Journal of Clinical Pharmacology* 1992;43:667–669.

30. Johnston CJ, Meyer CG, Srilakshmi JC. Vitamin C elevates red blood cell glutathione in healthy adults. *The American Journal of Clinical Nutrition* 1993;58: 103–105.

31. Jain A, Buist NR, Kennaaway NG, et al. Effect of ascorbate or N-acetylcysteine treatment in a patient with hereditary glutathione synthetase deficiency. *Journal of Pediatrics* 1994;124: 229–233.

32. Kleinveld HA, Demacker PNM, Stalenhoef AFH. Failure of N-acetylcysteine to reduce low-density lipoprotein oxidizability in healthy subjects. *European Journal of Clinical Pharmacology* 1992;43:639–642.

33. Quick AJ. Clinical value of the test for hippuric acid in cases of disease of the liver. *Archives of Internal Medicine* 1936;57: 544–556.

34. Frezza M, Pozzato G, Chiesa L, et al. Reversal of intrahepatic cholestasis of pregnancy in women after high dose S-adenosyl-L-methionine (SAMe) administration. *Hepatology* 1984; 4:274–278.

35. Gregus S, Oguro T, Klaassen CD. Nutritionally and chemically induced impairment of sulfate activation and sulfation of xenobiotics in vivo. *Chemico-Biological Interactions* 1994;92: 169–177.

36. Barzatt R, Beckman JD. Inhibition of phenol sulfotransferase by pyridoxal phosphate. *Biochemical Pharmacology* 1994; 47:2087–2095.

37. Skvortsova RI, Pzniakovskii VM, Agarkova IA. [Role of the vitamin factor in preventing phenol poisoning.] *Voprosy Pitaniia* 1981;2:32–35.

38. Bombardieri G. Effects of S-adenosyl-methionine (SAMe) in the treatment of Gilbert's

syndrome. *Current Therapeutic Research* 1985;37:580–585.

39. Birkmayer JGD, Beyer W. Biological and clinical relevance of trace elements. *Ärztl Lab* 1990; 36:284–287.

40. Di Padova C, Triapepe T, Di Padova F, et al. S-adenosyl-L-methionine antagonizes oral contraceptive-induced bile cholesterol supersaturation in healthy women: preliminary report of a controlled randomized trial. *The American Journal of Gastroenterology* 1984; 79:941–944.

41. Flora SJS, Singh S, Tandon SK. Prevention of lead intoxication by vitamin B complex. *Zeitschrift für die Gesamte Hygiene und Ihre Grenzgebiete* 1984;30:409–411.

42. Shakman RA. Nutritional influences on the toxicity of environmental pollutants: a review. *Archives of Environmental Health* 1974;28:105–133.

43. Flora SJS, Jain VK, Behari JR, Tandon SK. Protective role of trace metals in lead intoxication. *Toxicology Letters* 1982;13:51–56.

44. Wisniewska-Knypl J, Sokal JA, Klimczark J, et al. Protective effect of methionine against vinyl chloride-mediated depression of non-protein sulfhydryls and cytochrome P-450. *Toxicology Letters* 1981;8:147–152.

45. Barak AJ, Beckenhauer HC, Junnila M, Tuma DJ. Dietary betaine promotes generation of hepatic S-adenosylmethionine and protects the liver from ethanol-induced fatty infiltration. *Alcoholism: Clinical and Experimental Research* 1993;17: 552–555.

46. Zeisel SH, Da Costa KA, Franklin PD, et al. Choline, an essential nutrient for humans. *The FASEB Journal* 1991;5:2093–2098.

47. Hikino H, Kiso Y, Wagner H, Fiebig M. Antihepatotoxic actions of flavonolignans from Si-lybum marianum fruits. *Planta Medica* 1984;50:248–250.

48. Vogel G, Trost W. Studies on pharmacodynamics, site and mechanism of action of silymarin, the antihepatotoxic principle from *Silybum marianum* (L.) Gaert. *Arzneimittelforschung* 1975;25:179–185.

49. Valenzuela A, Aspillaga M, Vial S, Guerra R. Selectivity of silymarin on the increase of the glutathione content in different tissues of the rat. *Planta Medica* 1989;55:420–422.

50. Sarre H. Experience in the treatment of chronic hepatopathies with silymarin. *Arzneimittelforschung* 1971;21: 1209–1212.

51. Canini F, Bartolucci L, Cristallini E, et al. [Use of silymarin in the treatment of alcoholic hepatic steatosis.] *La Clinica Terapeutica* 1985;114:307–314.

52. Salmi HA, Sarna S. Effect of silymarin on chemical, functional, and morphological alteration of the liver. A double-blind controlled study. *Scandinavian Journal of Gastroenterology* 1982;17:417–421.

53. Boari C, Gennari P, Violante FS, et al. Occupational toxic liver diseases. Therapeutic effects of silymarin. *Minnesota Medicine* 1985;72:2679–2688.

54. Ferenci P, Dragosics H, Frank H, et al. Randomized controlled trial of silymarin treatment in patients with cirrhosis of the liver. *Journal of Hepatology* 1989;9:105–113.

55. Imamura M, Tung T. A trial of fasting cure for PCB poisoned patients in Taiwan. *American Journal of Industrial Medicine* 1984;5:147–153.

56. Kilburn K, Warsaw RH, Shields MG. Neurobehavioral dysfunction in firemen exposed to polychlorinated biphenyls (PCBs). Possible improvement after detoxification. *Archives of Environmental Health* 1989;44: 345–350.

Digestion and Elimination

1. McCarthy DM. Adverse effects of proton pump inhibitor drugs: clues and conclusions. *Current Opinion in Gastroenterology* 2010 Nov;26(6):624–631.

2. Tran T, Lowry AM, El-Serag HB. Meta-analysis: the efficacy of over-the-counter gastro-oesophageal reflux disease therapies. *Alimentary Pharmacology & Therapeutics* 2007 Jan 15; 25(2):143–153.

3. Sun J. D-limonene: safety and clinical applications. *Alternative Medicine Review* 2007 Sep; 12(3):259–264.

4. Howden CW, Hunt RH. Spontaneous hypochlorhydria in man: possible causes and consequences. *Digestive Diseases* 1986;4(1):26–32.

5. Rawls WB, Ancona VC. Chronic urticaria associated with hypochlorhydria or achlorhydria. *The Review of Gastroenterology* 1951;18:267–271.

6. Giannella RA, Broitman SA, Zamcheck N. Influence of gastric acidity on bacterial and parasitic enteric infections: a perspective. *Annals of Internal Medicine* 1973;78:271–276.

7. De Witte TJ, Geerdink PJ, Lamers CB, et al. Hypochlorhydria and hypergastrinaemia in rheumatoid arthritis. *Annals of the Rheumatic Diseases* 1979; 38:14–17.

8. Ryle JA, Barber HW. Gastric analysis in acne rosacea. *The Lancet* 1920;2:1195–1196.

9. Ayres S. Gastric secretion in psoriasis, eczema and dermatitis herpetiformis. *Archives of Dermatology* 1929;Jul:854–859.

10. Dotevall G, Walan A. Gastric secretion of acid and intrinsic factor in patients with hyper and hypothyroidism. *Acta Medica Scandinavica* 1969;186: 529–533.

11. Howitz J, Schwartz M. Vitiligo, achlorhydria, and pernicious anemia. *The Lancet* 1971;1: 1331–1334.

12. Howden CW, Hunt RH. Relationship between gastric secretion and infection. *Gut* 1987;28: 96–107.

13. Rafsky HA, Weingarten M. A study of the gastric secretory response in the aged. *Gastroenterology* 1947 May:348–352.

14. Davies D, James TG. An investigation into the gastric secretion of a hundred normal persons over the age of sixty. *British Medical Journal* 1930;1:1–14.

15. Baron JH. Studies of basal and peak acid output with an augmented histamine test. *Gut* 1963;4:136–144.

16. Mojaverian P, Ferguson RK, Vlasses PH, et al. Estimation of gastric residence time of the Heidelberg capsule in humans: effect of varying food composition. *Gastroenterology* 1985;89: 392–397.

17. Atherton JC. The pathogenesis of *Helicobacter pylori*–induced gastro-duodenal diseases. *Annual Review of Pathology* 2006; 1:63–96.

18. Ghoshal UC, Chourasia D. Gastroesophageal reflux disease and *Helicobacter pylori:* what may be the relationship? *Journal of Neurogastroenterology & Motility* 2010 Jul;16(3):243–250.

19. Sarker SA, Gyr K. Non-immunological defense mechanisms of the gut. *Gut* 1992;33:987–993.

20. Williams C. Occurrence and significance of gastric colonization during acid-inhibitory therapy. *Best Practice & Research: Clinical Gastroenterology* 2001 Jun;15(3):511–521.

21. Shibata T, Imoto I, Taguchi Y, et al. High acid secretion may protect the gastric mucosa from injury caused by ammonia produced by *Helicobacter pylori* in duodenal ulcer patients. *Journal of Gastroenterology and Hepatology* 1996;11:674–680.

22. Rokkas T, Papatheodorou G, Karameris A, et al. *Helicobacter pylori* infection and gastric juice vitamin C levels: impact of eradication. *Digestive Diseases and Sciences* 1995;40:615–621.

23. Phull PS, Price AB, Thorniley MS, et al. Vitamin E concentrations in the human stomach and duodenum: correlation with *Helicobacter pylori* infection. *Gut* 1996;39:31–35.

24. Baik SC, Youn HS, Chung MH, et al. Increased oxidative DNA damage in *Helicobacter pylori*–infected human gastric mucosa. *Cancer Research* 1996;56:1279–1282.

25. Beil W, Birkholz C, Sewing KF. Effects of flavonoids on parietal cell acid secretion, gastric mucosal prostaglandin production and helicobacter pylori growth. *Arzneimittelforschung* 1995;45: 697–700.

26. Marshall BJ, Valenzuela JE, McCallum RW, et al. Bismuth subsalicylate suppression of *Helicobacter pylori* in nonulcer dyspepsia. A double-blind placebo-controlled trial. *Digestive Diseases and Sciences* 1993;38:1674–1680.

27. Kang JY, Tay HH, Wee A, et al. Effect of colloidal bismuth subcitrate on symptoms and gastric histology in non-ulcer dyspepsia: a double blind placebo controlled study. *Gut* 1990;31: 476–480.

28. May B, Kuntz HD, Kieser M, et al. Efficacy of a fixed peppermint oil/caraway oil combination in non-ulcer dyspepsia. *Arzneimittelforschung* 1996;46: 1149–1153.

29. May B, Kohler S, Schneider B. Efficacy and tolerability of a fixed combination of peppermint oil and caraway oil in patients suffering from functional dyspepsia. *Alimentary Pharmacology & Therapeutics* 2000;14: 1671–1677.

30. Taylor JR, Gardner TB, Waljee AK, et al. Systematic review: efficacy and safety of pancreatic enzyme supplements for exocrine pancreatic insufficiency. *Alimentary Pharmacology & Therapeutics* 2010 Jan;31(1): 57–72.

31. Schneider MU, Knoll-Ruzicka ML, Domschke S, et al. Pancreatic enzyme replacement therapy: comparative effects of conventional and enteric-coated microspheric pancreatin and acid-stable fungal enzyme preparations on steatorrhoea in chronic pancreatitis. *Hepatogastroenterology* 1985;32:97–102.

32. Raithel M, Weidenhiller M, Schwab D, et al. Pancreatic enzymes: a new group of antiallergic drugs? *Inflammation Research* 2002 Apr;51 suppl 1: S13–S14.

33. Bures J, Cyrany J, Kohoutova D, et al. Small intestinal bacterial overgrowth syndrome. *World Journal of Gastroenterology* 2010 Jun 28;16(24):2978–2990.

34. Watanabe A, Obata T, Nagashima H. Berberine therapy of hypertyraminemia in patients with liver cirrhosis. *Acta Medica Okayama* 1982;36:277–281.

Heart and Cardiovascular Health

1. Viles-Gonzalez JF, Anand SX, Valdiviezo C, et al. Update in atherothrombotic disease. *Mount Sinai Journal of Medicine* 2004; 71:197–208.

2. Qiao Q, Tervahauta M, Nissinen A, et al. Mortality from all causes and from coronary heart disease related to smoking and changes in smoking during a 35-year follow-up of middle-aged Finnish men. *European Heart Journal* 2000;21:1621–1626.

3. Imamura H, Tanaka K, Hirae C, et al. Relationship of cigarette smoking to blood pressure and serum lipids and lipoproteins in men. *Clinical and Experimental Pharmacology and Physiology* 1996;23:397–402.

4. Levenson J, Simon AC, Cambien FA. Cigarette smoking and hypertension. Factors independently associated with blood hy-

perviscosity and arterial rigidity. *Arteriosclerosis* 1987;7:572–577.

5. Kritz H, Schmid P, Sinzinger H. Passive smoking and cardiovascular risk. *Archives of Internal Medicine* 1995;155:1942–1948.

6. Critchley JA, Capewell S. Mortality risk reduction associated with smoking cessation in patients with coronary heart disease: a systematic review. *JAMA, The Journal of the American Medical Association* 2003;290:86–97.

7. Law M, Tang JL. An analysis of the effectiveness of interventions intended to help people stop smoking. *Archives of Internal Medicine* 1995;155:1933–1941.

8. Ip S, Lichtenstein AH, Chung M, Systematic review: association of low-density lipoprotein subfractions with cardiovascular outcomes. *Annals of Internal Medicine* 2009 Apr 7; 150(7):474–484.

9. Davidson MH. Apolipoprotein measurements: is more widespread use clinically indicated? *Clinical Cardiology* 2009 Sep; 32(9):482–486.

10. Centers for Disease Control and Prevention (CDC). Trends in leisure-time physical inactivity by age, sex, and race/ethnicity—United States, 1994–2004. *Morbidity and Mortality Weekly Report* 2005 Oct 7;54(39):991–994.

11. Danesh J, Whincup P, Walker M, et al. Low grade inflammation and coronary heart disease: prospective study and updated meta-analysis. *BMJ* 2000;321:199–204.

12. Ridker PM, Rifai N, Rose L, et al. Comparison of C-reactive protein and low-density lipoprotein cholesterol levels in the prediction of first cardiovascular events. *The New England Journal of Medicine* 2002;347: 1557–1565.

13. Lee WY, Park JS, Noh SY, et al. C-reactive protein concentrations are related to insulin resis-tance and metabolic syndrome as defined by the ATP III report. *International Journal of Cardiology* 2004;97:101–106.

14. Khaw KT, Wareham N, Bingham S, et al. Combined impact of health behaviours and mortality in men and women: the EPIC-Norfolk prospective population study. PLoS Medicine 2008 Jan 8;5(1):e12.

15. De Lorgeril M, Salen P, Martin J-L, et al. Mediterranean diet, traditional risk factors, and the rate of cardiovascular complications after myocardial infarction: final report of the Lyon Diet Heart Study. *Circulation* 1999;99:779–785.

16. Esposito K, Marfella R, Ciotola M, et al. Effect of a Mediterranean-style diet on endothelial dysfunction and markers of vascular inflammation in the metabolic syndrome: a randomized trial. *JAMA, The Journal of the American Medical Association* 2004;292:1440–1446.

17. Martinez-González MA, Sánchez-Villegas A. The emerging role of Mediterranean diets in cardiovascular epidemiology: monounsaturated fats, olive oil, red wine or the whole pattern? *European Journal of Epidemiology* 2004;19:9–13.

18. Sieri S, Krogh V, Berrino F, et al. Dietary glycemic load and index and risk of coronary heart disease in a large Italian cohort: the EPICOR study. *Archives of Internal Medicine* 2010 Apr 12; 170(7):640–647.

19. Alarcon de la Lastra C, Barranco MD, Motilva V, et al. Mediterranean diet and health: biological importance of olive oil. *Current Pharmaceutical Design* 2001;7:933–950.

20. Bucher HC, Hengstler P, Schindler C, et al. N-3 polyunsaturated fatty acids in coronary heart disease: a meta-analysis of randomized controlled trials. *The American Journal of Medicine* 2002;112:298–304.

21. Harris WS, Von Schacky C. The omega-3 index: a new risk factor for death from coronary heart disease? *Preventive Medicine* 2004;39:212–220.

22. Harris WS. The omega-3 index as a risk factor for coronary heart disease. *The American Journal of Clinical Nutrition* 2008 Jun;87(6):1997S–2002S.

23. Hu FB, Bronner L, Willett WC, et al. Fish and omega-3 fatty acid intake and risk of coronary heart disease in women. *JAMA, The Journal of the American Medical Association* 2002;287: 1815–1821.

24. Albert CM, Campos H, Stampfer MJ, et al. Blood levels of long-chain n-3 fatty acids and the risk of sudden death. *The New England Journal of Medicine* 2002;346:1113–1118.

25. Skulas-Ray AC, Kris-Etherton PM, Harris WS, et al. Dose-response effects of omega-3 fatty acids on triglycerides, inflammation, and endothelial function in healthy persons with moderate hypertriglyceridemia. *The American Journal of Clinical Nutrition* 2011 Feb;93(2): 243–252.

26. Sandker GW, Kromhout D, Aravanis C. Serum cholesterol ester fatty acids and their relation with serum lipids in elderly men in Crete and the Netherlands. *European Journal of Clinical Nutrition* 1993;47:201–208.

27. Kagawa Y, Nishizawa M, Suzuki M, et al. Eicosapolyenoic acids of serum lipids of Japanese islanders with low incidence of cardiovascular diseases. *Journal of Nutritional Science and Vitaminology* 1982;28:441–453.

28. Hu FB, Stampfer MJ. Nut consumption and risk of coronary heart disease: a review of epidemiologic evidence. *Current Atherosclerosis Reports* 1999;1: 204–209.

29. Ros E, Nunez I, Perez-Heras A, et al. A walnut diet improves endothelial function in hypercholesterolemic subjects: a

randomized crossover trial. *Circulation* 2004;109:1609–1614.

30. Ford ES, Liu S, Mannino DM, et al. C-reactive protein concentration and concentrations of blood vitamins, carotenoids, and selenium among United States adults. *European Journal of Clinical Nutrition* 2003;57: 1157–1163.

31. Weisburger JH. Lycopene and tomato products in health promotion. *Advances in Experimental Medicine and Biology* 2002;227:924–927.

32. Williams MJ, Sutherland WH, Whelan AP, et al. Acute effect of drinking red and white wines on circulating levels of inflammation-sensitive molecules in men with coronary artery disease. *Metabolism* 2004;53: 318–323.

33. Rimm EB, Williams P, Fosher K, et al. Moderate alcohol intake and lower risk of coronary heart disease: meta-analysis of effects on lipids and haemostatic factors. *BMJ* 1999; 319:1523–1528.

34. Skaltsounis AL, Kremastinos DT. Polyphenolic compounds from red grapes acutely improve endothelial function in patients with coronary heart disease. *European Journal of Cardiovascular Prevention & Rehabilitation* 2005;12(6):596–600.

35. Oak MH, El Bedoui J, Schini-Kerth VB. Antiangiogenic properties of natural polyphenols from red wine and green tea. *The Journal of Nutritional Biochemistry* 2005;16(1):1–8.

36. Sumner MD, Elliott-Eller M, Weidner G, et al. Effects of pomegranate juice consumption on myocardial perfusion in patients with coronary heart disease. *American Journal of Cardiology* 2005;96(6):810–814.

37. Aviram M, Rosenblat M, Gaitini D, et al. Pomegranate juice consumption for 3 years by patients with carotid artery stenosis reduces common carotid intima-media thickness, blood pressure

and LDL oxidation. *Clinical Nutrition* 2004;23(3):423–433.

38. Esmaillzadeh A, Tahbaz F, Gaieni I, et al. Concentrated pomegranate juice improves lipid profiles in diabetic patients with hyperlipidemia. *Journal of Medicinal Food* 2004;7(3): 305–308.

39. Clarke R, Armitage J. Antioxidant vitamins and risk of cardiovascular disease. Review of large-scale randomised trials. *Cardiovascular Drugs and Therapy* 2002;16:411–415.

40. Vivekananthan DP, Penn MS, Sapp SK, et al. Use of antioxidant vitamins for the prevention of cardiovascular disease: meta-analysis of randomised trials. *The Lancet* 2003;361: 2017–2023.

41. Salonen RM, Nyyssonen K, Kaikkonen J, et al. Six-year effect of combined vitamin C and E supplementation on atherosclerotic progression: the Antioxidant Supplementation in Atherosclerosis Prevention (ASAP) Study. *Circulation* 2003;107:947–953.

42. Lowe GM, Bilton RF, Davies IG. Carotenoid composition and antioxidant potential in subfractions of human low-density lipoprotein. *Annals of Clinical Biochemistry* 1999;36:323–332.

43. Church TS, Earnest CP, Wood KA, et al. Reduction of C-reactive protein levels through use of a multivitamin. *The American Journal of Medicine* 2003; 115:702–707.

44. Princen HM, Van Duyvenvoorde W, Buytenhek R, et al. Supplementation with low doses of vitamin E protects LDL from lipid peroxidation in men and women. *Arteriosclerosis, Thrombosis, and Vascular Biology* 1995;15:325–333.

45. Gey KF, Puska P, Jordan P. Inverse correlation between plasma vitamin E and mortality from ischemic heart disease in cross-cultural epidemiology. *The American Journal of Clinical Nutrition* 1991;53:326S–334S.

46. Bellizzi MC, Franklin MF, Duthie GG. Vitamin E and coronary heart disease: the European paradox. *European Journal of Clinical Nutrition* 1994;48:822–831.

47. Stampfer MJ, Hennekens CH, Manson JE. Vitamin E consumption and the risk of coronary disease in women. *The New England Journal of Medicine* 1993;328:1444–1449.

48. Rimm EB, Stampfer MJ, Ascherio A. Vitamin E consumption and the risk of coronary heart disease in men. *The New England Journal of Medicine* 1993; 328:1450–1456.

49. Saremi A, Arora R. Vitamin E and cardiovascular disease. *American Journal of Therapeutics* 2010 May–Jun; 17(3):e56–e65.

50. Kaikkonen J, Nyyssonen K, Tomasi A, et al. Antioxidative efficacy of parallel and combined supplementation with coenzyme Q10 and d-alpha-tocopherol in mildly hypercholesterolemic subjects: a randomized placebo-controlled clinical study. *Free Radical Research* 2000;33:329–340.

51. Wang XL, Rainwater DL, Mahaney MC, et al. Cosupplementation with vitamin E and coenzyme Q10 reduces circulating markers of inflammation in baboons. *The American Journal of Clinical Nutrition* 2004;80: 649–655.

52. Thomas SR, Leichtweis SB, Pettersson K, et al. Dietary cosupplementation with vitamin E and coenzyme Q(10) inhibits atherosclerosis in apolipoprotein E gene knockout mice. *Arteriosclerosis, Thrombosis, and Vascular Biology* 2001;21:585–593.

53. Yegin A, Yegin H, Aliciguzel Y, et al. Erythrocyte selenium-glutathione peroxidase activity is lower in patients with coronary atherosclerosis. *Japanese Heart Journal* 1997;38:793–798.

54. Bor MV, Cevik C, Uslu I, et al.

Selenium levels and glutathione peroxidase activities in patients with acute myocardial infarction. *Acta Cardiologica* 1999; 54:271–276.

55. Frei B, England L, Ames BN. Ascorbate is an outstanding antioxidant in human blood plasma. *Proceedings of the National Academy of Sciences of the United States of America* 1989;86:6377–6381.

56. Harats D, Ben-Naim M, Dabach Y. Effect of vitamin C and E supplementation on susceptibility of plasma lipoproteins to peroxidation induced by acute smoking. *Atherosclerosis* 1990; 85:47–54.

57. Salonen RM, Nyyssonen K, Kaikkonen J, et al. Six-year effect of combined vitamin C and E supplementation on atherosclerotic progression: the Antioxidant Supplementation Atherosclerosis Prevention (ASAP) study. *Circulation* 2003;107:947–953.

58. Simon JA. Vitamin C and cardiovascular disease. a review. *Journal of the American College of Nutrition* 1992;11:107–125.

59. Howard PA, Meyers DG. Effect of vitamin C on plasma lipids. *The Annals of Pharmacotherapy* 1995;29:1129–1136.

60. Jacques PF, Sulsky SI, Perrone GA. Ascorbic acid and plasma lipids. *Epidemiology* 1994;5: 19–26.

61. Hallfrisch J, Singh VN, Muller DC, et al. High plasma vitamin C associated with high plasma HDL- and HDL2 cholesterol. *The American Journal of Clinical Nutrition* 1994;60:100–105.

62. Padayatty SJ, Katz A, Wang Y, et al. Vitamin C as an antioxidant: evaluation of its role in disease prevention. *Journal of the American College of Nutrition* 2003;22:18–35.

63. Tousoulis D, Antoniades C, Tountas C, et al. Vitamin C affects thrombosis/fibrinolysis system and reactive hyperemia in patients with type 2 diabetes and coronary artery disease.

Diabetes Care 2003;26:2749–2753.

64. Shi J, Yu J, Pohorly JE, et al. Polyphenolics in grape seeds—biochemistry and functionality. *Journal of Medicinal Food* 2003;6:291–299.

65. Rohdewald P. A review of the French maritime pine bark extract (Pycnogenol), a herbal medication with a diverse clinical pharmacology. *Int J Clin Pharmacol Ther* 2002;40:158–168.

66. Freese R, Mutanen M. Alpha-linolenic acid and marine long-chain n-3 fatty acids differ only slightly in their effects on hemostatic factors in healthy subjects. *The American Journal of Clinical Nutrition* 1997;66:591–598.

67. Smith RD, Kelly CN, Fielding BA, et al. Long-term monounsaturated fatty acid diets reduce platelet aggregation in healthy young subjects. *British Journal of Nutrition* 2003;90:597–606.

68. Lam SC, Harfenist EJ, Packham MA, et al. Investigation of possible mechanisms of pyridoxal 5-phosphate inhibition of platelet reactions. *Thrombosis Research* 1980;20:633–645.

69. Sermet A, Aybak M, Ulak G. Effect of oral pyridoxine hydrochloride supplementation on in vitro platelet sensitivity to different agonists. *Arzneimittelforschung* 1995;45:19–21.

70. Friso S, Girelli D, Martinelli N, et al. Low plasma vitamin B-6 concentrations and modulation of coronary artery disease risk. *The American Journal of Clinical Nutrition* 2004;79:992–998.

71. Kiesewetter H, Jung F, Pindur G. Effect of garlic on thrombocyte aggregation, microcirculation, and other risk factors. *International Journal of Clinical Pharmacology, Therapy and Toxicology* 1991;29: 151–155.

72. Ernst E. Fibrinogen: an important risk factor for atherothrombotic diseases. *Annals of Medicine* 1994;26:15–22.

73. Hsia CH, Shen MC, Lin JS, et al. Nattokinase decreases plasma levels of fibrinogen, factor VII, and factor VIII in human subjects. *Nutrition Research* 2009 Mar;29(3):190–196.

74. Chrysohoou C, Panagiotakos DB, Pitsavos C, et al. Adherence to the Mediterranean diet attenuates inflammation and coagulation process in healthy adults: the ATTICA Study. *Journal of the American College of Cardiology* 2004;44:152–158.

75. Boushey C, Beresford S, Omenn G, et al. A quantitative assessment of plasma homocysteine as a risk factor for vascular disease. Probable benefits of increasing folic acid intakes. *JAMA, The Journal of the American Medical Association* 1995;274: 1049–1057.

76. Gauthier GM, Keevil JG, McBride PE. The association of homocysteine and coronary artery disease. *Clinical Cardiology* 2003;26:563–568.

77. Bozkurt E, Keles S, Acikel M, et al. Plasma homocysteine level and the angiographic extent of coronary artery disease. *Angiology* 2004;55:265–270.

78. Humphrey LL, Fu R, Rogers K, et al. Homocysteine level and CHD incidence: a systematic review and meta-analysis. *Mayo Clinic Proceedings* 2008 Nov; 83(11):1203–1212.

79. Ubbink JB, Vermaak WJ, wan der Merwe A, et al. Vitamin B-12, vitamin B-6, and folate nutritional status in men with hyperhomocysteinemia. *The American Journal of Clinical Nutrition* 1993;57: 47–53.

80. Anderson JL, Jensen KR, Carlquist JF, et al. Effect of folic acid fortification of food on homocysteine-related mortality. *The American Journal of Medicine* 2004;116:158–164.

81. Matthews KA, Haynes SG. Type A behavior pattern and coronary disease risk. *American Journal of Epidemiology* 1986; 123:923–960.

82. Muller MM, Rau H, Brody S. The relationship between habitual anger coping style and serum lipid and lipoprotein concentrations. *Biological Psychology* 1995;41:69–81.

83. Strike PC, Steptoe A. Psychosocial factors in the development of coronary artery disease. *Progress in Cardiovascular Diseases* 2004;46:337–347.

84. Suarez EC. C-reactive protein is associated with psychological risk factors of cardiovascular disease in apparently healthy adults. *Psychosomatic Medicine* 2004;66:684–691.

85. Maier JA. Low magnesium and atherosclerosis: an evidence-based link. *Molecular Aspects of Medicine* 2003;24:137–146.

86. Maier JA, Malpuech-Brugere C, Zimowska W, et al. Low magnesium promotes endothelial cell dysfunction: implications for atherosclerosis, inflammation and thrombosis. *Biochimica et Biophysica Acta* 2004;1689:13–21.

87. Hampton EM, Whang DD, Whang R. Intravenous magnesium therapy in acute myocardial infarction. *The Annals of Pharmacotherapy* 1994;28: 212–219.

88. Teo KK, Yusuf S. Role of magnesium in reducing mortality in acute myocardial infarction. A review of the evidence. *Drugs* 1993;46:347–359.

89. Schecter M, Kaplinsky E, Rabinowitz B. The rationale of magnesium supplementation in acute myocardial infarction. A review of the literature. *Archives of Internal Medicine* 1992;152:2189–2196.

90. Kim DH, Sabour S, Sagar UN, et al. Prevalence of hypovitaminosis D in cardiovascular diseases (from the National Health and Nutrition Examination Survey 2001 to 2004). *American Journal of Cardiology* 2008 Dec 1;102(11):1540–1544.

91. Dobnig H, Pilz S, Scharnagl H, et al. Independent association of low serum 25-hydroxyvitamin d and 1,25-dihydroxyvitamin d levels with all-cause and cardiovascular mortality. *Archives of Internal Medicine*. 2008 Jun 23;168(12): 1340–1349.

92. Eidelman RS, Hebert PR, Weisman SM, et al. An update on aspirin in the primary prevention of cardiovascular disease. *Archives of Internal Medicine* 2003;163:2006–2010.

93. Weisman SM, Graham DY. Evaluation of the benefits and risks of low-dose aspirin in the secondary prevention of cardiovascular and cerebrovascular events. *Archives of Internal Medicine* 2002;162:2197–2202.

94. Willard JE, Lange RA, Hillis LD. The use of aspirin in ischemic heart disease. *The New England Journal of Medicine* 1992;327:175–181.

95. Weil J, Colin-Jones D, Langman M. Prophylactic aspirin and risk of peptic ulcer bleeding. *BMJ* 1995;310:827–830.

96. Ornish D. Can lifestyle changes reverse coronary heart disease? *The Lancet* 1990;336:129–133.

97. Burr ML, Fehily AM, Gilbert JF, et al. Effects of changes in fat, fish, and fiber intakes on death and myocardial reinfarction: Diet and Reinfarction Trial (DART). *The Lancet* 1989;2: 757–761.

98. de Lorgeril M, Renaud S, Mamelle N, et al. Mediterranean alpha-linolenic acid-rich diet in secondary prevention of coronary heart disease. *The Lancet* 1994;343:1454–1459.

99. Elliott WJ. Ear lobe crease and coronary artery disease. *The American Journal of Medicine* 1983;75:1024–1032.

100. Elliott WJ, Powell LH. Diagonal earlobe creases and prognosis in patients with suspected coronary artery disease. *The American Journal of Medicine* 1996;100:205–211.

Immune System Support

1. Campeau S, Day HE, Helmreich DL, et al. Principles of psychoneuroendocrinology. *Psychiatric Clinics of North America* 1998;21:259–276.

2. Bartrop RW, Luckhurst E, Lazarus L, et al. Depressed lymphocyte function after bereavement. *The Lancet* 1977;1: 834–836.

3. Padgett DA, Glaser R. How stress influences the immune response. *Trends in Immunology* 2003;24:444–448.

4. Cousins N. *Anatomy of an illness.* New York: Bantam, 1979.

5. Dillon KM, Minchoff B. Positive emotional states and enhancement of the immune system. *International Journal of Psychiatry in Medicine* 1986;15: 13–17.

6. Martin RA, Dobbin JP. Sense of humor, hassles, and immunoglobulin A: evidence for a stress-moderating effect of humor. *International Journal of Psychiatry in Medicine* 1988;18: 93–105.

7. Kiecolt-Glaser JK, Glaser R. Psychoneuroimmunology: can psychological interventions modulate immunity? *Journal of Consulting and Clinical Psychology* 1992;60: 569–575.

8. Mulla A, Buckingham JC. Regulation of the hypothalamo-pituitary-adrenal axis by cytokines. *Baillière's Best Practice and Research: Clinical Endocrinology & Metabolism* 1999;13:503–521.

9. Matalka KZ. Neuroendocrine and cytokines-induced responses to minutes, hours, and days of mental stress. *Neuroendocrinology Letters* 2003;24:283–292.

10. Elenkov IJ. Glucocorticoids and the Th1/Th2 balance. *Annals of the New York Academy of Sciences* 2004;1024:138–146.

11. Kiecolt-Glaser JK, Glaser R, Gravenstein S, et al. Chronic stress alters the immune response to influenza virus vaccine in older adults. *Proceedings of the National Academy of Sciences of the United States of America* 1996;93:3043–3047.

12. Burns VE, Carroll D, Drayson M,

et al. Life events, perceived stress and antibody response to influenza vaccination in young, healthy adults. *Journal of Psychosomatic Research* 2003;55: 569–572.

13. MacDonald CM. A chuckle a day keeps the doctor away: therapeutic humor and laughter. *Journal of Psychosocial Nursing and Mental Health Services* 2004;42:18–25.

14. Kusaka Y, Kondou H, Morimoto K. Healthy lifestyles are associated with higher natural killer cell activity. *Preventive Medicine* 1992;21:602–615.

15. Nakachi K, Imai K. Environmental and physiological influences on human natural killer cell activity in relation to good health practices. *Japan Journal of Cancer Research* 1992;83: 789–805.

16. Morimoto K, Takeshita T, Inoue-Sakurai C, et al. Lifestyles and mental health status are associated with natural killer cell and lymphokine-activated killer cell activities. *Science of the Total Environment* 2001;270:3–11.

17. Heiser P, Dickhaus B, Opper C, et al. Alterations of host defence system after sleep deprivation are followed by impaired mood and psychosocial functioning. *World Journal of Biological Psychiatry* 2001;2:89–94.

18. Marcos A, Nova E, Montero A. Changes in the immune system are conditioned by nutrition. *European Journal of Clinical Nutrition* 2003;57 suppl 1:S66–S69.

19. Chandra RK. Nutrition and the immune system from birth to old age. *European Journal of Clinical Nutrition* 2002;56 suppl 3:S73–S76.

20. Chandra RK. Impact of nutritional status and nutrient supplements on immune responses and incidence of infection in older individuals. *Ageing Research Reviews* 2004;3:91–104.

21. Sanchez A, Reeser J, Lau H,

et al. Role of sugars in human neutrophilic phagocytosis. *The American Journal of Clinical Nutrition* 1973;26:1180–1184.

22. Ringsdorf WM Jr, Cheraskin E, Ramsay RR Jr. Sucrose, neutrophilic phagocytosis and resistance to disease. *Dental Survey* 1976;52:46–48.

23. Nauss K, Bernstein J, Alpert S, et al. Depressed lymphocyte transformation in a whole blood culture system after oral glucose ingestion. *Nutrition Research* 1984;4:819–822.

24. Mann G. Hypothesis: the role of vitamin C in diabetic angiopathy. *Perspectives in Biology and Medicine* 1974;17:210–217.

25. Mann G, Newton P. The membrane transport of ascorbic acid. *Annals of the New York Academy of Sciences* 1975;258: 243–252.

26. Martí A, Marcos A, Martínez JA. Obesity and immune function relationships. *Obesity Reviews* 2001 May;2(2):131–134.

27. Hersoug LG, Linneberg A. The link between the epidemics of obesity and allergic diseases: does obesity induce decreased immune tolerance? *Allergy* 2007 Oct;62(10):1205–1213.

28. Waddell CC, Taunton OD, Twomey JJ. Inhibition of lymphoproliferation by hyperlipoproteinemic plasma. *Journal of Clinical Investigation* 1976;58: 950–954.

29. Dianzani M, Torrielli M, Canuto R, et al. The influence of enrichment with cholesterol on the phagocytic activity of rat macrophages. *The Journal of Pathology* 1976;118:193–199.

30. De Simone C, Ferrari M, Lozzi A, et al. Vitamins and immunity. II. Influence of l-carnitine on the immune system. *Acta Vitaminologica et Enzymologica* 1982;4:135–140.

31. Frank J, Witte K, Schrodl W, et al. Chronic alcoholism causes deleterious conditioning of innate immunity. *Alcohol and Alcoholism* 2004; 39:386–392.

32. Semba RD. Vitamin A, immunity, and infection. *Clinical Infectious Diseases* 1994;19: 489–499.

33. Seifter E, Rettura G, Seiter J, et al. Thymotrophic action of vitamin A. *Federation Proceedings* 1973;32:947.

34. Bendich A. Vitamin C and immune responses. *Food Technology* 1987;41:112–114.

35. Scott J. On the biochemical similarities of ascorbic acid and interferon. *Journal of Theoretical Biology* 1982;98:235–238.

36. Bendich A, Langseth L. The health effects of vitamin C supplementation: a review. *Journal of the American College of Nutrition* 1995;14:124–136.

37. Jacob RA, Sotoudeh G. Vitamin C function and status in chronic disease. *Nutrition in Clinical Care* 2002;5:66–74.

38. Di Carlo G, Mascolo N, Izzo AA, et al. Flavonoids: old and new aspects of a class of natural therapeutic drugs. *Life Sciences* 1999;65:337–353.

39. Kamen DL, Tangpricha V. Vitamin D and molecular actions on the immune system: modulation of innate and autoimmunity. *Journal of Molecular Medicine* 2010 May;88(5):441–450.

40. Hewison M. Vitamin D and the immune system: new perspectives on an old theme. *Endocrinology Metabolism Clinics of North America* 2010 Jun;39(2): 365–379.

41. Hayes CE, Nashold FE, Spach KM, Pedersen LB. The immunological functions of the vitamin D endocrine system. *Cellular and Molecular Biology* 2003 Mar;49(2):277–300.

42. Baeke F, Takiishi T, Korf H, et al. Vitamin D: modulator of the immune system. *Current Opinion in Pharmacology* 2010 Aug; 10(4):482–496.

43. Maruotti N, Cantatore FP. Vitamin D and the immune system. *The Journal of Rheumatology* 2010 Mar;37(3):491–495.

44. Yamshchikov AV, Desai NS,

Blumberg HM, et al. Vitamin D for treatment and prevention of infectious diseases: a systematic review of randomized controlled trials. *Endocrine Practice* 2009 Jul–Aug;15(5):438–449.

45. Kelleher J. Vitamin E and the immune response. *Proceedings of the Nutrition Society* 1991; 50:245–249.

46. Meydani SN, Meydani M, Blumberg JB, et al. Vitamin E supplementation and in vivo immune response in healthy elderly subjects: a randomized controlled trial. *JAMA, The Journal of the American Medical Association* 1997;277:1380–1386.

47. Meydani SN, Leka LS, Fine BC, et al. Vitamin E and respiratory tract infections in elderly nursing home residents: a randomized controlled trial. *JAMA, The Journal of the American Medical Association* 2004;292: 828–836.

48. Stockman J. Infections and iron: too much of a good thing? *American Journal of Diseases of Children* 1981;135:18–20.

49. Hadden JW. The treatment of zinc deficiency is an immunotherapy. *International Journal of Immunopharmacology* 1995; 17:697–701.

50. Walker CF, Black RE. Zinc and the risk for infectious disease. *Annual Review of Nutrition* 2004;24:255–275.

51. Eby GA, Davis DR, Halcomb WW. Reduction in duration of common colds by zinc gluconate lozenges in a double-blind study. *Antimicrobial Agents and Chemotherapy* 1984;25:20–24.

52. Mossad SB, Macknin ML, Medendorp SV, et al. Zinc gluconate lozenges for treating the common cold: a randomized, double-blind, placebo-controlled study. *Annals of Internal Medicine* 1996;125:81–88.

53. Kiremidjian-Schumacher L, Stotzky G. Selenium and immune responses. *Environmental Research* 1987;42:277–303.

54. Kiremidjian-Schumacher L, Roy M, Wishe HI, et al. Supplementation with selenium and human immune cell functions. II. Effect on cytotoxic lymphocytes and natural killer cells. *Biological Trace Element Research* 1994;41:115–127.

55. Roy M, Kiremidjian-Schumacher L, Wishe HI, et al. Supplementation with selenium and human immune cell functions. I. Effect on lymphocyte proliferation and interleukin 2 receptor expression. *Biological Trace Element Research* 1994; 41:103–114.

56. Broome CS, McArdle F, Kyle JA, et al. An increase in selenium intake improves immune function and poliovirus handling in adults with marginal selenium status. *The American Journal of Clinical Nutrition* 2004;80:154–162.

57. Dardenne M, Pleau JM, Nabarra B, et al. Contribution of zinc and other metals to the biological activity of the serum thymic factor. *Proceedings of the National Academy of Sciences of the United States of America* 1982;9:5370–5373.

58. Bogden JD, Oleske JM, Munves EM, et al. Zinc and immunocompetence in the elderly: baseline data on zinc nutriture and immunity in unsupplemented subjects. *The American Journal of Clinical Nutrition* 1987;46: 101–109.

59. Chang HM, But PPH, eds. *Pharmacology and applications of Chinese materia medica*. Singapore: World Scientific, 1986, 1041–1046.

60. Block KI, Mead MN. Immune system effects of echinacea, ginseng, and astragalus: a review. *Integrative Cancer Therapies* 2003;2:247–267.

61. Zhao KS, Mancini C, Doria G. Enhancement of the immune response in mice by *Astragalus membranaceus* extracts. *Immunopharmacology* 1990;20: 225–233.

62. Chu DT, Wong WL, Mavligit GM. Immunotherapy with Chinese medicinal herbs. I. Immune restoration of local xenogeneic graft-versus-host reaction in cancer patients by fractionated *Astragalus membranaceus* in vitro. *Journal of Clinical Laboratory & Immunology* 1988;25:119–123.

63. Goodridge HS, Wolf AJ, Underhill DM. Beta-glucan recognition by the innate immune system. *Immunological Reviews* 2009 Jul;230(1):38–50.

64. Volman JJ, Ramakers JD, Plat J. Dietary modulation of immune function by beta-glucans. *Physiology & Behavior* 2008 May 23; 94(2):276–284.

65. Talbott S, Talbott J. Effect of beta 1,3/1, 6 glucan on upper respiratory tract infection symptoms and mood state in marathon athletes. *Journal of Sports Science and Medicine* 2009;8: 509–515.

66. Feldman S, Schwartz H, Kalman D, et al. Randomized phase II clinical trials of Wellmune WGP® for immune support during cold and flu season. *Journal of Applied Research* 2009;9:20–42.

67. Talbott S, Talbott J. Beta 1,3/1,6 glucan decreases upper respiratory tract infection symptoms and improves psychological wellbeing in moderate to highly-stressed subjects. *Agro Food Industry Hi-Tech* 2010;21:21–24.

Longevity and Life Extension

1. Kochanek KD, Xu J, Murphy SL, et al. Deaths: preliminary data for 2009. *National Vital Statistics Reports* 2011;59(4): 1–51.

2. Jia H, Lubetkin EI. Trends in quality-adjusted life-years lost contributed by smoking and obesity. *American Journal of Preventive Medicine* 2010 Feb; 38(2):138–44.

3. Mazess RB, Forman SH. Longevity and age exaggeration in Vilcabamba, Ecuador. *The Jour-*

nals of Gerontology 1979;34: 94–98.

4. Medvedev ZA. Myths about the Caucasian mountain centers of longevity. *Geriatric Medicine Today* 1982;5:96–112.

5. Young RD, Desjardins B, McLaughlin K, Poulain M, Perls TT. Typologies of extreme longevity myths. *Current Gerontology and Geriatrics Research* 2010;2010:423087.

6. Taubman LB. Theories of aging. *Resident and Staff Physician* 1986;32:31–37.

7. Hayflick L. The cell biology of human aging. *The New England Journal of Medicine* 1976;295: 302–308.

8. Harley CB, Futcher AB, Greider CW. Telomeres shorten during aging of human fibroblasts. *Nature* 1990;345:458–460.

9. Ahmed A, Tollefsbol T. Telomeres and telomerase: basic science implications for aging. *Journal of the American Geriatrics Society* 2001 Aug;49(8): 1105–1109.

10. Ornish D, Lin J, Daubenmier J, et al. Increased telomerase activity and comprehensive lifestyle changes: a pilot study. *The Lancet Oncology* 2008 Nov; 9(11):1048–1057.

11. Cherkas LF, Hunkin JL, Kato BS, et al. The association between physical activity in leisure time and leukocyte telomere length. *Archives of Internal Medicine* 2008 Jan 28;168(2): 154–158.

12. Epel E, Daubenmier J, Moskowitz JT. Can meditation slow rate of cellular aging? Cognitive stress, mindfulness, and telomeres. *Annals of the New York Academy of Sciences* 2009 Aug; 1172:34–53.

13. Richards JB, Valdes AM, Gardner JP, et al. Higher serum vitamin D concentrations are associated with longer leukocyte telomere length in women. *The American Journal of Clinical Nutrition* 2007 Nov;86(5): 1420–1425.

14. Rubio MA, Davalos AR, Campisi J. Telomere length mediates the effects of telomerase on the cellular response to genotoxic stress. *Experimental Cell Research* 2004 Aug 1;298(1):17–27.

15. Harman D. Free radical theory of aging: the free radical diseases. *Age* 1984;7:111–131.

16. Finkel T, Holbrook NJ. Oxidants, oxidative stress and the biology of ageing. *Nature* 2000 Nov 9;408(6809):239–247.

17. Cutler RG. Peroxide-producing potential of tissues: inverse correlation with longevity of mammalian species. *Proceedings of the National Academy of Sciences of the United States of America* 1985;82:4798–4802.

18. Grillo MA, Colombatto S. Advanced glycation end-products (AGEs): involvement in aging and in neurodegenerative diseases. *Amino Acids* 2008 Jun; 35(1):29–36.

19. Cantó C, Auwerx J. Caloric restriction, SIRT1 and longevity. *Trends in Endocrinology & Metabolism* 2009 Sep;20(7): 325–331.

20. Visser M, Schaap LA. Consequences of sarcopenia. *Clinics in Geriatric Medicine* 2011 Aug;27(3):387–399.

21. Boirie Y. Physiopathological mechanism of sarcopenia. *Journal of Nutrition, Health & Aging* 2009 Oct;13(8):717–723.

22. Morley JE, Argiles JM, Evans WJ, et al. Nutritional recommendations for the management of sarcopenia. *Journal of the American Medical Directors Association* 2010 Jul;11(6):391–614.

23. Pennings B, Boirie Y, Senden JM, et al. Whey protein stimulates postprandial muscle protein accretion more effectively than do casein and casein hydrolysate in older men. *The American Journal of Clinical Nutrition* 2011 May;93(5):997–1005.

24. Schneider EL, Reed JD. Life extension. *The New England*

Journal of Medicine 1985;312: 1159–1168.

25. Cutler RG. Peroxide-producing potential of tissues: inverse correlation with longevity of mammalian species. *Proceedings of the National Academy of Sciences of the United States of America* 1985;82:4798–4802.

26. Cutler RG. Carotenoids and retinol: their possible importance in determining longevity of primate species. *Proceedings of the National Academy of Sciences of the United States of America* 1984;81:7627–7631.

27. de la Iglesia R, Milagro FI, Campión J, et al. Healthy properties of proanthocyanidins. *Biofactors* 2010 May–Jun;36(3): 159–168.

28. Khan N, Mukhtar H. Tea polyphenols for health promotion. *Life Sciences* 2007 Jul 26;81(7): 519–533.

29. Gertz HJ, Kiefer M. Review about *Ginkgo biloba* special extract EGb 761 (ginkgo). *Current Pharmaceutical Design* 2004; 10(3):261–264.

30. Kaschel R. *Ginkgo biloba*: specificity of neuropsychological improvement—a selective review in search of differential effects. *Human Psychopharmacology* 2009 Jul;24(5):345–370.

31. Agarwal B, Baur JA. Resveratrol and life extension. *Annals of the New York Academy of Sciences* 2011 Jan;1215:138–143.

32. Patel KR, Scott E, Brown VA, et al. Clinical trials of resveratrol. *Annals of the New York Academy of Sciences* 2011 Jan;1215: 161–169.

33. Autier P, Gandini S. Vitamin D supplementation and total mortality: a meta-analysis of randomized controlled trials. *Archives of Internal Medicine* 2007;167(16):1730–1737.

34. Holick MF. The vitamin D epidemic and its health consequences. *Journal of Nutrition* 2005;135(11):2739S–2748S.

35. Richards JB, Valdes AM, Gardner JP, et al. Higher serum

vitamin D concentrations are associated with longer leukocyte telomere length in women. *The American Journal of Clinical Nutrition* 2007;86(5):1420–1425.

36. Baker WL, Karan S, Kenny AM. Effect of dehydroepiandrosterone on muscle strength and physical function in older adults: a systematic review. *Journal of the American Geriatrics Society* 2011 Jun;59(6):997–1002.

37. Sorwell KG, Urbanski HF. Dehydroepiandrosterone and age-related cognitive decline. *Age (Dordrecht)* 2010 Mar;32(1):61–67.

38. Buford TW, Willoughby DS. Impact of DHEA(S) and cortisol on immune function in aging: a brief review. *Applied Physiology, Nutrition, and Metabolism* 2008 Jun;33(3):429–433.

39. Weiss EP, Villareal DT, Fontana L, et al. Dehydroepiandrosterone (DHEA) replacement decreases insulin resistance and lowers inflammatory cytokines in aging humans. *Aging* 2011 May;3(5):533–542.

40. Karasek M. Does melatonin play a role in aging processes? *Journal of Physiology and Pharmacology* 2007;58 suppl:105–113.

41. Chokroverty S. Sleep and neurodegenerative diseases. *Seminars in Neurology* 2009 Sep;29(4):446–467.

42. Dhand R, Sohal H. Good sleep, bad sleep! The role of daytime naps in healthy adults. *Current Opinion in Pulmonary Medicine* 2006 Nov;12(6):379–382.

43. Tanaka H, Shirakawa S. Sleep health, lifestyle and mental health in the Japanese elderly: ensuring sleep to promote a healthy brain and mind. *Journal of Psychosomatic Research* 2004 May;56(5):465–477.

Silent Inflammation

1. Windgassen EB, Funtowicz L, Lunsford TN, et al. C-reactive protein and high-sensitivity C-reactive protein: an update for clinicians. *Postgraduate Medicine* 2011 Jan;123(1):114–119.

2. Cushman M, Arnold AM, Psaty BM, et al. C-reactive protein and the 10-year incidence of coronary heart disease in older men and women: the Cardiovascular Health Study. *Circulation* 2005 Jul 5;112(1):25–31.

3. Dayer E, Dayer JM, Roux-Lombard P. Primer: the practical use of biological markers of rheumatic and systemic inflammatory diseases. *Nature Clinical Practice Rheumatology* 2007 Sep;3(9):512–520.

4. Hamer M, Stamatakis E. The accumulative effects of modifiable risk factors on inflammation and haemostasis. *Brain, Behavior, and Immunity* 2008 Oct;22(7):1041–1043.

5. Brooks GC, Blaha MJ, Blumenthal RS. Relation of C-reactive protein to abdominal adiposity. *American Journal of Cardiology* 2010 Jul 1;106(1):56–61.

6. Liu S, Manson JE, Buring JE, et al. Relation between a diet with a high glycemic load and plasma concentrations of high-sensitivity C-reactive protein in middle-aged women. *The American Journal of Clinical Nutrition* 2002 Mar;75(3):492–498.

7. Chrysohoou C, Panagiotakos DB, Pitsavos C, et al. Adherence to the Mediterranean diet attenuates inflammation and coagulation process in healthy adults: the ATTICA Study. *Journal of the American College of Cardiology* 2004 Jul 7;44(1):152–158.

8. Nanri A, Yoshida D, Yamaji T, et al. Dietary patterns and C-reactive protein in Japanese men and women. *The American Journal of Clinical Nutrition* 2008 May;87(5):1488–1496.

9. Chun OK, Chung SJ, Claycombe KJ. Serum C-reactive protein concentrations are inversely associated with dietary flavonoid intake in U.S. adults. *Journal of Nutrition* 2008 Apr;138(4):753–760.

10. Simopoulos AP. The importance of the omega-6/omega-3 fatty acid ratio in cardiovascular disease and other chronic diseases. *Experimental Medicine and Biology (Maywood)* 2008 Jun;233(6):674–688.

11. Schmitz G, Ecker J. The opposing effects of omega-3 and omega-6 fatty acids. *Progress in Lipid Research* 2008 Mar;47(2):147–155.

12. Handschin C, Spiegelman BM. The role of exercise and PGC1alpha in inflammation and chronic disease. *Nature* 2008 Jul 24;454(7203):463–469.

13. Nicklas BJ, Hsu FC, Brinkley TJ, et al. Exercise training and plasma C-reactive protein and interleukin-6 in elderly people. *Journal of the American Geriatrics Society* 2008 Nov;56(11):2045–2052.

14. Campbell KL, Campbell PT, Ulrich CM, et al. No reduction in C-reactive protein following a 12-month randomized controlled trial of exercise in men and women. *Cancer Epidemiology, Biomarkers & Prevention* 2008 Jul;17(7):1714–1718.

15. Belcaro G, Cesarone MR, Errichi S, et al. Variations in C-reactive protein, plasma free radicals and fibrinogen values in patients with osteoarthritis treated with Pycnogenol. *Redox Report* 2008;13(6):271–276.

16. Kar P, Laight D, Rooprai HK, et al. Effects of grape seed extract in type 2 diabetic subjects at high cardiovascular risk: a double blind randomized placebo controlled trial examining metabolic markers, vascular tone, inflammation, oxidative stress and insulin sensitivity. *Diabetic Medicine* 2009 May;26(5):526–531.

17. Jurenka JS. Anti-inflammatory properties of curcumin, a major constituent of *Curcuma longa:* a review of preclinical and clinical research. *Alternative Medicine Review* 2009 Jun;14(2):141–153.

18. Marczylo TH, Verschoyle RD,

Cooke DN, et al. Comparison of systemic availability of curcumin with that of curcumin formulated with phosphatidylcholine. *Cancer Chemotherapy and Pharmacology* 2007 Jul;60(2):171–177.

19. Appendino G, Belcaro G, Cesarone MR, et al. Efficacy and safety of Meriva, a curcumin-phosphatidylcholine complex, during extended administration in osteoarthritis patients. *Alternative Medicine Review* 2010 Dec;15(4):337–344.

20. Sasaki H, Sunagawa Y, Takahashi K, et al. Innovative preparation of curcumin for improved oral bioavailability. *Biological and Pharmaceutical Bulletin* 2011;34(5):660–665.

Stress Management

1. Benson H. *The relaxation response.* New York: William Morrow, 1975.

2. Selye H. *The stress of life.* New York: McGraw-Hill, 1978.

3. Holmes TH, Rahe RH. The social readjustment rating scale. *Journal of Psychosomatic Research* 1967;11:213–218.

4. Törnhage CJ. Salivary cortisol for assessment of hypothalamic-pituitary-adrenal axis function. *Neuroimmunomodulation* 2009;16(5):284–289.

5. Lewis JG. Steroid analysis in saliva: an overview. *The Clinical Biochemist Reviews* 2006 Aug;27(3):139–146.

6. Stetler C, Miller GE. Blunted cortisol response to awakening in mild to moderate depression: regulatory influences of sleep patterns and social contacts. *Journal of Abnormal Psychology* 2005 Nov;114(4):697–705.

7. Backhaus J, Junghanns K, Hohagen F. Sleep disturbances are correlated with decreased morning awakening salivary cortisol. *Psychoneuroendocrinology* 2004 Oct;29(9):1184–1191.

8. Steptoe A, Butler N. Sports participation and emotional wellbeing in adolescents. *The Lancet* 1996;347:1789–1792.

9. Chou T. Wake up and smell the coffee: caffeine, coffee, and the medical consequences. *Western Journal of Medicine* 1992;157:544–553.

10. Monteiro MG, Schuckit MA, Irwin M. Subjective feelings of anxiety in young men after ethanol and diazepam infusions. *Journal of Clinical Psychiatry* 1990;51:12–16.

11. Winokur A, Maislin G, Phillips JL, et al. Insulin resistance after oral glucose tolerance testing in patients with major depression. *The American Journal of Psychiatry* 1988;145:325–330.

12. Wright JH, Jacisin JJ, Radin NS, et al. Glucose metabolism in unipolar depression. *The British Journal of Psychiatry* 1978;132:386–393.

13. Rowe AH, Rowe A Jr. *Food allergy: its manifestations and control and the elimination diets: a compendium.* Springfield, Ill.: Charles C. Thomas, 1972.

14. Abdoua AM; Higashiguchia S, Horiea K, et al. Relaxation and immunity enhancement effects of gamma-aminobutyric acid (GABA) administration in humans. *Biofactors* 2006;26:201–208.

15. Bhattacharya SK, Mitra SK. Anxiolytic activity of *Panax ginseng* roots: an experimental study. *Journal of Ethnopharmacology* 1991;34:87–92.

16. Davydov M, Krikorian AD. *Eleutherococcus senticosus* (Rupr. & Maxim.) Maxim. (Araliaceae) as an adaptogen: a closer look. *Journal of Ethnopharmacology* 2000;72:345–393.

17. Hallstrom C, Fulder S, Carruthers M. Effect of ginseng on the performance of nurses on night duty. *Comparative Medicine East & West* 1982;6:277–282.

18. Shevtsov VA, Zholus BI, Shervarly VI, et al. A randomized trial of two different doses of a SHR-5 *Rhodiola rosea* extract versus placebo and control of capacity for mental work. *Phytomedicine* 2003;10:95–105.

19. Darbinyan V, Kteyan A, Panossian A, et al. *Rhodiola rosea* in stress induced fatigue—a double blind cross-over study of a standardized extract SHR-5 with a repeated low-dose regimen on the mental performance of healthy physicians during night duty. *Phytomedicine* 2000;7:365–371.

20. Spasov AA, Wikman GK, Mandrikov VB, et al. A double-blind, placebo-controlled pilot study of the stimulating and adaptogenic effect of *Rhodiola rosea* SHR-5 extract on the fatigue of students caused by stress during an examination period with a repeated low-dose regimen. *Phytomedicine* 2000;7:85–89.

21. Olsson EM, von Schéele B, Panossian AG. A randomised, double-blind, placebo-controlled, parallel-group study of the standardised extract shr-5 of the roots of *Rhodiola rosea* in the treatment of subjects with stress-related fatigue. *Planta Medica* 2009 Feb;75(2):105–112.

22. Auddy B, Hazra J, Mitra A, et al. A standardized *Withania somnifera* extract significantly reduces stress-related parameters in chronically stressed humans: a double-blind, randomized, placebo-controlled study. *Journal of the American Neutraceutical Association* 2008;11:50–56.

23. Buford TW, Willoughby DS. Impact of DHEA(S) and cortisol on immune function in aging: a brief review. *Applied Physiology, Nutrition, and Metabolism* 2008 Jun;33(3):429–433.

24. Bellarosa C, Chen PY. The effectiveness and practicality of occupational stress management interventions: a survey of subject matter expert opinions. *Journal of Occupational Health Psychology* 1997;2:247–262.

25. Williams KA, Kolar MM, Reger BE, et al. Evaluation of

a wellness-based mindfulness stress reduction intervention: a controlled trial. *American Journal of Health Promotion* 2001; 15:422–432.

Obesity and Weight Management

1. Centers for Disease Control and Prevention. Vital signs: state-specific obesity prevalence among adults—United States, 2009. *Morbidity and Mortality Weekly Report* 2010;59:951–955.

2. Flegal KM, Carroll MD, Ogden CL, Curtin LR. Prevalence and trends in obesity among U.S. adults, 1999–2008. *JAMA, The Journal of the American Medical Association* 2010;303(3): 235–241.

3. Ogden CL, Carroll MD, Curtin LR, et al. Prevalence of high body mass index in U.S. children and adolescents, 2007–2008. *JAMA, The Journal of the American Medical Association* 2010;303(3):242–249.

4. Jia H, Lubetkin EI. Trends in quality-adjusted life-years lost contributed by smoking and obesity. *American Journal of Preventive Medicine* 2010 Feb; 38(2):138–144.

5. Jia H, Lubetkin EI. Obesity-related quality-adjusted life years lost in the U.S. from 1993 to 2008. *American Journal of Preventive Medicine* 2010 Sep; 39(3):220–227.

6. Finkelstein EA, Trogdon JG, Cohen JW, Dietz W. Annual medical spending attributable to obesity: payer- and service-specific estimates. *Health Affairs* 2009:5:w822–w831.

7. Hancox RJ, Milne BJ, Poulton R. Association between child and adolescent television viewing and adult health: a longitudinal birth cohort study. *The Lancet* 2004;364:257–262.

8. Hu FB, Li TY, Colditz GA, et al. Television watching and other sedentary behaviors in relation to risk of obesity and type 2 diabetes mellitus in women. *JAMA,*

The Journal of the American Medical Association 2003;289: 1785–1791.

9. Havel PJ. Update on adipocyte hormones: regulation of energy balance and carbohydrate/lipid metabolism. *Diabetes* 2004;53 suppl 1:S143–S151.

10. Jazet IM, Pijl H, Meinders AE. Adipose tissue as an endocrine organ: impact on insulin resistance. *Netherlands Journal of Medicine* 2003;61:194–212.

11. Small CJ, Bloom SR. Gut hormones and the control of appetite. *Trends in Endocrinology & Metabolism* 2004;15:259–263.

12. Batterham RL, Cohen MA, Ellis SM, et al. Inhibition of food intake in obese subjects by peptide YY3-36. *The New England Journal of Medicine* 2003; 349:941–948.

13. Cummings DE, Weigle DS, Frayo RS, et al. Plasma ghrelin levels after diet-induced weight loss or gastric bypass surgery. *The New England Journal of Medicine* 2002;346:1623–1630.

14. Laville M, Cornu C, Normand S, et al. Decreased glucose-induced thermogenesis at the onset of obesity. *The American Journal of Clinical Nutrition* 1993;57: 851–856.

15. Ravussin E, Acheson KJ, Vernet O, et al. Evidence that insulin resistance is responsible for the decreased thermic effect of glucose in human obesity. *Journal of Clinical Investigation* 1985; 76:1268–1273.

16. Nelson KM, Weinsier RL, James LD, et al. Effect of weight reduction on resting energy expenditure, substrate utilization, and the thermic effect of food in moderately obese women. *The American Journal of Clinical Nutrition* 1992;55:924–933.

17. Schulz LO. Brown adipose tissue: regulation of thermogenesis and implications for obesity. *Journal of the American Dietetic Association* 1987;87:761–764.

18. Sims EA, Danforth E Jr., Hor-

ton ES, et al. Endocrine and metabolic effects of experimental obesity in man. *Recent Progress in Hormone Research* 1973; 29:457–496.

19. Leibel RL, Hirsch J. Diminished energy requirements in reduced obese patients. *Metabolism* 1984;33:164–170.

20. Eck LH, Klesges RC, Hanson CL, et al. Children at familial risk for obesity: an examination of dietary intake, physical activity, and weight status. *International Journal of Obesity and Related Metabolic Disorders* 1992;16:71–78.

21. Wurtman RJ, Wurtman JJ. Brain serotonin, carbohydrate-craving, obesity and depression. *Advances in Experimental Medicine and Biology* 1996;398: 35–41.

22. Wurtman J, Suffes S. *The serotonin solution.* New York: Fawcett Columbine, 1996.

23. Goodwin GM, Cowen PJ, Fairburn CG, et al. Plasma concentrations of tryptophan and dieting. *BMJ* 1990;300:1499–1500.

24. Villareal DT, Chode S, Parimi N, et al. Weight loss, exercise, or both and physical function in obese older adults. *The New England Journal of Medicine* 2011 Mar 31;364(13):1218–1229.

25. Hunter GR, Brock DW, Byrne NM, et al. Exercise training prevents regain of visceral fat for 1 year following weight loss. *Obesity* 2010 Apr;18(4):690–695.

26. Wing RR, Phelan S. Long-term weight loss maintenance. *The American Journal of Clinical Nutrition.* 2005 Jul;82(1 suppl): 222S–225S.

27. Larsen TM, Dalskov SM, van Baak M, et al. Diets with high or low protein content and glycemic index for weight-loss maintenance. *The New England Journal of Medicine* 2010 Nov 25;363(22):2102–2113.

28. Dennis EA, Dengo AL, Comber DL, et al. Water consumption

increases weight loss during a hypocaloric diet intervention in middle-aged and older adults. *Obesity* 2010 Feb;18(2):300–307.

29. Foster GD, Wyatt HR, Hill JO, et al. A randomized trial of a low-carbohydrate diet for obesity. *The New England Journal of Medicine* 2003;348:2082–2090.

30. Hays NP, Starling RD, Liu X, et al. Effects of an ad libitum low-fat, high-carbohydrate diet on body weight, body composition, and fat distribution in older men and women. *Archives of Internal Medicine* 2004;164:210–217.

31. Stern L, Iqbal N, Seshadri P, et al. The effects of low-carbohydrate versus conventional weight loss diets in severely obese adults: one-year follow-up of a randomized trial. *Annals of Internal Medicine* 2004;140:769–777.

32. Yancy WS Jr, Olsen MK, Guyton JR, et al. A low-carbohydrate, ketogenic diet versus a low-fat diet to treat obesity and hyperlipidemia. *Annals of Internal Medicine* 2004;140:769–777.

33. Howarth NC, Saltzman E, Roberts SB. Dietary fiber and weight regulation. *Nutrition Reviews* 2001;59:129–139.

34. Spiller GA. *Dietary fiber in health and nutrition.* Boca Raton, Fla.: CRC Press, 1994.

35. Krotkiewski M. Effect of guar on body weight, hunger ratings and metabolism in obese subjects. *British Journal of Nutrition* 1984;52:97–105.

36. Walsh DE, Yaghoubian V, Behforooz A. Effect of glucomannan on obese patients: a clinical study. *International Journal of Obesity* 1984;8:289–293.

37. Biancardi G, Palmiero L, Ghirardi PE. Glucomannan in the treatment of overweight patients with osteoarthrosis. *Current Therapeutic Research* 1989;46:908–912.

38. El-Shebini SM, Hanna LM, Topouzada ST, et al. The role of pectin as a slimming agent. *Journal of Clinical Biochemistry and Nutrition* 1988;4:255–262.

39. Rossner S, von Zwigbergk D, Ohlin A, et al. Weight reduction with dietary fibre supplements. Results of two double-blind studies. *Acta Medica Scandinavica* 1987;222:83–88.

40. Rigaud D, Ryttig KR, Leeds AR, et al. Mild overweight treated with energy restriction and a dietary fiber supplement: a 6-month randomized, double-blind, placebo-controlled trial. *International Journal of Obesity* 1990;14:763–771.

41. Abdelhameed AS, Ang S, Morris GA, et al. An analytical ultracentrifuge study on ternary mixtures of konjac glucomannan supplemented with sodium alginate and xanthan gum. *Carbohydrate Polymers* 2010;81:141–148.

42. Harding SE, Smith IH, Lawson CJ, et al. Studies on macromolecular interactions in ternary mixtures of konjac glucomannan, xanthan gum and sodium alginate. *Carbohydrate Polymers* 2010;10:1016–1020.

43. Brand-Miller JC, Atkinson FS, Gahler RJ, et al. Effects of PGX, a novel functional fibre, on acute and delayed postprandial glycaemia. *European Journal of Clinical Nutrition* 2010 Dec;64(12):1488–1493.

44. Jenkins AL, Kacinik V, Lyon MR, Wolever TMS. Reduction of postprandial glycemia by the novel viscous polysaccharide PGX in a dose-dependent manner, independent of food form. *Journal of the American College of Nutrition* 2010;29(2):92–98.

45. Vuksan V, Sievenpiper JL, Owen R, et al. Beneficial effects of viscous dietary fiber from konjac-mannan in subjects with the insulin resistance syndrome: results of a controlled metabolic trial. *Diabetes Care* 2000;23:9–14.

46. Reimer RA, Pelletier X, Carabin IG, et al. Increased plasma PYY levels following supplementation with the functional fiber PolyGlycopleX in healthy adults. *European Journal of Clinical Nutrition* 2010 Oct;64(10):1186–1191.

47. Lyon MR, Reichert RG. The effect of a novel viscous polysaccharide along with lifestyle changes on short-term weight loss and associated risk factors in overweight and obese adults: an observational retrospective clinical program analysis. *Alternative Medicine Review* 2010 Apr;15(1):68–75.

48. Noakes M, Foster PR, Keogh JB, et al. Meal replacements are as effective as structured weight-loss diets for treating obesity in adults with features of metabolic syndrome. *Journal of Nutrition* 2004;134:1894–1899.

49. Ashley JM, St Jeor ST, Perumean-Chaney S, et al. Meal replacements in weight intervention. *Obesity Research* 2001;9 suppl 4:312S–320S.

50. Ditschuneit HH, Flechtner-Mors M. Value of structured meals for weight management: risk factors and long-term weight maintenance. *Obesity Research* 2001;9 suppl 4:284S–289S.

51. Allison DB, Gadbury G, Schwartz LG, et al. A novel soy-based meal replacement formula for weight loss among obese individuals: a randomized controlled clinical trial. *European Journal of Clinical Nutrition* 2003;57:514–522.

52. Treyzon L, Chen S, Hong K, et al. A controlled trial of protein enrichment of meal replacements for weight reduction with retention of lean body mass. *Nutrition Journal* 2008 Aug 27;7:23.

53. Davis LM, Coleman C, Kiel J, et al. Efficacy of a meal replacement diet plan compared to a food-based diet plan after

a period of weight loss and weight maintenance: a randomized controlled trial. *Nutrition Journal* 2010 Mar 11;9:11.

54. Mertz W. Chromium in human nutrition: a review. *Journal of Nutrition* 1993;123:626–633.

55. Anderson RA. Chromium, glucose tolerance, and diabetes. *Biological Trace Element Research* 1992;32:19–24.

56. Anderson RA, Polansky MM, Bryden NA, et al. Effects of supplemental chromium on patients with symptoms of reactive hypoglycemia. *Metabolism* 1987;36:351–355.

57. McCarthy MF. Hypothesis: sensitization of insulin-dependent hypothalamic glucoreceptors may account for the fat-reducing effects of chromium picolinate. *Journal of Optimal Nutrition* 1993;21:36–53.

58. Evans GW, Pouchnik DJ. Composition and biological activity of chromium-pyridine carboxylate complexes. *Journal of Inorganic Biochemistry* 1993;49: 177–187.

59. Evans GW. Chromium picolinate is an efficacious and safe supplement. *International Journal of Sport Nutrition* 1993;3: 117–122.

60. Campbell WW, Joseph LJ, Anderson RA, et al. Effects of resistive training and chromium picolinate on body composition and skeletal muscle size in older women. *International Journal of Sport Nutrition and Exercise Metabolism* 2002;12:125–135.

61. Volpe SL, Huang HW, Larpadisorn K, et al. Effect of chromium supplementation and exercise on body composition, resting metabolic rate and selected biochemical parameters in moderately obese women following an exercise program. *Journal of the American College of Nutrition* 2001;20:293–306.

62. Ceci F, Cangiano C, Cairella M, et al. The effects of oral 5-hydroxytryptophan administration on feeding behavior in obese adult female subjects. *Journal of Neural Transmission* 1989;76:109–117.

63. Ceci F, Cangiano C, Cairella M, et al. Effects of 5-hydroxytryptophan on eating behavior and adherence to dietary prescriptions in obese adult subjects. *Advances in Experimental Medicine and Biology* 1991;294: 591–593.

64. Cangiano C, Ceci F, Cascino A, et al. Eating behavior and adherence to dietary prescriptions in obese adult subjects treated with 5-hydroxytryptophan. *The American Journal of Clinical Nutrition* 1992;56:863–867.

65. Chee H, Romsos DR, Leveille GA. Influence of (-)-hydroxycitrate on lipogenesis in chickens and rats. *Journal of Nutrition* 1977;107:112–119.

66. Sullivan AC, Triscari J, Hamilton JG, et al. Effect of (-)-hydroxycitrate upon the accumulation of lipid in the rat. I. Lipogenesis. *Lipids* 1974;9: 121–128.

67. Rao RN, Sakariah KK. Lipid-lowering and antiobesity effect of (-)-hydroxycitric acid. *Nutrition Research* 1988;8:209–212.

68. Preuss HG, Garis RI, Bramble JD, et al. Efficacy of a novel calcium/potassium salt of (-)-hydroxycitric acid in weight control. *International Journal of Clinical Pharmacology Research* 2005;25(3):133–144.

69. Baba N, Bracco EF, Hashim SA. Enhanced thermogenesis and diminished deposition of fat in response to overfeeding with diet containing medium chain triglyceride. *The American Journal of Clinical Nutrition* 1982;35:678–682.

70. St-Onge MP, Jones PJ. Greater rise in fat oxidation with medium-chain triglyceride consumption relative to long-chain triglyceride is associated with lower initial body weight and greater loss of subcutaneous adipose tissue. *International Journal of Obesity and Related Metabolic Disorders* 2003;27: 1565–1571.

71. St-Onge MP, Ross R, Parsons WD, et al. Medium-chain triglycerides increase energy expenditure and decrease adiposity in overweight men. *Obesity Researchearch* 2003;11: 395–402.

72. Seaton TB, Welle SL, Warenko MK, et al. Thermic effect of medium-chain and long-chain triglycerides in man. *The American Journal of Clinical Nutrition* 1986;44:630–634.

73. Hill JO, Peters JC, Yang D, et al. Thermogenesis in humans during overfeeding with medium-chain triglycerides. *Metabolism* 1989;38:641–648.

Acne

1. Pochi PE. Acne: endocrinologic aspects. *Cutis* 1982;30:212–214, 216–217, 219.

2. Schiavone FE, Rietschel RL, Squotas D, Harris R. Elevated free testosterone levels in women with acne. *Archives of Dermatology* 1983;119:799–802.

3. Darley CR, Moore JW, Besser GM, et al. Androgen status in women with late onset or persistent acne vulgaris. *Clinical and Experimental Dermatology* 1984;9:28–35.

4. Takayasu S, Wakimoto H, Itami S, Sano S. Activity of testosterone 5-alpha-reductase in various tissues of human skin. *Journal of Investigative Dermatology* 1980;74:187–191.

5. Sansone G, Reisner RM. Differential rates of conversion of testosterone to dihydrotestosterone in acne and normal human skin—a possible pathogenic factor in acne. *Journal of Investigative Dermatology* 1971;56: 366–372.

6. Goulden V, McGeown CH, Cunliffe WJ. The familial risk of adult acne: a comparison between first-degree relatives

of affected and unaffected individuals. *British Journal of Dermatology* 1999 Aug;141(2): 297–300.

7. Juhlin L, Michaelsson G. Fibrin microclot formation in patients with acne. *Acta Dermato-Venereologica* 1983;63:538–540.

8. Bowe WP, Logan AC. Acne vulgaris, probiotics and the gut-brain-skin axis—back to the future? *Gut Pathogens* 2011 Jan 31;3(1):1.

9. Cordain L, Lindeberg S, Hurtado M, et al. Acne vulgaris: a disease of Western civilization. *Archives of Dermatology* 2002;138:1584–1590.

10. Danby FW. Nutrition and acne. *Clinics in Dermatology* 2010 Nov–Dec;28(6):598–604.

11. Pappas A. The relationship of diet and acne: a review. *Dermatoendocrinology* 2009 Sep;1(5): 262–267.

12. Spencer EH, Ferdowsian HR, Barnard ND. Diet and acne: a review of the evidence. *International Journal of Dermatology* 2009 Apr;48(4):339–347.

13. Melnik BC, Schmitz G. Role of insulin, insulin-like growth factor-1, hyperglycaemic food and milk consumption in the pathogenesis of acne vulgaris. *Experimental Dermatology* 2009 Oct; 18(10):833–841.

14. Semon H, Herrmann F. Some observations on the sugar metabolism in acne vulgaris, and its treatment by insulin. *British Journal of Dermatology* 1940; 52:123–128.

15. Grover RW, Arikan N. The effect of intralesional insulin and glucagon in acne vulgaris. *Journal of Investigative Dermatology* 1963;40:259–261.

16. Kader MM, El-Mofty AM, Ismail AA, Bassili F. Glucose tolerance in blood and skin of patients with acne vulgaris. *Indian Journal of Dermatology* 1977;22:139–149.

17. Berra B, Rizzo AM. Glycemic index, glycemic load: new evidence for a link with acne. *Journal of the American College of Nutrition* 2009 Aug;28 suppl: 450S–454S.

18. Kappas A, Anderson K, Conney A, et al. Nutrition-endocrine interactions: induction of reciprocal changes in the delta 4–5 alpha-reduction of testosterone and the cytochrome P-450-dependent oxidation of estradiol by dietary macronutrients in man. *Proceedings of the National Academy of Sciences of the United States of America* 1983;80:7646–7649.

19. Offenbacher EG, Pi-Sunyer FX. Beneficial effect of chromium-rich yeast on glucose tolerance and blood lipids in elderly patients. *Diabetes* 1980;29:919–925.

20. McCarty M. High-chromium yeast for acne? *Medical Hypotheses* 1984;14:307–310.

21. Kilgman AM, Mills OH Jr, Leyden JJ, et al. Oral vitamin A in acne vulgaris: a preliminary report. *International Journal of Dermatology* 1981;20:278–285.

22. Michaelsson G, Juhlin L, Ljunghall K. A double-blind study of the effect of zinc and oxytetracycline in acne vulgaris. *British Journal of Dermatology* 1977; 97:561–566.

23. Weimar VM, Puhl SC, Smith WH, tenBroeke JE. Zinc sulphate in acne vulgaris. *Archives of Dermatology* 1978;114:1776–1778.

24. Dreno B, Amblard P, Agache P, Litoux P. Low doses of zinc gluconate for inflammatory acne. *Acta Dermato-Venereologica* 1989;69: 541–543.

25. Meynadier J. Efficacy and safety study of two zinc gluconate regimens in the treatment of inflammatory acne. *European Journal of Dermatology* 2000; 10:269–273.

26. Kobayashi H, Aiba S, Tagami H. Successful treatment of dissecting cellulitis and acne conglobata with oral zinc. *British Journal of Dermatology* 1999;141:1137–1138.

27. Michaelsson G, Juhlin L, Vahlquist A. Effects of oral zinc and vitamin A in acne. *Archives of Dermatology* 1977;113:31–36.

28. Leake A, Chisholm GD, Habib FK. The effect of zinc on the 5-alpha-reduction of testosterone by the hyperplastic human prostate gland. *Journal of Steroid Biochemistry* 1984;20: 651–655.

29. Michaelsson G, Vahlquist A, Juhlin L. Serum zinc and retinol-binding protein in acne. *British Journal of Dermatology* 1977;96:283–286.

30. Michaelsson G, Edqvist L. Erythrocyte glutathione peroxidase activity in acne vulgaris and the effect of selenium and vitamin E treatment. *Acta Dermato-Venereologica* 1984; 64:9–14.

31. Carson CF, Riley TV. The antimicrobial activity of tea tree oil. *The Medical Journal of Australia* 1994;160:236.

32. Bassett IB, Pannowitz DL, Barnetson RS. A comparative study of tea-tree oil versus benzoyl peroxide in the treatment of acne. *The Medical Journal of Australia* 1990;153:455–458.

33. Nazzaro-Porro M. Azelaic acid. *Journal of the American Academy of Dermatology* 1987;17: 1033–1041.

34. Nguyen QH, Bui TP. Azelaic acid. Pharmacokinetic and pharmacodynamic properties and its therapeutic role in hyperpigmentary disorders and acne. *International Journal of Dermatology* 1995;34:75–84.

Acquired Immunodeficiency Syndrome (AIDS) and HIV Infection

1. Simon V, Ho DD, Abdool Karim Q. HIV/AIDS epidemiology, pathogenesis, prevention, and treatment. *The Lancet* 2006 Aug 5;368(9534):489–504.

2. Casey KM. Malnutrition associated with HIV/AIDS. Part one: definition and scope, epidemiology, and pathophysiology. *Jour-*

nal of the Association of Nurses in AIDS Care 1997;8:24–32.

3. Babameto G, Kotler DP. Malnutrition in HIV infection. *Gastroenterology Clinics of North America* 1997;26:393–415.

4. Baum MK, Shor-Posner G, Lu Y, et al. Micronutrients and HIV-1 disease progression. *AIDS* 1995 Sep;9(9):1051–1056.

5. Jiamton S, Pepin J, Suttent R, et al. A randomized trial of the impact of multiple micronutrient supplementation on mortality among HIV-infected individuals living in Bangkok. *AIDS* 2003; 17:2461–2469.

6. Fawzi W, Msamanga G. Micronutrients and adverse pregnancy outcomes in the context of HIV infection. *Nutrition Reviews* 2004;62:269–275.

7. Rabeneck L, Palmer A, Knowles JB, et al. A randomized controlled trial evaluating nutrition counseling with or without oral supplementation in malnourished HIV-infected patients. *Journal of the American Dietetic Association* 1998;98: 434–438.

8. Fawzi WW, Msamanga GI, Spiegelman D, et al. A randomized trial of multivitamin supplements and HIV disease progression and mortality. *The New England Journal of Medicine* 2004;351:23–32.

9. Winkler P, Ellinger S, Boetzer AM, et al. Lymphocyte proliferation and apoptosis in HIV-seropositive and healthy subjects during long-term ingestion of fruit juices or a fruit-vegetable-concentrate rich in polyphenols and antioxidant vitamins. *European Journal of Clinical Nutrition* 2004;58: 317–325.

10. Arendt BM, Boetzer AM, Lemoch H, et al. Plasma antioxidant capacity of HIV-seropositive and healthy subjects during long-term ingestion of fruit juices or a fruit-vegetable-concentrate containing antioxidant polyphenols. *European*

Journal of Clinical Nutrition 2001;55:786–792.

11. Ichimura T, Otake T, Mori H, Maruyama S. HIV-1 protease inhibition and anti-HIV effect of natural and synthetic water-soluble lignin-like substances. *Bioscience, Biotechnology, and Biodiversity* 1999;63:2202–2204.

12. Hendricks KM, Dong KR, Tang AM, et al. High-fiber diet in HIV-positive men is associated with lower risk of developing fat deposition. *The American Journal of Clinical Nutrition* 2003; 78:790–795.

13. Carroccio A, Di Prima L, Di Grigoli C, et al. Exocrine pancreatic function and fat malabsorption in human immunodeficiency virus-infected patients. *Scandinavian Journal of Gastroenterology* 1999;34: 729–734.

14. Koch J, Garcia-Shelton YL, Neal EA, et al. Steatorrhea: a common manifestation in patients with HIV/AIDS. *Nutrition* 1996;12:507–510.

15. Quinones-Galvan A, Lifshitz-Guinzberg A, Ruiz-Arguelles GJ. Gluten-free diet for AIDS-associated enteropathy. *Annals of Internal Medicine* 1990;113: 806–807.

16. Monachese M, Cunningham-Rundles S, Diaz MA, et al. Probiotics and prebiotics to combat enteric infections and HIV in the developing world: a consensus report. *Gut Microbes* 2011 May–Jun;2(3):198–207.

17. Hummelen R, Changalucha J, Butamanya NL, et al. Effect of 25 weeks probiotic supplementation on immune function of HIV patients. *Gut Microbes* 2011 Mar–Apr;2(2):80–85.

18. Williams SB, Bartsch G, Muurahainen N, et al. Protein intake is positively associated with body cell mass in weight-stable HIV-infected men. *Journal of Nutrition* 2003;133:1143–1146.

19. Agin D, Gallagher D, Wang J, et al. Effects of whey protein

and resistance exercise on body cell mass, muscle strength, and quality of life in women with HIV. *AIDS* 2001;15:2431–2440.

20. Micke P, Beeh KM, Buhl R. Effects of long-term supplementation with whey proteins on plasma glutathione levels of HIV-infected patients. *European Journal of Nutrition* 2002; 41:12–18.

21. Villamor E, Mbise R, Spiegelman D, et al. Vitamin A supplements ameliorate the adverse effect of HIV-1, malaria, and diarrheal infections on child growth. *Pediatrics* 2002;109:E6.

22. Filteau SM, Rollins NC, Coutsoudis A, et al. The effect of antenatal vitamin A and beta-carotene supplementation on gut integrity of infants of HIV-infected South African women. *Journal of Pediatric Gastroenterology and Nutrition* 2001;32: 464–470.

23. Coodley GO, Nelson HD, Loveless MO, Folk C. Beta-carotene and HIV infection. *Journal of Acquired Immune Deficiency Syndromes* 1993;6:272–276.

24. Ullrich R, Schneider T, Heise W, et al. Serum carotene deficiency in HIV-infected patients. Berlin Diarrhoea/Wasting Syndrome Study Group. *AIDS* 1994;8:661–665.

25. Falguera M, Perez-Mur J, Piug T, Cao G. Study of the role of vitamin B12 and folinic acid supplementation in preventing hemologic toxicity of zidovudine. *European Journal of Haematology* 1995;55:97–102.

26. Herzlich BC, Ranginwala M, Nawabi I, Herbert V. Synergy of inhibition of DNA synthesis in human bone marrow by azidothymidine plus deficiency of folate and/or vitamin B12? *American Journal of Hematology* 1990;33:177–183.

27. Arici C, Tebaldi A, Quinzan GP, et al. Severe lactic acidosis and thiamine administration in an HIV-infected patient on HAART. *International Journal*

of *STD & AIDS* 2001;12:407–409.

28. Shoji S, Furuishi K, Misumi S, et al. Thiamine disulfide as a potent inhibitor of human immunodeficiency virus (type-1) production. *Biochemical and Biophysical Research Communications* 1994;205:967–975.

29. Muri RM, Von Overbeck J, Furrer J, Ballmer PE. Thiamin deficiency in HIV-positive patients: evaluation by erythrocyte transketolase activity and thiamin pyrophosphate effect. *Clinical Nutrition* 1999;18:375–378.

30. Baum MK, Mantero-Atienza E, Shor-Posner G, et al. Association of vitamin B6 status with parameters of immune function in early HIV-1 infection. *Journal of Acquired Immune Deficiency Syndromes* 1991;4:1122–1132.

31. Trakatellis A, Dimitriadou A, Trakatelli M. Pyridoxine deficiency: new approaches in immunosuppression and chemotherapy. *Postgraduate Medicine J* 1997;73:617–622.

32. Folkers K, Morita M, McRee J Jr. The activities of coenzyme Q10 and vitamin B6 for immune responses. *Biochemical and Biophysical Research Communications* 1993;193:88–92.

33. Tamura J, Kubota K, Murakami H, et al. Immunomodulation by vitamin B12: augmentation of CD8+ T lymphocytes and natural killer (NK) cell activity in vitamin B12–deficient patients by methyl-B12 treatment. *Clinical & Experimental Immunology* 1999;116:28–32.

34. Herzlich BC, Schiano TD. Reversal of apparent AIDS dementia complex following treatment with vitamin B12. *Journal of Internal Medicine* 1993;233:495–497.

35. Tang AM, Graham NM, Chandra RK, Saah AJ. Low serum vitamin B-12 concentrations are associated with faster human immunodeficiency virus

type 1 (HIV-1) disease progression. *Journal of Nutrition* 1997;127:345–351.

36. Rule SA, Hooker M, Costello C, et al. Serum vitamin B12 and transcobalamin levels in early HIV disease. *American Journal of Hematology* 1994;47:167–171.

37. Burkes RL, Cohen H, Krailo M, et al. Low serum cobalamin levels occur frequently in the acquired immune deficiency syndrome and related disorders. *European Journal of Haematology* 1987;38:141–147.

38. Harakeh S, Jariwalla RJ. Ascorbate effect on cytokine stimulation of HIV production. *Nutrition* 1995;11 suppl 5:684–687.

39. Allard JP, Aghdassi E, Chau J, et al. Effects of vitamin E supplementation on oxidative stress and viral load in HIV-infected subjects. *AIDS* 1998;12:1653–1659.

40. Edeas MA, Claise C, Vergnes L, et al. Protective effects of the lipophilic redox conjugate tocopheryl succinyl-ethyl ferulate on HIV replication. *FEBS Letters* 1997;418:15–18.

41. de la Asunción JG, Del Olmo ML, Gómez-Cambronero LG, et al. AZT induces oxidative damage to cardiac mitochondria: protective effect of vitamins C and E. *Life Sciences* 2004;76:47–56.

42. Tang AM, Graham NM, Semba RD, Saah AJ. Association between serum vitamin A and E levels and HIV-1 disease progression. *AIDS* 1997;11:613–620.

43. Pacht ER, Diaz P, Clanton T, et al. Serum vitamin E decreases in HIV-seropositive subjects over time. *Journal of Laboratory and Clinical Medicine* 1997;130:293–296.

44. Wasserman P, Rubin DS. Highly prevalent vitamin D deficiency and insufficiency in an urban cohort of HIV-infected men under care. *AIDS Patient Care and STDs* 2010 Apr;24(4):223–227.

45. Haug CJ, Aukrust, Haug P, et al. Severe deficiency of 1,25-dihydroxyvitamin D3 in human immunodeficiency virus infection: association with immunological hyperactivity and only minor changes in calcium homeostasis. *The Journal of Clinical Endocrinology & Metabolism* 1998 Nov;83(11):3832–3838.

46. Davis DA, Branca AA, Pallenberg AJ, et al. Inhibition of the human immunodeficiency virus–1 protease and human immuno-deficiency virus–1 replication by bathocuproine disulfonic acid CU¹⁺. *Archives of Biochemistry and Biophysics* 1995;322:127–134.

47. Baum MK, Javier JJ, Mantero-Atienza E, et al. Zidovudine-associated adverse reactions in a longitudinal study of asymptomatic HIV-1-infected homosexual males. *Journal of Acquired Immune Deficiency Syndromes* 1991;4:1218–1226.

48. Beach RS, Mantero-Atienza E, Shor-Posner G, et al. Specific nutrient abnormalities in asymptomatic HIV-1 infection. *AIDS* 1992;6:701–708.

49. Moreno Díaz MT, Ruiz López MD, Navarro Alarcón M, et al. [Magnesium deficiency in patients with HIV-AIDS.] *Nutrición Hospitalaria* 1997;12:304–308.

50. Seguro AC, de Araujo M, Seguro FS, et al. Effects of hypokalemia and hypomagnesemia on zidovudine (AZT) and didanosine (ddI) nephrotoxicity in rats. *Clinical Nephrology* 2003;59:267–272.

51. Hurwitz BE, Klaus JR. Suppression of human immunodeficiency virus type 1 viral load with selenium supplementation: a randomized controlled trial. *Archives of Internal Medicine* 2007 Jan 22;167(2):148–154.

52. Baum MK, Shor-Posner G, Lai S, et al. High risk of HIV-related mortality is associated with selenium deficiency. *Journal of Acquired Immune Defi-*

ciency Syndromes and Human Retrovirology 1997;15:370–374.

53. Shor-Posner G, Lecusay R, Miguez MJ, et al. Psychological burden in the era of HAART: impact of selenium therapy. International Journal of Psychiatry in Medicine 2003;33:55–69.

54. Burbano X, Miguez-Burbano MJ, McCollister K, et al. Impact of a selenium chemoprevention clinical trial on hospital admissions of HIV-infected participants. HIV Clinical Trials 2002; 3:483–491.

55. Rayman MP. The argument for increasing selenium intake. Proceedings of the Nutrition Society 2002;61:203–215.

56. Mocchegiani E, Muzzioli M. Therapeutic application of zinc in human immunodeficiency virus against opportunistic infections. Journal of Nutrition 2000; 130 suppl 5S:1424S–1431S.

57. Koch J, Neal EA, Schlott MJ, et al. Zinc levels and infections in hospitalized patients with AIDS. Nutrition 1996;12: 515–518.

58. Mocchegiani E, Veccia S, Ancarani F, et al. Benefit of oral zinc supplementation as an adjunct to zidovudine (AZT) therapy against opportunistic infections in AIDS. International Journal of Immunopharmacology 1995; 17:719–727.

59. Pace GW, Leaf CD. The role of oxidative stress in HIV disease. Free Radical Biology & Medicine 1995;19:523–528.

60. de la Asunción JG, Del Olmo ML, Sastre J, et al. AZT treatment induces molecular and ultrastructural oxidative damage to muscle mitochondria. Prevention by antioxidant vitamins. Journal of Clinical Investigation 1998;102:4–9.

61. de la Asunción JG, Del Olmo ML, Gómez-Cambronero LG, et al. AZT induces oxidative damage to cardiac mitochondria: protective effect of vitamins C and E. Life Sciences 2004;76:47–56.

62. Breitkreutz R, Pittack N, Nebe CT, et al. Improvement of immune functions in HIV infection by sulfur supplementation: two randomized trials. Journal of Molecular Medicine 2000;78: 55–62.

63. Akerlund B, Jarstrand C, Lindeke B, et al. Effect of N-acetylcysteine (NAC) treatment on HIV-1 infection: a double-blind placebo-controlled trial. European Journal of Clinical Pharmacology 1996;50: 457–461.

64. Spada C, Treitinger A, Reis M, et al. The effect of N-acetylcysteine supplementation upon viral load, CD4, CD8, total lymphocyte count and hematocrit in individuals undergoing antiretroviral treatment. Clinical Chemistry and Laboratory Medicine 2002;40:452–455.

65. Witschi A, Junker E, Schranz C, et al. Supplementation of N-acetylcysteine fails to increase glutathione in lymphocytes and plasma of patients with AIDS. AIDS Research and Human Retroviruses 1995;11: 141–143.

66. Grieb G. [Alpha-lipoic acid inhibits HIV replication.] Medizinische Monatsschrift fur Pharmazeuten 1992;15:243–244.

67. Suzuki YJ, Aggarwal BB, Packer L. Alpha-lipoic acid is a potent inhibitor of NF-kappa B activation in human T cells. Biochemical and Biophysical Research Communications 1992; 189:1709–1715.

68. Fuchs J, Schofer H, Milbradt R, et al. Studies on lipoate effects on blood redox state in human immunodeficiency virus infected patients. Arzneimittelforschung 1993;43:1359–1362.

69. Folkers K, Langsjoen P, Nara Y, et al. Biochemical deficiencies of coenzyme Q10 in HIV-infection and exploratory treatment. Biochemical and Biophysical Research Communications 1988;153:888–896.

70. Folkers K, Hanioka T, Xia LJ, et al. Coenzyme Q10 increases T4/T8 ratios of lymphcytes in ordinary subjects and relevance to patients having the AIDS related complex. Biochemical and Biophysical Research Communications 1991;176:786–791.

71. Mintz M. Carnitine in human immunodeficiency virus type 1 infection/acquired immune deficiency syndrome. Journal of Child Neurology 1995;10 suppl 2:S40–S44.

72. De Simone C, Famularo G, Tzantzoglou S, et al. Carnitine depletion in peripheral blood mononuclear cells from patients with AIDS: effect of oral L-carnitine. AIDS 1994;8:655–660.

73. Virmani MA, Biselli R, Spadoni A, et al. Protective actions of L-carnitine and acetyl-L-carnitine on the neurotoxicity evoked by mitochondrial uncoupling or inhibitors. Pharmacological Research 1995;32:383–389.

74. Claessens YE, Cariou A, Monchi M, et al. Detecting life-threatening lactic acidosis related to nucleoside-analog treatment of human immunodeficiency virus-infected patients, and treatment with L-carnitine. Critical Care Medicine 2003;31:1042–1047.

75. De Simone C, Tzantzoglou S, Famularo G, et al. High dose L-carnitine improves immunologic and metabolic parameters in AIDS patients. Immunopharmacology and Immunotoxicology 1993;15:1–12.

76. Scarpini E, Sacilotto G, Baron P, et al. Effect of acetyl-L-carnitine in the treatment of painful peripheral neuropathies in HIV+ patients. Journal of the Peripheral Nervous System 1997;2:250–252.

77. Li CJ, Zhang LJ, Dezube BJ, et al. Three inhibitors of human type 1 immunodeficiency virus: long terminal repeat, directed gene expression, and virus replication. Proceedings of the National Academy of Sciences of the United States of America 1993;90:1839–1841.

78. Mazumder A, Raghavan K, Weinstein J, et al. Inhibition of human immunodeficiency virus type-1 integrase by curcumin. *Biochemical Pharmacology* 49: 1165–1170, 1995.

79. Vajragupta O, Boonchoong P, Morris GM, Olson AJ. Active site binding modes of curcumin in HIV-1 protease and integrase. *Bioorganic & Medicinal Chemistry Letters* 2005 Jul 15; 15(14):3364–3368.

80. Jiang MC, Lin JK, Chen SS. Inhibition of HIV-1 Tat-mediated transactivation by quinacrine and chloroquine. *Biochemical and Biophysical Research Communications* 1996 Sep;4;226(1): 1–7.

81. Chan MM. Inhibition of tumor necrosis factor by curcumin, a phytochemical. *Biochemical Pharmacology* 1995;49(11): 1551–1556.

82. Singh S, Aggarwal BB. Activation of transcription factor NF-kappa B is suppressed by curcumin (diferulolymethane). *The Journal of Biological Chemistry* 1995;270(42): 24995–25000.

83. Copeland R, Baker D, Wilson H. Curcumin therapy in HIV-infected patients. International Conference on AIDS 1994;10:216.

84. Conteas CN, Panossian AM, Tran TT, Singh HM. Treatment of HIV-associated diarrhea with curcumin. *Digestive Diseases and Sciences* 2009 Oct;54(10): 2188–2191.

85. Marczylo TH, Verschoyle RD, Cooke DN, et al. Comparison of systemic availability of curcumin with that of curcumin formulated with phosphatidylcholine. *Cancer Chemotherapy and Pharmacology* 2007 Jul; 60(2):171–177.

86. Sasaki H, Sunagawa Y, Takahashi K, et al. Innovative preparation of curcumin for improved oral bioavailability. *Biological and Pharmaceutical Bulletin* 2011;34(5):660–665.

87. Ikegami N, Akatani K, Imai M, et al. Prophylactic effect of long-term oral administration of glycyrrhizin on AIDS development of asymptomatic patients. International Conference on AIDS 1993;9(1):234.

88. Mori K, Sakai H, Suzuki S, et al. Effects of glycyrrhizin (SNMC: Stronger Neo-Minophagen C) in hemophilia patients with HIV-1 infection. *The Tohoku Journal of Experimental Medicine* 162: 183–93, 1990.

89. Yamamoto Y, Yasuoka A, Tachikawa N, et al. Mitigation of hepato-cellular injury caused by HAART with glycyrrhizin compound in patients co-infected with HIV and HCV. *Japanese Journal of Infectious Diseases* 1999 Dec;52(6):248–249.

90. Ullum H, Palmo J, Halkjaer-Kristensen J, et al. The effect of acute exercise on lymphocyte subsets, natural killer cells, proliferative responses, and cytokines in HIV-seropositive persons. *Journal of Acquired Immune Deficiency Syndromes* 1994;7:1122–1133.

91. LaPerriere A, Antoni MH, Ironson G, et al. Effects of aerobic exercise training on lymphocyte subpopulations. *International Journal of Sports Medicine* 1994;15:S127–S130.

92. Galantino ML, Findley T, Krafft L, et al. Blending traditional and alternative strategies for rehabilitation: measuring functional outcomes and quality of life issues in an AIDS population, The Eighth World Congress of International Rehabilitation Medicine Association. *Monduzzi Editore* 1997;1: 713–716.

93. Rehse A. Body movement workshop for people with HIV/AIDS. Internaitonal Conference on AIDS 1992;8:126.

Alcohol Dependence

1. Hasin DS, Stinson FS, Ogburn E, Grant BF. Prevalence, correlates, disability, and co-morbidity of DSM-IV alcohol abuse and dependence in the United States: results from the National Epidemiologic Survey on Alcohol and Related Conditions. *Archives of General Psychiatry* 2007 Jul;64(7):830–842.

2. Enoch MA, Goldman D. Problem drinking and alcoholism: diagnosis and treatment. *American Family Physician* 2002;65: 441–448.

3. Rohde P, Lewinsohn PM, Kahler CW, et al. Natural course of alcohol use disorders from adolescence to young adulthood. *Journal of the American Academy of Child and Adolescent Psychiatry* 2001;40: 83–90.

4. Day CP. Who gets alcoholic liver disease: nature or nurture? *Journal of the Royal College of Physicians London* 2000;34: 557–562.

5. Kimura M, Higuchi S. Genetics of alcohol dependence. *Psychiatry and Clinical Neurosciences* 2011 Apr;65(3):213–225.

6. Pohorecky LA, Brick J. Pharmacology of ethanol. *Pharmacology & Therapeutics* 1988;36: 335–427.

7. Tipton KF, Heneman GTM, McCrodden JM. Metabolic and nutritional aspects of alcohol. *Biochemical Society Transactions* 1983;11:59–61.

8. Lieber CS. Alcohol, liver, and nutrition. *Journal of the American College of Nutrition* 1991; 10:602–632.

9. Piche T, Vandenbos F, Abakar-Mahamat A, et al. The severity of liver fibrosis is associated with high leptin levels in chronic hepatitis C. *Journal of Viral Hepatitis* 2004;11:91–96.

10. Nicolás JM, Fernández-Solà J, Fatjó F, et al. Increased circulating leptin levels in chronic alcoholism. *Alcoholism: Clinical and Experimental Research* 2001;25:83–88.

11. Das I, Burch RE, Hahn HK.

Effects of zinc deficiency on ethanol metabolism and alcohol and aldehyde dehydrogenase activities. *Journal of Laboratory and Clinical Medicine* 1984; 104:610–617.

12. Wu CT, Lee JN, Shen WW, et al. Serum zinc, copper, and ceruloplasmin levels in male alcoholics. *Biological Psychiatry* 1984;19:1333–1338.

13. Schölmerich J, Löhle E, Köttgen E, Gerok W. Zinc and vitamin A deficiency in liver cirrhosis. *Hepatogastroenterology* 1983;30:119–125.

14. Yunice AA, Lindeman RD. Effect of ascorbic acid and zinc sulphate on ethanol toxicity and metabolism. *Proceedings of the Society for Experimental Biology and Medicine* 1977; 154: 146–150.

15. Messiha FS. Vitamin A, gender and ethanol interactions. *Neurobehavioral Toxicology and Teratology* 1983;5:233–236.

16. Morin LP, Forger NG. Endocrine control of ethanol intake by rats or hamsters: relative contributions of the ovaries, adrenals and steroids. *Pharmacology Biochemistry and Behavior* 1982;17:529–537.

17. Lecomte E, Herbeth B, Pirollet P. Effect of alcohol consumption of blood antioxidant nutrients and oxidative stress indicators. *The American Journal of Clinical Nutrition* 1994; 60:255–261.

18. Sher L. Role of selenium depletion in the etiopathogenesis of depression in patients with alcoholism. *Medical Hypotheses* 2002;59: 330–333.

19. Suematsu T, Matsumura T, Sato N, et al. Lipid peroxidation in alcoholic liver disease in humans. *Alcoholism: Clinical and Experimental Research* 1981;5: 427–430.

20. DiLuzio NR. A mechanism of the acute ethanol-induced fatty liver and the modification of liver injury by antioxidants. *American Journal of Pharmacy and the Sciences Supporting Public Health* 1966;15:50–63.

21. Stanko RT, Mendelow H, Shinozuka H, et al. Prevention of alcohol-induced fatty liver by natural metabolites and riboflavin. *Journal of Laboratory and Clinical Medicine* 1978;91: 228–235.

22. Hartroft WS, Porta EA, Suzuki M. Effects of choline chloride on hepatic lipids after acute ethanol intoxication. *Journal of Studies on Alcohol and Drugs* 1964;25:427–437.

23. Sachan DS, Rhew TH, Ruark RA. Ameliorating effects of carnitine and its precursors on alcohol-induced fatty liver. *The American Journal of Clinical Nutrition* 1984;39:738–744.

24. Sachan DA, Rhew TH. Lipotropic effect of carnitine on alcohol-induced hepatic stenosis. *Nutrition Reports International* 1983;27:1221–1226.

25. Majumdar SK, Shaw GK, Thomson AD. Changes in plasma amino acid patterns in chronic alcoholic patients during ethanol withdrawal syndrome: their clinical implications. *Medical Hypotheses* 1983;12:239–251.

26. Branchey L, Branchey M, Shaw S, et al. Relationship between changes in plasma amino acids and depression in alcoholic patients. *The American Journal of Psychiatry* 1984;141: 1212–1215.

27. Rosen HM, Yoshimura N, Hodgman JM, et al. Plasma amino acid patterns in hepatic encephalopathy of differing etiology. *Gastroenterology* 1977; 72:483–487.

28. Fischer JE, Rosen HM, Ebeid AM, et al. The effect of normalization of plasma amino acids on hepatic encephalopathy. *Surgery* 1976;80:77–91.

29. Lieber CS. Hepatic, metabolic, and nutritional disorders of alcoholism: from pathogenesis to therapy. *Critical Reviews in Clinical Laboratory Sciences* 2000;37:551–584.

30. Baines M. Detection and incidence of B and C vitamin deficiency in alcohol-related illness. *Annals of Clinical Biochemistry* 1978;15:307–312.

31. Yunice AA, Hsu JM, Fahmy A, et al. Ethanol-ascorbate interrelationship in acute and chronic alcoholism in the guinea pig. *Proceedings of the Society for Experimental Biology and Medicine* 1984;177:262–271.

32. Finley JW, Penland JG. Adequacy or deprivation of dietary selenium in healthy men: clinical and psychological findings. *The Journal of Trace Elements in Experimental Medicine* 1998; 11:11–27.

33. Cornelius JR, Salloum IM, Mezzich J, et al. Disproportionate suicidality in patients with comorbid major depression and alcoholism. *The American Journal of Psychiatry* 1995;152: 358–364.

34. Koike H, Mori K, Misu K, et al. Painful alcoholic polyneuropathy with predominant small-fiber loss and normal thiamine status. *Neurology* 2001;56: 1727–1732.

35. Zimatkin SM, Zimatkina TI. Thiamine deficiency as predisposition to, and consequence of, increased alcohol consumption. *Alcohol and Alcoholism* 1996; 31:421–427.

36. Thomson AD. Mechanisms of vitamin deficiency in chronic alcohol misusers and the development of the Wernicke-Korsakoff syndrome. *Alcohol and Alcoholism* 2000;35 suppl 1:2–7.

37. Lumeng L. The role of acetaldehyde in mediating the deleterious effect of ethanol on pyridoxal 5-phosphate metabolism. *Journal of Clinical Investigation* 1978;62:286–293.

38. McMartin KE, Collins TD, Bairnsfather L. Cumulative excess urinary excretion of folate in rats after repeated ethanol treatment. *Journal of Nutrition* 1986;116:1316–1325.

39. Abbott L, Nadler J, Rude RK.

Magnesium deficiency in alcoholism: possible contribution to osteoporosis and cardiovascular disease in alcoholics. *Alcoholism: Clinical and Experimental Research* 1994;18:1076–1082.

40. Reitz RC. Dietary fatty acids and alcohol: effects on cellular membranes. *Alcohol and Alcoholism* 1993 Jan;28(1):59–71.

41. Pawlosky RJ, Bacher J, Salem N Jr. Ethanol consumption alters electroretinograms and depletes neural tissues of docosahexaenoic acid in rhesus monkeys: nutritional consequences of a low n-3 fatty acid diet. *Alcoholism: Clinical and Experimental Research* 2001;25:1758–1765.

42. Rogers LL, Pelton RB, Williams RJ. Voluntary alcohol consumption by rats following administration of glutamine. *The Journal of Biological Chemistry* 1955; 214:503–506.

43. Rogers LL, Pelton RB. Glutamine in the treatment of alcoholism. *Journal of Studies on Alcohol and Drugs* 1957;18: 581–587.

44. Ravel JM, Felsing B, Lansford EM Jr., et al. Reversal of alcohol toxicity by glutamine. *The Journal of Biological Chemistry* 1955;214:497–501.

45. Branchey L, Shaw S, Lieber CS. Ethanol impairs tryptophan transport into the brain and depresses serotonin. *Life Sciences* 1981;29:2751–2755.

46. Ireland MA, Vandongen R, Davidson L, et al. Acute effects of moderate alcohol consumption on blood pressure and plasma catecholamines. *Clinical Science* 1984;66:643–648.

47. Bode JC, Bode C, Heidelbach R, et al. Jejunal microflora in patients with chronic alcohol abuse. *Hepatogastroenterology* 1984;31:30–34.

48. Worthington BS, Meserole L, Syrotuck JA. Effect of daily ethanol ingestion on intestinal permeability to macromolecules. *American Journal of Digestive Diseases* 1978;23:23–32.

49. Sinyor D, Brown T, Rostant L, et al. The role of a physical fitness program in the treatment of alcoholism. *Journal of Studies on Alcohol* 1982;43:380–386.

50. Keung WM, Vallee BL. Kudzu root: an ancient Chinese source of modern antidipsotropic agents. *Phytochemistry* 1998 Feb;47(4): 499–506.

51. Arolfo MP, Overstreet DH, Yao L, et al. Suppression of heavy drinking and alcohol seeking by a selective ALDH–2 inhibitor. *Alcoholism: Clinical and Experimental Research* 2009 Nov;33(11):1935–1944.

52. Lukas SE, Penetar D, Berko J, et al. An extract of the Chinese herbal root kudzu reduces alcohol drinking by heavy drinkers in a naturalistic setting. *Alcoholism: Clinical and Experimental Research* 2005 May; 29(5):756–762.

53. Shebek J, Rindone JP. A pilot study exploring the effect of kudzu root on the drinking habits of patients with chronic alcoholism. *The Journal of Alternative and Complementary Medicine* 2000 Feb;6(1):45–48.

54. Ferenci P, Dragosics B, Dittrich H. Randomized controlled trial of silymarin treatment in patients with cirrhosis of the liver. *Journal of Hepatology* 1989;9:105–113.

55. Deak G, Muzes G, Lang I, et al. [Immunomodulator effect of silymarin therapy in chronic alcoholic liver diseases.] *Orvosi Hetilap* 1990;131:1291–1292,1295–1296.

Alzheimer's Disease

1. Ballard C, Gauthier S, Corbett A, et al. Alzheimer's disease. *The Lancet* 2011 Mar 19; 377(9770):1019–1013.

2. Wick G, Berger P, Jansen-Durr P, Grubeck-Loebenstein B. A Darwinian-evolutionary concept of age-related diseases. *Experimental Gerontology* 2003; 38:13–25.

3. Fu HJ, Liu B, Frost JL, Le-

mere CA. Amyloid-beta immunotherapy for Alzheimer's disease. *CNS & Neurological Disorders—Drug Targets* 2010 Apr;9(2):197–206.

4. Solfrizzi V, Panza F, Capurso A. The role of diet in cognitive decline. *Journal of Neural Transmission* 2003;110:95–110.

5. Grant WB, Campbell A, Itzhaki RF, Savory J. The significance of environmental factors in the etiology of Alzheimer's disease. *Journal of Alzheimer's Disease* 2002;4:179–189.

6. Bonda DJ, Wang X, Perry G, et al. Oxidative stress in Alzheimer disease: a possibility for prevention. *Neuropharmacology* 2010 Sep–Oct;59(4–5):290–294.

7. Craft S. Insulin resistance and Alzheimer's disease pathogenesis: potential mechanisms and implications for treatment. *Current Alzheimer Research* 2007 Apr;4(2):147–152.

8. Luchsinger JA, Small S, Biessels GJ. Should we target insulin resistance to prevent dementia due to Alzheimer disease? *Archives of Neurology* 2011 Jan; 68(1):17–18.

9. Feldman HH, Jacova C, Robillard A, et al. Diagnosis and treatment of dementia. 2. Diagnosis. *Canadian Medical Association Journal* 2008 Mar 25; 178(7):825–836.

10. Weinreb HJ. Fingerprint patterns in Alzheimer's disease. *Archives of Neurology* 1985;42: 50–54.

11. Solfrizzi V, Panza F, Frisardi V, et al. Diet and Alzheimer's disease risk factors or prevention: the current evidence. *Expert Review of Neurotherapeutics* 2011 May;11(5):677–708.

12. Frisardi V, Panza F, Seripa D, et al. Nutraceutical properties of Mediterranean diet and cognitive decline: possible underlying mechanisms. *Journal of Alzheimer's Disease* 2010 Jan 1; 22(3):715–740.

13. Gu Y, Luchsinger JA, Stern Y, Scarmeas N. Mediterranean

diet, inflammatory and metabolic biomarkers, and risk of Alzheimer's disease. *Journal of Alzheimer's Disease* 2010;22(2): 483–492.

14. Darvesh AS, Carroll RT, Bishayee A, et al. Oxidative stress and Alzheimer's disease: dietary polyphenols as potential therapeutic agents. *Expert Review of Neurotherapeutics* 2010 May; 10(5):729–745.

15. Hamaguchi T, Ono K, Murase A, Yamada M. Phenolic compounds prevent Alzheimer's pathology through different effects on the amyloid-beta aggregation pathway. *The American Journal of Pathology* 2009 Dec; 175(6):2557–2565.

16. Liu RH. Health benefits of fruit and vegetables are from additive and synergistic combinations of phytochemicals. *The American Journal of Clinical Nutrition* 2003;78 suppl 3:517S–520S.

17. Kim J, Lee HJ, Lee KW. Naturally occurring phytochemicals for the prevention of Alzheimer's disease. *Journal of Neurochemistry* 2010 Mar; 112(6):1415–1430.

18. Hamaguchi T, Ono K, Murase A, Yamada M. Phenolic compounds prevent Alzheimer's pathology through different effects on the amyloid-beta aggregation pathway. *The American Journal of Pathology* 2009 Dec; 175(6):2557–2565.

19. Williams P, Sorribas A, Howes MJ. Natural products as a source of Alzheimer's drug leads. *Natural Product Reports* 2011 Jan 17;28(1):48–77.

20. Wang YJ, Thomas P, Zhong JH, et al. Consumption of grape seed extract prevents amyloid-beta deposition and attenuates inflammation in brain of an Alzheimer's disease mouse. *Neurotoxicity Research* 2009 Jan; 15(1):3–14.

21. Wang J, Santa-Maria I, Ho L, et al. Grape derived polyphenols attenuate tau neuropathology in a mouse model of Alzheimer's disease. *Journal of Alzheimer's Disease* 2010;22(2):653–661.

22. Janle EM, Lila MA, Grannan M, et al. Pharmacokinetics and tissue distribution of 14C-labeled grape polyphenols in the periphery and the central nervous system following oral administration. *Journal of Medicinal Food* 2010 Aug;13(4): 926–933.

23. Peng Y, Sun J, Hon S, et al. L-3-n-butylphthalide improves cognitive impairment and reduces amyloid-beta in a transgenic model of Alzheimer's disease. *The Journal of Neuroscience* 2010 Jun 16;30(24): 8180–8189.

24. Henderson VW. Action of estrogens in the aging brain: dementia and cognitive aging. *Biochimica et Biophysica Acta* 2010 Oct;1800(10):1077–1083.

25. Matthews KA, Kuller LH, Wing RR, et al. Prior to use of estrogen replacement therapy, are users healthier than nonusers? *American Journal of Epidemiology* 1996;143:971–978.

26. Craig MC, Maki PM, Murphy DG. The Women's Health Initiative Memory Study: findings and implications for treatment. *The Lancet Neurology* 2005 Mar;4(3):190–194.

27. Almeida OP, Flicker L. Association between hormone replacement therapy and dementia: is it time to forget? *International Psychogeriatrics* 2005 Jun;17(2): 155–164.

28. Craig MC, Murphy DG. Estrogen therapy and Alzheimer's dementia. *Annals of the New York Academy of Sciences.* 2010 Sep;1205:245–253.

29. Hogervorst E, Yaffe K, Richards M, Huppert FA. Hormone replacement therapy to maintain cognitive function in women with dementia. Cochrane Database of Systematic Reviews 2009 Jan 21;1:CD003799.

30. Shin RW. Interaction of aluminum with paired helical filament tau is involved in neurofibrillary pathology of Alzheimer's disease. *Gerontology* 1997;43 suppl 1:16–23.

31. Zapatero MD, Garcia de Jalon A, Pascual F, et al. Serum aluminum levels in Alzheimer's disease and other senile dementias. *Biological Trace Element Research* 1995;47:235–240.

32. Walton J, Tuniz C, Fink D, et al. Uptake of trace amounts of aluminum into the brain from drinking water. *Neurotoxicology* 1995;16:187–190.

33. Nolan CR, DeGoes JJ, Alfrey AC. Aluminum and lead absorption from dietary sources in women ingesting calcium citrate. *Southern Medical Journal* 1994;87:894–898.

34. Glick JL. Dementias: the role of magnesium deficiency and hypothesis concerning the pathogenesis of Alzheimer's disease. *Medical Hypotheses* 1990;31: 211–225.

35. Tucker DM, Penland JG, Sandstead HH, et al. Nutrition status and brain function in aging. *The American Journal of Clinical Nutrition* 1990;52:93–102.

36. Praticò D. Oxidative stress hypothesis in Alzheimer's disease: a reappraisal. *Trends in Pharmacological Sciences* 2008 Dec; 29(12):609–615.

37. Gella A, Durany N. Oxidative stress in Alzheimer disease. *Cell Adhesion & Migration* 2009 Jan–Mar;3(1):88–93.

38. Jama JW, Launer LJ, Witteman JC, et al. Dietary antioxidants and cognitive function in a population-based sample of older persons. *American Journal of Epidemiology* 1996;144: 275–280.

39. Luchsinger JA, Tang MX, Shea S, Mayeux R. Antioxidant vitamin intake and risk of Alzheimer disease. *Archives of Neurology* 2003 Feb;60(2): 203–208.

40. Masaki KH, Losonczy KG, Izmirlian G, et al. Association of vitamin E and C supplement use with cognitive function and

dementia in elderly men. *Neurology* 2000;54:1265–1272.

41. Klatte ET, Scharre DW, Nagaraja HN, et al. Combination therapy of donepezil and vitamin E in Alzheimer disease. *Alzheimer Disease & Associated Disorders* 2003;17:113–116.

42. Gray SL, Anderson ML, Crane PK, et al. Antioxidant vitamin supplement use and risk of dementia or Alzheimer's disease in older adults. *Journal of the American Geriatrics Society* 2008;56:291–295.

43. Chen MF, Chen LT, Gold M, et al. Plasma and erythrocyte thiamin concentration in geriatric outpatients. *Journal of the American College of Nutrition* 1996;15:231–236.

44. Meador KJ, Nichols ME, Franke P, et al. Evidence for a central cholinergic effect of high dose thiamine. *Annals of Neurology* 1993;34:724–726.

45. Meador K, Loring D, Nichols M, et al. Preliminary findings of high-dose thiamine in dementia of Alzheimer's type. *Journal of Geriatric Psychiatry and Neurology* 1993;6:222–229.

46. Benton D, Fordy J, Haller J. The impact of long-term vitamin supplementation on cognitive functioning. *Psychopharmacology* 1995;117:298–305.

47. van Goor L, Woiski MD, Lagaay AM, et al. Review: cobalamin deficiency and mental impairment in elderly people. *Age and Ageing* 1995;24:536–542.

48. Shevell MI, Rosenblatt DS. The neurology of cobalamin. *Canadian Journal of Neurological Sciences* 1992;19:472–486.

49. Yao Y, Lu-Yao G, Mesches DN, Lou W. Decline of serum cobalamin levels with increasing age among geriatric outpatients. *Archives of Family Medicine* 1994;3:918–922.

50. Aronow WS. Homocysteine. The association with atherosclerotic vascular disease in older persons. *Geriatrics* 2003;58: 22–24,27–28.

51. Savage DG, Lindenbaum J, Stabler SP, Allen RH. Sensitivity of serum methylmalonic acid and total homocysteine determinations for diagnosing cobalamin deficiency. *The American Journal of Medicine* 1994;96:239–246.

52. Norman EJ, Morrison JA. Screening elderly populations for cobalamin (vitamin B12) deficiency using the urinary methylmalonic acid assay by gas chromatography mass spectrophotometry. *The American Journal of Medicine* 1993;94:589–594.

53. Seshadri S, Beiser A, Selhub J, et al. Plasma homocysteine as a risk factor for dementia and Alzheimer's disease. *The New England Journal of Medicine* 2002;346:476–483.

54. Nilsson K, Gustafson L, Faldt R, Gustafson L. Plasma homocysteine in relation to serum cobalamin and blood folate in a psychogeriatric population. *European Journal of Clinical Investigation* 1994;24:600–606.

55. Healton EB, Savage DH, Brust JC, et al. Neurologic aspects of cobalamin deficiency. *Medicine* 1991;70:229–245.

56. Martin DC, Francis J, Protetch J, Huff FJ. Time dependency of cognitive recovery with cobalamin replacement. A report of a pilot study. *Journal of the American Geriatrics Society* 1992;40:168–172.

57. Levitt AJ, Karlinsky H. Folate, vitamin B12 and cognitive impairment in patients with Alzheimer's disease. *Acta Psychiatrica Scandinavica* 1992; 86:301–305.

58. Kristensen MO, Gulmann MC, Christensen JE, et al. Serum cobalamin and methylmalonic acid in Alzheimer dementia. *Acta Neurologica Scandinavica* 1993;87:475–481.

59. Seal EC, Metz J, Flicker L, Melny J. A randomized, double-blind, placebo-controlled study of oral vitamin B12 supplementation in older patients with subnormal or borderline serum vitamin B12 concentrations. *Journal of the American Geriatrics Society* 2002;50:146–151.

60. van Dyck CH, Lyness JM, Rohrbaugh RM, Siegal AP. Cognitive and psychiatric effects of vitamin B12 replacement in dementia with low serum B12 levels: a nursing home study. *International Psychogeriatrics* 2009 Feb;21(1): 138–147.

61. Constantinidis J. The hypothesis of zinc deficiency in the pathogenesis of neurofibrillary tangles. *Medical Hypotheses* 1991;35:319–323.

62. Burnet FM. A possible role of zinc in the pathology of dementia. *The Lancet* 1981;1:186–188.

63. Tully CL, Snowdon DA, Markesbery WR. Serum zinc, senile plaques, and neurofibrillary tangles: findings from the Nun Study. *Neuroreport* 1995; 6:2105–2108.

64. Constantinidis J. Treatment of Alzheimer's disease by zinc compounds. *Drug Development Research* 1992;27:1–14.

65. Cuajungco MP, Faget KY. Zinc takes the center stage: its paradoxical role in Alzheimer's disease. *Brain Research Reviews* 2003;41:44–56.

66. Cuajungco MP, Lees GJ. Zinc and Alzheimer's disease: is there a direct link? *Brain Research Reviews* 1997;23:219–236.

67. Furuta A, Price DL, Pardo CA, et al. Localization of superoxide dismutases in Alzheimer's disease and Down's syndrome neocortex and hippocampus. *The American Journal of Pathology* 1995;146:357–367.

68. Walter A, Korth U, Hilgert M, et al. Glycerophosphocholine is elevated in cerebrospinal fluid of Alzheimer patients. *Neurobiology of Aging* 2004 Nov–Dec; 25(10):1299–1303.

69. Rosenberg G, Davis KL. The use of cholinergic precursors in neuropsychiatric diseases. *The*

American Journal of Clinical Nutrition 1982;36:709–720.

70. Levy R, Little A, Chuaqui P, Reith M. Early results from double-blind, placebo controlled trial of high dose phosphatidylcholine in Alzheimer's disease. *The Lancet* 1983;1:987–988.

71. Sitaram N, Weingartner B, Caine ED, Gillin JC. Choline: selective enhancement of serial learning and encoding of low imagery words in man. *Life Sciences* 1978;22:1555–1560.

72. Higgins JP, Flicker L. Lecithin for dementia and cognitive impairment. Cochrane Database of Systematic Reviews 2003;3:CD001015.

73. Amenta F, Parnetti L, Gallai V, Wallin A. Treatment of cognitive dysfunction associated with Alzheimer's disease with cholinergic precursors. Ineffective treatments or inappropriate approaches? *Mechanisms of Ageing and Development* 2001;122:2025–2040.

74. De Jesus Moreno Moreno M. Cognitive improvement in mild to moderate Alzheimer's dementia after treatment with the acetylcholine precursor choline alfoscerate: a multicenter, double-blind, randomized, placebo-controlled trial. *Clinical Therapeutics* 2003 Jan;25(1):178–193.

75. Caamano J, Gomez MJ, Franco A, et al. Effects of CDP-choline on cognition and cerebral hemodynamics in patients with Alzheimer's disease. *Methods & Findings in Experimental & Clinical Pharmacology* 1994;16:211–218.

76. Parnetti L, Amenta F, Gallai V. Choline alphoscerate in cognitive decline and in acute cerebrovascular disease: an analysis of published clinical data. *Mechanisms of Ageing and Development* 2001;122:2041–2055.

77. Cenacchi T, Bertoldin T, Farina C, et al. Cognitive decline in the elderly. A double-blind, placebo-controlled multicenter study on efficacy of phosphatidylserine administration. *Aging* (Milano) 1993;5:123–133.

78. Engel RR, Satzger W, Günther W, et al. Double-blind cross-over study of phosphatidylserine vs. placebo in patients with early dementia of the Alzheimer type. *European Neuropsychopharmacology* 1992;2:149–155.

79. Crook T, Petri W, Wells C, Massari DC. Effects of phosphatidylserine in Alzheimer's disease. *Psychopharmacology Bulletin* 1992;28:61–66.

80. Crook TH, Tinklenberg J, Yesavage J, et al. Effects of phosphatidylserine in age-associated memory impairment. *Neurology* 1991;41:644–649.

81. Funfgeld EW, Baggen M, Nedwidek P, et al. Double-blind study with phosphatidylserine (PS) in Parkinsonian patients with senile dementia of Alzheimer's type (SDAT). *Progress in Clinical and Biological Research* 1989;317:1235–1246.

82. Amaducci L. Phosphatidylserine in the treatment of Alzheimer's disease: results of a multicenter study. *Psychopharmacology Bulletin* 1988;24:1030–1034.

83. Nerozzi D, Aceti F, Melia E, et al. [Phosphatidylserine and memory disorders in the aged.] *La Clinica Terapeutica* 1987;120:399–404.

84. Palmieri G, Palmieri R, Inzoli MR, et al. Double-blind controlled trial of phosphatidylserine in patients with senile mental deterioration. *Clinical Trials* 1987;24:73–78.

85. Villardita C, Grioli S, Salmeri G, et al. Multicentre clinical trial of brain phosphatidylserine in elderly patients with intellectual deterioration. *Clinical Trials* 1987;24:84–93.

86. Delwaide PJ, Gyselynck-Mambourg AM, Hurlet A, Ylieff M. Double-blind randomized controlled study of phosphatidylserine in demented patients. *Acta Neurologica Scandinavica* 1986;73:136–140.

87. Bowman B. Acetyl-carnitine and Alzheimer's disease. *Nutrition Reviews* 1992;50:142–144.

88. Carta A, Calvani M, Bravi D, Bhuachalla SN. Acetyl-L-carnitine and Alzheimer's disease. Pharmacological considerations beyond the cholinergic sphere. *Annals of the New York Academy of Sciences* 1993;695:324–326.

89. Calvani M, Carta A, Caruso G, et al. Action of acetyl-L-carnitine in neurodegeneration and Alzheimer's disease. *Annals of the New York Academy of Sciences* 1992;663:483–486.

90. Montgomery SA, Thal LJ, Amrein R. Meta-analysis of double blind randomized controlled clinical trials of acetyl-L-carnitine versus placebo in the treatment of mild cognitive impairment and mild Alzheimer's disease. *International Clinical Psychopharmacology* 2003;18:61–71.

91. Bianchetti A, Rozzini R, Trabucchi M. Effects of acetyl-L-carnitine in Alzheimer's disease patients unresponsive to acetylcholinesterase inhibitors. *Current Medical Research & Opinion* 2003;19:350–353.

92. Vecchi GP, Chiari G, Cipolli C, et al. Acetyl-L-carnitine treatment of mental impairment in the elderly. Evidence from a multicenter study. *Archives of Gerontology and Geriatrics* 1991;2:159–168.

93. Salvioli G, Neri M. L-acetylcarnitine treatment of mental decline in the elderly. *Drugs Under Experimental and Clinical Research* 1994;20:169–176.

94. Cipolli C, Chiari G. [Effects of L-acetylcarnitine on mental deterioration in the aged. Initial results.] *La Clinica Terapeutica* 1990;132 suppl 6:479–510.

95. Yamada S, Akishita M, Fukai S. Effects of dehydroepiandrosterone supplementation on cog-

nitive function and activities of daily living in older women with mild to moderate cognitive impairment. *Geriatrics & Gerontology International* 2010 Oct; 10(4):280–287.

96. Kritz-Silverstein D, von Mühlen D, Laughlin GA, Bettencourt R. Effects of dehydroepiandrosterone supplementation on cognitive function and quality of life: the DHEA and Well-Ness (DAWN) Trial. *Journal of the American Geriatrics Society* 2008 Jul;56(7): 1292–1298.

97. Grimley Evans J, Malouf R, Huppert F, van Niekerk JK. Dehydroepiandrosterone (DHEA) supplementation for cognitive function in healthy elderly people. Cochrane Database of Systematic Reviews 2006 Oct 18;4: CD006221.

98. Wolkowitz OM, Kramer JH, Reus VI, et al. DHEA treatment of Alzheimer's disease: a randomized, double-blind, placebo-controlled study. *Neurology* 2003;60:1071–1076.

99. Olivieri G, Hess C, Savaskan E, et al. Melatonin protects SHSY5Y neuroblastoma cells from cobalt-induced oxidative stress, neurotoxicity and increased beta-amyloid secretion. *Journal of Pineal Research* 2001;31:320–325.

100. Asayama K, Yamadera H, Ito T, et al. Double blind study of melatonin effects on the sleep-wake rhythm, cognitive and non-cognitive functions in Alzheimer type dementia. *Journal of Nippon Medical School* 2003;70: 334–341.

101. Burns A, Allen H, Tomenson B, et al. Bright light therapy for agitation in dementia: a randomized controlled trial. *International Psychogeriatrics* 2009 Aug;21(4):711–721.

102. Dowling GA, Mastick J, Hubbard EM, et al. Effect of timed bright light treatment for rest-activity disruption in institutionalized patients with Alzheimer's

disease. *International Journal of Geriatric Psychiatry* 2005 Aug;20(8):738–743.

103. Ancoli-Israel S, Gehrman P, Martin JL, et al. Increased light exposure consolidates sleep and strengthens circadian rhythms in severe Alzheimer's disease patients. *Behavioral Sleep Medicine* 2003;1(1):22–36.

104. Dowling GA, Burr RL, Van Someren EJ, et al. Melatonin and bright-light treatment for rest-activity disruption in institutionalized patients with Alzheimer's disease. *Journal of the American Geriatrics Society* 2008 Feb;56(2):239–246.

105. Shi C, Liu J, Wu F, Yew DT. *Ginkgo biloba* extract in Alzheimer's disease: from action mechanisms to medical practice. *International Journal of Molecular Sciences* 2010 Jan 8; 11(1):107–123.

106. Weinmann S, Roll S, Schwarzbach C, et al. Effects of *Ginkgo biloba* in dementia: systematic review and meta-analysis. *BMC Geriatrics* 2010 Mar 17;10:14.

107. Ihl R, Bachinskaya N, Korczyn AD, et al. Efficacy and safety of a once-daily formulation of *Ginkgo biloba* extract EGb 761 in dementia with neuropsychiatric features: a randomized controlled trial. *International Journal of Geriatric Psychiatry* 2011 Nov;26(11):1186–1194.

108. Dodge HH, Zitzelberger T, Oken BS, et al. A randomized placebo-controlled trial of *Ginkgo biloba* for the prevention of cognitive decline. *Neurology* 2008 May 6;70(19 part 2): 1809–1817.

109. Wang BS, Wang H, Song YY, et al. Effectiveness of standardized ginkgo biloba extract on cognitive symptoms of dementia with a six-month treatment: a bivariate random effect meta-analysis. *Pharmacopsychiatry* 2010 May;43(3):86–91.

110. Kanowski S, Hermann WM, Stephan K, et al. Proof of ef-

ficacy of the *Ginkgo biloba* special extract EGb 761 in outpatients suffering from mild to moderate primary degenerative dementia of the Alzheimer type or multi-infarct dementia. *Phytomedicine* 1997;4:3–13.

111. Le Bars PL, Katz MM, Berman N, et al. A placebo-controlled, double-blind, randomized trial of an extract of *Ginkgo biloba* for dementia. North American EGb Study Group. *JAMA, The Journal of the American Medical Association* 1997;278: 1327–1332.

112. Bachinskava N, Hoerr R, Ihl R. Alleviating neuropsychiatric symptoms in dementia: the effects of *Ginkgo biloba* extract EGb 761. Findings from a randomized controlled trial. *Neuropsychiatric Disease and Treatment* 2011;7:209–215.

113. Wettstein A. Cholinesterase inhibitors and ginkgo extracts—are they comparable in the treatment of dementia? Comparison of published placebo-controlled efficacy studies of at least six months' duration. *Phytomedicine* 2000;6:393–401.

114. Oken BS, Storzbach DM, Kaye JA. The efficacy of *Ginkgo biloba* on cognitive function in Alzheimer disease. *Archives of Neurology* 1998;55:1409–1415.

115. Skolnick A. Old Chinese herbal medicine used for fever yields possible new Alzheimer disease therapy. *JAMA, The Journal of the American Medical Association* 1997;277:776.

116. Xu SS, Gao ZX, Weng Z, et al. Efficacy of tablet huperzine-A on memory, cognition and behavior in Alzheimer's disease. *Zhongguo Yao Li Xue Bao* 1995; 16:391–395.

117. Rafii MS, Walsh S, Little JT, et al. A phase II trial of huperzine A in mild to moderate Alzheimer disease. *Neurology* 2011 Apr 19;76(16):1389–1394.

118. Hamaguchi T, Ono K, Yamada M. Curcumin and

Alzheimer's disease. *CNS Neuroscience & Therapeutics* 2010 Oct;16(5):285–97.

119. Marczylo TH, Verschoyle RD, Cooke DN, et al. Comparison of systemic availability of curcumin with that of curcumin formulated with phosphatidylcholine. *Cancer Chemotherapy and Pharmacology* 2007 Jul; 60(2):171–177.

120. Sasaki H, Sunagawa Y, Takahashi K, et al. Innovative preparation of curcumin for improved oral bioavailability. *Biological and Pharmaceutical Bulletin* 2011;34(5):660–665.

Anemia

1. Killip S, Bennett JM, Chambers MD. Iron deficiency anemia. *American Family Physician* 2007 Mar 1;75(5):671–678.

2. Arvidsson B, Ekenved G, Rybo G, Solvell L. Iron prophylaxis in menorrhagia. *Acta Obstetricia et Gynecologica Scandinavica* 1981;60:157–160.

3. Taymor ML, Sturgis SH, Yahia C. The etiological role of chronic iron deficiency in production of menorrhagia. *JAMA, The Journal of the American Medical Association* 1964;187: 323–327.

4. Sharp PA. Intestinal iron absorption: regulation by dietary and systemic factors. *International Journal for Vitamin and Nutrition Research* 2010 Oct; 80(4–5):231–242.

5. Fidler MC, Walczyk T, Davidsson L, et al. A micronised, dispersible ferric pyrophosphate with high relative bioavailability in man. *British Journal of Nutrition* 2004 Jan;91(1):107–112.

6. Andrès E, Dali-Youcef N, Vogel T, et al. Oral cobalamin (vitamin B12) treatment: an update. *International Journal of Laboratory Hematology* 2009 Feb; 31(1):1–8.

7. Berlin R, Berlin H, Brante G, Pilbrant A. Vitamin B12 body stores during oral and parenteral treatment of pernicious anaemia. *Acta Medica Scandinavica* 1978;204(1–2):81–84.

8. Pietrzik K, Bailey L, Shane B. Folic acid and L-5-methyltetrahydrofolate: comparison of clinical pharmacokinetics and pharmacodynamics. *Clinical Pharmacokinetics* 2010 Aug 1; 49(8):535–548.

Angina

1. Bansal S, Toh SH, LaBresh KA. Chest pain as a presentation of reactive hypoglycemia. *Chest* 1983;84:641–662.

2. Hueb W, Soares PR, Gersh BJ, et al. The medicine, angioplasty, or surgery study (MASS-II): a randomized, controlled clinical trial of three therapeutic strategies for multivessel coronary artery disease: one-year results. *Journal of the American College of Cardiology* 2004;43: 1743–1751.

3. Graboys TB, Headley A, Lown B, et al. Results of a second opinion program for coronary artery bypass surgery. *JAMA, The Journal of the American Medical Association* 1987;258:1611–1614.

4. Alderman EL, Bourassa MG, Cohen LS, et al. Ten-year follow-up of survival and myocardial infarction in the randomized Coronary Artery Surgery Study. *Circulation* 1990;82:1629–1646.

5. Myocardial infarction and mortality in the coronary artery surgery study (CASS) randomized trial. *The New England Journal of Medicine* 1984;310:750–758.

6. Winslow CM, Kosecoff JB, Chassin M, et al. The appropriateness of performing coronary artery bypass surgery. *JAMA, The Journal of the American Medical Association* 1988;260: 505–509.

7. White CW, Wright CB, Doty DB, et al. Does visual interpretation of the coronary angiogram predict the physiologic importance of a coronary stenosis. *The New England Journal of Medicine* 1984;310:819–824.

8. Boden WE, O'Rourke RA, Teo KK, et al. Impact of optimal medical therapy with or without percutaneous coronary intervention on long-term cardiovascular end points in patients with stable coronary artery disease (from the COURAGE Trial). *American Journal of Cardiology* 2009 Jul 1;104(1):1–4.

9. Ballmer PE, Reinhart WH, Jordan P, et al. Depletion of plasma vitamin C but not vitamin E in response to cardiac operations. *The Journal of Thoracic and Cardiovascular Surgery* 1994; 108:311–320.

10. Chello M, Mastroroberto P, Romano R, et al. Protection of coenzyme Q10 from myocardial reperfusion injury during coronary artery bypass grafting. *The Annals of Thoracic Surgery* 1994;58:1427–1432.

11. Kostner K, Hornykewycz S, Yang P, et al. Is oxidative stress causally linked to unstable angina pectoris? A study in 100 CAD patients and matched controls. *Cardiovascular Research* 1997;36:330–336.

12. Vita JA, Keaney JF Jr, Raby KE, et al. Low plasma ascorbic acid independently predicts the presence of an unstable coronary syndrome. *Journal of the American College of Cardiology* 1998;31:980–986.

13. Watanabe H, Kakihana M, Ohtsuka S, et al. Randomized, double-blind, placebo-controlled study of ascorbate on the preventive effect of nitrate tolerance in patients with congestive heart failure. *Circulation* 1998; 97:886–891.

14. Watanabe H, Kakihana M, Ohtsuka S, et al. Randomized, double-blind, placebo-controlled study of supplemental vitamin E on attenuation of the development of nitrate tolerance. *Circulation* 1997;96:2545–2550.

15. Lagioia R, Scritinio D, Mangini SG, et al. Propionyl-L-carnitine: a new compound in the metabolic approach to the treatment

of effort angina. *International Journal of Cardiology* 1992;34: 167–172.

16. Bartels GL, Remme WJ, Pillay M, et al. Effects of L-propionyl-carnitine on ischemia-induced myocardial dysfunction in men with angina pectoris. *American Journal of Cardiology* 1994;74: 125–130.

17. Cacciatore L, Cerio R, Ciarimboli M, et al. The therapeutic effect of L-carnitine in patients with exercise-induced stable angina. A controlled study. *Drugs Under Experimental and Clinical Research* 1991;17:225–235.

18. Davini P, Bigalli A, Lamanna F. Controlled study on L-carnitine therapeutic efficacy in post-infarction. *Drugs Under Experimental and Clinical Research* 1992;18:355–365.

19. Kamikawa T, Suzuki Y, Kobayashi A, et al. Effects of L-carnitine on exercise tolerance in patients with stable angina pectoris. *Japanese Heart Journal* 1984;25:587–597.

20. Rebuzzi AG, Schiavoni G, Amico CM, et al. Beneficial effects of L-carnitine in the reduction of the necrotic area in acute myocardial infarction. *Drugs Under Experimental and Clinical Research* 1984;10:219–223.

21. Arsenio L, Bodria P, Magnati G, et al. Effectiveness of long-term treatment with pantethine in patients with dyslipidemias. *Clinical Therapeutics* 1986;8: 537–545.

22. Miccoli R, Marchetti P, Sampietro T, et al. Effects of pantethine on lipids and apolipoproteins in hypercholesterolemic diabetic and non-diabetic patients. *Current Therapeutic Research* 1984;36:545–549.

23. Gaddi A, Descovich GC, Noseda G, et al. Controlled evaluation of pantethine, a natural hypolipidemic compound, in patients with different forms of hyperlipoproteinemia. *Atherosclerosis* 1984;50:73–83.

24. Hayashi H, Kobayashi A, Terad H, et al. Effects of pantethine on action potential of canine papillary muscle during hypoxic perfusion. *Japanese Heart Journal* 1985;26:289–296.

25. Folkers K, Yamamura Y, eds. *Biomedical and clinical aspects of coenzyme Q: proceedings of the International Symposium on Coenzyme Q*, vols. 1–4. Amsterdam: Elsevier Scientific, 1977 (vol. 1), 1980 (vol. 2), 1982 (vol. 3), 1984 (vol. 4).

26. Kamikawa T, Kobayashi A, Yamashita T, et al. Effects of coenzyme Q10 on exercise tolerance in chronic stable angina pectoris. *American Journal of Cardiology* 1985;56:247–251.

27. Turlapaty PD, Altura BM. Magnesium deficiency produces spasms of coronary arteries. Relationship to etiology of sudden death ischemic heart disease. *Science* 1980;208:198–200.

28. Altura BM. Ischemic heart disease and magnesium. *Magnesium* 1988;7:57–67.

29. McLean RM. Magnesium and its therapeutic uses: a review. *The American Journal of Medicine* 1994;96:63–76.

30. Purvis JR, Movahed A. Magnesium disorders and cardiovascular disease. *Clinical Cardiology* 1992;15:556–568.

31. Hampton EM, Whang DD, Whang R. Intravenous magnesium therapy in acute myocardial infarction. *The Annals of Pharmacotherapy* 1994;28: 220–226.

32. Teo KK, Yusuf S. Role of magnesium in reducing mortality in acute myocardial infarction: a review of the evidence. *Drugs* 1993;46:347–359.

33. Schecter M, Kaplinsky E, Rabinowitz B. The rationale of magnesium supplementation in acute myocardial infarction: a review of the literature. *Archives of Internal Medicine* 1992;152:2189–2196.

34. Bednarz B, Wolk R, Chamiec T, et al. Effects of oral L-arginine supplementation on exercise-induced QT dispersion and exercise tolerance in stable angina pectoris. *International Journal of Cardiology* 2000 Sep 15; 75(2–3):205–210.

35. Kobayashi N, Nakamura M, Hiramori K. Effects of infusion of L-arginine on exercise-induced myocardial ischemic ST-segment changes and capacity to exercise of patients with stable angina pectoris. *Coronary Artery Disease* 1999 Jul;10(5): 321–326.

36. Ceremuzyński L, Chamiec T, Herbaczyńska-Cedro K. Effect of supplemental oral L-arginine on exercise capacity in patients with stable angina pectoris. *American Journal of Cardiology* 1997 Aug 1;80(3):331–333.

37. Tripathi P, Chandra M, Misra MK. Oral administration of L-arginine in patients with angina or following myocardial infarction may be protective by increasing plasma superoxide dismutase and total thiols with reduction in serum cholesterol and xanthine oxidase. *Oxidative Medicine and Cellular Longevity* 2009 Sep–Oct;2(4):231–237.

38. Schulman SP, Becker LC, Kass DA, et al. L-arginine therapy in acute myocardial infarction: the Vascular Interaction with Age in Myocardial Infarction (VINTAGE MI) randomized clinical trial. *JAMA, The Journal of the American Medical Association* 2006 Jan 4;295(1):58–64.

39. Rigelsky JM, Sweet BV. Hawthorn: pharmacology and therapeutic uses. *American Journal of Health-System Pharmacy* 2002;59:417–422.

40. Walker AF, Marakis G, Morris AP, Robinson PA. Promising hypotensive effect of hawthorn extract: a randomized double-blind pilot study of mild, essential hypertension. *Phytotherapy Research* 2002;16:48–54.

41. Holubarsch CJ, Colucci WS, Meinertz T, et al. The efficacy and safety of *Crataegus* extract

WS 1442 in patients with heart failure: the SPICE trial. *European Journal of Heart Failure* 2008 Dec;10(12):1255–1263.

42. Osher HL, Katz KH, Wagner DJ. Khellin in the treatment of angina pectoris. *The New England Journal of Medicine* 1951; 244:315–321.

43. Anrep GV, Kenawy MR, Barsoum GS. Coronary vasodilator action of khellin. *American Heart Journal* 1949;37:531–542.

44. Conn JJ, Kissane RW, Koons RA, et al. Treatment of angina pectoris with khellin. *Annals of Internal Medicine* 1952;36: 1173–1178.

45. Ballegaard S, Karpatschoff B, Holck JA, et al. Acupuncture in angina pectoris: do psychosocial and neurophysiological factors relate to the effect? *Acupuncture & Electro-Therapeutics Research* 1995;20:101–116.

46. Meng J. The effects of acupuncture in treatment of coronary heart diseases. *Journal of Traditional Chinese Medicine* 2004; 24:16–19.

47. Ballegaard S, Jensen G, Pedersen F, et al. Acupuncture in severe, stable angina pectoris: a randomized trial. *Acta Medica Scandinavica* 1986; 220:307–313.

48. Richter A, Herlitz J, Hjalmarson A. Effect of acupuncture in patients with angina pectoris. *European Heart Journal* 1991; 12:175–178.

49. Gilbert C. Clinical applications of breathing regulation. Beyond anxiety management. *Behavior Modification* 2003;27:692–709.

50. Cunningham C, Brown S, Kaski JC. Effects of transcendental meditation on symptoms and electrocardiographic changes in patients with cardiac syndrome X. *American Journal of Cardiology* 2000;85:653–655,A10.

51. Clarke CN, Clarke NE, Mosher RE. Treatment of angina pectoris with disodium ethylene diamine tetraacetic acid. *The American Journal of the Medical Sciences* 1956;232:654–666.

52. Clarke NE Sr. Atherosclerosis, occlusive vascular disease and EDTA. *American Journal of Cardiology* 1960;6:233–236.

53. Steinberg D, Parthasarathy S, Carew TE, et al. Beyond cholesterol. Modifications of low-density lipoprotein that increase its atherogenicity. *The New England Journal of Medicine* 1989; 320:915–924.

54. Cranton EM, Frackelton JP. Current status of EDTA chelation therapy in occlusive arterial disease. *Journal of Advancement in Medicine* 1989;2:107–119.

55. Olszewer E, Carter JP. EDTA chelation therapy. A retrospective study of 2,870 patients. *Journal of Advancement in Medicine* 1989;2:197–211.

56. Olszewer E, Sabbag FC, Carter JP. A pilot double-blind study of sodium-magnesium EDTA in peripheral vascular disease. *Journal of the National Medical Association* 1990;82:173–177.

57. Olszewer E, Carter JP. EDTA chelation therapy in chronic degenerative disease. *Medical Hypotheses* 1988;27:41–49.

58. Casdorph HR. EDTA chelation therapy, efficacy in arteriosclerotic heart disease. *Journal of Holistic Medicine* 1981;3:53–59.

59. Villarruz MV, Dans A, Tan F. Chelation therapy for atherosclerotic cardiovascular disease. *Cochrane Database of Systematic Reviews* 2002;4:CD002785.

Anxiety

1. M. Werbach. *Nutritional influences on mental illness: a sourcebook of clinical research.* Tarzana, Calif.: Third Line Press, 1991.

2. Bruce M, Lader M. Caffeine abstention in the management of anxiety disorders. *Psychological Medicine* 1989;19: 211–214.

3. Green P, Hermesh H, Monselise A, et al. Red cell membrane omega-3 fatty acids are decreased in nondepressed patients with social anxiety disorder. *European Neuropsychopharmacology* 2006;16:107–113.

4. Buydens-Branchey L, Branchey M, Hibbeln JR. Associations between increases in plasma n-3 polyunsaturated fatty acids following supplementation and decreases in anger and anxiety in substance abusers. *Progress in Neuro-Psychopharmacology and Biological Psychiatry* 2008; 32:568–575.

5. Kiecolt-Glaser JK, Belury MA, Andridge R, et al. Omega-3 supplementation lowers inflammation and anxiety in medical students: a randomized controlled trial. *Brain, Behavior, and Immunity* 2011 Nov;25(8): 1725–1734.

6. Rudin DO. The major psychoses and neuroses as omega-3 essential fatty acid deficiency syndrome: substrate pellagra. *Biological Psychiatry* 1981;16: 837–850.

7. Kinzler E, Kromer J, Lehmann E. Clinical efficacy of a kava extract in patients with anxiety syndrome. Double-blind placebo controlled study over 4 weeks. *Arzneimittelforschung* 1991;41:584–588.

8. Boerner RJ, Sommer H, Berger W, et al. Kava-kava extract LI 150 is as effective as opipramol and buspirone in generalised anxiety disorder—an 8-week randomized, double-blind multi-centre clinical trial in 129 out-patients. *Phytomedicine* 2003;10 suppl 4:38–49.

9. Cagnacci A, Arangino S, Renzi A, et al. Kava-kava administration reduces anxiety in perimenopausal women. *Maturitas* 2003;44:103–109.

10. De Leo V, la Marca A, Morgante G, et al. Evaluation of combining kava extract with hormone replacement therapy in the treatment of postmenopausal anxiety. *Maturitas* 2001;39:185–188.

11. Warnecke G. [Psychosomatic

dysfunctions in the female climacteric. Clinical effectiveness and tolerance of kava extract WS 1490.] *Fortschritte der Medizin* 1991;109:119–122.

12. Herberg KW. Effect of kava-special extract WS 1490 combined with ethyl alcohol on safety-relevant performance parameters. *Blutalkohol* 1993;30:96–105.

13. Munte TF, Heinze HJ, Matzke M, et al. Effects of oxazepam and an extract of kava roots (*Piper methysticum*) on event-related potentials in a word recognition task. *Neuropyschobiology* 1993;27:46–53.

14. Sarris J, Kavanagh DJ, Byrne G, et al. The Kava Anxiety Depression Spectrum Study (KADSS): a randomized, placebo-controlled crossover trial using an aqueous extract of *Piper methysticum*. *Psychopharmacology* 2009 Aug;205(3):399–407.

15. Ernst E. A re-evaluation of kava (*Piper methysticum*). *British Journal of Clinical Pharmacology* 2007 Oct;64(4):415–417.

16. Teschke R, Sarris J, Lebot V. Kava hepatotoxicity solution: a six-point plan for new kava standardization. *Phytomedicine* 2011 Jan 15;18(2–3):96–103.

17. World Health Organization. *Assessments of the risk of hepatotoxicity with kava products*. Geneva, Switzerland, WHO Document Production Services, 2007.

18. Schröder-Bernhardi D, Dietlein G. Compliance with prescription recommendations by physicians in practices. *International Journal of Clinical Pharmacology and Therapeutics* 2001;39:477–479.

19. Escher M, Desmeules J, Giostra E, Mentha G. Hepatitis associated with kava, a herbal remedy for anxiety. *BMJ* 2001;322:139.

20. Teschke R, Genthner A, Wolff A. Kava hepatotoxicity: comparison of aqueous, ethanolic, acetonic kava extracts and kava-herbs mixtures. *Journal of Ethnopharmacology* 2009 Jun 25;123(3):378–384.

21. Mathews JM, Etheridge AS, Black SR. Inhibition of human cytochrome P450 activities by kava extract and kavalactones. *Drug Metabolism and Disposition* 2002;30:1153–1157.

22. Schelosky L, Raffauf C, Jendroska K, et al. Kava and dopamine antagonism [letter]. *Journal of Neurology, Neurosurgery & Psychiatry* 1995;58:639–640.

Asthma

1. Fanta CH. Asthma. *The New England Journal of Medicine* 2009;360(10):1002–1014.

2. Murphy DM, O'Byrne PM. Recent advances in the pathophysiology of asthma. *Chest* 2010 Jun;137(6):1417–1426.

3. Joos L, Carlen Brutsche IE, Laule-Kilian K, et al. Systemic Th1- and Th2-gene signals in atopy and asthma. *Swiss Medical Weekly* 2004;134:159–164.

4. McGeady SJ. Immunocompetence and allergy. *Pediatrics* 2004;113 suppl 4:1107–1113.

5. Yen SS, Morris HG. An imbalance of arachidonic acid metabolism in asthma. *Biochemical and Biophysical Research Communications* 1981;103:774–779.

6. Tan Y, Collins-Williams C. Aspirin-induced asthma in children. *Annals of Allergy, Asthma & Immunology* 1982;48:1–5.

7. Vanderhoek JY, Ekborg SL, Bailey JM. Nonsteroidal anti-inflammatory drugs stimulate 15-lipoxygenase/leukotriene pathway in human polymorphonuclear leukocytes. *Journal of Allergy and Clinical Immunology* 1984;74:412–417.

8. Scanlon RT. Asthma. A panoramic view and a hypothesis. *Annals of Allergy, Asthma & Immunology* 1984;53:203–212.

9. Odent MR, Culpin EE, Kimmel T. Pertussis vaccination and asthma. Is there a link? *JAMA, The Journal of the American Medical Association* 1994;72:592–593.

10. Bergen R, Black S, Shinefield H, et al. Safety of cold-adapted live attenuated influenza vaccine in a large cohort of children and adolescents. *The Pediatric Infectious Disease Journal* 2004;23:138–144.

11. Marra F, Lynb L, Coombes M, et al. Does antibiotic exposure during infancy lead to development of asthma? A systematic review and meta-analysis. *Chest* 2006;129:610–618.

12. Kukkonen K, Kuitunen M, Haahtela T, et al. High intestinal IgA associates with reduced risk of IgE-associated allergic diseases. *Pediatric Allergy and Immunology* 2010 Feb;21(1 part 1):67–73.

13. Hide DW, Matthews S, Matthews L, et al. Effect of allergen avoidance in infancy on allergic manifestations at age two years. *Journal of Allergy and Clinical Immunology* 1994;93:842–846.

14. Romieu I, Werneck G, Ruiz Velasco S, et al. Breastfeeding and asthma among Brazilian children. *Journal of Asthma* 2000;37:575–583.

15. Becker A, Watson W, Ferguson A, et al. The Canadian Asthma Primary Prevention Study: outcomes at 2 years of age. *Journal of Allergy and Clinical Immunology* 2004;113:650–656.

16. Bock, SA. Food-related asthma and basic nutrition. *Journal of Asthma* 1983;20:377–381.

17. Ogle KA, Bullocks JD. Children with allergic rhinitis and/or bronchial asthma treated with elimination diet. A five-year follow-up. *Annals of Allergy, Asthma & Immunology* 1980;44:273.

18. Businco L, Falconieri P, Giampietro P, et al. Food allergy and asthma. *Pediatric Pulmonology* 1995;11 suppl:59–60.

19. Bircher AJ, Van Melle G, Haller E, et al. IgE to food allergens are highly prevalent in patients allergic to pollens, with and without symptoms of food

allergy. *Clinical & Experimental Allergy* 1994;24:367–374.

20. Hodge L, Yan KY, Loblay RL. Assessment of food chemical intolerance in adult asthmatic subjects. *Thorax* 1996;51:805–809.

21. Bray GW. The hypochlorhydria of asthma in childhood. *Quarterly Journal of Medicine* 1931; 24:181–197.

22. Benard A, Desreumeaux P, Huglo D, et al. Increased intestinal permeability in bronchial asthma. *Journal of Allergy and Clinical Immunology* 1996;97: 1173–1178.

23. Akiyama K, Shida T, Yasueda H, et al. Atopic asthma caused by *Candida albicans* acid protease: case reports. *Allergy* 1994;49: 778–781.

24. Freedman BJ. A diet free from additives in the management of allergic disease. *Clinical Allergy* 1977;7:417–421.

25. Stevenson DD, Simon RA. Sensitivity to ingested metabisulfites in asthmatic subjects. *Journal of Allergy and Clinical Immunology* 1981;68:26–32.

26. Papaioannou R, Pfeiffer CC. Sulfite sensitivity—unrecognized threat. Is molybdenum deficiency the cause? *Journal of Orthomolecular Psychiatry* 1984;13:105–110.

27. Carrey OJ, Locke C, Cookson JB. Effect of alterations of dietary sodium on the severity of asthma in men. *Thorax* 1993;48: 714–718.

28. Burney PG. A diet rich in sodium may potentiate asthma. Epidemiologic evidence for a new hypothesis. *Chest* 1987;91: 143–148.

29. Denny SI, Thompson RL, Margetts BM. Dietary factors in the pathogenesis of asthma and chronic obstructive pulmonary disease. *Current Allergy and Asthma Reports* 2003;3:130–136.

30. McKeever TM, Scrivener S, Broadfield E, et al. Prospective study of diet and decline in lung function in a general population. *American Journal of Respiratory and Critical Care Medicine* 2002;165:1299–1303.

31. Tabak C, Smit HA, Heederik D, et al. Diet and chronic obstructive pulmonary disease: independent beneficial effects of fruits, whole grains, and alcohol (the MORGEN study). *Clinical & Experimental Allergy* 2001; 31:747–755.

32. Romieu I, Trenga C. Diet and obstructive lung diseases. *Epidemiologic Reviews* 2001;23: 268–287.

33. Kelly Y, Sacker A, Marmot M. Nutrition and respiratory health in adults: findings from the health survey for Scotland. *European Respiratory Journal* 2003;21:664–671.

34. Shaheen SO, Sterne JA, Thompson RL, et al. Dietary antioxidants and asthma in adults: population-based case-control study. *American Journal of Respiratory and Critical Care Medicine* 2001;164:1823–1828.

35. Smith LJ, Holbrook JT, Wise R, et al. Dietary intake of soy genistein is associated with lung function in patients with asthma. *Journal of Asthma* 2004;41(8):833–843.

36. Kalhan R, Smith LJ, Nlend MC, et al. A mechanism of benefit of soy genistein in asthma: inhibition of eosinophil p38-dependent leukotriene synthesis. *Clinical & Experimental Allergy* 2008 Jan;38(1):103–112.

37. Liu XJ, Zhao J, Gu XY. The effects of genistein and puerarin on the activation of nuclear factor-kappaB and the production of tumor necrosis factor-alpha in asthma patients. *Pharmazie* 2010 Feb;65(2):127–131.

38. Lindahl O, Lindwall L, Spangberg A, et al. Vegan diet regimen with reduced medication in the treatment of bronchial asthma. *Journal of Asthma* 1985;22:45–55.

39. Hodge L, Salome CM, Peat JK, et al. Consumption of oily fish and childhood asthma risk. *The Medical Journal of Australia* 1996;164:137–140.

40. Arm JP, Horton CE, Spur BW, et al. The effects of dietary supplementation with fish oil lipids on the airway response to inhaled allergen in bronchial asthma. *American Review of Respiratory Disease* 1989;139: 1395–1400.

41. Dry J, Vincent D. Effect of a fish oil diet on asthma. Results of a 1-year double-blind study. *International Archives of Allergy & Applied Immunology* 1991;95:156–157.

42. Broughton KS, Johnson CS, Pace BK, et al. Reduced asthma symptoms with n-3 fatty acid ingestion are related to 5-series leukotriene production. *The American Journal of Clinical Nutrition* 1997;65:1011–1017.

43. Unge G, Grubbström J, Olsson P, et al. Effects of dietary tryptophan restrictions on clinical symptoms in patients with endogenous asthma. *Allergy* 1983;38:211–212.

44. Reynolds RD, Natta CL. Depressed plasma pyridoxal phosphate concentrations in adult asthmatics. *The American Journal of Clinical Nutrition* 1985; 41:684–688.

45. Collipp PJ, Goldzier S III, Weiss N, et al. Pyridoxine treatment of childhood asthma. *Annals of Allergy, Asthma & Immunology* 1975;35:93–97.

46. Sur S, Camara M, Buchmeier A, et al. Double-blind trial of pyridoxine (vitamin B6) in the treatment of steroid-dependent asthma. *Annals of Allergy, Asthma & Immunology* 1993; 70:147–152.

47. Shimizu T, Maeda S, Mochizuki H, et al. Theophylline attenuates circulating vitamin B6 levels in children with asthma. *Pharmacology* 1994;49: 392–397.

48. Bartel PR, Ubbink JB, Delport R, et al. Vitamin B6 supplementation and theophyl-

line-related effects in humans. *The American Journal of Clinical Nutrition* 1994;60:93–99.

49. Seaton A, Godden DJ, Brown K. Increase in asthma: a more toxic environment or a more susceptible population. *Thorax* 1994; 49:171–174.

50. Katsoulis K, Kontakiotis T, Leonardopoulos I, et al. Serum total antioxidant status in severe exacerbation of asthma: correlation with the severity of the disease. *Journal of Asthma* 2003; 40:847–854.

51. Romieu I, Sienra-Monge JJ, Ramírez-Aguilar M, et al. Antioxidant supplementation and lung functions among children with asthma exposed to high levels of air pollutants. *American Journal of Respiratory and Critical Care Medicine* 2002; 166:703–709.

52. Hatch GE. Asthma, inhaled oxidants, and dietary antioxidants. *The American Journal of Clinical Nutrition* 1995;61: 625S–630S.

53. Ford ES, Mannino DM, Redd SC. Serum antioxidant concentrations among U.S. adults with self-reported asthma. *Journal of Asthma* 2004;41:179–187.

54. Bielory L, Gandhi R. Asthma and vitamin C. *Annals of Allergy, Asthma & Immunology* 1994;73:89–96.

55. Johnston CS, Martin LJ, Cai X. Antihistamine effect of supplemental ascorbic acid and neutrophil chemotaxis. *Journal of the American College of Nutrition* 1992;11:172–176.

56. Tecklenburg SL, Mickleborough TD, Fly AD, et al. Ascorbic acid supplementation attenuates exercise-induced bronchoconstriction in patients with asthma. *Respiratory Medicine* 2007 Aug;101(8):1770–1778.

57. Hope WC, Welton AF, Fiedler-Nagy C, et al. In vitro inhibition of the biosynthesis of slow reacting substance of anaphylaxis (SRS-A) and lipoxygenase activity by quercetin. *Biochemical Pharmacology* 1983;32:367–371.

58. Middleton E Jr, Drzewiecki G, Krishnarao D. Quercetin. An inhibitor of antigen-induced human basophil histamine release. *The Journal of Immunology* 1981;127:546–550.

59. Foreman JC. Mast cells and the actions of flavonoids. *Journal of Allergy and Clinical Immunology* 1984;73:769–774.

60. Loke WM, Proudfoot JM, Stewart S, et al. Metabolic transformation has a profound effect on anti-inflammatory activity of flavonoids such as quercetin: lack of association between antioxidant and lipoxygenase inhibitory activity. *Biochemical Pharmacology* 2008 Mar 1; 75(5):1045–53..

61. Lau BH, Riesen SK, Truong KP, et al. Pycnogenol as an adjunct in the management of childhood asthma. *Journal of Asthma* 2004;41(8):825–832.

62. Watson RR, Zibadi S, Rafatpanah H, et al. Oral administration of the purple passion fruit peel extract reduces wheeze and cough and improves shortness of breath in adults with asthma. *Nutrition Research* 2008 Mar; 28(3):166–171.

63. Grosch W, Laskawy G. Co-oxidation of carotenes requires one soybean lipoxygenase isoenzyme. *Biochimica et Biophysica Acta* 1979;575: 439–445.

64. Wood LG, Gibson PG. Reduced circulating antioxidant defences are associated with airway hyper-responsiveness, poor control and severe disease pattern in asthma. *British Journal of Nutrition* 2010 Mar;103(5):735–741.

65. Riccioni G, Bucciarelli T, Mancini B, et al. Plasma lycopene and antioxidant vitamins in asthma: the PLAVA study. *Journal of Asthma* 2007 Jul–Aug; 44(6):429–432.

66. Hazlewood LC, Wood LG, Hansbro PM, Foster PS. Dietary lycopene supplementation suppresses Th2 responses and lung eosinophilia in a mouse model of allergic asthma. *The Journal of Nutritional Biochemistry* 2011 Jan;22(1):95–100.

67. Wood LG, Garg ML, Powell H, Gibson PG. Lycopene-rich treatments modify noneosinophilic airway inflammation in asthma: proof of concept. *Free Radical Research* 2008 Jan;42(1):94–102.

68. Falk B, Gorev R, Zigel L, et al. Effect of lycopene supplementation on lung function after exercise in young athletes who complain of exercise-induced bronchoconstriction symptoms. *Annals of Allergy, Asthma & Immunology* 2005 Apr;94(4): 480–485.

69. Neuman I, Nahum H, Ben-Amotz A. Reduction of exercise-induced asthma oxidative stress by lycopene, a natural antioxidant. *Allergy* 2000 Dec;55(12): 1184–1189.

70. Misso NL, Powers KA, Gillon RL, et al. Reduced platelet glutathione peroxidase activity and serum selenium concentration in atopic asthmatic patients. *Clinical & Experimental Allergy* 1996;26:838–847.

71. Stone J, Hinks LJ, Beasley R, et al. Reduced selenium status of patients with asthma. *Clinical Science* 1989;77:495–500.

72. Kadrabova J, Mad'aric A, Kovacikova Z, et al. Selenium status is decreased in patients with intrinsic asthma. *Biological Trace Element Research* 1996; 52:241–248.

73. Wright JV. Treatment of childhood asthma with parenteral vitamin B12, gastric re-acidification, and attention to food allergy, magnesium, and pyridoxine: three case reports with background and an integrated hypothesis. *Journal of Nutritional and Environmental Medicine* 1990;1:277–282.

74. Simon SW. Vitamin B12 therapy in allergy and chronic dermatoses. *Journal of Allergy* 1951;2: 183–185.

75. Trendelenburg P. Physiologische und pharmakologische untersuchungen an der isolierten bronchial muskulatur. *Archives of Experimental Pharmacology and Therapy* 1912;69:79.

76. Haury VG. Blood serum magnesium in bronchial asthma and its treatment by the administration of magnesium sulfate. *Journal of Laboratory and Clinical Medicine* 1940;26:340–344.

77. Skobeloff EM, Spivey WH, McNamara RM, et al. Intravenous magnesium sulfate for the treatment of acute asthma in the emergency department. *JAMA, The Journal of the American Medical Association* 1989;262: 1210–1213.

78. Okayama H, Aikawa T, Okayama M, et al. Bronchodilating effect of intravenous magnesium sulfate in bronchial asthma. *JAMA, The Journal of the American Medical Association* 1987;257:1076–1078.

79. Noppeen M, Vanmaele L, Impens N, et al. Bronchodilating effect of intravenous magnesium sulfate in acute severe bronchial asthma. *Chest* 1990; 97:373–376.

80. Skorodin MS, Tenholder MF, Yetter B, et al. Magnesium sulfate in exacerbations of chronic obstructive pulmonary disease. *Archives of Internal Medicine* 1995;155:496–500.

81. McLean RM. Magnesium and its therapeutic uses: a review. *The American Journal of Medicine* 1994;96:63–76.

82. Gullestad L, Oystein Dolva L, Birkeland K, et al. Oral versus intravenous magnesium supplementation in patients with magnesium deficiency. *Magnesium and Trace Elements* 1991–92; 10:11–16.

83. Oladipo OO, Chukwu CC, Ajala MO, et al. Plasma magnesium in adult asthmatics at the Lagos University Teaching Hospital, Nigeria. *East African Medical Journal* 2003;80:488–491.

84. Britton J, Pavord I, Richards K, et al. Dietary magnesium, lung function, wheezing, and airway hyper-reactivity in a random adult population sample. *The Lancet* 1994;344:357–362.

85. Gontijo-Amaral C, Ribeiro MA, Gontijo LS, et al. Oral magnesium supplementation in asthmatic children: a double-blind randomized placebo-controlled trial. *European Journal of Clinical Nutrition* 2007 Jan;61(1): 54–60.

86. Bede O, Nagy D, Surányi A, et al. Effects of magnesium supplementation on the glutathione redox system in atopic asthmatic children. *Inflammation Research* 2008 Jun;57(6):279–286.

87. Kazaks AG, Uriu-Adams JY, Albertson TE, et al. Effect of oral magnesium supplementation on measures of airway resistance and subjective assessment of asthma control and quality of life in men and women with mild to moderate asthma: a randomized placebo controlled trial. *Journal of Asthma* 2010 Feb;47(1):83–92.

88. Hughes R, Goldkorn A, Masoli M, et al. Use of isotonic nebulised magnesium sulphate as an adjuvant to salbutamol in treatment of severe asthma in adults: randomised placebo-controlled trial. *The Lancet* 2003;361:2114–2117.

89. Mak G, Hanania NA. Vitamin D and asthma. *Current Opinion in Pulmonary Medicine* 2011 Jan;17(1):1–5.

90. Brehm JM, Schuemann B, Fuhlbrigge AL, et al. Serum vitamin D levels and severe asthma exacerbations in the Childhood Asthma Management Program study. *Journal of Allergy and Clinical Immunology* 2010 Jul;126(1):52–58.

91. Urashima M, Segawa T, Okazaki M, et al. Randomized trial of vitamin D supplementation to prevent seasonal influenza A in schoolchildren. *The American Journal of Clinical Nutrition* 2010 May;91(5):1255–60.

92. Blanc PD, Kuschner WG, Katz PP, et al. Use of herbal products, coffee or black tea, and over-the-counter medications as self-treatments among adults with asthma. *Journal of Allergy and Clinical Immunology* 1997;100: 789–791.

93. American Pharmaceutical Association. *Handbook of nonprescription drugs*, 8th ed. Washington, D.C.: American Pharmaceutical Association, 1986.

94. Sieben A, Prenner L, Sorkalla T, et al. Alpha-hederin, but not hederacoside C and hederagenin from *Hedera helix*, affects the binding behavior, dynamics, and regulation of beta 2-adrenergic receptors. *Biochemistry* 2009 Apr 21;48(15): 3477–3482.

95. Hofmann D, Hecker M, Völp A. Efficacy of dry extract of ivy leaves in children with bronchial asthma—a review of randomized controlled trials. *Phytomedicine* 2003 Mar; 10(2–3):213–220.

96. Okimasu E, Moromizato Y, Watanabe S, et al. Inhibition of phospholipase A2 and platelet aggregation by glycyrrhizin, an anti-inflammatory drug. *Acta Medica Okayama* 1983;37:385–391.

97. Lundberg JM, Saria A. Capsaicin-induced desensitization of airway mucosa to cigarette smoke, mechanical and chemical irritants. *Nature* 1983;302: 251–253.

98. Payan DG, Levine JD, Goetzl EJ. Modulation of immunity and hypersensitivity by sensory neuropeptides. *The Journal of Immunology* 1984;132:1601–1604.

99. Cyong J, Otsuka Y. A pharmacological study of the anti-inflammatory activity of Chinese herbs. *Acupuncture & Electro-Therapeutics Research* 1982;7: 173–202.

100. Hanabusa K, Cyong J, Takahashi M. High-level of cyclic AMP in jujube plum. *Planta Medica* 1981;42:380–384.

101. Udupa AL, Udupa SL, Guruswamy MN. The possible site of anti-asthmatic action of *Tylophora asthmatica* on pituitary-adrenal axis in albino rats. *Planta Medica* 1991;57:409–413.

102. Gopalkrishnan C, Shankaranarayanan D, Nazimudeen SK, et al. Effect of tylophorine, a major alkaloid of *Tylophora indica,* on immunopathological and inflammatory reactions. *Indian Journal of Medical Research* 1980;71:940–948.

103. Gupta S, George P, Gupta V, et al. *Tylophora indica* in bronchial asthma—a double blind study. *Indian Journal of Medical Research* 1979;69:981–989.

104. Thiruvengadam KV, Haranath K, Sudarsan S, et al. *Tylophora indica* in bronchial asthma (a controlled comparison with a standard anti-asthmatic drug). *Journal of Indian Medical Association* 1978;71:172–176.

105. Shivpuri DN, Singhal SC, Prakash D. Treatment of asthma with an alcoholic extract of *Tylophora indica:* a cross-over, double-blind study. *Annals of Allergy, Asthma & Immunology* 1972;30:407–412.

106. Shivpuri DN, Menon MP, Prakash D. A crossover double-blind study on *Tylophora indica* in the treatment of asthma and allergic rhinitis. *Journal of Allergy* 1969;43:145–150.

107. Wilkens JH, Wilkens H, Uffmann J, et al. Effects of a PAF-antagonist (BN 52063) on bronchoconstriction and platelet activation during exercise induced asthma. *British Journal of Clinical Pharmacology* 1990; 29:85–91.

108. Guinot P, Brambilla C, Duchier J, et al. Effect of BN 52063, a specific PAF-acether antagonist, on bronchial provocation test to allergens in asthmatic patients: a preliminary study. *Prostaglandins* 1987;34:723–731.

109. Shida T, Tagi A, Nishimura H, et al. Effect of aloe extract on peripheral phagocytosis in adult bronchial asthma. *Planta Medica* 1985;51:273–275.

110. Lichey J, Friedrich T, Priesnitz M, et al. Effect of forskolin on methacholine-induced bronchoconstriction in extrinsic asthmatics. *The Lancet* 1984;2:167.

111. Bauer K, Dietersdorfer F, Sertl K, et al. Pharmacodynamic effects of inhaled dry powder formulations of fenoterol and colforsin in asthma. *Clinical Pharmacology & Therapeutics* 1993;53:76–83.

112. Wildfeuer A, Neu IS, Safayhi H, et al. Effects of boswellic acids extracted from a herbal medicine on the biosynthesis of leukotrienes and the course of experimental autoimmune encephalomyelitis. *Arzneimittelforschung* 1998;48:668–674.

113. Maa SH, Sun MF, Hsu KH, et al. Effect of acupuncture or acupressure on quality of life of patients with chronic obstructive asthma: a pilot study. *The Journal of Alternative and Complementary Medicine* 2003;9:659–670.

114. Wu HS, Wu SC, Lin JG, et al. Effectiveness of acupressure in improving dyspnoea in chronic obstructive pulmonary disease. *Journal of Advanced Nursing* 2004;45:252–259.

Attention Deficit/ Hyperactivity Disorder

1. Centers for Disease Control and Prevention (CDC). Increasing prevalence of parent-reported attention-deficit/hyperactivity disorder among children— United States, 2003 and 2007. *Morbidity and Mortality Weekly Report* 2010 Nov 12;59(44): 1439–1443.

2. Khan SA, Faraone SV. The genetics of attention-deficit/hyperactivity disorder: a literature review of 2005. *Current Psychiatry Reports* 2006 Oct;8: 393–397.

3. Wigal SB. Efficacy and safety limitations of attention-deficit hyperactivity disorder pharmacotherapy in children and adults. *CNS Drugs* 2009;23 suppl 1:21–31.

4. Berman S, Kuczenski R, McCracken J, London E. Potential adverse effects of amphetamine treatment on brain and behavior: a review. *Molecular Psychiatry* 2009 Feb;14(2):123–142.

5. Advokat C. Update on amphetamine neurotoxicity and its relevance to the treatment of ADHD. *Journal of Attention Disorders* 2007 Jul;11(1):8–16.

6. Bangs ME, Tauscher-Wisniewski S, Polzer J, et al. Meta-analysis of suicide-related behavior events in patients treated with atomoxetine. *Journal of the American Academy of Child and Adolescent Psychiatry* 2008 Feb;47(2):209–218.

7. Xu X, Nembhard W, Kan H, et al. Urinary trichlorophenol levels and increased risk of attention deficit hyperactivity disorder among US school-aged children. *Occupational and Environmental Medicine* August 2011;68(8):557–561.

8. Eubig PA, Aguiar A, Schantz SL. Lead and PCBs as risk factors for attention deficit/hyperactivity disorder. *Environmental Health Perspectives* 2010 Dec;118(12):1654–1667.

9. Milberger S, Biederman J, Faraone S, et al. Further evidence of an association between attention-deficit/hyperactivity disorder and cigarette smoking: findings from a high-risk sample of siblings. *American Journal on Addictions* 1997;6:205–217.

10. Wiliams G, O'Callaghan M, Najman J, et al. Maternal cigarette smoking and child psychiatric morbidity: a longitudinal study. *Pediatrics* 1998;102(1):e11.

11. Froehlich T, Lanphear B, Kahn R, et al. Association of tobacco and lead exposures with attention-deficit/hyperactivity disorder. *Pediatrics* 2009 Dec; 124(6):e1054–e1063.

12. Centers for Disease Control and

Prevention. Preventing Lead Poisoning in Young Children. www.cdc.gov/nceh/lead/publications/prevleadpoisoning.pdf.

13. Brockel B, Cory SD. Lead, attention, and impulsive behavior: changes in a fixed-ratio waiting-for-reward paradigm. *Pharmacology Biochemistry and Behavior* 1998;60:545–552.

14. David O, Hoffman S, Sverd J, et al. Lead and hyperactivity. Behavioral response to chelation: a pilot study. *The American Journal of Psychiatry* 1976;133:1155–1158.

15. Kenney J, Groth E, Benbrook C. *Worst first: high risk insecticide uses, children's foods and safer alternatives*. Washington, D.C.: Consumers Union of the United States, 1999.

16. Bouchard MF, Bellinger DC, Wright RO, Weisskopf MG. Attention-deficit/hyperactivity disorder and urinary metabolites of organophosphate pesticides. *Pediatrics* 2010;125: e1270–1277.

17. Curl CL, Fenske RA, Elgethun K. Organophosphorus pesticide exposure of urban and suburban preschool children with organic and conventional diets. *Environmental Health Perspectives* 2003;111:377–382.

18. Feingold B. *Why your child is hyperactive*. New York: Random House, 1975.

19. Rippere V. Food additives and hyperactive children: a critique of Conners. *British Journal of Clinical Psychology* 1983;22:19–32.

20. Rimland B. The Feingold diet: an assessment of the reviews by Mattes, by Kavale and Forness and others. *Journal of Learning Disabilities* 1983;16:331–333.

21. McCann D, Barrett A, Cooper A, et al. Food additives and hyperactive behaviour in 3-year-old and 8/9-year-old children in the community: a randomised, double-blinded, placebo-controlled trial. *The Lancet* 2007 Nov 3;370(9598):1560–1567.

22. Prinz R, Roberts W, Hantman E. Dietary correlates of hyperactive behavior in children. *Journal of Consulting and Clinical Psychology* 1980;48:760–769.

23. Langseth L, Dowd J. Glucose tolerance and hyperkinesis. *Food and Cosmetics Toxicology* 1978;16:129–133.

24. Bloch M, Qawasmi A. Omega-3 fatty acid supplementation for the treatment of children with attention-deficit/hyperactivity disorder symptomatology: systematic review and meta-analysis. *Journal of the American Academy of Child and Adolescent Psychiatry* 2011 Oct; 50(10):991–1000.

25. Transler C, Eilander A, Mitchell S, van de Meer N. The impact of polyunsaturated fatty acids in reducing child attention deficit and hyperactivity disorders. *Journal of Attention Disorders* 2010 Nov;14(3):232–246.

26. Hussain S, Roots B. Effect of essential fatty acid deficiency and immunopathological stresses on blood brain barrier (B-BB) in Lewis rats: a biochemical study. *Biochemical Society Transactions* 1994;3:338.

27. Uauy R, De Andraca I. Human milk and breast feeding for optimal mental development. *Journal of Nutrition* 1995;125: 2278S–2280S.

28. Sinn N. Nutritional and dietary influences on attention deficit hyperactivity disorder. *Nutrition Reviews* 2008 Oct;66(10): 558–568.

29. Schnoll R, Burshteyn D, Cea-Aravena J. Nutrition in the treatment of attention-deficit hyperactivity disorder: a neglected but important aspect. *Applied Psychophysiology and Biofeedback* 2003;28:63–75.

30. Kozielec T, Starobrat HB. Assessment of magnesium levels in children with attention deficit hyperactivity disorder (ADHD). *Magnesium Research* 1997;10: 143–148.

31. Starobrat HB, Kozielec T. The effects of magnesium physiological supplementation on hyperactivity in children with attention deficit hyperactivity disorder (ADHD). Positive response to magnesium oral loading test. *Magnesium Research* 1997;10:149–156.

32. Arnold L, Votolato N, Kleykamp D, et al. Does hair zinc predict amphetamine improvement of ADD/hyperactivity? *International Journal of Neuroscience* 1990;50:103–107.

33. Bekaroglu M, Aslan Y, Gedik Y, et al. Relationships between serum free fatty acids and zinc, and attention deficit hyperactivity disorder: a research note. *The Journal of Child Psychology and Psychiatry* 1996;37:225–227.

34. Bilici M, Yildirim F, Kandil S, et al. Double-blind, placebo-controlled study of zinc sulfate in the treatment of attention deficit hyperactivity disorder. *Progress in Neuro-Psychopharmacology and Biological Psychiatry* 2004;28:181–190.

35. Arnold LE, DiSilvestro RA. Zinc in attention-deficit/hyperactivity disorder. *Journal of Child and Adolescent Psychopharmacology* 2005;15:619–627.

36. Konofal E, Lecendreux M, Arnulf I, Mouren M. Iron deficiency in children with attention-deficit/hyperactivity disorder. *Archives of Pediatrics and Adolescent Medicine* 2004 Dec;158(12):1113–1115.

37. Sever Y, Ashkenazi A, Tyano S, Weizman A. Iron treatment in children with attention deficit hyperactivity disorder. A preliminary report. *Neuropsychobiology* 1997;35:178–180.

38. Konofal E, Lecendreux M, Arnulf I, et al. Effects of iron supplementation on attention deficit hyperactivity disorder in children. *Pediatric Neurology* 2008 Jan;38(1):20–26.

39. Pelsser L, Buitelaar J, Savelkoul H. ADHD as a (non) allergic hypersensitivity disorder: a hypothesis. *Pediatric Allergy and*

Immunology 2009 Mar;20(2): 107–112.

40. Tryphonas H, Trites R. Food allergy in children with hyperactivity, learning disabilities and/or minimal brain dysfunction. *Annals of Allergy, Asthma & Immunology* 1979;42:22–27.

41. Carter C, Urbanowicz M, Hemsley R, et al. Effects of a few food diet in attention deficit disorder. *Archives of Disease in Childhood* 1993;69:564–568.

42. Boris M. Foods and food additives are common causes of the attention deficit hyperactivity disorder in children. *Annals of Allergy, Asthma & Immunology* 1994;72:462–468.

43. Uhlig T, Merkenschlager A, Brandmaier R, Egger J. Topographic mapping of brain electrical activity in children with food-induced attention deficit hyperkinetic disorder. *European Journal of Pediatrics* 1997; 156:557–561.

44. Nsouli T, Nsouli S, Linde R, et al. Role of food allergy in serous otitis media. *Annals of Allergy, Asthma & Immunology* 1994; 73:215–219.

45. Hagerman RJ, Falkenstein MA. An association between recurrent otitis media in infancy and later hyperactivity. *Clinical Pediatrics* 1987;26:253–257.

46. Marcotte A, Thacher P, Butters M, et al. Parental report of sleep problems in children with attentional and learning disorders. *Journal of Developmental & Behavioral Pediatrics* 1998; 19:178–186.

47. McColley S, Carroll J, Curtis S, et al. High prevalence of allergic sensitization in children with habitual snoring and obstructive sleep apnea. *Chest* 1997;111: 170–173.

48. Kaplan B, McNicol J, Conte R, Moghadam H. Sleep disturbance in preschool-aged hyperactive and nonhyperactive children. *Pediatrics* 1987;80: 839–844.

49. Kaplan BJ. Dietary replacement in preschool-aged hyperactive boys. *Pediatrics* 1989;83:7–17.

50. Egger J, Carter C, Graham P, et al. Controlled trial of oligoantigenic treatment in the hyperkinetic syndrome. *The Lancet* 1985;1:540–545.

51. Schulte-Körne G, Deimel W, Gutenbrunner C, et al. [Effect of an oligo-antigen diet on the behavior of hyperkinetic children.] *Zeitschrift für Kinder-und Jugendpsychiatrie und Psychotherapie* 1996;3:176–183.

52. Egger J, Stolla A, McEwen L. Controlled trial of hyposensitisation in children with food-induced hyperkinetic syndrome. *The Lancet* 1992;339:1150–1153.

53. Salminen S, Isolauri E, Salminen E. Clinical uses of probiotics for stabilizing the gut mucosal barrier: successful strains and future challenges. *Antonie Van Leeuwenhoek* 1996;70:347–358.

54. Majamaa H, Isolauri E. Probiotics: a novel approach in the management of food allergy. *Journal of Allergy and Clinical Immunology* 1997;99:179–185.

55. Dvoráková M, Sivonová M, Trebatická J, et al. The effect of polyphenolic extract from pine bark, pycnogenol on the level of glutathione in children suffering from attention deficit hyperactivity disorder (ADHD). *Redox Report* 2006;11(4):163–172.

56. Chovanová Z, Muchová J, Sivonová M, et al. Effect of polyphenolic extract, pycnogenol, on the level of 8-oxoguanine in children suffering from attention deficit/hyperactivity disorder. *Free Radical Research* 2006 Sep;40(9):1003–1010.

57. Dvoráková M, Jezová D, Blazícek P, et al. Urinary catecholamines in children with attention deficit hyperactivity disorder (ADHD): modulation by a polyphenolic extract from pine bark (pycnogenol). *Nutritional Neuroscience* 2007 Jun–Aug;10(3–4):151–157.

58. Trebatická J, Kopasová S, Hradecná Z, et al. Treatment of ADHD with French maritime pine bark extract, pycnogenol. *European Child & Adolescent Psychiatry* 2006 Sep;15(6):329–335.

59. Lyon MR, Cline JC, Totosy de Zepetnek J, et al. Effect of the herbal extract combination *Panax quinquefolium* and *Ginkgo biloba* on attention-deficit hyperactivity disorder: a pilot study. *Journal of Psychiatry & Neuroscience* 2001;26: 221–228.

60. Niederhofer H. *Ginkgo biloba* treating patients with attention-deficit disorder. *Phytotherapy Research* 2010 Jan;24(1):26–27.

61. Lyon M, Kapoor MP, Juneja LR. The effects of L-theanine (Suntheanine®) in boys with attention deficit hyperactivity disorder (ADHD): a randomized, double-blind, placebo-controlled clinical trial. *Alternative Medicine Review* 2011;16(4);348–354.

62. Gevensleben H, Holl B, Heinrich H, et al. Neurofeedback training in children with ADHD: 6-month follow-up of a randomised controlled trial. *European Child & Adolescent Psychiatry* 2010 Sep;19(9):715–724.

63. Bakhshayesh A, Hansch S, Wyschkon A, Rezai M, Esser G. Neurofeedback in ADHD: a single-blind randomized controlled trial. *European Child & Adolescent Psychiatry* 2011 Sep;20(9):481–491.

64. Monastra VJ, Monastra DM, George S. The effects of stimulant therapy, EEG biofeedback, and parenting style on the primary symptoms of attention-deficit/hyperactivity disorder. *Applied Psychophysiology and Biofeedback* 2002;27:231–249.

65. Fuchs T, Birbaumer N, Lutzenberger W, et al. Neurofeedback treatment for attention-deficit/hyperactivity disorder in children: a comparison with methylphenidate. *Applied Psychophysiology and Biofeedback* 2003;28:1–12.

Autism Spectrum Disorder

1. Elder JH. The gluten-free, casein-free diet in autism: an overview with clinical implications. *Nutrition in Clinical Practice* 2008 Dec–2009 Jan; 23(6):583–588.

2. Millward C, Ferriter M, Calver S, Connell-Jones G. Gluten- and casein-free diets for autistic spectrum disorder. Cochrane Database of Systematic Reviews 2008 Apr 16;2:CD003498.

3. Elder JH, Shankar M, Shuster J, et al. The gluten-free, casein-free diet in autism: results of a preliminary double blind clinical trial. *Journal of Autism and Developmental Disorders* 2006 Apr;36(3):413–420.

4. Reichelt KL, Knivsberg AM. The possibility and probability of a gut-to-brain connection in autism. *Annals of Clinical Psychiatry* 2009 Oct–Dec;21(4): 205–211.

5. de Magistris L, Familiari V, Pascotto A, et al. Alterations of the intestinal barrier in patients with autism spectrum disorders and in their first-degree relatives. *Journal of Pediatric Gastroenterology and Nutrition* 2010 Oct;51(4):418–24.

6. Bent S, Bertoglio K, Hendren RL. Omega-3 fatty acids for autistic spectrum disorder: a systematic review. *Journal of Autism and Developmental Disorders* 2009;39(8):1135–1154.

7. Amminger GP, Berger GE, Schäfer MR, et al. Omega-3 fatty acids supplementation in children with autism: a double-blind randomized, placebo-controlled pilot study. *Biological Psychiatry* 2007 Feb 15;61(4): 551–553.

8. Bent S, Bertoglio K, Ashwood P, et al. A pilot randomized controlled trial of omega-3 fatty acids for autism spectrum disorder. *Journal of Autism and Developmental Disorders* 2011 May;41(5):545–554.

9. Politi P, Cena H, Comelli M, et al. Behavioral effects of omega-3 fatty acid supplementation in young adults with severe autism: an open label study. *Archives of Medical Research* 2008 Oct;39(7):682–685.

10. Rimland B, Callaway E, Dreyfuss P. The effects of high doses of vitamin B6 on autistic children: a double-blind crossover study. *The American Journal of Psychiatry* 1979;135:472–475.

11. Lelord G, Callaway E, Muh J. Clinical and biological effects of high doses of vitamin B6 and magnesium on autistic children. *Acta Vitaminologica et Enzymologica* 1982;4:27–44.

12. Barthelemy C, Garreau B, Ernouf D, et al. Behavioral and biochemical effects of oral magnesium, vitamin B6 and magnesium. Vitamin B6 administration in autistic children. *Magnesium Bulletin* 1981;3: 23–24.

13. Martineau J, Barthelemy C, Garreau B, Lelord G. Vitamin B6, magnesium, and combined B6-Mg: therapeutic effects in childhood autism. *Biological Psychiatry* 1985 May;20(5): 467–478.

14. Murza KA, Pavelko SL, Malani MD, Nye C. Vitamin B6–magnesium treatment for autism: the current status of the research. *Magnesium Research* 2010 Jun;23(2):115–117.

15. Frye RE, Huffman LC, Elliott GR. Tetrahydrobiopterin as a novel therapeutic intervention for autism. *Neurotherapeutics* 2010 Jul;7(3):241–249.

16. Doyen C, Mighiu D, Kaye K, et al. Melatonin in children with autistic spectrum disorders: recent and practical data. *European Child & Adolescent Psychiatry* 2011 May;20(5):231–239.

17. Rossignol DA, Frye RE. Melatonin in autism spectrum disorders: a systematic review and meta-analysis. *Developmental Medicine & Child Neurology* 2011 Sep;53(9):783–792.

18. Wright B, Sims D, Smart S, et al. Melatonin versus placebo in children with autism spectrum conditions and severe sleep problems not amenable to behaviour management strategies: a randomised controlled crossover trial. *Journal of Autism and Developmental Disorders* 2011 Feb;41(2):175–184.

19. Wirojanan J, Jacquemont S, Diaz R, et al. The efficacy of melatonin for sleep problems in children with autism, fragile X syndrome, or autism and fragile X syndrome. *Journal of Clinical Sleep Medicine* 2009 Apr 15; 5(2):145–150.

20. Garstang J, Wallis M. Randomized controlled trial of melatonin for children with autistic spectrum disorders and sleep problems. *Child: Care, Health and Development* 2006 Sep; 32(5):585–589.

21. Andersen IM, Kaczmarska J, McGrew SG, Malow BA. Melatonin for insomnia in children with autism spectrum disorders. *Journal of Child Neurology* 2008 May;23(5):482–485.

22. Chez MG, Buchanan CP, Aimonovitch MC, et al. Double-blind, placebo-controlled study of L-carnosine supplementation in children with autistic spectrum disorders. *Journal of Child Neurology* 2002;17:833–837.

23. Horvath K, Stefanatos G, Sokolski K, et al. Improved social and language skills after secretin administration in patients with autistic spectrum disorders. *Journal of the Association for Academic Minority Physicians* 1998;9:9–15.

24. Levy SE, Hyman SL. Novel treatments for autistic spectrum disorders. *Mental Retardation and Developmental Disabilities Research Reviews* 2005;11: 131–142.

25. Williams KW, Wray JJ, Wheeler DM. Intravenous secretin for autism spectrum disorder. Cochrane Database of Systematic Reviews 2005 Mar 24;3: CD003495.

Boils

1. Altman PM. Australian tea tree oil. *Australian Journal of Pharmacy* 1988;69:276–278.
2. Feinblatt HM. Cajeput-type oil for the treatment of furunculosis. *Journal of the National Medical Association* 1960;52:32–34.
3. Hahn FE, Ciak J. Berberine. *Antibiotics* 1976;3:577–588.
4. Johnson CC, Johnson G, Poe CF. Toxicity of alkaloids to certain bacteria. *Acta Pharmacologica et Toxicologica* 1952;8:71–78.

Breast Cancer (Prevention)

1. Miller AB, To T, Baines CJ, Wall C. Canadian National Breast Screening Study—2: 13-year results of a randomized trial in women aged 50–59 years. *Journal of the National Cancer Institute* 2000 Sep 20; 92(18):1490–1499.
2. Gøtzsche PC, Nielsen M. Screening for breast cancer with mammography. *Cochrane Database of Systematic Reviews* 2011 Jan 19;1:CD001877.
3. Lipworth L, Bailey LR, Trichopoulos D. History of breastfeeding in relation to breast cancer risk: a review of the epidemiologic literature. *Journal of the National Cancer Institute* 2000 Feb 16;92(4):302–312.
4. Haller CA, Simpser E. Breastfeeding: 1999 perspective. *Current Opinion in Pediatrics* 1999;11:379–383.
5. Lynch BM, Neilson HK, Friedenreich CM. Physical activity and breast cancer prevention. *Recent Results in Cancer Research* 2011;186:13–42.
6. Schmitz KH. Exercise for secondary prevention of breast cancer: moving from evidence to changing clinical practice. *Cancer Prevention Research* 2011 Apr;4(4):476–480.
7. Mock V, Dow KH, Meares CJ, et al. Effects of exercise on fatigue, physical functioning, and emotional distress during radiation therapy for breast cancer.

Oncology Nursing Forum 1997; 24:991–1000.
8. Schwartz AL, Mori M, Gao R, et al. Exercise reduces daily fatigue in women with breast cancer receiving chemotherapy. *Medicine & Science in Sports & Exercise* 2001;33:718–723.
9. Demark-Wahnefried W, Rimer BK, Winer EP. Weight gain in women diagnosed with breast cancer. *Journal of the American Dietetic Association* 1997;97:519–526.
10. Hauner H, Hauner D. The impact of nutrition on the development and prognosis of breast cancer. *Breast Care* 2010;5(6):377–381.
11. Hebert J, Rosen A. Nutritional, socioeconomic, and reproductive factors in relation to female breast cancer mortality: findings from a cross-national study. *Cancer Detection and Prevention* 1996;20:234–244.
12. Zheng W, Gustafson DR, Sinha R, et al. Well-done meat intake and the risk of breast cancer. *Journal of the National Cancer Institute* 1998;90:1724–1729.
13. Wendel M, Heller AR. Anticancer actions of omega-3 fatty acids—current state and future perspectives. *Anti-Cancer Agents in Medicinal Chemistry* 2009 May;9(4):457–470.
14. Bartsch H, Nair J, Owen RW. Dietary polyunsaturated fatty acids and cancers of the breast and colorectum: emerging evidence for their role as risk modifiers. *Carcinogenesis* 1999; 20:2209–2218.
15. Rose DP. Dietary fatty acids and breast cancer. *The American Journal of Clinical Nutrition* 1998;66 suppl:998S–1003S.
16. Bougnoux P, Maillard V, Chajes V. Omega-6/omega-3 polyunsaturated fatty acids ratio and breast cancer. *World Review of Nutrition and Dietetics* 2005;94:158–165.
17. Klein V, Chajes V, Germain E, et al. Low alpha-linolenic acid

content of adipose breast tissue is associated with an increased risk of breast cancer. *European Journal of Cancer* 2000;36:335–340.
18. Bougnoux P, Koscielny S, Chajes V, et al. Alpha-linolenic acid content of adipose breast tissue: a host determinant of the risk of early metastasis in breast cancer. *British Journal of Cancer* 1994;70:330–334.
19. Thompson LU, Seidl MM, Rickard SE, et al. Antitumorigenic effect of a mammalian lignan precursor from flaxseed. *Nutrition and Cancer* 1996;26:159–165.
20. Saarinen NM, Wärri A, Airio M, et al. Role of dietary lignans in the reduction of breast cancer risk. *Molecular Nutrition & Food Research* 2007 Jul;51(7):857–866.
21. Haggans CJ, Hutchins AM, Olson BA, et al. Effect of flaxseed consumption on urinary estrogen metabolites in postmenopausal women. *Nutrition and Cancer* 1999;33:188–195.
22. Thompson LU, Chen JM, Li T, et al. Dietary flaxseed alters tumor biological markers in postmenopausal breast cancer. *Clinical Cancer Research* 2005 May 15;11(10):3828–3835.
23. Dong JY, Qin LQ. Soy isoflavones consumption and risk of breast cancer incidence or recurrence: a meta-analysis of prospective studies. *Breast Cancer Research and Treatment* 2011 Jan;125(2):315–323.
24. Nagata C. Factors to consider in the association between soy isoflavone intake and breast cancer risk. *Journal of Epidemiology* 2010;20(2):83–79.
25. Messina M. Soy, soy phytoestrogens (isoflavones), and breast cancer. *The American Journal of Clinical Nutrition* 1999;70:574–75.
26. Zeligs M. Diet and estrogen status: the cruciferous connection. *Journal of Medicinal Food* 1998;1:67–81.

27. Shertzer HG, Senft AP. The micronutrient indole-3-carbinol: implications for disease and chemoprevention. *Drug Metabolism and Drug Interactions* 2000;17:159–188.

28. Michnovicz JJ. Increased estrogen 2-hydroxylation in obese women using oral indole-3-carbinol. *International Journal of Obesity and Related Metabolic Disorders* 1998;22 (3):227–229.

29. Del Priore G, Gudipudi DK, Montemarano N, et al. Oral diindolylmethane (DIM): pilot evaluation of a nonsurgical treatment for cervical dysplasia. *Gynecology Oncology* 2010 Mar;116(3):464–467.

30. Walaszek Z, Szemraj J, Narog M, et al. Metabolism, uptake, and excretion of a D-glucaric acid salt and its potential use in cancer prevention. *Cancer Detection and Prevention* 1997;21:178–190.

31. Walaszek Z. Potential use of D-glucaric acid derivatives in cancer prevention. *Cancer Letters* 1990;54:1–8.

32. Kolstad HA. Nightshift work and risk of breast cancer and other cancers—a critical review of the epidemiologic evidence. *Scandinavian Journal of Work, Environment & Health* 2008 Feb;34(1):5–22.

33. Schernhammer ES, Laden F, Speizer FE, et al. Rotating night shifts and risk of breast cancer in women participating in the nurses' health study. *Journal of the National Cancer Institute* 2001;93:1563–1568.

34. Davis S, Mirick DK, Stevens RG. Night shift work, light at night, and risk of breast cancer. *Journal of the National Cancer Institute* 2001;93:1557–1562.

35. Ogunleye AA, Xue F, Michels KB. Green tea consumption and breast cancer risk or recurrence: a meta-analysis. *Breast Cancer Research and Treatment* 2010 Jan;119(2):477–484.

Bronchitis and Pneumonia

1. Centers for Disease Control and Prevention. *National Vital Statistics Reports* 2003 Nov; 52(9):9.

2. Nuorti JC, Butler JC, Farley MM, et al. Cigarette smoking and invasive pneumococcal disease. *The New England Journal of Medicine* 2000;342:681–689.

3. Bauer T, Ewig S, Marcos MA, et al. Streptococcus pneumoniae in community-acquired pneumonia: how important is drug resistance? *Medical Clinics of North America* 2001;85:1367–1379.

4. Cunha BA. Clinical relevance of penicillin-resistant *Streptococcus pneumoniae*. *Seminars in Respiratory Infections* 2002;17: 204–214.

5. Garau J. Treatment of drug-resistant pneumococcal pneumonia. *The Lancet Infectious Diseases* 2002;2:404–415.

6. Felmingham D. Evolving resistance patterns in community-acquired respiratory tract pathogens: first results from the PROTEKT global surveillance study. Prospective resistant organism tracking and epidemiology for the ketolide telithromycin. *Journal of Infection* 2002;44 suppl A:3–10.

7. Jacobs MR, Felmingham D, Appelbaum PC, et al. The Alexander Project 1998–2000: susceptibility of pathogens isolated from community-acquired lower respiratory tract infection to commonly used antimicrobial agents. *Journal of Antimicrobial Chemotherapy* 2003;52: 229–246.

8. Braman SS. Chronic cough due to acute bronchitis: ACCP evidence-based clinical practice guidelines. *Chest* 2006;129(1 suppl):95S–103S.

9. Gonzales R, Sande M. What will it take to stop physicians from prescribing antibiotics in acute bronchitis? *The Lancet* 1995;345(8951):665–666.

10. Niimi A, Matsumoto H, Ueda T, et al. Impaired cough reflex in patients with recurrent pneumonia. *Thorax* 2003;58:152–153.

11. Cambar PJ, Shore SR, Aviado DM. Bronchopulmonary and gastrointestinal effects of lobeline. *Archives Internationales de Pharmacodynamie et de Thérapie* 1969;177:1–27.

12. Brendler T, van Wyk BE. A historical, scientific and commercial perspective on the medicinal use of *Pelargonium sidoides* (Geraniaceae). *Journal of Ethnopharmacology* 2008 Oct 28;119(3):420–433.

13. Kim CE, Griffiths WJ, Taylor PW. Components derived from *Pelargonium* stimulate macrophage killing of *Mycobacterium* species. *Journal of Applied Microbiology* Apr 2009;106(4): 1184–1193.

14. Michaelis M, Doerr HW, Cinatl J Jr. Investigation of the influence of EPs® 7630, a herbal drug preparation from *Pelargonium sidoides*, on replication of a broad panel of respiratory viruses. *Phytomedicine* 2011 Mar 15;18(5):384–386.

15. Agbabiaka TB, Guo R, Ernst E. *Pelargonium sidoides* for acute bronchitis: a systematic review and meta-analysis. *Phytomedicine* May 2008;15(5):378–385.

16. Matthys H, Lizogub VG, Malek FA, Kieser M. Efficacy and tolerability of EPs 7630 tablets in patients with acute bronchitis: a randomised, double-blind, placebo-controlled dose-finding study with a herbal drug preparation from *Pelargonium sidoides*. *Current Medical Research & Opinion* 2010 Jun; 26(6):1413–1422.

17. Kamin W, Maydannik V, Malek FA, Kieser M. Efficacy and tolerability of EPs 7630 in children and adolescents with acute bronchitis: a randomized, double-blind, placebo-controlled multicenter trial with a herbal drug preparation from *Pelargonium sidoides* roots. *Inter-*

national *Journal of Clinical Pharmacology and Therapeutics* 2010 Mar;48(3):184–191.

18. Sieben A, Prenner L, Sorkalla T, et al. Alpha-hederin, but not hederacoside C and hederagenin from *Hedera helix,* affects the binding behavior, dynamics, and regulation of beta 2-adrenergic receptors. *Biochemistry* 2009 Apr 21;48(15): 3477–3482.

19. Stauss-Grabo M, Atiye S, Warnke A, et al. Observational study on the tolerability and safety of film-coated tablets containing ivy extract (Prospan® cough tablets) in the treatment of colds accompanied by coughing. *Phytomedicine* 2011 Apr 15;18(6):433–436.

20. Hecker M, Runkel F, Voelp A. [Treatment of chronic bronchitis with ivy leaf special extract—multicenter postmarketing surveillance study in 1,350 patients.] *Forschende Komplementärmedizin und Klassische Naturheilkunde* 2002 Apr;9(2):77–84.

21. Kemmerich B, Eberhardt R, Stammer H. Efficacy and tolerability of a fluid extract combination of thyme herb and ivy leaves and matched placebo in adults suffering from acute bronchitis with productive cough: a prospective, double-blind, placebo-controlled clinical trial. *Arzneimittelforschung* 2006;56(9):652–660.

22. Grandjean EM, Berthet P, Ruffmann R, Leuenberger P. Efficacy of oral long-term N-acetylcysteine in chronic bronchopulmonary disease: a meta-analysis of published double-blind, placebo-controlled clinical trials. *Clinical Therapeutics* 2000;22:209–221.

23. Kelly GS. Bromelain. A literature review and discussion of its therapeutic applications. *Alternative Medicine Review* 1996;1: 243–257.

24. Rimoldi R, Ginesu F, Giura R. The use of bromelain in pneumological therapy. *Drugs Under Experimental and Clinical Research* 1978;4:55–66.

25. Klenner FR. Virus pneumonia and its treatment with vitamin C. *Southern Medicine and Surgery* 1948 Feb;110(2):36–38.

26. Hunt C, Chakravorty NK, Annan G, et al. The clinical effects of vitamin C supplementation in elderly hospitalized patients with acute respiratory infections. *International Journal for Vitamin and Nutrition Research* 1994;64:212–219.

27. Stephensen CB, Alvarez JO, Kohatsec J. Vitamin A is excreted in the urine during acute infection. *The American Journal of Clinical Nutrition* 1994;60:88–92.

28. Hussey GD, Klein M. A randomized, controlled trial of vitamin A in children with severe measles. *The New England Journal of Medicine* 1990;323: 160–164.

29. Kjolhede CL, Chew FJ, Gadomski AM, et al. Clinical trial of vitamin A as adjuvant treatment for lower respiratory tract infections. *Journal of Pediatrics* 1995;126:807–812.

30. Bhandari N, Bahl R, Taneja S, et al. Effect of routine zinc supplementation on pneumonia in children aged 6 months to 3 years: randomised controlled trial in an urban slum. *BMJ* 2002;324:1358.

31. Bjorkqvist M, Wiberg B, Bodin L, et al. Bottle-blowing in hospital-treated patients with community-acquired pneumonia. *Scandinavian Journal of Infectious Diseases* 1997;29:77–82.

32. Westerdahl E, Lindmark B, Almgren SO, et al. Chest physiotherapy after coronary artery bypass graft surgery—a comparison of three different deep breathing techniques. *Journal of Rehabilitation Medicine* 2001; 33:79–84.

Candidiasis, Chronic

1. Truss CO. *The missing diagnosis.* Birmingham, Ala.: self-published, 1983.

2. Crook WG. *The yeast connection,* 2nd ed. Jackson, Tenn.: Professional Books, 1984.

3. Kroker GF. Chronic candidiasis and allergy. In *Food allergy and intolerance,* ed. Brostoff J, Challacombe SJ. Philadelphia: W. B. Saunders, 1987, 850–872.

4. Crook WG. *The yeast connection and the woman.* Jackson, Tenn.: Professional Books, 1995.

5. Bauman DS, Hagglund HE. Correlation between certain polysystem chronic complaints and an enzyme immunoassay with antigens of *Candida albicans. Journal of Advancement in Medicine* 1991;4:5–19.

6. Boero M, Pera A, Andriulli A, et al. *Candida* overgrowth in gastric juice of peptic ulcer subjects on short- and long-term treatment with H₂-receptor antagonists. *Digestion* 1983;28: 158–163.

7. Rubinstein E, Mark Z, Haspel J, et al. Antibacterial activity of the pancreatic fluid. *Gastroenterology* 1985;88:927–932.

8. Sarker SA, Gyr K. Non-immunological defence mechanisms of the gut. *Gut* 1992;33:987–993.

9. Iwata K. Toxins produced by *Candida albicans. Contributions to Microbiology & Immunology* 1977;4:77–85.

10. Axelsen NH. Analysis of human *Candida precipitins* by quantitative immunoelectrophoresis: a model for analysis of complex microbial antigen-antibody systems. *Scandinavian Journal of Immunology* 1976;5:177–190.

11. Farah CS, Elahi S, Drysdale K, et al. Primary role for CD4+ T lymphocytes in recovery from oropharyngeal candidiasis. *Infection and Immunity* 2002;70: 724–731.

12. Fidel PL Jr. Immunity to *Candida. Oral Diseases* 2002;8 suppl 2:69–75.

13. Klein A, Pappas SC, Gordon P, et al. The effect of nonviral liver damage on the T-lymphocyte helper/suppressor ratio. *Clinical*

Immunology and Immunopathology 1988;46:214–220.

14. Abe F, Nagata S, Hotchi M. Experimental candidiasis in liver injury. *Mycopathologia* 1987;100:37–42.

15. Barak AJ, Beckenhauer HC, Junnila M, et al. Dietary betaine promotes generation of hepatic S-adenosylmethionine and protects the liver from ethanol-induced fatty infiltration. *Alcoholism: Clinical and Experimental Research* 1993;17:552–555.

16. Zeisel SH, Da Costa KA, Franklin PD, et al. Choline, an essential nutrient for humans. *The FASEB Journal* 1991;5:2093–2098.

17. Isolauri E. Probiotics in human disease. *The American Journal of Clinical Nutrition* 2001; 73:1142S–1146S.

18. Sullivan A, Nord CE. The place of probiotics in human intestinal infections. *International Journal of Antimicrobial Agents* 2002;20:313–319.

19. Hahn FE, Ciak J. Berberine. *Antibiotics* 1976;3:577–588.

20. Amin AH, Subbaiah TV, Abbasi KM. Berberine sulfate. Antimicrobial activity, bioassay, and mode of action. *Canadian Journal of Microbiology* 1969; 15:1067–1076.

21. Johnson CC, Johnson G, Poe CF. Toxicity of alkaloids to certain bacteria. II. Berberine, physostigmine, and sanguinarine. *Acta Pharmacologica et Toxicologica* 1952;8:71–78.

22. Kaneda Y, Torii M, Tanaka T, et al. In vitro effects of berberine sulphate on the growth of *Entamoeba histolytica, Giardia lamblia* and *Trichomonas vaginalis. Annals of Tropical Medicine and Parasitology* 1991;85:417–425.

23. Subbaiah TV, Amin AH. Effect of berberine sulphate on *Entamoeba histolytica. Nature* 1967;215:527–528.

24. Ghosh AK, Rakshit MM, Ghosh DK. Effect of berberine chloride on *Leishmania donovani. Indian Journal of Medical Research* 1983;78:407–416.

25. Mahajan VM, Sharma A, Rattan A. Antimycotic activity of berberine sulphate. An alkaloid from an Indian medicinal herb. *Sabouraudia* 1982;20:79–81.

26. Gupte S. Use of berberine in treatment of giardiasis. *American Journal of Diseases of Children* 1975;129:866.

27. Bhakat MP, Nandi N, Pal HK, et al. Therapeutic trial of berberine sulphate in non-specific gastroenteritis. *Indian Medical Journal* 1974;68:19–23.

28. Kamat SA. Clinical trial with berberine hydrochloride for the control of diarrhoea in acute gastroenteritis. *Journal of the Association of Physicians of India* 1967;15:525–529.

29. Desai AB, Shah KM, Shah DM. Berberine in the treatment of diarrhoea. *Indian Pediatrics* 1971;8:462–465.

30. Sharma R, Joshi CK, Goyal RK. Berberine tannate in acute diarrhoea. *Indian Pediatrics* 1970;7:496–501.

31. Choudhry VP, Sabir M, Bhide VN. Berberine in giardiasis. *Indian Pediatrics* 1972;9:143–146.

32. Rabbani GH, Butler T, Knight J, et al. Randomized controlled trial of berberine sulfate therapy for diarrhea due to enterotoxigenic *Escherichia coli* and *Vibrio cholerae. Journal of Infectious Diseases* 1987;155:979–984.

33. Kowalewski Z, Mrozikiewicz A, Bobkiewicz T, et al. [Toxicity of berberine sulfate.] *Acta Poloniae Pharmaceutica* 1975;32:113–120.

34. Moore GS, Atkins RD. The fungicidal and fungistatic effects of an aqueous garlic extract on medically important yeast-like fungi. *Mycologia* 1977;69:341–348.

35. Sandhu DK, Warraich MK, Singh S. Sensitivity of yeasts isolated from cases of vaginitis to aqueous extracts of garlic. *Mykosen* 1980;23:691–698.

36. Prasad G, Sharma VD. Efficacy of garlic (*Allium sativum*) treatment against experimental candidiasis in chicks. *British Veterinary Journal* 1980;136:448–451.

37. Stiles JC, Sparks W, Ronzio RA. The inhibition of *Candida albicans* by oregano. *Journal of Applied Nutrition* 1995;47:96–102.

38. Vazquez JA, Zawawi AA. Efficacy of alcohol-based and alcohol-free melaleuca oral solution for the treatment of fluconazole-refractory oropharyngeal candidiasis in patients with AIDS. *HIV Clinical Trials* 2002;3:379–385.

39. Stepanovic S, Antic N, Dakic I, et al. In vitro antimicrobial activity of propolis and synergism between propolis and antimicrobial drugs. *Microbiological Research* 2003;158:353–357.

40. Ota C, Unterkircher C, Fantinato V, et al. Antifungal activity of propolis on different species of *Candida. Mycoses* 2001;44:375–378.

41. D'Auria FD, Tecca M, Scazzocchio F, et al. Effect of propolis on virulence factors of *Candida albicans. Journal of Chemotherapy* 2003;15:454–460.

42. Martins RS, Pereira ES Jr, Lima SM, et al. Effect of commercial ethanol propolis extract on the in vitro growth of *Candida albicans* collected from HIV-seropositive and HIV-seronegative Brazilian patients with oral candidiasis. *Journal of Oral Science* 2002;44:41–48.

Canker Sores

1. Albanidou-Farmaki E, Poulopoulos AK, Epivatianos A, et al. Increased anxiety level and high salivary and serum cortisol concentrations in patients with recurrent aphthous stomatitis. *The Tohoku Journal of Experimental Medicine.* Apr 2008; 214(4):291–296.

2. Hasan AA, Ciancio S. Association between ingestion of nonsteroidal anti-inflammatory drugs and the

emergence of aphthous-like ulcers. *Journal of the International Academy of Periodontology* 2009 Jan;11(1):155–159.

3. Wilson CWM. Food sensitivities, taste changes, aphthous ulcers and atopic symptoms in allergic disease. *Annals of Allergy, Asthma & Immunology* 1980;44:302–307.

4. Bays RA, Hamerlinck F, Cormane RH. Immunoglobulin-bearing lymphocytes and polymorphonuclear leukocytes in recurrent aphthous ulcers in man. *Archives of Oral Biology* 1977;22:147–153.

5. Wray D, Vlagopoulos TP, Siraganian RP. Food allergens and basophil histamine release in recurrent aphthous stomatitis. *Oral Surgery, Oral Medicine, Oral Pathology* 1982;54:388–395.

6. Nolan A, Lamey PJ, Milligan KA. Recurrent aphthous ulceration and food sensitivity. *Journal of Oral Pathology & Medicine* 1991;20:473–475.

7. Ferguson R, Basu MK, Asquith P, Cooke WT. Jejunal mucosal abnormalities in patients with recurrent aphthous ulceration. *British Medical Journal* 1976;1:11–13.

8. Ferguson MM, Wray D, Carmichael HA, et al. Celiac disease associated with recurrent aphthae. *Gut* 1980;21:223–226.

9. Wray D. Gluten-sensitive recurrent aphthous stomatitis. *Digestive Diseases and Sciences* 1981; 26:737–740.

10. Besu I, Jankovic L, Magdu IU et al. Humoral immunity to cow's milk proteins and gliadin within the etiology of recurrent aphthous ulcers? *Oral Diseases* 2009 Nov;15(8):560–564.

11. O'Farrelly C, O'Mahony D, Graeme-Cook F, et al. Gliadin antibodies identify gluten-sensitive oral ulceration in the absences of villous atrophy. *Journal of Oral Pathology & Medicine* 1991;20:476–478.

12. Haisraeli-Shalish M, Livneh A,

Katz J. Recurrent aphthous stomatitis and thiamine deficiency. *Oral Surgery, Oral Medicine, Oral Pathology, Oral Radiology & Endodontics* 1996;82: 634–636.

13. Wray D, Ferguson MM, Hutcheon AW, Daag JH. Nutritional deficiencies in recurrent aphthae. *Journal of Oral Pathology* 1978;7:418–423.

14. Nolan A, McIntosh WB, Allam BF, Lamey PJ. Recurrent aphthous ulceration. Vitamin B_1, B_2, and B_6 status and response to replacement therapy. *Journal of Oral Pathology & Medicine* 1991;20:389–391.

15. Arikan S, Durusoy C, Akalin N, et al. Oxidant/antioxidant status in recurrent aphthous stomatitis. *Oral Diseases* Oct 2009; 15(7):512–515.

16. Hay KD, Reade PC. The use of an elimination diet in the treatment of recurrent aphthous ulceration of the oral cavity. *Oral Surgery, Oral Medicine, Oral Pathology* 1984;57:504–507.

17. Wright A, Ryan FP, Willingham SE, et al. Food allergy or intolerance in severe recurrent aphthous ulceration of the mouth. *British Medical Journal* (Clinical Research Edition). 1986 May 10;292(6530):1237–1238.

18. Wray D, Ferguson MM, Mason DK, et al. Recurrent aphthae: treatment with vitamin B_{12}, folic acid, and iron. *British Medical Journal* 1975;2:490–493.

19. Carrozzo M. Vitamin B12 for the treatment of recurrent aphthous stomatitis. *Evidence-Based Dentistry* 2009;10(4):114–115.

20. Orbak R, Cicek Y, Tezel A, Dogru Y. Effects of zinc treatment in patients with recurrent aphthous stomatitis. *Dental Materials Journal* 2003; 22:21–29.

21. Yasui K, Kurata T, Yashiro M, et al. The effect of ascorbate on minor recurrent aphthous stomatitis. *Acta Paediatrica* 2010 Mar;99(3):442–445.

22. Das SK, Das V, Gulati AK, Singh VP. Deglycyrrhizinated

liquorice in aphthous ulcers. *Journal of the Association of Physicians of India* 1989;37:647.

Carpal Tunnel Syndrome

1. Stevens JC, Sun S, Beard CM, et al. Carpal tunnel syndrome in Rochester, Minnesota, 1961 to 1980. *Neurology* 1988;38: 134–138.

2. Viera AJ. Management of carpal tunnel syndrome. *American Family Physician* 2003:68: 265–72,279–80.

3. O'Connor D, Marshall S, Massy-Westropp N. Non-surgical treatment (other than steroid injection) for carpal tunnel syndrome. *Cochrane Database of Systematic Reviews* 2003(1): CD003219.

4. Cook AC, Szabo RM, Birkholz SW, King EF. Early mobilization following carpal tunnel release. A prospective randomized study. *The Journal of Hand Surgery: British & European Volume* 1995 Apr;20(2):228–230.

5. Jeffrey SL, Belcher HJ. Use of arnica to relieve pain after carpal-tunnel release surgery. *Alternative Therapies in Health and Medicine* 2002 Mar–Apr; 8(2):66–68.

6. Hochberg J. A randomized prospective study to assess the efficacy of two cold-therapy treatments following carpal tunnel release. *Journal of Hand Therapy* 2001 Jul–Sep;14(3): 208–215.

7. Gravlee, JR, Van Durme DJ. Braces and splints for musculoskeletal conditions. *American Family Physician* 2007 Feb 1; 75(3):342–348.

8. Walker WC, Metzler M, Cifu DX, Swartz Z. Neutral wrist splinting in carpal tunnel syndrome: a comparison of nighttime only versus full-time wear instructions. *Archives of Physical Medicine and Rehabilitation* 2000;81:424–429.

9. Ellis JM, Folkers K. Clinical aspects of treatment of carpal tunnel syndrome with vita-

min B6. *Annals of the New York Academy of Sciences* 1990;585: 302–320.

10. Folkers K, Ellis J. Successful therapy with vitamin B6 and vitamin B2 of the carpal tunnel syndrome and need for determination of the RDA's for vitamin B6 and B2 disease states. *Annals of the New York Academy of Sciences* 1990;585: 295–301.

11. Folkers K, Wolaniuk A, Vadhanavikit S. Enzymology of the response of carpal tunnel syndrome to riboflavin and to combined riboflavin and pyridoxine. *Proceedings of the National Academy of Sciences of the United States of America* 1984; 81:7076–7078.

12. Spooner GR, Desai HB, Angel JF, et al. Using pyridoxine to treat carpal tunnel syndrome: randomized control trial. *Canadian Family Physician* 1993;39: 2122–2127.

13. Stransky M, Rubin A, Lava NS, Lazaro RP. Treatment of carpal tunnel syndrome with vitamin B6: a double-blind study. *Southern Medical Journal* 1989; 82:841–842.

14. Yang CP, Hsieh CL, Wang NH, et al. Acupuncture in patients with carpal tunnel syndrome: a randomized controlled trial. *The Clinical Journal of Pain* 2009 May;25(4):327–333.

15. Chen GS. The effect of acupuncture treatment on carpal tunnel syndrome. *American Journal of Acupuncture* 1990; 18:5–9.

Cataracts

1. Bouton S. Vitamin C and the aging eye. *Archives of Internal Medicine* 1939;63:930–945.

2. Ringvold A, Johnsen H, Blika S. Senile cataract and ascorbic acid loading. *Acta Ophthalmologica* 1985;63:277–280.

3. Atkinson DT. Malnutrition as an etiological factor in senile cataract. *Eye, Ear, Nose & Throat Monthly* 1952;31:79–83.

4. Rathbun W, Hanson S. Glutathione metabolic pathway as a scavenging system in the lens. *Ophthalmic Research* 1979;11: 172–176.

5. Swanson AA, Truesdale AW. Elemental analysis in normal and cataractous human lens tissue. *Biochemical and Biophysical Research Communications* 1971;45:1488–1496.

6. Karaküçük S, Ertugrul Mirza G, Faruk Ekinciler O. Selenium concentrations in serum, lens, and aqueous humour of patients with senile cataract. *Acta Ophthalmologica Scandinavica* 1995;73:329–332.

7. Taylor A. Cataract: relationships between nutrition and oxidation. *Journal of the American College of Nutrition* 1993;12: 138–146.

8. Taylor A, Jacques PF, Chylack LT Jr, et al. Long-term intake of vitamins and carotenoids and odds of early age-related cortical and posterior subcapsular lens opacities. *The American Journal of Clinical Nutrition* 2002;75:540–549.

9. Jacques PF, Chylack LT Jr, Hankinson SE, et al. Long-term nutrient intake and early age-related nuclear lens opacities. *Archives of Ophthalmology* 2001;119:1009–1019.

10. Kuzniarz M, Mitchell P, Cumming RG, et al. Use of vitamin supplements and cataract: the Blue Mountains Eye Study. *American Journal of Ophthalmology* 2001;132:19–26.

11. Valero MP, Fletcher AE, De Stavola BL, et al. Vitamin C is associated with reduced risk of cataract in a Mediterranean population. *Journal of Nutrition* 2002;132:1299–1306.

12. Granado F, Olmedilla B, Blanco I. Nutritional and clinical relevance of lutein in human health. *British Journal of Nutrition* 2003;90:487–502.

13. Hankinson SE, Stampfer MJ, Seddon JM, et al. Nutrient intake and cataract extraction in women: a prospective study. *BMJ* 1992;305:335–339.

14. Brown L, Rimm EB, Seddon JM, et al. A prospective study of carotenoid intake and risk of cataract extraction in US men. *The American Journal of Clinical Nutrition* 1999;70:517–524.

15. Chasan-Taber L, Willett WC, Seddon JM, et al. A prospective study of carotenoid and vitamin A intakes and risk of cataract extraction in US women. *The American Journal of Clinical Nutrition* 1999;70:509–516.

16. Lyle BJ, Mares-Perlman JA, Klein BE, et al. Antioxidant intake and risk of incident age-related nuclear cataracts in the Beaver Dam Eye Study. *American Journal of Epidemiology* 1999;149:801–809.

17. Olmedilla B, Granado F, Blanco I, et al. Lutein, but not alpha-tocopherol, supplementation improves visual function in patients with age-related cataracts: a 2-y double-blind, placebo-controlled pilot study. *Nutrition* 2003;19:21–24.

18. Christen WG, Glynn RJ, Sesso HD, et al. Age-related cataract in a randomized trial of vitamins E and C in men. *Archives of Ophthalmology* 2010 Nov; 128(11):1397–1405.

19. McNeil JJ, Robman L, Tikellis G, et al. Vitamin E supplementation and cataract: randomized controlled trial. *Ophthalmology* 2004;111:75–84.

20. A randomized, placebo-controlled, clinical trial of high-dose supplementation with vitamins C and E and beta carotene for age-related cataract and vision loss: AREDS report no. 9. Age-Related Eye Disease Study Research Group. *Archives of Ophthalmology* 2001;119:1439–1452.

21. Whanger P, Weswig P. Effects of selenium, chromium and antioxidants on growth, eye cataracts, plasma cholesterol and blood glucose in selenium deficient, vitamin E supplemented

rats. *Nutrition Reports International* 1975;12:345–358.

22. Rao GN, Cotlier E. The enzymatic activities of GTP cyclohydrolase, sepiapterin reductase, dihydropteridine reductase and dihydrofolate reductase; and tetrahydrobiopterin content in mammalian ocular tissues and in human senile cataracts. *Comparative Biochemistry and Physiology—Part B: Biochemistry & Molecular Biology* 1985;80B:61–66.

23. Skalka H, Prchal J. Cataracts and riboflavin deficiency. *The American Journal of Clinical Nutrition* 1981;34:861–863.

24. Prchal JT, Conrad ME, Skalka HW. Association of pre-senile cataracts with heterozygosity for galactosemic states and riboflavin deficiency. *The Lancet* 1978;1:12–13.

25. Rathbun WB. Influence on lenticular glutathione research. *Ophthalmic Research* 1995;27 suppl 1:13–17.

26. Burton GW, Ingold KU. Beta-carotene: an unusual type of lipid antioxidant. *Science* 1984;224:569–573.

27. Christen W, Glynn R, Sperduto R, et al. Age-related cataract in a randomized trial of beta-carotene in women. *Ophthalmic Epidemiology* 2004 Dec;11(5):401–12.

28. Christen WG, Manson JE, Glynn RJ, et al. A randomized trial of beta carotene and age-related cataract in US physicians. *Archives of Ophthalmology* 2003 Mar;121(3):372–378.

29. Hess HH, Knapka JJ, Newsome DA, et al. Dietary prevention of cataracts in the pink-eyed RCS rat. *Laboratory Animal Science* 1985;35:47–53.

30. Bravetti G. [Preventive medical treatment of senile cataract with vitamin E and anthocyanosides: clinical evaluation.] *Annali di Ottalmologia e Clinica Oculistica* 1989;115:109.

Celiac Disease

1. Rubio-Tapia A, Murray JA. Celiac disease. *Current Opinion in Gastroenterology* 2010 Mar;26(2):116–122.

2. Rewers M. Epidemiology of celiac disease: what are the prevalence, incidence, and progression of celiac disease? *Gastroenterology* 2005 Apr;128(4 suppl 1):S47–S51.

3. Tack GJ, Verbeek WH, Schreurs MW, Mulder CJ. The spectrum of celiac disease: epidemiology, clinical aspects and treatment. *Nature Reviews Gastroenterology & Hepatology* 2010 Apr;7(4):204–13

4. Dewar D, Pereira SP, Ciclitira PJ. The pathogenesis of coeliac disease. *The International Journal of Biochemistry & Cell Biology* 2004;36:17–24.

5. Persson LA, Ivarsson A, Hernell O. Breast-feeding protects against celiac disease in childhood—epidemiological evidence. *Advances in Experimental Medicine and Biology* 2002;503:115–123.

6. Ivarsson A, Hernell O, Stenlund H, et al. Breast-feeding protects against celiac disease. *The American Journal of Clinical Nutrition* 2002;75:914–921.

7. Faellstroem SP, Winberg J, Andersen HJ. Cow's milk induced malabsorption as a precursor of gluten intolerance. *Acta Paediatrica Scandinavica* 1965;54:101–115.

8. Ludvigsson JF, Montgomery SM, Ekbom A, et al. Small-intestinal histopathology and mortality risk in celiac disease. *JAMA, The Journal of the American Medical Association* 2009 Sep 16;302(11):1171–1178.

9. Rubio-Tapia A, Kyle RA, Kaplan EL, et al. Increased prevalence and mortality in undiagnosed celiac disease. *Gastroenterology* 2009 Jul;137(1):88–93.

10. Green PH, Fleischauer AT, Bhagat G, et al. Risk of malignancy in patients with celiac disease.

The American Journal of Medicine 2003;115:191–195.

11. Dohan FC, Harper EH, Clark MH, et al. Is schizophrenia rare if grain is rare? *Biological Psychiatry* 1984;19:385–399.

12. Dohan FC, Gasberger JC. Relapsed schizophrenics: earlier discharge from the hospital after cereal-free, milk-free diet. *The American Journal of Psychiatry* 1973;130:685–688.

13. Ludvigsson JF, Osby U, Ekbom A, Montgomery SM. Coeliac disease and risk of schizophrenia and other psychosis: a general population cohort study. *Scandinavian Journal of Gastroenterology* 2007 Feb;42(2):179–185.

14. Paroli E. Opioid peptides from food (the exorphins). *World Review of Nutrition and Dietetics* 1988;55:58–97.

15. Ludvigsson JF, Reutfors J, Osby U, et al. Coeliac disease and risk of mood disorders—a general population-based cohort study. *Journal of Affective Disorders* 2007 Apr;99(1–3):117–126.

16. Hu WT, Murray JA, Greenaway MC, et al. Cognitive impairment and celiac disease. *Archives of Neurology* 2006 Oct;63(10):1440–6.

17. Millward C, Ferriter M, Calver S, Connell-Jones G. Gluten- and casein-free diets for autistic spectrum disorder. *Cochrane Database of Systematic Reviews* 2004;2:CD003498.

18. Saalman R, Dahlgren UI, Fallstrom SP, et al. Avidity progression of dietary antibodies in healthy and coeliac children. *Clinical & Experimental Immunology* 2003;134:328–334.

19. Hallert C, Svensson M, Tholstrup J, Hultberg B. Clinical trial: B vitamins improve health in patients with coeliac disease living on a gluten-free diet. *Alimentary Pharmacology & Therapeutics* 2009 Apr 15;29(8):811–816.

20. Janatuinen EK, Kemppainen TA, Julkunen RJ, et al. No harm from five year ingestion of oats in coeliac disease. *Gut* 2002; 50(3):332–335.

21. Hollen E, Holmgren Peterson K, Sundqvist T, et al. Coeliac children on a gluten-free diet with or without oats display equal anti-avenin antibody titres. *Scandinavian Journal of Gastroenterology* 2006;41(1): 42–47.

22. Hogberg L, Laurin P, Falth-Magnusson K. Oats to children with newly diagnosed coeliac disease: a randomised double blind study. *Gut* 2004;53(5): 649–54.

23. Srinivasan U, Jones E, Carolan J, Feighery C. Immunohistochemical analysis of coeliac mucosa following ingestion of oats. *Clinical & Experimental Immunology* 2006;144(2):197–203.

24. Peraaho M, Kaukinen K, Mustalahti K, et al. Effect of an oats-containing gluten-free diet on symptoms and quality of life in coeliac disease: a randomized study. *Scandinavian Journal of Gastroenterology* 2004;39(1): 27–31.

25. Love AHG, Elmes M, Golden M, et al. Zinc deficiency and celiac disease. In *Perspectives in coeliac disease. Proceedings of the 3rd International Symposium on Coeliac Disease*, ed. McNicholl B, McCarthy CF, Fottrell PF. Baltimore: University Press, 1978, 335–342.

26. Carroccio A, Iacono G, Montalto G, et al. Pancreatic enzyme therapy in childhood celiac disease. A double-blind prospective randomized study. *Digestive Diseases and Sciences* 1995;40:2555–2560.

Cerebral Vascular Insufficiency

1. Mahe G, Ronziere T, Laviolle B, et al. An unfavorable dietary pattern is associated with symptomatic ischemic stroke and carotid atherosclerosis. *Journal of Vascular Surgery* 2010 Jul; 52(1):62–68.

2. Barnett HJM, Barnes RW, Robertson JT. The uncertainties surrounding carotid endarterectomy. *JAMA, The Journal of the American Medical Association* 1992;268:3120–3121.

3. NASCET Collaborators. Beneficial effect of carotid endarterectomy in symptomatic patients with high-grade carotid stenosis. *The New England Journal of Medicine* 1991;325:445–453.

4. Easton JD, Wilterdink JL. Carotid endarterectomy: trials and tribulations. *Annals of Neurology* 1994;35:5–17.

5. Ederle J, Dobson J, Featherstone RL, et al. Carotid artery stenting compared with endarterectomy in patients with symptomatic carotid stenosis (International Carotid Stenting Study): an interim analysis of a randomised controlled trial. *The Lancet* 2010 Mar 20;375(9719): 985–997.

6. Ederle J, Bonati LH, Dobson J, et al. Endovascular treatment with angioplasty or stenting versus endarterectomy in patients with carotid artery stenosis in the Carotid and Vertebral Artery Transluminal Angioplasty Study (CAVATAS): long-term follow-up of a randomised trial. *The Lancet Neurology* 2009 Oct;8(10):898–907.

7. Bazan HA, Lu Y, Thoppil D, et al. Diminished omega-3 fatty acids are associated with carotid plaques from neurologically symptomatic patients: implications for carotid interventions. *Vascular Pharmacology* 2009 Nov–Dec;51(5–6):331–336.

8. Cawood AL, Ding R, Napper FL, et al. Eicosapentaenoic acid (EPA) from highly concentrated n-3 fatty acid ethyl esters is incorporated into advanced atherosclerotic plaques and higher plaque EPA is associated with decreased plaque inflammation and increased stability. *Atherosclerosis* 2010 Sep;212(1):252–259.

9. Kleijnen J, Knipschild P. *Ginkgo biloba* for cerebral insufficiency. *British Journal of Clinical Pharmacology* 1992;34:352–358.

10. Engelsen J, Nielsen JD, Winther K. Effect of coenzyme Q10 and *Ginkgo biloba* on warfarin dosage in stable, long-term warfarin treated outpatients: a randomised, double blind, placebo-crossover trial. *Thrombosis and Haemostasis* 2002;87: 1075–1076.

11. Bone KM. Potential interaction of *Ginkgo biloba* leaf with antiplatelet or anticoagulant drugs: what is the evidence? *Molecular Nutrition & Food Research* 2008 Jul;52(7):764–771.

Cervical Dysplasia

1. de Vet HC, Sturmans F. Risk factors for cervical dysplasia: implications for prevention. *Public Health* 1994;108:241–249.

2. Moore TO, Moore AY, Carrasco D. Human papillomavirus, smoking, and cancer. *Journal of Cutaneous Medicine and Surgery* 2001 Jul–Aug;5(4): 323–328.

3. Clarke EA, Morgan RW, Newman AM. Smoking as a risk factor in cancer of the cervix: additional evidence from a case-control study. *American Journal of Epidemiology* 1982;115: 59–66.

4. Lyon JL, Gardner JW, West DW, et al. Smoking and carcinoma in situ of the uterine cervix. *The American Journal of Public Health* 1983;73:558–562.

5. Marshall JR, Graham S, Byers T, et al. Diet and smoking in the epidemiology of cancer of the cervix. *Journal of the National Cancer Institute* 1983;70: 847–851.

6. Clarke EA, Hatcher J, McKeown-

Eyssen GE, Lickrish GM. Cervical dysplasia: association with sexual behavior, smoking, and oral contraceptive use? *American Journal of Obstetrics & Gynecology* 1985;151: 612–616.

7. Orr JW Jr, Wilson K, Bodiford C, et al. Nutritional status of patients with untreated cervical cancer. II. Vitamin assessment. *American Journal of Obstetrics & Gynecology* 1985; 151:632–635.

8. Orr JW Jr, Wilson K, Bodiford C, et al. Nutritional status of patients with untreated cervical cancer. I. Biochemical and immunologic assessment. *American Journal of Obstetrics & Gynecology* 1985;151:625–631.

9. Tomita L, Filho A, Costa M, et al. Diet and serum micronutrients in relation to cervical neoplasia and cancer among low-income Brazilian women. *International Journal of Cancer* 2009;126:703–714.

10. Ghosh C, Baker J, Moysich K, et al. Dietary intakes of selected nutrients and food groups and risk of cervical cancer. *Nutrition and Cancer* 2008;60(3): 331–341.

11. Hwang J, Kim M, Lee J. Dietary supplements reduce the risk of cervical intraepithelial neoplasia. *International Journal of Gynecological Cancer* 2010; 20(3):398–403.

12. La Vecchia C, Franceschi S, Decarli A, et al. Dietary vitamin A and the risk of invasive cervical cancer. *International Journal of Cancer* 1984;34:319–322.

13. Romney SL, Palan PR, Duttagupta C, et al. Retinoids and the prevention of cervical dysplasias. *American Journal of Obstetrics & Gynecology* 1981; 141:890–894.

14. Wylie-Rosett JA, Romney SL, Slagle NS, et al. Influence of vitamin A on cervical dysplasia and carcinoma in situ. *Nutrition and Cancer* 1984;6:49–57.

15. Dawson E, Nosovitch J, Hanni-

gan E. Serum vitamin and selenium changes in cervical dysplasia. *Federation Proceedings* 1984;43:612.

16. Romney SL, Palan PR, Basu J, Mikhail M. Nutrients antioxidants in the pathogenesis and prevention of cervical dysplasias and cancer. *Journal of Cellular Biochemistry* 1995;23 suppl:96–103.

17. Keefe K, Schell M, Brewer C, et al. A randomized, double blind, phase III trial using oral beta-carotene supplementation for women with high-grade cervical intraepithelial neoplasia. *Cancer Epidemiology* 2001;10: 1029–1035.

18. Romeny, S, Ho, G, Palan P, et al. Effects of beta-carotene and other factors on outcome of cervical dysplasia and human papillomavirus infection. *Gynecology Oncology* 1997;65: 483–492.

19. Fairley, C, Tabrizi S, Chen S, et al. A randomized clinical trial of beta-carotene vs. placebo for the treatment of cervical HPV infections. *International Journal of Gynecological Cancer* 1996;6:225–230.

20. de Vet, H, Knipschild P, Willebrand D, et al. The effect of beta-carotene on the regression and progression of cervical dysplasia: a clinical experiement. *Journal of Clinical Epidemiology* 1991;44:273–283.

21. Mackerras, D, Irwig L, Simpson J, et al. Randomized double-blind trial of beta-carotene and vitamin C in women with minor cervical abnormalities. *British Journal of Cancer* 1999;79: 1448–1453.

22. Meyskens FL Jr, Surwit E, Moon TE, et al. Enhancement of regression of cervical intraepithelial neoplasia II (moderate dysplasia) with topically applied all-trans-retinoic acid: a randomized trial. *Journal of the National Cancer Institute* 1994; 86:539–543.

23. Graham V, Surwit ES, Weiner S,

Meyskens FL Jr. Phase II trial of beta-all-trans-retinoic acid for cervical intraepithelial neoplasia delivered via a collagen sponge and cervical cap. *Western Journal of Medicine* 1986; 145:192–195.

24. Wassertheil-Smoller S, Romney SL, Wylie-Rosett J, et al. Dietary vitamin C and uterine cervical dysplasia. *American Journal of Epidemiology* 1981; 114:714–724.

25. Romney SL, Duttagupta C, Basu J, et al. Plasma vitamin C and uterine cervical dysplasia. *American Journal of Obstetrics & Gynecology* 1985;151: 978–980.

26. Kim SY, Kim JW, Ko YS, et al. Changes in lipid peroxidation and antioxidant trace elements in serum of women with cervical intraepithelial neoplasia and invasive cancer. *Nutrition and Cancer* 2003;47(2):126–130.

27. Van Niekerk W. Cervical cytological abnormalities caused by folic acid deficiency. *Acta Cytologica* 1966;10:67–73.

28. Kitay DZ, Wentz WB. Cervical cytology in folic acid deficiency of pregnancy. *American Journal of Obstetrics & Gynecology* 1969;104:931–938.

29. Streiff RR. Folate deficiency and oral contraceptives. *JAMA, The Journal of the American Medical Association* 1970;214: 105–108.

30. Whitehead N, Reyner F, Lindenbaum J. Megaloblastic changes in the cervical epithelium: association with oral contraceptive therapy and reversal with folic acid. *JAMA, The Journal of the American Medical Association* 1973;226:1421–1424.

31. Butterworth CE Jr, Hatch KD, Macaluso M, et al. Folate deficiency and cervical dysplasia. *JAMA, The Journal of the American Medical Association* 1992;267:528–533.

32. Harper JM, Levine AJ, Rosenthal DL, et al. Erythrocyte folate levels, oral contraceptive

use and abnormal cervical cytology. *Acta Cytologica* 1994;38:324–330.

33. Butterworth CE Jr, Hatch KD, Soong SJ, et al. Oral folic acid supplementation for cervical dysplasia. A clinical intervention trial. *American Journal of Obstetrics & Gynecology* 1992;166:803–809.

34. Butterworth CE Jr, Hatch KD, Gore H, et al. Improvement in cervical dysplasia associated with folic acid therapy in users of oral contraceptives. *The American Journal of Clinical Nutrition* 1982;35:73–82.

35. Flatley JE, McNeir K, Balasubramani L, et al. Folate status and aberrant DNA methylation are associated with HPV infection and cervical pathogenesis. *Cancer Epidemiology, Biomarkers & Prevention* 2009 Oct;18(10):2782–2789.

36. Piyathilake CJ, Macaluso M, Alvarez RD, et al. Lower risk of cervical intraepithelial neoplasia in women with high plasma folate and sufficient vitamin B12 in the post–folic acid fortification era. *Cancer Prevention Research*. 2009 Jul;2(7):658–664.

37. Zeligs M. Diet and estrogen status: the cruciferous connection. *Journal of Medicinal Food* 1998;1:67–81.

38. Newfield L, Goldsmith A, Bradlow H, Auborn K. Estrogen metabolism and human papillomavirus-induced tumors of the larynx: chemo-prophylaxis with indole-3-carbinol. *Anticancer Research* 1993;13:337–341.

39. Bell M, Crowley-Nowick P, Bradlow H, et al. Placebo-controlled trial of indole-3-carbinol in the treatment of CIN. *Gynecology Oncology* 2000;78:123–129.

40. Del Priore G, Gudipudi DK, Montemarano N, et al. Oral diindolylmethane (DIM): pilot evaluation of a nonsurgical treatment for cervical dysplasia. *Gynecology Oncology* 2010 Mar;116(3):464–467.

41. Ahn WS, Yoo J, Huh SW, et al. Protective effects of green tea extracts (polyphenon E and EGCG) on human cervical lesions. *European Journal of Cancer Prevention* 2003 Oct;12(5):383–390.

Chronic Fatigue Syndrome

1. Holmes GP, Kaplan J, Gantz N, et al. Chronic fatigue syndrome: a working case definition. *Annals of Internal Medicine* 1988;108:387–389.

2. Bates DW, Schmitt W, Buchwald D, et al. Prevalence of fatigue and chronic fatigue syndrome in a Primary Care practice. *Archives of Internal Medicine* 1993;153(24)2759–2765.

3. Reid S, Chalder T, Cleare A, et al. Chronic fatigue syndrome. *Clinical Evidence* 2008;08:1101–1115.

4. Kyle DV, deShazo RD. Chronic fatigue syndrome: a conundrum. *The American Journal of the Medical Sciences* 1992;303:28–34.

5. Caligiuri M, Murray C, Buchwald D, et al. Phenotypic and functional deficiency of natural killer cells in patients with chronic fatigue syndrome. *The Journal of Immunology* 1987;139:3306–3313.

6. Gupta S, Vayuvegula B. A comprehensive immunological analysis in chronic fatigue syndrome. *Scandinavian Journal of Immunology* 1991;33:319–327.

7. Komaroff AI, Goldenberg D. The chronic fatigue syndrome: definition, current studies and lessons for fibromyalgia research. *The Journal of Rheumatology* 1989;16:23–27.

8. Buchwald D, Garrity DL. Comparison of patients with chronic fatigue syndrome, fibromyalgia and multiple chemical sensitivities. *Archives of Internal Medicine* 1994;154:2049–2053.

9. Prins JB, Bos E, Huibers MJ, et al. Social support and the persistence of complaints in chronic fatigue syndrome. *Psychotherapy and Psychosomatics* 2004;73:174–182.

10. Sharpe M, Hawton K, Simkin S, et al. Cognitive behavior therapy for the chronic fatigue syndrome: a randomized controlled trial. *BMJ* 1996;312:22–26.

11. Deale A, Chalder T, Marks L, et al. Cognitive behavior therapy for chronic fatigue syndrome: a randomized controlled trial. *The American Journal of Psychiatry* 1997;154:408–414.

12. Tintera JW. The hypoadrenocortical state and its management. *New York State Journal of Medicine* 1955;55:1869–1876.

13. Demitrack MA. Chronic fatigue syndrome: a disease of the hypothalamic-pituitary-adrenal axis? *Annals of Medicine* 1994;26:1–3.

14. Roberts AD, Wessely S, Chalder T, et al. Salivary cortisol response to awakening in chronic fatigue syndrome. *The British Journal of Psychiatry* 2004;184:136–141.

15. Cleare AJ. The HPA axis and the genesis of chronic fatigue syndrome. *Trends in Endocrinology & Metabolism* 2004;15:55–59.

16. Demitrack MA, Dale JK, Straus SE, et al. Evidence for impaired activation of hypothalamic-pituitary-adrenal axis in patients with chronic fatigue syndrome. *The Journal of Clinical Endocrinology & Metabolism* 1991;73:1224–1234.

17. Seaton A, Jeelinek EH, Kennedy P. Major neurological disease and occupational exposure to organic solvents. *Quarterly Journal of Medicine* 1992;305:707–712.

18. Rutter M, Russell-Jones R, eds. *Lead versus health: sources and effects of low level lead exposure*. New York: John Wiley, 1983.

19. Bland JS, Barrager E, Reedy RG, et al. A medical food-supplemented detoxification program in the management of

chronic health problems. *Alternative Therapies in Health and Medicine* 1995;1:62–71.

20. Rigden S, Barrager E, Bland JS. Evaluation of the effect of a modified entero-hepatic resuscitation program in chronic fatigue syndrome patients. *Journal of Advancement in Medicine* 1998;11(4):247–262.

21. Rowe AH, Rowe A Jr. *Food allergy: its manifestations and control and the elimination diets: a compendium.* Springfield, Ill.: Charles C. Thomas, 1972.

22. Breneman JC. *Basics of food allergy.* Springfield, Ill.: Charles C. Thomas, 1977.

23. Estler CJ, Ammon HP, Herzog C. Swimming capacity of mice after prolonged treatment with psychostimulants. I. Effects of caffeine on swimming performance and cold stress. *Psychopharmacology* 1978;58: 161–166.

24. Greden JF, Fontaine P, Lubetsky M, et al. Anxiety and depression associated with caffeinism among psychiatric inpatients. *The American Journal of Psychiatry* 1978;135:963–966.

25. Chou T. Wake up and smell the coffee. Caffeine, coffee, and the medical consequences. *Western Journal of Medicine* 1992;157: 544–553.

26. Hughes JR, Higgins ST, Bickel WK, et al. Caffeine self-administration, withdrawal, and adverse effects among coffee drinkers. *Archives of General Psychiatry* 1991;48:611–617.

27. Behan PO, Behan WM, Horrobin D. Effect of high doses of essential fatty acids on the postviral fatigue syndrome. *Acta Neurologica Scandinavica* 1990;82:209–216.

28. Puri BK, Holmes J, Hamilton G. Eicosapentaenoic acid-rich essential fatty acid supplementation in chronic fatigue syndrome associated with symptom remission and structural brain changes. *International Journal*

of *Clinical Practice* 2004;58: 297–299.

29. Manuel Y, Keenoy B, Moorkens G, et al. Magnesium status and parameters of the oxidant-antioxidant balance in patients with chronic fatigue: effects of supplementation with magnesium. *Journal of the American College of Nutrition* 2000;19: 374–382.

30. Cox IM, Campbell MJ, Dowson D. Red blood cell magnesium and chronic fatigue syndrome. *The Lancet* 1991;337: 757–760.

31. Ahlborg H, Ekelund LG, Nilsson CG. Effect of potassium-magnesium aspartate on the capacity for prolonged exercise in man. *Acta Physiologica Scandinavica* 1968;74:238–245.

32. Hicks JT. Treatment of fatigue in general practice: a double blind study. *Clinical Medicine* 1964 Jan;71:85–90.

33. Friedlander HS. Fatigue as a presenting symptom: management in general practice. *Current Therapeutic Research* 1962;4:441–449.

34. Shaw DL Jr, Chesney MA, Tullis IF, et al. Management of fatigue: a physiologic approach. *The American Journal of the Medical Sciences* 1962;243: 758–769.

35. Gullestad L, Oystein Dolva L, Birkeland K, et al. Oral versus intravenous magnesium supplementation in patients with magnesium deficiency. *Magnesium and Trace Elements* 1991;10: 11–16.

36. Lindberg JS, Zobitz MM, Poindexter JR, et al. Magnesium bioavailability from magnesium citrate and magnesium oxide. *Journal of the American College of Nutrition* 1990;9:48–45.

37. Plioplys AV, Plioplys S. Amantadine and L-carnitine treatment of chronic fatigue syndrome. *Neuropsychobiology* 1997;35: 16–23.

38. Maes M, Mihaylova I, Kubera M, et al. Coenzyme Q10

deficiency in myalgic encephalomyelitis/chronic fatigue syndrome (ME/CFS) is related to fatigue, autonomic and neurocognitive symptoms and is another factor explaining the early mortality in ME/CFS due to cardiovascular disorder. *Neuroendocrinology Letters* 2009; 30(4):470–476.

39. LaManca JJ, Sisto SA, DeLuca J, et al. Influence of exhaustive treadmill exercise on cognitive functioning in chronic fatigue syndrome. *The American Journal of Medicine* 1998; 105:S59–S65.

40. Farmer ME, Locke BZ, Moscicki EK, et al. Physical activity and depressive symptoms: the NHANES 1 Epidemiologic Follow-up Study. *American Journal of Epidemiology* 1988; 1328:1340–1351.

41. Fiatarone MA, Morley JE, Bloom ET, et al. The effect of exercise on natural killer cell activity in young and old subjects. *The Journals of Gerontology* 1989;44:M37–M45.

42. Makinnon LT. Exercise and natural killer cells. What is their relationship? *Sports Medicine* 1989;7:141–149.

43. Sun XS, Xu Y, Xia YJ. Determination of E-rosette-forming lymphocytes in aged subjects with taichiquan exercise. *International Journal of Sports Medicine* 1989;10:217–219.

44. Friedberg F. Does graded activity increase activity? A case study of chronic fatigue syndrome. *Journal of Behavior Therapy and Experimental Psychiatry* 2002;33:203–215.

45. Wallman KE, Morton AR, Goodman C, et al. Randomised controlled trial of graded exercise in chronic fatigue syndrome. *The Medical Journal of Australia* 2004;180: 444–448.

46. Bohn B, Nebe CT, Birr C. Flow-cytometric studies with *Eleutherococcus senticosus* extract as an immunomodulatory

agent. *Arzneimittelforschung* 1987;37:1193–1196.

47. Olsson EM, von Schéele B, Panossian AG. A randomised, double-blind, placebo-controlled, parallel-group study of the standardised extract shr-5 of the roots of *Rhodiola rosea* in the treatment of subjects with stress-related fatigue. *Planta Medica* 2009 Feb;75(2):105–512.

Chronic Obstructive Pulmonary Disease

1. Hoogendoorn M, Feenstra TL, Hoogenveen RT, Rutten-van Mölken MPMH. Long-term effectiveness and cost-effectiveness of smoking cessation interventions in patients with COPD. *Thorax* 2010;65(8):711–718.

2. Stav D, Raz M. Effect of N-acetylcysteine on air trapping in COPD: a randomized placebo-controlled study. *Chest* 2009 Aug;136(2):381–386.

3. Rolla G, Bucca C, Bugiani M, et al. Hypomagnesemia in chronic obstructive lung disease: effect of therapy. *Magnesium and Trace Elements* 1990;9:132–136.

4. Fiaccadori E, Del Canale S, Coffrini E, et al. Muscle and serum magnesium in pulmonary intensive care unit patients. *Critical Care Medicine* 1988;16:751–760.

5. Skorodin MS, Tenholder MF, Yetter B, et al. Magnesium sulfate in exacerbations of chronic obstructive pulmonary disease. *Archives of Internal Medicine* 1995;155:496–500.

Common Cold

1. Sanchez A, Reeser J, Lau H, et al. Role of sugars in human neutrophilic phagocytosis. *The American Journal of Clinical Nutrition* 1973;26:1180–1184.

2. Ringsdorf WM Jr, Cheraskin E, Ramsay RR Jr. Sucrose, neutrophilic phagocytosis and resistance to disease. *Dental Survey* 1976;52:46–48.

3. Bernstein J, Alpert S, Nauss K, et al. Depression of lymphocyte transformation following oral glucose ingestion. *The American Journal of Clinical Nutrition* 1977;30:613

4. Pauling L. *Vitamin C and the common cold.* San Francisco: Freeman, 1970.

5. Douglas RM, Hemilä H, Chalker E, Treacy B. Vitamin C for preventing and treating the common cold. Cochrane Database of Systematic Reviews 2007 Jul 18;3:CD000980.

6. Katz E, Margalith E. Inhibition of vaccinia virus maturation by zinc chloride. *Antimicrobial Agents and Chemotherapy* 1981;19:213–217.

7. Hemilä H. Zinc lozenges may shorten the duration of colds: a systematic review. *The Open Respiratory Medicine Journal* 2011;5:51–58.

8. Mossad SB, Macknin ML, Medendorp SV, Mason P. Zinc gluconate lozenges for treating the common cold. A randomized, double-blind, placebo-controlled study. *Annals of Internal Medicine* 1996;125:142–144.

9. Zarembo JE, Godfrey JC, Godfrey NJ. Zinc (II) in saliva: determination of concentrations produced by different formulations of zinc gluconate lozenges containing common excipients. *Journal of Pharmaceutical Sciences* 1992;81:128–130.

10. Turner RB, Riker DK, Gangemi JD. Ineffectiveness of echinacea for prevention of experimental rhinovirus colds. *Antimicrobial Agents and Chemotherapy* 2000;44:1708–1709.

11. Goel V, Lovlin R, Barton R, et al. Efficacy of a standardized echinacea preparation (Echinilin) for the treatment of the common cold: a randomized, double-blind, placebo-controlled trial. *Journal of Clinical Pharmacy and Therapeutics* 2004;29:75–83.

12. Melchart D, Linde K, Worku F, et al. Immunomodulation with Echinacea—a systematic review of controlled clinical trials. *Phytomedicine* 1994;1:245–254.

13. Barrett B, Brown R, Rakel D, et al. Echinacea for treating the common cold: a randomized trial. *Annals of Internal Medicine* 2010 Dec 21;153(12):769–777.

14. Melchart D, Linde K, Fischer P, et al. Echinacea for preventing and treating the common cold. Cochrane Database of Systematic Reviews 2000;2:CD000530.

15. Schoneberger D. The influence of immune-stimulating effects of pressed juice from *Echinacea purpurea* on the course and severity of colds. Results of a double-blind study. *Forum Immunologie* 1992;8:2–12.

16. Hoheisel O, Sandberg M, Bertram S, et al. Echinagard treatment shortens the course of the common cold: a double-blind, placebo-controlled clinical trial. *European Journal of Clinical Research* 1997;9:261–268.

17. Taylor JA, Weber W, Standish L, et al. Efficacy and safety of echinacea in treating upper respiratory tract infections in children: a randomized controlled trial. *JAMA, The Journal of the American Medical Association* 2003;290:2824–2830.

18. Yale SH, Liu K. *Echinacea purpurea* therapy for the treatment of the common cold: a randomized, double-blind, placebo-controlled clinical trial. *Archives of Internal Medicine* 2004;164:1237–1241.

19. Sperber SJ, Shah LP, Gilbert RD, et al. *Echinacea purpurea* for prevention of experimental rhinovirus colds. *Clinical Infectious Diseases* 2004;38:1367–1371.

20. Lizogub VG, Riley DS, Heger M. Efficacy of a *Pelargonium sidoides* preparation in patients with the common cold: a randomized, double blind, placebo-controlled clinical trial. *Explore: The Journal of Science*

and Healing 2007 Nov–Dec; 3(6):573–584.

Congestive Heart Failure

1. Gorelik O, Almoznino-Sarafian D, Feder I, et al. Dietary intake of various nutrients in older patients with congestive heart failure. *Cardiology* 2003; 99:177–181.

2. Gottlieb SS, Baruch L, Kukin ML. Prognostic importance of serum magnesium concentration in patients with congestive heart failure. *Journal of the American College of Cardiology* 1990;16:827–831.

3. Gottlieb SS. Importance of magnesium in congestive heart failure. *American Journal of Cardiology* 1989;63:39G–42G.

4. Cohen N, Almoznino-Sarafian D, Zaidenstein R, et al. Serum magnesium aberrations in furosemide (frusemide) treated patients with congestive heart failure: pathophysiological correlates and prognostic evaluation. *Heart* 2003;89:411–416.

5. Oladapo OO, Falase AO. Serum and urinary magnesium during treatment of patients with chronic congestive heart failure. *African Journal of Medicine and Medical Sciences* 2000;29: 301–303.

6. Cohen N, Alon I, Almoznino-Sarafian D, et al. Metabolic and clinical effects of oral magnesium supplementation in furosemide-treated patients with severe congestive heart failure. *Clinical Cardiology* 2000;23:433–436.

7. Crippa G, Sverzellati E, Giorgi-Pierfranceschi M, et al. Magnesium and cardiovascular drugs: interactions and therapeutic role. *Annali Italiani di Medicina Interna* 1999;14:40–45.

8. Chen MF, Chen LT, Gold M. Plasma and erythrocyte thiamin concentration in geriatric outpatients. *Journal of the American College of Nutrition* 1996;15: 231–236.

9. Leslie D, Gheorghiade M. Is there a role for thiamine supplementation in the management of heart failure. *American Heart Journal* 1996;131:1248–1250.

10. Mendoza CE, Rodriguez F, Rosenberg DG. Reversal of refractory congestive heart failure after thiamine supplementation: report of a case and review of literature. *Journal of Cardiovascular Pharmacology and Therapeutics* 2003;8:313–316.

11. Zenuk C, Healey J, Donnelly J, et al. Thiamine deficiency in congestive heart failure patients receiving long term furosemide therapy. *The Canadian Journal of Clinical Pharmacology* 2003; 10:184–188.

12. Goa KL, Brogden RN. L-carnitine: a preliminary review of its pharmacokinetics, and its therapeutic use in ischemic cardiac disease and primary and secondary carnitine deficiencies in relationship to its role in fatty acid metabolism. *Drugs* 1987;34:1–24.

13. Mancini M, Rengo F, Lingetti M, et al. Controlled study on the therapeutic efficacy of propionyl-L-carnitine in patients with congestive heart failure. *Arzneimittelforschung* 1992;42:1101–1104.

14. Pucciarelli G, Matsursi M, Latte S, et al. [The clinical and hemodynamic effects of propionyl-L-carnitine in the treatment of congestive heart failure.] *La Clinica Terapeutica* 1992;141: 379–384.

15. Rizos I. Three-year survival of patients with heart failure caused by dilated cardiomyopathy and L-carnitine administration. *American Heart Journal* 2000;139(2 part 3):S120–S123.

16. Ishiyama T, Morital Y, Toyama S, et al. A clinical study of the effect of coenzyme Q on congestive heart failure. *Japanese Heart Journal* 1976;17:32–42.

17. Tsuyusaki T, Noro C, Kikawada R. Mechanocardiography of ischemic or hypertensive heart failure. In *Biomedical and clinical aspects of coenzyme Q*, vol. 2, ed. Yamamura Y, Folkers K, Ito Y. Amsterdam: Elsevier/North-Holland Biomedical Press, 1980, 273–288.

18. Judy WV, Stogsdill WW, Folkers K. Myocardial effects of co-enzyme Q_{10} in primary heart failure. In *Biomedical and clinical aspects of coenzyme Q*, vol. 4, ed. Folkers K, Yamamura Y. Amsterdam: Elsevier Science, 1984, 353–367.

19. Vanfraechem JHP, Picalausa C, Folkers K. Coenzyme Q_{10} and physical performance in myocardial failure. In *Biomedical and clinical aspects of coenzyme Q*, vol. 4, ed. Folkers K, Yamamura Y. Amsterdam: Elsevier Science, 1984:281–290.

20. Hofman-Bang C, Rehnquist N, Swedberg K, et al. Coenzyme Q_{10} as an adjunctive treatment of congestive heart failure. *Journal of Cardiac Failure* 1995;1: 101–107.

21. Morisco C, Trimarco B, Condorelli M. Effect of coenzyme Q_{10} therapy in patients with congestive heart failure. A long-term multicenter randomized study. *Clinical Investigation* 1993;71(8 suppl):S134–S136.

22. Baggio E, Gandini R, Plancher AC. Italian multicenter study on the safety and efficacy of coenzyme Q_{10} as adjunctive therapy in heart failure. *Molecular Aspects of Medicine* 1994;15: S287–S294.

23. Khatta M, Alexander BS, Krichten CM, et al. The effect of coenzyme Q10 in patients with congestive heart failure. *Annals of Internal Medicine* 2000;132: 636–640.

24. Langsjoen PH, Langsjoen AM. Supplemental ubiquinol in patients with advanced congestive heart failure. *Biofactors* 2008; 32(1–4):119–128.

25. Rector TS, Bank A, Mullen KA, et al. Randomized, double-blind, placebo-controlled study of supplemental oral L-arginine in

patients with heart failure. *Circulation* 1996; 93:2135–2141.

26. Hambrecht R, Hilbrich L, Erbs S, et al. Correction of endothelial dysfunction in chronic heart failure: additional effects of exercise training and oral L-arginine supplementation. *Journal of the American College of Cardiology* 2000;35:706–713.

27. Watanabe G, Tomiyama H, Doba N. Effects of oral administration of L-arginine on renal function in patients with heart failure. *Journal of Hypertension* 2000;18:229–234.

28. Schulman SP, Becker LC, Kass DA, et al. L-arginine therapy in acute myocardial infarction: the Vascular Interaction with Age in Myocardial Infarction (VINTAGE MI) randomized clinical trial. *JAMA, The Journal of the American Medical Association* 2006 Jan 4;295(1):58–64.

29. Leuchtgens H. Crataegus Special Extract WS 1442 in NYHA II heart failure: a placebo controlled randomized double-blind study. *Fortschritte der Medizin* 1993;111:352–354.

30. Tauchert M, Ploch M, Hubner WD. Effectiveness of the Hawthorn Extract LI 132 compared to ACE inhibitor Captopril: multicentre double-blind study with 132 NYHA Stage II. *Münchener Medizinische Wochenschrift* 1994;136 suppl 1:S27–S33.

31. Zick SM, Vautaw BM, Gillespie B, Aaronson KD. Hawthorn Extract Randomized Blinded Chronic Heart Failure (HERB CHF) trial. *European Journal of Heart Failure* 2009 Oct; 11(10):990–999.

32. Bharani A, Ganguly A, Bhargava KD. Salutary effect of *Terminalia arjuna* in patients with severe refractory heart failure. *International Journal of Cardiology* 1995;49:191–199.

Constipation

1. Suares NC, Ford AC. Systematic review: the effects of fibre in the management of chronic idiopathic constipation. *Alimentary Pharmacology & Therapeutics* 2011 Apr;33(8):895–901.

2. Attaluri A, Donahoe R, Valestin J, Brown K, Rao SS. Randomised clinical trial: dried plums (prunes) vs. psyllium for constipation. *Alimentary Pharmacology & Therapeutics* 2011 Apr;33(7):822–828.

3. Iacono G, Cavataio F, Montalto G, et al. Intolerance of cow's milk and chronic constipation in children. *The New England Journal of Medicine* 1998; 339(16):1100–1104.

Crohn's Disease and Ulcerative Colitis (Inflammatory Bowel Disease)

1. Jung C, Hugot JP. Inflammatory bowel diseases: the genetic revolution. *Gastroentérologie Clinique et Biologique* 2009 Jun;33 suppl 3:S123–S130.

2. Khor B, Gardet A, Xavier RJ. Genetics and pathogenesis of inflammatory bowel disease. *Nature* 2011 Jun 15;474(7351): 307–317.

3. Chassaing B, Darfeuille-Michaud A. The commensal microbiota and enteropathogens in the pathogenesis of inflammatory bowel diseases. *Gastroenterology* 2011 May;140(6): 1720–1728.

4. Shaw SY, Blanchard JF, Bernstein CN. Association between the use of antibiotics and new diagnoses of Crohn's disease and ulcerative colitis. *The American Journal of Gastroenterology* 2011 Dec;106(12): 2133–2142.

5. Hou JK, Abraham B, El-Serag H. Dietary intake and risk of developing inflammatory bowel disease: a systematic review of the literature. *The American Journal of Gastroenterology* 2011 Apr;106(4): 563–573.

6. Asakura H, Suzuki K, Kitahora T, Morizane T. Is there a link between food and intestinal microbes and the occurrence of Crohn's disease and ulcerative colitis? *Journal of Gastroenterology and Hepatology* 2008 Dec;23(12):1794–1801.

7. Cashman KD, Shanahan F. Is nutrition an aetiological factor for inflammatory bowel disease? *European Journal of Gastroenterology & Hepatology* 2003 Jun;15(6):607–613.

8. Thornton JR, Emmett PM, Heaton KW. Diet and Crohn's disease: characteristics of the pre-illness diet. *British Medical Journal* 1979;279:762–764.

9. Reif S, Klein I, Lubin F, et al. Pre-illness dietary factors in inflammatory bowel disease. *Gut* 1997;40:754–760.

10. Sakamoto N, Kono S, Wakai K, et al. Dietary risk factors for inflammatory bowel disease: a multicenter case-control study in Japan. *Inflammatory Bowel Diseases* 2005 Feb;11(2):154– 163.

11. Persson PG, Ahlbom A, Hellers G. Diet and inflammatory bowel disease: a case-control study. *Epidemiology* 1992;3: 47–52.

12. Shoda R, Matsueda K, Yamato S, Umeda N. Epidemiologic analysis of Crohn's disease in Japan. Increased dietary intake of w-6 polyunsaturated fatty acids and animal protein relates to the increased incidence of Crohn's disease in Japan. *The American Journal of Clinical Nutrition* 1996;63:741–745.

13. Meyers S, Janowitz HD. "Natural history" of Crohn's disease: an analytical review of the placebo lesson. *Gastroenterology* 1984;87:1189–1192.

14. Mekhjian HS, Switz DM, Melnyk CS, et al. Clinical features and natural history of Crohn's disease. *Gastroenterology* 1979; 77:898–906.

15. Malchow H, Ewe K, Brandes JW, et al. European Cooperative Crohn's Disease Study (ECCDS): results of drug treat-

ment. *Gastroenterology* 1984; 86:249–266.

16. Calder PC. Polyunsaturated fatty acids, inflammatory processes and inflammatory bowel diseases. *Molecular Nutrition & Food Research* 2008 Aug;52(8): 885–897.

17. Belluzzi A, Brignola C, Compieri M, et al. Effect of an enteric-coated fish oil preparation on relapses in Crohn's disease. *The New England Journal of Medicine* 1996;334: 1557–1560.

18. Loeschke K, Ueberschaer B, Pietsch A, et al. W-3 fatty acids only delay early relapse of ulcerative colitis in remission. *Digestive Diseases and Sciences* 1996;41:2087–2094.

19. Feagan BG, Sandborn WJ, Mittmann U, et al. Omega-3 free fatty acids for the maintenance of remission in Crohn disease: the EPIC Randomized Controlled Trials. *JAMA, The Journal of the American Medical Association* 2008 Apr 9;299(14): 1690–1697.

20. Podolsky DK, Isselbacher KJ. Glycoprotein composition of colonic mucosa. Specific alterations in ulcerative colitis. *Gastroenterology* 1984;87:991–998.

21. Kim YS, Byrd JC. Ulcerative colitis: a specific mucin defect? *Gastroenterology* 1984;87:1193–1195.

22. Boland CR, Lance P, Levin B, et al. Abnormal goblet cell glycoconjugates in rectal biopsies associated with an increased risk of neoplasia in patients with ulcerative colitis: early results of a prospective study. *Gut* 1984; 25:1364–1371.

23. Hentges DJ, ed. *Human intestinal microflora in health and disease.* New York: Academic Press, 1983.

24. Mottet NK. On animal models for inflammatory bowel disease [editorial]. *Gastroenterology* 1972;62:1269–1271.

25. Bentiz KR, Goldberg L, Coulston F. Intestinal effect

of carrageenans in the rhesus monkey (*Macaca mulatta*). *Food and Cosmetics Toxicology* 1973; 11:565–575.

26. Bonfils S. Carrageenan and the human gut. *The Lancet* 1970;2: 414.

27. Saller R, Meier R, Brignoli R. The use of silymarin in the treatment of liver diseases. *Drugs* 2001;61:2035–2063.

28. Valentini L, Schulzke JD. Mundane, yet challenging: the assessment of malnutrition in inflammatory bowel disease. *European Journal of Internal Medicine* 2011 Feb;22(1):13–15.

29. Zachos M, Tondeur M, Griffiths AM. Enteral nutritional therapy for inducing remission of Crohn's disease. Cochrane Database of Systematic Reviews 2001;3:CD000542.

30. Rajendran N, Kumar D. Role of diet in the management of inflammatory bowel disease. *World Journal of Gastroenterology* 2010 Mar 28;16(12): 1442–1448.

31. Mishkin S. Dairy sensitivity, lactose malabsorption, and elimination diets in inflammatory bowel disease. *The American Journal of Clinical Nutrition* 1997 Feb;65(2):564–567.

32. Voitk AJ, Echave V, Feller JH, et al. Experience with elemental diet in the treatment of inflammatory bowel disease. Is this primary therapy? *Archives of Surgery* 1973;107:329–333.

33. Borok G, Segal I. Inflammatory bowel disease. Individualized dietary therapy. *South African Family Practice* 1995;16:393–399.

34. Jones VA, Workman E, Freeman AH, et al. Crohn's disease: maintenance of remission by diet. *The Lancet* 1985;2:177–180.

35. Galvez J, Rodríguez-Cabezas ME, Zarzuelo A. Effects of dietary fiber on inflammatory bowel disease. *Molecular Nutrition & Food Research* 2005 Jun; 49(6):601–608.

36. Lih-Brody L, Powell SR, Collier

KP, et al. Increased oxidative stress and decreased antioxidant defenses in mucosa of inflammatory bowel disease. *Digestive Diseases and Sciences* 1996 Oct;41(10):2078–2086.

37. Romier B, Schneider YJ, Larondelle Y, During A. Dietary polyphenols can modulate the intestinal inflammatory response. *Nutrition Reviews* 2009 Jul;67(7):363–378.

38. Fleming CR, Huizenga KA, McCall JT, et al. Zinc nutrition in Crohn's disease. *Digestive Diseases and Sciences* 1981;26: 865–870.

39. Scrimgeour AG, Condlin ML. Zinc and micronutrient combinations to combat gastrointestinal inflammation. *Current Opinion in Clinical Nutrition and Metabolic Care* 2009 Nov; 12(6):653–660.

40. Franklin JL, Rosenberg IH. Impaired folic acid absorption in inflammatory bowel disease: effects of salicylazosulfapyridine (Azulfidine). *Gastroenterology* 1973;64:517–525.

41. Carruthers LB. Chronic diarrhea treated with folic acid. *The Lancet* 1946;1:849–850.

42. Filipsson S, Hulten L, Lindstedt G. Malabsorption of fat and vitamin B12 before and after intestinal resection for Crohn's disease. *Scandinavian Journal of Gastroenterology* 1978;13: 529–536.

43. Harries AD, Brown R, Heatley RV, et al. Vitamin D status in Crohn's disease: association with nutrition and disease activity. *Gut* 1985; 26:1197–1203.

44. Jørgensen SP, Agnholt J, Glerup H, et al. Clinical trial: vitamin D3 treatment in Crohn's disease—a randomized double-blind placebo-controlled study. *Alimentary Pharmacology & Therapeutics* 2010 Aug; 32(3):377–383.

45. Hallert C, Bjorck I, Nyman M, et al. Increasing fecal butyrate in ulcerative colitis patients by diet: controlled pilot study.

Inflammatory Bowel Diseases 2003 Mar;9(2):116–121.

46. Seidner DLH, Lashner BAH, Brzezinski AH, et al. An oral supplement enriched with fish oil, soluble fiber, and antioxidants for corticosteroid sparing in ulcerative colitis: a randomized, controlled trial. *Clinical Gastroenterology and Hepatology* 2005 Apr;3(4):358–369.

47. Bamba T, Kanauchi O, Andoh A, Fujiyama Y. A new prebiotic from germinated barley for nutraceutical treatment of ulcerative colitis. *Journal of Gastroenterology and Hepatology* 2002 Aug;17(8):818–824.

48. Kanauchi O, Mitsuyama K, Homma T, et al. Treatment of ulcerative colitis patients by long-term administration of germinated barley foodstuff: multicenter open trial. *International Journal of Molecular Medicine* 2003 Nov;12(5):701–704.

49. Hanai H, Kanauchi O, Mitsuyama K, et al. Germinated barley foodstuff prolongs remission in patients with ulcerative colitis. *International Journal of Molecular Medicine* 2004 May; 13(5):643–647.

50. Furrie E, Macfarlane S, Kennedy A, et al. Synbiotic therapy (*Bifidobacterium longum*/Synergy 1) initiates resolution of inflammation in patients with active ulcerative colitis: a randomised controlled pilot trial. *Gut* 2005 Feb;54(2):242–249.

51. Cain AM, Karpa KD. Clinical utility of probiotics in inflammatory bowel disease. *Alternative Therapies in Health and Medicine* 2011 Jan–Feb;17(1):72–79.

52. Guandalini S. Update on the role of probiotics in the therapy of pediatric inflammatory bowel disease. *Expert Review of Clinical Immunology* 2010 Jan;6(1): 47–54.

53. Hegazy SK, El-Bedewy MM. Effect of probiotics on proinflammatory cytokines and NF-kappaB activation in ulcerative colitis. *World Journal of Gastroenterology* 2010 Sep 7; 16(33):4145–4151.

54. Sood A, Midha V, Makharia GK, et al. The probiotic preparation VSL#3 induces remission in patients with mild-to-moderately active ulcerative colitis. *Clinical Gastroenterology and Hepatology* 2009 Nov;7(11): 1202–1209.

55. Fujimori S, Gudis K, Mitsui K, et al. A randomized controlled trial on the efficacy of synbiotic versus probiotic or prebiotic treatment to improve the quality of life in patients with ulcerative colitis. *Nutrition* 2009 May;25(5):520–525.

56. Tsuda Y, Yoshimatsu Y, Aoki H, et al. Clinical effectiveness of probiotics therapy (BIO-THREE) in patients with ulcerative colitis refractory to conventional therapy. *Scandinavian Journal of Gastroenterology* 2007 Nov;42(11): 1306–1311.

57. Guslandi M, Mezzi G, Sorghi M, Testoni PA. *Saccharomyces boulardii* in maintenance treatment of Crohn's disease. *Digestive Diseases and Sciences* 2000;45:1462–1464.

58. Guandalini S. Use of *Lactobacillus*-GG in paediatric Crohn's disease. *Digestive and Liver Disease* 2002;34 suppl 2:S63–S65.

59. Wahed M, Corser M, Goodhand JR, Rampton DS. Does psychological counseling alter the natural history of inflammatory bowel disease? *Inflammatory Bowel Diseases* 2010 Apr;16(4): 664–669.

60. Jobin C, Bradham CA, Russo MP, et al. Curcumin blocks cytokine-mediated NF-kappa B activation and proinflammatory gene expression by inhibiting inhibitory factor I-kappa B kinase activity. *The Journal of Immunology* 1999;163(6):3474–3483.

61. Sugimoto K, Hanai H, Tozawa K, et al. Curcumin prevents and ameliorates trinitrobenzene sulfonic acid-induced colitis in mice. *Gastroenterology* 2002; 123(6):1912–1922.

62. Jian YT, Mai GF, Wang JD, et al. Preventive and therapeutic effects of NF-kappaB inhibitor curcumin in rats colitis induced by trinitrobenzene sulfonic acid. *World Journal of Gastroenterology* 2005;11(12):1747–1752.

63. Zhang M, Deng C, Zheng J, et al. Curcumin inhibits trinitrobenzene sulphonic acid-induced colitis in rats by activation of peroxisome proliferator-activated receptor gamma. *International Immunopharmacology* 2006; 6(8):1233–1242.

64. Holt PR, Katz S, Kirshoff R. Curcumin therapy in inflammatory bowel disease: a pilot study. *Digestive Diseases and Sciences* 2005;50(11):2191–2193.

65. Hanai H, Iida T, Takeuchi K, et al. Curcumin maintenance therapy for ulcerative colitis: randomized, multicenter, double-blind, placebo-controlled trial. *Clinical Gastroenterology and Hepatology* 2006;4(12): 1502–1506.

66. Ammon HPH. [Boswellic acids (components of frankincense) as the active principle in treatment of chronic inflammatory diseases.] *Wiener Medizinische Wochenschrift* 2002;152(15–16):373–378.

67. Gupta I, Parihar A, Malhotra P, et al. Effects of gum resin of *Boswellia serrata* in patients with chronic colitis. *Planta Medica* 2001 Jul;67(5):391–395.

68. Gupta I, Parihar A, Malhotra P, et al. Effects of *Boswellia serrata* gum resin in patients with ulcerative colitis. *European Journal of Medical Research* 1997 Jan;2(1):37–43.

69. Gerhardt H, Seifert F, Buvari P, et al. [Therapy of active Crohn disease with *Boswellia serrata* extract H 15.] *Zeitschrift für Gastroenterologie* 2001 Jan; 39(1):11–17.

70. Langmead L, Makins RJ, Rampton DS. Anti-inflammatory effects of aloe vera gel

in human colorectal mucosa in vitro. *Alimentary Pharmacology & Therapeutics* 2004 Mar 1;19(5):521–527.

71. Langmead L, Feakins RM, Goldthorpe S, et al. Randomized, double-blind, placebo-controlled trial of oral aloe vera gel for active ulcerative colitis. *Alimentary Pharmacology & Therapeutics* 2004 Apr 1;19(7): 739–747.

72. Robinson M. Medical therapy of inflammatory bowel disease for the 21st century. *European Journal of Surgery* 1998 suppl; 582:90–98.

73. Tibble JA, Bjarnason I. Noninvasive investigation of inflammatory bowel disease. *World Journal of Gastroenterology* 2001;7:460–465.

74. Best WR, Becktel JM, Singleton JW, Kern F. Development of a Crohn's disease activity index. *Gastroenterology* 1976;70:439–444.

Cystitis and Interstitial Cystitis/Painful Bladder

1. Nickel JC. Interstitial cystitis: a chronic pelvic pain syndrome. *Medical Clinics of North America* 2004;88:467–481.

2. Bogart LM, Berry SH, Clemens JQ. Symptoms of interstitial cystitis, painful bladder syndrome and similar diseases in women: a systematic review. *Journal of Urology* 2007;177:450–456.

3. Driscoll A, Teichman JMH. How do patients with interstitial cystitis present? *Journal of Urology* 2001;166:2118–2120.

4. Herati A, Shorter B, Tai J, et al. Differences in food sensitivities between IC/PBS and CP/CPPS. *Journal of Urology* 2009;181 suppl 4:60.

5. Shorter B, Lesser M, Moldwin R, Kushner, L. Effect of comestibles on symptoms of interstitial cystitis. *Journal of Urology* 2007;178(1):145–152.

6. Aziz-Fam A. Use of titrated extract of *Centella asiatica* (TECA) in bilharzial bladder

lesions. *International Surgery* 1973;58:451–452.

7. Etrebi A, Ibrahim A and Zaki K. Treatment of bladder ulcer with asiaticoside. *The Journal of the Egyptian Medical Association* 1975;58:324–327.

8. Munday PE, Savage S. Cymalon in the management of urinary tract symptoms. *Genitourinary Medicine* 1990;66:461.

9. Spooner JB. Alkalinization in the management of cystitis. *Journal of International Medical Research* 1984;12:30–34.

10. Guay DR. Cranberry and urinary tract infections. *Drugs* 2009;69:775–807.

11. Sobota AE. Inhibition of bacterial adherence by cranberry juice: potential use for the treatment of urinary tract infections. *Journal of Urology* 1984;131: 1013–1016.

12. Schmidt DR, Sobota AE. An examination of the anti-adherence activity of cranberry juice on urinary and nonurinary bacterial isolates. *Microbios* 1988;55: 173–181.

13. Habash MB, Van der Mei HC, Busscher HJ, et al. The effect of water, ascorbic acid, and cranberry derived supplementation on human urine and uropathogen adhesion to silicone rubber. *Canadian Journal of Microbiology* 1999;45:691–694.

14. Sharon N, Ofek I. Fighting infectious diseases with inhibitors of microbial adhesion to host tissues. *Critical Reviews in Food Science and Nutrition* 2002;42 suppl:267–272.

15. Stothers L. A randomized trial to evaluate effectiveness and cost effectiveness of naturopathic cranberry products as prophylaxis against urinary tract infection in women. *The Canadian Journal of Urology* 2002;9: 1558–1562.

16. Avorn J, Monane M, Gurwitz JH, et al. Reduction of bacteriuria and pyuria after ingestion of cranberry juice. *JAMA, The Journal of the American*

Medical Association 1994;271: 751–754.

17. Barbosa-Cesnik C, Brown MB, Buxton M, et al. Cranberry juice fails to prevent recurrent urinary tract infection: results from a randomized placebo-controlled trial. *Clinical Infectious Diseases* 2011 Jan;52(1): 23–30.

18. Kraemer RJ. Cranberry juice and the reduction of ammoniacal odor of urine. *Southwest Medicine* 1964;45:211–212.

19. DuGan CR, Cardaciotto PS. Reduction of ammoniacal urinary odors by the sustained feeding of cranberry juice. *Journal of Psychiatric Nursing* 1966; 8:467–470.

20. Parejo I, Viladomat F, Bastida J, et al. A single extraction step in the quantitative analysis of arbutin in bearberry (*Arctostaphylos uva-ursi*) leaves by high-performance liquid chromatography. *Phytochemical Analysis* 2001;12: 336–339.

21. Larsson B, Jonasson A, Fianu S. Prophylactic effect of UVA-E in women with recurrent cystitis: a preliminary report. *Current Therapeutic Research* 1993;53: 441–443.

22. Amin AH, Subbaiah TV, Abbasi KM. Berberine sulfate: antimicrobial activity, bioassay, and mode of action. *Canadian Journal of Microbiology* 1969;15: 1067–1076.

23. Johnson CC, Johnson G, Poe CF. Toxicity of alkaloids to certain bacteria. II. Berberine, physostigmine, and sanguinarine. *Acta Pharmacologica et Toxicologica* 1952;8:71–78.

Depression

1. Seligman M. *Learned optimism*. New York: Knopf, 1991.

2. Peterson C, Seligman M, Vaillant G. Pessimistic explanatory style is a risk factor for physical illness: a thirty-five year longitudinal study. *Journal of Personality and Social Psychology* 1988; 55:23–27.

3. Moncrieff J, Cohen D. Do antidepressants cure or create abnormal brain states? *PLoS Med* 2006 Jul;3(7):e240.

4. Middleton H, Moncrieff J. "They won't do any harm and might do some good": time to think again on the use of antidepressants? *British Journal of General Practice* 2011 Jan;61(582):47–49.

5. Möller HJ. Is there evidence for negative effects of antidepressants on suicidality in depressive patients? A systematic review. *European Archives of Psychiatry and Clinical Neuroscience* 2006 Dec;256(8):476–496.

6. Fournier JC, DeRubeis RJ, Hollon SD, et al. Antidepressant drug effects and depression severity: a patient-level meta-analysis. *JAMA, The Journal of the American Medical Association* 2010;303(1):47–53.

7. Schwartz TL, Nihalani N, Jindal S, et al. Psychiatric medication-induced obesity: a review. *Obesity Reviews* 2004;5(2):115–121.

8. Raeder MB, Bjelland I, Emil Vollset S, Steen VM. Obesity, dyslipidemia, and diabetes with selective serotonin reuptake inhibitors: the Hordaland Health Study. *Journal of Clinical Psychiatry* 2006;67(12):1974

9. Jarrett RB, Rush AJ. Short-term psychotherapy of depressive disorders: current status and future directions. *Psychiatry* 1994;57:115–132.

10. Robins CJ, Hayes AM. An appraisal of cognitive therapy. *Journal of Consulting and Clinical Psychology* 1993;61:205–214.

11. Evans M, Hollon SD, DeRubeis RJ, et al. Differential relapse following cognitive therapy and pharmacotherapy for depression. *Archives of General Psychiatry* 1992;49:802–808.

12. Gold M, Pottash A, Extein I. Hypothyroidism and depression, evidence from complete thyroid function evaluation. *JAMA, The Journal of the American Medical Association* 1981;245:1919–1922.

13. Joffe R, Roy-Byrne P, Udhe T, et al. Thyroid function and affective illness: a reappraisal. *Biological Psychiatry* 1984;19:1685–1691.

14. Altar C, Bennett B, Wallace R, et al. Glucocorticoid induction of tryptophan oxygenase. Attenuation by intragastrically administered carbohydrates and metabolites. *Biochemical Pharmacology* 1983;32:979–984.

15. Schottenfeld RS, Cullen MR. Organic affective illness associated with lead intoxication. *The American Journal of Psychiatry* 1984;141:1423–1426.

16. Rutter M, Russell-Jones R, eds. *Lead versus health: sources and effects of low level lead exposure.* New York: John Wiley, 1983.

17. Seaton A, Jellinek EH, Kennedy P. Major neurological disease and occupational exposure to organic solvents. *Quarterly Journal of Medicine* 1992;305:707–712.

18. Nunes EV, Levin FR. Treatment of depression in patients with alcohol or other drug dependence: a meta-analysis. *JAMA, The Journal of the American Medical Association* 2004;291:1887–1896.

19. Chou T. Wake up and smell the coffee: caffeine, coffee, and the medical consequences. *Western Journal of Medicine* 1992;157:544–553.

20. Gilliland K, Bullock W. Caffeine: a potential drug of abuse. *Advances in Alcohol & Substance Abuse* 1984;3:53–73.

21. Greden J, Fontaine P, Lubetsky M, et al. Anxiety and depression associated with caffeinism among psychiatric inpatients. *The American Journal of Psychiatry* 1978;135:963–966.

22. Neil JF, Himmelhoch JM, Mallinger AG, et al. Caffeinism complicating hypersomnic depressive episodes. *Comprehensive Psychiatry* 1978;19:377–385.

23. Charney D, Heninger G, Jatlow P. Increased anxiogenic effects of caffeine in panic disorders. *Archives of General Psychiatry* 1985;42:233–243.

24. Bolton S, Null G. Caffeine, psychological effects, use and abuse. *Orthomolecular Psychiatry* 1981;10:202–211.

25. Kreitsch K. Prevalence, presenting symptoms, and psychological characteristics of individuals experiencing a diet-related mood disturbance. *Behavior Therapy* 1985;19:593–594.

26. Christensen L. Psychological distress and diet—effects of sucrose and caffeine. *Journal of Applied Nutrition* 1988;40:44–50.

27. Martin JE, Dubbert PM. Exercise applications and promotion in behavioral medicine: current status and future directions. *Journal of Consulting and Clinical Psychology* 1982;50:1004–1017.

28. Onyike CU, Crum RM, Lee HB, et al. Is obesity associated with major depression? Results from the Third National Health and Nutrition Examination Survey. *American Journal of Epidemiology* 2003;158:1139–1147.

29. Weyerer S, Kupfer B. Physical exercise and psychological health. *Sports Medicine* 1994;17:108–116.

30. Carr DB, Bullen BA, Skrinar GS, et al. Physical conditioning facilitates the exercise-induced secretion of beta-endorphin and beta-lipotropin in women. *The New England Journal of Medicine* 1981;305:560–563.

31. Lobstein DD, Mosbacher BJ, Ismail AH. Depression as a powerful discriminator between physically active and sedentary middle-aged men. *Journal of Psychosomatic Research* 1983;27:69–76.

32. Folkins CH, Sime WE. Physical fitness training and mental health. *American Psychologist* 1981;36:373–389.

33. Martinsen EW. The role of aerobic exercise in the treatment of depression. *Stress Medicine* 1987;3:93–100.

34. Byrne A, Byrne DG. The effect of exercise on depression, anxiety and other mood states: a review. *Journal of Psychosomatic Research* 1993;37:565–574.

35. Casper RC. Exercise and mood. *World Review of Nutrition and Dietetics* 1993;71:115–143.

36. Sánchez-Villegas A, Delgado-Rodríguez M, Alonso A, et al. Association of the Mediterranean dietary pattern with the incidence of depression. *Archives of General Psychiatry* 2009;66(10):1090–1098.

37. Hadji-Georgopoulus A, Schmidt MI, Margolis S, et al. Elevated hypoglycemic index and late hyperinsulinism in symptomatic postprandial hypoglycemia. *The Journal of Clinical Endocrinology & Metabolism* 1980;50:371–376.

38. Fabrykant M. The problem of functional hyperinsulinism on functional hypoglycemia attributed to nervous causes. 1. Laboratory and clinical correlations. *Metabolism* 1955;4:469–479.

39. Westover AN, Marangell LB. A cross-national relationship between sugar consumption and major depression? *Depression and Anxiety* 2002;16:118–120.

40. Werbach M. *Nutritional influences on mental illness: a sourcebook of clinical research.* Tarzana, Calif.: Third Line Press, 1991.

41. Crellin R, Bottiglieri T, Reynolds EH. Folates and psychiatric disorders: clinical potential. *Drugs* 1993;45:623–636.

42. Carney MW, Chary TK, Laundy M, et al. Red cell folate concentrations in psychiatric patients. *Journal of Affective Disorders* 1990;19:207–213.

43. Godfrey PS, Toone BK, Carney MW, et al. Enhancement of recovery from psychiatric illness by methylfolate. *The Lancet* 1990;336:392–395.

44. Reynolds E, Preece J, Bailey J, et al. Folate deficiency in depressive illness. *The British Journal of Psychiatry* 1970;117:287–292.

45. Thornton WE, Thornton BP. Geriatric mental function and serum folate: a review and survey. *Southern Medical Journal* 1977;70:919–922.

46. Abalan F, Subra G, Picard M, et al. [Incidence of vitamin B12 and folic acid deficiencies in old aged psychiatric patients.] *L'Encéphale* 1984;10:9–12.

47. Zucker D, Livingston R, Nakra R, et al. B12 deficiency and psychiatric disorders: case report and literature review. *Biological Psychiatry* 1981;16:197–205.

48. Kivela SL, Pahkala K, Eronen A. Depression in the aged: relation to folate and vitamins C and B12. *Biological Psychiatry* 1989;26:210–213.

49. Curtius H, Niederwieser A, Levine R, et al. Successful treatment of depression with tetrahydrobiopterin. *The Lancet* 1983;1:657–658.

50. Leeming R, Harpey J, Brown S, et al. Tetrahydrofolate and hydroxocobalamin in the management of dihydropteridine reductase deficiency. *Journal of Mental Deficiency Research* 1982;26:21–25.

51. Botez M, Young S, Bachevalier J, et al. Effect of folic acid and vitamin B12 deficiencies on 5-hydroxyindoleacetic acid in human cerebrospinal fluid. *Annals of Neurology* 1982;12:479–484.

52. Reynolds E, Stramentinoli G. Folic acid, S-adenosylmethionine and affective disorder. *Psychological Medicine* 1983;13:705–710.

53. Reynolds E, Carney M, Toone B. Methylation and mood. *The Lancet* 1984;2:196–198.

54. Taylor MJ, Carney S, Geddes J, et al. Folate for depressive disorders. Cochrane Database of Systematic Reviews 2003;2:CD003390.

55. Crellin R, Bottiglieri T, Reynolds EH. Folates and psychiatric disorders: clinical potential. *Drugs* 1993;45:623–636.

56. Russ C, Hendricks T, Chrisley B, et al. Vitamin B6 status of depressed and obsessive-compulsive patients. *Nutrition Reports International* 1983;27:867–873.

57. Carney MW, Williams DG, Sheffield BF. Thiamine and pyridoxine lack in newly-admitted psychiatric patients. *The British Journal of Psychiatry* 1979;135:249–254.

58. Nobbs B. Letter: Pyridoxal phosphate status in clinical depression. *The Lancet* 1974;1:405–406.

59. Carney MW, Williams DG, Sheffield BF. Thiamine and pyridoxine lack newly-admitted psychiatric patients. *The British Journal of Psychiatry* 1979;135:249–254.

60. Stewart JW, Harrison W, Quitkin F, et al. Low B6 levels in depressed outpatients. *Biological Psychiatry* 1984;19:613–616.

61. Prasad AS. Clinical, biochemical and nutritional spectrum of zinc deficiency in human subjects: an update. *Nutrition Reviews* 1983;41:197–208.

62. Nowak G, Schlegel-Zawadzka M. Alterations in serum and brain trace element levels after antidepressant treatment. Part I. Zinc. *Biological Trace Element Research* 1999;67:85–92.

63. Nowak G, Szewczyk B. Mechanism contributing to antidepressant zinc actions. *Polish Journal of Pharmacology* 2002;54:587–592.

64. Nowak G, Siwek M, Dudek D, et al. Effect of zinc supplementation on antidepressant therapy in unipolar depression: a preliminary placebo-controlled study. *Polish Journal of Pharmacology* 2003;55:1143–1147.

65. Sher L. Role of selenium depletion in the etiopathogenesis of depression in patient with alcoholism. *Medical Hypotheses* 2002;59:330–333.

66. Finley JW, Penland JG. Adequacy or deprivation of dietary selenium in healthy men: clinical and psychological findings. *The Journal of Trace Elements in Experimental Medicine* 1998; 11:11–27.

67. Davidson JR, Abraham K, Connor KM, et al. Effectiveness of chromium in atypical depression: a placebo-controlled trial. *Biological Psychiatry* 2003;53: 261–264.

68. McLeod MN, Golden RN. Chromium treatment of depression. *The International Journal of Neuropsychopharmacology* 2000;3:311–314.

69. Harms LR, Burne TH, Eyles DW, McGrath JJ. Vitamin D and the brain. *Best Practice & Research: Clinical Endocrinology & Metabolism* 2011;25(4): 657–669.

70. Jordea R, Snevea M, Figenschaua Y, et al. Effects of vitamin D supplementation on symptoms of depression in obese subjects: randomized double blind trial. *Journal of Internal Medicine* 2008;264(6): 599–609.

71. Hoang MT, Defina LF, Willis BL, et al. Association between low serum 25-hydroxyvitamin d and depression in a large sample of healthy adults: the Cooper Center Longitudinal Study. *Mayo Clinic Proceedings* 2011 Nov;86(11):1050–1055.

72. Arvold DS, Odean MJ, Dornfeld MP, et al. Correlation of symptoms with vitamin D deficiency and symptom response to cholecalciferol treatment: a randomized controlled trial. *Endocrine Practice* 2009 Apr; 15(3):203–212.

73. Sanders KM, Stuart AL, Williamson EJ, et al. Annual high-dose vitamin D3 and mental wellbeing: randomised controlled trial. *The British Journal of Psychiatry* 2011 May;198(5): 357–364.

74. Freeman MP, Rapaport MH. Omega-3 fatty acids and depression: from cellular mechanisms to clinical care. *Journal of Clinical Psychiatry* 2011 Feb; 72(2):258–259.

75. Maes M, Christophe A, Delanghe J, et al. Lowered omega-3 polyunsaturated fatty acids in serum phospholipids and cholesteryl esters of depressed patients. *Psychiatry Research* 1999;85:275–291.

76. Nemets B, Stahl Z, Belmaker RH. Addition of omega-3 fatty acid to maintenance medication treatment for recurrent unipolar depressive disorder. *The American Journal of Psychiatry* 2002; 159:477–479.

77. Severus WE, Ahrens B, Stoll AL. Omega-3 fatty acids: the missing link? *Archives of General Psychiatry* 1999;56:380–381.

78. Baldessarini RJ. Neuropharmacology of S-adenosyl-L-methionine. *The American Journal of Medicine* 1987;83 suppl 5A: 95–103.

79. Reynolds E, Carney M, Toone B. Methylation and mood. *The Lancet* 1984;2:196–198.

80. Bottiglieri T, Laundy M, Martin R, et al. S-adenosylmethionine influences monoamine metabolism. *The Lancet* 1984;2:224.

81. Janicak PG, Lipinski J, Davis JM, et al. Parenteral S-adenosyl-methionine (SAMe) in depression: literature review and preliminary data. *Psychopharmacology Bulletin* 1989;25: 238–242.

82. Friedel HA, Goa KL, Benfield P. S-adenosyl-L-methionine. *Drugs* 1989;38:389–416.

83. Carney MW, Toone BK, Reynolds EH. S-adenosylmethionine and affective disorder. *The American Journal of Medicine* 1987;83 suppl 5A:104–106.

84. Vahora SA, Malek-Ahmadi P. S-adenosylmethionine in the treatment of depression. *Neuroscience & Biobehavioral Reviews* 1988;12:139–141.

85. Nguyen M, Gregan A. S-adenosylmethionine and depression. *Australian Family Physician* 2002;31:339–343.

86. Kagan BL, Sultzer DL, Rosenlicht N, et al. Oral S-adenosylmethionine in depression: a randomized, double-blind, placebo-controlled trial. *The American Journal of Psychiatry* 1990;147:591–595.

87. Rosenbaum JF, Fava M, Falk WE, et al. An open-label pilot study of oral S-adenosyl-L-methionine in major depression: interim results. *Psychopharmacology Bulletin* 1988;24:189–194.

88. De Vanna M, Rigamonti R. Oral S-adenosyl-L-methionine in depression. *Current Therapeutic Research* 1992;52:478–485.

89. Salmaggi P, Bressa GM, Nicchia G, et al. Double-blind, placebo-controlled study of S-adenosyl-L-methionine in depressed postmenopausal women. *Psychotherapy and Psychosomatics* 1993;59:34–40.

90. Bell KM, Potkin SG, Carreon D, et al. S-adenosylmethionine blood levels in major depression: changes with drug treatment. *Acta Neurologica Scandinavica* 1994 suppl;154: 15–18.

91. Rowe AH, Rowe A, Jr. *Food allergy: its manifestations and control and the elimination diets: a compendium.* Springfield, Ill.: Charles C. Thomas, 1972.

92. Brostoff J, Challacombe SJ, eds. *Food allergy and intolerance.* Philadelphia: W. B. Saunders, 1987.

93. Hertzman PA, Blevins WL, Mayer J, et al. Association of the eosinophilia-myalgia syndrome with the ingestion of tryptophan. *The New England Journal of Medicine* 1990;322:869–873.

94. Kilbourne EM. Eosinophilia-myalgia syndrome: coming to grips with a new illness. *Epidemiologic Reviews* 1992;14: 16–36.

95. Kilbourne EM, Philen RM, Kamb ML, et al. Tryptophan

produced by Showa Denko and epidemic eosinophilia-myalgia syndrome. *The Journal of Rheumatology* 1996 suppl;46:81–88.

96. Filippini GA, Costa CVL, Bertazzo A, eds. *Recent advances in tryptophan research: tryptophan and serotonin pathways.* New York: Plenum Press, 1996.

97. Eosinophilic-myalgia syndrome: review and reappraisal of Clinical, Epidemiologic and Animal Studies Symposium. Washington, D.C., December 7–8, 1994. Proceedings. *The Journal of Rheumatology* 1996 Oct;46 suppl:1–110.

98. Belongia EA, Hedberg CW, Gleich GJ, et al. An investigation of the cause of the eosinophilia-myalgia syndrome associated with tryptophan use. *The New England Journal of Medicine* 1990;323:357–365.

99. Silver RM, McKinley K, Smith EA, et al. Tryptophan metabolism via the kynurenine pathway in patients with the eosinophilia-myalgia syndrome. *Arthritis & Rheumatism* 1992; 35:1097–1105.

100. Hertzman PA. The eosinophilia-myalgia syndrome and the toxic oil syndrome. Pursuing parallels. *Advances in Experimental Medicine and Biology* 1996; 398:339–342.

101. Hatch DL, Goldman LR. Reduced severity of eosinophilia-myalgia syndrome associated with the consumption of vitamin-containing supplements before illness. *Archives of Internal Medicine* 1993;153:2368–2373.

102. Boman B. L-tryptophan: a rational anti-depressant and a natural hypnotic? *Australian and New Zealand Journal of Psychiatry* 1988;22:83–97.

103. Moller S, Kirk L, Brandrup E, et al. Tryptophan availability in endogenous depression—relation to efficacy of L-tryptophan treatment. *Advances in Biological Psychiatry* 1983;10:30–46.

104. d'Elia G, Hanson L, Raotma H. L-tryptophan and 5-hydroxy-tryptophan in the treatment of depression. A review. *Acta Psychiatrica Scandinavica* 1978;57:239–252.

105. Carroll BJ. Monoamine precursors in the treatment of depression. *Clinical Pharmacology & Therapeutics* 1971;12:743–761.

106. van Praag HM. Studies in the mechanism of action of serotonin precursors in depression. *Psychopharmacology Bulletin* 1984;20:599–602.

107. van Praag HM. Central monoamine metabolism in depressions. I. Serotonin and related compounds. *Comprehensive Psychiatry* 1980;21:30–43.

108. Agazzi A, De Ponti F, De Giorgio R, et al. Review of the implications of dietary tryptophan intake in patients with irritable bowel syndrome and psychiatric disorders. *Digestive and Liver Disease* 2003;35:590–595.

109. van Hiele LJ. 1–5-Hydroxytryptophan in depression: the first substitution therapy in psychiatry? The treatment of 99 outpatients with "therapy-resistant" depressions. *Neuropsychobiology* 1980;6:230–240.

110. Byerley WF, Judd LL, Reimherr FW, et al. 5-hydroxytryptophan: a review of its antidepressant efficacy and adverse effects. *Journal of Clinical Psychopharmacology* 1987;7:127–137.

111. van Praag HM. Management of depression with serotonin precursors. *Biological Psychiatry* 1981;16:291–310.

112. Poldinger W, Calanchini B, Schwarz W. A functional-dimensional approach to depression: serotonin deficiency as a target syndrome in a comparison of 5-hydroxytryptophan and fluvoxamine. *Psychopathology* 1991;24:53–81.

113. van Praag HM, Lemus C. Monoamine precursors in the treatment of psychiatric disorders. In *Nutrition and the brain*, vol. 7, ed. Wurtman RJ, Wurtman JJ. New York: Raven Press, 1986, 89–139.

114. Takahashi S, Kondo H, Kato N. Effect of L-5-hydroxytryptophan on brain monoamine metabolism and evaluation of its clinical effect in depressed patients. *Journal of Psychiatric Research* 1975;12:177–187.

115. Fujiwara J, Otsuki S. Subtype of affective psychosis classified by response on amine precursors and monoamine metabolism. *Journal of Oral Pathology* 1973; 2:93–100.

116. Nakajima T, Kudo Y, Kaneko Z. Clinical evaluation of 5-hydroxy-L-tryptophan as an antidepressant drug. *Folia Psychiatrica et Neurologica Japonica* 1978;32: 223–230.

117. Kaneko M, Kumashiro H, Takahashi Y, Hoshino Y. L-5-HTP treatment and serum 5-HTP level after L-5-HTP loading on depressed patients. *Neuropsychobiology* 1979;5:232–240.

118. Alino JJ, Gutierrez JL, Iglesias ML. 5-hydroxytryptophan (5-HTP) and a MAOI (nialamide) in the treatment of depressions. A double-blind controlled study. *International Pharmacopsychiatry* 1976;11:8–15.

119. van Praag HM, Korf J. 5-hydroxytryptophan as an antidepressant. The predictive value of the probenecid test. *The Journal of Nervous and Mental Disease* 1974; 158:331–337.

120. van Praag HM, Korf J. Serotonin metabolism in depression: clinical application of the probenecid test. *International Pharmacopsychiatry* 1974;9: 35–51.

121. Kielholz P. Treatment for therapy-resistant depression. *Psychopathology* 1986;19:194–200.

122. Linde K. St. John's wort—an overview. *Forschende Komplementärmedizin* 2009 Jun;16(3): 146–155.

123. Linde K, Berner MM, Kriston L. St John's wort for major depression. Cochrane Database of Systematic Reviews 2008 Oct 8;4:CD000448.

124. Kasper S, Caraci F, Forti B,

Drago F, Aguglia E. Efficacy and tolerability of *Hypericum* extract for the treatment of mild to moderate depression. *European Neuropsychopharmacology* 2010 Nov;20(11):747–765.

125. Trautmann-Sponsel RD, Dienel A. Safety of *Hypericum* extract in mildly to moderately depressed outpatients: a review based on data from three randomized, placebo-controlled trials. *Journal of Affective Disorders* 2004 Oct 15;82(2):303–307.

126. Solomon D, Ford E, Adams J, Graves N. Potential of St John's wort for the treatment of depression: the economic perspective. *Australian and New Zealand Journal of Psychiatry* 2011 Feb;45(2):123–130.

127. Hypericum Depression Trial Study Group. Effect of *Hypericum perforatum* (St John's wort) in major depressive disorder: a randomized controlled trial. *JAMA, The Journal of the American Medical Association* 2002;287(14):1807–1814.

128. Gastpar M, Singer A, Zeller K. Efficacy and tolerability of hypericum extract STW3 in long-term treatment with a once-daily dosage in comparison with sertraline. *Pharmacopsychiatry* 2005;38(2):78–86.

129. Szegedi A, Kohnen R, Dienel A, Kieser M. Acute treatment of moderate to severe depression with hypericum extract WS 5570 (St John's wort): randomised controlled double blind non-inferiority trial versus paroxetine. *BMJ* 2005;330(7490):503.

130. DeFeudis FV, ed. Ginkgo biloba extract (EGb 761): pharmacological activities and clinical applications. Paris: Elsevier, 1991.

131. Funfgeld EW, ed. *Rokan (Ginkgo biloba): recent results in pharmacology and clinic.* New York: Springer-Verlag, 1988.

132. Kleijnen J, Knipschild P. *Ginkgo biloba. The Lancet* 1992;340:1136–1139.

133. Kleijnen J, Knipschild P. *Ginkgo biloba* for cerebral insufficiency. *British Journal of Clinical Pharmacology* 1992;34:352–358.

134. Schubert H, Halama P. [Depressive episode primarily unresponsive to therapy in elderly patients: efficacy of *Ginkgo biloba* (Egb 761) in combination with antidepressants.] *Geriatric Forschung* 1993;3:45–53.

135. Huguet F, Drieu K, Piriou A, et al. Decreased cerebral 5-HT1a receptors during aging: reversal by *Ginkgo biloba* extract (EGb 761). *Journal of Pharmacy and Pharmacology* 1994;46:316–318.

136. Noorbala AA, Akhondzadeh S. Hydro-alcoholic extract of *Crocus sativus* L. versus fluoxetine in the treatment of mild to moderate depression: a double-blind, randomized pilot trial. *Journal of Ethnopharmacology* 2005 Feb 28;97(2):281–284.

137. Akhondzadeh S, Fallah-Pour H. Comparison of *Crocus sativus* L. and imipramine in the treatment of mild to moderate depression: a pilot double-blind randomized trial [ISRCTN45683816]. *BMC Complementary and Alternative Medicine* 2004 Sep 2;4:12.

138. Moshiri E, Basti AA, Noorbala AA, et al. *Crocus sativus* L. (petal) in the treatment of mild-to-moderate depression: a double-blind, randomized and placebo-controlled trial. *Phytomedicine* 2006;13:607–611.

139. Akhondzadeh Basti A, Moshiri E. Comparison of petal of *Crocus sativus* L. and fluoxetine in the treatment of depressed outpatients: a pilot double-blind randomized trial. *Progress in Neuro-Psychopharmacology and Biological Psychiatry* 2007 Mar 30;31(2):439–442.

140. Akhondzadeh S, Kashani L, Fotouhi A, et al. Comparison of *Lavandula angustifolia* Mill. tincture and imipramine in the treatment of mild to moderate depression: a double-blind, randomized trial. *Progress in Neuro-Psychopharmacology and Biological Psychiatry* 2003; 27:123–127.

Diabetes

1. Ford ES. Prevalence of the metabolic syndrome defined by the International Diabetes Federation among adults in the U.S. *Diabetes Care* 2005 Nov;28(11):2745–2749.

2. Cook S, Auinger P, Li C, et al. Metabolic syndrome rates in United States adolescents, from the National Health and Nutrition Examination Survey, 1999–2002. *Journal of Pediatrics* 2008 Feb;152(2):165–170.

3. Ford ES, Li C. Metabolic syndrome and health-related quality of life among U.S. adults. *Annals of Epidemiology* 2008 Mar;18(3):165–171.

4. Perry RC, Shankar RR, Fineberg N, et al. HbA1C measurement improves the detection of type 2 diabetes in high-risk individuals with nondiagnositc levels of fasting plasma glucose: the Early Diabetes Intervention Program (EDIP). *Diabetes Care* 2001;24:465–471.

5. Kelly MA, Mijovic CH, Barnett AH. Genetics of type 1 diabetes. *Best Practice & Research: Clinical Endocrinology & Metabolism* 2001;15:279–291.

6. Akerblom HK, Vaarala O, Hyoty H, et al. Environmental factors in the etiology of Type 1 diabetes. *American Journal of Medical Genetics* 2002;115:18–29.

7. Knip M, Akerblom HK. Environmental factors in the pathogenesis of Type 1 diabetes mellitus. *Experimental and Clinical Endocrinology & Diabetes* 1999;107 suppl 3:S93–S100.

8. Kaprio J, Tuomilehto J, Koskenvuo M, et al. Concordance for type 1 (insulin-dependent) and type 2 (non-insulin-dependent) diabetes mellitus in a population-based cohort of twins in Finland. *Diabetologia* 1992;35:1060–1067.

9. Redondo MJ, Yu L, Hawa M, et al. Heterogeneity of type 1 diabetes: analysis of monozygotic twins in Great Britain and the United States. *Diabetologia* 2001;44:354–362. [Erratum in *Diabetologia* 2001;44:927.]

10. Metcalfe KA, Hitman GA, Rowe RE, et al. Concordance for type 1 diabetes in identical twins is affected by insulin genotype. *Diabetes Care* 2001; 24:838–842.

11. Onkamo P, Vaananen S, Karvonen M, et al. Worldwide increase in incidence of type 1 diabetes—the analysis of the data on published incidence trends. *Diabetologia* 1999;42: 1395–1403. [Erratum in *Diabetologia* 2000;43:685.]

12. Feltbower RG, Bodansky HJ, McKinney PA, et al. Trends in the incidence of childhood diabetes in south Asians and other children in Bradford, UK. *Diabetic Medicine* 2002;19: 162–166.

13. Bodansky HJ, Staines A, Stephenson C, et al. Evidence for an environmental effect in the aetiology of insulin dependent diabetes in a transmigratory population. *BMJ* 1992;304: 1020–1022.

14. Elliott RB. Epidemiology of diabetes in Polynesia and New Zealand. *Pediatric and Adolescent Endocrinology* 1992;21: 66–71.

15. Vaarala O. The gut immune system and type 1 diabetes. *Annals of the New York Academy of Sciences* 2002;958:39–46.

16. Hypponen E, Kenward MG, Virtanen SM, et al. Infant feeding, early weight gain, and risk of Type 1 diabetes. Childhood Diabetes in Finland (DiMe) Study Group. *Diabetes Care* 1999;22:1961–1965.

17. Monetini L, Cavallo MG, Manfrini S, et al. Antibodies to bovine beta-casein in diabetes and other autoimmune diseases. *Hormone and Metabolic Research* 2002;34:455–459.

18. Hyoty H. Enterovirus infections and type 1 diabetes. *Annals of Medicine* 2002;34:138–147.

19. Roivainen M. Enteroviruses: new findings on the role of enteroviruses in type 1 diabetes. *The International Journal of Biochemistry & Cell Biology* 2006;38(5–6):721–725.

20. Vitamin D supplement in early childhood and risk for type 1 (insulin-dependent) diabetes mellitus. The EURODIAB Substudy 2 Study Group. *Diabetologia* 1999;42:51–54.

21. Hypponen E, Laara E, Reunanen A, et al. Intake of vitamin D and risk of type 1 diabetes: a birth-cohort study. *The Lancet* 2001;358:1500–1503.

22. Stene LC, Ulriksen J, Magnus P, et al. Use of cod liver oil during pregnancy associated with lower risk of type 1 diabetes in the offspring. *Diabetologia* 2000;43: 1093–1098.

23. Brekke HK, Ludvigsson J. Vitamin D supplementation and diabetes-related autoimmunity in the ABIS study. *Pediatric Diabetes* 2007 Feb;8(1):11–14.

24. Norris JM, Yin X, Lamb MM, et al. Omega-3 polyunsaturated fatty acid intake and islet autoimmunity in children at increased risk for Type 1 diabetes. *JAMA, The Journal of the American Medical Association* 2007 Sep 26;298(12): 1420–1428.

25. Krishna Mohan I, Das UN. Prevention of chemically induced diabetes mellitus in experimental animals by polyunsaturated fatty acids. *Nutrition* 2001;17: 126–151.

26. Zhao HX, Mold MD, Stenhouse EA, et al. Drinking water composition and childhood-onset type 1 diabetes mellitus in Devon and Cornwall, England. *Diabetic Medicine* 2001;18:709–717.

27. Parslow RC, McKinney PA, Law GR, et al. Incidence of childhood diabetes mellitus in Yorkshire, northern England, is associated with nitrate in drinking water: an ecological analysis. *Diabetologia* 1997;40:550–556.

28. Kretowski A, Mysliwiec J, Szelachowska M, et al. Nicotinamide inhibits enhanced in vitro production of interleukin-12 and tumour necrosis factor-alpha in peripheral whole blood of people at high risk of developing type 1 diabetes and people with newly diagnosed type 1 diabetes. *Diabetes Research and Clinical Practice* 2000;47: 81–86.

29. Kolb H, Burkart V. Nicotinamide in type 1 diabetes: mechanism of action revisited. *Diabetes Care* 1999;22 suppl 2: B16–B20.

30. Cleary JP. Vitamin B3 in the treatment of diabetes mellitus: case reports and review of the literature. *Journal of Nutritional and Environmental Medicine* 1990;1:217–225.

31. Pocoit F, Reimers JI, Andersen HU. Nicotinamide—biological actions and therapeutic potential in diabetes prevention. *Diabetologia* 1993;36:574–576.

32. Pozzilli P, Andreani D. The potential role of nicotinamide in the secondary prevention of IDDM. *Diabetes/Metabolism Reviews* 1993;9:219–230.

33. Visalli N, Cavallo MG, Signore A, et al. A multi-centre randomized trial of two different doses of nicotinamide in patients with recent-onset type 1 diabetes (the IMDIAB VI). *Diabetes/Metabolism Research and Reviews* 1999; 15:181–185.

34. Crino A, Schiaffini R, Manfrini S, et al. A randomized trial of nicotinamide and vitamin E in children with recent onset type 1 diabetes (IMDIAB IX). *European Journal of Endocrinology* 2004;150:719–724.

35. Schatz DA, Bingley PJ. Update on major trials for the prevention of type 1 diabetes mellitus: the American Diabetes Prevention Trial (DPT-1) and the European Nicotinamide

Diabetes Intervention Trial (ENDIT). *Journal of Pediatric Endocrinology & Metabolism* 2001;14 suppl 1:619–622.

36. Gale EA, Bingley PJ, Emmett CL; European Nicotinamide Diabetes Intervention Trial (ENDIT) Group. European Nicotinamide Diabetes Intervention Trial (ENDIT): a randomised controlled trial of intervention before the onset of type 1 diabetes. *The Lancet* 2004;363:925–931.

37. Kretowski A, Mysliwiec J, Szelachowska M, et al. Nicotinamide inhibits enhanced in vitro production of interleukin-12 and tumour necrosis factor-alpha in peripheral whole blood of people at high risk of developing type 1 diabetes and people with newly diagnosed type 1 diabetes. *Diabetes Research and Clinical Practice* 2000;47: 81–86.

38. Chakravarthy BK, Gupta S, Gode KD. Functional beta cell regeneration in the islets of pancreas in alloxan induced diabetic rats by (-)-epicatechin. *Life Sciences* 1982;31:2693–2697.

39. Mukoyama A, Ushijima H, Nishimura S, et al. Inhibition of rotavirus and enterovirus infections by tea extracts. *Japanese Journal of Medical Science & Biology* 1991;44:181–186.

40. Guerre-Millo M. Adipose tissue hormones. *Journal of Endocrinological Investigation* 2002;25: 855–861.

41. Trayhurn P, Beattie JH. Physiological role of adipose tissue: white adipose tissue as an endocrine and secretory organ. *Proceedings of the Nutrition Society* 2001;60:329–339.

42. Tschritter O, Fritsche A, Thamer C, et al. Plasma adiponectin concentrations predict insulin sensitivity of both glucose and lipid metabolism. *Diabetes* 2003;52:239–243.

43. Spranger J, Kroke A, Mohlig M, et al. Adiponectin and protec-tion against type 2 diabetes mellitus. *The Lancet* 2003;361: 226–228.

44. Gloyn AL, McCarthy MI. The genetics of type 2 diabetes. *Best Practice & Research: Clinical Endocrinology & Metabolism* 2001;15:293–308.

45. Bennett PH. Type 2 diabetes among the Pima Indians of Arizona: an epidemic attributable to environmental change? *Nutrition Reviews* 1999;57:S51–S54.

46. Nelson KM, Reiber G, Boyko EJ. Diet and exercise among adults with type 2 diabetes: findings from the Third National Health and Nutrition Examination Survey (NHANES III). *Diabetes Care* 2002;25: 1722–1728.

47. Snitker S, Mitchell BD, Shuldiner AR. Physical activity and prevention of type 2 diabetes. *The Lancet* 2003;361:87–88.

48. Hsueh WC, Mitchell BD, Aburomia R, et al. Diabetes in the Old Order Amish: characterization and heritability analysis of the Amish Family Diabetes Study. *Diabetes Care* 2000;23: 595–601.

49. The Diabetes Prevention Program (DPP): description of lifestyle intervention. *Diabetes Care* 2002;25:2165–2171.

50. Willett W, Manson J, Liu S. Glycemic index, glycemic load, and risk of type 2 diabetes. *The American Journal of Clinical Nutrition* 2002;76:274S–280S.

51. Jenkins DJ, Kendall CW, Augustin LS, et al. Glycemic index: overview of implications in health and disease. *The American Journal of Clinical Nutrition* 2002;76:266S–273S.

52. Riccardi G, Rivellese AA, Giacco R. Role of glycemic index and glycemic load in the healthy state, in prediabetes, and in diabetes. *The American Journal of Clinical Nutrition* 2008 Jan; 87(1):269S–274S.

53. Liu S, Willett WC, Stampfer MJ, et al. A prospective study of dietary glycemic load, carbohydrate intake, and risk of coronary heart disease in US women. *The American Journal of Clinical Nutrition* 2000;71: 1455–1461.

54. Wursch P, Pi-Sunyer FX. The role of viscous soluble fiber in the metabolic control of diabetes. A review with special emphasis on cereals rich in beta-glucan. *Diabetes Care* 1997;20:1774–1780.

55. Slama G. Dietary therapy in Type 2 diabetes oriented towards postprandial blood glucose improvement. *Diabetes/ Metabolism Reviews* 1998;14 suppl 1:S19–S24.

56. Montonen J, Knekt P, Jarvinen R, et al. Whole-grain and fiber intake and the incidence of type 2 diabetes. *The American Journal of Clinical Nutrition* 2003;77:622–629.

57. Fung TT, Hu FB, Pereira MA, et al. Whole-grain intake and the risk of type 2 diabetes: a prospective study in men. *The American Journal of Clinical Nutrition* 2002;76:535–540.

58. Hung T, Sievenpiper JL, Marchie A, et al. Fat versus carbohydrate in insulin resistance, obesity, diabetes and cardiovascular disease. *Current Opinion in Clinical Nutrition and Metabolic Care* 2003;6:165–176.

59. Salmeron J, Hu FB, Manson JE, et al. Dietary fat intake and risk of type 2 diabetes in women. *The American Journal of Clinical Nutrition* 2001;73: 1019–1026.

60. Rivellese AA, De Natale C, Lilli S. Type of dietary fat and insulin resistance. *Annals of the New York Academy of Sciences* 2002;967:329–335.

61. Jiang R, Manson JE, Stampfer MJ, et al. Nut and peanut butter consumption and risk of type 2 diabetes in women. *JAMA, The Journal of the American Medical Association* 2002;288:2554–2560.

62. Sargeant LA, Khaw KT, Bingham S, et al. Fruit and vegetable

intake and population glycosylated haemoglobin levels: the EPIC-Norfolk Study. *European Journal of Clinical Nutrition* 2001;55:342–348.

63. Williams DE, Wareham NJ, Cox BD, et al. Frequent salad vegetable consumption is associated with a reduction in the risk of diabetes mellitus. *Journal of Clinical Epidemiology* 1999;52: 329–335.

64. Reunanen A, Knekt P, Aaran RK, et al. Serum antioxidants and risk of non-insulin dependent diabetes mellitus. *European Journal of Clinical Nutrition* 1998;52:89–93.

65. Feskens EJ, Virtanen SM, Rasanen L, et al. Dietary factors determining diabetes and impaired glucose tolerance. A 20-year follow-up of the Finnish and Dutch cohorts of the Seven Countries Study. *Diabetes Care* 1995;18:1104–1112.

66. Ruhe RC, McDonald RB. Use of antioxidant nutrients in the prevention and treatment of type 2 diabetes. *Journal of the American College of Nutrition* 2001;5:363S–369S.

67. Facchini FS, Humphreys MH, DoNascimento CA, et al. Relation between insulin resistance and plasma concentrations of lipid hydroperoxides, carotenoids, and tocopherols. *The American Journal of Clinical Nutrition* 2000;72:776–779.

68. Salonen JT, Nyyssonen K, Tuomainen TP. Increased risk of non-insulin diabetes mellitus at low plasma vitamin E concentrations. A four year follow-up study in men. *BMJ* 1995;311: 1124–1127.

69. Maritim AC, Sanders RA, Watkins JB III. Diabetes, oxidative stress, and antioxidants: a review. *Journal of Biochemical and Molecular Toxicology* 2003; 17:24–38.

70. Evans JL, Goldfine ID, Maddux BA, et al. Are oxidative stress-activated signaling pathways mediators of insulin resistance and beta-cell dysfunction? *Diabetes* 2003;52:1–8.

71. Lee DH, Lee IK, Song K, et al. A strong dose-response relation between serum concentrations of persistent organic pollutants and diabetes: results from the National Health and Examination Survey 1999–2002. *Diabetes Care* 2006 Jul;29(7): 1638–1644.

72. Lee DH, Lee IK, Song K, et al. Relationship between serum concentrations of persistent organic pollutants and the prevalence of metabolic syndrome among non-diabetic adults: results from the National Health and Nutrition Examination Survey 1999–2002. *Diabetologia* 2007 Sep;50(9):1841–1851.

73. Lee DH, Ha MH, Kim JH, et al. Gamma-glutamyltransferase and diabetes—a 4 year follow-up study. *Diabetologia* 2003;46: 359–364.

74. Knowler WC, Barrett-Connor E, Fowler SE, et al. Reduction in the incidence of type 2 diabetes with lifestyle intervention or metformin. *The New England Journal of Medicine* 2002;346: 393–403.

75. Goldstein DE, Little RR. Monitoring glycemia in diabetes: short-term assessment. *Endocrinology Metabolism Clinics of North America* 1997;26: 475–486.

76. American Diabetes Association. Tests of glycemia in diabetes (position statement). *Diabetes Care* 1997;20 suppl 1:518–520.

77. DCCT Research Group. The effect of intensive treatment of diabetes on the development and progression of long-term complications in insulin-dependent diabetes mellitus. *The New England Journal of Medicine* 1993;329:977.

78. UK Prospective Diabetes Study (UKPDS) Group. Intensive blood-glucose control with sulphonylureas or insulin compared with conventional treatment and risk of complications in patients with type 2 diabetes (UKPDS 33). *The Lancet* 1998; 352:837–853.

79. Bertrand S, Aris-Jilwan N, Reddy S, et al. Recommendations for the use of self-monitoring of blood glucose (SMBG) in diabetes mellitus. *Diabetes Care* 1992;20:14–16.

80. DAFNE Study Group. Training in flexible, intensive insulin management to enable dietary freedom in people with type 1 diabetes: dose adjustment for normal eating (DAFNE) randomized controlled trial. *BMJ* 2002;325:746.

81. Ohkubo Y, Kishikawa H, Araki E, et al. Intensive insulin therapy prevents the progression of diabetic microvascular complications in Japanese patients with non-insulin-dependent diabetes mellitus: a randomized prospective 6-year study. *Diabetes Research and Clinical Practice* 1995;28: 103–117.

82. Lingenfelser T, Overkamp D, Renn W, et al. Insulin-associated modulation of neuro-endocrine counterregulation, hypoglycemia perception, and cerebral function in insulin-dependent diabetes mellitus: evidence for an intrinsic effect of insulin on the central nervous system. *The Journal of Clinical Endocrinology & Metabolism* 1996;81:1197–1205.

83. Maxwell SR, Thomason H, Sandler D, et al. Antioxidant status in patients with uncomplicated insulin-dependent and non-insulin-dependent diabetes mellitus. *European Journal of Clinical Investigation* 1997;27: 484–490.

84. Skrha J, Hodinar A, Kvasnicka J, et al. Relationship of oxidative stress and fibrinolysis in diabetes mellitus. *Diabetic Medicine* 1996;13:800–805.

85. Hoogeveen EK, Kostense PJ, Eysink PE, et al. Hyperhomocysteinemia is associated with the presence of retinopathy in type 2 diabetes mellitus. *Ar-*

chives of Internal Medicine 2000;160:2984–2990.

86. De Mattia G, Laurenti O, Fava D. Diabetic endothelial dysfunction: effect of free radical scavenging in type 2 diabetic patients. *Journal of Diabetes and Its Complications* 2003;17 suppl 2:30–35.

87. Price KD, Price CS, Reynolds RD. Hyperglycemia-induced ascorbic acid deficiency promotes endothelial dysfunction and the development of atherosclerosis. *Atherosclerosis* 2001; 158:1–12.

88. Heitzer T, Finckh B, Albers S, et al. Beneficial effects of alpha-lipoic acid and ascorbic acid on endothelium-dependent, nitric oxide-mediated vasodilation in diabetic patients: relation to parameters of oxidative stress. *Free Radical Biology & Medicine* 2001;31:53–61.

89. Carr A, Frei B. The role of natural antioxidants in preserving the biological activity of endothelium-derived nitric oxide. *Free Radical Biology & Medicine* 2000;28:1806–1814.

90. Gilbertson HR, Brand-Miller JC, Thorburn AW, et al. The effect of flexible low glycemic index dietary advice versus measured carbohydrate exchange diets on glycemic control in children with type 1 diabetes. *Diabetes Care* 2001;24:1137–1143.

91. Giacco R, Parillo M, Rivellese AA, et al. Long-term dietary treatment with increased amounts of fiber-rich low-glycemic index natural foods improves blood glucose control and reduces the number of hypoglycemic events in type 1 diabetic patients. *Diabetes Care* 2000;23:1461–1466.

92. Buyken AE, Toeller M, Heitkamp G, et al. Glycemic index in the diet of European outpatients with type 1 diabetes: relations to glycated hemoglobin and serum lipids. *The American Journal of Clinical Nutrition* 2001;73:574–581.

93. Toeller M, Buyken AE, Heitkamp G, et al. Prevalence of chronic complications, metabolic control and nutritional intake in type 1 diabetes: comparison between different European regions. EURODIAB Complications Study Group. *Hormone and Metabolic Research* 1999; 31:680–685.

94. Kalkwarf HJ, Bell RC, Khoury JC, et al. Dietary fiber intakes and insulin requirements in pregnant women with type 1 diabetes. *Journal of the American Dietetic Association* 2001; 101:305–310.

95. Hung T, Sievenpiper JL, Marchie A, et al. Fat versus carbohydrate in insulin resistance, obesity, diabetes and cardiovascular disease. *Current Opinion in Clinical Nutrition and Metabolic Care* 2003;6:165–176.

96. Chandalia M, Garg A, Lutjohann D, et al. Beneficial effects of high dietary fiber intake in patients with Type 2 diabetes mellitus. *The New England Journal of Medicine* 2000;342: 1392–1398.

97. Jarvi AE, Karlstrom BE, Granfeldt YE, et al. Improved glycemic control and lipid profile and normalized fibrinolytic activity on a low-glycemic index diet in Type 2 diabetic patients. *Diabetes Care* 1999;22:10–18.

98. Brynes AE, Lee JL, Brighton RE, et al. A low glycemic diet significantly improves the 24-h blood glucose profile in people with Type 2 diabetes, as assessed using the continuous glucose MiniMed monitor. *Diabetes Care* 2003;26:548–549.

99. Grey M, Boland EA, Davidson M, et al. Coping skills training for youths with diabetes on intensive therapy. *Applied Nursing Research* 1999;12:3–12.

100. Barglow P, Hatcher R, Edidin DV, et al. Stress and metabolic control in diabetes: psychosomatic evidence and evaluation of methods. *Psychosomatic Medicine* 1984;46:127–144.

101. McGrady A, Bailey BK, Good MP. Controlled study of biofeedback-assisted relaxation in type 1 diabetes. *Diabetes Care* 1991;14:360–365.

102. Lane JD, McCaskill CC, Ross SL, et al. Relaxation training for NIDDM: predicting who may benefit. *Diabetes Care* 1993;16: 1087–1094.

103. Boule NG, Haddad E, Kenny GP, et al. Effects of exercise on glycemic control and body mass in type 2 diabetes mellitus: a meta-analysis of controlled clinical trials. *JAMA, The Journal of the American Medical Association* 2001;286:1218–1227.

104. Pronk NO, Wing RR. Physical activity and long term maintenance of weight loss. *Obesity Research* 1994;2:587–589.

105. Barringer T, Kirk J, Santaniello A, et al. Effects of a multivitamin and mineral supplement on infection and quality of life. *Annals of Internal Medicine* 2003;138:365–371.

106. Althuis MD, Jordan NE, Ludington EA, et al. Glucose and insulin responses to dietary chromium supplements: a meta-analysis. *The American Journal of Clinical Nutrition* 2002;76: 148–155.

107. Kleefstra N, Houweling ST, Bakker SJ, et al. Chromium treatment has no effect in patients with type 2 diabetes in a Western population: a randomized, double-blind, placebo-controlled trial. *Diabetes Care* 2007 May;30(5):1092–1096.

108. Albarracin CA, Fuqua BC, Evans JL, Goldfine ID. Chromium picolinate and biotin combination improves glucose metabolism in treated, uncontrolled overweight to obese patients with type 2 diabetes. *Diabetes/Metabolism Research and Reviews* 2008 Jan–Feb; 24(1):41–51.

109. Geohas J, Daly A, Juturu V, et al. Chromium picolinate and biotin combination reduces atherogenic index of plasma in patients with

type 2 diabetes mellitus: a placebo-controlled, double-blinded, randomized clinical trial. *The American Journal of the Medical Sciences* 2007 Mar;333(3): 145–153.

110. Cunningham JJ. The glucose/insulin system and vitamin C: implications in insulin-dependent diabetes mellitus. *Journal of the American College of Nutrition* 1998;17:105–108.

111. Eriksson J, Kohvakka A. Magnesium and ascorbic acid supplementation in diabetes mellitus. *Annals of Nutrition and Metabolism* 1995;39:217–223.

112. Mullan BA, Young IS, Fee H, et al. Ascorbic acid reduces blood pressure and arterial stiffness in type 2 diabetes. *Hypertension* 2002;40:804–809.

113. Vincent TE, Mendiratta S, May JM. Inhibition of aldose reductase in human erythrocytes by vitamin C. *Diabetes Research and Clinical Practice* 1999;43: 1–8.

114. Anderson JW, Gowri MS, Turner J, et al. Antioxidant supplementation effects on low-density lipoprotein oxidation for individuals with type 2 diabetes mellitus. *Journal of the American College of Nutrition* 1999; 18:451–461.

115. Astley S, Langrish-Smith A, Southon S, et al. Vitamin E supplementation and oxidative damage to DNA and plasma LDL in type 1 diabetes. *Diabetes Care* 1999;22:1626–1631.

116. Pinkney JH, Downs L, Hopton M, et al. Endothelial dysfunction in type 1 diabetes mellitus: relationship with LDL oxidation and the effects of vitamin E. *Diabetic Medicine* 1999; 16:993–999.

117. Skyrme-Jones RA, O'Brien RC, Berry KL, et al. Vitamin E supplementation improves endothelial function in type 1 diabetes mellitus: a randomized, placebo-controlled study. *Journal of the American College of Cardiology* 2000;36:94–102.

118. Gazis A, White DJ, Page SR, et al. Effect of oral vitamin E (alpha-tocopherol) supplementation on vascular endothelial function in type 2 diabetes mellitus. *Diabetic Medicine* 1999; 16:304–311.

119. Paolisso G, Tagliamonte MR, Barbieri M, et al. Chronic vitamin E administration improves brachial reactivity and increases intracellular magnesium concentration in type 2 diabetic patients. *The Journal of Clinical Endocrinology & Metabolism* 2000;85:109–115.

120. Barbagallo M, Dominguez LJ, Tagliamonte MR, et al. Effects of vitamin E and glutathione on glucose metabolism: role of magnesium. *Hypertension* 1999;34: 1002–1006.

121. Upritchard JE, Sutherland WH, Mann JI. Effect of supplementation with tomato juice, vitamin E, and vitamin C on LDL oxidation and products of inflammatory activity in type 2 diabetes. *Diabetes Care* 2000; 23:733–738.

122. Devaraj S, Jialal I. Alpha tocopherol supplementation decreases serum C-reactive protein and monocyte interleukin-6 levels in normal volunteers and type 2 diabetic patients. *Free Radical Biology & Medicine* 2000;29: 790–792.

123. Gokkusu C, Palanduz S, Ademoglu E, et al. Oxidant and antioxidant systems in NIDDM patients: influence of vitamin E supplementation. *Endocrine Research* 2001;27: 377–386.

124. Tutuncu NB, Bayraktar M, Varli K. Reversal of defective nerve conduction with vitamin E supplementation in type 2 diabetes: a preliminary study. *Diabetes Care* 1998;21: 1915–1918.

125. Bursell SE, Clermont AC, Aiello LP, et al. High-dose vitamin E supplementation normalizes retinal blood flow and creatinine clearance in patients with type 1 diabetes. *Diabetes Care* 1999; 22:1245–1251.

126. Milman U, Blum S, Shapira C, et al. Vitamin E supplementation reduces cardiovascular events in a subgroup of middle-aged individuals with both type 2 diabetes mellitus and the haptoglobin 2-2 genotype: a prospective double-blinded clinical trial. *Arteriosclerosis, Thrombosis, and Vascular Biology* 2008 Feb;28(2):341–347.

127. Ward NC, Wu JH, Clarke MW, et al. The effect of vitamin E on blood pressure in individuals with type 2 diabetes: a randomized, double-blind, placebo-controlled trial. *Journal of Hypertension* 2007 Jan;25(1): 227–234.

128. Polo V, Saibene A, Pontiroli AE. Nicotinamide improves insulin secretion and metabolic control in lean type 2 diabetic patients with secondary failure to sulphonylureas. *Acta Diabetologica* 1998;35:61–64.

129. Jones CL, Gonzalez V. Pyridoxine deficiency: a new factor in diabetic neuropathy. *Journal of the American Podiatry Association* 1978;68:646–653.

130. Solomon LR, Cohen K. Erythrocyte O2 transport and metabolism and effects of vitamin B6 therapy in type 2 diabetes mellitus. *Diabetes* 1989;38:881–886.

131. Coelingh-Bennick HJT, Schreurs WHP. Improvement of oral glucose tolerance in gestational diabetes. *British Medical Journal* 1975;3:13–15.

132. Barbagallo M, Dominguez LJ, Galioto A, et al. Role of magnesium in insulin action, diabetes and cardio-metabolic syndrome X. *Molecular Aspects of Medicine* 2003;24:39–52.

133. Lima Mde L, Cruz T, Pousada JC, et al. The effect of magnesium supplementation in increasing doses on the control of type 2 diabetes. *Diabetes Care* 1998;21:682–686.

134. White JR, Campbell RK. Magnesium and diabetes: a review.

The Annals of Pharmacotherapy 1993;27:775–780.

135. Salgueiro MJ, Krebs N, Zubillaga MB, et al. Zinc and diabetes mellitus: is there a need of zinc supplementation in diabetes mellitus patients? *Biological Trace Element Research* 2001; 81:215–228.

136. Maebashi M, Makino Y, Furukawa Y, et al. Therapeutic evaluation of the effect of biotin on hyperglycemia in patients with non-insulin dependent diabetes mellitus. *Journal of Clinical Biochemistry and Nutrition* 1993;14:211–218.

137. Koutsikos D, Agroyannis B, Tzanatos-Exarchou H. Biotin for diabetic peripheral neuropathy. *Biomedicine & Pharmacotherapy* 1990;44:511–514.

138. Farmer A, Montori V, Dinneen S, et al. Fish oil in people with type 2 diabetes mellitus. Cochrane Database of Systematic Reviews 2001;3:CD003205.

139. Montori VM, Farmer A, Wollan PC, et al. Fish oil supplementation in type 2 diabetes: a quantitative systematic review. *Diabetes Care* 2000;23:1407–1415.

140. Woodman RJ, Mori TA, Burke V, et al. Effects of purified eicosapentaenoic and docosahexaenoic acids on glycemic control, blood pressure, and serum lipids in type 2 diabetic patients with treated hypertension. *The American Journal of Clinical Nutrition* 2002;76: 1007–1015.

141. Bell DS. Importance of postprandial glucose control. *Southern Medical Journal* 2001;94: 804–809.

142. Vuksan V, Jenkins DJ, Spadafora P, et al. Konjac-mannan (glucomannan) improves glycemia and other associated risk factors for coronary heart disease in type 2 diabetes. A randomized controlled metabolic trial. *Diabetes Care* 1999;22:913–919.

143. Jenkins DJ, Kendall CW, Axelsen M, et al. Viscous and nonviscous fibres, nonabsorbable and low glycaemic index carbohydrates, blood lipids and coronary heart disease. *Current Opinion in Lipidology* 2000;11: 49–56.

144. Marlett JA, McBurney MI, Slavin JL. Position of the American Dietetic Association: health implications of dietary fiber. *Journal of the American Dietetic Association* 2002;102: 993–1000.

145. Abdelhameed AS, Ang S, Morris GA, et al. An analytical ultracentrifuge study on ternary mixtures of konjac glucomannan supplemented with sodium alginate and xanthan gum. *Carbohydrate Polymers* 2010;81: 141–148.

146. Harding SE, Smith IH, Lawson CJ, Gahler RJ, Wood S. Studies on macromolecular interactions in ternary mixtures of konjac glucomannan, xanthan gum and sodium alginate. *Carbohydrate Polymers* 2010;10:1016–1020.

147. Brand-Miller JC, Atkinson FS, Gahler RJ, et al. Effects of PGX, a novel functional fibre, on acute and delayed postprandial glycaemia. *European Journal of Clinical Nutrition* 2010 Dec; 64(12):1488–1493.

148. Jenkins AL, Kacinik V, Lyon MR, Wolever TMS. Reduction of postprandial glycemia by the novel viscous polysaccharide PGX in a dose-dependent manner, independent of food form. *Journal of the American College of Nutrition* 2010;29(2):92–98.

149. Vuksan V, Sievenpiper JL, Owen R, et al. Beneficial effects of viscous dietary fiber from konjac-mannan in subjects with the insulin resistance syndrome: results of a controlled metabolic trial. *Diabetes Care* 2000;23: 9–14.

150. Vuksan V, Lyon M, Breitman P, et al. 3-week consumption of a highly viscous dietary fibre blend results in improvements in insulin sensitivity and reductions in body fat. Results of a double blind, placebo controlled trial. Presented at the 64th Annual Meeting of the American Diabetes Association, Orlando, Fla., June 4–8, 2004.

151. Fujita H, Yamagami T, Ohshima K. Fermented soybean-derived water-soluble touchi extract inhibits alpha-glucosidase and is antiglycemic in rats and humans after single oral treatments. *Journal of Nutrition* 2001; 131:1211–1213.

152. Hiroyuki F, Tomohide Y, Kazunori O. Efficacy and safety of touchi extract, an alpha-glucosidase inhibitor derived from fermented soybeans, in non-insulin-dependent diabetic mellitus. *The Journal of Nutritional Biochemistry* 2001;12:351–356.

153. Fujita H, Yamagami T, Ohshima K. Long-term ingestion of a fermented soybean-derived touchi-extract with alpha-glucosidase inhibitory activity is safe and effective in humans with borderline and mild type-2 diabetes. *Journal of Nutrition* 2001;131:2105–2108.

154. Asano N, Oseki K, Tomioka E, et al. N-containing sugars from *Morus alba* and their glycosidase inhibitory activities. *Carbohydrate Research* 1994;259: 243–255.

155. Chen F, Nakashima N, Kimura I, et al. Hypoglycemic activity and mechanisms of extracts from mulberry leaves (folium mori) and cortex mori radicis in streptozotocin-induced diabetic mice. *Yakugaku Zasshi* 1995;115:476–482.

156. Andallu B, Suryakantham V, Lakshmi Srikanthi B, et al. Effect of mulberry (*Morus indica* L.) therapy on plasma and erythrocyte membrane lipids in patients with type 2 diabetes. *Clinica Chimica Acta* 2001;314: 47–53.

157. Porchezhian E, Dobriyal RM. An overview on the advances of *Gymnema sylvestre*: chemistry, pharmacology and patents. *Pharmazie* 2003;58:5–12.

158. Shanmugasundaram ER, Rajeswari G, Baskaran K, et al. Use of *Gymnema sylvestre* leaf extract in the control of blood glucose in insulin-dependent diabetes mellitus. *Journal of Ethnopharmacology* 1990;30:281–294.

159. Baskaran K, Ahamath BK, Shanmugasundaram KR, et al. Antidiabetic effect of a leaf extract from *Gymnema sylvestre* in non-insulin dependent diabetes mellitus patients. *Journal of Ethnopharmacology* 1990;30: 295–305.

160. Srivastava Y, Venkatakrishna-Bhatt H, Verma Y, et al. Antidiabetic and adaptogenic properties of *Momordica charantia* extract: an experimental and clinical evaluation. *Phytotherapy Research* 1993;7:285–289.

161. Welihinda J, Karunanaya EH, Sheriff MHR, et al. Effect of *Momordica charantia* on the glucose tolerance in maturity onset diabetes. *Journal of Ethnopharmacology* 1986;17:277–282.

162. Vuksan V, Stavro MP, Sievenpiper J, et al. American ginseng (*Panax quinquefolius*) reduces postproandial glycemia in non-diabetic subjects with type 2 diabetes mellitus. *Archives of Internal Medicine* 2000;160: 1009–1013.

163. Vuksan V, Stavro MP, Sievenpiper J, et al. Similar postprandial glycemic reductions with escalation of dose and administration time of American ginseng in Type 2 diabetes. *Diabetes Care* 2000;23:1221–1226.

164. Vuksan V, Sievenpiper J, Wong J, et al. American ginseng (*Panax quinquefolius*) attenuates postprandial glycemia in a time dependent but not dose dependent manner in healthy individuals. *The American Journal of Clinical Nutrition* 2001; 73:753–758.

165. Vuksan V, Stavro MP, Sievenpiper J, et al. American ginseng improves glycemia in individuals with normal glucose tolerance: effect of dose and time escalation. *Journal of the American College of Nutrition* 2000; 19:738–744.

166. Sievenpiper J, Arnason JT, Leiter LA, et al. Variable effects of American ginseng: a batch of American ginseng (*Panax quinquefolius*) with a depressed ginsenoside profile does not affect postprandial glycemia. *European Journal of Clinical Nutrition* 2003;57:243–248.

167. Franz MJ, Bantle JP, Beebe CA, et al. Evidence-based nutrition principles and recommendations for the treatment and prevention of diabetes and related complications. *Diabetes Care* 2002;25:148–198.

168. Sotaniemi EA, Haapakoski E, Rautio A. Ginseng therapy in non-insulin-dependent diabetic patients. *Diabetes Care* 1995;18: 1373–1375.

169. Sharma RD, Raghuram TC, Rao NS. Effect of fenugreek seeds on blood glucose and serum lipids in type 1 diabetes. *European Journal of Clinical Nutrition* 1990;44:301–306.

170. Mada Z, Abel R, Samish S, et al. Glucose-lowering effect of fenugreek in non-insulin dependent diabetics. *European Journal of Clinical Nutrition* 1988;42: 51–54.

171. Gupta A, Gupta R, Lal B. Effect of *Trigonella foenum-graecum* (fenugreek) seeds on glycaemic control and insulin resistance in type 2 diabetes mellitus: a double blind placebo controlled study. *Journal of the Association of Physicians of India* 2001;49: 1057–1061.

172. Sharma KK, Gupta RK, Gupta S, et al. Antihyperglycemic effect of onion: effect on fasting blood sugar and induced hyperglycemia in man. *Indian Journal of Medical Research* 1977;65:422–429.

173. Manuel y Keenoy B, Vertommen J, et al. The effect of flavonoid treatment on the glycation and antioxidant status in type 1 diabetic patients. *Diabetes, Nutrition & Metabolism* 1999;12: 256–263.

174. Reljanovic M, Reichel G, Rett K, et al. Treatment of diabetic polyneuropathy with the antioxidant thioctic acid (alpha-lipoic acid): a two year multicenter randomized double-blind placebo-controlled trial (ALADIN II). Alpha Lipoic Acid in Diabetic Neuropathy. *Free Radical Research* 1999;31:171–179.

175. Jacob S, Ruus P, Hermann R, et al. Oral administration of RAC-alpha-lipoic acid modulates insulin sensitivity in patients with type-2 diabetes mellitus: a placebo-controlled pilot trial. *Free Radical Biology & Medicine* 1999;27:309–314.

176. Rindone JP, Achacoso S. Effect of low-dose niacin on glucose control in patients with non-insulin-dependent diabetes mellitus and hyperlipidemia. *American Journal of Therapeutics* 1996;3:637–639.

177. Grundy SM, Vega GL, McGovern ME, et al. Efficacy, safety, and tolerability of once-daily niacin for the treatment of dyslipidemia associated with type 2 diabetes: results of the assessment of diabetes control and evaluation of the efficacy of niaspan trial. *Archives of Internal Medicine* 2002;162: 1568–1576.

178. Kane MP, Hamilton RA, Addesse E, et al. Cholesterol and glycemic effects of Niaspan in patients with type 2 diabetes. *Pharmacotherapy* 2001;21: 1473–1478.

179. El-Enein AMA, Hafez YS, Salem H, et al. The role of nicotinic acid and inositol hexaniacinate as anticholesterolemic and antilipemic agents. *Nutrition Reports International* 1983;28: 899–911.

180. Schonlau F, Rohdewald P. Pycnogenol for diabetic retinopathy. A review. *International Opthalmology* 2001;24:161–171.

181. Passariello N, Bisesti V, Sgam-

bato S. [Influence of anthocyanosides on the microcirculation and lipid picture in diabetic and dyslipidic subjects.] *Gazzetta Medica Italiana* 1979;138:563–566.

182. Stirban A, Negrean M, Stratmann B, et al. Benfotiamine prevents macro- and microvascular endothelial dysfunction and oxidative stress following a meal rich in advanced glycation end products in individuals with type 2 diabetes. *Diabetes Care* 2006 Sep;29(9):2064–2071.

183. Stracke H, Gaus W, Achenbach U, Federlin K, Bretzel RG. Benfotiamine in Diabetic Polyneuropathy (BENDIP): results of a randomised, double blind, placebo-controlled clinical study. *Experimental and Clinical Endocrinology & Diabetes* 2008 Nov;116(10):600–605.

184. Alkhalaf A, Klooster A, van Oeveren W, et al. A double-blind, randomized, placebo-controlled clinical trial on benfotiamine treatment in patients with diabetic nephropathy. *Diabetes Care* 2010 Jul;33(7):1598–1601.

185. Du X, Edelstein D, Brownlee M. Oral benfotiamine plus alpha-lipoic acid normalises complication-causing pathways in type 1 diabetes. *Diabetologia* 2008 Oct;51(10):1930–1932.

186. Forst T, Pohlmann T, Kunt T, et al. The influence of local capsaicin treatment on small nerve fibre function and neurovascular control in symptomatic diabetic neuropathy. *Acta Diabetologica* 2002;39:1–6.

187. Rains C, Bryson HM. Topical capsaicin: a review of its pharmacological properties and therapeutic potential in postherpetic neuralgia, diabetic neuropathy and osteoarthritis. *Drugs & Aging* 1995;7:317–328.

188. Hu H. A review of treatment of diabetes by acupuncture during the past forty years. *Journal of Traditional Chinese Medicine* 1995;15:145–154.

189. Abuaisha BB, Costanzi JB, Boulton AJ. Acupuncture for the treatment of chronic painful peripheral diabetic neuropathy: a long-term study. *Diabetes Research and Clinical Practice* 1998;39:115–121.

190. Younes H, Alphonse JC, Behr S, et al. Role of fermentable carbohydrate supplements with a low-protein diet in the course of chronic renal failure: experimental bases. *American Journal of Kidney Diseases* 1999;33:633–646.

191. Gaede P, Poulsen HE, Parving HH, et al. Double-blind, randomised study of the effect of combined treatment with vitamin C and E on albuminuria in type 2 diabetic patients. *Diabetic Medicine* 2001;18:756–760.

192. Parving HH, Hovind P. Microalbuminuria in type 1 and type 2 diabetes mellitus: evidence with angiotensin converting enzyme inhibitors and angiotensin II receptor blockers for treating early and preventing clinical nephropathy. *Current Hypertension Reports* 2002;4:387–393.

Diarrhea

1. Leob H, Vandenplas Y, Wursch P, Guesry P. Tannin-rich carob pod for the treatment of acute-onset diarrhea. J Pediatr Gastroenterol Nutr = *Journal of Pediatric Gastroenterology and Nutrition* 1989;8:480–485.

2. Hostettler M, Steffen R, Tschopp A. Efficacy of tolerability of insoluble carob fraction in the treatment of travellers' diarrhea. *Journal of Diarrhoeal Diseases Research* 1995;13:155–158.

3. Majamaa H, Isolauri E, Saxelin M, et al. Lactic acid bacteria in the treatment of acute rotavirus gastroenteritis. *Journal of Pediatric Gastroenterology and Nutrition* 1995;20:333–338.

4. Goossens D, Jonkers D, Stobberingh E, et al. Probiotics in gastroenterology: indications and future perspectives. *Scan-*

dinavian Journal of Gastroenterology 2003 suppl;239:15–23.

5. Guandalini S. Probiotics for prevention and treatment of diarrhea. *Journal of Clinical Gastroenterology* 2011 Nov;45 suppl:S149–S153.

6. Allen SJ, Martinez EG, Gregorio GV, Dans LF. Probiotics for treating acute infectious diarrhoea. Cochrane Database of Systematic Reviews 2010 Nov 10;11:CD003048.

7. Zoppi G, Deganello A, Benoni G, et al. Oral bacteriotherapy in clinical practice. I. The use of different preparations in infants treated with antibiotics. *European Journal of Pediatrics* 1982;139:18–21.

8. Gotz VP, Romankiewics JA, Moss J. Prophylaxis against ampicillin-associated diarrhea with a lactobacillus preparation. *American Journal of Hospital Pharmacy* 1979;36:754–757.

9. Ahuja MC, Khamar B. Antibiotic associated diarrhoea: a controlled study comparing plain antibiotic with those containing protected lactobacilli. *Journal of Indian Medical Association* 2002;100:334–335.

10. Na X, Kelly C. Probiotics in *Clostridium difficile* infection. *Journal of Clinical Gastroenterology*. 2011 Nov;45 suppl:S154–S158

11. Gupte S. Use of berberine in the treatment of giardiasis. *American Journal of Diseases of Children* 1975;129:866.

12. Bhakat MP. Therapeutic trial of Berberine sulphate in nonspecific gastroenteritis. *Indian Medical Journal* 1974;68:19–23.

13. Kamat SA. Clinical trial with berberine hydrochloride for the control of diarrhoea in acute gastroenteritis. *Journal of the Association of Physicians of India* 1967;15:525–529.

14. Desai AB, Shah KM, Shah DM. Berberine in the treatment of diarrhoea. *Indian Pediatrics* 1971;8:462–465.

15. Sharma R, Joshi CK, Goyal RK.

Berberine tannate in acute diarrhea. *Indian Pediatrics* 1970;7:496–501.

16. Choudry VP, Sabir M, Bhide VN. Berberine in giardiasis. *Indian Pediatrics* 1972;9:143–146.

17. Rabbani GH, Butler T, Knight J, et al. Randomized controlled trial of berberine sulfate therapy for diarrhea due to enterotoxigenic *Escherichia coli* and *Vibrio cholerae. Journal of Infectious Diseases* 1987;155:979–984.

18. Tai YH, Feser JF, Mernane WG, et al. Antisecretory effects of berberine in rat ileum. *American Journal of Physiology* 1981;241:G253–G258.

19. Swabb EA, Tai YH, Jordan L. Reversal of cholera toxin-induced secretion in rat ileum by luminal berberine. *American Journal of Physiology* 1981;241:G248–G252.

20. Akhter MH, Sabir M, Bhide NK. Possible mechanism of antidiarrhoeal effect of berberine. *Indian Journal of Medical Research* 1979;70:233–241.

21. Joshi PV, Shirkhedkar AA, Prakash K, Maheshwari VL. Antidiarrheal activity, chemical and toxicity profile of *Berberis aristata. Pharmacology and Biology.* 2011 Jan;49(1):94–100.

22. Subbotina MD, Timchenko VN, Vorobyov MM, et al. Effect of oral administration of tormentil root extract (*Potentilla tormentilla*) on rotavirus diarrhea in children: a randomized, double blind, controlled trial. *The Pediatric Infectious Disease Journal* 2003;22:706–711.

Ear Infection (Otitis Media)

1. MacIntyre EA, Chen CM, Herbarth O, Early-life otitis media and incident atopic disease at school age in a birth cohort. *The Pediatric Infectious Disease Journal* 2010 Dec;29(12):e96–e99.

2. Kleinman LC, Kosecoff J, Dubois RW, et al. The medical appropriateness of tympanostomy tubes proposed for children younger than 16 years in the United States. *JAMA, The Journal of the American Medical Association* 1994;271:1250–1255.

3. Bluestone CD. Otitis media in children: to treat or not to treat? *The New England Journal of Medicine* 1982;306:1399–1404.

4. van Buchem FL, Dunk JH, van't Hof MA. Therapy of acute otitis media: myringotomy, antibiotics, or neither? *The Lancet* 1981;2:883–887.

5. Williams RL, Chalmers TC, Stange KC, et al. Use of antibiotics in preventing recurrent acute otitis media and in treating otitis media with effusion. A meta-analytic attempt to resolve the brouhaha. *JAMA, The Journal of the American Medical Association* 1993;270:1344–1351.

6. Rosenfeld RM, Vertrees JE, Carr J, et al. Clinical efficacy of antimicrobial drugs for acute otitis media: metaanalysis of 5400 children from thirty-three randomized trials. *Journal of Pediatrics* 1994;124:355–367.

7. Froom J, Culpepper L, Jacobs M, et al. Antimicrobials for acute otitis media? A review from the International Primary Care Network. *British Medical Journal* 1997;315:98–102.

8. Del Castillo F, Baquero-Artigao F, Garcia-Perea A. Influence of recent antibiotic therapy on antimicrobial resistance of *Streptococcus pneumoniae* in children with acute otitis media in Spain. *The Pediatric Infectious Disease Journal* 1998;17:94–97.

9. Rovers MM, Schilder AG, Zielhuis GA, et al. Otitis media. *The Lancet* 2004;363:465–473.

10. Mandel EM, Casselbrant ML, Rockette HE, et al. Systemic steroid for chronic otitis media with effusion in children. *Pediatrics* 2002;110:1071–1080.

11. Hannley MT, Denneny JC III, Holzer SS. Use of ototopical antibiotics in treating three common ear diseases. *Otolaryngology—Head and Neck Surgery* 2000;122:934–940.

12. Woodhead M. Antibiotic resistance. *British Journal of Hospital Medicine* 1996;56:314–315.

13. Cates C. An evidence based approach to reducing antibiotic use in children with acute otitis media: controlled before and after study. *BMJ* 1999;318:715–716.

14. Saarinen UM. Prolonged breast feeding as prophylaxis for recurrent otitis media. *Acta Paediatrica Scandinavica* 1982;71:567–571.

15. Uhari M, Mäntysaari K, Niemelä M. A meta-analytic review of the risk factors for acute otitis media. *Clinical Infectious Diseases* 1996;22:1079–1083.

16. Editor. Breast feeding prevents otitis media. *Nutrition Reviews* 1983;41:241–242.

17. Hasselbalch H, Jeppesen DL, Engelmann MD, et al. Decreased thymus size in formula-fed infants compared with breastfed infants. *Acta Paedriatrica* 1996;85:1029–1032.

18. Ramakrishnan JB. The role of food allergy in otolaryngology disorders. *Current Opinion in Otolaryngology & Head and Neck Surgery* 2010 Jun;18(3):195–199.

19. McMahan JT, Calenoff E, Croft DJ, et al. Chronic otitis media with effusion and allergy: modified RAST analysis of 119 cases. *Otolaryngology—Head and Neck Surgery* 1981;89:427–431.

20. Van Cauwenberge PB. The role of allergy in otitis media with effusion. *Therapeutische Umschau* 1982;39:1011–1016.

21. Bellionin P, Cantani A, Salvinelli F. Allergy: a leading role in otitis media with effusion. *Allergologia et Immunopathologia* 1987;15:205–208.

22. Hurst DS. Association of otitis media with effusion and allergy as demonstrated by intradermal skin testing and eosinophil protein levels in both middle ear

effusions and mucosal biopsies. *The Laryngoscope* 1996;106: 1128–1137.

23. Nsouli TM, Nsouli SM, Linde RE, et al. Role of food allergy in serous otitis media. *Annals of Allergy, Asthma & Immunology* 1994;73:215–219.

24. Sarrell EM, Cohen HA, Kahan E. Naturopathic treatment for ear pain in children. *Pediatrics* 2003;111:574–579.

25. Sarrell EM, Mandelberg A, Cohen HA. Efficacy of naturopathic extracts in the management of ear pain associated with acute otitis media. *Archives of Pediatrics & Adolescent Medicine* 2001;155:796–799.

26. Uhari M, Kontiokari T, Koskela M, et al. Xylitol chewing gum in prevention of acute otitis media: double blind randomised trial. *BMJ* 1996;313:1180–1184.

27. Uhari M, Kontiokari T, Niemela M. A novel use of xylitol sugar in preventing acute otitis media. *Pediatrics* 1998; 102:879–884.

28. Lovejoy HM, McGuirt WF, Ayres PH, et al. Effects of low humidity on the rat middle ear. *The Laryngoscope* 1994;104: 1055–1058.

Endometriosis

1. Giudice LC. Clinical practice. Endometriosis. *The New England Journal of Medicine* 2010 Jun 24;362(25):2389–2398.

2. Weuve J, Hauser R, Calafat AM, et al. Association of exposure to phthalates with endometriosis and uterine leiomyomata: findings from NHANES, 1999–2004. *Environmental Health Perspectives* 2010 Jun;118(6): 825–832.

3. Missmer SA, Chavarro JE, Malspeis S, et al. A prospective study of dietary fat consumption and endometriosis risk. *Human Reproduction* 2010 Jun;25(6): 1528–1535.

4. Gazvani MR, Smith L, Haggarty P, et al. High omega-3: omega-6 fatty acid ratios in culture medium reduce endometrial-cell survival in combined endometrial gland and stromal cell cultures from women with and without endometriosis. *Fertility and Sterility* 2001;76: 717–722.

5. Kappas A, Anderson KE, Conney AH, et al. Nutrition-endocrine interactions: induction of reciprocal changes in the delta 4-5 alpha-reduction of testosterone and the cytochrome P-450-dependent oxidation of estradiol by dietary macronutrients in man. *Proceedings of the National Academy of Sciences of the United States of America* 1983;80:7646–7649.

6. Goldin BR, Adlercreutz H, Dwyer JT, et al. Effect of diet on excretion of estrogens in pre- and postmenopausal women. *Cancer Research* 1981;41:3771–3773.

7. Michnovicz JJ, Bradlow HL. Altered estrogen metabolism and excretion in humans following consumption of indole-3-carbinol. *Nutrition and Cancer* 1991; 16:59–66.

8. Leibovitz BE, Mueller JA. Bioflavonoids and polyphenols: medical applications. *Journal of Optimal Nutrition* 1993;2: 17–35.

9. Nagata C, Takatsuka N, Kawakami N, Shimizu H. Soy product intake and premenopausal hysterectomy in a follow-up study of Japanese women. *European Journal of Clinical Nutrition* 2001 Sep;55(9):773–777.

10. Tremblay L. Reproductive toxins conference—pollution prevention network. *Endometriosis Association Newsletter* 1996;17: 13–15.

11. Mathias JR, Franklin R, Quast DC, et al. Relation of endometriosis and neuromuscular disease of the gastrointestinal tract: new insights. *Fertility and Sterility* 1998 Jul;70(1):81–88.

12. Grodstein F, Goldman MB, Ryan L, Cramer DW. Relation of female infertility to consumption of caffeinated beverages. *American Journal of Epidemiology* 1993;137:1353–1360.

13. Kohama T, Herai K, Inoue M. Effect of French maritime pine bark extract on endometriosis as compared with leuprorelin acetate. *The Journal of Reproductive Medicine* 2007;52(8): 703–708.

14. Wuttke W, Jarry H, Christoffel V, et al. Chaste tree (*Vitex agnus-castus*)—pharmacology and clinical indications. *Phytomedicine* 2003 May;10(4):348–357.

Erectile Dysfunction

1. Hatzimouratidis K. Epidemiology of male sexual dysfunction. *American Journal of Men's Health* 2007 Jun;1(2):103–125.

2. Shin D, Pregenzer G Jr, Gardin JM. Erectile dysfunction: a disease marker for cardiovascular disease. *Cardiology in Review* 2011 Jan–Feb;19(1):5–11.

3. Heidelbaugh JJ. Management of erectile dysfunction. *American Family Physician* 2010 Feb 1; 81(3):305–312.

4. Safarinejad MR. Safety and efficacy of coenzyme Q10 supplementation in early chronic Peyronie's disease: a double-blind, placebo-controlled randomized study. *International Journal of Impotence Research* 2010 Sep–Oct;22(5):298–309.

5. White JR, Case DA, McWhirter D, Mattisson AM. Enhanced sexual behavior in exercising men. *Archives of Sexual Behavior* 1990;19:193–209.

6. Sommer F, Goldstein I, Korda JB. Bicycle riding and erectile dysfunction: a review. *The Journal of Sexual Medicine* 2010 Jul; 7(7):2346–2358.

7. Chen J, Wollman Y, Chernichovsky T, Effect of oral administration of high-dose nitric oxide donor L-arginine in men with organic erectile dysfunction: results of a double-blind, randomized, placebo-controlled study.

BJU International 1999 Feb; 83(3):269–273.

8. Stanislavov R, Nikolova V, Rohdewald P. Improvement of erectile function with Prelox: a randomized, double-blind, placebo-controlled, crossover trial. *International Journal of Impotence Research* 2008 Mar–Apr; 20(2):173–180.

9. Ledda A, Belcaro G, Cesarone MR, et al. Investigation of a complex plant extract for mild to moderate erectile dysfunction in a randomized, double-blind, placebo-controlled, parallel-arm study. *BJU International* 2010 Oct;106(7):1030–1033.

10. Aoki H, Nagao J, Ueda T, et al. Clinical assessment of a supplement of Pycnogenol® and l-arginine in Japanese patients with mild to moderate erectile dysfunction. *Phytotherapy Research* 2012 Feb;26(2):204–207.

11. Cormio L, De Siati M, Lorusso F, et al. Oral L-citrulline supplementation improves erection hardness in men with mild erectile dysfunction. *Urology* 2011 Jan;77(1):119–122.

12. Ernst E, Pittler MH. Yohimbine for erectile dysfunction: a systematic review and meta-analysis of randomized clinical trials. *Journal of Urology* 1998; 159:433–436.

13. Betz J, White KD, der Marderosian AH. Chemical analysis of 26 commercial yohimbe products. *Journal of AOAC International* 1995;78(5):1189–1194.

14. Waynberg J. Aphrodisiacs: contribution to the clinical validation of the traditional use of *Ptychopetalum guyanna*. Presented at the First International Congress on Ethnopharmacology, Strasbourg, France, June 5–9, 1990.

15. Jang DJ, Lee MS, Shin BC, et al. Red ginseng for treating erectile dysfunction: a systematic review. *British Journal of Clinical Pharmacology* 2008 Oct;66(4):444–450.

16. Hong B, Ji YH, Hong JH, et al.

A double-blind crossover study evaluating the efficacy of Korean red ginseng in patients with erectile dysfunction: a preliminary report. *Journal of Urology* 2002;168:2070–2073.

17. Zanoli P, Zavatti M, Montanari C, Baraldi M. Influence of Eurycoma longifolia on the copulatory activity of sexually sluggish and impotent male rats. *Journal of Ethnopharmacology* 2009 Nov 12;126(2):308–313.

18. Ang HH, Lee KL, Kiyoshi M. Sexual arousal in sexually sluggish old male rats after oral administration of *Eurycoma longifolia* Jack. *Journal of Basic and Clinical Physiology and Pharmacology* 2004;15(3–4): 303–309.

19. Hamzah S, Yusof A. The ergogenic effects of *Eurycoma longifolia* Jack: a pilot study. *British Journal of Sports Medicine* 2003;37: 464–470.

20. Gauthaman K, Ganesan AP. The hormonal effects of *Tribulus terrestris* and its role in the management of male erectile dysfunction—an evaluation using primates, rabbit and rat. *Phytomedicine* 2008;15(1–2): 44–54.

21. Rogerson S, Riches CJ, Jennings C, et al. The effect of five weeks of *Tribulus terrestris* supplementation on muscle strength and body composition during preseason training in elite rugby league players. *The Journal of Strength and Conditioning Research* 2007;21(2): 348–353.

22. Steels E, Rao A, Vitetta L. Physiological aspects of male libido enhanced by standardized *Trigonella foenum-graecum* extract and mineral formulation. *Phytotherapy Research* 2011 Sep;25(9):1294–1300.

23. Sikora R, Sohn M, Deutz et al. *Ginkgo biloba* extract in the therapy of erectile dysfunction. *Journal of Urology* 1989;141: 188A.

24. Sohn M, Sikora R. *Ginkgo biloba* extract in the therapy of erectile dysfunction. *Journal of Sex Education and Therapy* 1991;17:53–61.

25. Cohen AJ, Bartlik B. *Ginkgo biloba* for antidepressant-induced sexual dysfunction. *Journal of Sex & Marital Therapy* 1998;24: 139–143.

26. Kang BJ, Lee SJ, Kim MD, Cho MJ. A placebo-controlled, double-blind trial of *Ginkgo biloba* for antidepressant-induced sexual dysfunction. *Human Psychopharmacology* 2002 Aug; 17(6):279–284.

Eczema (Atopic Dermatitis)

1. Barnes, KC. An update on the genetics of atopic dermatitis: scratching the surface in 2009. *Journal of Allergy and Clinical Immunology* 2010 Jan;125(1): 16–29.

2. Saarinen UM, Kajosaari M. Breastfeeding as prophylaxis against atopic disease: prospective follow-up study until 17 years old. *The Lancet* 1995;346: 1065–1069.

3. Isolauri E, Tahvanainen A, Peltola T, et al. Breast-feeding of allergic infants. *Journal of Pediatrics* 1999;134:27–32.

4. Arvola T, Moilanen E, Vuento R, et al. Weaning to hypoallergenic formula improves gut barrier function in breast-fed infants with atopic eczema. *Journal of Pediatric Gastroenterology and Nutrition* 2004;38: 92–96.

5. Cant AJ, Bailes JA, et al. Effect of maternal dietary exclusion on breast fed infants with eczema: two controlled studies. *British Medical Journal* 1986;293:231–233.

6. Burks AW, Williams LW, Mallory SB, et al. Peanut protein as a major cause of adverse food reaction in patients with atopic dermatitis. *Allergy Proceedings* 1989;10:265–269.

7. Lever R, MacDonald C, Waugh P, et al. Randomised controlled trial of advice on an egg

exclusion diet in young children with atopic eczema and sensitivity to eggs. *Pediatric Allergy and Immunology* 1998;9:13–19.

8. de Maat-Bleeker F, Bruijnzeel-Koomen C. Food allergy in adults with atopic dermatitis. *Monographs in Allergy* 1996;32: 157–163.

9. Van Bever HP, Docx M, Stevens WJ. Food and food additives in severe atopic dermatitis. *Allergy* 1989;44:588–594.

10. Sampson HA, Scanlon SM. Natural history of food hypersensitivity in children with atopic dermatitis. *Journal of Pediatrics* 1989;115:23–27.

11. Savolainen J, Lammintausta K, Kalimo K, et al. Candida albicans and atopic dermatitis. *Clinical & Experimental Allergy* 1993;23:332–339.

12. Adachi A, Horikawa T, Ichihashi M, et al. [Role of *Candida* allergen in atopic dermatitis and efficacy of oral therapy with various antifungal agents.] *Arerugi* 1999 Jul;48(7):719–725.

13. Isolauri E, Arvola T, Sutas Y, et al. Probiotics in the management of atopic eczema. *Clinical & Experimental Allergy* 2000; 30:1604–1610.

14. Majamaa H, Isolauri E. Probiotics: a novel approach in the management of food allergy. *Journal of Allergy and Clinical Immunology* 1997;99:179–185.

15. Rosenfeldt V, Benfeldt E, Nielsen SD, et al. Effect of probiotic *Lactobacillus* strains in children with atopic dermatitis. *Journal of Allergy and Clinical Immunology* 2003;111:389–395.

16. Osborn DA, Sinn JK. Probiotics in infants for prevention of allergic disease and food hypersensitivity. Cochrane Database of Systematic Reviews 2007 Oct 17;4:CD006475.

17. Stewart JCM, Morse PF, Moss M, et al. Treatment of severe and moderately severe atopic dermatitis with evening primrose oil (Epogam): a multicenter study. *Journal of Nutritional and Environmental Medicine* 1991;2:9–15.

18. Hederos CA, Berg A. Epogam evening primrose oil treatment in atopic dermatitis and asthma. *Archives of Disease in Childhood* 1996;75:494–497.

19. Fiocchi A, Sala M, Signoroni P, et al. The efficacy and safety of gamma-linolenic acid in the treatment of infantile atopic dermatitis. *Journal of International Medical Research* 1994; 22:24–32.

20. Berth-Jones J, Graham-Brown RA. Placebo-controlled trial of essential fatty acid supplementation in atopic dermatitis. *The Lancet* 1993;341:1557–1560.

21. Takwale A, Tan E, Agarwal S, et al. Efficacy and tolerability of borage oil in adults and children with atopic eczema: randomised, double blind, placebo controlled, parallel group trial. *BMJ* 2003;327:1385.

22. Soyland E, Funk J, Rajka G, et al. Dietary supplementation with very long-chain n-3 fatty acids in patients with atopic dermatitis. A double-blind, multicentre study. *British Journal of Dermatology* 1994;130:757–764.

23. Kremmyda LS, Vlachava M, Noakes PS, et al. Atopy risk in infants and children in relation to early exposure to fish, oily fish, or long-chain omega-3 fatty acids: a systematic review. *Clinical Reviews in Allergy and Immunology* 2011 Aug;41(1): 36–66.

24. Atherton DJ, Sheehan MP, Rustin MH, et al. Treatment of atopic eczema with traditional Chinese medicinal plants. *Pediatric Dermatology* 1992;9: 373–375.

25. Sheehan MP, Rustin MH, Atherton DJ, et al. Efficacy of traditional Chinese herbal therapy in adult atopic dermatitis. *The Lancet* 1992;340:13–17.

26. Sheehan MP, Atherton DJ. A controlled trial of traditional Chinese medicinal plants in widespread non-exudative atopic eczema. *British Journal of Dermatology* 1992;126:179–184.

27. Evans FQ. The rational use of glycyrrhetinic acid in dermatology. *The British Journal of Clinical Practice* 1958;12:269–274.

Fibrocystic Breast Disease

1. Peters F, Schuth W, Scheurich B, Breckwoldt M. Serum prolactin levels in patients with fibrocystic breast disease. *Obstetrics & Gynecology* 1984;64: 381–385

2. Boyle CA, Berkowitz GS, LiVolsi VA, et al. Caffeine consumption and fibrocystic breast disease: a case-control epidemiologic study. *Journal of the National Cancer Institute* 1984; 72:1015–1019.

3. Minton JP, Abou-Issa H, Reiches N, Roseman JM. Clinical and biochemical studies on methylxanthine-related fibrocystic breast disease. *Surgery* 1981;90:299–304.

4. Minton JP, Foecking MK, Webster DJT, Matthews RH. Caffeine, cyclic nucleotides, and breast disease. *Surgery* 1979;86: 105–109.

5. Ernster VL, Mason L, Goodson WH III, et al. Effects of caffeine-free diet on benign breast disease: a random trial. *Surgery* 1982;91:263–267.

6. Lubin F, Ron E, Wax Y, et al. A case-control study of caffeine and methylxanthine in benign breast disease. *JAMA, The Journal of the American Medical Association* 1985;253:2388–2392.

7. Shairer C, Brinton LA, Hoover RN. Methylxanthine and benign breast disease. *American Journal of Epidemiology* 1986;124: 603–611.

8. Marshall J, Graham S, Swanson M. Caffeine consumption and benign breast disease: a case-control comparison. *The American Journal of Public Health* 1982;72:610–612.

9. Baghurst PA, Rohan TE. Dietary fiber and risk of benign proliferative epithelial disor-

ders of the breast. *International Journal of Cancer* 1995;63:481–485.

10. Petrakis NL, King EB. Cytological abnormalities in nipple aspirates of breast fluid from women with severe constipation. *The Lancet* 1981;2:1203–1204.

11. Goldin B, Aldercreutz H, Dwyer JT, et al. Effect of diet on excretion of estrogens in pre- and post-menopausal women. *Cancer Research* 1981;41:3771–3773.

12. Goldin B, Gorback S. The effect of milk and lactobacillus feeding on human intestinal bacterial enzyme activity. *The American Journal of Clinical Nutrition* 1984;39:756–761.

13. Boyd NF, McGuire V, Shannon P, et al. Effect of a low-fat high-carbohydrate diet on symptoms of cyclical mastopathy. *The Lancet* 1988;2:128–132.

14. Rose DP, Boyar AP, Cohen C, Strong LE. Effect of a low-fat diet on hormone levels in women with cystic breast disease. I. Serum steroids and gonadotropins. *Journal of the National Cancer Institute* 1987;78:623–626.

15. Pye J, Mansel RE, Hughes LE. Clinical experience of drug treatment for mastalgia. *The Lancet* 1985;2:373–377.

16. Pashby N, Mansel RE, Hughes LE, et al. A clinical trial of evening primrose oil in mastalgia. *British Journal of Surgery* 1981; 68:801–824.

17. Shannon J, King IB, Lampe JW, et al. Erythrocyte fatty acids and risk of proliferative and nonproliferative fibrocystic disease in women in Shanghai, China. *The American Journal of Clinical Nutrition* 2009 Jan; 89(1):265–276.

18. London RS, Sundaram G, Manimekalai S, et al. The effect of alpha-tocopherol on pre-menstrual symptomatology: a double-blind study. II. Endocrine correlates. *Journal of the American College of Nutrition* 1984;3:351–356.

19. London R, Sundaram G, Manimekalai S, et al. Mammary dysplasia: endocrine parameters and tocopherol therapy. *Nutrition Research* 1982;7:243.

20. London R, Sundaram GS, Schultz M, et al. Endocrine parameters and alpha-tocopherol therapy of patients with mammary dysplasia. *Cancer Research* 1981;41:3811–3813.

21. Myer EC, Sommers DK, Reitz CJ, Mentis H. Vitamin E and benign breast disease. *Surgery* 1990;107:549–551.

22. London RS, Sundaram GS, Murphy L, et al. The effect of vitamin E on mammary dysplasia: a double-blind study. *Obstetrics & Gynecology* 1985;65:104–106.

23. Bespalov V, Barash N, Ivanova O, et al. [Study of an antioxidant dietary supplement "Karinat" in patients with benign breast disease.] *Voprosy Onkologii* 2004;50:467–472.

24. Eskin BA, Bartushka DG, Dunn MR, et al. Mammary gland dysplasia in iodine deficiency. *JAMA, The Journal of the American Medical Association* 1967;200:691–695.

25. Ghent WR, Eskin BA, Low DA, Hill LP. Iodine replacement in fibrocystic disease of the breast. *Canadian Journal of Surgery* 1993;36:453–460.

26. Mielens ZE, Rozitis J Jr, Sansone VJ Jr. The effect of oral iodides on inflammation. *Texas Reports on Biology & Medicine* 1968;26:117–121.

27. Estes NC. Mastodynia due to fibrocystic disease of the breast controlled with thyroid hormone. *The American Journal of Surgery* 1981;142:764–766.

28. Loch E, Selle H, Boblitz N. Treatment of premenstrual syndrome with a phytopharmaceutical formulation containing *Vitex agnus castus*. *Journal of Women's Health and Gender-Based Medicine* 2000;9:315–320.

29. Halaska M, Beles P, Gorkow C, Sieder C. Treatment of cyclical mastalgia with a solution containing a *Vitex agnus castus* extract: results of a placebo-controlled double-blind study. *Breast* 1000;8:175–181.

30. Atmaca M, Kumru S, Tezcan E. Fluoxetine versus *Vitex agnus castus* extract in the treatment of premenstrual dysphoric disorder. *Human Psychopharmacology* 2003;18:191–195.

31. Schellenberg R. Treatment for the premenstrual syndrome with agnus castus fruit extract: prospective, randomised, placebo controlled study. *British Medical Journal* 2001;322:134–137.

Food Allergy

1. Adams F. *The genuine works of Hippocrates*. Baltimore: Williams & Williams, 1939.

2. Sampson HA. Update on food allergy. *Journal of Allergy and Clinical Immunology* 2004;113:805–819.

3. Sicherer S, Sampson H. Food allergy. *Journal of Allergy and Clinical Immunology* 2006;117:S470–S475.

4. Osterballe M, Hansen TK, Mortz CG, et al. The prevalence of food hypersensitivity in an unselected population of children and adults. *Pediatric Allergy and Immunology* 2005;16:567–573.

5. Andre FA, Andre C, Colin L, et al. Role of new allergens and of allergens consumption in the increased incidence of food sensitizations in France. *Toxicology* 1994;93:77–83.

6. Sicherer SH. Manifestations of food allergy: evaluation and management. *American Family Physician* 1999;59:415–424, 429–430.

7. Rowe AH, Rowe A. *Food allergy: its manifestations and control and the elimination diets*. Springfield, Ill.: Charles C. Thomas, 1972.

8. Dockhorn RJ, Smith TC. Use

of a chemically defined hypoallergenic diet in the management of patients with suspected food allergy. *Annals of Allergy, Asthma & Immunology* 1981;47: 264–266.

9. Metcalfe D. Food hypersensitivity. *Journal of Allergy and Clinical Immunology* 1984;73: 749–761.

10. AAAI Board of Directors. Measurement of specific and nonspecific IgG4 levels as diagnostic and prognostic tests for clinical allergy. *Journal of Allergy and Clinical Immunology* 1995;95:652–654.

11. Gwynn CM, Ingram J, Almousawi T, Stanworth DR. Bronchial provocation tests in atopic patients with allergen-specific IgG4 antibodies. *The Lancet* 1982;1(8266):254–256.

12. Shakib F, Brown HM, Phelps A, Redhead R. Study of IgG subclass antibodies in patients with milk intolerance. *Clinical Allergy* 1986 Sep;16(5):451–458.

13. el Rafei A, Peters SM, Harris N, Bellanti JA. Diagnostic value of IgG4 measurements in patients with food allergy. *Annals of Allergy, Asthma & Immunology* 1989;62(2):94–99.

14. Hamilton R. Clinical laboratory assessment of IgE-dependent hypersensitivity. *Journal of Allergy and Clinical Immunology* 2003 Feb;111:S687–S701.

15. Biagini RE, MacKenzie BA, Sammons DL, et al. Latex specific IgE: performance characteristics of the IMMULITE 2000 3gAllergy assay compared with skin testing. *Annals of Allergy, Asthma & Immunology* 2006;97:196–202.

16. Cox L, Williams B, Sicherer S, et al. Pearls and pitfalls of allergy diagnostic testing: report from the American College of Allergy, Asthma and Immunology/American Academy of Allergy, Asthma and Immunology Specific IgE Test Task Force. *Annals of Allergy, Asthma & Immunology* 2008;101:580–592.

17. Niggemann B, Gruber C. Unproven diagnostic procedures in IgE-mediated allergic diseases. *Allergy* 2004;59:806–808.

18. Bindslev-Jensen C, Poulsen LK. What do we at present know about the ALCAT test and what is lacking? *Monographs in Allergy* 1996;32:228–232.

19. Lieberman P, Crawford L, Bjelland J, et al. Controlled study of the cytotoxic food test. *JAMA, The Journal of the American Medical Association* 1975;231 (7):728–730.

20. Beyer K, Teuber SS. Food allergy diagnostics: scientific and unproven procedures. *Current Opinion in Allergy and Clinical Immunology* 2005;5:261–266.

21. Gerez IF, Shek LP, Chng HH, Lee BW. Diagnostic tests for food allergy. *Singapore Medical Journal* 2010;51:4–9.

22. Teuber SS, Porch-Curren C. Unproved diagnostic and therapeutic approaches to food allergy and intolerance. *Current Opinion in Allergy and Clinical Immunology* 2003;3:217–221.

23. Wuthrich B. Unproven techniques in allergy diagnosis. *Journal of Investigative Allergology and Clinical Immunology* 2005;15:86–90.

24. Hodsdon W, Zwickey H. NMJ original research: reproducibility and reliability of two food allergy testing methods. *Natural Medicine Journal* 2010;2: 8–13.

25. Rinkel HJ. Food allergy. IV. The function and clinical application of the rotary diversified diet. *Journal of Pediatrics* 1948;32: 266–274.

26. Oelgoetz AW, Oelgoetz PA, Wittenkind J. The treatment of food allergy and indigestion of pancreatic origin with pancreatic enzymes. *American Journal of Digestive Diseases* 1935;2: 422–426.

27. Raithel M, Weidenhiller M, Schwab D, et al. Pancreatic enzymes: a new group of antiallergic drugs? *Inflammation Research* 2002;51 suppl 1:S13–S14.

28. Zuercher AW, Holvoet S, Weiss M, Mercenier A. Polyphenol-enriched apple extract attenuates food allergy in mice. *Clinical & Experimental Allergy* 2010 Jun;40(6):942–950.

29. Akiyama H, Sato Y, Watanabe T, et al. Dietary unripe apple polyphenol inhibits the development of food allergies in murine models. *FEBS Letters* 2005 Aug 15; 579(20):4485–4491.

Gallstones

1. Trowell H, Burkitt D, Heaton K, eds. *Dietary fibre, fibre-depleted foods and disease*. London: Academic Press, 1985, 289–304.

2. Kalloo AN, Kantsevoy SV. Gallstones and biliary disease. *Primary Care* 2001;28:591–606,vii.

3. Ruhl CE, Everhart JE. Gallstone disease is associated with increased mortality in the United States. *Gastroenterology* 2011 Feb;140(2):508–516.

4. Vitetta L, Sali A, Little P, et al. Gallstones and gall bladder carcinoma. *ANZ Journal of Surgery* 2000;70:667–673.

5. Festi D, Colecchia A, Larocca A, et al. Review: low caloric intake and gallbladder motor function. *Alimentary Pharmacology & Therapeutics* 2000;14 suppl 2: 51–53.

6. Mathus-Vliegen EM, Van Ierland-Van Leeuwen ML, Terpstra A. Determinants of gallbladder kinetics in obesity. *Digestive Diseases and Sciences* 2004;49:9–16.

7. Akin ML, Uluutku H, Erenoglu C, et al. Tamoxifen and gallstone formation in postmenopausal breast cancer patients: retrospective cohort study. *World Journal of Surgery* 2003;27:395–399.

8. Wang DQ. Aging per se is an independent risk factor for cholesterol gallstone formation in gallstone susceptible mice. *The*

Journal of Lipid Research 2002; 43:1950–1959.

9. Pandey M, Shukla VK. Diet and gallbladder cancer: a case-control study. *European Journal of Cancer Prevention* 2002;11: 365–368.

10. Marks JW, Cleary PA, Albers JJ. Lack of correlation between serum lipoproteins and biliary cholesterol saturation in patients with gallstones. *Digestive Diseases and Sciences* 1984;29: 1118–1122.

11. Van der Linder W, Bergman F. An analysis of data on human hepatic bile. Relationship between main bile components, serum cholesterol and serum triglycerides. *Scandinavian Journal of Clinical & Laboratory Investigation* 1977;37:741–747.

12. Smelt AH. Triglycerides and gallstone formation. *Clinica Chimica Acta* 2010 Nov 11; 411(21–22):1625–1631.

13. Nervi F, Covarrubias C, Bravo P, et al. Influence of legume intake on biliary lipids and cholesterol saturation in young Chilean men. *Gastroenterology* 1989;96: 825–830.

14. Thijs C, Knipschild P. Legume intake and gallstone risk: results from a case-control study. *International Journal of Epidemiology* 1990 Sep;19(3):660–663.

15. Pixley F, Wilson D, McPherson K, et al. Effect of vegetarianism on development of gallstones in women. *British Medical Journal* 1985;291:11–12.

16. Kritchevsky D, Klurfeld DM. Gallstone formation in hamsters: effect of varying animal and vegetable protein levels. *The American Journal of Clinical Nutrition* 1983;37: 802–804.

17. Breneman JC. Allergy elimination diet as the most effective gallbladder diet. *Annals of Allergy, Asthma & Immunology* 1968;26:83–87.

18. Necheles H, Rappaport BZ, Green R, et al. Allergy of the gallbladder. *American Journal of Digestive Diseases* 1949;7: 238–241.

19. Walzer M, Gray I, Harten M, et al. The allergic reaction in the gallbladder: experimental studies in rhesus monkeys. *Gastroenterology* 1943;1:565–572.

20. De Muro P, Ficari A. Experimental studies on allergic cholecystitis. *Gastroenterology* 1946; 6:302–314.

21. Tomotake H, Shimaoka I, Kayashita J, et al. A buckwheat protein product suppresses gallstone formation and plasma cholesterol more strongly than soy protein isolate in hamsters. *Journal of Nutrition* 2000;130: 1670–1674.

22. Kritchevsky D, Klurfeld DM. Influence of vegetable protein on gallstone formation in hamsters. *The American Journal of Clinical Nutrition* 1979;32: 2174–2176.

23. Tomotake H, Shimaoka I, Kayashita J, et al. Stronger suppression of plasma cholesterol and enhancement of the fecal excretion of steroids by a buckwheat protein product than by a soy protein isolate in rats fed on a cholesterol-free diet. *Bioscience, Biotechnology, and Biodiversity* 2001;65:1412–1414.

24. Liu Z, Ishikawa W, Huang X, et al. A buckwheat protein product suppresses 1,2-dimethylhydrazine-induced colon carcinogenesis in rats by reducing cell proliferation. *Journal of Nutrition* 2001;131:1850–1853.

25. Thornton JR, Emmett PM, Heaton KW. Diet and gall stones: effects of refined and unrefined carbohydrate diets on bile cholesterol saturation and bile acid metabolism. *Gut* 1983;24:2–6.

26. Tsai CJ, Leitzmann MF, Willett WC, Giovannucci EL. Glycemic load, glycemic index, and carbohydrate intake in relation to risk of cholecystectomy in women. *Gastroenterology* 2005 Jul;129(1):105–112.

27. Moerman CJ, Bueno de Mesquita HB, Runia S. Dietary sugar intake in the etiology of biliary tract cancer. *International Journal of Epidemiology* 1993;22:207–214.

28. Moerman CJ, Smeets FW, Kromhout D. Dietary risk factors for clinically diagnosed gallstones in middle-aged men: a 25-year follow-up study (the Zutphen Study). *Annals of Epidemiology* 1994;4:248–254.

29. Tandon RK, Saraya A, Paul S, et al. Dietary habits of gallstone patients in northern India: a case control study. *Journal of Clinical Gastroenterology* 1996; 22:23–27.

30. Caroli-Bosc FX, Deveau C, Peten EP, et al. Cholelithiasis and dietary risk factors: an epidemiologic investigation in Vidauban, southeast France. General Practitioners' Group of Vidauban. *Digestive Diseases and Sciences* 1998;43:2131–2137.

31. Kamrath RO, Plummer LF, Sadur CN. Cholelithiasis in patients treated with a very-low-calorie diet. *The American Journal of Clinical Nutrition* 1992;56:255S–257S.

32. van Erpecum KJ, van Berge Henegouwen GP. Intestinal aspects of cholesterol gallstone formation. *Digestive and Liver Disease* 2003;35 suppl 3:S8–S11.

33. Spirt BA, Graves LW, Weinstock R. Gallstone formation in obese women treated by a low-calorie diet. *International Journal of Obesity and Related Metabolic Disorders* 1995;19: 593–595.

34. Douglas BR, Jansen JB, Tham RT. Coffee stimulation of cholecystokinin release and gallbladder contraction in humans. *The American Journal of Clinical Nutrition* 1990;52:553–556.

35. Leitzmann MF, Stampfer MJ, Willett WC, et al. Coffee intake is associated with lower risk of symptomatic gallstone disease in women. *Gastroenterology* 2002;123:1823–1830.

36. Kasbo J, Tuchweber B, Perwaiz S, et al. Phosphatidylcho-

line-enriched diet prevents gallstone formation in mice susceptible to cholelithiasis. *The Journal of Lipid Research* 2003; 44:2297–2303.

37. Tuzhilin SA, Drieling DA, Narodetskaja RV, et al. The treatment of patients with gallstones by lecithin. *The American Journal of Gastroenterology* 1976;65:231–235.

38. Hanin I, Ansell GB. *Lecithin: technological, biological, and therapeutic aspects.* New York: Plenum Press, 1987.

39. Jenkins SA. Vitamin C and gallstone formation: a preliminary report. *Experientia* 1977;33: 1616–1617.

40. Dam H, Christensen F. Alimentary production of gallstones in hamsters. *Acta Pathologica et Microbiologica Scandinavica* 1952;30:236–242.

41. Sies CW, Brooker J. Could these be gallstones? *The Lancet* 2005 Apr 16–22;365(9468):1388.

42. Lee SP, Tassman-Jones C, Carlisle V. Oleic acid–induced cholelithiasis in rabbits. *The American Journal of Pathology* 1986;124:18–24.

43. Beynen AC. Dietary monounsaturated fatty acids and liver cholesterol. *Artery* 1988;15: 170–175.

44. Baggio G, Pagnan A, Muraca M, et al. Olive-oil-enriched diet: effect on serum lipoprotein levels and biliary cholesterol saturation. *The American Journal of Clinical Nutrition* 1988;47: 960–964.

45. Scobey MW, Johnson FL, Parks JS. Dietary fish oil effects on biliary lipid secretion and cholesterol gallstone formation in the African green monkey. *Hepatology* 1991;14(4 part 1): 679–684.

46. Magnuson TH, Lillemoe KD, High RC, et al. Dietary fish oil inhibits cholesterol monohydrate crystal nucleation and gallstone formation in the prairie dog. *Surgery* 1995;118:517–523.

47. Jonkers IJ, Smelt AH, Princen HM, et al. Fish oil increases bile acid synthesis in male patients with hypertriglyceridemia. *Journal of Nutrition* 2006 Apr;136(4): 987–991.

48. Méndez-Sánchez N, González V, Aguayo P, et al. Fish oil (n-3) polyunsaturated fatty acids beneficially affect biliary cholesterol nucleation time in obese women losing weight. *Journal of Nutrition* 2001 Sep;131(9):2300–2303.

49. Hussain MS, Chandrasekhara N. Effect on curcumin on cholesterol gall-stone induction in mice. *Indian Journal of Medical Research* 1992;96:288–291.

50. Portincasa P, Di Ciaula A, Wang HH, et al. Medicinal treatments of cholesterol gallstones: old, current and new perspectives. *Current Medicinal Chemistry* 2009;16(12):1531–1542.

51. Di Ciaula A, Wang DQ, Wang HH, et al. Targets for current pharmacologic therapy in cholesterol gallstone disease. *Gastroenterology Clinics of North America* 2010 Jun;39(2): 245–264.

52. Hordinsky BZ. Terpenes in the treatment of gallstones. *Minnesota Medicine* 1971;54:649–652.

53. Bell GD, Doran J. Gallstone dissolution in man using an essential oil preparation. *British Medical Journal* 1979;1:24.

54. Doran J, Keighley RB, Bell GD. Rowachol—a possible treatment for cholesterol gallstones. *Gut* 1979;20:312–317.

55. Ellis WR, Bell GD. Treatment of biliary duct stones with a terpene preparation. *British Medical Journal* (Clinical Research Edition) 1981;282:611.

56. Somerville KW, Ellis WR, Whitten BH, et al. Stones in the common bile duct: experience with medical dissolution therapy. *Postgraduate Medical Journal* 1985;61:313–316.

57. Ellis WR, Bell GD, Middleton B, et al. Adjunct to bile-acid treatment for gall-stone dissolution: low-dose chenodeoxycholic acid combined with a terpene preparation. *British Medical Journal* 1981;282:611–612.

58. Ellis WR, Somerville KW, Whitten BH, Bell GD. Pilot study of combination treatment for gall stones with medium dose chenodeoxycholic acid and a terpene preparation. *British Medical Journal* 1984;289:153–156.

Glaucoma

1. Distelhorst JS, Hughes GM. Open-angle glaucoma. *American Family Physician* 2003;67: 1937–1944.

2. Tengroth B, Ammitzboll T. Changes in the content and composition of collagen in the glaucomatous eye—basis for a new hypothesis for the genesis of chronic open-angle glaucoma. *Acta Ophthalmologica* 1984;62: 999–1008.

3. Weiss J, Jayson M. *Collagen in health and disease.* Edinburgh and New York: Churchill Livingstone, 1982, 388–403.

4. Quigley H, Addicks E. Regional differences in the structure of the lamina cribrosa and their relation to glaucomatous optic nerve damage. *Archives of Ophthalmology* 1981;99:137–143.

5. Krakau T, Bengtsson B, Holmin C. The glaucoma theory updated. *Acta Ophthalmologica* 1983;61:737–741.

6. Rohen JW. Why is intraocular pressure elevated in chronic simple glaucoma? Anatomical considerations. *Ophthalmology* 1983;90: 758–765.

7. Raymond LF. Allergy and chronic simple glaucoma. *Annals of Allergy, Asthma & Immunology* 1964;22:146–150.

8. Bietti G. Further contributions on the value of osmotic substances as means to reduce intra-ocular pressure. *Transactions of the Ophthalmological Society of Australia* 1967;26: 61–71.

9. Fishbein S, Goodstein S. The

pressure lowering effect of ascorbic acid. *Annals of Ophthalmology* 1972;4:487–491.

10. Linner E. The pressure lowering effect of ascorbic acid in ocular hypertension. *Acta Ophthalmologica* 1969;47:685–689.

11. Shen TM, Yu MC. Clinical evaluation of glycerin-sodium ascorbate solution in lowering intraocular pressure. *Chinese Medical Journal* 1975;1:64–68.

12. Virno M, Bucci M, Pecori-Giraldi J, et al. Oral treatment of glaucoma with vitamin C. *Eye, Ear, Nose & Throat Monthly* 1967;46:1502–1508.

13. Gabor M. Pharmacologic effects of flavonoids on blood vessels. *Angiologica* 1972;9:355–374.

14. Monboisse J, Braquet P, Borel J. Oxygen-free radicals as mediators of collagen breakage. *Agents & Actions* 1984;15:49–50.

15. Hagerman A, Butler L. The specificity of proanthocyanidin-protein interactions. *The Journal of Biological Chemistry* 1981;256:4494–4497.

16. Steigerwalt RD, Gianni B, Paolo M, et al. Effects of Mirtogenol on ocular blood flow and intraocular hypertension in asymptomatic subjects. *Molecular Vision* 2008 Jul 10;14: 1288–1292.

17. Stocker F. New ways of influencing the intraocular pressure. *New York State Journal of Medicine* 1949;49:58–63.

18. Chung HS, Harris A, Kristinsson JK, et al. *Ginkgo biloba* extract increases ocular blood flow velocity. *Journal of Ocular Pharmacology and Therapeutics* 1999 Jun;15(3):233–240.

19. Quaranta L, Bettelli S, Uva MG, et al. Effect of *Ginkgo biloba* extract on preexisting visual field damage in normal tension glaucoma. *Ophthalmology* 2003 Feb;110(2):359–362.

20. Gaspar AZ, Gasser P, Flammer J. The influence of magnesium on visual field and peripheral vasospasm in glaucoma. *Ophthalmologica* 1995;209:11–13.

21. Aydin B, Onol M, Hondur A, et al. The effect of oral magnesium therapy on visual field and ocular blood flow in normotensive glaucoma. *Eur J Ophthalmol* 2010 Jan–Feb;20(1):131–135.

22. Lane BC. Diet and glaucomas. *Journal of the American College of Nutrition* 1991;10:536.

23. McGuire R. Fish oil cuts lower ocular pressure. *Medical Tribune* 1991;19:25.

24. Cellini M, Caramazza N, Mangiafico P, et al. Fatty acid use in glaucomatous optic neuropathy treatment. *Acta Ophthalmologica Scandinavica* 1998 suppl; 227:41–42.

25. Avisar R, Avisar E, Weinberger D. Effect of coffee consumption on intraocular pressure. *The Annals of Pharmacotherapy* 2002;36:992–995.

26. Qureshi IA. The effects of mild, moderate, and severe exercise on intraocular pressure in glaucoma patients. *The Japanese Journal of Physiology* 1995;45: 561–569.

27. Qureshi IA. Effects of exercise on intraocular pressure in physically fit subjects. *Clinical and Experimental Pharmacology and Physiology* 1996;23: 648–652.

28. Era P, Parssinen O, Kallinen M, et al. Effect of bicycle ergometer test on intraocular pressure in elderly athletes and controls. *Acta Ophthalmologica* 1993;71: 301–307.

Gout

1. Richette P, Bardin T. Gout. *The Lancet* 2010 Jan 23;375(9711): 318–328.

2. Brook RA, Forsythe A, Smeeding JE, Lawrence Edwards N. Chronic gout: epidemiology, disease progression, treatment and disease burden. *Current Medical Research & Opinion* 2010 Dec;26(12):2813–2821.

3. Hernández-Cuevas CB, Roque LH, Huerta-Sil G, et al. First acute gout attacks commonly precede features of the metabolic syndrome. *Journal of Clinical Rheumatology* 2009 Mar; 15(2):65–67.

4. Choi HK, De Vera MA, Krishnan E. Gout and the risk of type 2 diabetes among men with a high cardiovascular risk profile. *Rheumatology* 2008 Oct;47(10):1567–1570.

5. Singh JA, Reddy SG, Kundukulam J. Risk factors for gout and prevention: a systematic review of the literature. *Current Opinion in Rheumatology* 2011 Mar; 23(2):192–202.

6. Schumacher HR Jr, Becker MA, Wortmann RL, et al. Effects of febuxostat versus allopurinol and placebo in reducing serum urate in subjects with hyperuricemia and gout: a 28-week, phase III, randomized, double-blind, parallel-group trial. *Arthritis & Rheumatism* 2008 Nov 15;59(11):1540–1548.

7. Graziano JH, Blum C. Lead exposure from lead crystal. *The Lancet* 1991;337:141–142.

8. Kanbara A, Hakoda M, Seyama I. Urine alkalization facilitates uric acid excretion. *Nutrition Journal* 2010 Oct 19;9:45.

9. Dessein PH, Shipton EA, Stanwix AE, et al. Beneficial effects of weight loss associated with moderate calorie/carbohydrate restriction, and increased proportional intake of protein and unsaturated fat on serum urate and lipoprotein levels in gout: a pilot study. *Annals of the Rheumatic Diseases* 2000;59: 539–543.

10. Lewis AS, Murphy L, McCalla C, et al. Inhibition of mammalian xanthine oxidase by folate compounds and amethopterin. *The Journal of Biological Chemistry* 1984;259:12–15.

11. Oster KA. Folic acid and xanthine oxidase. *Annals of Internal Medicine* 1977;86:367.

12. Flouvier B, Devulder B. Folic acid, xanthine oxidase, and uric acid. *Annals of Internal Medicine* 1978 Feb;88(2):269.

13. Bindoli A, Valente M, Caval-

lini L. Inhibitory action of quercetin on xanthine oxidase and xanthine dehydrogenase activity. *Pharmacological Research Commununications* 1985;17:831–839.

14. Busse WW, Kopp DE, Middleton E Jr. Flavonoid modulation of human neutrophil function. *Journal of Allergy and Clinical Immunology* 1984;73:801–809.

15. Yoshimoto T, Furukawa M, Yamamoto S, et al. Flavonoids: potent inhibitors of arachidonate 5-lipoxygenase. *Biochemical and Biophysical Research Communications* 1983;116:612–618.

16. Stein HB, Hasan A, Fox IH. Ascorbic acid-induced uricosuria. A consequence of megavitamin therapy. *Annals of Internal Medicine* 1976;84:385–388.

17. Gershon SL, Fox IH. Pharmacologic effects of nicotinic acid on human purine metabolism. *Journal of Laboratory and Clinical Medicine* 1974;84:179–186.

18. Blau LW. Cherry diet control for gout and arthritis. *Texas Reports on Biology & Medicine* 1950;8:309–311.

19. Jacob RA, Spinozzi GM, Simon VA, et al. Consumption of cherries lowers plasma urate in healthy women. *Journal of Nutrition* 2003;133:1826–1829.

20. Soundararajan S, Daunter B. Ajvine: pilot biomedical study for pain relief in rheumatic pain. School of Medicine, The University of Queensland, Brisbane, Queensland, Australia, 1991–1992.

21. Venkat S, Soundararajan S, Daunter B, Madhusudhan S. Use of Ayurvedic medicine in the treatment of rheumatic illness. Department of Orthopaedics, Kovai Medical Center and Hospitals, Coimbatore, India, 1995.

22. Hu D, Huang XX, Feng YP. [Effect of dl-3-n-butylphthalide (NBP) on purine metabolites in striatum extracellular fluid in four-vessel occlusion rats.] *Yao Hsueh Hsueh Pao* 1996;31:13–17.

Hair Loss in Women

1. Mounsey AL, Reed SW. Diagnosing and treating hair loss. *American Family Physician* 2009 Aug 15;80(4):356–362.

2. Azziz R, Sanchez LA, Knochenhauer ES, et al. Androgen excess in women: experience with over 1000 consecutive patients. *The Journal of Clinical Endocrinology & Metabolism* 2004; 89:453–462.

3. Price VH. Androgenetic alopecia in women. *Journal of Investigative Dermatology Symposium Proceedings* 2003;8:24–27.

4. Birch MP, Lalla SC, Messenger AG. Female pattern hair loss. *Clinical and Experimental Dermatology* 2002;27:383–388.

5. Giralt M, Cervello I, Nogues MR, et al. Glutathione, glutathione S-transferase and reactive oxygen species of human scalp sebaceous glands in male pattern baldness. *Journal of Investigative Dermatology* 1996;107:154–158.

6. Legro RS, Carmina E, Stanczyk FZ, et al. Alterations in androgen conjugate levels in women and men with alopecia. *Fertility and Sterility* 1994;62:744–750.

7. Cela E, Robertson C, Rush K, et al. Prevalence of polycystic ovaries in women with androgenic alopecia. *European Journal of Endocrinology* 2003;149:439–442.

8. Matilainen V, Laakso M, Hirsso P, et al. Hair loss, insulin resistance, and heredity in middle-aged women. A population-based study. *Journal of Cardiovascular Risk* 2003;10:227–231.

9. Shum KW, Cullen DR, Messenger AG. Hair loss in women with hyperandrogenism: four cases responding to finasteride. *Journal of the American Academy of Dermatology* 2002;47:733–739.

10. Kantor J, Kessler LJ, Brooks DG, et al. Decreased serum ferritin is associated with alopecia in women. *Journal of Investigative Dermatology* 2003;12:985–988.

11. Moeinvaziri M, Mansoori P, Holakooee K, et al. Iron status in diffuse telogen hair loss among women. *Acta Dermatovenerologica Croatica* 2009; 17(4):279–284.

12. Deloche C, Bastien P, Chadoutaud S, et al. Low iron stores: a risk factor for excessive hair loss in non-menopausal women. *European Journal of Dermatology* 2007 Nov–Dec;17(6):507–512.

13. Wickett RR, Kossmann E, Barel A, et al. Effect of oral intake of choline-stabilized orthosilicic acid on hair tensile strength and morphology in women with fine hair. *Archives of Dermatological Research* 2007 Dec;299(10):499–505.

14. Corazza GR, Andreani ML, Venturo N, et al. Celiac disease and alopecia areata: report of a new association. *Gastroenterology* 1995;109:1333–1337.

Hay Fever

1. Cox L, Wallace D. Specific allergy immunotherapy for allergic rhinitis: subcutaneous and sublingual. *Immunology and Allergy Clinics of North America* 2011 Aug;31(3):561–599.

2. Sieber J, Shah-Hosseini K, Mösges R. Specific immunotherapy for allergic rhinitis to grass and tree pollens in daily medical practice—symptom load with sublingual immunotherapy compared to subcutaneous immunotherapy. *Annals of Medicine* 2011;43(6):418–424.

3. Egert S, Wolffram S, Bosy-Westphal A, et al. Daily quercetin supplementation dose-dependently increases plasma quercetin concentrations in healthy humans. *Journal of Nutrition* 2008 Sep;138(9):1615–1621.

4. Jin F, Nieman DC, Shanely RA, et al. The variable plasma quercetin response to 12-week quercetin supplementation in

humans. *European Journal of Clinical Nutrition* 2010 Jul;64(7):692–697.

5. Kawai M, Hirano T, Arimitsu J, et al. Effect of enzymatically modified isoquercitrin, a flavonoid, on symptoms of Japanese cedar pollinosis: a randomized double-blind placebo-controlled trial. *International Archives of Allergy and Immunology* 2009;149(4):359–368.

6. Hirano T, Kawai M, Arimitsu J, et al. Preventative effect of a flavonoid, enzymatically modified isoquercitrin on ocular symptoms of Japanese cedar pollinosis. *Allergology International* 2009 Sep;58(3):373–382.

7. Kishi K, Saito M, Saito T, et al. Clinical efficacy of apple polyphenol for treating cedar pollinosis. *Bioscience, Biotechnology, and Biodiversity* 2005 Apr;69(4):829–832.

8. Enomoto T, Nagasako-Akazome Y, Kanda T, et al. Clinical effects of apple polyphenols on persistent allergic rhinitis: a randomized double-blind placebo-controlled parallel arm study. *Journal of Investigative Allergology and Clinical Immunology* 2006;16(5):283–289.

Headache, Nonmigraine Tension Type

1. Mathew NT. Chronic refractory headache. *Neurology* 1993;43 suppl 3:S26–S33.

2. Hurwitz EL, PD Aker, AH Adams, et al. Manipulation and mobilization of the cervical spine. A systematic review of literature. *Spine* 1996;21:1746–1760.

3. Haas M, Bronfort G, Evans RL. Chiropractic clinical research: progress and recommendations. *Journal of Manipulative and Physiological Therapeutics* 2006;29(9):695–706.

4. Biondi DM. Physical treatments for headache: a structured review. *Headache* 2005;45(6):738–746.

5. Lenssinck ML, Damen L,

Verhagen AP, et al. The effectiveness of physiotherapy and manipulation in patients with tension-type headache: a systematic review. *Pain* 2004;112(3):381–388.

6. Larsson B and Carlsson J. A school-based, nurse-administered relaxation training for children with chronic tension-type headache. *Journal of Pediatric Psychology* 1996;21:603–614.

7. Larsson B, Carlsson J, Fichtel A, Melin L. Relaxation treatment of adolescent headache sufferers: results from a school-based replication series. *Headache* 2005;45(6):692–704.

8. Grazzi L, Andrasik F, Usai S, Bussone G. Magnesium as a preventive treatment for paediatric episodic tension-type headache: results at 1-year follow-up. *Neurological Sciences* 2007 Jun;28(3):148–150.

9. Grazzi L, Andrasik F, Usai S, Bussone G. Magnesium as a treatment for paediatric tension-type headache: a clinical replication series. *Neurological Sciences* 2005 Feb;25(6):338–341.

Heart Arrhythmias

1. Onalan O, Crystal E, Daoulah A, et al. Meta-analysis of magnesium therapy for the acute management of rapid atrial fibrillation. *American Journal of Cardiology* 2007 Jun 15;99(12):1726–1732.

2. Ho KM, Sheridan DJ, Paterson T. Use of intravenous magnesium to treat acute onset atrial fibrillation: a meta-analysis. *Heart* 2007 Nov;93(11):1433–1440.

3. McLean RM. Magnesium and its therapeutic uses: a review. *The American Journal of Medicine* 1994;96:63–76.

4. Brodsky MA, Orlov MV, Capparelli EV, et al. Magnesium therapy in new-onset atrial fibrillation. *American Journal of Cardiology* 1994 Jun 15;73(16):1227–1229.

Hemorrhoids

1. Trowell H, Burkitt D, Heaton K. *Dietary fibre, fibre-depleted foods and disease.* London: Academic Press, 1985.

2. Moesgaard F, Nielsen ML, Hansen JB, Knudsen JT. High-fiber diet reduces bleeding and pain in patients with hemorrhoids. *Diseases of the Colon & Rectum* 1982;25:454–456.

3. Alonso-Coello P, Mills E, Heels-Ansdell D, López-Yarto M. Fiber for the treatment of hemorrhoids complications: a systematic review and meta-analysis. *The American Journal of Gastroenterology* 2006 Jan;101(1):181–188.

4. Annoni F, Boccasanta P, Chiurazzi D, et al. [Treatment of acute symptoms of hemorrhoid disease with high dose oral O-(beta-hydroxyethyl)-rutosides.] *Minerva Medica* 1986;77:1663–1668.

5. Wijayanegara H, Mose JC, Achmad L, et al. A clinical trial of hydroxyethylrutosides in the treatment of haemorrhoids of pregnancy. *Journal of International Medical Research* 1992;20:54–60.

6. Bennani A, Biadillah MC, Cherkaoui A, Sebti M. Acute attack of hemorrhoids: efficacy of Cyclo 3 Fort based on results in 124 cases reported by specialists. *Phlebologie* 1999;52:89–93.

Hepatitis

1. Schuppan D, Krebs A, Bauer M, et al. Hepatitis C and liver fibrosis. *Cell Death & Differentiation* 2003;10 suppl 1:S59–S67.

2. Centers for Disease Control and Prevention. Prevention of hepatitis A through active or passive immunization: recommendations of the Advisory Committee on Immunization Practices (ACIP). *Morbidity and Mortality Weekly Report Recommendations and Reports* 1999;48:1–37.

3. McMahon BJ, Beller M, Williams J, et al. A program to con-

trol an outbreak of hepatitis A in Alaska by using an inactivated hepatitis A vaccine. *Archives of Pediatrics & Adolescent Medicine* 1996;150:733–739.

4. Marsano LS. Hepatitis. *Primary Care* 2003;30:81–107.

5. Cathcart RF. The third face of vitamin C. *Journal of Orthomolecular Medicine* 1993;7: 197–200.

6. Cathcart RF. The method of determining proper doses of vitamin C for the treatment of disease by titrating to bowel tolerance. *Journal of Orthomolecular Psychiatry* 1981;10: 125–132.

7. Klenner FR. Observations on the dose of administration of ascorbic acid when employed beyond the range of a vitamin in human pathology. *Journal of Applied Nutrition* 1971;23:61–88.

8. Baetgen D. [Results of treatment of epidemic hepatitis in childhood with high doses of ascorbic acid in the years 1957–1958.] *Medizinische Monatsschrift* 1961;15:30–36.

9. Baur H, Staub H. Treatment of hepatitis with infusions of ascorbic acid: comparison with other therapies. *JAMA, The Journal of the American Medical Association* 1954;156:565.

10. Murata A. Virucidal activity of vitamin C: vitamin C for prevention and treatment of viral diseases. In *Proceedings of the First Intersectional Congress of the International Association of the Microbiological Society*, vol. 3, ed. Hasegawa T. Tokyo: Tokyo University Press, 1975, 432–442.

11. Czuczejko J, Zachara BA, Staubach-Topczewska E, et al. Selenium, glutathione and glutathione peroxidases in blood of patients with chronic liver diseases. *Acta Biochimica Polonica* 2003;50:1147–1154.

12. Irmak MB, Ince G, Ozturk M, et al. Acquired tolerance of hepatocellular carcinoma cells to selenium deficiency: a selective

survival mechanism? *Cancer Research* 2003;63:6707–6715.

13. Jain SK, Pemberton PW, Smith A, et al. Oxidative stress in chronic hepatitis C: not just a feature of late stage disease. *Journal of Hepatology* 2002;36: 805–811.

14. Evans JL, Goldfine ID. Alpha-lipoic acid: a multifunctional antioxidant that improves insulin sensitivity in patients with type 2 diabetes. *Diabetes Technology & Therapeutics* 2000;2: 401–413.

15. Bustamante J, Lodge JK, Marcocci L, et al. Alpha-lipoic acid in liver metabolism and disease. *Free Radical Biology & Medicine* 1998;24:1023–1039.

16. Berkson BM. A conservative triple antioxidant approach to the treatment of hepatitis C. Combination of alpha lipoic acid (thioctic acid), silymarin, and selenium: three case histories. *Medizinische Klinik (Munich)* 1999;94 suppl 3:84–89.

17. Gal-Tanamy M, Bachmetov L, Ravid A, et al. Vitamin D: an innate antiviral agent suppressing hepatitis C virus in human hepatocytes. *Hepatology* 2011 Nov;54(5):1570–1579.

18. Bitetto D, Fabris C, Fornasiere E, et al. Vitamin D supplementation improves response to antiviral treatment for recurrent hepatitis C. *Transplant International* 2011 Jan;24(1):43–50.

19. Lange CM, Bojunga J, Ramos-Lopez E, et al. Vitamin D deficiency and a CYP27B1–1260 promoter polymorphism are associated with chronic hepatitis C and poor response to interferon-alfa based therapy. *Journal of Hepatology* 2011 May;54(5):887–893.

20. Arteh J, Narra S, Nair S. Prevalence of vitamin D deficiency in chronic liver disease. *Digestive Diseases and Sciences* 2010 Sep;55(9):2624–2628.

21. Milne A, Hopkirk N, Lucas CR, et al. Failure of New Zealand hepatitis B carriers to respond

to *Phyllanthus amarus. New Zealand Medical Journal* 1994; 107:243.

22. Suzuki H, Ohta Y, Takino T, et al. Effects of glycyrrhizin on biochemical tests in patients with chronic hepatitis—double blind trial. *Asian Medical Journal* 1984;26:423–438.

23. Mori K, Sakai H, Suzuki S, et al. Effects of glycyrrhizin (SNMC. Stronger Neo-Minophagen C) in hemophilia patients with HIV-1 infection. *The Tohoku Journal of Experimental Medicine* 1990; 162:183–193.

24. Eisenburg J. [Treatment of chronic hepatitis B. Part 2. Effect of glycyrrhizic acid on the course of illness.] *Fortschritte der Medizin* 1992;110:395–398.

25. Acharya SK, Dasarathy S, Tandon A, et al. A preliminary open trial on interferon stimulator (SNMC) derived from *Glycyrrhiza glabra* in the treatment of subacute hepatic failure. *Indian Journal of Medical Research* 1993;98:69–74.

26. Arase Y, Ikeda K, Murashima N, et al. The long term efficacy of glycyrrhizin in chronic hepatitis C patients. *Cancer* 1997;79: 1494–1500.

27. Farese RV Jr, Biglieri EG, Shackleton CH, et al. Licorice-induced hypermineralocorticoidism. *The New England Journal of Medicine* 1991;325:1223–1227.

28. Deak G, Muzes G, Lang I, et al. [Immunomodulator effect of silymarin therapy in chronic alcoholic liver diseases.] *Orvosi Hetilap* 1990;131:1291–1292,1295–1296.

29. Magliulo E, Gagliardi B, Fiori GP. [Results of a double blind study on the effect of silymarin in the treatment of acute viral hepatitis, carried out at two medical centres.] *Med Klin* 1978;73:1060–1065.

30. Schandalik R, Gatti G, Perucca E. Pharmacokinetics of silybin in bile following administration of silipide and silymarin in cholecystectomy patients.

Arzneimittelforschung 1992;42: 964–968.

31. Barzaghi N, Crema F, Gatti G, et al. Pharmacokinetic studies on IdB 1016, a silybin-phosphatidylcholine complex, in healthy human subjects. *European Journal of Drug Metabolism and Pharmacokinetics* 1990;15: 333–338.

32. Vailati A, Aristia L, Sozze E, et al. Randomized open study of the dose-effect relationship of a short course of IdB 1016 in patients with viral or alcoholic hepatitis. *Fitoterapia* 1993;44: 219–228.

33. Moscarella S, Giusti A, Marra F, et al. Therapeutic and antilipoperoxidant effects of silybin-phosphatidylcholine complex in chronic liver disease: preliminary results. *Current Therapeutic Research* 1993;53:98–102.

34. Buzzelli G, Moscarella S, Giusti A, et al. A pilot study on the liver protective effect of silybin-phosphatidylcholine complex (IdB 1016) in chronic active hepatitis. *International Journal of Clinical Pharmacology, Therapy and Toxicology* 1993;31:456–460.

35. Marena C, Lampertico M. Preliminary clinical development of silipide: a new complex of silybin in toxic liver disorders. *Planta Medica* 1991;57 suppl 2: A124–A125.

Herpes

1. Malkin JE. Epidemiology of genital herpes simplex virus infection in developed countries. *Herpes* 2004;11 suppl 1: 2A–23A.

2. Lafferty WE. The changing epidemiology of HSV-1 and HSV-2 and implications for serological testing. *Herpes* 2002;9:51–55.

3. Roberts CM, Pfister JR, Spear SJ. Increasing proportion of herpes simplex virus type 1 as a cause of genital herpes infection in college students. *Sexually Transmitted Diseases* 2003;30: 797–800.

4. Fitzherbert J. Genital herpes and zinc. *The Medical Journal of Australia* 1979;1:399.

5. Brody I. Topical treatment of recurrent herpes simplex and post-herpetic erythema multiforme with low concentrations of zinc sulphate solution. *British Journal of Dermatology* 1981; 104:191–213.

6. Hovi T, Hirvimies A, Stenvik M, et al. Topical treatment of recurrent mucocutaneous herpes with ascorbic acid-containing solution. *Antiviral Research* 1995; 27:263–270.

7. The use of water-soluble bioflavinoid-ascorbic acid complex in the treatment of recurrent herpes labialis. *Oral Surgery, Oral Medicine, Oral Pathology* 1978 Jan;45(1):56–62.

8. Cathcart RF. Vitamin C in the treatment of acquired immune deficiency syndrome (AIDS). *Medical Hypotheses* 1984;14: 423–433.

9. Griffith R, DeLong DC, Nelson JD. Relation of arginine-lysine antagonism to herpes simplex growth in tissue culture. *Chemotherapy* 1981;27:209–213.

10. DiGiovanna JJ, Blank H. Failure of lysine in frequently recurrent herpes simplex infection. *Archives of Dermatology* 1984;120:48–51.

11. Griffith R, Norins A, Kagan C. A multicentered study of lysine therapy in herpes simplex infection. *Dermatologica* 1978;156: 257–267.

12. McCune MA, Perry HO, Muller SA. Treatment of recurrent herpes simplex infections with L-lysine monohydrochlorite. *Cutis* 1984;34:366–373.

13. Griffith RS, Walsh DE, Myrmel KH, et al. Success of L-lysine therapy in frequently recurrent herpes simplex infection. *Dermatologica* 1987;175:183–190.

14. Gaby, A. Natural remedies for herpes simplex. *Alternative Medicine Review* 2006 Jun; 11(2):93–101.

15. Wolbling RH, Leonhardt K. Local therapy of herpes simplex with dried extract from *Melissa officinalis*. *Phytomedicine* 1994; 1:25–31.

16. Koytchev R, Alken RG, Dundarov S. Balm mint extract (Lo-701) for topical treatment of recurring herpes labialis. *Phytomedicine* 1999;6:225–230.

17. Nolkemper S, Reichling J, Stintzing FC, et al. Antiviral effect of aqueous extracts from species of the Lamiaceae family against *Herpes simplex* virus type 1 and type 2 in vitro. *Planta Medica* 2006 Dec;72(15): 1378–1382.

18. Pompei R, Pani A, Flore O, et al. Antiviral activity of glycyrrhizic acid. *Experientia* 1980; 36:304.

19. Partridge M, Poswillo D. Topical carbenoxolone sodium in the management of herpes simplex infection. *British Journal of Oral and Maxillofacial Surgery* 1984;22:138–145.

20. Csonka G, Tyrrell D. Treatment of herpes genitalis with carbenoxolone and cicloxolone creams: a double blind placebo controlled trial. *The British Journal of Venereal Diseases* 1984;60: 178–181.

21. Ikeda T, Yokomizo K, Okawa M, et al. Anti-herpes virus type 1 activity of oleanane-type tripterpenoids. *Biological and Pharmaceutical Bulletin* 2005 Sep;28(9):1779–1781.

High Blood Pressure

1. Nawrot TS, Thijs L, Den Hond EM, et al. An epidemiological re-appraisal of the association between blood pressure and blood lead: a meta-analysis. *Journal of Human Hypertension* 2002;16:123–131.

2. Pizent A, Jurasovie J, Telisman S. Blood pressure in relation to dietary calcium intake, alcohol consumption, blood lead, and blood cadmium in female nonsmokers. *Journal of Trace Elements in Medicine and Biology* 2001;15:123–130.

3. Telisman S, Jurasovic J, Pizent A, Cvitkovic P. Blood pressure in relation to biomarkers of lead, cadmium, copper, zinc, and selenium in men without occupational exposure to metals. *Environmental Research* 2001;87:57–68.

4. Martin D, Glass TA, Bandeen-Roche K, et al. Association of blood lead and tibia lead with blood pressure and hypertension in a community sample of older adults. *American Journal of Epidemiology* 2006;163(5): 467–478.

5. Chrysant SG. Treatment of white coat hypertension. *Current Hypertension Reports* 2000;2:412–417.

6. Munakata M, Saito Y, Nunokawa T, et al. Clinical significance of blood pressure response triggered by a doctor's visit in patients with essential hypertension. *Hypertension Research* 2002;25:343–349.

7. Strandberg TE, Salomaa V. White coat effect, blood pressure and mortality in men: prospective cohort study. *European Heart Journal* 2000;21: 1714–1718.

8. Addison C, Varney S, Coats A. The use of ambulatory blood pressure monitoring in managing hypertension according to different treatment guidelines. *Journal of Human Hypertension* 2001;15:535–538.

9. Blumenthal JA, Sherwood A, Gullette EC, et al. Biobehavioral approaches to the treatment of essential hypertension. *Journal of Consulting and Clinical Psychology* 2002;70: 569–589.

10. Grossman E, Grossman A, Schein MH, et al. Breathing-control lowers blood pressure. *Journal of Human Hypertension* 2001;15:263–269.

11. Driscoll D, Dicicco G. The effects of metronome breathing on the variability of autonomic activity measurements. *Journal of Manipulative and Physio-*logical *Therapeutics* 2000;23: 610–614.

12. Schein MH, Gavish B, Herz M, et al. Treating hypertension with a device that slows and regularises breathing: a randomised, double-blind controlled study. *Journal of Human Hypertension* 2001;15:271–278.

13. Anderson DE, Bagrov AY, Austin JL. Inhibited breathing decreases renal sodium excretion. *Psychosomatic Medicine* 1995; 57:373–380.

14. Bernardi L, Porta C, Spicuzza L, et al. Slow breathing increases arterial baroreflex sensitivity in patients with chronic heart failure. *Circulation* 2002; 105:143–145.

15. Schein MH, Gavish B, Baevsky T, et al. Treating hypertension in type II diabetic patients with device-guided breathing: a randomized controlled trial. *Journal of Human Hypertension* 2009 May;23(5): 325–331.

16. Arakawa K. Exercise, a measure to lower blood pressure and reduce other risks. *Clinical and Experimental Hypertension* 1999;21:797–803.

17. Lesniak KT, Dubbert PM. Exercise and hypertension. *Current Opinion in Cardiology* 2001;16: 356–359.

18. Ohkubo T, Hozawa A, Nagatomi R, et al. Effects of exercise training on home blood pressure values in older adults: a randomized controlled trial. *Journal of Hypertension* 2001; 19:1045–1052.

19. Blumenthal JA, Sherwood A, Gullette EC, et al. Exercise and weight loss reduce blood pressure in men and women with mild hypertension: effects on cardiovascular, metabolic, and hemodynamic functioning. *Archives of Internal Medicine* 2000;160:1947–1958.

20. Moreira WD, Fuchs FD, Ribeiro JP, Appel LJ. The effects of two aerobic training intensities on ambulatory blood pres-sure in hypertensive patients: results of a randomized trial. *Journal of Clinical Epidemiology* 1999;52:637–642.

21. Fogari R, Zoppi A, Corradi L, et al. Effect of body weight loss and normalization on blood pressure in overweight non-obese patients with stage 1 hypertension. *Hypertension Research* 2010 Mar; 33(3):236–242.

22. Navaneethan SD, Yehnert H, Moustarah F, et al. Weight loss interventions in chronic kidney disease: a systematic review and meta-analysis. *Clinical Journal of the American Society of Nephrology* 2009 Oct;4(10): 1565–1574.

23. Rouse IL, Beilin LJ, Mahoney DP, et al. Vegetarian diet and blood pressure. *The Lancet* 1983;2:742–743.

24. John JH, Ziebland S, Yudkin P, et al. Effects of fruit and vegetable consumption on plasma antioxidant concentrations and blood pressure: a randomised controlled trial. *The Lancet* 2002; 359:1969–1974.

25. Yasunari K, Maeda K, Nakamura M, Yoshikawa J. Oxidative stress in leukocytes is a possible link between blood pressure, blood glucose, and C-reacting protein. *Hypertension* 2002;39: 777–780.

26. Ortiz MC, Manriquez MC, Romero JC, Juncos LA. Antioxidants block angiotensin II-induced increases in blood pressure and endothelin. *Hypertension* 2001;38:655–659.

27. Tsi D, Tan BKH. Cardiovascular pharmacology of 3-n-butylphthalide in spontaneously hypertensive rats. *Phytotherapy Research* 1997;11:576–582.

28. Silagy CA, Neil HA. A meta-analysis of the effect of garlic on blood pressure. *Journal of Hypertension* 1994;12:463–468.

29. Appel LJ, Moore TJ, Obarzanek E, et al. A clinical trial of the effects of dietary patterns on blood pressure. DASH Collaborative Research Group. *The*

New England Journal of Medicine 1997;336:1117–1124.

30. Moore TJ, Conlin PR, Ard J, Svetkey LP. DASH (Dietary Approaches to Stop Hypertension) diet is effective treatment for stage 1 isolated systolic hypertension. *Hypertension* 2001;38: 155–158.

31. Sacks FM, Svetkey LP, Vollmer WM, et al. Effects on blood pressure of reduced dietary sodium and the Dietary Approaches to Stop Hypertension (DASH) diet. DASH-Sodium Collaborative Research Group. *The New England Journal of Medicine* 2001;344:3–10.

32. Jansson B. Dietary, total body, and intracellular potassium-to-sodium ratios and their influence on cancer. *Cancer Detection and Prevention* 1990;14:563–565.

33. Khaw KT, Barrett-Connor E. Dietary potassium and stroke-associated mortality. A 12-year prospective population study. *The New England Journal of Medicine* 1987;316:235–240.

34. He FJ, MacGregor GA. Salt, blood pressure and cardiovascular disease. *Current Opinion in Cardiology* 2007 Jul;22(4): 298–305.

35. Whelton PK, He J. Potassium in preventing and treating high blood pressure. *Seminars in Nephrology* 1999;19:494–499.

36. Patki PS, Singh J, Gokhale SV, et al. Efficacy of potassium and magnesium in essential hypertension: a double-blind, placebo-controlled, crossover study. *BMJ* 1990;301:521–523.

37. Fotherby MD, Potter JF. Potassium supplementation reduces clinic and ambulatory blood pressure in elderly hypertensive patients. *Journal of Hypertension* 1992;10:1403–1408.

38. Thijs L, Amery A, Birkenhager W, et al. Age-related effects of placebo and active treatment in patients beyond the age of 60 years: the need for a proper control group. *Journal of Hypertension* 1990;8:997–1002.

39. Nurminen ML, Niittynen L, Korpela R, Vapaatalo H. Coffee, caffeine and blood pressure: a critical review. *European Journal of Clinical Nutrition* 1999; 53:831–839.

40. Hodgson JM, Puddey IB, Burke V, et al. Effects on blood pressure of drinking green and black tea. *Journal of Hypertension* 1999;17:457–463.

41. Jee SH, He J, Whelton PK, et al. The effect of chronic coffee drinking on blood pressure: a meta-analysis of controlled clinical trials. *Hypertension* 1999; 33:647–652.

42. Hartley TR, Lovallo WR, Whitsett TL, et al. Caffeine and stress: implications for risk, assessment, and management of hypertension. *Journal of Clinical Hypertension* (Greenwich) 2001 Nov–Dec;3(6):354–361.

43. Jee SH, Miller ER III, Guallar E, et al. The effect of magnesium supplementation on blood pressure: a meta-analysis of randomized clinical trials. *American Journal of Hypertension* 2002;15:691–696.

44. Motoyama T, Sano H, Fukuzaki H. Oral magnesium supplementation in patients with essential hypertension. *Hypertension* 1989;13:227–232.

45. Whelton PK, Klag MJ. Magnesium and blood pressure: review of the epidemiologic and clinical trial experience. *American Journal of Cardiology* 1989;63: 26G–30G.

46. Joffres MR, Reed DM, Yano K. Relationship of magnesium intake and other dietary factors to blood pressure. The Honolulu Heart Study. *The American Journal of Clinical Nutrition* 1987;45:469–475.

47. Lindberg JS, Zobitz MM, Poindexter JR, Pak CY. Magnesium bioavailability from magnesium citrate and magnesium oxide. *Journal of the American College of Nutrition* 1990;9:48–55.

48. Bohmer T, Roseth A, Holm H, et al. Bioavailability of oral magne-

sium supplementation in female students evaluated from elimination of magnesium in 24-hour urine. *Magnesium and Trace Elements* 1990;9:272–278.

49. Cappuccio FP, Elliott P, Allender PS, et al. Epidemiologic association between dietary calcium intake and blood pressure: a meta-analysis of published data. *American Journal of Epidemiology* 1995;142:935–945.

50. Meese RB, Gonzales DG, Casparian JM, et al. The inconsistent effects of calcium supplements upon blood pressure in primary hypertension. *The American Journal of the Medical Sciences* 1987;294:219–224.

51. Sowers JR, Zemel MB, Standley PR, Zemel PC. Calcium and hypertension. *Journal of Laboratory and Clinical Medicine* 1989;114:338–348.

52. Takagi Y, Fukase M, Takata S, et al. Calcium treatment of essential hypertension in elderly patients evaluated by 24 H monitoring. *American Journal of Hypertension* 1991;4:836–839.

53. Hajjar IM, George V, Sasse EA, Kochar MS. A randomized, double-blind, controlled trial of vitamin C in the management of hypertension and lipids. *American Journal of Therapeutics* 2002;9:289–293.

54. Fotherby MD, Williams JC, Forster LA, et al. Effect of vitamin C on ambulatory blood pressure and plasma lipids in older persons. *Journal of Hypertension* 2000;18:411–415.

55. Galley HF, Thornton J, Howdle PD, et al. Combination oral antioxidant supplementation reduces blood pressure. *Clinical Science* 1997;92:361–365.

56. van Dijk RA, Rauwerda JA, Steyn M, et al. Long-term homocysteine-lowering treatment with folic acid plus pyridoxine is associated with decreased blood pressure but not with improved brachial artery endothelium-dependent vasodilation or ca-

rotid artery stiffness: a 2-year, randomized, placebo-controlled trial. *Arteriosclerosis, Thrombosis, and Vascular Biology* 2001;21:2072–2079.

57. Aybak M, Sermet A, Ayyildiz MO, Karakilcik AZ. Effect of oral pyridoxine hydrochloride supplementation on arterial blood pressure in patients with essential hypertension. *Arzneimittelforschung* 1995;45:1271–1273.

58. Geleijnse JM, Giltay EJ, Grobbee DE, et al. Blood pressure response to fish oil supplementation: metaregression analysis of randomized trials. *Journal of Hypertension* 2002;20:1493–1499.

59. Cicero AF, Ertek S, Borghi C. Omega-3 polyunsaturated fatty acids: their potential role in blood pressure prevention and management. *Current Vascular Pharmacology* 2009 Jul;7(3):330–337.

60. Singer P. Alpha-linolenic acid vs. long-chain n-3 fatty acids in hypertension and hyperlipidemia. *Nutrition* 1992;8:133–135.

61. Berry EM, Hirsch J. Does dietary linolenic acid influence blood pressure? *The American Journal of Clinical Nutrition* 1986;44:336–340.

62. Kelly BS, Alexander JW, Dreyer D, et al. Oral arginine improves blood pressure in renal transplant and hemodialysis patients. *Journal of Parenteral and Enteral Nutrition* 2001;25:194–202.

63. Kelly JJ, Williamson P, Martin A, Whitworth JA. Effects of oral L-arginine on plasma nitrate and blood pressure in cortisol-treated humans. *Journal of Hypertension* 2001;19:263–268.

64. Ast J, Jablecka A, Bogdanski P, et al. Evaluation of the antihypertensive effect of L-arginine supplementation in patients with mild hypertension assessed with ambulatory blood pressure monitoring. *Medical Science Monitor* 2010 Apr 28;16(5):CR266–CR271.

65. Campo C, Lahera V, Garcia-Robles R, et al. Aging abolishes the renal response to L-arginine infusion in essential hypertension. *Kidney International* 1996;55 suppl:S126–128.

66. Fujita H, Yoshikawa M. LKPNM: a prodrug-type ACE-inhibitory peptide derived from fish protein. *Immunopharmacology* 1999;44:123–127.

67. Fujita H, Yamagami T, Ohshima K. Effects of an ACE-inhibitory agent, katsuobushi oligopeptide, in the spontaneously hypertensive rat and in borderline and mildly hypertensive subjects. *Nutrition Research* 2001;21:1149–1158.

68. Fujita H, Yasumoto R, Hasegawa M, Ohshima K. Antihypertensive activity of "Katsuobushi Oligopeptide" in hypertensive and borderline hypertensive subjects. *Japan Pharmacology & Therapeutics* 1997;25:147–151.

69. Fujita H, Yasumoto R, Hasegawa M, Ohshima K. Antihypertensive activity of "Katsuobushi Oligopeptide" in hypertensive and borderline hypertensive subjects. *Japan Pharmacology & Therapeutics* 1997;25:153–157.

70. Kawasaki T, Seki E, Osajima K, et al. Antihypertensive effect of valyl-tyrosine, a short chain peptide derived from sardine muscle hydrolysate, on mild hypertensive subjects. *Journal of Human Hypertension* 2000;14:519–523.

71. Ho MJ, Bellusci A, Wright JM. Blood pressure lowering efficacy of coenzyme Q10 for primary hypertension. Cochrane Database of Systematic Reviews 2009 Oct 7;4:CD007435.

72. Langsjoen P, Langsjoen P, Willis R, Folkers K. Treatment of essential hypertension with coenzyme Q10. *Molecular Aspects of Medicine* 1994;15 suppl:S265–S272.

73. Digiesi V, Cantini F, Bisi G, et al. Mechanism of action of coenzyme Q10 in essential hypertension. *Current Therapeutic Research* 1992;51:668–672.

74. Walker AF, Marakis G, Morris AP, Robinson PA. Promising hypotensive effect of hawthorn extract: a randomized double-blind pilot study of mild, essential hypertension. *Phytotherapy Research* 2002;16:48–54.

75. Walker AF, Marakis G, Simpson E, et al. Hypotensive effects of hawthorn for patients with diabetes taking prescription drugs: a randomised controlled trial. *British Journal of General Practice* 2006 Jun;56(527):437–443.

76. Scheffler A, Rauwald HW, Kampa B, et al. *Olea europaea* leaf extract exerts L-type Ca(2+) channel antagonistic effects. *Journal of Ethnopharmacology* 2008 Nov 20;120(2):233–240.

77. Cherif S, Rahal N, Haouala M, et al. [A clinical trial of a titrated Olea extract in the treatment of essential arterial hypertension.] *J Pharm Belg* 1996;51:69–71.

78. Perrinjaquet-Moccetti T, Busjahn A, Schmidlin C, et al. Food supplementation with an olive (*Olea europaea* L.) leaf extract reduces blood pressure in borderline hypertensive monozygotic twins. *Phytotherapy Research* 2008 Sep;22(9):1239–1242.

79. Susalit E, Agus N, Effendi I, et al. Olive (*Olea europaea*) leaf extract effective in patients with stage-1 hypertension: comparison with Captopril. *Phytomedicine* 2011 Feb 15;18(4):251–258.

80. McKay DL, Chen CY, Saltzman E, Blumberg JB. *Hibiscus sabdariffa* L. tea (tisane) lowers blood pressure in prehypertensive and mildly hypertensive adults. *Journal of Nutrition* 2010 Feb;140(2):298–303.

81. Mozaffari-Khosravi H, Jalali-Khanabadi BA, Afkhami-Ardekani M, et al. The effects of sour tea (*Hibiscus sabdariffa*)

on hypertension in patients with type II diabetes. *Journal of Human Hypertension* 2009 Jan; 23(1):48–54.

82. Haji Faraji M, Haji Tarkhani A. The effect of sour tea (*Hibiscus sabdariffa*) on essential hypertension. *Journal of Ethnopharmacology* 1999 Jun;65(3): 231–236.

83. Herrera-Arellano A, Miranda-Sánchez J, Avila-Castro P, et al. Clinical effects produced by a standardized herbal medicinal product of *Hibiscus sabdariffa* on patients with hypertension. A randomized, double-blind, lisinopril-controlled clinical trial. *Planta Medica* 2007 Jan;73(1): 6–12.

84. Herrera-Arellano A, Flores-Romero S, Chávez-Soto MA, Tortoriello J. Effectiveness and tolerability of a standardized extract from *Hibiscus sabdariffa* in patients with mild to moderate hypertension: a controlled and randomized clinical trial. *Phytomedicine* 2004 Jul;11(5): 375–382.

High Cholesterol and/or Triglycerides

1. Wilson PW. High-density lipoprotein, low-density lipoprotein and coronary artery disease. *American Journal of Cardiology* 1990;66:7A–10A.

2. Ip S, Lichtenstein AH, Chung M, Systematic review: association of low-density lipoprotein subfractions with cardiovascular outcomes. *Annals of Internal Medicine* 2009 Apr 7; 150(7):474–484.

3. Davidson MH. Apolipoprotein measurements: is more widespread use clinically indicated? *Clinical Cardiology* 2009 Sep; 32(9):482–486.

4. Schaefer EJ, Lamon-Fava S, Jenner JL, et al. Lipoprotein(a) levels and risk of coronary heart disease in men. The Lipid Research Clinics Coronary Primary Prevention Trial. *JAMA, The Journal of the American*

Medical Association 1994;271: 999–1003.

5. Kannel WB, Vasan RS. Triglycerides as vascular risk factors: new epidemiologic insights. *Current Opinion in Cardiology* 2009 Jul;24(4):345–350.

6. Stalenhoef AF, de Graaf J. Association of fasting and non-fasting serum triglycerides with cardiovascular disease and the role of remnant-like lipoproteins and small dense LDL. *Current Opinion in Lipidology* 2008 Aug;19(4):355–361.

7. Pedersen TR. Pro and con: low-density lipoprotein cholesterol lowering is and will be the key to the future of lipid management. *American Journal of Cardiology* 2001;87:8B–12B.

8. Ong HT. The statin studies: from targeting hypercholesterolaemia to targeting the high-risk patient. *QJM* 2005 Aug; 98(8):599–614.

9. Jenkins DJ, Kendall CW, Marchie A, et al. Effects of a dietary portfolio of cholesterol-lowering foods vs lovastatin on serum lipids and C-reactive protein. *JAMA, The Journal of the American Medical Association* 2003;290:502–510.

10. Jenkins DJ, Kendall CW, Faulkner DA, et al. Long-term effects of a plant-based dietary portfolio of cholesterol-lowering foods on blood pressure. *European Journal of Clinical Nutrition* 2008 Jun;62(6):781–788.

11. Gigleux I, Jenkins DJ, Kendall CW, et al. Comparison of a dietary portfolio diet of cholesterol-lowering foods and a statin on LDL particle size phenotype in hypercholesterolaemic participants. *British Journal of Nutrition* 2007 Dec;98(6): 1229–1236.

12. Reynolds K, Chin A, Lees KA, et al. A meta-analysis of the effect of soy protein supplementation on serum lipids. *American Journal of Cardiology* 2006; 98(5):633–640.

13. Anderson JW, Johnstone BM,

Cook-Newell ME. Meta-analysis of the effects of soy protein intake on serum lipids. *The New England Journal of Medicine* 1995;333:276–282.

14. Langsjoen PH, Langsjoen AM. The clinical use of HMG CoA-reductase inhibitors and the associated depletion of coenzyme Q10. A review of animal and human publications. *Biofactors* 2003;18:101–111.

15. Rundek T, Naini A, Sacco R, et al. Atorvastatin decreases the coenzyme Q10 level in the blood of patients at risk for cardiovascular disease and stroke. *Archives of Neurology* 2004;61: 889–892.

16. McNamara DJ. Dietary cholesterol and atherosclerosis. *Biochimica et Biophysica Acta* 2000 Dec 15;1529(1–3):310–320.

17. Glore SR, Van Treeck D, Knehans AW, et al. Soluble fiber and serum lipids: a literature review. *Journal of the American Dietetic Association* 1994;94: 425–436.

18. Vuksan V, Jenkins DJ, Spadafora P, et al. Konjac-mannan (glucomannan) improves glycemia and other associated risk factors for coronary heart disease in type 2 diabetes. A randomized controlled metabolic trial. *Diabetes Care* 1999;22: 913–919.

19. Vuksan V, Sievenpiper JL, Owen R, et al. Beneficial effects of viscous dietary fiber from konjac-mannan in subjects with the insulin resistance syndrome: results of a controlled metabolic trial. *Diabetes Care* 2000;23: 9–14.

20. Ripsin CM, Keenan JM, Jacobs DR, et al. Oat products and lipid lowering, a meta-analysis. *JAMA, The Journal of the American Medical Association* 1992;267:3317–3325.

21. Ajani UA, Ford ES, Mokdad AH. Dietary fiber and C-reactive protein: findings from national health and nutrition examination survey data. *Jour-*

nal of Nutrition 2004;134:1181–1185.

22. Weitz D, Weintraub H, Fisher E, Schwartzbard AZ. Fish oil for the treatment of cardiovascular disease. *Cardiology in Review* 2010 Sep–Oct;18(5):258–263.

23. McKenney JM, Sica D. Role of prescription omega-3 fatty acids in the treatment of hypertriglyceridemia. *Pharmacotherapy* 2007 May;27(5):715–728.

24. Musa-Veloso K, Binns MA, Kocenas AC, et al. Long-chain omega-3 fatty acids eicosapentaenoic acid and docosahexaenoic acid dose-dependently reduce fasting serum triglycerides. *Nutrition Reviews* 2010 Mar;68(3):155–167.

25. Skulas-Ray AC, Kris-Etherton PM, Harris WS, et al. Dose-response effects of omega-3 fatty acids on triglycerides, inflammation, and endothelial function in healthy persons with moderate hypertriglyceridemia. *The American Journal of Clinical Nutrition* 2011 Feb;93(2):243–252.

26. Davidson MH. Mechanisms for the hypotriglyceridemic effect of marine omega-3 fatty acids. *American Journal of Cardiology* 2006 Aug 21;98(4A):27i–33i.

27. Canner PL, Berge KG, Wenger NK. Fifteen year mortality in Coronary Drug Project patients: long-term benefit with niacin. *Journal of the American College of Cardiology* 1986;8:1245–1255.

28. DiPalma JR, Thayer WS. Use of niacin as a drug. *Annual Review of Nutrition* 1991;11:169–187.

29. Illingworth DR, Stein EA, Mitchel YB, et al. Comparative effects of lovastatin and niacin in primary hypercholesterolemia. *Archives of Internal Medicine* 1994;14:1586–1595.

30. Carlson LA, Hamsten A, Asplund A. Pronounced lowering of serum levels of lipoprotein Lp(a) in hyperlipidaemic subjects treated with nicotinic

acid. *Journal of Internal Medicine* 1989;226:271–276.

31. Pan J, Lin M, Kesala RL, et al. Niacin treatment of the atherogenic lipid profile and Lp(a) in diabetes. *Diabetes, Obesity and Metabolism* 2002;4:255–261.

32. Vega GL, Grundy SM. Lipoprotein responses to treatment with lovastatin, gemfibrozil, and nicotinic acid in normolipidemic patients with hypoalphalipoproteinemia. *Archives of Internal Medicine* 1994;154:73–82.

33. Van JT, Pan J, Wasty T, et al. Comparison of extended-release niacin and atorvastatin monotherapies and combination treatment of the atherogenic lipid profile in diabetes mellitus. *American Journal of Cardiology* 2002;89:1306–1308.

34. Rindone JP, Achacoso S. Effect of low-dose niacin on glucose control in patients with non–insulin-dependent diabetes mellitus and hyperlipidemia. *American Journal of Therapeutics* 1996;3:637–639.

35. Kane MP, Hamilton RA, Addesse E, et al. Cholesterol and glycemic effects of Niaspan in patients with type 2 diabetes. *Pharmacotherapy* 2001;21:1473–1478.

36. Kuvin JT, Dave DM, Sliney KA, et al. Effects of extended-release niacin on lipoprotein particle size, distribution, and inflammatory markers in patients with coronary artery disease. *American Journal of Cardiology.* 2006;98(6):743–745.

37. McKenney JM, Proctor JD, Harris S, et al. A comparison of the efficacy and toxic effects of sustained- vs immediate-release niacin in hypercholesterolemic patients. *JAMA, The Journal of the American Medical Association* 1994;271:672–677.

38. Goldberg AC. A meta-analysis of randomized controlled studies on the effects of extended-release niacin in women. *American Journal of Cardiology* 2004;94:121–124.

39. Guyton JR. Extended-release

niacin for modifying the lipoprotein profile. *Expert Opin Pharmacother* 2004;5:1385–1398.

40. Rubenfire M. Impact of Medical Subspecialty on Patient Compliance to Treatment Study Group. Safety and compliance with once-daily niacin extended-release/lovastatin as initial therapy in the Impact of Medical Subspecialty on Patient Compliance to Treatment (IMPACT) study. *American Journal of Cardiology* 2004;94:306–311.

41. Vogt A, Kassner U, Hostalek U, et al. Evaluation of the safety and tolerability of prolonged-release nicotinic acid in a usual care setting: the NAUTILUS study. *Current Medical Research & Opinion* 2006;22(2):417–425.

42. Welsh AL, Ede M. Inositol hexanicotinate for improved nicotinic acid therapy. *International Record of Medicine* 1961;174:9–15.

43. El-Enein AMA, Hafez YS, Salem H, et al. The role of nicotinic acid and inositol hexaniacinate as anticholesterolemic and antilipemic agents. *Nutrition Reports International* 1983;28:899–911.

44. Ostlund RE Jr. Phytosterols and cholesterol metabolism. *Current Opinion in Lipidology* 2004;15:37–41.

45. Miettinen TA, Gylling H. Plant stanol and sterol esters in prevention of cardiovascular diseases. *Annals of Medicine* 2004;36:126–134.

46. Kozlowska-Wojciechowska M, Jastrzebska M, Naruszewicz M, et al. Impact of margarine enriched with plant sterols on blood lipids, platelet function, and fibrinogen level in young men. *Metabolism* 2003;52:1373–1378.

47. Yoshida Y, Niki E. Antioxidant effects of phytosterol and its components. *Journal of Nutritional Science and Vitaminology* 2003 Aug;49 (4):277–280.

48. de Jong A, Plat J, Mensink RP. Metabolic effects of plant ste-

rols and stanols. *The Journal of Nutritional Biochemistry* 2003; 14:362–369.

49. Arsenio L, Bodria P, Magnati G, et al. Effectiveness of long-term treatment with pantethine in patients with dyslipidemias. *Clinical Therapeutics* 1986;8: 537–545.

50. Gaddi A, Descovich GC, Noseda P, et al. Controlled evaluation of pantethine, a natural hypolipidemic compound, in patients with different forms of hyperlipoproteinemia. *Atherosclerosis* 1984; 50:73–83.

51. Coronel F, Tomero F, Torrente J, et al. Treatment of hyperlipemia in diabetic patients on dialysis with a physiological substance. *American Journal of Nephrology* 1991;11:32–36.

52. Donati C, Bertieri RS, Barbi G. Pantethine, diabetes mellitus and atherosclerosis: clinical study of 1045 patients. *La Clinica Terapeutica* 1989; 128:411–422.

53. Hiramatsu K, Nozaki H, Arimori S. Influence of pantethine on platelet volume, microviscosity, lipid composition and functions in diabetes mellitus with hyperlipidemia. *The Tokai Journal of Experimental and Clinical Medicine* 1981;6:49–57.

54. Lawson LD, Wang ZJ, Papdimitrou D. Allicin release under simulated gastrointestinal conditions from garlic powder tablets employed in clinical trials on serum cholesterol. *Planta Medica* 2001;67:13–18.

55. Lawson LD, Wang ZJ. Tablet quality: a major problem in clinical trials with garlic supplements. *Forsch Komplmentaermed* 2000;7:45.

56. Banerjee SK, Maulik SK. Effect of garlic on cardiovascular disorders: a review. *Nutrition Journal* 2002;1:4.

57. Alder R, Lookinland S, Berry JA, et al. A systematic review of the effectiveness of garlic as an anti-hyperlipidemic agent.

Journal of American Academy of Nurse Practitioners 2003;15: 120–129.

58. Stevinson C, Pittler MH, Erst E. Garlic for treating hypercholesterolemia: a meta-analysis of randomized clinical trials. *Annals of Internal Medicine* 2000;133:420–429.

Hives (Urticaria)

1. Muller BA. Urticaria and angioedema: a practical approach. *American Family Physician* 2004;69:1123–1128.

2. Dreskin S. Urticaria. *Immunology and Allergy Clinics of North America* 2004;24;xi.

3. Ormerod AD, Reid TM, Main RA. Penicillin in milk—its importance in urticaria. *Clinical Allergy* 1987;17:229–234.

4. Wicher K, Reisman RE. Anaphylactic reaction to penicillin in a soft drink. *Journal of Allergy and Clinical Immunology* 1980;66:155–157.

5. Schwartz HJ, Sher TH. Anaphylaxis to penicillin in a frozen dinner. *Annals of Allergy, Asthma & Immunology* 1984; 52:342–343.

6. Boonk WJ, Van Ketel WG. The role of penicillin in the pathogenesis of chronic urticaria. *British Journal of Dermatology* 1982;106:183–190.

7. Lindemayr H, Knobler R, Kraft D, et al. Challenge of penicillin allergic volunteers with penicillin contaminated meat. *Allergy* 1981;36:471–478.

8. Settipane RA, Constantine HP, Settipane GA. Aspirin intolerance and recurrent urticaria in normal adults and children. *Allergy* 1980;35:149–154.

9. Warin RP. The effect of aspirin in chronic urticaria. *British Journal of Dermatology* 1960; 72:350–351.

10. Moore-Robinson M, Warin RP. Effects of salicylates in urticaria. *British Medical Journal* 1967;4:262–264.

11. Champion RH, Roberts SO,

Carpenter RG, et al. Urticaria and angio-oedema. A review of 554 patients. *British Journal of Dermatology* 1969;81:588–597.

12. James J, Warin RP. Chronic urticaria: the effect of aspirin. *British Journal of Dermatology* 1970;82:204–205.

13. Grattan CE. Aspirin sensitivity and urticaria. *Clinical and Experimental Dermatology* 2003; 28:123–127.

14. Rawls WB, Ancona VC. Chronic urticaria associated with hypochlorhydria or achlorhydria. *The Review of Gastroenterology* 1951;18:267–271.

15. Baird PC. Etiology and treatment of urticaria: diagnosis, prevention and treatment of poison-ivy dermatitis. *The New England Journal of Medicine* 1941;224:649–658.

16. Allison JR. The relation of hydrochloric acid and vitamin B complex deficiency in certain skin diseases. *Southern Medical Journal* 1945;38:235–241.

17. Zuberbier T, Chantraine-Hess S, Hartmann K, et al. Pseudoallergen-free diet in the treatment of chronic urticaria. A prospective study. *Acta Dermato-Venereologica* (Stockholm) 1995;75: 484–487.

18. Collins-Williams C. Clinical spectrum of adverse reactions to tartrazine. *Journal of Asthma* 1985;22:139–143.

19. Lessof MH. Reactions to food additives. *Clinical & Experimental Allergy* 1995;25 suppl 1: 27–28.

20. Natbony SF, Phillips ME, Elias JM, et al. Histologic studies of chronic idiopathic urticaria. *Journal of Allergy and Clinical Immunology* 1983;71:177–183.

21. Swain AR, Dutton SP, Truswell AS. Salicylates in foods. *Journal of the American Dietetic Association* 1985;85:950–960.

22. Kulczycki A. Aspartame-induced urticaria. *Annals of Internal Medicine* 1986;104:207–208.

23. Moneret-Vautrin DA, Faure G,

Bene MC. Chewing-gum preservative induced toxidermic vasculitis. *Allergy* 1986;41:546–548.

24. Vally H, Misso NL, Madan V. Clinical effects of sulphite additives. *Clinical & Experimental Allergy* 2009 Nov;39(11):1643–1651.

25. Birkmayer JGD, Beyer W. Biological and clinical relevance of trace elements. *Ärtzl Lab* 1990; 36:284–287.

26. Serrano H. [Hypersensitivity to "candida albicans" and other fungi in patients with chronic urticaria.] *Allergol Immunopathol* 1975;3:289–298.

27. James J, Warin RP. An assessment of the role of *Candida albicans* and food yeast in chronic urticaria. *British Journal of Dermatology* 1971;84:227–237.

28. Rives H, Pellerat J, Thivolet J. [Chronic urticaria and Quincke's oedema. 100 case reports. Allergology and therapeutic results.] *Dermatologica* 1972;144:193–204.

29. Green G, Koelsche G, Kierland R. Etiology and pathogenesis of chronic urticaria. *Annals of Allergy, Asthma & Immunology* 1965;23:30–36.

30. Shertzer CL, Lookingbill DP. Effects of relaxation therapy and hypnotizability in chronic urticaria. *Archives of Dermatology* 1987;123:913–916.

31. Hannuksela M, Kokkonen EL. Ultraviolet light therapy in chronic urticaria. *Acta Dermato-Venereologica* 1985;65: 449–450.

32. Olafsson JH, Larko O, Roupe G, et al. Treatment of chronic urticaria with PUVA or UVA plus placebo: a double-blind study. *Archives of Dermatological Research* 1986;278:228–231.

33. Johnston CS, Martin LJ, Cai X. Antihistamine effect of supplemental ascorbic acid and neutrophil chemotaxis. *Journal of the American College of Nutrition* 1992;11:172–176.

34. Simon SW. Vitamin B12 therapy in allergy and chronic dermatoses. *Journal of Allergy* 1951;22: 183–185.

35. Simon SW. Edmonds P. Cyanocobalamin (B12): Comparison of aqueous and repository preparations in urticaria; possible mode of action. *Journal of the American Geriatrics Society* 1964;12: 79–85.

36. Healy E, Newell L, Howarth P, Friedmann PS. Control of salicylate intolerance with fish oils. *British Journal of Dermatology.* 2008 Dec;159(6):1368–1369.

37. Cusack C, Gorman DJ. Role of thyroxine in chronic urticaria and angio-oedema. *J R Soc Med* 2004;97:257.

38. Leznoff A, Sussman GL. Syndrome of idiopathic chronic urticaria and angioedema with thyroid autoimmunity: a study of 90 patients. *Journal of Allergy and Clinical Immunology* 1989;84:66–71.

Hyperthyroidism

1. Larson PR, Ingbar SH. The thyroid gland. In *Williams' textbook of endocrinology,* 8th ed., ed. Wilson JD, Foster DW. Philadelphia: W. B. Saunders, 1992, 367–487.

2. Sonino N, Girelli ME, Boscaro M, et al. Life events in the pathogenesis of Graves' disease. A controlled study. *Acta Endocrinologica* 1993;128:293–296.

3. Radosavljević VR, Janković SM, Marinković JM. Stressful life events in the pathogenesis of Graves' disease. *European Journal of Endocrinology* 1996 Jun; 134(6):699–701.

4. Winsa B, Karlsson A. Graves' disease, endocrine ophthalmopathy and smoking. *Acta Endocrinologica* 1993;128:156–160.

5. Bartalena L, Bogazzi F, Tanda ML, et al. Cigarette smoking and the thyroid. *European Journal of Endocrinology* 1995;133: 507–512.

6. Shine B, Fells P, Edwards OM, et al. Association between Graves' ophthalmopathy and smoking. *The Lancet* 1990;335: 1261–1263.

7. Galofre JC, Fernandez-Calvet L, Rios M, et al. Increased incidence of thyrotoxicosis after iodine supplementation in an iodine sufficient area. *Journal of Endocrinological Investigation* 1994;17:23–27.

8. Benvenga S, Ruggeri RM, Russo A, et al. Usefulness of L-carnitine, a naturally occurring peripheral antagonist of thyroid hormone action, in iatrogenic hyperthyroidism: a randomized, double-blind, placebo-controlled clinical trial. *The Journal of Clinical Endocrinology & Metabolism* 2001;86:3579–3594.

Hypoglycemia

1. Chalew SA, Koetter H, Hoffman S, et al. Diagnosis of reactive hypoglycemia. Pitfalls in the use of the oral glucose tolerance test. *Southern Medical Journal* 1986;79:285–287.

2. Palardy J, Havrankova J, Lepage R, et al. Blood glucose measurements during symptomatic episodes in patients with suspected postprandial hypoglycemia. *The New England Journal of Medicine* 1989;321: 1421–1425.

3. Kwentus JA, Achilles JT, Goyer PF. Hypoglycemia: etiologic and psychosomatic aspects of diagnosis. *Postgraduate Medicine* 1982;71:99–104.

4. Yogev Y, Ben-Haroush A, Chen R, et al. Undiagnosed asymptomatic hypoglycemia: diet, insulin, and glyburide for gestational diabetic pregnancy. *Obstetrics & Gynecology* 2004;104: 88–93.

5. Galloway PJ, Thomson GA, Fisher BM, et al. Insulin-induced hypoglycemia induces a rise in C-reactive protein. *Diabetes Care* 2000;23:861–862.

6. Gross TM, Mastrototaro JJ. Efficacy and reliability of the

continuous glucose monitoring system. *Diabetes Technology & Therapeutics* 2000;2 suppl 1: S19–S26.

7. Murray MT, Lyon MR. *Hunger free forever.* New York: Atria, 2008.

8. Statement on hypoglycemia. *JAMA, The Journal of the American Medical Association* 1973;223:682.

9. Cahill GF Jr, Soeldner JS. A non-editorial on non-hypoglycemia. *The New England Journal of Medicine* 1974;291:905–906.

10. Hofeldt FD. Patients with bona fide meal-related hypoglycemia should be treated primarily with dietary restriction of refined carbohydrate. *Endocrinology Metabolism Clinics of North America* 1989;18:185–201.

11. Sanders LR, Hofeldt FD, Kirk MC, Levin J. Refined carbohydrate as a contributing factor in reactive hypoglycemia. *Southern Medical Journal* 1982;75: 1072–1075.

12. National Research Council. *Diet and health: implications for reducing chronic disease risk.* Washington, D.C.: National Academy Press, 1989.

13. Winokur A, Maislin G, Phillips JL, Amsterdam JD. Insulin resistance after glucose tolerance testing in patients with major depression. *The American Journal of Psychiatry* 1988;145:325–330.

14. Wright JH, Jacisin JJ, Radin NS, et al. Glucose metabolism in unipolar depression. *The British Journal of Psychiatry* 1978;132: 386–393.

15. Schauss AG. Nutrition and behavior: complex interdisciplinary research. *Nutrition and Health* 1984;3:9–37.

16. Benton D. Hypoglycemia and aggression: a review. *The Journal of Neuroscience* 1988;41: 163–168.

17. Virkkunen M. Reactive hypoglycemic tendency among arsonists. *Acta Psychiatrica Scandinavica* 1984;69:445–452.

18. Schoenthaler SJ. Diet and crime: an empirical examination of the value of nutrition in the control and treatment of incarcerated juvenile offenders. *International Journal of Biosocial Research* 1983;4:25–39.

19. Schoenthaler SJ. The northern California diet-behavior program. An empirical evaluation of 3,000 incarcerated juveniles in Stanislaus County Juvenile Hall. *International Journal of Biosocial Research* 1983;5:99–106.

20. Abraham GE. Nutritional factors in the etiology of the premenstrual tension syndromes. *The Journal of Reproductive Medicine* 1983;28:446–464.

21. Walsh CH, O'Sullivan DJ. Studies of glucose tolerance, insulin and growth hormone secretion during the menstrual cycle in healthy women. *Irish Journal of Medical Sciences* 1975;144: 18–24.

22. Critchley M. Migraine. *The Lancet* 1933;1:123–126.

23. Dexter JD, Roberts J, Byer JA. The five hour glucose tolerance test and effect of low sucrose diet in migraine. *Headache* 1978;18:91–94.

24. Mykkanen L, Laakso M, Pyorala K. High plasma insulin levels associated with coronary heart disease in the elderly. *American Journal of Epidemiology* 1993;137:1190–1202.

25. Yudkin J. Metabolic changes induced by sugar in relation to coronary heart disease and diabetes. *Nutrition and Health* 1987;5:5–8.

26. Pyorala K. Relationship of glucose tolerance and plasma insulin to the incidence of coronary heart disease: results from two population studies in Finland. *Diabetes Care* 1979;2:131–141.

27. Bansal S, Toh SH, LaBresh KA. Chest pain as a presentation of reactive hypoglycemia. *Chest* 1983;84:641–642.

28. Hanson M, Bergentz SE, Ericsson BF, et al. The oral glucose tolerance test in men under 55 years of age with intermittent claudication. *Angiology* 1987;38: 469–473.

29. Jenkins DJ, Wolever TM, Taylor RH, et al. Glycemic index of foods: a physiological basis for carbohydrate exchange. *The American Journal of Clinical Nutrition* 1981;34:362–366.

30. Jenkins AL, Kacinik V, Lyon M, Wolever TM. Effect of adding the novel fiber, PGX®, to commonly consumed foods on glycemic response, glycemic index and GRIP: a simple and effective strategy for reducing post prandial blood glucose levels—a randomized, controlled trial. *Nutrition Journal* 2010 Nov 22;9:58.

31. Brand-Miller JC, Atkinson FS, Gahler RJ, et al. Effects of PGX, a novel functional fibre, on acute and delayed postprandial glycaemia. *European Journal of Clinical Nutrition* 2010 Dec; 64(12):1488–1493.

32. Jenkins AL, Kacinik V, Lyon MR, Wolever TM. Reduction of postprandial glycemia by the novel viscous polysaccharide PGX, in a dose-dependent manner, independent of food form. *Journal of the American College of Nutrition* 2010 Apr;29(2): 92–98.

33. Anderson RA. Chromium, glucose tolerance, and diabetes. *Biological Trace Element Research* 1992;32:19–24.

34. Anderson RA, Polansky MM, Bryden NA, et al. Effects of supplemental chromium on patients with symptoms of reactive hypoglycemia. *Metabolism* 1987;36:351–355.

35. McCarty MF. Chromium and other insulin sensitizers may enhance glucagon secretion: implications for hypoglycemia and weight control. *Medical Hypotheses* 1996;46:77–80.

36. Anderson RA. Nutritional factors influencing glucose/insulin system: chromium. *Journal of the American College of Nutrition* 1997;16:404–410.

37. Hirata Y. Diabetes and alcohol. *Asian Med J* 1988;31:564–569.

38. Selby JV, Newman B, King MC, et al. Environmental and behavioral determinants of fasting plasma glucose in women: a matched co-twin analysis. *American Journal of Epidemiology* 1987;125:979–988.

39. Vallerand AL, Cuerrier JP, Shapcott D, et al. Influence of exercise training on tissue chromium concentrations in the rat. *The American Journal of Clinical Nutrition* 1984;39:402–409.

40. Sato Y, Nagasaki M, Nakai N, Fushimi M. Physical exercise improves glucose metabolism in lifestyle-related diseases. *Experimental Medicine and Biology (Maywood)* 2003 Nov; 228(10):1208–1212.

Hypothyroidism

1. Wang C, Crapo LM. The epidemiology of thyroid disease and implications for screening. *Endocrinology Metabolism Clinics of North America* 1997;26: 189–218.

2. Weetman AP. Hypothyroidism: screening and subclinical disease. *BMJ* 1997;314:1175–1178.

3. Banovac K, Zakarija M, McKenzie JM. Experience with routine thyroid function testing: abnormal results in "normal" populations. *J Fla Med Assoc* 1985;72: 835–839.

4. Arem R, Escalante D. Subclinical hypothyroidism: epidemiology, diagnosis, and significance. *Adv Internal Medicine* 1996;41: 213–250.

5. Canaris GJ, Manowitz NR, Mayor G, et al. The Colorado Thyroid Disease Prevalence Study. *Archives of Internal Medicine* 2000;160:526–534.

6. Aoki Y, Belin RM, Clickner R, Jeffries R, Phillips L, Mahaffey KR. Serum TSH and total T4 in the United States population and their association with participant characteristics: National Health and Nutrition Examination Survey (NHANES 1999–

2002). *Thyroid* 2007 Dec;17(12): 1211–1223.

7. Barnes BO, Galton L. *Hypothyroidism: the unsuspected illness.* New York: Crowell, 1976.

8. Langer SE, Scheer JF. *Solved: the riddle of illness.* New Canaan, Conn.: Keats, 1984.

9. Evans TC. Thyroid disease. *Primary Care* 2003;30:625–640.

10. Gold MS, Pottash AL, Extein I. Hypothyroidism and depression, evidence from complete thyroid function evaluation. *JAMA, The Journal of the American Medical Association* 1981;245:1919–1922.

11. Esposito S, Prange AJ Jr, Golden RN. The thyroid axis and mood disorders: overview and future prospects. *Psychopharmacology Bulletin* 1997;33:205–217.

12. Cappola AR, Ladenson PW. Hypothyroidism and atherosclerosis. *The Journal of Clinical Endocrinology & Metabolism* 2003;88:2438–2444.

13. Razvi S, Weaver JU, Vanderpump MP, Pearce SH. The incidence of ischemic heart disease and mortality in people with subclinical hypothyroidism: reanalysis of the Whickham Survey cohort. *The Journal of Clinical Endocrinology & Metabolism* 2010 Apr;95(4):1734–1740.

14. Althaus U, Staub JJ, Ryff-De Leche A, et al. LDL/HDL-changes in subclinical hypothyroidism: possible risk factors for coronary heart disease. *Clinical Endocrinology* 1988;28:157–163.

15. Krupsky M, Flatan E, Yarom R, et al. Musculoskeletal symptoms as a presenting sign of long-standing hypothyroidism. *Israel Journal of Medical Sciences* 1987;23:1110–1113.

16. Hochberg MC, Koppes GM, Edwards CQ, et al. Hypothyroidism presenting as a polymyositis-like syndrome. *Arthritis & Rheumatism* 1976;19:1363–1366.

17. Prasad A. Clinical, biochemical and nutritional spectrum of zinc deficiency in human subjects:

an update. *Nutrition Reviews* 1983;41:197–208.

18. Nishiyama S, Futagoishi-Suginohara Y, Matsukura M, et al. Zinc supplementation alters thyroid hormone metabolism in disabled patients with zinc deficiency. *Journal of the American College of Nutrition* 1994;13:62–67.

19. Toro T. Selenium's role in thyroid found. *New Scientist* 1991; 129:27.

20. Meinhold H, Campos-Barros A, Behne D, et al. Effects of selenium and iodine deficiency on iodothyronine deiodinases in brain, thyroid and peripheral tissue. *Acta Medica Austriaca* 1992;19:8–12.

21. Berry MJ, Larsen PR. The role of selenium in thyroid hormone action. *Endocrine Reviews* 1992;13:207–219.

22. Gärtner R, Gasnier BCH, Dietrich JW, et al. Selenium supplementation in patients with autoimmune thyroiditis decreases thyroid peroxidase antibodies concentrations. *The Journal of Clinical Endocrinology & Metabolism* 2002;87: 1687–1691.

23. van Vollenhoven RF. Dehydroepiandrosterone for the treatment of systemic lupus erythematosus. *Expert Opin Pharmacother* 2002;3:23–31.

24. Lennon D, Nagle F, Stratman F, et al. Diet and exercise training effects on resting metabolic rate. *International Journal of Obesity* 1985;9:39–47.

25. Mainardi E, Montanelli A, Dotti M, et al. Thyroid-related autoantibodies and celiac disease: a role for a gluten-free diet? *Journal of Clinical Gastroenterology* 2002;35:245–248.

Infertility (Female)

1. Gnoth C, Godehardt E, Frank-Hermann P, Freundi G. Time to pregnancy: results of the German prospective study and impact on the management of infertility. *Human Reproduction* 2003;18:1959–1966.

2. te Velde ER, Pearson PL. The variability of female reproduction ageing. *Human Reproduction* Update 2002;8(2):141–154.

3. Wood JW. Fecundity and natural fertility in humans. *Oxford Reviews of Reproductive Biology* 1989;11:61–109.

4. Noord-Zaadstra BM, Looman CW, Alsbach H, et al. Delaying childbearing: effect of age on fecundity and outcome of pregnancy. *British Medical Journal* 1991 Jun 8;302(6789):1361–1365.

5. Heffner LJ. Advanced maternal age—how old is too old? *The New England Journal of Medicine* 2004 Nov 4;351(19):1927–1929.

6. Balasch J, Gratacós E. Delayed childbearing: effects on fertility and the outcome of pregnancy. *Fetal Diagnosis and Therapy* 2011;29(4):263–73..

7. Jose-Miller A, Boyden JW, Frey KA. Infertility. *American Family Physician* 2007;75:849–856,857–858.

8. Levitas E, Lunenefeld E, Weiss N, et al. Relationship between the duration of sexual abstinence and semen quality: analysis of 9,489 semen samples. *Fertility and Sterility* 2005;83:1680–1686.

9. Wilcox AJ, Weinberg CR, Baird DD. Timing of sexual intercourse in relation to ovulation—effects on the probability of conception, survival of the pregnancy and sex of the baby. *The New England Journal of Medicine* 1995;333:1517–1521.

10. Bolúmar F, Olsen J, Rebagliato M, et al. Body mass index and delayed conception: a European multicentre study on infertility and subfecundity. *American Journal of Epidemiology* 2000;151(11):1072–1079.

11. ESHRE Capri Workshop Group. Nutrition and reproduction in women. *Human Reproduction Update* 2006;12(3):193–207.

12. Shiloh H, Lahav Baratz S, Koif-man M, et al. The impact of cigarette smoking on zona pellucida thickness of oocytes and embryos prior to transfer into the uterine cavity. *Human Reproduction* 2004 Jan;19(1):157–159.

13. Waylen AL, Jones GL, Ledger WL. Effect of cigarette smoking upon reproductive hormones in women of reproductive age: a retrospective analysis. *Reproductive BioMedicine Online* 2010 Jun;20(6):861–865.

14. Anderson K, Norman RJ, Middleton P. Preconception lifestyle advice for people with subfertility. Cochrane Database of Systematic Reviews 2010 Apr 14;4:CD008189.

15. Bolúmar F, Olsen J, Rebagliato M, Bisanti L. Caffeine intake and delayed conception: a European multicenter study on infertility and subfecundity. *American Journal of Epidemiology* 1997;145(4):324–334.

16. Wilcox AJ, Weinberg C, Baird DD. Caffeinated beverages and decreased fertility. *The Lancet* 1988;2(8626–8627):1453–1456.

17. Stanton CK, Gray RH. Effects of caffeine consumption on delayed conception. *American Journal of Epidemiology* 1995;142(12):1322–1329.

18. Hofman GF, Davies M, Norman R. The impact of lifestyle factors on reproductive performance in the general population and those undergoing infertility treatment: a review. *Human Reproduction Update* 2007;13(3):209–223.

19. Lucero J, Harlow BL, Barbieri RL, et al. Early follicular phase hormone levels in relation to patterns of alcohol, tobacco, and coffee use. *Fertility and Sterility* 2001;76:723–729.

20. Hakim RB, Gray RH, Zacur H. Alcohol and caffeine consumption and decreased fertility *Fertility and Sterility* 1998 Oct;70(4):632–637.

21. Mendelson JH. Alcohol effects on reproductive function in women. *Psychiatry Letter* 1986;4(7):35–38.

22. Gill J. The effects of moderate alcohol consumption on female hormone levels and reproductive function *Alcohol and Alcoholism* 2000 Sep–Oct;35(5):417–423.

23. Windham GC, Fenster L, Swan SH. Moderate maternal and paternal alcohol consumption and the risk of spontaneous abortion. *Epidemiology* 1992;3:364–370.

24. Chavarro JE, Rich-Edwards JW, Rosner BA, Willett WC. Diet and lifestyle in the prevention of ovulatory disorder infertility. *Obstetrics & Gynecology* 2007;110:1050–1058.

25. Chavarro JE, Rich-Edwards JW, Rosner BA, Willett WC. Dietary fatty acids intakes and the risk of ovulatory infertility. *The American Journal of Clinical Nutrition* 2007;85:231–237.

26. Chavarro JE, Rich-Edwards JW, Rosner BA, Willett WC. Protein intake and ovulatory infertility. *American Journal of Obstetrics and Gynecology* 2008;198(2):210.e1–e7.

27. Vujkovic M, de Vries JH, Lindemans J, et al. The preconception Mediterranean dietary pattern in couples undergoing in vitro fertilization/intracytoplasmic sperm injection treatment increases the chance of pregnancy. *Fertility and Sterility* 2010 Nov;94(6):2096–2101.

28. Allen LH. Multiple micronutrients in pregnancy and lactation: an overview. *ACJN* 2005;81(5):1206S–1212S.

29. Cetin I, Berti C, Calabrese S. Role of micronutrients in the periconceptional period *Human Reproduction Update* 2010 Jan–Feb;16(1):80–95.

30. Chavarro JE, Rich-Edwards JW, Rosner BA, Willett WC. Iron intake and risk of ovulatory infertility. *Obstetrics & Gynecology* 2006;108:1145–1152.

31. Stankiewicz M, Smith C, Alvino H, Norman R. The use of

complementary medicine and therapies by patients attending a reproductive medicine unit in South Australia: a prospective survey. *Aust NZ J Obstet Gynaecol* 2007;47(2):145–149.

32. Rumhold A, Middleton P, Crowther CA. Vitamin supplementation for preventing miscarriage. *Cochrane Database of Systematic Reviews* 2005;2: CD004073.

33. Ruder EH, Hartman TJ, Blumberg J, Goldman MB. Oxidative stress and antioxidants: exposure and impact on female fertility. *Human Reproduction Update* 2008 Jul–Aug;14(4): 345–357.

34. Agarwal A, Gupta S, Sharma RK. Role of oxidative stress in female reproduction. *Reproductive Biology and Endocrinology* 2005 Jul 14;3:28.

35. Mansour G, Abdelrazik H, Sharma RK, et al. L-carnitine supplementation reduces oocyte cytoskeleton damage and embryo apoptosis induced by incubation in peritoneal fluid from patients with endometriosis. *Fertility and Sterility* 2009 May; 91(5 suppl):2079–2086.

36. Wu G. Amino acids: metabolism, functions, and nutrition. *Amino Acids* 2009 May;37(1):1–17.

37. Battaglia C, Salvatori M, Maxia N, et al. Adjuvant L-arginine treatment for in-vitro fertilization in poor responder patients. *Human Reproduction* 1999 Jul;14(7):1690–1697.

38. Goldenberg RL, Hauth JC, Andrews WW. Intrauterine infection and preterm delivery. *The New England Journal of Medicine* 2000;342:1500–1507.

39. Verstraelen H, Verhelst R, Roelens K, et al. Modified classification of Gram-stained vaginal smears to predict spontaneous preterm birth: a prospective cohort study. *American Journal of Obstetrics & Gynecology* 2007 Jun;196(6):528.e1–e6.

40. Peters-Welte C, Albrecht M. Menstrual-cycle disorders and

PMS: study on the use of *Vitex-agnus castus*. *TW Gynäkologie* 1994;7(1):49–52.

41. Amann W. [Amenorrhoea. Favourable effect of *Agnus castus* (Agnolyt®) on amenorrhea.] *Zeitschrift für Allgemeine Medizin* 1982;58(4):228–31.

42. Roeder D. Therapy of cyclical disorders with *Vitex agnus castus*. *Z Phytotherapie* 1994;15(3): 157–163.

43. Gerhard II, Patek A, Monga B, et al. Mastodynon® in female infertility. *Forschende Komplementärmedizin* 1998;5 (6):272–278.

Infertility (Male)

1. Brugh VM 3rd, Lipshultz LI. Male factor infertility: evaluation and management. *Medical Clinics of North America* 2004; 88:367–385.

2. Zorgniotti AW, Cohen MS, Sealfon AI. Chronic scrotal hypothermia: results in 90 infertile couples. *Journal of Urology* 1986;135:944–947.

3. Purvis K, Christiansen E. Review: infection in the male reproductive tract. Impact, diagnosis and treatment in relation to male infertility. *International Journal of Andrology* 1993;16:1–13.

4. Sharpe RM, Skakkebaek NE. Are oestrogens involved in falling sperm counts and disorders of the male reproduction tract? *The Lancet* 1993;341: 1392–1395.

5. Field B, Selub M, Hughes CL. Reproductive effects of environmental agents. *Seminars in Reproductive Endocrinology* 1990;8:44–54.

6. Joffe M. Infertility and environmental pollutants. *British Medical Bulletin* 2003;68:47–70.

7. Skakkebaek NE, Jørgensen N, Main NE, et al. Is human fecundity declining? *International Journal of Andrology* 2006;29:2–12.

8. Anway MD, Cupp AS, Uzumcu M, et al. Epigenetic

transgenerational actions of endocrine disruptors and male fertility. *Science* 2005;308: 1466–1469.

9. Joffe M. Infertility and environmental pollutants. *British Medical Bulletin* 2003;68:47–70.

10. British Medical Association Board of Science and Education. Mobile phones and health: an interim report. May 2001. www.bma.org.uk/images/Mobile phones_tcm41-20881.pdf.

11. Lai H, Singh NP. Single- and double-strand DNA breaks in rat brain cells after acute exposure to radiofrequency electromagnetic radiation. *International Journal of Radiation Biology* 1996;69:513–521.

12. Fejes Z, Zavaczki J, Szollosi S, et al. Is there a relationship between cell phone use and semen quality? *Archives of Andrology* 2005;51:385–393.

13. Davoudi M, Brossner C, Kuber W. The influence of electromagnetic waves on sperm motility. *Journal für Urologie und Urogynäkologie* 2002;19: 18–22.

14. Agarwal A, Deepinder F, Sahrma RK, et al. Effect of cell phone usage on semen analysis in men attending infertility clinic: an observational study. *Fertility and Sterility* 2008 Jan; 89(1):124–128.

15. Saleh RA, Agarwal A, Sharma RK, et al. Effect of cigarette smoking on levels of seminal oxidative stress in infertile men: a prospective study. *Fertility and Sterility* 2002 Sep;78:491–499.

16. Chohan KR, Badawy SZ. Cigarette smoking impairs sperm bioenergetics. *Int Braz J Urol* 2010 Jan–Feb;36(1):60–65.

17. Gaur DS, Talekar MS, Pathak VP. Alcohol intake and cigarette smoking: impact of two major lifestyle factors on male fertility *Indian Journal of Pathology and Microbiology* 2010 Jan–Mar; 53(1):35–40.

18. Battista N, Pasquariello N, Di Tommaso M, Maccarrone M.

Interplay between endocannabinoids, steroids and cytokines in the control of human reproduction. *Journal of Neuroendocrinology* 2008 May;20 suppl 1: 82–89.

19. Badawy ZS, Chohan KR, Whyte DA, et al. Cannabinoids inhibit the respiration of human sperm. *Fertility and Sterility* 2009 Jun; 91(6):2471–2476.

20. Rossato M. Endocannabinoids, sperm functions and energy metabolism. *Molecular and Cellular Endocrinology* 2008 Apr 16; 286(1–2 suppl 1):S31–S35.

21. Lighten A. A weighty issue: managing reproductive problems in the obese. *Conceptions* 2009 June;9.

22. Lenzi L, Gandini V, Maresca R, et al. Fatty acid composition of spermatozoa and immature germ cells. *Molecular Human Reproduction* 2000; 6(3):226–231.

23. Gulaya NM, Margitich VM, Govseeva NM, et al. Phospholipid composition of human sperm and seminal plasma in relation to sperm fertility. *Archives of Andrology* 2001;46(3): 169–175.

24. Safarinejad MR, Hosseini SY, Dadkhah F, Asgari MA. Relationship of omega-3 and omega-6 fatty acids with semen characteristics, and anti-oxidant status of seminal plasma: a comparison between fertile and infertile men. *Clinical Nutrition* 2010 Feb;29(1):100–105.

25. Weller DP, Zaneveld JD, Farnsworth NR. Gossypol: pharmacology and current status as a male contraceptive. *Economic and Medicinal Plant Research* 1985;1:87–112.

26. Showell MG, Brown J, Tazdani A, et al. Antioxidants for male subfertility. Cochrane Database of Systematic Reviews 2011 Jan 19;1:CD007411.

27. Agarwal A, Nallella KP, Allamaneni SS, et al. Role of antioxidants in treatment of male infertility: an overview of the literature. *Reproductive Bio-Medicine Online* 2004;8:616–627.

28. Zini A, de Lamirande E, Gagnon C. Reactive oxygen species in semen of infertile patients: levels of superoxide dismutase- and catalase-like activities in seminal plasma and spermatozoa. *International Journal of Andrology* 1993;16:183–188.

29. Pasqualotto FF, Sharma RK, Nelson DR, et al. Relationship between oxidative stress, semen characteristics, and clinical diagnosis in men undergoing infertility investigation. *Fertility and Sterility* 2000;73:459–464.

30. Akmal M, Qadri JQ, Al-Waili NS, Thangal S, Haq A, Saloom KY. Improvement in human semen quality after oral supplementation of vitamin C. *Journal of Medicinal Food* 2006 Fall; 9(3):440–442.

31. Colagar AH, Marzony ET. Ascorbic acid in human seminal plasma: determination and its relationship to sperm quality *Journal of Clinical Biochemistry and Nutrition* 2009 Sep; 45(2):144–149.

32. Patel SR, Sigman M. Antioxidant therapy in male infertility. *Urologic Clinics of North America* 2008;35:319–330.

33. Song GJ, Norkus EP, Lewis V. Relationship between seminal ascorbic acid and sperm DNA integrity in infertile men. *International Journal of Andrology* 2006 Dec;29(6):569–575.

34. Kao SH, Chao HT, Chen HW, et al. Increase of oxidative stress in human sperm with lower motility. *Fertility and Sterility* 2008 May;89(5):1183–1190.

35. Fraga CG, Motchnik PA, Shigenaga MK, et al. Ascorbic acid protects against endogenous oxidative DNA damage in human sperm. *Proceedings of the National Academy of Sciences of the United States of America* 1991;88:11003–11006.

36. Dawson EB, Harris WA, Teter MC, Powell LC. Effect of vitamin C supplementation on sperm quality of heavy smokers. *Fertility and Sterility* 1992; 58(5):1034–1039.

37. Dawson EB, Harris WA, Rankin WE, et al. Effect of ascorbic acid on male fertility. *Annals of the New York Academy of Sciences* 1987;498:312–323.

38. Aitken RJ, Clarkson JS, Hargreave TB, et al. Analysis of the relationship between defective sperm function and the generation of reactive oxygen species in cases of oligozoospermia. *Journal of Andrology* 1989;10: 214–220.

39. Suleiman SA, Ali ME, Zaki ZM, et al. Lipid peroxidation and human sperm mobility: protective role of vitamin E. *Journal of Andrology* 1996;17:530–537.

40. Geva E, Bartoov B, Zabludovsky N, et al. The effect of antioxidant treatment on human spermatozoa and fertilization rate in an in vitro fertilization program. *Fertility and Sterility* 1996 Sep;66(3):430–434.

41. Al-Azemi MK, Omu AE, Fatinikun T, et al. Factors contributing to gender differences in serum retinol and alpha-tocopherol in infertile couples. *Reproductive BioMedicine Online* 2009 Oct;19(4):583–590.

42. Morales A, Cavicchia JC. Spermatogenesis and blood-testis barrier in rats after long-term vitamin A deprivation. *Tissue and Cell* 2002 Oct;34(5):349–355.

43. Eskenazi B, Kidd SA, Marks AR, et al. Antioxidant intake is associated with semen quality in healthy men. *Human Reproduction* 2005;20(4):1006–1012.

44. Gupta NP, Kumar R. Lycopene therapy in idiopathic male infertility—a preliminary report. *International Urology and Nephrology* 2002;34:369–372.

45. Colagar AH, Marzony ET, Chaichi MJ. Zinc levels in seminal plasma are associated with sperm quality in fertile and infertile men. *Nutrition Research* 2009 Feb;29(2):82–88.

46. El-Tawil AM. Zinc deficiency in men with Crohn's disease may contribute to poor sperm function and male infertility. *Andrologia* 2003;35:337–341.

47. Chia SE, Ong C, Chua L, et al. Comparison of zinc concentration in blood and seminal plasma and various sperm parameters between fertile and infertile men. *Journal of Andrology* 2000;21:53–57.

48. Bjorndahl L, Kvist U. Importance of zinc for human sperm head-tail connection. *Acta Physiologica Scandinavica* 1982;126:51–55.

49. Carreras A, Mendoza C. Zinc levels in seminal plasma of infertile and fertile men. *Andrologia* 1990 May–Jun;22(3):279–283.

50. Takihara H, Cosentino MJ, Cockett AT. Zinc sulfate therapy for infertile males with or without varicocelectomy. *Urology* 1987;29:638–641.

51. Netter A, Hartoma R, Nakoul K. Effect of zinc administration on plasma testosterone, dihydrotestosterone and sperm count. *Archives of Andrology* 1981;7:69–73.

52. Wong WY, Merkus HM, Thomas CM, et al. Effects of folic acid and zinc sulfate on male factor subfertility: a double-blind, randomized, placebo-controlled trial. *Fertility and Sterility* 2002;77:491–498.

53. Tremellen K, Miari G, Froilan D, Thompson J. A randomized control trial examining the effect of an antioxidant (Menevit) on pregnancy outcome during IVF-ICSI treatment. *Australian and New Zealand Journal of Obstetrics and Gynaecology* 2007;47:216–221.

54. Ursini F, Heim S, Kiess M, et al. Dual function of the selenoprotein PHGPx during sperm maturation. *Science* 1999;285:1393.

55. Vézina D, Mauffette F, Roberts KD, Bleau G. Selenium-vitamin E supplementation in infertile men: effects on semen parameters and micronutrient levels and distribution. *Biological Trace Element Research* 1996 Summer;53(1–3):65–83.

56. Rayman MP, Rayman MP. The argument for increasing selenium intake. *Proceedings of the Nutrition Society* 2002;61:203–215.

57. Schneider M, Förster H, Boersma A, et al. Mitochondrial glutathione peroxidase 4 disruption causes male infertility. *The FASEB Journal* 2009 Sep;23(9):3233–242.

58. Scott R, MacPherson A, Yates RW, et al. The effect of oral selenium supplementation on human sperm motility. *British Journal of Urology* 1998 Jul;82(1):76–80.

59. Safarinejad MR, Safarinejad S. Efficacy of selenium and/or N-acetyl-cysteine for improving semen parameters in infertile men: a double-blind, placebo controlled, randomized study. *Journal of Urology* 2009 Feb;181(2):741–751.

60. Sandler B, Faragher B. Treatment of oligospermia with vitamin B12. *Infertility* 1984;7:133–138.

61. Boxmeer JC, Smit M, Weber RF, et al. Seminal plasma cobalamin significantly correlates with sperm concentration in men undergoing IVF or ICSI procedures. *Journal of Andrology* 2007 Jul–Aug;28(4):521–527.

62. Boxmeer JC, Smit M, Utomo E, et al. Low folate in seminal plasma is associated with increased sperm DNA damage. *Fertility and Sterility* 2009 Aug;92(2):548–556.

63. Sandler B, Faragher B. Treatment of oligospermia with vitamin B12. *Infertility* 1984;7:133–138.

64. Kumamoto Y, Maruta H, Ishigami J, et al. [Clinical efficacy of mecobalamin in treatment of oligozoospermia. Results of a double-blind comparative clinical study.] *Acta Urologica Japonica* 1988;34:1109–1132.

65. Bilska A, Włodek L. Lipoic acid—the drug of the future? *Phamacological Reports* 2005 Sep–Oct;57(5):570–577.

66. Selvakumar E, Prahalathan C, Sudharsan PT, Varalakshmi P. Chemoprotective effect of lipoic acid against cyclophosphamide-induced changes in the rat sperm. *Toxicology* 2006 Jan 5;217(1):71–78.

67. Prahalathan C, Selvakumar E, Varalakshmi P. Modulatory role of lipoic acid on adriamycin-induced testicular injury. *Chemico-Biological Interactions* 2006 Mar 25;160(2):108–114.

68. Ibrahim SF, Osman K, Das S, et al. A study of the antioxidant effect of alpha lipoic acids on sperm quality. *Clinics* 2008 Aug;63(4):545–550.

69. Ng CM, Blackman MR, Wang C, Swerdloff RS. The role of carnitine in the male reproductive system. *Annals of the New York Academy of Sciences* 2004 Nov;1033:177–178.

70. Costa M, Canale D, Filicori M, et al. L-carnitine in idiopathic asthenozoospermia: a multicenter study. Italian Study Group on Carnitine and Male Infertility. *Andrologia* 1994;26:155–159.

71. Vitali G, Parente R, Melotti C. Carnitine supplementation in human idiopathic asthenospermia: clinical results. *Drugs Under Experimental and Clinical Research* 1995;21:157–159.

72. Vicari E, La Vignera S, Calogero AE. Antioxidant treatment with carnitines is effective in infertile patients with prostatovesiculoepididymitis and elevated seminal leukocyte concentrations after treatment with nonsteroidal anti-inflammatory compounds. *Fertility and Sterility* 2002;78:1203–1208.

73. Lenzi A, Sgrò P, Salacone P, et al. A placebo-controlled double-blind randomized trial of the use of combined L-carnitine

and L-acetyl-carnitine treatment in men with asthenozoospermia. *Fertility and Sterility* 2004;81:1578–1584.

74. Lenzi A, Lombardo F, Sgro P, et al. Use of carnitine therapy in selected cases of male factor infertility: a double-blind crossover trial. *Fertility and Sterility* 2003;79:292–300.

75. Balercia G, Regoli F, Armeni T, et al. Placebo-controlled, double-blind, randomized trial on the use of L-carnitine, L-acetylcarnitine, or combined L-carnitine and L-acetylcarnitine in men with idiopathic asthenozoospermia. *Fertility and Sterility* 2005 Sep;84(3):662–671.

76. Mancini L, De Marinis A, Oradei E, et al. Coenzyme Q10 concentration in normal and pathological human seminal fluid. *Journal of Andrology* 1994;15:591–559.

77. Balercia G, Mosca F, Mantero F, et al. Coenzyme Q(10) supplementation in infertile men with idiopathic asthenozoospermia: an open, uncontrolled pilot study. *Fertility and Sterility* 2004 Jan;81(1):93–98.

78. Balercia G, Buldreghini E, Vignini A, et al. Coenzyme Q10 treatment in infertile men with idiopathic asthenozoospermia: a placebo-controlled, double-blind randomized trial. *Fertility and Sterility* 2009 May;91(5):1785–1792.

79. Schacter A, Goldman JA, Zukerman Z. Treatment of oligospermia with the amino acid arginine. *Journal of Urology* 1973;110:311–313.

80. Stanislavov R, Nikolova V, Rohdewald P. Improvement of seminal parameters with Prelox: a randomized, double-blind, placebo-controlled, cross-over trial. *Phytotherapy Research* 2009 Mar;23(3):297–302.

81. Roseff SJ. Improvement in sperm quality and function with French maritime pine tree bark extract. *The Journal of Reproductive Medicine* 2002;47:821–824.

82. Zhang H, Zhou QM, Li XD, et al. Ginsenoside R(e) increases fertile and asthenozoospermic infertile human sperm motility by induction of nitric oxide synthase. *Archives of Pharmacal Research* 2006 Feb;29(2):145–151.

83. Zhang H, Zhou Q, Li X, et al. Ginsenoside Re promotes human sperm capacitation through nitric oxide-dependent pathway. *Molecular Reproduction and Development* 2007 Apr;74(4):497–501.

84. Salvati G, Genovesi G, Marcellini L, et al. Effects of *Panax ginseng* saponins on male fertility. *Panminerva Medica* 1996 Dec;38(4):249–254.

85. Choi HK, Seong DH, Rha KH. Clinical efficacy of Korean red ginseng for erectile dysfunction. *International Journal of Impotence Research* 1995 Sep;7(3):181–186.

86. Lucchetta G, Weill A, Becker N, et al. Reactivation of the secretion from the prostatic gland in cases of reduced fertility: biological study of seminal fluid modifications. *Urologia Internationalis* 1984;39:222–224.

87. Menchini-Fabris GF, Giorgi P, Reini F, et al. [New perspectives on treatment of prostato-vesicular pathologies with *Pygeum africanum*.] *Archivio Italiano di Urologia, Nefrologia, Andrologia* 1988;60:313–322.

88. Clavert A, Cranz C, Riffaud JP, et al. [Effects of an extract of the bark of *Pygeum africanum* on prostatic secretions in the rat and man.] *Annales d'Urologie* 1986;20:341–343.

89. Carani C, Salvioli C, Scuteri A, et al. [Urological and sexual evaluation of treatment of benign prostatic disease using *Pygeum africanum* at high dose.] *Archivio Italiano di Urologia, Nefrologia, Andrologia* 1991;63:341–345.

90. Gauthaman K, Ganesan AP. The hormonal effects of *Tribulus terrestris* and its role in the management of male erectile dysfunction—an evaluation using primates, rabbit and rat. *Phytomedicine* 2008 Jan;15(1–2):44–54.

91. Neychev VK, Mitev VI. The aphrodisiac herb *Tribulus terrestris* does not influence the androgen production in young men. *Journal of Ethnopharmacology* 2005 Oct 3;101(1–3):319–323.

92. Adimoelja, A. Phytochemicals and the breakthrough of traditional herbs in the management of sexual dysfunctions. *International Journal of Andrology* 2000;23 suppl 2:82–84.

93. Tripathi YB, Upadhyay AK. Antioxidant property of *Mucuna pruriens*. *Current Science* 2001; 80:1377–1378.

94. Ahmad MK, Mahdi AA, Shukla KK, et al. Effect of *Mucuna pruriens* on semen profile and biochemical parameters in seminal plasma of infertile men. *Fertility and Sterility* 2008;90:627–635.

95. Ahmad MK, Mahdi AA, Shukla KK, et al. *Mucuna pruriens* improves male fertility by its action on the hypothalamus-pituitary-gonadal axis. *Fertility and Sterility* 2009;92:1934–1940.

96. Ahmad MK, Mahdi AA, Shukla KK, et al. *Withania somnifera* improves semen quality by regulating reproductive hormone levels and oxidative stress in seminal plasma of infertile males. *Fertility and Sterility* 2010 Aug;94(3):989–996.

Insomnia

1. Roth T, Roehrs T. Insomnia: epidemiology, characteristics, and consequences. *Clinical Cornerstone* 2003;5:5–15.

2. Vermeeren A. Residual effects of hypnotics: epidemiology and clinical implications. *CNS Drugs* 2004;18:297–328.

3. Montgomery P, Dennis J. A systematic review of non-pharmacological therapies for sleep problems in later life. *Sleep Medicine Reviews* 2004;8:47–62.

4. Victor LD. Treatment of obstructive sleep apnea in Primary Care. *American Family Physician* 2004;69:561–568.

5. Leproult R, Copinschi G, Buxton O, et al. Sleep loss results in an elevation of cortisol levels the next evening. *Sleep* 1997;20:865–870.

6. Hartmann E. L-tryptophan: a rational hypnotic with clinical potential. *The American Journal of Psychiatry* 1977;134:366–370.

7. George CF, Millar TW, Hanly PJ. The effect of L-tryptophan on daytime sleep latency in normals: correlation with blood levels. *Sleep* 1989;12:345–353.

8. Thorleifsdóttir B, Björnsson JK, Kjeld M, Kristbjarnarson H. Effects of L-tryptophan on daytime arousal. *Neuropsychobiology* 1989;21(3):170–176.

9. Hajak G, Huether G, Blanke J, et al. The influence of intravenous L-tryptophan on plasma melatonin and sleep in men. *Pharmacopsychiatry* 1991;24:17–20.

10. Zarcone VP Jr, Hoddes E. Effects of 5-hydroxytryptophan on fragmentation of REM sleep in alcoholics. *The American Journal of Psychiatry* 1975;132:74–76.

11. Soulairac A, Lambinet H. [Effect of 5-hydroxytryptophan, a serotonin precursor, on sleep disorders.] *Annales Medico-Psychologiques* 1977;1:792–798.

12. Hartmann E, Elion R. The insomnia of "sleeping in a strange place": effects of l-tryptophane. *Psychopharmacology* 1977;53:131–133.

13. Wyatt RJ. The serotonin-catecholamine-dream bicycle: a clinical study. *Biological Psychiatry* 1972;5:33–64.

14. Guilleminault C, Cathala HP, Castaigne P. Effects of 5-HTP on sleep of a patient with brain stem lesion. *Electroencephalography and Clinical Neurophysiology* 1973;34:177–184.

15. Wyatt RJ, Zarcone V, Engelman K. Effects of 5-hydroxytryptophan on the sleep of normal human subjects. *Electroencephalography and Clinical Neurophysiology* 1971;30:505–509.

16. Autret A, Minz M, Bussel B, et al. Human sleep and 5-HTP. Effects of repeated high doses and of association with benserazide. *Electroencephalography and Clinical Neurophysiology* 1976;41:408–413.

17. Nave R, Peled R, Lavie P. Melatonin improves evening napping. *European Journal of Pharmacology* 1995;275:213–216.

18. Olde Rikkert MG, Rigaud AS. Melatonin in elderly patients with insomnia: a systematic review. *Zeitschrift für Gerontologie und Geriatrie* 2001;34:491–497.

19. Haimov I, Lavie P, Laudon M, et al. Melatonin replacement therapy of elderly insomniacs. *Sleep* 1995;18:598–603.

20. Dollins AB, Zhdanova IV, Wurtman RJ, et al. Effect of inducing nocturnal serum melatonin concentrations in daytime on sleep, mood, body temperature, and performance. *Proceedings of the National Academy of Sciences of the United States of America* 1994;91:1824–1828.

21. Mallo C, Zaidan R, Faure A, et al. Effects of a four-day nocturnal melatonin treatment on the 24 h plasma melatonin, cortisol and prolactin profiles in humans. *Acta Endocrinologica* 1988;119:474–480.

22. Botez MI, Cadotte M, Beaulieu R, et al. Neurologic disorders responsive to folic acid therapy. *Canadian Medical Association Journal* 1976;115:217–223.

23. O'Keeffe ST, Gavin K, Lavan JN. Iron status and restless legs syndrome in the elderly. *Age and Ageing* 1994;23:200–203.

24. Hadley S, Petry JJ. Valerian. *American Family Physician* 2003;67:1755–1758.

25. Stevinson C, Ernst E. Valerian for insomnia: a systematic review of randomized clinical trials. *Sleep Medicine* 2000;1:91–99.

26. Kripke DF. Chronic hypnotic use: deadly risks, doubtful benefit. *Sleep Medicine Reviews* 2000 Feb;4(1):5–20.

27. Kripke DF. Do hypnotics cause death and cancer? The burden of proof. *Sleep Medicine* 2009 Mar;10(3):275–276.

28. Mallon L, Broman JE, Hetta J. Is usage of hypnotics associated with mortality? *Sleep Medicine* 2009 Mar;10(3):279–286.

29. Kripke DF, Langer RD, Kline LE. Hypnotics' association with mortality or cancer: A matched cohort study. *BMJ Open* 2012;2: e000850.

Irritable Bowel Syndrome

1. Simren M, Mansson A, Langkilde AM, et al. Food-related gastrointestinal symptoms in the irritable bowel syndrome. *Digestion* 2001;63:108–115.

2. Eswaran S, Tack J, Chey WD. Food: the forgotten factor in the irritable bowel syndrome. *Gastroenterology Clinics of North America* 2011 Mar;40(1):141–162.

3. Cann PA, Read NW, Holdsworth CD. What is the benefit of coarse wheat bran in patients with irritable bowel syndrome? *Gut* 1984;25:168–173.

4. Fielding JF, Kehoe M. Different dietary fibre formulations and the irritable bowel syndrome. *Irish Journal of Medical Sciences* 1984;153:178–180.

5. Chouinard LE. The role of psyllium fibre supplementation in treating irritable bowel syndrome. *Canadian Journal of Dietetic Practice and Research* 2011 Spring;72(1):e107–e114.

6. Slavin JL, Greenberg NA. Partially hydrolyzed guar gum: clinical nutrition uses. *Nutrition* 2003;19:549–552.

7. Hollander E. Mucous colitis due to food allergy. *The American*

Journal of the Medical Sciences 1927;174:495–500.

8. Gay L. Mucous colitis, complicated by colonic polyposis, relieved by allergic management. *American Journal of Digestive Diseases* 1937;3:326–329.

9. Jones VA, McLaughlan P, Shorthouse M, et al. Food intolerance: a major factor in the pathogenesis of irritable bowel syndrome. *The Lancet* 1982;2:1115–1117.

10. Petitpierre M, Gumowski P, Girard JP. Irritable bowel syndrome and hypersensitivity to food. *Annals of Allergy, Asthma & Immunology* 1985;54:538–540.

11. Nanda R, James R, Smith H, et al. Food intolerance and the irritable bowel syndrome. *Gut* 1989;30:1099–1104.

12. Gertner D, Powell-Tuck J. Irritable bowel syndrome and food intolerance. *Practitioner* 1994 Jul;238(1540):499–504.

13. Drisko J, Bischoff B, Hall M, McCallum R. Treating irritable bowel syndrome with a food elimination diet followed by food challenge and probiotics. *Journal of the American College of Nutrition* 2006 Dec;25(6):514–522.

14. Russo A, Fraser R, Horowitz M. The effect of acute hyperglycemia on small intestinal motility in normal subjects. *Diabetologia* 1996;39:984–989.

15. Shepherd SJ, Gibson PR. Fructose malabsorption and symptoms of irritable bowel syndrome: guidelines for effective dietary management. *Journal of the American Dietetic Association* 2006;106:1631–1639.

16. Shepherd SJ, Parker FC, Muir JG, et al. Dietary triggers of abdominal symptoms in patients with irritable bowel syndrome: randomised, placebo-controlled evidence. *Clinical Gastroenterology and Hepatology* 2008;6:765–771.

17. Brenner DM, Moeller MJ, Chey WD, Schoenfeld PS. The utility of probiotics in the treatment of irritable bowel syndrome: a systematic review. *The American Journal of Gastroenterology* 2009 Apr;104(4):1033–1049.

18. O'Mahony L, McCarthy J, Kelly P, et al. Lactobacillus and bifidobacterium in irritable bowel syndrome: symptom responses and relationship to cytokine profiles. *Gastroenterology* 2005 Mar;128(3):541–551.

19. Whorwell PJ, Altringer L, Morel J, et al. Efficacy of an encapsulated probiotic *Bifidobacterium infantis* 35624 in women with irritable bowel syndrome. *The American Journal of Gastroenterology* 2006 Jul;101(7):1581–1590.

20. Gawrońska A, Dziechciarz P, Horvath A, Szajewska H. A randomized double-blind placebo-controlled trial of *Lactobacillus* GG for abdominal pain disorders in children. *Alimentary Pharmacology & Therapeutics* 2007 Jan 15;25(2):177–184.

21. Niedzielin K, Kordecki H, Birkenfeld B. A controlled, double-blind, randomized study on the efficacy of *Lactobacillus plantarum* 299V in patients with irritable bowel syndrome. *European Journal of Gastroenterology & Hepatology* 2001;13:1143–1147.

22. Kajander K, Hatakka K, Poussa T, et al. A probiotic mixture alleviates symptoms in irritable bowel syndrome patients: a controlled 6-month intervention. *Alimentary Pharmacology & Therapeutics* 2005;22(5):387–394.

23. Kim HJ, Vazquez Roque MI, Camilleri M, et al. A randomized controlled trial of a probiotic combination VSL# 3 and placebo in irritable bowel syndrome with bloating. *Neurogastroenterology & Motility* 2005;17(5):687–696.

24. Kajander K, Krogius-Kurikka L, Rinttilä T, et al. Effects of multispecies probiotic supplementation on intestinal microbiota in irritable bowel syndrome. *Alimentary Pharmacology & Therapeutics* 2007;26(3):463–473.

25. Kajander K, Myllyluoma E, Rajilić-Stojanović M, et al. Clinical trial: multispecies probiotic supplementation alleviates the symptoms of irritable bowel syndrome and stabilizes intestinal microbiota. *Alimentary Pharmacology & Therapeutics* 2008 Jan 1;27(1):48–45.

26. Leicester RJ, Hunt RH. Peppermint oil to reduce colonic spasm during endoscopy. *The Lancet* 1982;2:989.

27. Somerville KW, Richmond CR, Bell GD. Delayed release peppermint oil capsules (Colpermin) for the spastic colon syndrome: a pharmacokinetic study. *British Journal of Clinical Pharmacology* 1984;18:638–640.

28. Rees WD, Evans BK, Rhodes J. Treating irritable bowel syndrome with peppermint oil. *British Medical Journal* 1979;2:835–836.

29. Pittler MH, Ernst E. Peppermint oil for irritable bowel syndrome: a critical review and metaanalysis. *The American Journal of Gastroenterology* 1998;93:1131–1135.

30. Liu JH, Chen GH, Yeh HZ, et al. Enteric-coated peppermint oil capsules in the treatment of irritable bowel syndrome: a prospective, randomized trial. *Journal of Gastroenterology* 1997;32:765–768.

31. Stiles JC, Sparks W, Ronzio RA. The inhibition of *Candida albicans* by oregano. *Journal of Applied Nutrition* 1995;47:96–102.

32. Kline RM, Kline JJ, Di Palma J, et al. Enteric-coated, pH-dependent peppermint oil capsules for the treatment of irritable bowel syndrome in children. *Journal of Pediatrics* 2001;138:125–128.

33. Goldsmith G, Levin JS. Effect of sleep quality on symptoms of irritable bowel syndrome. *Di-*

gestive *Diseases and Sciences* 1993;38:1809–1814.

34. Narducci F, Snape WJ Jr, Battle WM, et al. Increased colonic motility during exposure to a stressful situation. *Digestive Diseases and Sciences* 1985;30: 40–44.

35. Blanchard EB, Greene B, Scharff L, et al. Relaxation training as a treatment for irritable bowel syndrome. *Biofeedback & Self Regulation* 1993;18: 125–132.

36. Goldsmith G, Patterson M. Irritable bowel syndrome: treatment update. *American Family Physician* 1985;31:191–195.

37. Schwarz SP, Taylor AE, Scharff L, et al. Behaviorally treated irritable bowel syndrome patients: a four-year follow-up. *Behaviour Research and Therapy* 1990;28:331–335.

38. Shaw G, Srivastava ED, Sadlier M, et al. Stress management for irritable bowel syndrome: a controlled trial. *Digestion* 1991; 50:36–42.

Kidney Stones

1. Griffith HM, O'Shea B, Maguire M, Koegh B, Kevany JP. A case-control study of dietary intake of renal stone patients. II. Urine biochemistry and stone analysis. *Urological Research* 1986;14(2):75–82.

2. Thom J, Morris J, Bishop A, et al. The influence of refined carbohydrate on urinary calcium excretion. *British Journal of Urology* 1978;50:459–464.

3. Lemann J, Piering W, Lennon E. Possible role of carbohydrate-induced calciuria in calcium oxalate kidney-stone formation. *The New England Journal of Medicine* 1969;280: 232–237.

4. Zechner O, Latal D, Pfluger H, et al. Nutritional risk factors in urinary stone disease. *Journal of Urology* 1981;125:51–54.

5. Robertson W, Peacock M, Marshall D. Prevalence of urinary stone disease in vegetarians. *European Urology* 1982;8:334–339.

6. Griffith H, O'Shea B, Kevany J, et al. A control study of dietary factors in renal stone formation. *British Journal of Urology* 1981; 53:416–420.

7. Shuster J, Jenkins A, Logan C, et al. Soft drink consumption and urinary stone recurrence: a randomized prevention trial, *Journal of Clinical Epidemiology* 1992;45:911–916.

8. Siener R, Hesse A. The effect of a vegetarian and different omnivorous diets on urinary risk factors for uric acid stone formation. *European Journal of Nutrition* 2003;42:332–337.

9. Shah P, Williams G, Green N. Idiopathic hypercalciuria: its control with unprocessed bran. *British Journal of Urology* 1980;52:426–429.

10. Rose G, Westbury E. The influence of calcium content of water, intake of vegetables and fruit and of other food factors upon the incidence of renal calculi. *Urological Research* 1975; 3:61–66.

11. Kessler T, Jansen B, Hesse A. Effect of blackcurrant-, cranberry- and plum-juice consumption on risk factors associated with kidney stone formation. *European Journal of Clinical Nutrition* 2002;56:1020–1023.

12. Light I, Gursel E, Zinnser HH. Urinary ionized calcium in urolithiasis. Effect of cranberry juice. *Urology* 1:67–70, 1973.

13. Borghi L, Meschi T, Amato F, et al. Urinary volume, water and recurrences in idiopathic calcium nephrolithiasis: a 5-year randomized prospective study. *Journal of Urology* 1966 Mar; 155(3):839–843.

14. Nouvenne A, Meschi T, Prati B, et al. Effects of low salt diet on idiopathic hypercalciuria in calcium oxalate stone formers: a 3-mo randomized controlled trial. *The American Journal of Clinical Nutrition* 2010;91:565–570.

15. Ulmann A, Aubert J, Bourdeau A, et al. Effects of weight and glucose ingestion on urinary calcium and phosphate excretion: implications for calcium urolithiasis. *The Journal of Clinical Endocrinology & Metabolism* 1982;54:1063–1068.

16. Rao N, Gordon C, Davies D, et al. Are stone formers maladaptive to refined carbohydrates? *British Journal of Urology* 1982;54:575–577.

17. Blacklock NJ. Sucrose and idiopathic renal stone. *Nutrition and Health* 1987;5:9–17.

18. Rushton H, Spector M. Effects of magnesium deficiency on intratubular calcium oxalate formation and crystalluria in hyperoxaluric rats. *Journal of Urology* 1982;127:598–604.

19. Wunderlich W. Aspects of the influence of magnesium ions on the formation of calcium oxalate. *Urological Research* 1981; 9:157–161.

20. Hallson P, Rose G, Sulaiman SM. Magnesium reduces calcium oxalate crystal formation in human whole urine. *Clinical Science* 1982;62:17–19.

21. Johansson G, Backman U, Danielson B, et al. Magnesium metabolism in renal stone formers. Effects of therapy with magnesium hydroxide. *Scandinavian Journal of Urology and Nephrology* 1980;53 suppl:125–134.

22. Prien E, Gershoff S. Magnesium oxide-pyridoxine therapy for recurrent calcium oxalate calculi. *Journal of Urology* 1974; 112:509–512.

23. Gershoff S, Prien E. Effect of daily MgO and vitamin B6 administration to patients with recurring calcium oxalate kidney stones. *The American Journal of Clinical Nutrition* 1967;20: 393–399.

24. Will E, Bijvoet O. Primary oxalosis: clinical and biochemical response to high-dose pyridoxine therapy. *Metabolism* 1979; 28:542–548.

25. Lyon E, Borden T, Ellis J, et al. Calcium oxalate lithiasis produced by pyridoxine deficiency and inhibition with high magnesium diets. *Investigative Urology* 1966;4:133–142.

26. Murthy M, Farooqui S, Talwar H, et al. Effect of pyridoxine supplementation on recurrent stone formers. *International Journal of Clinical Pharmacology, Therapy and Toxicology* 1982;20:434–437.

27. Liebman M, Chai W. Effect of dietary calcium on urinary oxalate excretion after oxalate loads. *The American Journal of Clinical Nutrition* 1997;65: 1453–1459.

28. Usui Y, Matsuzaki S, Matsushita K, et al. Urinary citrate in kidney stone disease. *The Tokai Journal of Experimental and Clinical Medicine* 2003;28: 65–70.

29. Pak CY, Fuller C. Idiopathic hypocitraturic calcium-oxalate nephrolithiasis successfully treated with potassium citrate. *Annals of Internal Medicine* 1986;104:33–37.

30. Whalley NA, Meyers AM, Martins M, et al. Long-term effects of potassium citrate therapy on the formation of new stones in groups of recurrent stone formers with hypocitraturia. *British Journal of Urology* 1996;78: 10–14.

31. Barcelo P, Wuhl O, Servitge E, et al. Randomized double-blind study of potassium citrate in idiopathic hypocitraturic calcium nephrolithiasis. *Journal of Urology* 1993;150:1761,1764.

32. Nakagawa Y, Margolis H, Yokoyama S, et al. Purification and characterization of a calcium oxalate monohydrate crystal growth inhibitor from human kidney tissue culture medium. *The Journal of Biological Chemistry* 1981;256:3936–3944.

33. Dharmsathaphorn K, Freeman D, Binder H, et al. Increased risk of nephrolithiasis in patients with steatorrhea. *Digestive Diseases and Sciences* 1982;27:401–405.

34. Coe F, Moran E, Kavalich A. The contribution of dietary purine over-consumption to hyperuricosuria in calcium oxalate stone formers. *Journal of Chronic Diseases* 1976;29: 793–800.

35. Holmes RP, Goodman HO, Assimos DG, et al. Contribution of dietary oxalate to urinary oxalate excretion. *Kidney International* 2001;59:270.

36. Assimos DG, Holmes RP. Role of diet in the therapy of urolithiasis. *Urologic Clinics of North America* 2000;27:255–268.

37. Borghi L, Schianchi T, Meschi T, et al. Comparison of two diets for the prevention of recurrent stones in idiopathic hypercalciuria. *The New England Journal of Medicine* 2002;346: 77–84.

38. Rivers JM. Safety of high-level vitamin C ingestion. *International Journal for Vitamin and Nutrition Research* 1989 suppl; 30:95–102.

39. Wandzilak TR, D'Andre SD, Davis PA, et al. Effect of high dose vitamin C on urinary oxalate levels. *Journal of Urology* 1994;151:834–837.

40. Massey LK, Liebman M, Kynast-Gales SA., Ascorbate increases human oxaluria and kidney stone risk. *Journal of Nutrition* 2005 Jul;135(7):1673–1677.

41. Moyad MA, Combs MA, Crowley DC, et al. Vitamin C with metabolites reduce oxalate levels compared to ascorbic acid: a preliminary and novel clinical urologic finding. *Urologic Nursing* 2009 Mar–Apr;29(2): 95–102.

42. Grases F, Costa-Bauza A. Phytate (IP6) is a powerful agent for preventing calcifications in biological fluids: usefulness in renal lithiasis treatment. *Anticancer Research* 1999;19:3717–3722.

43. Anton R, Haag-Berrurier M. Therapeutic use of natural anthraquinone for other than laxative actions. *Pharmacology* 1980;20:104–112.

44. Berg W, Hesse A, Hensel K, et al. [Influence of anthraquinones on the formation of urinary calculi in experimental animals.] *Urologe A* 1976;15:188–191.

Macular Degeneration

1. de Jong PT. Age-related macular degeneration. *The New England Journal of Medicine* 2006;355(14):1474–1485.

2. Kaufman SR. Developments in age-related macular degeneration: diagnosis and treatment. *Geriatrics* 2009 Mar;64(3):16–19.

3. Chakravarthy U, Wong TY, Fletcher A, et al. Clinical risk factors for age-related macular degeneration: a systematic review and meta-analysis. *BMC Ophthalmology* 2010 Dec 13; 10:31.

4. Vinderling JR, Dielemans I, Bots ML. Age-related macular degeneration is associated with atherosclerosis. The Rotterdam Study. *American Journal of Epidemiology* 1995;142:404–409.

5. Chung M, Lotery AJ. Genetics update of macular diseases. *Ophthalmology Clinics of North America* 2002;15:459–465.

6. Hall NF, Gale CR, Syddall H, et al. Relation between size at birth and risk of age-related macular degeneration. *Investigative Ophthalmology & Visual Science* 2002;43:3641–3645.

7. Antioxidant status and neovascular age-related macular degeneration. Eye Disease Case-Control Study Group. *Archives of Ophthalmology* 1993; 111:104–109.

8. Snodderly DM. Evidence for protection against age-related macular degeneration by carotenoids and antioxidant vitamins. *The American Journal of Clinical Nutrition* 1995;62:1448S–1461S.

9. Mares-Perlman JA, Brady WE, Klein R, et al. Serum antioxi-

dants and age-related macular degeneration in a population-based case-control study. *Archives of Ophthalmology* 1995; 113:1518–1523.

10. Landrum JT, Bone RA, Kilburn MD. The macular pigment: a possible role in protection from age-related macular degeneration. *Advances in Pharmacology* 1997;38:537–556.

11. Carpentier S, Knaus M, Suh M. Associations between lutein, zeaxanthin, and age-related macular degeneration: an overview. *Critical Reviews in Food Science and Nutrition* 2009 Apr;49(4):313–326.

12. Obisesan TO, Hirsch R, Kosoko O, et al. Moderate wine consumption is associated with decreased odds of developing age-related macular degeneration in NHANES-1. *Journal of the American Geriatrics Society* 1998;46:1–7.

13. Ritter LL, Klein R, Klein BE, et al. Alcohol use and age-related maculopathy in the Beaver Dam Eye Study. *American Journal of Ophthalmology* 1995;120: 190–196.

14. Seddon JM, Cote J, Rosner B. Progression of age-related macular degeneration: association with dietary fat, transunsaturated fat, nuts, and fish intake. *Archives of Ophthalmology* 2003;121:1728–1737.

15. Merle B, Delyfer MN, Korobelnik JF, et al. Dietary omega-3 fatty acids and the risk for age-related maculopathy: the Alienor Study. *Investigative Ophthalmology and Visual Sciences.* 2011 Jul;52(8):6004–11.

16. SanGiovanni JP, Chew EY, Agrón E, et al. The relationship of dietary omega-3 long-chain polyunsaturated fatty acid intake with incident age-related macular degeneration: AREDS report no. 23. *Archives of Ophthalmology* 2008 Sep;126(9): 1274–1279.

17. SanGiovanni JP, Agrón E, Clemons TE, Chew EY. Omega-3 long-chain polyunsaturated fatty acid intake inversely associated with 12-year progression to advanced age-related macular degeneration. *Archives of Ophthalmology* 2009 Jan;127(1): 110–112.

18. AREDS Research Group. A randomized, placebo-controlled, clinical trial of high-dose supplementation with vitamins C and E, beta carotene, and zinc for age-related macular degeneration and vision loss. *Archives of Ophthalmology* 2001;119:1417–1436.

19. Richer S. Multicenter ophthalmic and nutritional age-related macular degeneration study. Part 1. Design, subjects and procedures. *Journal of the American Optometric Association* 1996;67:12–29.

20. Richer S. Multicenter ophthalmic and nutritional age-related macular degeneration study. Part 2. Antioxidant intervention and conclusions. *Journal of the American Optometric Association* 1996;67:30–49.

21. Bartlett H, Eperjesi F. Age-related macular degeneration and nutritional supplementation: a review of randomised controlled trials. *Ophthalmic and Physiological Optics* 2003;23:383–399.

22. Christen WG, Glynn RJ, Chew EY, et al. Folic acid, pyridoxine, and cyanocobalamin combination treatment and age-related macular degeneration in women: the Women's Antioxidant and Folic Acid Cardiovascular Study. *Archives of Internal Medicine* 2009 Feb 23; 169(4):335–341.

23. Richer S, Stiles W, Statkute L, et al. Double-masked, placebo-controlled, randomized trial of lutein and antioxidant supplementation in the intervention of atrophic age-related macular degeneration: the Veterans LAST study (Lutein Antioxidant Supplementation Trial). *Optometry* 2004;75:216–230.

24. Parisi V, Tedeschi M, Gallinaro G, et al. Carotenoids and antioxidants in age-related maculopathy Italian study: multifocal electroretinogram modifications after 1 year. *Ophthalmology* 2008 Feb;115(2):324–333.

25. Newsome DA, Swartz M, Leone NC, et al. Oral zinc in macular degeneration. *Archives of Ophthalmology* 1988;106:192–198.

26. Newsome DA. A randomized, prospective, placebo-controlled clinical trial of a novel zinc-monocysteine compound in age-related macular degeneration. *Current Eye Research* 2008 Jul; 33(7):591–598.

27. Scharrer A, Ober M. [Anthocyanosides in the treatment of retinopathies.] *Klinische Monatsblätter für Augenheilkunde* 1981;178:386–389.

28. Caselli L. Clinical and electroretinographic study on the activity of anthocyanosides. *Archivio di Medicina Interna* 1985;37:29–35.

29. Lebuisson DA, Leroy L, Rigal G. [Treatment of senile macular degeneration with *Ginkgo biloba* extract. A preliminary double-blind, drug vs. placebo study.] *La Presse Médicale* 1986;15:1556–1558.

30. Corbe C, Boisin JP, Siou A. [Light vision and chorioretinal circulation. Study of the effect of procyanidolic oligomers (Endotelon).] *Journal Français d'Ophtalmologie* 1988;11:453–460.

31. Rein DB, Saaddine JB, Wittenborn JS, et al. Cost-effectiveness of vitamin therapy for age-related macular degeneration. *Ophthalmology* 2007 Jul;114(7): 1319–1326.

Menopause

1. Theisen SC, Mansfield PK. Menopause: social construction or biological destiny? *Journal of Health Education* 1993;24: 209–213.

2. Martin MC, Block JE, Sanchez SD, et al. Menopause without symptoms: the endocrinology of menopause among rural Mayan

Indians. *American Journal of Obstetrics & Gynecology* 1993; 168:1839–1845.

3. Rossouw JE, Anderson GL, Prentice RL, et al. Risks and benefits of estrogen plus progestin in healthy postmenopausal women: principal results from the Women's Health Initiative randomized controlled trial. *JAMA, The Journal of the American Medical Association* 2002; 288:321–333.

4. Hulley S, Grady D, Bush T, et al. Randomized trial of estrogen plus progestin for secondary prevention of coronary heart disease in postmenopausal women. Heart and Estrogen/Progestin Replacement Study (HERS) Research Group. *JAMA, The Journal of the American Medical Association* 1998;280:605–613.

5. Heckbert SR, Weiss NS, Koepsell TD, et al. Duration of estrogen replacement therapy in relation to the risk of incident myocardial infarction in postmenopausal women. *Archives of Internal Medicine* 1997;157: 1330–1336.

6. Grodstein F, Manson JE, Stampfer MJ. Postmenopausal hormone use and secondary prevention of coronary events in the Nurses' Health Study: a prospective, observational study. *Annals of Internal Medicine* 2001;135:1–8.

7. Grady D, Herrington D, Bittner V, et al. Cardiovascular disease outcomes during 6.8 years of hormone therapy: Heart and Estrogen/Progestin Replacement Study follow-up (HERS II). *JAMA, The Journal of the American Medical Association* 2002;288:49–57.

8. Colditz GA, Rosner B. Cumulative risk of breast cancer to age 70 years according to risk factor status: data from the Nurses' Health Study. *American Journal of Epidemiology* 2000;152: 950–964.

9. Berry DA, Ravdin PM. Breast cancer trends: a marriage between clinical trial evidence and epidemiology. *Journal of the National Cancer Institute* 2007; 99(15):1139–1141.

10. Hammar M, Berg G, Lindgren R. Does physical exercise influence the frequency of postmenopausal hot flushes? *Acta Obstetricia et Gynecologica Scandinavica* 1990;69:409–412.

11. Manson J, Greenland P, LaCroix AZ, et al. Walking compared with vigorous exercise for the prevention of cardiovascular events in women. *The New England Journal of Medicine* 2002; 347:716–725.

12. McTiernan A, Kooperberg C, White E, et al. Recreational physical activity and the risk of breast cancer in postmenopausal women: the Women's Health Initiative Cohort Study. *JAMA, The Journal of the American Medical Association* 2003;290:1331–1336.

13. Kemmler W, Engelke K, Weineck J, et al. The Erlangen Fitness Osteoporosis Prevention Study: a controlled exercise trial in early postmenopausal women with low bone density-first year results. *Archives of Physical Medicine and Rehabilitation* 2003;84:673–682.

14. Dalais FS, Rice GE, Wahlqvist ML, et al. Effects of dietary phytoestrogens in postmenopausal women. *Climacteric* 1998;1(2): 124–129.

15. Albertazzi P, Pansini F, Bonaccorsi G, et al. The effect of dietary soy supplementation on hot flushes. *Obstetrics & Gynecology* 1998;91:6–11.

16. Messina M, Hughes C. Efficacy of soy foods and soybean isoflavone supplements for alleviating menopausal symptoms is positively related to initial hot flush frequency. *Journal of Medicinal Food* 2003;6(1):1–11.

17. Upmalis DH, Lobo R, Bradley L, et al. Vasomotor symptom relief by soy isoflavone extract tablets in postmenopausal women: a multicenter, double-blind, randomized, placebo-controlled study. *Menopause* 2000;7:236–242.

18. Huntley A, Ernst E. Soy for the treatment of perimenopausal symptoms—a systematic review. *Maturitas* 2004;47:1–9.

19. Krebs E, Ensrud K, MacDonald R, Wilt T. Phytoestrogens for treatment of menopausal symptoms: a systematic review. *Obstetrics & Gynecology* 2004; 104:824–836.

20. Jou HJ, Wu SS, Change FW, et al. Effect of intestinal production of equol on menopausal symptoms in women treated with soy isoflavones. *International Journal of Gynecology & Obstetrics* 2008 Jul;102(1): 44–49.

21. Haggans CJ, Hutchins AM, Olson BA, et al. Effect of flaxseed consumption on urinary estrogen metabolites in postmenopausal women. *Nutrition and Cancer* 1999;33(2):188–195.

22. Haggans CJ, Travelli EJ, Thomas W, et al. The effect of flaxseed and wheat bran consumption on urinary estrogen metabolites in premenopausal women. *Cancer Epidemiology, Biomarkers & Prevention* 2000; 9(7):719–725.

23. Pruthi SL, Thompson PJ, Novotny DL, et al. Pilot evaluation of flaxseed for the management of hot flashes. *Journal of the Society for Integrative Oncology* 2007;5(3):106–112.

24. Lucas M, Asselin G, Merette C, et al. Effects of ethyl-eicosapentaenoic acid omega-3 fatty acid supplementation on hot flashes and quality of life among middle-aged women: a double-blind, placebo-controlled, randomized clinical trial. *Menopause* 2009; 16(2):357–366.

25. Smith CJ. Non-hormonal control of vaso-motor flushing in menopausal patients. *Chicago Medicine* 1964;67:193–195.

26. Yang HM, Liao MF, Zhu SY, et al. A randomised, double-blind, placebo-controlled trial on the effect of Pycnogenol

on the climacteric syndrome in peri-menopausal women. *Acta Obstetricia et Gynecologica Scandinavica* 2007;86:978–985.

27. Murase Y, Iishima H. Clinical studies of oral administration of gamma-oryzanol on climacteric complaints and its syndrome. *Obstetrics and Gynecology Practice* 1963;12:147–149.

28. Ishihara M. Effect of gamma-oryzanol on serum lipid peroxide levels and climacteric disturbances. *Asia-Oceania Journal of Obstetrics and Gynaecology* 1984;10:317–323.

29. Yoshino G, Kazumi T, Amano M, et al. Effects of gamma-oryzanol on hyperlipidemic subjects. *Current Therapeutic Research, Clinical and Experimental* 1989;45:543–552.

30. Christy CJ. Vitamin E in menopause. *American Journal of Obstetrics & Gynecology* 1945;50:84–87.

31. McLaren HC. Vitamin E in the menopause. *British Medical Journal* 1949;2:1378–1381.

32. Finkler RS. The effect of vitamin E in the menopause. *The Journal of Clinical Endocrinology & Metabolism* 1949;9:89–94.

33. Borrelli F, Ernst E. *Cimicifuga racemosa:* a systematic review of its clinical efficacy. *European Journal of Clinical Pharmacology* 2002;58:235–241.

34. Stolze H. An alternative to treat menopausal complaints. *Gyne* 1982;3:14–16.

35. Wuttke W, Seidlova-Wuttke D, Gorkow C. The *Cimicifuga* preparation BNO 1055 vs. conjugated estrogens in a double-blind placebo-controlled study: effects on menopause symptoms and bone markers. *Maturitas* 2003;44:S67–S77.

36. Chung D, Kim H, Park K, et al. Black cohosh and St. John's wort (GYNO-Plus) for climacteric symptoms. *Yonsei Medical Journal* 2007;48(2):289–294.

37. Cancellieri F, De Leo V, Genazzani A, et al. Efficacy on menopausal neurovegetative symptoms and some plasma lipids blood levels of an herbal product containing isoflavones and other plant extracts. *Maturitas* 2007;56:249–256.

38. Meissner H, Mscisz A, Reich-Bilinska R, et al. Hormone-balancing effect of pre-gelatinized organic maca (*Lepidium peruvianum* Chacon). III. Clinical response of early-postmenopausal women to maca in a double blind, randomized, placebo-controlled, crossover configuration, outpatient study. *International Journal of Biomedical Science* 2006;2(4):375–394.

39. Dini A, Migliuolo G, Rastrelli L, et al. Chemical composition of *Lepidium meyenii*. *Food Chemistry* 1994;49:347.

40. Ganzera M, Zhao J, Muhammad I, Khan I. Chemical profiling and standardization of *Lepidium meyenii* (maca) by reversed phase high performance liquid chromatography. *Chemical and Pharmaceutical Bulletin* 2002;50:988.

41. Brooks N, Wilcox G, Walker K, et al. Beneficial effects of *Lepidium meyenii* (maca) on psychological symptoms and measures of sexual dysfunction in postmenopausal women are not related to estrogen or androgen content. *Menopause* 2008;15(6):1157–1162.

42. Thompson Coon J, Pittler M, Ernst E. *Trifolium pretense* isoflavones in the treatment of menopausal hot flushes: a systematic review and meta-analysis. *Phytomedicine* 2007;14:153–159

43. Baber RJ, Templeman C, Morton T, et al. Randomized placebo-controlled trial of an isoflavone supplement and menopausal symptoms in women. *Climacteric* 1999;2:85–92.

44. Knight D, Howes J, Eden J. The effect of Promensil, an isoflavone extract, on menopausal symptoms. *Climacteric* 1999;2:79–84.

45. Jeri A, deRomana C. The effect of isoflavone phytoestrogens in relieving hot flushes in Peruvian post-menopausal women. *Proceedings of the 9th International Menopause Society World Congress on the Menopause,* Yokohama, Japan, 1999.

46. Nachtigall L, La Grega L, Lee W, Fenichel R. The effects of isoflavones derived from red clover on vasomotor symptoms and endometrial thickness. *Proceedings of the 9th International Menopause Society World Congress on the Menopause,* Yokohama, Japan, 1999.

47. van de Weijer P, Barentsen R. Isoflavones from red clover (Promensil) significantly reduce menopausal hot flush symptoms compared with placebo. *Maturitas* 2002;42:187–193.

48. Tice J, Ettinger B, Ensrud K, et al. Phytoestrogen supplements for the treatment of hot flashes: the isoflavone clover extract (ICE) study. *JAMA, The Journal of the American Medical Association* 2003;290:207–214.

49. Hirata JD, Swiersz LM, Zell B, et al. Does dong quai have estrogenic effects in postmenopausal women? A double-blind, placebo-controlled trial. *Fertility and Sterility* 1997;68:981–986.

50. Chang HM, But PPH, eds. *Pharmacology and applications of Chinese materia medica,* vol. 1. Singapore: World Scientific, 1987, 489–505.

51. Yang Q, Populo SM, Zhang J, et al. Effect of *Angelica sinensis* on the proliferation of human bone cells. *Clinica Chimica Acta* 2002;324:89–97.

52. Abdali K, Khajehei M, Tabatabaee R. Effect of St. John's wort on severity, frequency, and duration of hot flashes in premenopausal, perimenopausal and postmenopausal women: a randomized, double-blind, placebo-controlled study. *Menopause* 2010;17(2): 326–331.

53. Al-Akoum M, Maunsell E, Verreault R, et al. Effects of *Hypericum perforatum* (St. John's wort) on hot flashes and quality of life in perimenopausal women: a randomized pilot trial. *Menopause* 2009 Mar-Apr; 16(2):307–314.

54. Grube B, Walper A, Whatley D. St. John's wort extract: efficacy for menopausal symptoms of psychological origin. *Advances in Therapy* 1999;16:177.

55. Chang A, Kwak BY, Yi K, Kim JS. The effect of herbal extract (EstroG-100) on pre-, peri- and post-menopausal women: a randomized double-blind, placebo-controlled study. *Phytotherapy Research* 2011 Sep 2; doi: 10.1002/ptr.3597.

Menstrual Blood Loss, Excessive (Menorrhagia)

1. Hallberg L, Hogdahl AM, Nilsson L, Rybo G. Menstrual blood loss—a population study. Variation at different ages and attempts to define normality. *Acta Obstetricia et Gynecologica Scandinavica* 1966;45:320–351.

2. Chimbira TH, Anderson AB, Turnbull A. Relation between measured blood loss and patients' subjective assessment of loss, duration of bleeding, number of sanitary towels used, uterine weight and endometrial surface area. *British Journal of Obstetrics and Gynaecology* 1980;87:603–609.

3. Downing I, Hutchon DJ, Poyser NL. Uptake of [3H]-arachidonic acid by human endometrium. Differences between normal and menorrhagic tissue. *Prostaglandins* 1983;26:55–69.

4. Kelly RW, Lumsden MA, Abel MH, Baird DT. The relationship between menstrual blood loss and prostaglandin production in the human: evidence for increased availability of arachidonic acid in women suffering from menorrhagia. *Prostaglandins, Leukotrienes, and Medicine* 1984;16:69–78.

5. Stoffer SS. Menstrual disorders and mild thyroid insufficiency: intriguing cases suggesting an association. *Postgraduate Medicine* 1982;72:75–82.

6. Stott PC. The outcome of menorrhagia: a retrospective case control study. *The Journal of the Royal College of General Practitioners* 1983;33:715–720.

7. Taymor ML, Sturgis SH, Yahia C. The etiological role of chronic iron deficiency in production of menorrhagia. *JAMA, The Journal of the American Medical Association* 1964;187:323–327.

8. Arvidsson B, Ekenved G, Rybo G, Solvell L. Iron prophylaxis in menorrhagia. *Acta Obstetricia et Gynecologica Scandinavica* 1981;60:157–160.

9. Lewis GJ. Do women with menorrhagia need iron? *British Medical Journal* (Clinical Research Edition) 1982;284:1158.

10. Cohen JD, Rubin HW. Functional menorrhagia: treatment with bioflavonoids and vitamin C. *Current Therapeutic Research* 1960;2:539–542.

11. Schumann E. Newer concepts of blood coagulation and control of hemorrhage. *American Journal of Obstetrics & Gynecology* 1939;38:1002–1007.

12. Gubner R, Ungerleider HE. Vitamin K therapy in menorrhagia. *Southern Medical Journal* 1944;37:556–558.

13. Biskind M. Nutritional deficiency in the etiology of menorrhagia, metrorrhagia, cystic mastitis and premenstrual tension: treatment with vitamin B complex. *The Journal of Clinical Endocrinology & Metabolism* 1943;3:227–234.

14. Bleier W. [Phytotherapy in irregular menstrual cycles or bleeding periods and other gynecological disorders of endocrine origin.] *Zentralblatt für Gynäkologie* 1959;81:701–709.

Migraine Headache

1. Goadsby P, Lipton R, Ferrari M. Migraine—current understanding and treatment. *The New England Journal of Medicine* 2002; 346;4:257–270.

2. Lanzi G, Grandi AM, Gamba G, et al. Migraine, mitral valve prolapse and platelet function in the pediatric age group. *Headache* 1986;26:142–145.

3. Isler H. Migraine treatment as a cause of chronic migraine. In *Advances in migraine research and therapy*, ed. Rose FC. New York: Raven Press, 1982, 159–164.

4. Olesen J. Analgesic headache. *BMJ* 1995;310:479–480.

5. Mansfield LE, Vaughan TR, Waller SF, et al. Food allergy and adult migraine: double-blind and mediator confirmation of an allergic etiology. *Annals of Allergy, Asthma & Immunology* 1985;55:126–129.

6. Carter CM, Egger J, Soothill JF. A dietary management of severe childhood migraine. *Human Nutrition—Applied Nutrition* 1985;39:294–303.

7. Hughes EC, Gott PS, Weinstein RC, Binggeli R. Migraine: a diagnostic test for etiology of food sensitivity by a nutritionally supported fast and confirmed by long-term report. *Annals of Allergy, Asthma & Immunology* 1985;55:28–32.

8. Egger J, Carter CM, Wilson J, et al. Is migraine food allergy? A double-blind controlled trial of oligoantigenic diet treatment. *The Lancet* 1983;2:865–869.

9. Monro J, Brostoff J, Carini C, Zilkha K. Food allergy in migraine: study of dietary exclusion and RAST. *The Lancet* 1980;2:1–4.

10. Grant EC. Food allergies and migraine. *The Lancet* 1979;1: 966–969.

11. Little CH, Stewart AG, Fennessy MR. Platelet serotonin release in rheumatoid arthritis: a study in food-intolerant patients. *The Lancet* 1983;2:297–299.

12. Peatfield RC. Relationship between food, wine, and beer-precipitated migrainous headaches. *Headache* 1995;35:355–357.

13. Jarisch R, Wantke F. Wine and headache. *International Archives of Allergy and Immunology* 1996;110:7–12.

14. Wantke F, Gotz M, Jarisch R. Histamine free diet: treatment of choice for histamine-induced food intolerance and supporting treatment for chronic headaches. *Clinical & Experimental Allergy* 1993;23:982–985.

15. Jarman J, Glover V, Sandler M. Release of (^{14}C)5-hydroxytryptamine from human platelets by red wine. *Life Sciences* 1991;48: 2297–2300.

16. Martner-Hewes PM, Hunt IF, Murphy NJ, et al. Vitamin B-6 nutriture and plasma diamine oxidase activity in pregnant Hispanic teenagers. *The American Journal of Clinical Nutrition* 1988;44:907–913.

17. Sabbah A, Heulin M, Drouet M, et al. [Antihistaminic or antidegranulating activity of pregnancy serum.] *Allergie et Immunologie* 1988;20:236–240.

18. Lindberg S. 14-C-histamine elimination from blood of pregnant and non-pregnant women with special reference to the uterus. *Acta Obstetricia et Gynecologica Scandinavica* 1963; 42 suppl 1:3–25.

19. Wilkinson CF Jr. Recurrent migrainoid headaches associated with spontaneous hypoglycemia. *The American Journal of the Medical Sciences* 1949;218: 209–212.

20. Dexter JD, Roberts J, Byer JA. The five hour glucose tolerance test and effect of low sucrose diet in migraine. *Headache* 1978;18:91–94.

21. Brainard JB. Angiotensin and aldosterone elevation in salt-induced migraine. *Headache* 1981;21:222–226.

22. Ratner D, Shoshani E, Dubnov B. Milk protein-free diet for nonseasonal asthma and migraine in lactase-deficient patients. *Israel Journal of Medical Sciences* 1983;19:806–809.

23. Koehler SM, Glaros A. The effect of aspartame on migraine headache. *Headache* 1988;28: 10–14.

24. Blumenthal HR, Vance DA. Chewing gum headaches. *Headache* 1997;37:665–666.

25. Gerrard JM, White JG, Krivit W. Labile aggregation stimulating substance, free fatty acids and platelet aggregation. *Journal of Laboratory and Clinical Medicine* 1976;87:73–82.

26. Sanders TA, Roshanai F. The influence of different types of omega–3 polyunsaturated fatty acids on blood lipids and platelet function in healthy volunteers. *Clinical Science* 1983;64: 91–99.

27. Woodcock BE, Smith E, Lambert WH, et al. Beneficial effect of fish oil on blood viscosity in peripheral vascular disease. *British Medical Journal* 1984; 288:592–594.

28. McCarren T, Hitzemann R, Allen C, et al. Amelioration of severe migraine by fish oil (w-3) fatty acids. *The American Journal of Clinical Nutrition* 1985; 41:874.

29. Glueck CJ, McCarren T, Hitzemann R, et al. Amelioration of severe migraine with omega-3 fatty acids: a double-blind, placebo-controlled clinical trial. *The American Journal of Clinical Nutrition* 1986;43:710.

30. Harel Z, Gascon G, Riggs S, et al. Supplementation with omega-3 polyunsaturated fatty acids in the management of recurrent migraines in adolescents. *Journal of Adolescent Health* 2002;31:154–161.

31. Titus F, Davalos A, Alom J, Codina A. 5-hydroxytryptophan versus methysergide in the prophylaxis of migraine. Randomized clinical trial. *European Neurology* 1986;25:327–329.

32. Bono G, Criscuoli M, Martignoni E, et al. Serotonin precursors in migraine prophylaxis. *Advances in Neurology* 1982; 33:357–363.

33. Maissen CP, Ludin HP. [Comparison of the effect of 5-hydroxytryptophan and propranolol in the interval treatment of migraine.] *Schweizerische Medizinische Wochenschrift* 1991;121:1585–1590.

34. Montagna P, Sacquegna T, Cortelli P, Lugaresi E. Migraine as a defect of brain oxidative metabolism: a hypothesis. *Journal of Neurology* 1989;236:124–125.

35. Schoenen J, Jacquy J, Lenaerts M. Effectiveness of high-dose riboflavin in migraine prophylaxis. A randomized controlled trial. *Neurology* 1998;50: 466–470.

36. Welch KMA, Levine SR, D'Andrea G, et al. Preliminary observations on brain energy metabolism in migraine studied studied by in vivo phosphorus 31 NMR spectroscopy. *Neurology* 1989;39:538–541.

37. Sandor, PS, Afra J, Ambrosini A, Schoenen J. Prophylactic treatment of migraine with beta blockers and riboflavin: differential effects on the intensity dependence of auditory evoked cortical potentials. *Headache* 2000;40:30–35.

38. Schoenen J, Lenaerts M, Bastings E. High-dose riboflavin as a prophylactic treatment of migraine: results of an open pilot study. *Cephalalgia* 1994; 14:328–329.

39. Kopjas TL. The use of folic acid in vascular headache of the migraine type. *Headache* 1969;8: 167–170.

40. Altura BM, Brodsky MA, Elin RJ, et al. Magnesium: growing in clinical importance. *Patient Care* 1994;10:130–150.

41. Johnson S. The multifaceted and widespread pathology of magnesium deficiency. *Medical Hypotheses* 2001;56:163–170.

42. Swanson DR. Migraine and magnesium: eleven neglected connections. *Perspectives in Biology and Medicine* 1988;31: 526–557.

43. Ramadan NM, Halvorson H,

Vande-Linde A, et al. Low brain magnesium in migraine. *Headache* 1989;29:590–593.

44. Gallai V, Sarchielli P, Morucci P, Abbritti G. Magnesium content of mononuclear blood cells in migraine patients. *Headache* 1994;34:160–165.

45. Mazzotta G, Sarchielli P, Alberti A, Gallai V. Electromyographical ischemic test and intracellular and extracellular magnesium concentration in migraine and tension-type headache patients. *Headache* 1996; 36:357–361.

46. Pfaffenrath V, Wessely P, Meyer C, et al. Magnesium in the prophylaxis of migraine—a double-blind placebo-controlled study. *Cephalalgia* 1996;16:436–440.

47. Peikert A, Wilimzig C, Kohne-Volland R. Prophylaxis of migraine with oral magnesium: results from a prospective, multi-center, placebo-controlled and double-blind randomized study. *Cephalalgia* 1996;16: 257–263.

48. Mauskop A, Altura BT, Cracco RQ, et al. Intravenous magnesium sulphate relieves migraine attacks in patients with low serum ionized magnesium levels: a pilot study. *Clinical Science* 1995;89:633–636.

49. Mauskop A, Altura BM. Role of magnesium in the pathogenesis and treatment of migraines. *Clinical Neuroscience* 1998;5: 24–27.

50. Galland LD, Baker SM, McLellan RK. Magnesium deficiency in the pathogenesis of mitral valve prolapse. *Magnesium* 1986;5:165–174.

51. Lindberg JS, Zobitz MM, Poindexter JR, Pak CY. Magnesium bioavailability from magnesium citrate and magnesium oxide. *Journal of the American College of Nutrition* 1990;9:48–55.

52. Majumdar P, Boylan M. Alteration of tissue magnesium levels in rats by dietary vitamin B6 supplementation. *International Journal for Vitamin and Nutrition Research* 1989;59:300–303.

53. Johnson ES, Kadam NP, Hylands DM, Hylands PJ. Efficacy of feverfew as prophylactic treatment of migraine. *British Medical Journal* 1985;291:569–573.

54. Murphy JJ, Heptinstall S, Mitchell JR. Randomised double-blind placebo-controlled trial of feverfew in migraine prevention. *The Lancet* 1988;2:189–192.

55. Barsby RW, Salan U, Knight BW, Hoult JR. Feverfew and vascular smooth muscle: extracts from fresh and dried plants show opposing pharmacological profiles, dependent upon sesquiterpene lactone content. *Planta Medica* 1993;59:20–25.

56. Heptinstall S, Awang DV, Dawson BA, et al. Parthenolide content and bioactivity of feverfew (*Tanacetum parthenium* [L.] Schultz-Bip.). Estimation of commercial and authenticated feverfew products. *Journal of Pharmacy and Pharmacology* 1992;44:391–395.

57. Ernst E, Pittler MH. The efficacy and safety of feverfew (*Tanacetum parthenium* L.): an update of a systematic review. *Public Health Nutrition* 2000;3: 509–514.

58. Grossman M, Schmidramsl H. An extract of *Petasites hybridus* is effective in the prophylaxis of migraine. *International Journal of Clinical Pharmacy* 2000;38: 430–435.

59. Eaton J. Butterbur, herbal help for migraine. *Natural Pharmacy* 1998;2:23–24.

60. Mustafa T, Srivastava KC. Ginger (*Zingiber officinale*) in migraine headaches. *Journal of Ethnopharmacology* 1990;29: 267–273.

61. Kiuchi F, Iwakami S, Shibuya M et al. Inhibition of prostaglandin and leukotriene biosynthesis by gingerols and diarylheptanoids. *Chemical and Pharmaceutical Bulletin* 1992;40:387–391.

62. Srivastava KC. Isolation and effects of some ginger components on platelet aggregation and eicosanoid biosynthesis. *Prostaglandins, Leukotrienes, and Medicine* 1986;25:187–198.

63. Lindeberg T. Acupuncture in headache. *Cephalalgia* 1999;19 suppl 25:65–68.

64. Melchant D, Linde K, Fischer P, et al. Acupuncture for recurrent headache: a systematic review of randomized controlled trials. *Cephalalgia* 1999;19 suppl: 779–786.

65. Baischer W. Acupuncture in migraine: long-term outcome and predicting factors. *Headache* 1995;35:472–474.

66. Holroyd KA, Penzien DB. Pharmacological versus non-pharmacological prophylaxis of recurrent migraine headache: a meta-analytic review of clinical trials. *Pain* 1990;42:1–13.

67. Manias P, Tagaris G, Karageorgiou K. Acupuncture in headache: a critical review. *The Clinical Journal of Pain* 2000; 16:334–339.

Multiple Sclerosis

1. Noseworthy JH, Lucchinetti C, Rodriguez M, Weinshenker BG. Multiple sclerosis. *The New England Journal of Medicine* 2000;343:938–952.

2. Lublin FD, Reingold SC. Defining the clinical course of multiple sclerosis: results of an international survey. National Multiple Sclerosis Society (USA) Advisory Committee on Clinical Trials of New Agents in Multiple Sclerosis. *Neurology* 1996; 46:907–911.

3. Frank JA, Stone LA, Smith ME, et al. Serial contrast-enhanced magnetic resonance imaging in patients with early relapsing-remitting multiple sclerosis: implications for treatment trials. *Annals of Neurology* 1994;36: S86–S90.

4. Weinshenker BG. Epidemiology of multiple sclerosis. *Neurologic Clinics* 1996;14:291–308.

5. Hogancamp WE, Rodriguez M,

Weinshenker BG. The epidemiology of multiple sclerosis. *Mayo Clinic Proceedings* 1997; 72:871–878.

6. Sadovnick AD, Ebers GC. Epidemiology of multiple sclerosis: a critical overview. *Canadian Journal of Neurological Sciences* 1993;20:17–29.

7. Ebers GC, Sadovnick AD. The geographic distribution of multiple sclerosis: a review. *Neuroepidemiology* 1993;12:1–5.

8. Baranzini SE. Revealing the genetic basis of multiple sclerosis: are we there yet? *Current Opinion in Genetics & Development* 2011 Jun;21(3):317–324.

9. Sadovnick AD, Dyment D, Ebers GC. Genetic epidemiology of multiple sclerosis. *Epidemiologic Reviews* 1997;19: 99–106.

10. James WH. Review of the contribution of twin studies in the search for non-genetic causes of multiple sclerosis. *Neuroepidemiology* 1996;15:132–141.

11. Taylor BV. The major cause of multiple sclerosis is environmental: genetics has a minor role—Yes. *Multiple Sclerosis* 2011 Oct;17(10):1171–1173.

12. Lucchinetti CF, Rodriguez M. The controversy surrounding the pathogenesis of the multiple sclerosis lesion. *Mayo Clinic Proceedings* 1997;72:665–678.

13. Ascherio A, Munger KL. Environmental risk factors for multiple sclerosis. Part I. The role of infection. *Annals of Neurology* 2007 Apr;61(4):288–299.

14. Ascherio A, Munger KL. Environmental risk factors for multiple sclerosis. Part II. Non-infectious factors. *Annals of Neurology* 2007;61:504–513.

15. Fernandes de Abreu DA, Babron MC, Rebeix C, et al. Season of birth and not vitamin D receptor promoter polymorphisms is a risk factor for multiple sclerosis. *Multiple Sclerosis* 2009;15(10):1146–1152.

16. Lucas RM, Ponsonby AL, Dear K, et al. Sun exposure and vitamin D are independent risk factors for CNS demyelination. *Neurology* 2011 Feb 8;76(6): 540–548.

17. Swank RL, Lerstad O, Strom A, Backer J. Multiple sclerosis in rural Norway: its geographic distribution and occupational incidence in relation to nutrition. *The New England Journal of Medicine* 1952;246: 721–728.

18. Lauer K. Diet and multiple sclerosis. *Neurology* 1997;49(2 suppl 2):S55–S61.

19. Zhang SM, Willett WC, Hernan MA, et al. Dietary fat in relation to risk of multiple sclerosis among two large cohorts of women. *American Journal of Epidemiology* 2000;152:1056–1064.

20. Zhang SM, Hernan MA, Olek MJ, et al. Intakes of carotenoids, vitamin C, and vitamin E and MS risk among two large cohorts of women. *Neurology* 2001;57:75–80.

21. Ghadirian P, Jain M, Ducic S, et al. Nutritional factors in the aetiology of multiple sclerosis: a case-control study in Montreal, Canada. *International Journal of Epidemiology* 1998;27:845–852.

22. Polman CH, O'Conner PW, Havrdova E, et al. A randomized, placebo-controlled trial of natalizumab for relapsing remitting multiple sclerosis. *The New England Journal of Medicine* 2006; 354(9):899–910.

23. Miller DH, Soon D, Fernando KT, et al. MRI outcomes in a placebo controlled trial of natalizumab in relapsing MS. *Neurology* 2007;68(17):1390–1401.

24. The IFNB Multiple Sclerosis Study Group. Interferon beta-1b is effective in relapsing-remitting multiple sclerosis. I. Clinical results of a multicenter, randomized, double-blind, placebo-controlled trial. *Neurology* 1993;43:655–661.

25. Johnson KP, Brooks BR, Cohen JA, et al. Copolymer 1 reduces relapse rate and improves disability in relapsing-remitting multiple sclerosis: results of a phase III multicenter, double-blind placebo-controlled trial. The Copolymer 1 Multiple Sclerosis Study Group. *Neurology* 1995;45:1268–1276.

26. Jacobs LD, Cookfair DL, Rudick RA, et al. Intramuscular interferon beta-1a for disease progression in relapsing multiple sclerosis. The Multiple Sclerosis Collaborative Research Group (MSCRG). *Annals of Neurology* 1996;39:285–294.

27. PRISMS (Prevention of Relapses and Disability by Interferon beta-1a Subcutaneously in Multiple Sclerosis) Study Group. Randomised double-blind placebo-controlled study of interferon beta-1a in relapsing/remitting multiple sclerosis. *The Lancet* 1998;352:1498–1504.

28. Hartung HP, Gonsette R, Konig N, et al. Mitoxantrone in progressive multiple sclerosis: a placebo-controlled, double-blind, randomised, multicentre trial. *The Lancet* 2002;360: 2018–2025.

29. Swank RL. Multiple sclerosis: twenty years on low fat diet. *Archives of Neurology* 1970;23: 460–474.

30. Swank RL, Dugan BB. *The multiple sclerosis diet book: a low fat diet for the treatment of MS.* Garden City, N.Y.: Doubleday, 1987.

31. Swank RL, Dugan BB. Effect of low saturated fat diet in early and late cases of multiple sclerosis. *The Lancet* 1990;336:37–39.

32. Youdim KA, Martin A, Joseph JA. Essential fatty acids and the brain: possible health implications. *International Journal of Developmental Neuroscience* 2000;18:383–399.

33. Nordvik I, Myhr KM, Nyland H, Bjerve KS. Effect of dietary advice and n-3 supplementation in newly diagnosed MS patients. *Acta Neurologica Scandinavica* 2000;102:143–149.

34. Weinstock-Guttman B, Baier M, Park Y, et al. Low fat dietary intervention with omega-3 fatty acid supplementation in multiple sclerosis patients. *Prostaglandins, Leukotrienes and Essential Fatty Acids* 2005;73: 397–404.

35. Gallai V, Sarchielli P, Trequattrini A, et al. Cytokine secretion and eicosanoid production in the peripheral blood mononuclear cells of MS patients undergoing dietary supplementation with n-3 polyunsaturated fatty acids. *Journal of Neuroimmunology* 1995;56:143–153.

36. Bates D, Cartlidge NE, French JM, et al. A double-blind controlled trial of long chain n-3 polyunsaturated fatty acids in the treatment of multiple sclerosis. *Journal of Neurology, Neurosurgery & Psychiatry* 1989; 52:18–22.

37. Dworkin RH, Bates D, Millar JH, Paty DW. Linoleic acid and multiple sclerosis: a reanalysis of three double-blind trials. *Neurology* 1984;34:1441–1445.

38. Bates D, Fawcett PR, Shaw DA, Weightman D. Polyunsaturated fatty acids in treatment of acute remitting multiple sclerosis. *British Medical Journal* 1978;2: 1390–1391.

39. Solomon AJ. Multiple sclerosis and vitamin D. *Neurology* 2011 Oct 25;77(17):e99–e100.

40. Munger KL, Levin LI, Hollis BW, et al. Serum 25-hydroxyvitamin D levels and risk of multiple sclerosis. *JAMA, The Journal of the American Medical Association* 2006;296: 2832–2838.

41. Munger KL, Zhang SM, O'Reilly E, et al. Vitamin D intake and incidence of multiple sclerosis. *Neurology* 2004;62: 60–65.

42. Hiremath GS, Cettomai D, Baynes M, et al. Vitamin D status and effect of low-dose cholecalciferol and high-dose ergocalciferol supplementation in multiple sclerosis. *Multiple Sclerosis* 2009;15:735–740.

43. Lemire JM, Archer DC. 1,25-dihydroxyvitamin D3 prevents the in vivo induction of murine experimental autoimmune encephalomyelitis. *Journal of Clinical Investigation* 1991;87:1103–1107.

44. Cantorna MT, Humpal-Winter J, DeLuca HF. Dietary calcium is a major factor in 1,25-dihydroxycholecalciferol suppression of experimental autoimmune encephalomyelitis in mice. *Journal of Nutrition* 1999; 129:1966–1971.

45. Nashold FE, Miller DJ, Hayes CE. 1,25-dihydroxyvitamin D3 treatment decreases macrophage accumulation in the CNS of mice with experimental autoimmune encephalomyelitis. *Journal of Neuroimmunology* 2000;103: 171–179.

46. Kragt J, van Amerongen B, Killestein J, et al. Higher levels of 25-hydroxyvitamin D are associated with a lower incidence of multiple sclerosis only in women. *Multiple Sclerosis* 2009;15:9–15.

47. Smolders J, Thewissen M, Peelen E, et al. Vitamin D status is positively correlated with regulatory T cell function in patients with multiple sclerosis. *PLoS One* 2009;4:e6635.

48. Packer L, Roy S, Sen CK. Alpha-lipoic acid: a metabolic antioxidant and potential redox modulator of transcription. *Advances in Pharmacology* 1997; 38:79–101.

49. Moini H, Packer L, Saris NE. Antioxidant and prooxidant activities of alpha-lipoic acid and dihydrolipoic acid. *Toxicology and Applied Pharmacology* 2002;182:84–90.

50. Hagen TM, Liu J, Lykkesfeldt J, et al. Feeding acetyl-L-carnitine and lipoic acid to old rats significantly improves metabolic function while decreasing oxidative stress. *Proceedings of the National Academy of Sciences of the United States of America* 2002;99:1870–1875.

51. Marracci GH, Jones RE, McKeon GP, Bourdette DN. Alpha lipoic acid inhibits T cell migration into the spinal cord and suppresses and treats experimental autoimmune encephalomyelitis. *Journal of Neuroimmunology* 2002;131: 104–114.

52. Morini M, Roccatagliata L, Dell'Eva R, et al. α-lipoic acid is effective in prevention and treatment of experimental autoimmune encephalomyelitis. *Journal of Neuroimmunology* 2004;148:146–153.

53. Schriebelt G, Musters RJ, Reijerkerk A, et al. Lipoic acid affects cellular migration into the central nervous system and stabilizes blood-brain barrier integrity. *The Journal of Immunology* 2006;177:2630–2637.

54. Marracci GH, McKeon GP, Marquardt WE, et al. α-lipoic acid inhibits human T-cell migration: implications for multiple sclerosis. *Journal of Neuroscience Research* 2004;78:362–370.

55. Yadav V, Marracci G, Lover J, et al. Lipoic acid in multiple sclerosis: a pilot study. *Multiple Sclerosis* 2005;11:159–165.

56. Ransberger K, van Schaik W. Enzyme therapy in multiple sclerosis. *Der Kassenarzt* 1986; 41:42–45.

57. Amato MP, Ponziani G, Siracusa G, et al. Cognitive dysfunction in early-onset multiple sclerosis: a reappraisal after 10 years. *Archives of Neurology* 2001;58:1602–1606.

58. Lovera J, Bagert B, Smoot K, et al. *Ginkgo biloba* for the improvement of cognitive performance in multiple sclerosis: a randomized, placebo-controlled trial. *Multiple Sclerosis* 2007;13: 376–385.

59. Snook EM, Motl RW. Effect of exercise training on walking mobility in multiple sclerosis: a meta-analysis. *Neurohabilita-*

tion & Neural Repair 2009; 23(2):108–116.

60. Motl RW, Gosney JL. Effect of exercise training on quality of life in multiple sclerosis: a meta-analysis. Multiple Sclerosis 2008;14(1):129–135.

61. Sutherland G, Andersen MB. Exercise and multiple sclerosis: physiological, psychological, and quality of life issues. The Journal of Sports Medicine and Physical Fitness 2001;41:421–432.

62. Mostert S, Kesselring J. Effects of a short-term exercise training program on aerobic fitness, fatigue, health perception and activity level of subjects with multiple sclerosis. Multiple Sclerosis 2002;8:161–168.

63. Oken BS, Kishiyama S, Zajdel D, et al. Randomized controlled trial of yoga and exercise in multiple sclerosis. Neurology 2004;62(11):2058–2064.

64. Mills N, Allen J. Mindfulness of movement as a coping strategy in multiple sclerosis. A pilot study. General Hospital Psychiatry 2000;22:425–431.

65. Husted C, Pham L, Hekking A, Niederman R. Improving quality of life for people with chronic conditions: the example of t'ai chi and multiple sclerosis. Alternative Therapies in Health and Medicine 1999;5: 70–74.

66. Gehlsen GM, Grigsby SA, Winant DM. Effects of an aquatic fitness program on the muscular strength and endurance of patients with multiple sclerosis. Physical Therapy 1984;64: 653–657.

67. Mohr, DC. Stress and multiple sclerosis. Journal of Neurology 2007; 254 suppl 2: II65–II68.

68. Mohr DC, Goodkin DE, Bacchetti P, et al. Psychological stress and the subsequent appearance of new brain MRI lesions in MS. Neurology 2000; 55:55–61.

69. Fischler BH, Marks M, Reich T.

Hyperbaric-oxygen treatment of multiple sclerosis. The New England Journal of Medicine 1983; 308:181–186.

70. Kleijnen J, Knipschild P. Hyperbaric oxygen for multiple sclerosis: review of controlled trials. Acta Neurologica Scandinavica 1995;91:330–334.

71. Bennett M, Heard R. Hyperbaric oxygen therapy for multiple sclerosis. CNS Neuroscience & Therapeutics 2010 Apr;16(2): 115–124.

Nonalcoholic Fatty Liver Disease (NAFLD)/ Nonalcoholic Steatohepatitis (NASH)

1. Marchesini G, Brizi M, Morselli-Labate AM, et al. Association of nonalcoholic fatty liver disease with insulin resistance. The American Journal of Medicine 1999;107:450–455.

2. Comert B, Mas MR, Erdem H, et al. Insulin resistance in nonalcoholic steatohepatitis. Digestive and Liver Disease 2001;33: 353–358.

3. Sanyal AJ, Campbell-Sargent C, Mirshahi F, et al. Nonalcoholic steatohepatitis: association of insulin resistance and mitochondrial abnormalities. Gastroenterology 2001;120:1183–1192.

4. Tilg H, Moschen A. Weight loss: cornerstone in the treatment of non-alcoholic fatty liver disease. Minerva Gastroenterologica e Dietologica 2010 Jun;56(2):159–167.

5. Assy N, Nasser G, Kamayse I, et al. Soft drink consumption linked with fatty liver in the absence of traditional risk factors. Canadian Journal of Gastroenterology 2008 Oct;22(10): 811–816.

6. Younossi ZM, Gramlich T, Bacon BR, et al. Hepatic iron and nonalcoholic fatty liver disease. Hepatology 1999;30:847–850.

7. Bonkovsky HL, Jawaid Q, Tortorelli K, et al. Non-alcoholic

steatohepatitis and iron: increased prevalence of mutations of the HFE gene in non-alcoholic steatohepatitis. Journal of Hepatology 1999;31:421–429.

8. MacDonald GA, Ward PJ, George DK, Powell LW. Iron and fibrosis in nonalcoholic fatty liver disease. Hepatology 2000; 31:549–550.

9. Chang CY, Argo CK, Al-Osaimi AM, Caldwell SH. Therapy of NAFLD: antioxidants and cytoprotective agents. Journal of Clinical Gastroenterologyogy 2006 Mar;40 suppl 1:S51–S60.

10. Noto R, Maugeri A, Grasso R, et al. Free fatty acids and carnitine in patients with liver disease. Current Therapeutic Research 1986;40:35–39.

11. Sachan DS, Rhew TH, Ruark RA. Ameliorating effects of carnitine and its precursors on alcohol-induced fatty liver. The American Journal of Clinical Nutrition 1984;39:738–744.

12. Lim CY, Jun DW, Jang SS, et al. Effects of carnitine on peripheral blood mitochondrial DNA copy number and liver function in non-alcoholic fatty liver disease. The Korean Journal of Gastroenterology 2010 Jun; 55(6):384–389.

13. Ratziu V, de Ledinghen V, Oberti F, et al. A randomized controlled trial of high-dose ursodesoxycholic acid for nonalcoholic steatohepatitis. Journal of Hepatology 2011 May;54(5): 1011–1019.

Osteoarthritis

1. Lawrence RC, Helmick CG, Arnett FC, et al. Estimates of the prevalence of arthritis and selected musculoskeletal disorders in the United States. Arthritis & Rheumatism 1998;41:778–799.

2. Zhang Y, Jordan JM. Epidemiology of osteoarthritis. Clinics in Geriatric Medicine 2010 Aug; 26(3):355–369.

3. Grotle M, Hagen KB, Natvig B, et al. Obesity and osteoarthri-

tis in knee, hip and/or hand: an epidemiological study in the general population with 10 years follow-up. *BMC Musculoskeletal Disorders* 2008 Oct 2;9:132.

4. Hinton R, Moody RL, Davis AW, et al. Osteoarthritis: diagnosis and therapeutic considerations. *American Family Physician* 2002;65:841–848.

5. Summers MN, Haley WE, Reveille JD, et al. Radiographic assessment and psychologic variables as predictors of pain and functional impairment in osteoarthritis of the knee or hip. *Arthritis & Rheumatism* 1988; 31:204–209.

6. Heinegård D, Saxne T. The role of the cartilage matrix in osteoarthritis. *Nature Reviews Rheumatology* 2011 Jan;7(1):50–57.

7. Bland JH, Cooper SM. Osteoarthritis: a review of the cell biology involved and evidence for reversibility. Management rationally related to known genesis and pathophysiology. *Seminars in Arthritis and Rheumatism* 1984;14:106–133.

8. Perry GH, Smith MJ, Whiteside CG. Spontaneous recovery of the hip joint space in degenerative hip disease. *Annals of the Rheumatic Diseases* 1972;31: 440–448.

9. Shield MJ. Anti-inflammatory drugs and their effects on cartilage synthesis and renal function. *European Journal of Rheumatology and Inflammation* 1993;13:7–16.

10. Brooks PM, Potter SR, Buchanan WW. NSAID and osteoarthritis—help or hindrance? *The Journal of Rheumatology* 1982;9:3–5.

11. Newman NM, Ling RS. Acetabular bone destruction related to non-steroidal anti-inflammatory drugs. *The Lancet* 1985;2:11–13.

12. Solomon L. Drug induced arthropathy and necrosis of the femoral head. *Journal of Bone and Joint Surgery* 1973;55:246–261.

13. Ronningen H, Langeland N. Indomethacin treatment in osteoarthritis of the hip joint. *Acta Orthopaedica* 1979;50:169–174.

14. Katz JD, Agrawal S, Velasquez M. Getting to the heart of the matter: osteoarthritis takes its place as part of the metabolic syndrome. *Current Opinion in Rheumatology* 2010 Sep;22(5): 512–519.

15. Huang MH, Chen CH, Chen TW, et al. The effects of weight reduction on the rehabilitation of patients with knee osteoarthritis and obesity. *Arthritis Care & Research* 2000;13: 398–405.

16. Messier SP, Loeser RF, Miller GD, et al. Exercise and dietary weight loss in overweight and obese older adults with knee osteoarthritis: the Arthritis, Diet, and Activity Promotion Trial. *Arthritis & Rheumatism* 2004; 50:1501–1510.

17. Sköldstam L, Hagfors L, Johansson G. An experimental study of a Mediterranean diet intervention for patients with rheumatoid arthritis, *Annals of the Rheumatic Diseases* 2003; 62:208–214.

18. McKellar G, Morrison E, McEntegart A, et al. A pilot study of a Mediterranean-type diet intervention in female patients with rheumatoid arthritis living in areas of social deprivation in Glasgow. *Annals of the Rheumatic Diseases* 2007;66: 1239–1243.

19. Childers NF, Russo GM. *The nightshades and health.* Somerville, N.J.: Horticulture Publications, Somerset Press, 1977.

20. Crolle G, D'Este E. Glucosamine sulfate for the management of arthrosis: a controlled clinical investigation. *Current Medical Research & Opinion* 1980;7:104–109.

21. Pujalte JM, Llavore EP, Ylescupidez FR. Double-blind clinical evaluation of oral glucosamine sulphate in the basic treatment of osteoarthrosis. *Current Medi-*

ical Research & Opinion 1980;7: 110–114.

22. Drovanti A, Bignamini AA, Rovati AL. Therapeutic activity of oral glucosamine sulfate in osteoarthrosis: a placebo-controlled double-blind investigation. *Clinical Therapeutics* 1980;3:260–272.

23. D'Ambrosia E, Casa B, Bompani R, et al. Glucosamine sulphate: a controlled clinical investigation in arthrosis. *Pharmatherapeutica* 1982;2:504–508.

24. Braham R, Dawson B, Goodman C. The effect of glucosamine supplementation on people experiencing regular knee pain. *British Journal of Sports Medicine* 2003;37:45–49.

25. Christgau S, Henrotin Y, Tanko LB, et al. Osteoarthritic patients with high cartilage turnover show increased responsiveness to the cartilage protecting effects of glucosamine sulphate. *Clinical and Experimental Rheumatology* 2004;22:36–42.

26. Reginster JY, Deroisy R, Rovati LC, et al. Long-term effects of glucosamine sulphate on osteoarthritis progression: a randomised, placebo-controlled clinical trial. *The Lancet* 2001; 357:251–256.

27. Pavelka K, Gatterova J, Olejarova M, et al. Glucosamine sulfate use and delay of progression of knee osteoarthritis: a 3-year, randomized, placebo-controlled, double-blind study. *Archives of Internal Medicine* 2002;162:2113–2123.

28. Bruyere O, Honore A, Ethgen O, et al. Correlation between radiographic severity of knee osteoarthritis and future disease progression. Results from a 3-year prospective, placebo-controlled study evaluating the effect of glucosamine sulfate. *Osteoarthritis and Cartilage* 2003;1:1–5.

29. Bruyere O, Pavelka K, Rovati LC, et al. Glucosamine sulfate

reduces osteoarthritis progression in postmenopausal women with knee osteoarthritis: evidence from two 3-year studies. *Menopause* 2004 Mar-Apr; 11(2):138–43.

30. Bruyere O, Pavelka K, Rovati LC, et al. Total joint replacement after glucosamine sulphate treatment in knee osteoarthritis: results of a mean 8-year observation of patients from two previous 3-year, randomised, placebo-controlled trials. *Osteoarthritis and Cartilage* 2008 Feb;16(2):254–60.

31. Lopes Vaz A. Double-blind clinical evaluation of the relative efficacy of ibuprofen and glucosamine sulfate in the management of osteoarthrosis of the knee in out-patients. *Current Medical Research & Opinion* 1982;8:145–149.

32. Muller-Fassbender H, Bach GL, Haase W, et al. Glucosamine sulfate compared to ibuprofen in osteoarthritis of the knee. *Osteoarthritis and Cartilage* 1994;2:61–69.

33. Rovati LC, Giacovelli G, Annefeld M, et al. A large, randomized, placebo controlled, double-blind study of glucosamine sulfate vs piroxicam and vs their association, on the kinetics of the symptomatic effect in knee osteoarthritis. *Osteoarthritis and Cartilage* 1994;2 suppl 1:56.

34. Qiu GX, Gao SN, Giacovelli G, et al. Efficacy and safety of glucosamine sulfate versus ibuprofen in patients with knee osteoarthritis. *Arzneimittelforschung* 1998;48:469–474.

35. Thie NM, Prasad NG, Major PW. Evaluation of glucosamine sulfate compared to ibuprofen for the treatment of temporomandibular joint osteoarthritis: a randomized double blind controlled 3 month clinical trial. *The Journal of Rheumatology* 2001;28:1347–1355.

36. Herrero-Beaumont G, Ivorra JA, Del Carmen Trabado M, et al. Glucosamine sulfate in the treatment of knee osteoarthritis symptoms: a randomized, double-blind, placebo-controlled study using acetaminophen as a side comparator. *Arthritis & Rheumatism* 2007 Feb;56(2):555–567.

37. Petersen SG, Saxne T, Heinegard D, et al. Glucosamine but not ibuprofen alters cartilage turnover in osteoarthritis patients in response to physical training. *Osteoarthritis and Cartilage* 2010 Jan;18(1):34–40.

38. Hughes R, Carr A. A randomized, double-blind, placebo-controlled trial of glucosamine sulphate as an analgesic in osteoarthritis of the knee. *Rheumatology* 2002;41:279–284.

39. Rindone JP, Hiller D, Collacott E, et al. Randomized, controlled trial of glucosamine for treating osteoarthritis of the knee. *Western Journal of Medicine* 2000;172:91–94.

40. Rozendaal RM, Koes BW, van Osch GJ, et al. Effect of glucosamine sulfate on hip osteoarthritis: a randomized trial. *Annals of Internal Medicine* 2008 Feb 19;148(4):268–277.

41. Cibere J, Thorne A, Kopec JA, et al. Glucosamine sulfate and cartilage type II collagen degradation in patients with knee osteoarthritis: randomized discontinuation trial results employing biomarkers. *The Journal of Rheumatology* 2005 May; 32(5):896–902.

42. Tapadinhas MJ, Rivera IC, Bignamini AA. Oral glucosamine sulfate in the management of arthrosis: report on a multi-centre open investigation in Portugal. *Pharmatherapeutica* 1982;3:157–168.

43. Yoshimura M, Sakamoto K, Tsuruta A, et al. Evaluation of the effect of glucosamine administration on biomarkers for cartilage and bone metabolism in soccer players. *International Journal of Molecular Medicine* 2009 Oct;24(4):487–494.

44. Ostojic SM, Arsic M, Prodanovic S, Vukovic J, Zlatanovic M. Glucosamine administration in athletes: effects on recovery of acute knee injury. *Research in Sports Medicine* 2007 Apr–Jun; 15(2):113–124.

45. Sawitzke AD, Shi H, Finco MF, et al. The effect of glucosamine and/or chondroitin sulfate on the progression of knee osteoarthritis: a report from the glucosamine/chondroitin arthritis intervention trial. *Arthritis & Rheumatism* 2008 Oct;58(10): 3183–3191.

46. Sawitzke AD, Shi H, Finco MF, et al. Clinical efficacy and safety of glucosamine, chondroitin sulphate, their combination, celecoxib or placebo taken to treat osteoarthritis of the knee: 2-year results from GAIT. *Annals of the Rheumatic Diseases* 2010 Aug;69(8):1459–1464.

47. Monauni T, Zenti MG, Cretti A, et al. Effects of glucosamine infusion on insulin secretion and insulin action in humans. *Diabetes* 2000;49:926–935.

48. Scroggie DA, Albright A, Harris MD. The effect of glucosamine-chondroitin supplementation on glycosylated hemoglobin levels in patients with type 2 diabetes mellitus: a placebo-controlled, double-blinded, randomized clinical trial. *Archives of Internal Medicine* 2003;163:1587–1590.

49. Tannis AJ, Barban J, Conquer JA. Effect of glucosamine supplementation on fasting and non-fasting plasma glucose and serum insulin concentrations in healthy individuals. *Osteoarthritis and Cartilage* 2004 Jun; 12(6):506–11.

50. Simon RR, Marks V, Leeds AR, Anderson JW. A comprehensive review of oral glucosamine use and effects on glucose metabolism in normal and diabetic individuals. *Diabetes/Metabolism Research and Reviews* 2011 Jan; 27(1):14–22.

51. Knudsen JF, Sokol GH. Potential glucosamine-warfarin in-

teraction resulting in increased international normalized ratio: case report and review of the literature and MedWatch database. *Pharmacotherapy* 2008 Apr;28(4):540–548.

52. Baici A, Horler D, Moser B, et al. Analysis of glycosaminoglycans in human sera after oral administration of chondroitin sulfate. *Rheumatology International* 1992;12:81–88.

53. Conte A, Volpi N, Palmieri L, et al. Biochemical and pharmacokinetic aspects of oral treatment with chondroitin sulfate. *Arzneimittelforschung* 1995;45: 918–925.

54. Volpi N, Oral bioavailability of chondroitin sulfate (Condrosulf) and its constituents in healthy male volunteers. *Osteoarthritis and Cartilage* 2002;10:768–777.

55. Shinmei M, Kobayashi T, et al. Significance of the levels of carboxy terminal type II procollagen peptide, chondroitin sulfate isomers, tissue inhibitor of metalloproteinases, and metalloproteinases in osteoarthritis joint fluid. *The Journal of Rheumatology* 1995;43 suppl:78–81.

56. Conte A, de Bernardi M, Palmieri L, et al. Metabolic fate of exogenous chondroitin sulfate in man. *Arzneimittelforschung* 1991;41:768–772.

57. Baici A, Wagenhauser FJ. Bioavailability of oral chondroitin sulfate. *Rheumatology International* 1993;13:41–43.

58. Uebelhart D, Malaise M, Marcolongo R, et al. Intermittent treatment of knee osteoarthritis with oral chondroitin sulfate: a one-year, randomized, double-blind, multicenter study versus placebo. *Osteoarthritis and Cartilage* 2004;12:269–276.

59. Pipitone VR. Chondroprotection with chondroitin sulfate. *Drugs Under Experimental and Clinical Research* 1991;18:3–7.

60. L'Hirondel JL. [Double-blind clinical study with oral administration of chondroitin sulfate versus placebo in tibiofemoral gonarthrosis.] *Litera Rheumatologica* 1992;14:77–82.

61. Conrozier T, Vignon E. [The effect of chondroitin sulfate treatment in coxarthritis. A double-blind placebo study.] *Litera Rheumatologica* 1992;14:69–75.

62. Morreale P, Manopulo R, Galati M, et al. Comparision of the anti-inflammatory efficacy of chondroitinsulfate and diclofenac sodium in patients with knee osteoarthritis. *The Journal of Rheumatology* 1996; 23:1385–1391.

63. Mazières B, Hucher M, Zaïm M, Garnero P. Effect of chondroitin sulphate in symptomatic knee osteoarthritis: a multicentre, randomised, double-blind, placebo-controlled study. *Annals of the Rheumatic Diseases* 2007 May;66(5):639–645.

64. Kahan A, Uebelhart D, De Vathaire F, et al. Long-term effects of chondroitins 4 and 6 sulfate on knee osteoarthritis: the study on osteoarthritis progression prevention, a two-year, randomized, double-blind, placebo-controlled trial. *Arthritis & Rheumatism* 2009 Feb;60(2): 524–533.

65. Bellamy N, Campbell J, Robinson V, et al. Viscosupplementation for the treatment of osteoarthritis of the knee. Cochrane Database of Systematic Reviews 2006 Apr 19;2: CD005321.

66. Kalman DS, Heimer M, Valdeon A, et al. Effect of a natural extract of chicken combs with a high content of hyaluronic acid (Hyal-Joint) on pain relief and quality of life in subjects with knee osteoarthritis: a pilot randomized double-blind placebo-controlled trial. *Nutrition Journal* 2008 Jan 21;7:3.

67. Sato T, Iwaso H. An effectiveness study of hyaluronic acid (Hyabest® J) in the treatment of osteoarthritis of the knee on the patients in the United States. *Journal of New Remedies and Clinics* 2008;57(2):128–137

68. Kaufman W. *The common form of joint dysfunction: its incidence and treatment.* Brattleboro, Vt.: E. L. Hildreth, 1949.

69. Hoffer A. Treatment of arthritis by nicotinic acid and nicotinamide. *Canadian Medical Association Journal* 1959;81: 235–238.

70. Jonas WB, Rapoza CP, Blair WF. The effect of niacinamide on osteoarthritis: a pilot study. *Inflammation Research* 1996; 45:330–334.

71. Soeken KL, Lee WL, Bausell RB, et al. Safety and efficacy of S-adenosylmethionine (SAMe) for osteoarthritis. *The Journal of Family Practice* 2002;51: 425–430.

72. Harmand MF, Vilamitjana J, Maloche E, et al. Effects of S-adenosylmethionine on human articular chondrocyte differentiation: an in vitro study. *The American Journal of Medicine* 1987;83:48–54.

73. Konig H, Stahl H, Sieper J, et al. [Magnetic resonance tomography of finger polyarthritis: morphology and cartilage signals after ademetionine therapy.] *Aktuelle Radiologie* 1995; 5:36–40.

74. Muller-Fassbender H. Double-blind clinical trial of S-adenosylmethionine versus ibuprofen in the treatment of osteoarthritis. *The American Journal of Medicine* 1987;83:81–83.

75. Glorioso S, Todesco S, Mazzi A, et al. Double-blind multicentre study of the activity of S-adenosylmethionine in hip and knee osteoarthritis. *International Journal of Clinical Pharmacology Research* 1985;5:39–49.

76. Domljan Z, Vrhovac B, Durrigl T, et al. A double-blind trial of ademetionine vs naproxen in activated gonarthrosis. *International Journal of Clinical Pharmacology, Therapy and Toxicology* 1989;27:329–333.

77. Caruso I, Pietrogrande V. Italian double-blind multicenter study comparing S-adenosylme-

thionine, naproxen, and placebo in the treatment of degenerative joint disease. *The American Journal of Medicine* 1987;83:66–71.

78. Vetter G. Double-blind comparative clinical trial with S-adenosylmethionine and indomethacin in the treatment of osteoarthritis. *The American Journal of Medicine* 1987;83:78–80.

79. Maccagno A, DiGiorgio EE, Caston OL, et al. Double-blind controlled clinical trial of oral S-adenosylmethionine versus piroxicam in knee osteoarthritis. *The American Journal of Medicine* 1987;83:72–77.

80. Konig B. A long-term (two years) clinical trial with S-adenosylmethionine for the treatment of osteoarthritis. *The American Journal of Medicine* 1987;83:89–94.

81. Berger R, Nowak H. A new medical approach to the treatment of osteoarthritis. Report of an open phase IV study with ademetionine (Gumbaral). *The American Journal of Medicine* 1987;83:84–88.

82. Lund-Olesen K, Menander KB. Orgotein: a new anti-inflammatory metalloprotein drug. Preliminary evaluation of clinical efficacy and safety in degenerative joint disease. *Current Therapeutic Research Clin Exp* 1974;16:706–717.

83. McAlindon TE, Jacques P, Zhang Y, et al. Do antioxidant micronutrients protect against the development and progression of knee osteoarthritis? *Arthritis & Rheumatism* 1996;39:648–656.

84. Schwartz ER. The modulation of osteoarthritic development by vitamins C and E. *International Journal for Vitamin and Nutrition Research* 1984 suppl;26:141–146.

85. Bates CJ. Proline and hydroxyproline excretion and vitamin C status in elderly human subjects. *Clinical Science & Molecular Medicine* 1977;52:535–543.

86. Prins AP, Lipman JM, McDevitt CA, et al. Effect of purified growth factors on rabbit articular chondrocytes in monolayer culture. II. Sulfated proteoglycan synthesis. *Arthritis & Rheumatism* 1982;25:1228–1238.

87. Krystal G, Morris GM, Sokoloff L. Stimulation of DNA synthesis by ascorbate in cultures of articular chondrocytes. *Arthritis & Rheumatism* 1982;25:318–325.

88. Peregoy J, Wilder FV. The effects of vitamin C supplementation on incident and progressive knee osteoarthritis: a longitudinal study. *Public Health Nutrition* 2011 Apr;14(4):709–715.

89. McAlindon TE, Felson DT, Zhang Y, et al. Relation of dietary intake and serum levels of vitamin D to progression of osteoarthritis of the knees among participants in the Framingham Study. *Annals of Internal Medicine* 1996;125:353–359.

90. Heidari B, Heidari P, Hajian-Tilaki K. Association between serum vitamin D deficiency and knee osteoarthritis. *International Orthopaedics* 2011 Nov;35(11):1627–1631.

91. Nawabi DH, Chin KF, Keen RW, Haddad FS. Vitamin D deficiency in patients with osteoarthritis undergoing total hip replacement: a cause for concern? *Journal of Bone and Joint Surgery, British Volume* 2010 Apr;92(4):496–499.

92. Travers RL, Rennie GC, Newnham RE. Boron and arthritis. The results of a double-blind pilot study. *Journal of Nutritional and Environmental Medicine* 1990;1:127–132.

93. Newnham RE. Arthritis or skeletal fluorosis and boron. *Int Clinical Nutrition Reviews* 1991;11:68–70.

94. Oka H, Akune T, Muraki S, et al. Association of low dietary vitamin K intake with radiographic knee osteoarthritis in the Japanese elderly population: dietary survey in a population-based cohort of the ROAD study. *Journal of Orthopaedic Science* 2009 Nov;14(6):687–692.

95. Neogi T, Booth SL, Zhang YQ, et al. Low vitamin K status is associated with osteoarthritis in the hand and knee. *Arthritis & Rheumatism* 2006 Apr;54(4):1255–1261.

96. Jurenka JS. Anti-inflammatory properties of curcumin, a major constituent of *Curcuma longa:* a review of preclinical and clinical research. *Alternative Medicine Review* 2009 Jun;14(2):141–153.

97. Marczylo TH, Verschoyle RD, Cooke DN, et al. Comparison of systemic availability of curcumin with that of curcumin formulated with phosphatidylcholine. *Cancer Chemotherapy and Pharmacology* 2007 Jul;60(2):171–177.

98. Sasaki H, Sunagawa Y, Takahashi K, et al. Innovative preparation of curcumin for improved oral bioavailability. *Biological and Pharmaceutical Bulletin* 2011;34(5):660–665.

99. Belcaro G, Cesarone MR, Dugall M, et al. Product-evaluation registry of Meriva®, a curcumin-phosphatidylcholine complex, for the complementary management of osteoarthritis. *Panminerva Medica* 2010 Jun;52(2 suppl 1):55–62.

100. Appendino G, Belcaro G, Cesarone MR, et al. Efficacy and safety of Meriva, a curcumin-phosphatidylcholine complex, during extended administration in osteoarthritis patients. *Alternative Medicine Review* 2010 Dec;15(4):337–344.

101. Singh GB, Atal CK. Pharmacology of an extract of salai guggal ex-*Bosewellia serrata*, a new non-steroidal anti-inflammatory agent. *Agents & Actions* 1986;18:407–412.

102. Reddy GK, Chandrakasan G, Dhar SC. Studies on the metabolism of glycosaminoglycans under the influence of new herbal anti-inflammatory

agents. *Biochemical Pharmacology* 1989;38:3527–3534.

103. Kulkani RR, Patki PS, Jog VP, et al. Treatment of osteoarthritis with a herbomineral formulation: a double-blind, placebo-controlled, cross-over study. *Journal of Ethnopharmacology* 1991;33:91–95.

104. Sengupta K, Alluri KV, Satish AR, et al. A double blind, randomized, placebo controlled study of the efficacy and safety of 5-Loxin for treatment of osteoarthritis of the knee. *Arthritis Research & Therapy* 2008; 10(4):R85.

105. Sengupta K, Krishnaraju AV, Vishal AA, et al. Comparative efficacy and tolerability of 5-Loxin and Aflapin against osteoarthritis of the knee: a double blind, randomized, placebo controlled clinical study. *International Journal of Medical Sciences* 2010 Nov 1;7(6): 366–377.

106. Kimmatkar N, Thawani V, Hingorani L, Khiyani R. Efficacy and tolerability of *Boswellia serrata* extract in treatment of osteoarthritis of knee—a randomized double blind placebo controlled trial. *Phytomedicine* 2003 Jan;10(1):3–7.

107. Belcaro G, Cesarone MR, Errichi S, et al. Treatment of osteoarthritis with Pycnogenol. The SVOS (San Valentino Osteoarthrosis Study): evaluation of signs, symptoms, physical performance and vascular aspects. *Phytotherapy Research* 2008 Apr;22(4):518–523.

108. Cisár P, Jány R, Waczulíková I, et al. Effect of pine bark extract (Pycnogenol) on symptoms of knee osteoarthritis. *Phytotherapy Research* 2008 Aug;22(8): 1087–1092.

109. Altman RD, Marcussen KC. Effects of a ginger extract on knee pain in patients with osteoarthritis. *Arthritis & Rheumatism* 2001;44:2531–2538.

110. Bliddal H, Rosetzsky A, Schlichting P, et al. A randomized, placebo-controlled, cross-over study of ginger extracts and ibuprofen in osteoarthritis. *Osteoarthritis and Cartilage* 2000; 8:9–12.

111. Gagnier JJ, Chrubasik S, Manheimer E. *Harpagophytum procumbens* for osteoarthritis and low back pain: a systematic review. *BMC Complementary and Alternative Medicine* 2004; 4:13–23.

112. Lecomte A, Costa JP. [Harpagophytum and osteoarthritis: a double-blind placebo-controlled trial.] *Le Magazine* 1992;15:27–30.

113. Chantre P, Cappelaere A, Leblan D, et al. Efficacy and tolerance of Harpagophytum procumbens versus diacerhein in treatment of osteoarthritis. *Phytomedicine* 2000;7:177–183.

114. Vlachojannis J, Roufogalis BD, Chrubasik S. Systematic review on the safety of *Harpagophytum* preparations for osteoarthritic and low back pain. *Phytotherapy Research* 2008;22:149–152.

115. Hesslink R Jr, Armstrong D 3rd, Nagendran MV, et al. Cetylated fatty acids improve knee function in patients with osteoarthritis. *The Journal of Rheumatology* 2002;29(8):1708–1712.

116. Kraemer WJ, Ratamess NA, Anderson JM, et al. Effect of a cetylated fatty acid topical cream on functional mobility and quality of life of patients with osteoarthritis. *The Journal of Rheumatology* 2004;31(4): 767–774.

117. Kraemer WJ, Ratamess NA, Maresh CM, et al. Effects of treatment with a cetylated fatty acid topical cream on static postural stability and plantar pressure distribution in patients with knee osteoarthritis. *The Journal of Strength and Conditioning Research* 2005;19(1): 115–121.

118. Sharma L, Song J, Felson DT, et al. The role of knee alignment in disease progression and functional decline in knee osteoarthritis. *JAMA, The Journal of the American Medical Association* 2001;286:792.

119. Wright V. Treatment of osteoarthritis of the knees. *Annals of the Rheumatic Diseases* 1964; 23:389–391.

120. Clarke GR, Willis LA, Stenners L, et al. Evaluation of physiotherapy in the treatment of osteoarthrosis of the knee. *Rheumatology and Rehabilitation* 1974;13:190–197.

121. Vanharanta H. Effect of shortwave diathermy on mobility and radiological stage of the knee in the development of experimental osteoarthritis. *American Journal of Physical Medicine* 1982;61:59–65.

122. Falconer J, Hayes KW, Chang RW. Effect of ultrasound on mobility in osteoarthritis of the knee. A randomized clinical trial. *Arthritis Care & Research* 1992;5:29–35.

123. Stelian J, Gil I, Habot B, et al. Improvement of pain and disability in elderly patients with degenerative osteoarthritis of the knee treated with narrowband light therapy. *Journal of the American Geriatrics Society* 1992;40:23–26.

124. Fisher NM, Pendergast DR, Gresham GE. Muscle rehabilitation: its effects on muscular and functional performance of patients with knee osteoarthritis. *Archives of Physical Medicine and Rehabilitation* 1991;72: 367–374.

125. Kovar PA, Allegrante JP, MacKenzie CR, et al. Supervised fitness walking in patients with osteoarthritis of the knee. A randomized controlled trial. *Annals of Internal Medicine* 1992; 116:529–534.

126. Zelazny CM. Therapeutic instrumental music playing in hand rehabilitation for older adults with osteoarthritis: four case studies. *Journal of Music Therapy* 2001;38:97–113.

127. Vas J, Perea-Milla E, Mendez C.

Acupuncture and moxibustion as an adjunctive treatment for osteoarthritis of the knee—a large case series. *Acupuncture in Medicine* 2004;22:23–28.

128. Tukmachi E, Jubb R, Dempsey E, et al. The effect of acupuncture on the symptoms of knee osteoarthritis—an open randomised controlled study. *Acupuncture in Medicine* 2004; 22:14–22.

129. Ng MM, Leung MC, Poon DM. The effects of electro-acupuncture and transcutaneous electrical nerve stimulation on patients with painful osteoarthritic knees: a randomized controlled trial with follow-up evaluation. *The Journal of Alternative and Complementary Medicine* 2003;9:641–649.

130. Sangdee C, Teekachunhatean S, Sananpanich K. Electroacupuncture versus diclofenac in symptomatic treatment of osteoarthritis of the knee: a randomized controlled trial. *BMC Complementary and Alternative Medicine* 2002;2:3.

131. Panagos A, Jensen M, Cardenas DD. Treatment of myofascial shoulder pain in the spinal cord injured population using static magnetic fields: a case series. *The Journal of Spinal Cord Medicine* 2004;27:138–142.

132. Pipitone N, Scott DL. Magnetic pulse treatment for knee osteoarthritis: a randomised, double-blind, placebo-controlled study. *Current Medical Research & Opinion* 2001;17:190–196.

133. Wolsko PM, Eisenberg DM, Simon LS, et al. Double-blind placebo-controlled trial of static magnets for the treatment of osteoarthritis of the knee: results of a pilot study. *Alternative Therapies in Health and Medicine* 2004;10:36–43.

134. Jacobson JI, Gorman R, Yamanashi WS, et al. Low-amplitude, extremely low frequency magnetic fields for the treatment of osteoarthritic knees: a double-blind clinical study. *Alternative Therapies in Health and Medicine* 2001;7:54–64,66–69.

135. Nicolakis P, Kollmitzer J, Crevenna R, et al. Pulsed magnetic field therapy for osteoarthritis of the knee—a double-blind sham-controlled trial. *Wiener Klinische Wochenschrift* 2002; 114:678–684.

136. McCaffrey R, Freeman E. Effect of music on chronic osteoarthritis pain in older people. *Journal of Advanced Nursing* 2003;44:517–524.

Osteoporosis

1. Sweet MG, Sweet JM, Jeremiah MP, Galazka SS. Diagnosis and treatment of osteoporosis. *American Family Physician* 2009 Feb 1;79(3):193–200.

2. Kanis J. Assessment of fracture risk and its application to screening for postmenopausal osteoporosis: synopsis of a WHO report. WHO Study Group. *Osteoporosis International* 1994;4:368–381.

3. Looker A, Wahner H, Dunn W, et al. Updated data on proximal femur bone mineral levels of US adults. *Osteoporosis International* 1998;8:468–489.

4. Looker A, Orwoll E, Johnston C Jr, et al. Prevalence of low femoral bone density in older U.S. adults from NHANES. III. *Journal of Bone and Mineral Research* 1997;12:1761–1768.

5. Melton L, Thamer M, Ray N, et al. Fractures attributable to osteoporosis: report from the National Osteoporosis Foundation. *Journal of Bone and Mineral Research* 1997;12:16–23

6. Siris E, Chen Y, Abbott T, et al. Bone mineral density thresholds for pharmacological intervention to prevent fractures. *Archives of Internal Medicine* 2004;164:1108–1112.

7. Lindsay R, Silverman S, Cooper C, et al. Risk of new vertebral fracture in the year following a fracture. *JAMA, The Journal of the American Medical Association* 2001;285:320–323.

8. Klotzbuecher C, Ros P, Landsman P, et al. Patients with prior fractures have an increased risk of future fractures: a summary of the literature and statistical synthesis. *Journal of Bone and Mineral Research* 2000;15: 721–739.

9. Seeman E. Osteoporosis in men. *Baillière's Clinical Rheumatology* 1997 Aug;11(3):613–629.

10. Smith DM, Nance WE, Kang KW, et al. Genetic factors in determining bone mass. *Journal of Clinical Investigation* 1973; 52:2800–2808.

11. Slemenda CW, Christian JC, Williams CJ, et al. Genetic determinants of bone mass in adult women: a reevaluation of the twin model and the potential importance of gene interaction on heritability estimates. *Journal of Bone and Mineral Research* 1991;6:561–567.

12. Pocock NA, Eisman JA, Hopper JL, et al. Genetic determinants of bone mass in adults: a twin study. *Journal of Clinical Investigation* 1987;80:706–710.

13. Evans RA, Marel GM, Lancaster EK, et al. Bone mass is low in relatives of osteoporotic patients. *Annals of Internal Medicine* 1988;109:870–873.

14. Kanis J, De Laet C, Delmas P, et al. A meta-analysis of previous fracture and fracture risk. *Bone* 20045;35:375–382.

15. Bischoff-Ferrari HA, Giovannucci E, Willett WC, et al. Estimation of optimal serum concentrations of 25-hydroxyvitamin D for multiple health outcomes. *The American Journal of Clinical Nutrition* 2006;84: 18–26.

16. Nieves JW, Golden AL, Siris E, et al. Teenage and current calcium intake are related to bone mineral density of the hip and forearm in women aged 30–39 years. *American Journal of Epidemiology* 1995;141:342–351.

17. Feskanich D, Willett WC, Stampfer MJ, Colditz GA. Protein consumption and bone

fractures in women. *American Journal of Epidemiology* 1996; 143:472–479.

18. Slemenda CW, Hui SL, Longcope C, Johnston CC Jr. Cigarette smoking, obesity, and bone mass. *Journal of Bone and Mineral Research* 1989;4:737–741.

19. Krall EA, Dawson-Hughes B. Smoking and bone loss among postmenopausal women. *Journal of Bone and Mineral Research* 1991;6:331–338.

20. Seeman E, Melton LJ III, O'Fallon WM, Riggs BL. Risk factors for spinal osteoporosis in men. *The American Journal of Medicine* 1983;75:977–983.

21. Cummings S, Nevitt M, Browner W, et al. Risk factors for hip fracture in white women. Study of Osteoporotic Fractures Research Group. *The New England Journal of Medicine* 1995; 332:767–773.

22. Laitinen K, Valimaki M. Alcohol and bone. *Calcified Tissue International* 1991;49 suppl: S70–S73.

23. Rico H. Alcohol and bone disease. *Alcohol and Alcoholism* 1990;25:345–352.

24. Slemenda CW, Johnston CC. High intensity activities in young women: site specific bone mass effects among female figure skaters. *Bone and Mineral* 1993;20:125–132.

25. Donaldson CL, Hulley SB, Vogel JM, et al. Effect of prolonged bed rest on bone mineral. *Metabolism* 1970;19:1071–1084.

26. Lloyd T, Myers C, Buchanan JR, Demers LM. Collegiate women athletes with irregular menses during adolescence have decreased bone density. *Obstetrics & Gynecology* 1988;72: 639–642.

27. Kanis J. Bone density measurements and osteoporosis. *Journal of Internal Medicine* 1997;241: 173–175.

28. Chestnut CH III, Bell NH, Clark GS, et al. Hormone replacement therapy in postmenopausal women: urinary N-telopeptide of type I collagen monitors therapeutic effect and predicts response of bone mineral density. *The American Journal of Medicine* 1997;102: 29–37.

29. Schuit SC, van der Klift M, Weel AE, et al. Fracture incidence and association with bone mineral density in elderly men and women: the Rotterdam Study. *Bone* 2004;34(1): 195–202.

30. Robbins J, Aragaki AK, Kooperberg C, et al. Factors associated with 5-year risk of hip fracture in postmenopausal women. *JAMA, The Journal of the American Medical Association* 2007;298(20):2389–2398.

31. Sinaki M. Falls, fractures, and hip pads. *Current Osteoporosis Reports* 2004;2(4):131–137.

32. Wells G, Tugwell P, Shea B, et al, for the Osteoporosis Methodology Group and the Osteoporosis Research Advisory Group. Meta-analyses of therapies for postmenopausal osteoporosis. V. Meta-analysis of the efficacy of hormone replacement therapy in treating and preventing osteoporosis in postmenopausal women. *Endocrine Reviews* 2002;23:529–539.

33. Torgerson D, Bell-Syer S. Hormone replacement therapy and prevention of nonvertebral fractures: a meta-analysis of randomized trials. *JAMA, The Journal of the American Medical Association* 2001;285:2891–2897.

34. Black DM, Cummings SR, Karpf DB, et al. Randomised trial of effect of alendronate on risk of fracture in women with existing vertebral fractures. Fracture Intervention Trial Research Group. *The Lancet* 1996; 348(9041):1535–1541.

35. Stevenson M, Jones ML, De Nigris E, et al. A systematic review and economic evaluation of alendronate, etidronate, risedronate, raloxifene and teriparatide for the prevention and treatment of postmenopausal osteoporosis. *Health Technology Assessment* 2005;9(22):1–160.

36. Delmas P, Bjarnason N, Mitlak B, et al. Effects of raloxifene on bone mineral density, serum cholesterol concentrations and uterine endometrium in postmenopausal women. *The New England Journal of Medicine* 1997;337:1641–1647.

37. Ettinger B, Black D, Mitlack B, et al. Reduction of vertebral fracture risk in postmenopausal women with osteoporosis treated with raloxifene: results from a 3-year randomized clinical trial. Multiple Outcomes of Raloxifene Evaluation (MORE) investigators. *JAMA, The Journal of the American Medical Association* 1999;282:637–645.

38. Dempster D, Cosman F, Kurland E, et al. Effects of daily treatment with parathyroid hormone on bone microarchitecture and turnover in patients with osteoporosis: a paired biopsy study. *Journal of Bone and Mineral Research* 2001;16: 1846–1853.

39. Lindsay R, Nieves J, Formica C, et al. Randomised controlled study of effect of parathyroid hormone on vertebral-bone mass and fracture incidence among postmenopausal women on oestrogen with osteoporosis. *The Lancet* 1997;350:550–555.

40. Neer R, Arnaud C, Zanchetta J, et al. Effect of parathyroid hormone on fractures and bone mineral density in postmenopausal women with osteoporosis. *The New England Journal of Medicine* 2001;344:1434–1441.

41. Chestnut C, Silverman S, Andriano K, et al. A randomized trial of nasal spray salmon calcitonin in postmenopausal women with established osteoporosis: the Prevent Recurrence of Osteoporotic Fractures Study. PROOF Study Group. *The American Journal of Medicine* 2000;109: 267–276.

42. Slemenda C, Hui S, Long-

cope C, et al. Cigarette smoking, obesity, and bone mass. *Journal of Bone and Mineral Research* 1989;4:737–741.

43. Kato I, Toniolo P, Akhmedkhanov A, et al. Prospective study of factors influencing the onset of natural menopause. *Journal of Clinical Epidemiology* 1998; 51:1271–1276.

44. Krall E, Dawson-Hughes B. Smoking and bone loss among postmenopausal women. *Journal of Bone and Mineral Research* 1991;6:331–338.

45. Baron J, Farahmand B, Weiderpass E, et al. Cigarette smoking, alcohol consumption, and risk for hip fracture in women. *Archives of Internal Medicine* 2001;161:983–988

46. Law M, Hackshaw A. A meta-analysis of cigarette smoking, bone mineral density and risk of hip fracture: recognition of a major effect. *BMJ* 1997;315: 841–846.

47. Kanis J, Johnell O, Oden A, et al. Smoking and fracture risk: a meta-analysis. *Osteoporosis International* 2005;16:155–162.

48. Tucker K, Jugdaohsingh R, Powell J, et al. Effects of beer, wine, and liquor intakes on bone mineral density in older men and women. *The American Journal of Clinical Nutrition* 2009;89: 1188–1196.

49. Felson D, Zhang Y, Hannan M, et al. Alcohol intake and bone mineral density in elderly men and women: the Framingham Study. *American Journal of Epidemiology* 1995;142:485–492.

50. Felson D, Kiel D, Anderson J, Kannel W. Alcohol consumption and hip fractures: the Framingham Study. *American Journal of Epidemiology* 1988;128: 1102–1110.

51. Kanis J, Johansson H, Johnell O, et al. Alcohol intake as a risk factor for fracture. *Osteoporosis International* 2005;16:737–742.

52. Jaglar SB, Kreiger N, Darlington G. Past and recent physical activity and the risk of osteoporosis. *American Journal of Epidemiology* 1993;138:107–118.

53. Prior JC, Barr SI, Chow R, Faulkner RA. Prevention and management of osteoporosis: consensus statements from the Scientific Advisory Board of the Osteoporosis Society of Canada. 5. Physical activity as therapy for osteoporosis. *Canadian Medical Association Journal* 1996;155:940–944.

54. Marcus R, Drinkwater B, Dalsky G, et al. Osteoporosis and exercise in women. *Medicine & Science in Sports & Exercise* 1992;24 suppl 6:S301–S307.

55. Pocock NA, Eisman JA, Yeates MG, et al. Physical fitness is the major determinant of femoral neck and lumbar spine density. *Journal of Clinical Investigation* 1986;78:618–621.

56. Krolner B, Toft B, Pors Nielsen S, Tondevold E. Physical exercise as prophylaxis against involutional vertebral bone loss: a controlled trial. *Clinical Science* 1983;64:541–546.

57. Yeater RA, Martin RB. Senile osteoporosis: the effects of exercise. *Postgraduate Medicine* 1984;75:147–149.

58. Lunt M, Masaryk P, Scheidt-Nve C, et al. The effects of lifestyle, dietary dairy intake and diabetes on bone density and vertebral deformity prevalence: the EVOS study. *Osteoporosis International* 2001;12:688–698.

59. Wilsgaard T, Emaus N, Ahmed L, et al. Lifestyle impact on lifetime bone loss in women and men: the Tromsø Study. *American Journal of Epidemiology* 2009;169:877–886.

60. Dook J, James C, Henderson N, Price R. Exercise and bone mineral density in mature female athletes. *Medicine & Science in Sports & Exercise* 1997;29: 291–296.

61. Kelley G, Kelley K, Tran Z. Exercise and lumbar spine bone mineral density in postmenopausal women: a meta-analysis of individual patient data. *The Journals of Gerontology Series A: Biological Sciences and Medical Sciences* 2002;57:599–604.

62. Robertson M, Campbell A, Gardner M, Devlin N. Preventing injuries in older people by preventing falls: a meta-analysis of individual-level data. *Journal of the American Geriatrics Society* 2002;50:905–911.

63. Eaton-Evans J. Osteoporosis and the role of diet. *British Journal of Biomedical Science* 1994;51:358–370.

64. Saltman PD, Strause LG. The role of trace minerals in osteoporosis. *Journal of the American College of Nutrition* 1993; 12:384–389.

65. Hannan M, Tucker K, Dawson-Hughes B, et al. Effect of dietary protein on bone loss in elderly men and women: the Framingham Osteoporosis Study. *Journal of Bone and Mineral Research* 2000;15:2504–2512.

66. Ellis F, Holesh S, Ellis J. Incidence of osteoporosis in vegetarians and omnivores. *The American Journal of Clinical Nutrition* 1972;25:55–58.

67. Marsh AG, Sanchez TV, Chaffe FL, et al. Bone mineral mass in adult lacto-ovo-vegetarian and omnivorous adults. *The American Journal of Clinical Nutrition* 1983;37:453–456.

68. Licata AA, Bou E, Bartter FC, West F. Acute effects of dietary protein on calcium metabolism in patients with osteoporosis. *The Journals of Gerontology* 1981;36:14–19.

69. Heaney R, Layman D. Amount and type of protein influences bone health. *The American Journal of Clinical Nutrition* 2008;87:1567S–1570S.

70. Pizzorno J, Frassetto LA, Katzinger J. Diet-induced acidosis: is it real and clinically relevant? *British Journal of Nutrition* 2010;103:1185–1194.

71. Grossman M, Kirsner J, Gillespie I. Basal and histalog-stimulated gastric secretion in control subjects and in patients

with peptic ulcer or gastric cancer. *Gastroenterology* 1963;45: 15–26.

72. Wood RJ, Serfaty-Lacrosniere C. Gastric acidity, atrophic gastritis, and calcium absorption. *Nutrition Reviews* 1992;50:33–40.

73. Nicar MJ, Pak CY. Calcium bioavailability from calcium carbonate and calcium citrate. *The Journal of Clinical Endocrinology & Metabolism* 1985; 61:391–393.

74. Ngamruengphong S, Leontiadis GI, Radhi S, et al. Proton pump inhibitors and risk of fracture: a systematic review and meta-analysis of observational studies. *The American Journal of Gastroenterology* 2011 Jul;106(7): 1209–1218.

75. Kwok CS, Yeong JK, Loke YK. Meta-analysis: risk of fractures with acid-suppressing medication. *Bone* 2011 Apr 1;48(4): 768–776.

76. Thom JA, Morris JE, Bishop A, Blacklock NJ. The influence of refined carbohydrate on urinary calcium excretion. *British Journal of Urology* 1978;50: 459–464.

77. Mazariegos-Ramos E, Guerrero-Romero F, Rodriguez-Moran M, et al. Consumption of soft drinks with phosphoric acid as a risk factor for the development of hypocalcemia in children: a case-control study. *Journal of Pediatrics* 1995;126: 940–942.

78. Wyshak G, Frisch RE. Carbonated beverages, dietary calcium, the dietary calcium/phosphorus ratio, and bone fractures in girls and boys. *Journal of Adolescent Health* 1994;15:210–215.

79. Vermeer C, Gijsbers BL, Cracium AM, et al. Effects of vitamin K on bone mass and bone metabolism. *Journal of Nutrition* 1996;126(4 suppl):1187S–1191S.

80. Bitensky L, Hart JP, Catterall A, et al. Circulating vitamin K levels in patients with fractures. *Journal of Bone and Joint Surgery, British Volume* 1988;70: 663–664.

81. Feskanich D, Weber P, Willett WC, et al. Vitamin K intake and hip fractures in women: a prospective study. *The American Journal of Clinical Nutrition* 1999;69:74–79.

82. Kanai T, Takagi T, Masuhiro K, et al. Serum vitamin K level and bone mineral density in postmenopausal women. *International Journal of Gynecology & Obstetrics* 1997;56:25–30.

83. Booth SL, Tucker KL, Chen H, et al. Dietary vitamin K intakes are associated with hip fracture but not with bone mineral density in elderly men and women. *The American Journal of Clinical Nutrition* 2000;71: 1201–1208.

84. Neilsen FH, Hunt CD, Mullen LM, Hunt JR. Effect of dietary boron on mineral, estrogen, and testosterone metabolism in postmenopausal women. *The FASEB Journal* 1987 Nov 1;1(5): 394–397.

85. Nielsen FH, Gallagher SK, Johnson LK, Nielsen EJ. Boron enhances and mimics some of the effects of estrogen therapy in postmenopausal women. *The Journal of Trace Elements in Experimental Medicine* 1992;5: 237–246.

86. Stacewicz-Sapuntzakis M, Bowen PE, Hussain EA, et al. Chemical composition and potential health effects of prunes: a functional food? *Critical Reviews in Food Science and Nutrition* 2001;41(4): 251–286.

87. Setchell K. Soy isoflavones-benefits and risk from nature's selective estrogen receptor modulators (SERMS). *Journal of the American College of Nutrition* 2001;20:354S–362S.

88. Weaver C, Cheong J. Soy isoflavones and bone health: the relationship is still unclear. *Journal of Nutrition* 2005;135: 1243–1247.

89. Arjmandi B, Khalil D, Smith B, et al. Soy protein has a greater effect on bone in postmenopausal women not on hormone replacement therapy, as evidenced by reducing bone resorption and urinary calcium excretion. *The Journal of Clinical Endocrinology & Metabolism* 2003;88:1048–1054.

90. Greendale G, FitzGerald G, Huang M, et al. Dietary soy isoflavones and bone mineral density: results from the study of women's health across the nation. *American Journal of Epidemiology* 2002;155(8):746–754.

91. Somekawa Y, Chiguchi M, Ishibashi T, Takeshi A. Soy intake related to menopausal symptoms, serum lipids, and bone mineral density in postmenopausal Japanese women. *Obstetrics & Gynecology* 2001;97: 109–115.

92. Ma DF, Qin LQ, Want P-Y, Katoh R. Soy isoflavone intake inhibits bone resorption and stimulates bone formation in menopausal women: meta-analysis of randomized controlled trials. *European Journal of Clinical Nutrition* 2008; 62: 155–161.

93. Branca F. Dietary phyto-oestrogens and bone health. *Proceedings of the Nutrition Society* 2003;62:877–887.

94. Wangen K, Duncan A, Merz-Demlow B, et al. Effects of soy isoflavones on markers of bone turnover in premenopausal and postmenopausal women. *The Journal of Clinical Endocrinology & Metabolism* 2000;85: 3043–3048.

95. Mei J, Yeung S, Kung A. High dietary phytoestrogen intake is associated with higher bone mineral density in postmenopausal but not premenopausal women. *The Journal of Clinical Endocrinology & Metabolism* 2001;86:5217–5221.

96. Bischoff-Ferrari H, Dawson-Hughes B, Baron J, et al. Calcium intake and hip fracture

risk in men and women: a meta-analysis of prospective cohort studies and randomized controlled trials. *The American Journal of Clinical Nutrition* 2007;86:1780–1790.

97. Shea B, Wells G, Cranney A, et al. Meta-analyses of therapies for postmenopausal osteoporosis. VII. Meta-analysis of calcium supplementation for the prevention of postmenopausal osteoporosis. *Endocrine Reviews* 2002;23:552–559.

98. Jackson R, LaCroix A, Gass M, et al. for the Women's Health Initiative Investigators. Calcium plus vitamin D supplementation and the risk of fractures. *The New England Journal of Medicine* 2006;354:669–683.

99. Cumming RG. Calcium intake and bone mass: a quantitative review of the evidence. *Calcified Tissue International* 1990; 47:194–201.

100. Elders PJ, Netelenbos JC, Lips P, et al. Calcium supplementation reduces vertebral bone loss in perimenopausal women: a controlled trial in 248 women between 46 and 55 years of age. *The Journal of Clinical Endocrinology & Metabolism* 1991;73:533–540.

101. Heaney RP. Phosphorus nutrition and the treatment of osteoporosis. *Mayo Clinic Proceedings* 2004 Jan;79(1):91–7.

102. Heaney RP, Nordin BE. Calcium effects on phosphorus absorption: implications for the prevention and co-therapy of osteoporosis. *Journal of the American College of Nutrition* 2002 Jun;21(3):239–244.

103. Feskanich D, Willett WC, Stampfer MJ, Colditz GA. Milk, dietary calcium, and bone fractures in women: a 12-year prospective study. *The American Journal of Public Health* 1997; 87(6):992–997.

104. Grant A, Avenell A, Campbell M, et al. for the RECORD Trial Group. Oral vitamin D3 and calcium for secondary prevention of low-trauma fractures in elderly people (Randomised Evaluation of Calcium OR vitamin D, RECORD): a randomised placebo-controlled trial. *The Lancet* 2005;365:1621–1628.

105. Bischoff-Ferrari H, Willett W, Wong J, et al. Fracture prevention with vitamin D supplementation: a meta-analysis of randomized controlled trials. *JAMA, The Journal of the American Medical Association* 2005;293:2257–2264.

106. Bolton-Smith C, McMurdo M, Paterson C, et al. Two-year randomized controlled trial of vitamin K1 (phylloquinone) and vitamin D3 plus calcium on the bone health of older women. *Journal of Bone and Mineral Research* 2007;22:509–519.

107. Boonen S, Vanderschueren D, Haentjens P, Lips P. Calcium and vitamin D in the prevention and treatment of osteoporosis—a clinical update. *Journal of Internal Medicine* 2006;259(6):539–552.

108. Bischoff H, Stahelin H, Dick W, et al. Effects of vitamin D and calcium supplementation on falls: a randomized controlled trial. *Journal of Bone and Mineral Research* 2003;18:343–351.

109. Pfeifer M, Begerow B, Minne H, et al. Effects of a short-term vitamin D and calcium supplementation on body sway and secondary hyperparathyroidism in elderly women. *Journal of Bone and Mineral Research* 2000;15:1113–1118.

110. Bischoff-Ferrari H, Dawson-Hughes B, Willett W, et al. Effect of vitamin D on falls: a meta-analysis. *JAMA, The Journal of the American Medical Association* 2004;291:1999–2006.

111. Cohen L, Kitzes R. Infrared spectroscopy and magnesium content of bone mineral in osteoporotic women. *Israel Journal of Medical Sciences* 1981;17: 1123–1125.

112. Stendig-Lindberg G, Tepper R, Leichter I. Trabecular bone density in a two year controlled trial of peroral magnesium in osteoporosis. *Magnesium Research* 1993;6:155–163.

113. Palacios C. The role of nutrients in bone health, from A to Z. *Critical Reviews in Food Science and Nutrition* 2006;46(8): 621–628.

114. Follis RH Jr, Bush JA, Cartwright GE, Wintrobe MM. Studies on copper metabolism XVIII. Skeletal changes associated with copper deficiency in swine. *Bulletin of the Johns Hopkins Hospital* 1955;97:405–409.

115. Smith R, Smith J, Fields M, Reiser S. Mechanical properties of bone from copper deficient rats fed starch or fructose. *Federation Proceedings* 1985;44:541.

116. Eaton-Evans J, McIlrath EM, Jackson WE, et al. Copper supplementation and the maintenance of bone mineral density in middle-aged women. *The Journal of Trace Elements in Experimental Medicine* 1996;9:87–94.

117. Leach R, Muenster A, Weign E. Studies on the role of manganese in bone formation. II. Effect upon chondroitin sulfate synthesis in chick epiphyseal cartilage. *Archives of Biochemistry and Biophysics* 1969;133: 22–28.

118. Silicon and bone formation. *Nutrition Reviews* 1980; 38:194–195.

119. Hott M, de Pollak C, Modrowski D, Marie P. Short-term effects of organic silicon on trabecular bone in mature ovariectomized rats. *Calcified Tissue International* 1993;53:174–179.

120. Spector TD, Calomme MR, Anderson SH, et al. Choline-stabilized orthosilicic acid supplementation as an adjunct to calcium/vitamin D3 stimulates markers of bone formation in osteopenic females: a randomized, placebo-controlled trial. *BMC Musculoskeletal Disorders* 2008 Jun 11;9:85.

121. Van Neurs J, Dhonukshe-Rutten R, Pluijm S, et al. Homo-

cysteine levels and the risk of osteoporotic fractures. *The New England Journal of Medicine* 2004;350:2042–2090.

122. Hyams DE, Ross EJ. Scurvy, megaloblastic anemia and osteoporosis. *The British Journal of Clinical Practice* 1963;17:332–340.

123. Booth S, Dallal G, Shea K, et al. Effect of vitamin K supplementation on bone loss in elderly men and women. *The Journal of Clinical Endocrinology & Metabolism* 2008;93:1217–1223.

124. Cheung A, Tile L, Lee Y, et al. Vitamin K supplementation in postmenopausal women with osteopenia (ECKO Trial): a randomized controlled trial. *PLoS Medicine* 2008 Oct 14;5(10):e196.

125. Cockayne S, Adamson J, Lanham-New S, et al. Vitamin K and prevention of fractures: systematic review and meta-analysis of randomized controlled trials. *Archives of Internal Medicine* 2006;166:1256–1261.

126. Binkley N, Harke J, Krueger D, et al. Vitamin K treatment reduces undercarboxylated osteocalcin but does not alter bone turnover, density or geometry in healthy postmenopausal, North American women. *Journal of Bone and Mineral Research* 2009;24(6):983–991.

127. Braam L, Knapen M, Geusens P, et al. Vitamin K1 supplementation retards bone loss in postmenopausal women between 50 and 60 years of age. *Calcified Tissue International* 2003;73:21–26.

128. Schurgers LJ, Geleijnse JM, Grobbee DE, et al. Nutritional intake of vitamins K1 (phylloquinone) and K2 (menaquinone) in the Netherlands. *Journal of Nutritional and Environmental Medicine* 1999 June;9(2):115–122.

129. Schurgers LJ, Teunissen KJ, Hamulyák K, et al. Vitamin K–containing dietary supplements: comparison of synthetic vitamin K1 and natto-derived menaqui-none-7. *Blood* 2007 Apr 15;109 (8):3279–3283.

130. Schurgers LJ, Vermeer C. Differential lipoprotein transport pathways of K-vitamins in healthy subjects. *Biochimica et Biophysica Acta* 2002 Feb 15;1570(1):27–32.

131. Kaneki M, Hedges S, Hosoi T, et al. Japanese fermented soybean food as the major determinant of the large geographic difference in circulating levels of vitamin K2: possible implications for hip-fracture risk. *Nutrition* 2001;17:315–321.

132. Forli L, Bollerslev J, Simonsen S, et al. Dietary vitamin K2 supplement improves bone status after lung and heart transplantation. *Transplantation* 2010 Feb 27;89(4):458–464.

133. Emaus N, Gjesdal CG, Almås B, et al. Vitamin K2 supplementation does not influence bone loss in early menopausal women: a randomised double-blind placebo-controlled trial. *Osteoporosis International* 2010 Oct;21(10):1731–1740.

134. Mounier P, Roux R, Seaman E, et al. The effects of strontium ranelate on the risk of vertebral fracture in women with postmenopausal osteoporosis. *The New England Journal of Medicine* 2004 Jan 29;350:459–468.

135. Meunier, P, Slosman, D, Delmas, P, et al. Strontium ranelate: dose-dependent effects in established postmenopausal vertebral osteoporosis—a 2-year randomized placebo controlled trial. *The Journal of Clinical Endocrinology & Metabolism* 2002;87:2060–2066.

136. Moscarini M, Patacchiola F, Spacca G, et al. New perspectives in the treatment of postmenopausal osteoporosis: ipriflavone. *Gynecological Endocrinology* 1994 Sep;8(3):203–207.

137. Passeri M, Biondi M, Costi D, et al. Effect of ipriflavone on bone mass in elderly osteoporotic women. *Bone and Mineral* 1992;19 suppl 1:S57–S62.

138. Agnusdei D, Crepaldi G, Isaia G, et al. A double blind, placebo-controlled trial of ipriflavone for prevention of postmenopausal spinal bone loss. *Calcified Tissue International* 1997;61:142–147.

139. Adami S, Bufalino L, Cervetti R, DiMarco C, DiMunno O, Fantasia L, et al. Ipriflavone prevents radial bone loss in postmenopausal women with low bone mass over 2 years. *Osteoporosis International* 1997;7:119–125.

140. Melis GB, Paoletti AM, Cagnacci A, et al. Lack of any estrogenic effect of ipriflavone in postmenopausal women. *Journal of Endocrinological Investigation* 1992;15:755–761.

141. Alexandersen P, Toussaint A, Christiansen C, et al. Ipriflavone in the treatment of postmenopausal osteoporosis: a randomized controlled trial. *JAMA, The Journal of the American Medical Association* 2001;285:1482–1488.

142. Zhang X, Li SW, Wu JF, et al. Effects of ipriflavone on postmenopausal syndrome and osteoporosis. *Gynecological Endocrinology* 2010 Feb;26(2):76–80.

143. Halpner AD, Kellermann G, Ahlgrimm MJ, et al. The effect of an ipriflavone-containing supplement on urinary N-linked telopeptide levels in postmenopausal women. *Journal of Women's Health and Gender-Based Medicine* 2000 Nov;9(9):995–998.

144. Ohta H, Komukai S, Makita K, et al. Effects of 1-year ipriflavone treatment on lumbar bone mineral density and bone metabolic markers in postmenopausal women with low bone mass. *Hormone Research* 1999;51(4):178–183.

145. Muraki S, Yamamoto S, Ishibashi H, et al. Diet and lifestyle associated with increased bone mineral density: cross-sectional study of Japanese el-

derly women at an osteoporosis outpatient clinic. *Journal of Orthopaedic Science* 2007 Jul; 12(4):317–320.

146. Shen CL, Yeh JK, Cao JJ, et al. Green tea and bone health: evidence from laboratory studies. *Pharmacological Research* 2011 Aug;64(2):155–161.

147. Shen CL, Cao JJ, Dagda RY, et al. Supplementation with green tea polyphenols improves bone microstructure and quality in aged, orchidectomized rats. *Calcified Tissue International* 2011 Jun;88(6):455–463.

148. Shen CL, Yeh JK, Cao JJ, Wang JS. Green tea and bone metabolism. *Nutrition Research* 2009 Jul;29(7):437–456.

Parkinson's Disease

1. Samii A, Nutt JG, Ransom BR. Parkinson's disease. *The Lancet* 2004;363:1783–1793.

2. Calne DB, Langston JW, Martin WR, et al. Positron emission tomography after MPTP: observations relating to the cause of Parkinson's disease. *Nature* 1985;317:246–248.

3. Priyadarshi A, Khuder SA, Schaub EA, et al. Environmental risk factors and Parkinson's disease: a metaanalysis. *Environmental Research* 2001;86: 122–127.

4. Betarbet R, Sherer TB, MacKenzie G, et al. Chronic systemic pesticide exposure reproduces features of Parkinson's disease. *Nature Neuroscience* 2000;3:1301–1306.

5. Bashkatova V, Alam M, Vanin A, et al. Chronic administration of rotenone increases levels of nitric oxide and lipid peroxidation products in rat brain. *Experimental Neurology* 2004; 186:235–241.

6. Snyder SH, D'Amato RJ. Predicting Parkinson's disease. *Nature* 1985;317:198–199.

7. Di Monte DA. The environment and Parkinson's disease: Is the nigrostriatal system preferentially targeted by neurotoxins?

The Lancet Neurology 2003; 2: 531–538.

8. Olanow CW. Manganese-induced Parkinsonism and Parkinson's disease. *Annals of the New York Academy of Sciences* 2004;1012:209–223.

9. Logroscino G. The role of early life environmental risk factors in Parkinson disease: what is the evidence? *Environmental Health Perspectives* 2005;113: 1234–1238.

10. Landrigan PJ, Sonawane B, Butler RN, et al. Early environmental origins of neurodegenerative disease in later life. *Environmental Health Perspectives* 2005;113:1230–1233.

11. Siderowf A, Stern M. Update on Parkinson disease. *Annals of Internal Medicine* 2003;138: 651–658.

12. Nisticò R, Mehdawy B, Piccirilli S, Mercuri N. Paraquat- and rotenone-induced models of Parkinson's disease. *International Journal of Immunopathology and Pharmacology* 2011 Apr–Jun;24(2):313–322.

13. Vanacore N, Gasparini M, Brusa L, et al. A possible association between exposure to n-hexane and parkinsonism. *Neurological Sciences* 2000;21: 49–52.

14. McDonnell L, Maginnis C, Lewis S, et al. Occupational exposure to solvents and metals and Parkinson's disease. *Neurology* 2003;61:716–717.

15. Onyango IG. Mitochondrial dysfunction and oxidative stress in Parkinson's disease. *Neurochemical Research* 2008 Mar; 33(3):589–597.

16. Bharath S, Hsu M, Kaur D, et al. Glutathione, iron and Parkinson's disease. *Biochemical Pharmacology* 2002;64:1037–1048.

17. Büeler H. Impaired mitochondrial dynamics and function in the pathogenesis of Parkinson's disease. *Experimental Neurology* 2009 Aug;218(2):235–246.

18. Jankovic J. Levodopa strengths

and weaknesses. *Neurology* 2002;58(4 suppl 1):S19–S32.

19. Karstaedt PJ, Pincus JH. Protein redistribution diet remains effective in patients with fluctuating parkinsonism. *Archives of Neurology* 1992;49:149–151.

20. de Rijk MC, Breteler MM, den Breeijen JH, et al. Dietary antioxidants and Parkinson disease. The Rotterdam Study. *Archives of Neurology* 1997;54:762–765.

21. Scheider WL, Hershey LA, Vena JE, et al. Dietary antioxidants and other dietary factors in the etiology of Parkinson's disease. *Movement Disorders* 1997;12:190–196.

22. Vatassery GT, Fahn S, Kuskowski MA. Alpha tocopherol in CSF of subjects taking high-dose vitamin E in the DATATOP study. Parkinson Study Group. *Neurology* 1998; 50:1900–1902.

23. Fahn S. A pilot trial of highdose alpha-tocopherol and ascorbate in early Parkinson's disease. *Annals of Neurology* 1992;32:S128–S32.

24. Shoulson I. DATATOP: a decade of neuroprotective inquiry. Parkinson Study Group. Deprenyl and tocopherol antioxidative therapy of parkinsonism. *Annals of Neurology* 1998;44: S160–S166.

25. Zhang SM, Hernán MA, Chen H, et al. Intakes of vitamins E and C, carotenoids, vitamin supplements, and PD risk. *Neurology* 2002;59:1161–1169.

26. Shults CW, Haas RH, Beal MF. A possible role of coenzyme Q10 in the etiology and treatment of Parkinson's disease. *Biofactors* 1999;9:267–272.

27. Shults CW, Oakes D, Kieburtz K, et al. Effects of coenzyme Q10 in early Parkinson disease: evidence of slowing of the functional decline. *Archives of Neurology* 2002;59: 1541–1550.

28. NINDS Website (Accessed 06/15/2011 at http://www.ninds

.nih.gov/disorders/clinical_trials/CoQ10-Trial-Update.html.)

29. Swerdlow RH. Is NADH effective in the treatment of Parkinson's disease? *Drugs & Aging* 1998;13:263–268.

30. Birkmayer W, Birkmayer GJ. Nicotinamidadenindinucleotide (NADH): the new approach in the therapy of Parkinson's disease. *Annals of Clinical & Laboratory Science* 1989;19:38–43.

31. Kuhn W, Muller T, Winkel R, et al. Parenteral application of NADH in Parkinson's disease: clinical improvement partially due to stimulation of endogenous levodopa biosynthesis. *Journal of Neural Transmission* 1996;103:1187–1193.

32. Funfgeld EW, Baggen M, Nedwidek P, et al. Double-blind study with phosphatidylserine (PS) in Parkinsonian patients with senile dementia of Alzheimer's type (SDAT). *Progress in Clinical and Biological Research* 1989;317:1235–1246.

33. Mayeux R, Stern Y, Sano M, et al. The relationship of serotonin to depression in Parkinson's disease. *Movement Disorders* 1988;3:237–244.

34. Bastard J, Truelle JL, Émile J. [Effectiveness of 5 hydroxy-tryptophan in Parkinson's disease.] *La Nouvelle Presse Médicale* 1976 Sep 11;5(29):1836–1837.

35. Sano VI, Taniguchi K. L-5-hydroxytryptophan (L-5-HTP) therapy in Parkinson's disease, *Morbidity and Mortality Weekly Report* 1972;114:1717–1719.

36. Chase TN, Ng LK, Watanabe AM. Parkinson's disease: modification by 5-hydroxytryptophan. *Neurology* 1972;22:479–484.

37. Mendlewicz J, Youdim MB. Antidepressant potentiation of 5-hydroxytryptophan by L-deprenil in affective illness. *Journal of Affective Disorders* 1980;2:137–146.

38. Berman AE, Chan WY, Brennan AM, et al. N-acetylcysteine prevents loss of dopaminergic neurons in the EAAC1-/- mouse. *Annals of Neurology* 2011 Mar;69(3):509–520.

39. Hauser RA, Lyons KE, McClain T, et al. Randomized, double-blind, pilot evaluation of intravenous glutathione in Parkinson's disease. *Movement Disorders* 2009 May 15;24(7):979–983.

40. Pan T, Jankovic J, Le W. Potential therapeutic properties of green tea polyphenols in Parkinson's disease. *Drugs & Aging* 2003;20:711–721.

41. Weinreb O, Mandel S, Amit T, et al. Neurological mechanisms of green tea polyphenols in Alzheimer's and Parkinson's diseases. *The Journal of Nutritional Biochemistry* 2004;15:506–516.

42. Gessner B, Voelp A, Klasser M. Study of the long-term action of a *Ginkgo biloba* extract on vigilance and mental performance as determined by means of quantitative pharmaco-EEG and psychometric measurements. *Arzneimittelforschung* 1985;35:1459–1465.

43. Yang SF, Wu Q, Sun AS, et al. Protective effect and mechanism of *Ginkgo biloba* leaf extracts for Parkinson disease induced by 1-methyl-4-phenyl-1,2,3,6-tetrahydropyridine. *Acta Pharmacologica Sinica* 2001;22:1089–1093.

44. HP-200 in Parkinson's Disease Study Group. An alternative medicine treatment for Parkinson's disease: results of a multicenter clinical trial. *The Journal of Alternative and Complementary Medicine* 1995;1:249–255.

45. Katzenschlager R, Evans A, Manson A, Patsalos PN. *Mucuna pruriens* in Parkinson's disease: a double blind clinical and pharmacological study. *Journal of Neurology, Neurosurgery & Psychiatry* 2004 Dec;75(12):1672–1677.

46. Lieu CA, Kunselman AR, Manyam BV, et al. A water extract of *Mucuna pruriens* provides long-term amelioration of parkinsonism with reduced risk for dyskinesias. *Parkinsonism & Related Disorders* 2010 Aug;16(7):458–465.

47. Kasture S, Pontis S, Pinna A, et al. Assessment of symptomatic and neuroprotective efficacy of *Mucuna pruriens* seed extract in rodent model of Parkinson's disease. *Neurotoxicity Research* 2009 Feb;15(2):111–122.

48. Rabey JM, Vered Y, Shabtai H, et al. Broad bean (*Vicia faba*) consumption and Parkinson's disease. *Advances in Neurology* 1993;60:681–684.

Peptic Ulcer

1. Yeomans ND. The ulcer sleuths: the search for the cause of peptic ulcers. *Journal of Gastroenterology and Hepatology* 2011 Jan;26 suppl 1:35–41.

2. Berstad K, Berstad A. *Helicobacter pylori* infection in peptic ulcer disease. *Scandinavian Journal of Gastroenterology* 1993;28:561–567.

3. Weil J, Colin-Jones D, Langman M. Prophylactic aspirin and risk of peptic ulcer bleeding. *BMJ* 1995;310:827–830.

4. Feldman EJ, Sabovich KA. Stress and peptic ulcer disease. *Gastroenterology* 1980;78:1087–1089.

5. Anda RF, Williamson DF, Escobedo LG, et al. Self-perceived stress and the risk of peptic ulcer disease. A longitudinal study of US adults. *Archives of Internal Medicine* 1992;152:829–833.

6. Ogle CW. Smoking and gastric ulcers: the possible role of nicotine. *The Journal of Clinical Pharmacology* 1999 May;39(5):448–453.

7. Siegel J. Gastrointestinal ulcer—Arthus reaction! *Annals of Allergy, Asthma & Immunology* 1974;32:127–130.

8. Andre C, Moulinier B, Andre F, et al. Evidence for anaphylactic reactions in peptic ulcer and varioliform gastritis. *Annals of*

Allergy, Asthma & Immunology 1983;51:325–328.

9. Siegel J. Immunologic approach to the treatment and prevention of gastrointestinal ulcers. *Annals of Allergy, Asthma & Immunology* 1977;38:27–41.

10. Rebhun J. Duodenal ulceration in allergic children. *Annals of Allergy, Asthma & Immunology* 1975;34:145–149.

11. Kumar N, Kumar A, Broor SL, et al. Effect of milk on patients with duodenal ulcers. *British Medical Journal* 1986;293:666.

12. Rydning A, Berstad A, Aadland E, et al. Prophylactic effect of dietary fiber in duodenal ulcer disease. *The Lancet* 1982; 2:736–739.

13. Kang JY, Tay HH, Guan R, et al. Dietary supplementation with pectin in the maintenance treatment of duodenal ulcer: a controlled study. *Scandinavian Journal of Gastroenterology* 1988;23:95–99.

14. Harju E, Larmi TK. Effect of guar gum added to the diet of patients with duodenal ulcer. *Journal of Parenteral and Enteral Nutrition* 1985;9:496–500.

15. Cheney G. Rapid healing of peptic ulcers in patients receiving fresh cabbage juice. *California Medicine* 1949;70:10–14.

16. Cheney G. Anti–peptic ulcer dietary factor. *Journal of the American Dietetic Association* 1950;26:668–672.

17. Shive W, Snider RN, DuBilier B, et al. Glutamine in treatment of peptic ulcer; preliminary report. *Texas State Journal of Medicine* 1957;53: 840–842.

18. Yanaka A, Fahey JW, Fukumoto A, et al. Dietary sulforaphane-rich broccoli sprouts reduce colonization and attenuate gastritis in *Helicobacter pylori*–infected mice and humans. *Cancer Prevention Research* 2009 Apr;2(4):353–360.

19. Marshall BJ, Valenzuela JE, McCallum RW, et al. Bismuth subsalicylate suppression of *Helicobacter pylori* in nonulcer dyspepsia: a double-blind placebo-controlled trial. *Digestive Diseases and Sciences* 1993;38: 1674–1680.

20. Kang JY, Tay HH, Wee A, et al. Effect of colloidal bismuth subcitrate on symptoms and gastric histology in non-ulcer dyspepsia. A double blind placebo controlled study. *Gut* 1990;31: 476–480.

21. Loughlin MF. Novel therapeutic targets in *Helicobacter pylori*. *Expert Opinion on Therapeutic Targets* 2003;7:725–735.

22. Thyagarajan SP, Ray P, Das BK, et al. Geographical difference in antimicrobial resistance pattern of *Helicobacter pylori* clinical isolates from Indian patients: multicentric study. *Journal of Gastroenterology and Hepatology* 2003;18:1373–1378.

23. Schumpelick V, Farthmann E. [Study on the protective effect of vitamin A on stress ulcer of the rat.] *Arzneimittelforschung* 1976;26:386–388.

24. al-Moutairy AR, Tariq M. Effect of vitamin E and selenium on hypothermic restraint stress and chemically-induced ulcers. *Digestive Diseases and Sciences* 1996;41:1165–1171.

25. Patty I, Benedek S, Deák G, et al. Cytoprotective effect of vitamin A and its clinical importance in the treatment of patients with chronic gastric ulcer. *International Journal of Tissue Reactions* 1983;5(3):301–307.

26. Frommer DJ. The healing of gastric ulcers by zinc sulphate. *The Medical Journal of Australia* 1975;2:793–796.

27. Matsukura T, Tanaka H. Applicability of zinc complex of L-carnosine for medical use. *Biochemistry* (Moscow) 2000 Jul;65(7):817–823.

28. Morgan AG, McAdam WA, Pacsoo C, et al. Comparison between cimetidine and Caved-S in the treatment of gastric ulceration, and subsequent maintenance therapy. *Gut* 1982;23:545–551.

29. Tewari SN, Trembalowicz FC. Some experience with deglycyrrhizinated liquorice in the treatment of gastric and duodenal ulcers with special reference to its spasmolytic effect. *Gut* 1968; 9:48–51.

30. Balakrishnan V, Pillai MV, Raveendran PM, et al. Deglycyrrhizinated liquorice in the treatment of chronic duodenal ulcer. *Journal of the Association of Physicians of India* 1978;26: 811–814.

31. Rees WD, Rhodes J, Wright JE, et al. Effect of deglycyrrhizinated liquorice on gastric mucosal damage by aspirin. *Scandinavian Journal of Gastroenterology* 1979;14:605–607.

32. Fukai T, Marumo A, Kaitou K, et al. Anti–*Helicobacter pylori* flavonoids from licorice extract. *Life Sciences* 2002;71:1449–1463.

33. Al-Habbal MJ, Al-Habbal Z, Huwez FU. A double-blind controlled clinical trial of mastic and placebo in the treatment of duodenal ulcer. *Clinical and Experimental Pharmacology and Physiology* 1984 Sep–Oct;11(5): 541–544.

34. Dabos KJ, Sfika E, Vlatta LJ, Giannikopoulos G. The effect of mastic gum on *Helicobacter pylori*: a randomized pilot study. *Phytomedicine* 2010 Mar;17(3–4):296–299.

35. Zhou H, Jiao D. [312 cases of gastric and duodenal ulcer bleeding treated with 3 kinds of alcoholic extract rhubarb tablets.] *Zhong Xi Yi Jie He Za Zhi* 1990;10:150–151,131–132.

Periodontal Disease

1. Newman MG, Takei H, Klokkevold PR, Carranza F. *Carranza's Clinical Periodontology*, 11th ed. Philadelphia: W. B. Saunders, 2011.

2. Deliargyris EN, Madianos PN, Kadoma W, et al. Periodontal disease in patients with acute myocardial infarction: prevalence and contribution to el-

evated C-reactive protein levels. *American Heart Journal* 2004; 147:1005–1009.

3. Page RC, Schroeder HE. Current status of the host response in chronic marginal periodontitis. *Journal of Periodontology* 1981;52:477–491.

4. Hyyppa T. Gingival IgE and histamine concentrations in patients with asthma and in patients with periodontitis. *Journal of Clinical Periodontology* 1984; 11:132–137.

5. Addya S, Chakravarti K, Basu A, et al. Effects of mercuric chloride on several scavenging enzymes in rat kidney and influence of vitamin E supplementation. *Acta Vitaminologica et Enzymologica* 1984;6:103–107.

6. Bartold PM, Wiebkin OW, Thonard JC. The effect of oxygen-derived free radicals on gingival proteoglycans and hyaluronic acid. *Journal of Periodontal Research* 1984;19:390–400.

7. Schenkein HA, Gunsolley JC, Koertge TE, et al. Smoking and its effects on early-onset periodontitis. *The Journal of the American Dental Association* 1995;126:1107–1113.

8. Kaldahl WB, Johnson GK, Patil KD, et al. Levels of cigarette consumption and response to periodontal therapy. *Journal of Periodontology* 1996;67:675–681.

9. Pelletier O. Smoking and vitamin C levels in humans. *The American Journal of Clinical Nutrition* 1968;21:1259–1267.

10. Abbas F, van der Velden U, Hart AA. Relation between wound healing after surgery and susceptibility to periodontal disease. *Journal of Clinical Periodontology* 1984;11:221–229.

11. Alvares O, Altman LC, Springmeyer S, et al. The effect of subclinical ascorbate deficiency on periodontal health in nonhuman primates. *Journal of Periodontal Research* 1981;16:628–636.

12. Woolfe SN, Hume WR, Kenney EB. Ascorbic acid and periodontal disease: a review of the

literature. *The Journal of the Western Society of Periodontology/Periodontal Abstracts* 1980; 28:44–56.

13. Alfano MC, Miller SA, Drummond JF. Effect of ascorbic acid deficiency on the permeability and collagen biosynthesis of oral mucosal epithelium. *Annals of the New York Academy of Sciences* 1975;258:253–263.

14. Alvares O, Siegel I. Permeability of gingival sulcular epithelium in the development of scorbutic gingivitis. *Journal of Oral Pathology* 1981;10:40–48.

15. Ringsdorf WM Jr, Cheraskin E, Ramsay RR Jr. Sucrose, neutrophilic phagocytosis and resistance to disease. *Dental Survey* 1976;52:46–48.

16. Sanchez A, Reeser JL, Lau HS, et al. Role of sugars in human neutrophilic phagocytosis. *The American Journal of Clinical Nutrition* 1973;26:1180–1184.

17. Prasad AS. Clinical, biochemical and nutritional spectrum of zinc deficiency in human subjects: an update. *Nutrition Reviews* 1983;41:197–208.

18. Freeland JH, Cousins RJ, Schwartz R. Relationship of mineral status and intake to periodontal disease. *The American Journal of Clinical Nutrition* 1976;29:745–749.

19. Harrap GJ, Saxton CA, Best JS. Inhibition of plaque growth by zinc salts. *Journal of Periodontal Research* 1983;18:634–642.

20. Hsieh S, Hayali A, Navia J. Zinc. In *Trace elements in dental disease*, ed. Curzon M, Cutress T. Boston: John Wright PSG, 1983, 99–220.

21. Kim JE, Shklar G. The effect of vitamin E on the healing of gingival wounds in rats. *Journal of Periodontology* 1983;54: 305–308.

22. Folkers K, Yamamura Y. *Biomedical and clinical aspects of coenzyme Q*, vol. 1. Amsterdam: Elsevier/North Holland Biomedical Press, 1977, 294–311.

23. Folkers K, Yamamura Y. *Bio-

medical and clinical aspects of coenzyme Q*, vol. 3. Amsterdam: Elsevier/North Holland Biomedical Press, 1981, 109–125.

24. Rao CN, Rao VH, Steinmann B. Influence of bioflavonoids on the metabolism and crosslinking of collagen. *Italian Journal of Biochemistry* 1981;30:259–270.

25. Pearce FL, Befus AD, Bienenstock J. Mucosal mast cells. III. Effect of quercetin and other flavonoids on antigen-induced histamine secretion from rat intestinal mast cells. *Journal of Allergy and Clinical Immunology* 1984;73:819–823.

26. Busse WW, Kopp DE, Middleton E Jr. Flavonoid modulation of human neutrophil function. *Journal of Allergy and Clinical Immunology* 1984;73:801–809.

27. Petti S, Scully C. Polyphenols, oral health and disease: a review. *Journal of Dentistry* 2009 Jun;37(6):413–423.

28. Houde V, Grenier D, Chandad F. Protective effects of grape seed proanthocyanidins against oxidative stress induced by lipopolysaccharides of periodontopathogens. *Journal of Periodontology* 2006 Aug;77(8): 1371–1379.

29. Koyama Y, Kuriyama S, Aida J, et al. Association between green tea consumption and tooth loss: cross-sectional results from the Ohsaki Cohort 2006 Study. *Preventive Medicine* 2010 Apr; 50(4):173–179.

30. Hirasawa M, Takada K, Makimura M, et al. Improvement of periodontal status by green tea catechin using a local delivery system: a clinical pilot study. *Journal of Periodontal Research* 2002;37:433–438.

31. Krahwinkel T, Willershausen B. The effect of sugar-free green tea chew candies on the degree of inflammation of the gingiva. *European Journal of Medical Research* 2000;5:463–467.

32. Kimbrough C, Chun M, dela Roca G, et al. Pycnogenol chewing gum minimizes gingival

bleeding and plaque formation. *Phytomedicine* 2002;9:410–413.

33. Vogel RI, Fink RA, Schneider LC, et al. The effect of folic acid on gingival health. *Journal of Periodontology* 1976;47:667–668.

34. Vogel RI, Fink RA, Frank O, et al. The effect of topical application of folic acid on gingival health. *Journal of Oral Medicine* 1978;33:20–22.

35. Pack AR, Thomson ME. Effects of topical and systemic folic acid supplementation on gingivitis in pregnancy. *Journal of Clinical Periodontology* 1980;7:402–414.

36. Thomson ME, Pack AR. Effects of extended systemic and topical folate supplementation on gingivitis of pregnancy. *Journal of Clinical Periodontology* 1982;9:275–280.

37. Pack AR. Folate mouthwash: effects on established gingivitis in periodontal patients. *Journal of Clinical Periodontology* 1984;11:619–628.

38. Whitehead N, Reyner F, Lindenbaum J. Megaloblastic changes in the cervical epithelium association with oral contraceptive therapy and reversal with folic acid. *JAMA, The Journal of the American Medical Association* 1973;226:1421–1424.

39. Butterworth CE Jr, Hatch KD, Gore H, et al. Improvement in cervical dysplasia associated with folic acid therapy in users of oral contraceptives. *The American Journal of Clinical Nutrition* 1982;35:73–82.

40. da Costa M, Rothenberg SP. Appearance of a folate binder in leukocytes and serum of women who are pregnant or taking oral contraceptives. *Journal of Laboratory and Clinical Medicine* 1974;83:207–214.

41. Godowski KC. Antimicrobial action of sanguinarine. *The Journal of Clinical Dentistry* 1989;1:96–101.

42. Grossman E, Meckel AH, Isaacs RL, et al. A clinical comparison of antibacterial mouthrinses: effects of chlorhexidine, phenolics, and sanguinarine on dental plaque and gingivitis. *Journal of Periodontology* 1989;60:435–440.

43. Benedicenti A, Galli D, Merlini A. [The clinical therapy of periodontal disease, the use of potassium hydroxide and the water-alcohol extract of *Centella asiatica* in combination with laser therapy in the treatment of severe periodontal disease.] *Parodontologia e Stomatologia* 1985;24:11–26.

Premenstrual Syndrome

1. Biskind MS, Biskind GR. Diminution in ability of the liver to inactivate estrone in vitamin B complex deficiency. *Science* 1941;94:462.

2. Biskind MS. Nutritional deficiency in the etiology of menorrhagia, metrorrhagia, cystic mastitis and premenstrual tension; treatment with vitamin B complex. *The Journal of Clinical Endocrinology & Metabolism* 1943;3:227–234.

3. Facchinetti F, Nappi G, Petraglia F, et al. Oestradiol/progesterone imbalance and the premenstrual syndrome. *The Lancet* 1983;2:1302.

4. Chuong CJ, Hsi BP, Gibbons WE. Periovulatory beta-endorphin levels in premenstrual syndrome. *Obstetrics & Gynecology* 1994;83:755–760.

5. Wynn V, Adams PW, Folkard J, Seed M. Tryptophan, depression and steroidal contraception. *Journal of Steroid Biochemistry* 1975;6:965–970.

6. Bermond P. Therapy of side effects of oral contraceptive agents with vitamin B6. *Acta Vitaminologica et Enzymologica* 1982;4:45–54.

7. Abraham GE. Nutritional factors in the etiology of the premenstrual tension syndromes. *The Journal of Reproductive Medicine* 1983;28:446–464.

8. Goei G, Ralston J, Abraham G. Dietary patterns of patients with premenstrual tension. *Journal of Applied Nutrition* 1982;34:4.

9. Cross G, Marley J, Miles H, Wilson K. Changes in nutrient intake during the menstrual cycle of overweight women with premenstrual syndrome. *British Journal of Nutrition* 2001;5(4):475–482.

10. Wurtman J. Carbohydrate craving. Relationship between carbohydrate intake and disorders of mood. *Drugs* 1990;39 suppl 3:49–52.

11. Rossignol AM, Bonnlander H. Prevalence and severity of the premenstrual syndrome. Effects of foods and beverages that are sweet or high in sugar content. *The Journal of Reproductive Medicine* 1991;36:131–136.

12. Yudkin J, Eisa O. Dietary sucrose and oestradiol concentration in young men. *Annals of Nutrition and Metabolism* 1988;32:53–55.

13. Boyd N, McGuire V, Shannon P, et al. Effect of a low-fat high-carbohydrate diet on symptoms of cyclical mastopathy. *The Lancet* 1988;2(8603):128–132.

14. Puder JJ, Blum CA, Mueller B, et al. Menstrual cycle symptoms are associated with low-grade inflammation. *European Journal of Clinical Investigation* 2006;36:58–64.

15. Gorbach SL, Goldin BR. Diet and the excretion and enterohepatic cycling of estrogens. *Preventive Medicine* 1987;16:525–531.

16. Goldin BR, Adlercreutz H, Gorbach SL, et al. Estrogen patterns and plasma levels in vegetarian and omnivorous women. *The New England Journal of Medicine* 1982;307:1542–1547.

17. Longcope C, Gorbach S, Goldin B, et al. The effect of a low fat diet on estrogen metabolism. *The Journal of Clinical Endocrinology & Metabolism* 1987;64:1246–1250.

18. Woods MN, Gorbach SL,

Longcope C, et al. Low-fat, high-fiber diet and serum estrone sulfate in premenopausal women. *The American Journal of Clinical Nutrition* 1989;49: 1179–1183.

19. Jones DY. Influence of dietary fat on self-reported menstrual symptoms. *Physiology & Behavior* 1987;40:483–487.

20. Gold E, Bair Y, Block G, et al. Diet and lifestyle factors associated with premenstrual symptoms in a racially diverse community sample: Study of Women's Health Across the Nation (SWAN). *Journal of Women's Health* 2007 Jun;16(5): 641–656.

21. Brayshaw ND, Brayshaw DD. Thyroid hypofunction in premenstrual syndrome. *The New England Journal of Medicine* 1986;315:1486–1487.

22. Roy-Byrne PP, Rubinow DR, Hoban MC, et al. TSH and prolactin responses to TRH in patients with premenstrual syndrome. *The American Journal of Psychiatry* 1987;144:480–484.

23. Girdler SS, Pedersen CA, Light KC. Thyroid axis function during the menstrual cycle in women with premenstrual syndrome. *Psychoneuroendocrinology* 1995;20:395–403.

24. Schmidt PJ, Grover GN, Roy-Byrne PP, Rubinow DR. Thyroid function in women with premenstrual syndrome. *The Journal of Clinical Endocrinology & Metabolism* 1993;76: 671–674.

25. Rapkin A. The role of serotonin in premenstrual syndrome. *Clinical Obstetrics and Gynecology* 1992;35:629–636.

26. Kuczmierczyk AR, Johnson CC, Labrum AH. Coping styles in women with premenstrual syndrome. *Acta Psychiatrica Scandinavica* 1994;89:301–305.

27. Eriksson E, Alling C, Andersch B, et al. Cerebrospinal fluid levels of monoamine metabolites. A preliminary study of their relation to menstrual cycle phase, sex steroids, and pituitary hormones in healthy women and in women with premenstrual syndrome. *Neuropsychopharmacology* 1994;11:201–213.

28. Halbreich U, Petty F, Yonkers K, et al. Low plasma gamma-aminobutyric acid levels during the late luteal phase of women with premenstrual dysphoric disorder. *The American Journal of Psychiatry* 1996;153: 718–720.

29. Van Zak DB. Biofeedback treatments for premenstrual and premenstrual affective syndromes. *International Journal of Psychosomatics* 1994;41:53–60.

30. Kirkby RJ. Changes in premenstrual symptoms and irrational thinking following cognitive-behavioral coping skills training. *Journal of Consulting and Clinical Psychology* 1994;62: 1026–1032.

31. Aganoff JA, Boyle GJ. Aerobic exercise, mood states and menstrual cycle symptoms. *Journal of Psychosomatic Research* 1994;38:183–192.

32. Choi PY, Salmon P. Symptom changes across the menstrual cycle in competitive sportswomen, exercisers and sedentary women. *British Journal of Clinical Psychology* 1995;34: 447–460.

33. Steege JF, Blumenthal JA. The effects of aerobic exercise on premenstrual symptoms in middle-aged women. A preliminary study. *Journal of Psychosomatic Research* 1993;37:127–133.

34. Gannon L. The potential role of exercise in the alleviation of menstrual disorders and menopausal symptoms: a theoretical synthesis of recent research. *Women and Health* 1988;14: 105.

35. Kliejnen J, Ter Riet G, Knipschild P. Vitamin B6 in the treatment of premenstrual syndrome—a review. *British Journal of Obstetrics and Gynaecology* 1990;97:847–852.

36. Barr W. Pyridoxine supplements in the premenstrual syndrome. *Practitioner* 1984;228:425–427.

37. Doll H, Brown S, Thurston A, Vessey M. Pyridoxine (vitamin B6) and the premenstrual syndrome: a randomized crossover trial. *Journal of the Royal College of General Practitioners* 1989;39:364–368.

38. Berman MK, Taylor ML, Freeman E. Vitamin B6 in premenstrual syndrome. *Journal of the American Dietetic Association* 1990;90:859–861.

39. Zempleni J. Pharmacokinetics of vitamin B6 supplements in humans. *Journal of the American College of Nutrition* 1995; 14:579–586.

40. Majumdar P, Boylan M. Alteration of tissue magnesium levels in rats by dietary vitamin B6 supplementation. *International Journal for Vitamin and Nutrition Research* 1989;59:300–303.

41. Posaci C, Erten O, Uren A, Acar B. Plasma copper, zinc, and magnesium levels in patients with premenstrual tension syndrome. *Acta Obstetricia et Gynecologica Scandinavica* 1994;73:452–455.

42. Piesse JW. Nutritional factors in the premenstrual syndrome. *International Clinical Nutrition Review* 1984;4:54–81.

43. Facchinetti F, Borella P, Sances G, et al. Oral magnesium successfully relieves premenstrual mood changes. *Obstetrics & Gynecology* 1991;78:177–181.

44. Rosenstein DL, Elin RJ, Hosseini JM, et al. Magnesium measures across the menstrual cycle in premenstrual syndrome. *Biological Psychiatry* 1994;35: 557–561.

45. London RS, Bradley R, Chiamori NY. Effect of a nutritional supplement on premenstrual symptomatology in women with premenstrual syndrome: a double-blind longitudinal study. *Journal of the American College of Nutrition* 1991;10:494–499.

46. Stewart A. Clinical and bio-

chemical effects of nutritional supplementation on the premenstrual syndrome. *The Journal of Reproductive Medicine* 1987;32:435–441.

47. Lindberg JS, Zobitz MM, Poindexter JR, Pak CY. Magnesium bioavailability from magnesium citrate and magnesium oxide. *Journal of the American College of Nutrition* 1990;9:48–55.

48. Bohmer T, Roseth A, Holm H, et al. Bioavailability of oral magnesium supplementation in female students evaluated from elimination of magnesium in 24-hour urine. *Magnesium and Trace Elements* 1990;9:272–278.

49. Thys-Jacobs S, Starkey P, Bernstein D, Tian J. Calcium carbonate and the premenstrual syndrome: effects on premenstrual and menstrual symptoms. Premenstrual Syndrome Study Group. *American Journal of Obstetrics & Gynecology* 1998 Aug;179(2):444–452.

50. Penland JG, Johnson PE. Dietary calcium and manganese effects on menstrual cycle symptoms. *American Journal of Obstetrics & Gynecology* 1993; 168:1417–1423.

51. Thys-Jacobs S, Ceccarelli S, Bierman A. Calcium supplementation in premenstrual syndrome: a randomized crossover trial. *Journal of General Internal Medicine* 1989;4:183–189.

52. Chuong CJ, Dawson EB. Zinc and copper levels in premenstrual syndrome. *Fertility and Sterility* 1994;62:313–320.

53. Judd AM, Macleod RM, Login IS. Zinc acutely, selectively and reversibly inhibits pituitary prolactin secretion. *Brain Research* 1984;294:190–192.

54. London RS, Sundaram G, Manimekalai S, et al. The effect of alpha-tocopherol on premenstrual symptomatology: a double-blind study. II. Endocrine correlates. *Journal of the American College of Nutrition* 1984;3:351–356.

55. Horrobin DF, Manku M, Brush M, et al. Abnormalities in plasma essential fatty acid levels in women with premenstrual syndrome and with non-malignant breast disease. *Journal of Nutritional and Environmental Medicine* 1991;2:259–264.

56. Budeiri D, Li Wan Po A, Dornan JC. Is evening primrose oil of value in the treatment of premenstrual syndrome? *Controlled Clinical Trials* 1996;17: 60–68.

57. Khoo SK, Munro C, Battistutta D. Evening primrose oil and treatment of premenstrual syndrome. *The Medical Journal of Australia* 1990;153:189–192.

58. Steinberg S, Annable L, Young SN, Liyanage N. A placebo-controlled study of the effects of L-tryptophan in patients with premenstrual dysphoria. *Advances in Experimental Medicine and Biology* 1999;467: 85–88.

59. Steinberg S, Annable L, Young SN, Bélanger MC. Tryptophan in the treatment of late luteal phase dysphoric disorder: a pilot study. *Journal of Psychiatry & Neuroscience* 1994 Mar;19(2): 114–119.

60. Dittmar FW. [Premenstrual syndrome: treatment with a phytopharmaceutical.] *Therapiewoche Gynäkologie* 1992;5: 60–68.

61. Peteres-Welte C, Albrecht M. [Menstrual abnormalities and PMS. *Vitex agnus-castus*.] *Therapiewoche Gynäkologie* 1994;7: 49–52.

62. Schellenberg R. Treatment for the premenstrual syndrome with agnus castus fruit extract: prospective, randomized, placebo controlled study. *BMJ* 2001;322:134–137.

63. Atmaca M, Kumru S, Tezcan C. Fluoxetine versus *Vitex agnus castus* extract in the treatment of premenstrual dysphoric syndrome. *Human Psychopharmacology* 2003;3:191–5.

64. He Z, Chen R, Zhou Y, et al. Treatment for premenstrual syndrome with *Vitex agnus castus*: a prospective, randomized, multi-center placebo controlled study in China. *Maturitas* 2009; 63:99–103.

65. Van Die M, Bone K, Burger H, et al. Effects of a combination of *Hypericum perforatum* and *Vitex agnus-castus* on PMS-like symptoms in late-perimenopausal women: findings from a subpopulation analysis. *The Journal of Alternative and Complementary Medicine* 2009; 15(9):1045–1048.

66. Tamborini A, Taurelle R. [Value of standardized *Ginkgo biloba* extract in the management of congestive symptoms of premenstrual syndrome.] *Revue Française de Gynécologie et d'Obstetrique* 1993;88:447–457.

67. Ozgoli G, Selselei E, Mojab F, Majd H. A randomized, placebo-controlled trial of *Ginkgo biloba* L. in treatment of premenstrual syndrome. *The Journal of Alternative and Complementary Medicine* 2009 Aug;15(8):845–851.

68. Canning S, Waterman M, Orsi N, et al. The efficacy of *Hypericum perforatum* (St John's wort) for the treatment of premenstrual syndrome. *CNS Drugs* 2010; 24(3):207–225.

69. Stevinson C, Ernst E. A pilot study of *Hypericum perforatum* for the treatment of premenstrual syndrome. *British Journal of Obstetrics and Gynaecology* 2000;107:870–876.

70. Agha-Hosseini M, Kashani L, Aleyaseen A, et al. *Crocus sativus* L. (saffron) in the treatment of premenstrual syndrome: a double-blind, randomised and placebo-controlled trial. *British Journal of Obstetrics and Gynaecology* 2008;115:515–519.

Prostate Cancer (Prevention)

1. Ilic D, O'Connor D, Green S, Wilt TJ. Screening for prostate cancer: an updated Cochrane systematic review. *BJU Inter-*

national 2011 Mar;107(6):882–891.

2. Chou R, Croswell JM, Dana T, et al. Screening for prostate cancer: a review of the evidence for the U.S. Preventive Services Task Force. *Annals of Internal Medicine* 2011 Nov 4 [epub ahead of print].

3. Hawk E, Breslow RA, Graubard BI. Male pattern baldness and clinical prostate cancer in the epidemiologic follow-up of the first National Health and Nutrition Examination Survey. *Cancer Epidemiology, Biomarkers & Prevention* 2000;9:523–527.

4. Fair WR, Fleshner NE, Heston W. Cancer of the prostate: a nutritional disease? *Urology* 1997;50:840–848.

5. Hori S, Butler E, McLoughlin J. Prostate cancer and diet: food for thought? *BJU International* 2011 May;107(9):1348–1359.

6. Venkateswaran V, Klotz LH. Diet and prostate cancer: mechanisms of action and implications for chemoprevention. *Nature Reviews Urology* 2010 Aug;7(8): 442–453.

7. John EM, Stern MC, Sinha R, Koo J. Meat consumption, cooking practices, meat mutagens, and risk of prostate cancer. *Nutrition and Cancer* 2011 May; 63(4):525–537.

8. Raimondi S, Mabrouk JB, Shatenstein B, et al. Diet and prostate cancer risk with specific focus on dairy products and dietary calcium: a case-control study. *Prostate* 2010 Jul 1;70(10): 1054–1065.

9. Newmark HL, Heaney RP. Dairy products and prostate cancer risk. *Nutrition and Cancer* 2010;62(3):297–299.

10. Hardin J, Cheng I, Witte JS. Impact of consumption of vegetable, fruit, grain, and high glycemic index foods on aggressive prostate cancer risk. *Nutrition and Cancer* 2011;63(6): 860–872.

11. Itsiopoulos C, Hodge A, Kaimakamis M. Can the Medi-terranean diet prevent prostate cancer? *Molecular Nutrition & Food Research* 2009 Feb;53(2): 227–239.

12. Yan L, Spitznagel EL. Soy consumption and prostate cancer risk in men: a revisit of a meta-analysis. *The American Journal of Clinical Nutrition* 2009 Apr; 89(4):1155–1163.

13. Moyad MA. Soy, disease prevention, and prostate cancer. *Seminars in Urologic Oncology* 1999;17:97–102.

14. Jacobsen BK, Knutsen SF, Fraser GE. Does high soy milk intake reduce prostate cancer incidence? The Adventist Health Study (United States). *Cancer Causes and Control* 1998;9:553–557.

15. Travis RC, Spencer EA, Allen NE, et al. Plasma phyto-oestrogens and prostate cancer in the European Prospective Investigation into Cancer and Nutrition. *British Journal of Cancer* 2009 Jun 2;100(11):1817–1823.

16. Norrish AE, Skeaff CM, Arribas GL, et al. Prostate cancer risk and consumption of fish oils: a dietary biomarker-based case-control study. *British Journal of Cancer* 1999;81:1238–1242.

17. Williams CD, Whitley BM, Hoyo C, et al. A high ratio of dietary n-6/n-3 polyunsaturated fatty acids is associated with increased risk of prostate cancer. *Nutrition Research* 2011 Jan; 31(1):1–8.

18. Newcomer LM, King IB, Wicklund KG, Stanford JL. The association of fatty acids with prostate cancer risk. *Prostate* 2001;47:262–268.

19. Gann PH, Hennekens CH, Sacks FM, et al. Prospective study of plasma fatty acids and risk of prostate cancer. *Journal of the National Cancer Institute* 1994;86:281–286.

20. Giovannucci E, Rimm EB, Colditz GA, et al. A prospective study of dietary fat and risk of prostate cancer. *Journal of the National Cancer Institute* 1993; 85:1571–1579.

21. Simon JA, Chen YH, Bent S. The relation of alpha-linolenic acid to the risk of prostate cancer: a systematic review and meta-analysis. *The American Journal of Clinical Nutrition* 2009 May;89(5):1558S–1564S.

22. Hayes RB, Ziegler RG, Gridley G, et al. Dietary factors and risks for prostate cancer among blacks and whites in the United States. *Cancer Epidemiology, Biomarkers & Prevention* 1999; 8:25–34.

23. Demark-Wahnefried W, Price DT, Polascik TJ, et al. Pilot study of dietary fat restriction and flaxseed supplementation in men with prostate cancer before surgery: exploring the effects on hormonal levels, prostate-specific antigen, and histopathologic features. *Urology* 2001;58: 47–52.

24. Heinonen OP, Albanes D, Virtamo J, et al. Prostate cancer and supplementation with alpha-tocopherol and ß-carotene: incidence and mortality in a controlled trial. *Journal of the National Cancer Institute* 1998; 90:440–446.

25. Helzlsouer KJ, Huang HY, Alberg AJ, et al. Association between alpha-tocopherol, gamma-tocopherol, selenium, and subsequent prostate cancer. *Journal of the National Cancer Institute* 2000;92:2018–2023.

26. Clark LC, Combs GF Jr, Turnbull BW, et al. Effects of selenium supplementation for cancer prevention in patients with carcinoma of the skin. A randomized controlled trial. Nutritional Prevention of Cancer Study Group. *JAMA, The Journal of the American Medical Association* 1996 Dec 25; 276(24):1957–1963.

27. Lippman SM, Klein EA, Goodman PJ, et al. Effect of selenium and vitamin E on risk of prostate cancer and other cancers: the Selenium and Vitamin E

Cancer Prevention Trial (SE-LECT). *JAMA, The Journal of the American Medical Association* 2009 Jan 7;301(1):39–51.

28. Duffield-Lillico AJ, Dalkin BL, Reid ME, et al. Selenium supplementation, baseline plasma selenium status and incidence of prostate cancer: an analysis of the complete treatment period of the Nutritional Prevention of Cancer Trial. *BJU International* 2003;91(7):608–612.

29. Gann PH, Ma J, Giovannucci E, et al. Lower prostate cancer risk in men with elevated plasma lycopene levels: results of a prospective analysis. *Cancer Research* 1999;59:1225–1230.

30. Kucuk O, Sarkar FH, Sakr W, et al. Phase II randomized clinical trial of lycopene supplementation before radical prostatectomy. *Cancer Epidemiology, Biomarkers & Prevention* 2001;10:861–868.

31. Weisburger JH. Lycopene and tomato products in health promotion. *Advances in Experimental Medicine and Biology* 2002;227:924–927.

32. Pastori M, Pfander H, Boscoboinik D, Azzi A. Lycopene in association with alpha-tocopherol inhibits at physiological concentrations proliferation of prostate carcinoma cells. *Biochemical and Biophysical Research Communications* 1998; 250:582–585.

33. Gilbert R, Metcalfe C, Fraser WD, et al. Associations of circulating 25-hydroxyvitamin D with prostate cancer diagnosis, stage and grade. *International Journal of Cancer* 2011 Oct 27. DOI: 10.1002/ijc.27327. [Epub ahead of print.]

34. Seeram NP, Adams LS, Zhang Y, et al. Blackberry, black raspberry, blueberry, cranberry, red raspberry, and strawberry extracts inhibit growth and stimulate apoptosis of human cancer cells in vitro. *Journal of Agricultural and Food Chemistry* 2006 Dec 13;54(25):9329–9339.

35. Kampa M, Theodoropoulou K, Mavromati F, et al. Novel oligomeric proanthocyanidin derivatives interact with membrane androgen sites and induce regression of hormone-independent prostate cancer. *Journal of Pharmacology and Experimental Therapeutics* 2011 Apr; 337(1):24–32.

36. Shang XJ, Yao G, Ge JP, et al. Procyanidin induces apoptosis and necrosis of prostate cancer cell line PC-3 in a mitochondrion-dependent manner. *Journal of Andrology* 2009 Mar–Apr;30(2):122–126.

37. Adhami VM, Khan N, Mukhtar H. Cancer chemoprevention by pomegranate: laboratory and clinical evidence. *Nutrition and Cancer* 2009; 61(6):811–815.

38. Brasky TM, Kristal AR, Navarro SL, et al. Specialty supplements and prostate cancer risk in the VITamins and Lifestyle (VITAL) cohort. *Prostate* 2008 Nov 1;68(15):1647–1654.

39. Rossi M, Bosetti C, Negri E, et al. Flavonoids, proanthocyanidins, and cancer risk: a network of case-control studies from Italy. *Nutrition and Cancer* 2010;62(7):871–877.

40. Khan N, Adhami VM, Mukhtar H. Review: green tea polyphenols in chemoprevention of prostate cancer: preclinical and clinical studies. *Nutrition and Cancer* 2009;61(6):836–841.

41. Wang P, Aronson WJ, Huang M, et al. Green tea polyphenols and metabolites in prostatectomy tissue: implications for cancer prevention. *Cancer Prevention Research* 2010 Aug;3(8):985–993.

42. McLarty J, Bigelow RL, Smith M, et al. Tea polyphenols decrease serum levels of prostate-specific antigen, hepatocyte growth factor, and vascular endothelial growth factor in prostate cancer patients and inhibit production of hepatocyte growth factor and vascular en-dothelial growth factor in vitro. *Cancer Prevention Research* 2009 Jul;2(7):673–782.

43. Bettuzzi S, Brausi M, Rizzi F, et al. Chemoprevention of human prostate cancer by oral administration of green tea catechins in volunteers with high-grade prostate intraepithelial neoplasia: a preliminary report from a one-year proof-of-principle study. *Cancer Research* 2006 Jan 15;66(2):1234–1240.

44. Papaioannou M, Schleich S, Roell D, et al. NBBS isolated from *Pygeum africanum* bark exhibits androgen antagonistic activity, inhibits AR nuclear translocation and prostate cancer cell growth. *Investigational New Drugs* 2010 Dec;28(6): 729–743.

45. Quiles MT, Arbós MA, Fraga A, et al. Antiproliferative and apoptotic effects of the herbal agent *Pygeum africanum* on cultured prostate stromal cells from patients with benign prostatic hyperplasia (BPH). *Prostate* 2010 Jul 1;70(10):1044–1053.

Prostate Enlargement (BPH)

1. Bushman W. Etiology, epidemiology, and natural history of benign prostatic hyperplasia. *Urologic Clinics of North America* 2009 Nov;36(4):403–415.

2. Pearson JD, Lei HH, Beaty TH, et al. Familial aggregation of bothersome benign prostatic hyperplasia symptoms. *Urology* 2003; 61:781–785.

3. Habuchi T, Liqing Z, Suzuki T, et al. Increased risk of prostate cancer and benign prostatic hyperplasia associated with a CYP17 gene polymorphism with a gene dosage effect. *Cancer Research* 2000;60:5710–5713.

4. Horton R. Benign prostatic hyperplasia. A disorder of androgen metabolism in the male. *Journal of the American Geriatrics Society* 1984;32:380–385.

5. Dull P, Reagan RW Jr, Bahnson RR. Managing benign prostatic

hyperplasia. *American Family Physician* 2002;66:77–84.

6. Platz EA, Kawachi I, Rimm EB, et al. Physical activity and benign prostatic hyperplasia. *Archives of Internal Medicine* 1998 Nov 23;158:2349–2356.

7. Suzuki S, Platz EA, Kawachi I, et al. Intakes of energy and macronutrients and the risk of benign prostatic hyperplasia. *The American Journal of Clinical Nutrition* 2002;75:689–697.

8. Zhang SX, Yu B, Guo SL, et al. [Comparison of incidence of BPH and related factors between urban and rural inhabitants in district of Wannan.] *Zhonghua Nan Ke Xue* 2003;9:45–47.

9. Lagiou P, Wuu J, Trichopoulou A, et al. Diet and benign prostatic hyperplasia: a study in Greece. *Urology* 1999;54: 284–290.

10. Ambrosini GL, de Klerk NH, Mackerras D, et al. Dietary patterns and surgically treated benign prostatic hyperplasia: a case control study in Western Australia. *BJU International* 2008 Apr;101(7):853–860.

11. Gass R. Benign prostatic hyperplasia: the opposite effects of alcohol and coffee intake. *BJU International* 2002;90: 649–654.

12. Bush IM, Berman E, Nourkayhan S, et al. Zinc and the prostate. Presented at the annual meeting of the American Medical Association, Chicago, 1974.

13. Fahim M, Fahim Z, Der R, et al. Zinc treatment for the reduction of hyperplasia of the prostate. *Federation Proceedings* 1976;35:361.

14. Leake A, Chrisholm GD, Busuttil A, et al. Subcellular distribution of zinc in the benign and malignant human prostate: evidence for a direct zinc androgen interaction. *Acta Endocrinologica* 1984;105:281–288.

15. Zaichick VY, Sviridova TV, Zaichick SV. Zinc concentration in human prostatic fluid: normal, chronic prostatitis, ade-

noma and cancer. *International Urology and Nephrology* 1996; 28:687–694.

16. Leake A, Chisholm GD, Habib FK. The effect of zinc on the 5-alpha-reduction of testosterone by the hyperplastic human prostate gland. *Journal of Steroid Biochemistry* 1984;20: 651–655.

17. Wallace AM, Grant JK. Effect of zinc on androgen metabolism in the human hyperplastic prostate. *Biochemical Society Transactions* 1975;3:540–542.

18. Judd AM, Macleod RM, Login IS. Zinc acutely, selectively and reversibly inhibits pituitary prolactin secretion. *Brain Research* 1984;294:190–192.

19. Login IS, Thorner MO, MacLeod RM. Zinc may have a physiological role in regulating pituitary prolactin secretion. *Neuroendocrinology* 1983;37: 317–320.

20. Farnsworth WE, Slaunwhite WR, Sharma M, et al. Interaction of prolactin and testosterone in the human prostate. *Urological Research* 1981;9: 79–88.

21. Farrar DJ, Pryor JS. The effect of bromocriptine in patients with benign prostatic hyperplasia. *British Journal of Urology* 1976;48:73–75.

22. DeRosa G, Corsello SM, Ruffilli MP, et al. Prolactin secretion after beer. *The Lancet* 1981;2: 934.

23. Corenblum B, Whitaker M. Inhibition of stress-induced hyperprolactinaemia. *British Medical Journal* 1977;2:1328.

24. Chyou PH, Nomura AM, Stemmermann GN, et al. A prospective study of alcohol, diet, and other lifestyle factors in relation to obstructive uropathy. *Prostate* 1993;22:253–264.

25. Chyou PH, Nomura AM, Stemmermann GN, et al. A prospective study of alcohol, diet, and other lifestyle factors in relation to obstructive uropathy. *Prostate* 1993;22:253–264.

26. Damrau F. Benign prostatic hypertrophy: amino acid therapy for symptomatic relief. *Journal of the American Geriatrics Society* 1962;10:426–430.

27. Feinblatt HM, Gant JC. Palliative treatment of benign prostatic hypertrophy; value of glycine-alanine-glutamic acid combination. *The Journal of the Maine Medical Association* 1958;49:99–101.

28. Tilvis RS, Miettinen TA. Serum plant sterols and their relation to cholesterol absorption. *The American Journal of Clinical Nutrition* 1986;43:92–97.

29. Berges RR, Windeler J, Tramisch HJ, et al. Randomised, placebo-controlled, double-blind clinical trial of beta-sitosterol in patients with benign prostatic hyperplasia. Beta-sitosterol Study Group. *The Lancet* 1995; 345:1529–1532.

30. Buck AC. Phytotherapy for the prostate. *British Journal of Urology* 1996;78:325–336.

31. Wilt TJ, Ishani A, Stark G, et al. Saw palmetto extracts for treatment of benign prostatic hyperplasia: a systematic review. *JAMA, The Journal of the American Medical Association* 1998;280:1604–1609.

32. Wilt T, Ishani A, MacDonald R. *Serenoa repens* for benign prostatic hyperplasia. Cochrane Database of Systematic Reviews 2002;3:CD001423.

33. Wilt T, Ishani A, Stark G, et al. *Serenoa repens* for benign prostatic hyperplasia. Cochrane Database of Systematic Reviews 2000;2:CD001423.

34. Gordon AE, Shaughnessy AF. Saw palmetto for prostate disorders. *American Family Physician* 2003;67:1281–1283.

35. Bent S, Kane C, Shinohara K, et al. Saw palmetto for benign prostatic hyperplasia. *The New England Journal of Medicine* 2006;354(6):557–566.

36. Yasumoto R, Kawanishi H, Tsujino, et al. Clinical evaluation of long-term treatment using cer-

nitin pollen extract in patients with benign prostatic hyperplasia. *Clinical Therapeutics* 1995; 17:82–86.

37. Buck AC, Cox R, Rees RW, et al. Treatment of outflow tract obstruction due to benign prostatic hyperplasia with the pollen extract, cernilton. A double-blind, placebo-controlled study. *British Journal of Urology* 1990;66:398–404.

38. Dutkiewicz S. Usefulness of cernilton in the treatment of benign prostatic hyperplasia. *International Urology and Nephrology* 1996;28:49–53.

39. Habib FK, Ross M, Lawenstein A. Identification of a prostate inhibitory substance in a pollen extract. *Prostate* 1995;26: 133–139.

40. MacDonald R, Ishani A, Rutks I, et al. A systematic review of cernilton for the treatment of benign prostatic hyperplasia. *BJU International* 2000; 85:836–841.

41. Edgar AD, Levin R, Constantinou CE, Denis L. A critical review of the pharmacology of the plant extract of *Pygeum africanum* in the treatment of LUTS. *Neurourology and Urodynamics* 2007;26(4):458–463.

42. Duvia R, Radice GP, Galdini R. Advances in the phytotherapy of prostatic hypertrophy. *Mediz Praxis* 1983;4:143–148.

43. Belaiche P, Lievoux O. Clinical studies on the palliative treatment of prostatic adenoma with extract of *Urtica* root. *Phytotherapy Research* 1991;5:267–269.

44. Romics I. Observations with Bazoton in the management of prostatic hyperplasia. *International Urology and Nephrology* 1987;19:293–297.

45. Sokeland J. Combined sabal and urtica extract compared with finasteride in men with benign prostatic hyperplasia: analysis of prostate volume and therapeutic outcome. *BJU International* 2000;86:439–442.

46. Wagner H, Willer F, Samtleben R, et al. Search for the antiprostatic principle of stinging nettle (*Urtica dioica*) roots. *Phytomedicine* 1994;1:213–224.

47. Schottner M, Gansser D, Spiteller G. Lignans from the roots of *Urtica dioica* and their metabolites bind to human sex hormone binding globulin (SHBG). *Planta Medica* 1997; 63:529–532.

Psoriasis

1. Chandran V, Raychaudhuri SP. Geoepidemiology and environmental factors of psoriasis and psoriatic arthritis. *Journal of Autoimmunity* 2010 May;34(3): J314–J321.

2. Roberson ED, Bowcock AM. Psoriasis genetics: breaking the barrier. *Trends in Genetics* 2010 Sep;26(9):415–423.

3. Elder JT, Bruce AT, Gudjonsson JE, et al. Molecular dissection of psoriasis: integrating genetics and biology. *Journal of Investigative Dermatology* 2010 May; 130(5):1213–1226.

4. Nair RP, Ding J, Duffin KC, et al. Psoriasis bench to bedside: genetics meets immunology. *Archives of Dermatology* 2009 Apr;145(4):462–464.

5. Robert C, Kupper TS. Inflammatory skin diseases, T cells and immune surveillance. *The New England Journal of Medicine* 1999;341:1817–1878.

6. Traub, M, Marshall K. Psoriasis—pathophysiology, conventional, and alternative approaches to treatment. *Alternative Medicine Review* 2007 Dec;12(4):319–330.

7. Tonel G, Conrad C. Interplay between keratinocytes and immune cells—recent insights into psoriasis pathogenesis. *The International Journal of Biochemistry & Cell Biology* 2009 May; 41(5):963–968.

8. Wahie S, Alexandroff A, Reynolds NJ, Meggit SJ. Psoriasis occurring after myeloablative therapy and autologous stem cell transplantation. *British Journal of Dermatology* 2006; 154:194–195.

9. Eedy DJ, Burrows D, Bridges JM, Jones FG. Clearance of severe psoriasis after allogenic bone marrow transplantation. *BMJ* 1990;300:908.

10. Ojetti V, Aguilar Sanchez J, Guerriero C, et al. High prevalence of celiac disease in psoriasis. *The American Journal of Gastroenterology* 2003;98: 2574–2575.

11. Najarian DJ, Gottlieb AB. Connections between psoriasis and Crohn's disease. *Journal of the American Academy of Dermatology* 2003;48:805–821.

12. Gisondi P, Del Giglio M, Cozzi A, Girolomoni G. Psoriasis, the liver, and the gastrointestinal tract. *Dermatology and Therapy* 2010 Mar–Apr;23(2): 155–159.

13. Scarpa R, Manguso F, D'Arienzo A, et al. Microscopic inflammatory changes in colon of patients with both active psoriasis and psoriatic arthritis without bowel symptoms. *The Journal of Rheumatology* 2000;27:1241–1246.

14. Proctor M, Wilkenson D, Orenberg E, et al. Lowered cutaneous and urinary levels of polyamines with clinical improvement in treated psoriasis. *Archives of Dermatology* 1979; 115:945–949.

15. Voorhees JJ. Polyamines and psoriasis. *Archives of Dermatology* 1979;115:943–944.

16. McDonald CJ. Polyamines in psoriasis. *Journal of Investigative Dermatology* 1983;81:385–387.

17. Haddox M, Scott KF, Russel D. Retinol inhibition of ornithine decarboxylase induction and G1 progression in Chinese hamster ovary cells. *Cancer Research* 1979;39:4930–4938.

18. Kuwano S, Yamauchi K. Effect of berberine on tyrosine decarboxylase activity of *Streptococcus faecalis*. *Chemical and*

Pharmaceutical Bulletin 1960; 8:491–496.

19. Rosenberg E, Belew P. Microbial factors in psoriasis. *Archives of Dermatology* 1982; 118:1434–1444.

20. Rao M, Field M. Enterotoxins and ion transport. *Biochemical Society Transactions* 1984;12: 177–180.

21. Juhlin L, Vahlquist C. The influence of treatment and fibrin microclot generation in psoriasis. *British Journal of Dermatology* 1983;108:33–37.

22. Gyurcsovics K, Bertók L. Pathophysiology of psoriasis: coping endotoxins with bile acid therapy. *Pathophysiology* 2003;10: 57–61.

23. Thurmon FM. The treatment of psoriasis with sarsaparilla compound. *The New England Journal of Medicine* 1942;337: 128–133.

24. Weber G, Galle K. [The liver, a therapeutic target in dermatoses.] *Medizinische Welt* 1983;34: 108–111.

25. Pietrzak A, Lecewicz-Toruń B, Kadziela-Wypyska G. [Changes in the digestive system in patients suffering from psoriasis.] *Annales Universitatis Mariae Curie Sklodowska. Sectio D: Med* 1998;53:187–194.

26. Monk BE, Neill SM. Alcohol consumption and psoriasis. *Dermatologica* 1986;173:57–60.

27. Hikino H, Kiso Y, Wagner H, et al. Antihepatotoxic actions of flavonolignans from *Silybum marianum* fruits. *Planta Medica* 1984;50:248–250.

28. Adzet T. Polyphenolic compounds with biological and pharmacological activity. In *Herbs, spices, and medicinal plants*, vol. 1, ed. Craker LE, Simon JE. Binghamton, N.Y.: Food Products Press, 1986, 167–184.

29. Bittiner SB, Tucker WF, Cartwright I, et al. A double-blind, randomized, placebo-controlled trial of fish oil in psoriasis. *The Lancet* 1988;1:378–380.

30. Grimmunger F, Mayser P, Papavassilis C. A double-blind, randomized, placebo-controlled trial of N-3 fatty acid based lipid infusion in acute, extended guttate psoriasis. Rapid improvement of clinical manifestations and changes in neutrophil leukotriene profile. *Clinical Investigation* 1993;71:634–643.

31. Maurice PD, Allen BR, Barkley AS, et al. The effects of dietary supplementation with fish oil in patients with psoriasis. *British Journal of Dermatology* 1987; 1117:599–606.

32. Mayser P, Grimm H, Grimminger F. N-3 fatty acids in psoriasis. *British Journal of Nutrition* 2002;87:S77–S82.

33. Lithell H, Bruce A, Gustafsson IB, et al. A fasting and vegetarian diet treatment trial on chronic inflammatory disorders. *Acta Dermato-Venereologica* 1983;63:397–403.

34. Douglas JM. Psoriasis and diet. *California Medicine* 1980;133: 450.

35. Bazex A. Diet without gluten and psoriasis. *Annals of Dermatology Symposiums* 1976;103:648.

36. Aggarwal BB, Shishodia S. Suppression of the nuclear factor-kappaB activation pathway by spice-derived phytochemicals: reasoning for seasoning. *Annals of the New York Academy of Sciences* 2004;1030:434–441.

37. Majewski S, Janik P, Langer A, et al. Decreased levels of vitamin A in serum of patients with psoriasis. *Archives of Dermatological Research* 1989;280: 499–501.

38. Hinks LJ, Young S, Clayton B. Trace element status in eczema and psoriasis. *Clinical and Experimental Dermatology* 1987; 12:93–97.

39. Donadini A, Dazzaglia A, Desirello G. [Plasma levels of Zn, Cu and Ni in healthy controls and in psoriatic patients. Possible correlations with vitamins.] *Acta Vitaminologica et Enzymologica* 1980;1:9–16.

40. Fratino P, Pelfini C, Jucci A, et al. Glucose and insulin in psoriasis: the role of obesity and genetic history. *Panminerva Medica* 1979 Oct–Dec;21(4): 167–172.

41. Kimball AB, Wu Y. Cardiovascular disease and classic cardiovascular risk factors in patients with psoriasis. *International Journal of Dermatology* 2009 Nov;48(11):1147–1156.

42. Rocha-Pereira P, Santos-Silva A, Rebelo I, et al. Dyslipidemia and oxidative stress in mild and in severe psoriasis as a risk for cardiovascular disease. *Clinica Chimica Acta* 2001;303:33–39.

43. Ludwig RJ, Herzog C, Rostock A, et al. Psoriasis: a possible risk factor for development of coronary artery calcification. *British Journal of Dermatology* 2007;156:271–276.

44. Vanizor Kural B, Orem A, et al. Plasma homocysteine and its relationship with atherothrombotic markers in psoriatic patients. *Clinica Chimica Acta* 2003;332:23–30.

45. Malerba M, Gisondi P, Radaeli A, et al. Plasma homocysteine and folate levels in patients with chronic plaque psoriasis. *British Journal of Dermatology* 2006;155:1165–1169.

46. Juhlin L, Edqvist LE, Ekman LG, et al. Blood glutathione-peroxidase levels in skin diseases: effect of selenium and vitamin E treatment. *Acta Dermato-Venereologica* 1982;62: 211–214.

47. Serwin AB, Wasowicz W, Gromadzinska J, et al. Selenium status in psoriasis and its relations to the duration and severity of the disease. *Nutrition* 2003;19: 301–304.

48. Michaelsson G, Berne B, Calmark B, et al. Selenium in whole blood and plasma is decreased in patients with moderate and severe psoriasis. *Acta Dermato-Venereologica* 1989;69:29–34.

49. Staberg B, Oxholm A, Klemp P, Christiansen C. Abnormal vita-

min D metabolism in patients with psoriasis. *Acta Dermato-Venereologica* 1987;67:65–68.

50. Reichrath J. Vitamin D and the skin: an ancient friend, revisited. *Experimental Dermatology* 2007;16:618–625.

51. Mendonça CO, Burden AD. Current concepts in psoriasis and its treatment. *Pharmacology & Therapeutics* 2003;99: 133–147.

52. Peric M, Koglin S, Dombrowski Y, et al. Vitamin D analogs differentially control antimicrobial peptide/"alarmin" expression in psoriasis. *PLoS One* 2009 Jul 22:4(7):e6340.

53. Gorman S, Judge MA, Hart PH. Immune-modifying properties of topical vitamin D: focus on dendritic cells and T cells. *The Journal of Steroid Biochemistry and Molecular Biology* 2010 Jul; 121(1–2):247–249.

54. Okita H, Ohtsuka T, Yamakage A, Yamazaki S. Polymorphism of the vitamin D(3) receptor in patients with psoriasis. *Archives of Dermatological Research* 2002;294:159–162.

55. Jacobs ET, Alberts DS, Foote JA, et al. Vitamin D insufficiency in southern Arizona. *The American Journal of Clinical Nutrition* 2008 March;87(3): 608–613.

56. Grant WB, Holick MF. Benefits and requirements of vitamin D for optimal health: a review. *Alternative Medicine Review* 2005;10:94–111.

57. Altmeyer PJ, Matthes U, Pawlak F, et al. Antipsoriatic effect of fumaric acid derivatives. Results of a multicenter double-blind study in 100 patients. *Journal of the American Academy of Dermatology* 1994;30: 977–981.

58. Nieboer C, de Hoop D, van Loenen AC, et al. Systemic therapy with fumaric acid derivates: new possibilities in the treatment of psoriasis. *Journal of the American Academy of Dermatology* 1989;20:601–608.

59. Basavaraj KH, Navya MA, Rashmi R. Stress and quality of life in psoriasis: an update. *International Journal of Dermatology* 2011 Jul;50(7):783–792.

60. Kazandjieva J, Grozdev I, Darlenski R, Tsankov N. Climatotherapy of psoriasis. *Clinics in Dermatology* 2008;269(5): 477–485.

61. Ben-Amitai D, David M. Climatotherapy at the Dead Sea for pediatric-onset psoriasis vulgaris. *Pediatric Dermatology* 2009;26(1):103–104.

62. Snellman E, Lauharanta J, Reunanen A, et al. Effect of heliotherapy on skin and joint symptoms in psoriasis: a 6-month follow-up study. *British Journal of Dermatology* 1993;128:172–177.

63. Fleischer AB Jr, Feldman SR, Rapp SR, et al. Alternative therapies commonly used within a population of patients with psoriasis. *Cutis* 1996;58:216–220.

64. Fleischer AB Jr, Clark AR, Rapp SR, et al. Commercial tanning bed treatment is an effective psoriasis treatment: results from an uncontrolled clinical trial. *Journal of Investigative Dermatology* 1997;109:170–174.

64. Markham T, Rogers S, Collins P. Narrowband UV-B (TL-01) phototherapy vs oral 8-methoxypsoralen psoralen-UV-A for the treatment of chronic plaque psoriasis. *Archives of Dermatology* 2003;139:325–328.

66. Das S, Lloyd JJ, Walshaw D, et al. Response of psoriasis to sunbed treatment: comparison of conventional ultraviolet A lamps with new higher ultraviolet B-emitting lamps. *British Journal of Dermatology* 2002; 147:966–972.

67. Kudish AI, Abels D, Harari M. Ultraviolet radiation properties as applied to photoclimatherapy at the Dead Sea. *International Journal of Dermatology* 2003; 42:359–365.

68. Kushelevsky AP, Harari M, Kudish AI, et al. Safety of solar phototherapy at the Dead Sea. *Journal of the American Academy of Dermatology* 1998;38: 447–452.

69. Tanghetti EA. The role of topical vitamin D modulators in psoriasis therapy. *The Journal of Drugs in Dermatology* 2009 Aug;8(8 suppl):s4-s8.

70. Syed TA, Ahmad SA, Holt AH, et al. Management of psoriasis with *Aloe vera* extract in a hydrophilic cream: a placebo-controlled, double-blind study. *Tropical Medicine & International Health* 1996 Aug;1(4): 505–509.

71. Choonhakarn C, Busaracome P, Sripanidkulchai B, Sarakarn P. A prospective, randomized clinical trial comparing topical aloe vera with 0.1% triamcinolone acetonide in mild to moderate plaque psoriasis. *Journal of the European Academy of Dermatology and Venereology* 2010 Feb;24(2):168–172.

72. Ellis CN, Berberian B, Sulica VI, et al. A double-blind evaluation of topical capsaicin in pruritic psoriasis. *Journal of the American Academy of Dermatology* 1993;29:438–442.

73. Bernstein JE, Parish LC, Rapaport M, et al. Effects of topically applied capsaicin on moderate and severe psoriasis vulgaris. *Journal of the American Academy of Dermatology* 1986;15: 504–507.

74. Heng MC, Song MK, Harker J, Heng MK. Drug-induced suppression of phosphorylase kinase activity correlates with resolution of psoriasis as assessed by clinical, histological and immunohistochemical parameters. *British Journal of Dermatology*. 2000 Nov;143(5): 937–949.

75. Lew BL, Cho Y, Kim J, et al. Ceramides and cell signaling molecules in psoriatic epidermis: reduced levels of ceramides, PKC-alpha, and JNK. *J Korean Med Science* 2006 Feb; 21(1):95–99.

Rheumatoid Arthritis

1. Aletaha D, Neogi T, Silman AJ. Rheumatoid arthritis classification criteria: an American College of Rheumatology/European League Against Rheumatism collaborative initiative. *Annals of the Rheumatic Diseases* 2010 Sep;69(9):1580–1588.

2. Meda F, Folci M, Baccarelli A, Selmi C. The epigenetics of autoimmunity. *Cellular & Molecular Immunology* 2011 May;8(3):226–236.

3. van de Merwe J P, Stegeman J H, Hazenberg M P. The resident faecal flora is determined by genetic characteristics of the host. Implications for Crohn's disease? *Antonie van Leeuwenhoek* 1993;49:119–124.

4. Kobayashi S, Momohara S, Kamatani N, Okamoto H. Molecular aspects of rheumatoid arthritis: role of environmental factors. *FEBS Journal* 2008 Sep;275(18):4456–4462.

5. Stolt P, Bengtsson C, Nordmark B, et al. Quantification of the influence of cigarette smoking on rheumatoid arthritis: results from a population based case-control study, using incident cases. *Annals of the Rheumatic Diseases* 2003;62(9):835–841.

6. Symmons DP. Environmental factors and the outcome of rheumatoid arthritis. *Best Practice & Research: Clinical Rheumatology* 2003;17:717–727.

7. Strusberg I, Mendelberg RC, Serra HA, Strusberg AM. Influence of weather conditions on rheumatic pain. *The Journal of Rheumatology* 2002;29:335–338.

8. Ling S, Li Z, Borschukova O, et al. The rheumatoid arthritis shared epitope increases susceptibility to oxidative stress by antagonizing an adenosine-mediated anti-oxidative pathway. *Arthritis Research & Therapy* 2007;9(1):R5.

9. Tak PP. Rheumatoid arthritis and p53: how oxidative stress might alter the course of inflammatory diseases. *Immunology Today* 2000;21:78–82.

10. Karlson EW, Chibnik LB, Tworoger SS, et al. Biomarkers of inflammation and development of rheumatoid arthritis in women from two prospective cohorts. *Arthritis & Rheumatism* 2009 Mar;60(3):641–652.

11. van Gaalen F, Ion-Facsinay A, Huizinga TW, Toes RE. The devil in the details: the emerging role of anticitrulline autoimmunity in rheumatoid arthritis. *The Journal of Immunology* 2005;175:5575–5580.

12. Wyburn-Mason R. The naeglerial causation of rheumatoid disease and many human cancers: a new concept in medicine. *Medical Hypotheses* 1979;5:1237–1249.

13. Wojtulewski JA, Gow PJ, Walter J, et al. Clotriamzole in rheumatoid arthritis. *Annals of the Rheumatic Diseases* 1980;39(5):469–472.

14. Agarwal V, Singh R, Chauhan S. Remission of rheumatoid arthritis after acute disseminated varicella-zoster infection. *Clinical Rheumatology* 2007 May;26(5):779–780.

15. Ogrendik M. Efficacy of roxithromycin in adult patients with rheumatoid arthritis who had not received disease-modifying antirheumatic drugs: a 3-month, randomized, double-blind, placebo-controlled trial. *Clinical Therapeutics* 2009 Aug;31(8):1754–1764.

16. Stone M, Fortin PR, Pacheco-Tena C, Inman RD. Should tetracycline treatment be used more extensively for rheumatoid arthritis? Metaanalysis demonstrates clinical benefit with reduction in disease activity. *The Journal of Rheumatology* 2003 Oct;30(10):2112–2122.

17. Schipper LG, Fransen J, Barrera P, et al. Methotrexate therapy in rheumatoid arthritis after failure to sulphasalazine: to switch or to add? *Rheumatology* (Oxford) 2009 Oct;48(10):1247–1253.

18. Tilley BC, Alarcon GS, Heyse SP, et al. Minocycline in rheumatoid arthritis. A 48-week, double-blind, placebo-controlled trial. *Annals of Internal Medicine* 1995; 122(2):81–89.

19. Toivanen P, Vaahtovuo J, Eerola E. Influence of major histocompatibility complex on bacterial composition of fecal flora. *Infection and Immunity* 2001 Apr;69(4):2372–2377.

20. Sekirov I, Russell SL, Caetano L, et al. Gut microbiota in health and disease. *Physiology Reviews* 2010;90:859–904.

21. Hooper LV, Wong MH, Thelin A, et al. Olecular analysis of commensal host-microbial relationships in the intestine. *Science* 2001 Feb 2;291(5505):881–884.

22. Vaahtovuo J, Munukka E, Korkeamäki M, et al. Fecal microbiota in early rheumatoid arthritis. *The Journal of Rheumatology* 2008 Aug;35(8):1500–1505.

23. Peltonen R, Kjeldsen-Kvagh J, Haugen M, et al. Changes in faecal flora in rheumatoid arthritis during fasting and one-year vegetarian diet. *British Journal of Rheumatology* 1994 Jan;33(7):638–643.

24. Peltonen R, Nenonen M, Helve T, et al. Faecal microbial flora and disease activity in rheumatoid arthritis during a vegan diet. *British Journal of Rheumatology* 1997 Jan;36(1):64–68.

25. Henrikksson AE, Blomquist L, Nord CE, et al. Small intestinal bacterial overgrowth in patients with rheumatoid arthritis. *Annals of the Rheumatic Diseases* 1993 Jul;52(7):503–510.

26. Martinez-Martinez RE, Abud-Mendoza C, Patiño-Marin N, et al. Detection of periodontal bacterial DNA in serum and synovial fluid in refractory rheumatoid arthritis patients. *Jour-*

nal of Clinical Periodontology 2009 Dec;36(12):1004–1010.

27. Mercado FB, Marshall RI, Klestov AC, Bartold PM. Relationship between rheumatoid arthritis and periodontitis. *Journal of Periodontology* June 2001;72(6):779–787.

28. Hitchon CA, Chandad F, Ferucci ED, et al. Antibodies to porphyromonas gingivalis are associated with anticitrullinated protein antibodies in patients with rheumatoid arthritis and their relatives. *The Journal of Rheumatology* 2010 Jun;37(6): 1105–1112.

29. Chafen JJ, Newberry SJ, Riedl MA, et al. Diagnosing and managing common food allergies: a systematic review. *JAMA, The Journal of the American Medical Association* 2010 May 12; 303(18):1848–1856.

30. Karatay S, Erdem T, Yildirim K, et al. The effect of individualized diet challenges consisting of allergenic foods on TNF-α and IL-ß levels in patients with rheumatoid arthritis. *Rheumatology* 2004;43(11):1429–1433.

31. Cordian L, Toohey L, Smith MJ, Hickey MS. Modulation of immune function by dietary lectins in rheumatoid arthritis. *British Journal of Nutrition* 2000;83:207–217.

32. Havatum M, Kanerud L, Hällgren R, Brandtzaeg P. The gut-joint axis: cross-reactive food antibodies in rheumatoid arthritis. *Gut* 2006;55:1240–1247.

33. Pawlik A, Ostanek L, Brzosko I, et al. Increased genotype frequency of N-acetyltransferase 2 slow acetylation in patients with rheumatoid arthritis. *Clinical Pharmacology & Therapeutics* 2002 Sep;72(3):319–325.

34. Pawlik A, Ostanek L, Brzosko I, et al. The influence of N-acetyltransferase 2 polymorphism on rheumatoid arthritis activity. *Clinical and Experimental Rheumatology* 2004 Jan–Feb; 22(1):99–102.

35. Vojdani A, Bazargan M, Vojdani

E, et al. Heat shock protein and gliadin peptide promote development of peptidase antibodies in children with autism and patients with autoimmune disease. *Clinical and Diagnostic Laboratory Immunology* 2004 May;11(3):515–524.

36. Vojdani A, Pangborn JB, Vojdani E, Cooper EL. Infections, toxic chemicals and dietary peptides binding to lymphocyte receptors and tissue enzymes are major instigators of autoimmunity in autism. *International Journal of Immunopathology and Pharmacology* 2003 Sep–Dec;16(3):189–99.

37. Smith MD, Gibson RA, Brooks PM. Abnormal bowel permeability in ankylosing spondylitis and rheumatoid arthritis. *The Journal of Rheumatology* 1985; 12:299–305.

38. Zaphiropoulos GC. Rheumatoid arthritis and the gut. *British Journal of Rheumatology* 1986; 25:138–140.

39. Segal AW, Isenberg DA, Hajirousou V, et al. Preliminary evidence for gut involvement in the pathogenesis of rheumatoid arthritis. *British Journal of Rheumatology* 1986 May;25(2): 162–166.

40. Deitch EA, Specian RD, Berg RD. Endotoxin-induced bacterial translocation and mucosal permeability: role of xanthine oxidase, complement activation, and macrophage products. *Critical Care Medicine* 1991 Jun; 19(6):785–791.

41. Bjarnason I, Williams P, So A, et al. Intestinal permeability and inflammation in rheumatoid arthritis: effects of non-steroidal anti-inflammatory drugs. *The Lancet* 1984 Nov 24;2(8413): 1171–1174.

42. Bjarnason I, Peters TJ. Influence of anti-rheumatic drugs on gut permeability and on the gut associated lymphoid tissue. *Ballière's Clinical Rheumatology* 1996;10:165–176.

43. Berg RD. Bacterial transloca-

tion from the gastrointestinal tract. *Advances in Experimental Medicine and Biology* 1999;473: 11–30.

44. Tengstrand B, Carlstrom K, Fellander-Tsai L, Hafstrom I. Abnormal levels of serum dehydroepiandrosterone, estrone, and estradiol in men with rheumatoid arthritis: high correlation between serum estradiol and current degree of inflammation. *The Journal of Rheumatology* 2003 Nov;30(11): 2338–2343.

45. Straub RH, Scholmerich J, Zietz B. Replacement therapy with DHEA plus corticosteroids in patients with chronic inflammatory diseases—substitutes of adrenal and sex hormones. *Zeitschrift für Rheumatologie* 2000;59 suppl 2:II/108–II/118.

46. Kanik KS, Chrousos GP, Schumacher HR, et al. Adrenocorticotropin, glucocorticoid, and androgen secretion in patients with new onset synovitis/rheumatoid arthritis: relations with indices of inflammation. *The Journal of Clinical Endocrinology & Metabolism* 2000 Apr;85(4):1461–1466.

47. Cutolo M, Balleari E, Giusti M, et al. Androgen replacement therapy in male patients with rheumatoid arthritis. *Arthritis & Rheumatism* 1991 Jan;34(1): 1–5.

48. Doran MF, Crowson CS, O'Fallon WM, Gabriel SE. The effect of oral contraceptives and estrogen replacement therapy on the risk of rheumatoid arthritis: a population based study. *The Journal of Rheumatology* 2004;31:207–213.

49. K Forslind, I Hafström, M Ahlmén, B Svensson. Sex: a major predictor of remission in early rheumatoid arthritis? *Annals of the Rheumatic Diseases* 2007 Jan;66(1):46–52.

50. Brandt KD. Effects of nonsteriodal anti-inflammatory drugs on chondrocyte metabolism in vitro and in vivo. *The American*

Journal of Medicine 1987 Nov 20;83(5A):29–34.

51. Vidal y Plana RR, Bizzarri D, Rovati AL. Articular cartilage pharmacology. I. In vitro studies on glucoasamine and non steroidal anti-inflammatory drugs. *Pharmacological Research Commununications* 1978 Jun;10(6): 557–569.

52. Jenkins RT, Rooney PJ, Jones DB, et al. Increased intestinal permeability in patients with rheumatoid arthritis: a side effect of oral nonsteroidal anti-inflammatory drug therapy? *British Journal of Rheumatology* 1987 Apr;26(2):103–107.

53. Dearlove M, Barr K, Neuman V, et al. The effect of non-steroidal anti-inflammatory drugs of faecal flora and bacterial antibody levels in rheumatoid arthritis. *British Journal of Rheumatology* 1992; 31:443–447.

54. Wade CR, Jackson PG, Highton J, VanRij AM. Lipid peroxidation and malondialdehyde in the synovial fluid and plasma of patients with rheumatoid arthrits. *Clinica Chimica Acta* 1987;164:245–250.

55. Singh G. Recent considerations in nonsteroidal anti-inflammatory drug gastropathy. *The American Journal of Medicine* 1998 Jul 27;105(1B):31S–38S.

56. Lombardo L, Foti M, Ruggia O, Chiecchio A. Increased incidence of small intestinal bacterial overgrowth during proton pump inhibitor therapy. *Clinical Gastroenterology and Hepatology* 2010 Jun;8(6):504–508.

57. Laine L, Smith R, Min K, et al. Systematic review: the lower gastrointestinal adverse effects of non-steroidal anti-inflammatory drugs. *Alimentary Pharmacology & Therapeutics* 2006;24:751–767.

58. Mukherjee D, Nissen SE, Topol EJ. Risk of cardiovascular events associated with selective COX-2 inhibitors. *JAMA, The Journal of the American Medical Association* 2001 Aug 22–29;286(8): 954–959.

59. Inotai A, Mészáros A. Economic evaluation of nonsteroidal anti-inflammatory drug strategies in rheumatoid arthritis. *International Journal of Technological Assessment in Health Care* 2009 Apr;25(2):190–195.

60. Segasothy M, Chin GL, Sia KK, et al. Chronic nephrotoxicity of anti-inflammatory drugs used in the treatment of arthritis. *British Journal of Rheumatology* 1995 Feb;34(2):162–165.

61. Sihvonen S, Korpela M, Mustonen J, et al. Mortality in patients with rheumatoid arthritis treated with low-dose oral glucocorticoids. A population-based cohort study. *The Journal of Rheumatology* 2006 Sep; 33(9):1740–1746.

62. Seshadri V, Coyle CH, Chu CR. Lidocaine potentiates the chondrotoxicity of methylprednisolone. *Arthroscopy* 2009 Apr; 25(4):337–347.

63. Vosse D, de Vlam K. Osteoporosis in rheumatoid arthritis and ankylosing spondylitis. *Clinical and Experimental Rheumatology* 2009 Jul–Aug;27(4 suppl 55):S62–S67.

64. Mielants H, Goemaere S, De Vos M, et al. Intestinal mucosal permeability in inflammatory rheumatic diseases. I. Role of anti-inflammatory drugs. *The Journal of Rheumatology* 1991 Mar;18(3):389–393.

65. Chung CP, Avalos I, Raggi P, Stein CM. Atherosclerosis and inflammation: insights from rheumatoid arthritis. *Clinical Rheumatology* 2007 Aug;26(8): 1228–1233.

66. Belt NK, Kronholm E, Kauppl MJ. Sleep problems in fibromyalgia and rheumatoid arthritis compared with the general population. *Clinical and Experimental Rheumatology* 2009 Jan–Feb;27(10):35–41.

67. Mahowald MW, Mahowald ML, Bundlie SR, Ytterberg SR. Sleep fragmentation in rheumatoid arthritis. *Arthritis & Rheumatism* 1989 Aug;32(8):974–983.

68. Margaretten M, Yelin E, Imboden J, et al. Predictors of depression in a multiethnic cohort of patients with rheumatoid arthritis. *Arthritis & Rheumatism* 2009 Nov 15;61(11):1586–1591.

69. Gaujoux-Viala C, Smolen JS, Landewé R, et al. Synthetic disease-modifying antirheumatic drugs: a systematic literature review informing the EULAR recommendations for the management of rheumatoid arthritis. *Annals of the Rheumatic Diseases* 2010 Jun;69(6):1004–1009.

70. Curtis JR, Singh JA. Use of biologics in rheumatoid arthritis: current and emerging paradigms of care. *Clinical Therapeutics* 2011 Jun;33(6):679–707.

71. Winthrop KL. Serious infections with antirheumatic therapy: are biologicals worse? *Annals of the Rheumatic Diseases* 2006 Nov;65(suppl 3): iii54–iii57.

72. Dahlqvist SR, Engstrand S, Berglin E, Johnson O. Conversion toward an atherogenic lipid profile in rheumatoid arthritis patients during long-term infliximab therapy. *Scandinavian Journal of Rheumatology* 2006; 35:107–111.

73. Trowell H, Burkitt D. *Western diseases: their emergence and prevention.* Cambridge, Mass.: Harvard University Press, 1981.

74. Darlington LG, Ramsey NW. Clinical review: Review of dietary therapy for rheumatoid arthritis. *British Journal of Rheumatology* 1993;32:507–514.

75. Buchanan HM, Preston SJ, Brooks PM, Buchannan WW. Is diet important in rheumatoid arthritis? *British Journal of Rheumatology* 1991 Apr;30(2): 125–134.

76. McCrae F, Veerapen K, Dieppe P. Diet and arthritis. *Practitioner* 1986;230:359–361.

77. Kjeldsen-Kragh J. Rheumatoid arthritis treated with vegetarian diets. *The American Journal of Clinical Nutrition* 1999;70 suppl:594S–600S.

78. Darlington LG, Ramsey NW, Mansfield JR. Placebo-controlled, blind study of dietary manipulation therapy in rheumatoid arthritis. *The Lancet* 1986;1:236–238.

79. Hicklin JA, McEwen LM, Morgan JE. The effect of diet in rheumatoid arthritis. *Clinical Allergy* 1980;10:463–467.

80. Panush RS. Delayed reactions to foods. Food allergy and rheumatic disease. *Annals of Allergy, Asthma & Immunology* 1986;56:500–503.

81. Van de Laar MA, Ander Korst JK. Food intolerance in rheumatoid arthritis. I. A double-blind, controlled trial of the clinical effects of elimination of milk allergens and azo dyes. *Annals of the Rheumatic Diseases* 1992; 51:298–302.

82. Darlington LG. Dietary therapy for arthritis. *Rheumatic Disease Clinics of North America* 1991; 17:273–285.

83. Panush R, Carter RL, Katz P, et al. Diet therapy for rheumatoid arthritis. *Arthritis & Rheumatism* 1983 Apr;26(4):462–471.

84. Palmblad J, Hafström I, Ringertz B. Antirheumatic effects of fasting. *Rheumatic Disease Clinics of North America* 1991 May;17(2):351–362.

85. Fraser DA, Thoen J, Djøseland O, et al. Serum levels of interleukin-6 and dehydroepiandrosterone sulphate in response to either fasting or a ketogenic diet in rheumatoid arthritis patients. *Clinical and Experimental Rheumatology* 2000 May–Jun;18(3):357–362.

86. Sundqvist T, Lundström F, Magnusson KE, et al. Influence of fasting on intestinal permeability and disease activity in patients with rheumatoid arthritis. *Scandinavian Journal of Rheumatology* 1982;11(1):33–38.

87. Kjeldsen-Kragh J, Hougen M, Borchgrevink CF, et al. Controlled trial of fasting and one-year vegetarian diet in rheumatoid arthritis. *The Lancet* 1991 Oct 12;338(8772):899–902.

88. Skoldstam L, Larsson L, Lindstrom FD. Effects of fasting and lactovegetarian diet on rheumatoid arthritis. *Scandinavian Journal of Rheumatology* 1979; 8:249–255.

89. Kroker GF, Stroud RM, Marshall R, et al. Fasting and rheumatoid arthritis: a multicenter study. *Archives of Clinical Ecology* 1984;2:137–144.

90. Hafstrom I, Ringertz B, Gyllenhammar H, et al. Effects of fasting on disease activity, neutrophil function, fatty acid composition, and leukotriene biosynthesis in patients with rheumatoid arthritis. *Arthritis & Rheumatism* 1988 May;31(5): 585–592.

91. Muller H, de Toledo FW, Resch KL. Fasting followed by vegetarian diet in patients with rheumatoid arthritis: a systematic review. *Scandinavian Journal of Rheumatology* 2001; 30(1):1–10.

92. Kjeldsen-Kvagh J, Rashid T, Dybwald A, et al. Decrease in anti–*Proteus mirabilis* but not anti–*Escherichia coli* antibody levels in rheumatoid arthritis patients treated with fasting and a one year vegetarian diet. *Annals of the Rheumatic Diseases* 1995 Mar;54(3):221–224.

93. Darlington LG, Stone TW. Antioxidants and fatty acids in the amelioration of RA and related disorders. *British Journal of Nutrition* 2001;85:251–269.

94. Pattison DJ, Winyard PG. Dietary antioxidants in inflammatory arthritis: do they have any role in etiology or therapy? *Nature Clinical Practice Rheumatology* 2008 Nov;4(11):590–596.

95. Lucas P, Power L. Dietary fat aggravates active rheumatoid arthritis. *Clinical Research* 1981;29:754A.

96. Shapiro JA, Koepsell TD, Voigt LF, et al. Diet and rheumatoid arthritis in women. A possible protective effect of fish consumption. *Epidemiology* 1996 May;7(3):256–263.

97. Pattison DJ, Symmons DP, Lunt M, et al. Dietary risk factors for the development of inflammatory polyarthritis: evidence for a role of high level of red meat consumption. *Arthritis & Rheumatism* 2004 Dec; 50(12):3804–3812.

98. Grant WB. The role of meat in the expression of rheumatoid arthritis. *British Journal of Nutrition* 2000;84:589–595.

99. Waterman E, Lockwood B. Active components and clinical applications of olive oil. *Alternative Medicine Review* 2007; 12(4):331–342.

100. Pattison DJ, Winyard PG. Dietary antioxidants in inflammatory arthritis: do they have any role in etiology or therapy? *Nature Clinical Practice Rheumatology* 2008 Nov;4(11):590–596.

101. Pettersson T, Friman C, Abrahamsson L, et al. Serum homocysteine and methylmalonic acid in patients with rheumatoid arthritis and cobalaminopenia. *The Journal of Rheumatology* 1998 May;25(5):859–863.

102. Schumacher HR, Bernhart FW, György P. Vitamin B6 levels in rheumatoid arthritis: effect of treatment. *The American Journal of Clinical Nutrition* 1975 Nov;28(11):1200–1203.

103. Grennan DM, Knudson JM, Dunckley J, et al. Serum copper and zinc in rheumatoid arthritis and osteoarthritis. *New Zealand Medical Journal* 1980 Jan 23; 91(652):47–50.

104. Tarp U, Overvad K, Hansen JC, Thorling EB. Low selenium level in severe rheumatoid arthritis. *Scandinavian Journal of Rheumatology* 1985;14(2): 97–101.

105. Kremer JM, Bigaouette J. Nutrient intake of patients with rheumatoid arthritis is deficient in pyridoxine, zinc, copper, and magnesium. *The Journal of Rheumatology* 1996 Jun;23(6): 990–994.

106. Munthe E, Aaseth J, Jellum E. Trace elements and rheumatoid arthritis (RA)—pathogenetic and therapeutic aspects. *Acta Pharmacologica et Toxicologica* 1986;59 suppl 7:365–373.

107. Canter PH, Wider B, Ernst E. The antioxidant vitamins A, C, E and selenium in the treatment of arthritis: a systematic review of clinical trials. *Rheumatology* (Oxford) 2007 Aug;46(8):1223–1233.

108. Tarp U, Overvad K, Thorling EB, et al. Selenium treatment in rheumatoid arthritis. *Scandinavian Journal of Rheumatology* 1985;14(4):364–368.

109. Edmonds SE, Winyard PG, Guo R, et al. Putative analgesic activity of repeated oral doses of vitamin E in the treatment of rheumatoid arthritis. Results of a placebo controlled double blind trial. *Annals of the Rheumatic Diseases* 1997; 56:649–655.

110. Zoli A, Altomonte L, Caricchio R, et al. Serum zinc and copper in active rheumatoid arthritis: correlation with interleukin 1 beta and tumour necrosis factor alpha. *Clinical Rheumatology* 1998;17(5):378–382.

111. Peretz A, Neve J, Famaey JP. Effects of chronic and acute corticosteroid therapy on zinc and copper status in rheumatoid arthritis patients. *Journal of Trace Elements and Electrolytes in Health and Disease* 1989 Jun;3(2):103–108.

112. Pandley SP, Bhattacharya SK, Sundar S. Zinc in rheumatoid arthritis. *Indian Journal of Medical Research* 1985;81: 618–620.

113. Simkin PA. Treatment of rheumatoid arthritis with oral zinc sulfate. *Agents & Actions* suppl 1981;8:587–595.

114. Mattingly PC, Mowat AG. Zinc sulphate in rheumatoid arthritis. *Annals of the Rheumatic Diseases* 1982;41:456–457.

115. Pasquier C, Mach PS, Raichvarg D, et al. Manganese-containing superoxide-dismutase deficiency in polymorphonuclear leukocytes of adults with rheumatoid arthritis. *Inflammation* 1984 Mar;8(1):27–32.

116. Menander-Huber KB. Orgotein in the treatment of rheumatoid arthritis. *European Journal of Rheumatology and Inflammation* 1981;4:201–211.

117. Zidenberg-Cherr S, Keen CL, Lonnerdal B, Hurley LS. Dietary superoxide dismutase does not affect tissue levels. *The American Journal of Clinical Nutrition* 1983 Jan;37(1):5–7.

118. de Rosa GD, Keen CL, Leach RM, Hurley LS. Regulation of superoxide dismutase activity by dietary manganese. *Journal of Nutrition* 1980 Apr;110(4): 795–804.

119. Mullen A, Wilson CW. The metabolism of ascorbic acid in rheumatoid arthritis. *Proceedings of the Nutrition Society* 1976;35:8A–9A.

120. Subramanian N. Histamine degradative potential of ascorbic acid. *Agents & Actions* 1978; 8:484–487.

121. Levine M. New concepts in the biology and biochemistry of ascorbic acid. *The New England Journal of Medicine* 1986;314: 892–902.

122. Hagfors L, Leanderson P, Sköldstam L, et al. Antioxidant intake, plasma antioxidants and oxidative stress in a randomized, controlled, parallel, Mediterranean dietary intervention study on patients with rheumatoid arthritis. *Nutrition Journal* 2003 Jul 30;2:5.

123. Jacobsson L, Lindgärde F, Manthorpe R, Akesson B. Correlation of fatty acid composition of adipose tissue lipids and serum phosphatidylcholine and serum concentrations of micronutrients with disease duration in rheumatoid arthritis. *Annals of the Rheumatic Diseases* 1990 Nov;49(11):901–905.

124. Barton-Wright EC, Elliott WA. The pantothenic acid metabolism of rheumatoid arthritis. *The Lancet* 1963;2:862–863.

125. General Practitioner Research Group. Calcium pantothenate in arthritic conditions. *Practitioner* 1980;224:208–211.

126. Chiang EP, Bagley PJ, Selhub J, et al. Abnormal vitamin B6 status is associated with severity of symptoms in patients with rheumatoid arthritis. *The American Journal of Medicine* 2003 Mar; 114(4):283–287.

127. Woolf K, Manore MM. Elevated plasma homocysteine and low vitamin B-6 status in nonsupplementing older women with rheumatoid arthritis. *Journal of the American Dietetic Association* 2008 Mar;108(3):443–453.

128. Walker WR, Keats DM. An investigation of the therapeutic value of the "copper bracelet"—dermal assimilation of copper in arthritic/rheumatoid conditions. *Agents & Actions* 1976;6: 454–458.

129. Chung MH, Kessner L, Chan PC. Degradation of articular cartilage by copper and hydrogen peroxide. *Agents & Actions* 1984;15:328–335.

130. Adorini L, Penna G. Control of autoimmune diseases by the vitamin D endocrine system. *Nature Clinical Practice Rheumatology* 2008 Aug;4(8):404–412.

131. Cutolo M, Otsa K, Laas K, et al. Circannual vitamin D serum levels and disease activity in rheumatoid arthritis: northern versus southern Europe. *Clinical and Experimental Rheumatology* 2006 Nov–Dec;24(6): 702–704.

132. de Witte TJ, Geerdink PJ, Lamers CB, et al. Hypochlorhydria and hypergastrinaemia in rheumatoid arthritis. *Annals of the Rheumatic Diseases* 1979 Feb; 38(1):14–17.

133. Henriksson K, Uvnas-Moberg K, Nord CE, et al. Gastrin, gastric acid secretion, and gastric microflora in patients with rheumatoid arthritis. *Annals of*

the Rheumatic Diseases 1986 June;45(6):475–483.

134. Kanerud L, Hafström I, Berg A. Effects of antirheumatic treatment on gastric secretory function and salivary flow in patients with rheumatoid arthritis. *Clinical and Experimental Rheumatology* 1991;9:595–601.

135. Horger I. Enzyme therapy in multiple rheumatic diseases. *Therapiewoche* 1983;33:3948–3957.

136. Ransberger K. Enzyme treatment of immune complex diseases. *Arthritis & Rheumatism* 1986;8:16–19.

137. Kekkonen RA, Lummela N, Karjalainen H, et al. Probiotic intervention has strain-specific anti-inflammatory effects in healthy adults. *World Journal of Gastroenterology* 2008 Apr 7; 14(13):2029–2036.

138. Hatakka K, Martin J, Korpela M, et al. Effects of probiotic therapy on the activity and activation of mild rheumatoid arthritis—a pilot study. *Scandinavian Journal of Rheumatology* 2003;32(4):211–215.

139. Mandel DR, Eichas K, Holmes J. *Bacillus coagulans:* a viable adjunct therapy for relieving symptoms of rheumatoid arthritis according to a randomized, controlled trial. *BMC Complementary and Alternative Medicine* 2010 Jan 12;10:1.

140. James M, Proudman S, Cleland L. Fish oil and rheumatoid arthritis: past, present and future. *Proceedings of the Nutrition Society* 2010 Aug;69(3): 316–323.

141. van der Tempel H, Tulleken JE, et al. Effects of fish oil supplementation in rheumatoid arthritis. *Annals of the Rheumatic Diseases* 1990 Feb;49:76–80.

142. Kremer JM, Lawrence DA, Jubiz W, et al. Dietary fish oil and olive oil supplementation in patients with rheumatoid arthritis. Clinical and immunologic effects. *Arthritis & Rheumatism* 1990 Jun;33(6):810–820.

143. Lau CS, Morley KD, Belch JJ. Effects of fish oil supplementation on non-steroidal anti-inflammatory drug requirement in patients with mild rheumatoid arthritis—a double-blind placebo controlled study. *British Journal of Rheumatology* 1993; 32:982–989.

144. Nielsen GL, Faarvang KL, Thomsen BS, et al. The effects of dietary supplementation with ω-3 polyunsaturated fatty acids in patients with rheumatoid arthritis: a randomized, double-blind trial. *European Journal of Clinical Investigation* 1992 Oct; 22(10):687–691.

145. Volker D, Fitzgerald P, Major G, Garg M. Efficacy of fish oil concentrate in the treatment of rheumatoid arthritis. *The Journal of Rheumatology* 2000 Oct;27(10):2343–2346.

146. Ariza-Ariza R, Mestanza-Peralta M, Cardiel MH. Omega-3 fatty acids in rheumatoid arthritis: an overview. *Seminars in Arthritis and Rheumatism* 1998;27:366–370.

147. Galli C, Calder PC. Effects of fat and fatty acid intake on inflammatory and immune responses: a critical review. *Annals of Nutrition and Metabolism* 2009;55: 123–139.

148. Jurenka JS. Anti-inflammatory properties of curcumin, a major constituent of *Curcuma longa:* a review of preclinical and clinical research. *Alternative Medicine Review* 2009 Jun;14(2):141–153.

149. Deodhar SD, Sethi R, Srimal RC. Preliminary studies on antirheumatic activity of curcumin (diferuloyl methane). *Indian Journal of Medical Research* 1980;71:632–634.

150. Benny M, Antony B. Bioavailability of biocurcumax (BCM–095™). *Spice India* 2006 Sep 9; 19(9):11–15.

151. Marczylo TH, Verschoyle RD, Cooke DN, et al. Comparison of systemic availability of curcumin with that of curcumin formulated with phosphatidyl-choline. *Cancer Chemotherapy and Pharmacology* 2007 Jul; 60(2):171–177.

152. Sasaki H, Sunagawa Y, Takahashi K, et al. Innovative preparation of curcumin for improved oral bioavailability. *Biological and Pharmaceutical Bulletin* 2011;34(5):660–665.

153. Taussig S, Batkin S. Bromelain: the enzyme complex of pineapple (*Ananas comosus*) and its clinical application. An update. *Journal of Ethnopharmacology* 1988;22:191–203.

154. Cohen A, Goldman J. Bromelain therapy in rheumatoid arthritis. *Pennsylvania Medicine Journal* 1964;67:27–30.

155. Desser L, Holomanova D, Zavadova E, et al. Oral therapy with proteolytic enzymes decreases excessive TGF-beta levels in human blood. *Cancer Chemotherapy and Pharmacology* 2001 Jul;47 suppl:S10–S15.

156. Kim SY, Han SW, Kim GW, et al. TGF-beta1 polymorphism determines the progression of joint damage in rheumatoid arthritis. *Scandinavian Journal of Rheumatology* 2004;33(6): 389–394.

157. Srivastava KC, Mustafa T. Ginger (*Zingiber officinale*) and rheumatic disorders. *Medical Hypotheses* 1989;29:25–28.

158. Srivastava KC, Mustafa T. Ginger (*Zingiber officinale*) in rheumatism and musculoskeletal disorders. *Medical Hypotheses* 1992;39:342–348.

159. Leung A. *Encyclopedia of common natural ingredients used in food, drugs, and cosmetics.* New York: John Wiley, 1980.

160. Lundberg IE, Nader GA. Molecular effects of exercise in patients with inflammatory rheumatic disease. *Nature Clinical Practice Rheumatology* 2008 Nov;4(11):597–604.

161. de Jong Z, Munneke M, Zwinderman AH, et al. Is a long-term high-intensity exercise program effective and safe in patients with rheumatoid arthritis? Re-

sults of a randomized controlled trial. *Arthritis & Rheumatism* 2003 Sep;48(9):2415–2424.

162. Keefe FJ, Affleck G, Lefebvre J, et al. Living with rheumatoid arthritis: the role of daily spirituality and daily religious and spiritual coping. *The Journal of Pain* 2001 Apr;2(2): 101–110.

163. Kraaimaat FW, Van Dam-Baggen RM, Bijlsma JW. Association of social support and the spouse's reaction with psychological distress in male and female patients with rheumatoid arthritis. *The Journal of Rheumatology* 1995;22:644–648.

Rosacea

1. Wilkin J, Dahl M, Detmar M, et al. Standard classification of rosacea: Report of the National Rosacea Society Expert Committee on the Classification and Staging of Rosacea. *Journal of the American Academy of Dermatology* 2002;46:584–587.

2. Buechner SA. Rosacea: an update. *Dermatology* 2005;210(2): 100–108.

3. Szlachcic A, Sliwowski Z, Karczewska E, et al. *Helicobacter pylori* and its eradication in rosacea. *Journal of Physiology and Pharmacology* 1999;50: 777–786.

4. Ryle J, Barber H. Gastric analysis in acne rosacea. *The Lancet* 1920;2:1195–1196.

5. Poole W. Effect of vitamin B complex and S-factor on acne rosacea. *Southern Medical Journal* 1957;50:207–210.

6. Barba A, Rosa B, Angelini G, et al. Pancreatic exocrine function in rosacea. *Dermatologica* 1982; 165:601–606.

7. Baker B. *Helicobacter pylori* strikes again: this time it's rosacea. *Family Practice News* 1994 Sept;1:6.

8. Diaz C, O'Callaghan CJ, Khan A, Ilchyshyn A. Rosacea: a cutaneous marker of *Helicobacter pylori* infection? Results of a pilot study. *Acta Dermato-Venereologica* 2003;83:282–286.

9. Rebora A, Drago F, Parodi A. May *Helicobaeter pylori* be important for dermatologists? *Dermatology* 1995;191:6–8.

10. Sharma VK, Lynn A, Kaminski M, et al. A study of the prevalence of *Helicobacter pylori* infection and other markers of upper gastrointestinal tract disease in patients with rosacea. *The American Journal of Gastroenterology* 1998;93:220–222.

11. Tulipan L. Acne rosacea: a vitamin B complex deficiency. *New York State Journal of Medicine* 1929;29:1063–1064.

12. Johnson L, Eckardt R. Rosacea keratitis and conditions with vascularization of the cornea treated with riboflavin. *Archives of Ophthalmology* 1940;23:899.

13. Georgala S, Katoulis AC, Kylafis GD, et al. Increased density of *Demodex folliculorum* and evidence of delayed hypersensitivity reaction in subjects with papulopustular rosacea. *Journal of the European Academy of Dermatology and Venereology* 2001;15:441–444.

14. Sherertz E. Acneiform eruption due to "megadose" vitamins B6 and B12. *Cutis* 1991;48:119–120.

15. Sharquie KE, Najim RA, Al-Salman HN. Oral zinc sulfate in the treatment of rosacea: a double-blind, placebo-controlled study. *International Journal of Dermatology* 2006; 45(7):857–861.

16. Elewski B, Thiboutot D. A clinical overview of azelaic acid. *Cutis* 2006;77(2 suppl):12–16.

17. Liu RH, Smith MK, Basta SA, Farmer ER. Azelaic acid in the treatment of papulopustular rosacea: a systematic review of randomized controlled trials. *Archives of Dermatology* 2006; 142(8):1047–1052.

18. Czernielewski J, Liu Y. Comparison of 15% azelaic acid gel and 0.75% metronidazole gel for the topical treatment of papulopustular rosacea. *Archives*

of Dermatology 2004;140(10): 1282–1283.

Seborrheic Dermatitis

1. Eppig JJ. Seborrhea capitis in infants: a clinical experience in allergy therapy. *Annals of Allergy, Asthma & Immunology* 1971;29:323–324.

2. Nisenson A. Seborrheic dermatitis of infants and Leiner's disease: a biotin deficiency. *Journal of Pediatrics* 1957;51:537–548.

3. Nisenson A, Barness LA. Treatment of seborrheic dermatitis with biotin and vitamin B complex. *Journal of Pediatrics* 1972; 81:630–631.

4. Schreiner A, Slinger W, Hawkins V, et al. Seborrheic dermatitis. A local metabolic defect involving pyridoxine. *Journal of Laboratory and Clinical Medicine* 1952;40:121–130.

5. Callaghan T. The effect of folic acid on seborrheic dermatitis. *Cutis* 1967;3:584–588.

6. Andrews GC, Post CF, Domonkos AN. Seborrheic dermatitis: supplemental treatment with vitamin B12. *New York State Journal of Medicine* 1950; 50:1921–1925.

7. Vardy DA, Cohen AD, Tchetov T, et al. A double-blind, placebo-controlled trial of an aloe vera (*A. barbadensis*) emulsion in the treatment of seborrheic dermatitis. *Journal of Dermatological Treatment* 1999; 10:7–11.

8. Gupta AK, Nicol K, Batra R. Role of antifungal agents in the treatment of seborrheic dermatitis. *American Journal of Clinical Dermatology* 2004; 5(6):417–422.

9. Satchell AC, Sauragen A, Bell C, Barnetson RS. Treatment of dandruff with 5% tea tree oil shampoo. *Journal of the American Academy of Dermatology* 2002 Dec;47(6):852–825.

Sinus Infections

1. Stalman WA, van Essen GA, van der Graaf Y. Determinants for

the course of acute sinusitis in adult general practice patients. *Postgraduate Medical Journal* 2001;77:778–782.

2. Stalman W, van Essen GA, van der Graf Y. Maxillary sinusitis in adults: an evaluation of placebo-controlled double-blind trials. *Family Practice* 1997;14: 124–129.

3. Ahovuo-Saloranta A, Borisenko OV, et al. Antibiotics for acute maxillary sinusitis. *Otolaryngology—Head and Neck Surgery* 2008 Oct;139(4):486–489.

4. Cohen R. The antibiotic treatment of acute otitis media and sinusitis in children. *Diagnostic Microbiology and Infectious Disease* 1997;27:35–39.

5. Dohlman AW, Hamstreet MPB, Odrezin GT, Bartolucci AA. Subacute sinusitis: are antimicrobials necessary? *Journal of Allergy and Clinical Immunology* 1993;91:1015–1023.

6. Gutman M, Torres A, Keen KJ, Houser SM. Prevalence of allergy in patients with chronic rhinosinusitis. *Otolaryngology—Head and Neck Surgery* 2004; 130:545–552.

7. Emanuel IA, Shah SB. Chronic rhinosinusitis: allergy and sinus computed tomography relationships. *Otolaryngology—Head and Neck Surgery* 2000;123: 687–691.

8. Evans R III. Environmental control and immunotherapy for allergic disease. *Journal of Allergy and Clinical Immunology* 1992;90:462–468.

9. Majima Y. Mucoactive medications and airway disease. *Paediatric Respiratory Reviews* 2002;3:104–109.

10. Grandjean EM, Berthet P, Ruffmann R, Leuenberger P. Efficacy of oral long-term N-acetylcysteine in chronic bronchopulmonary disease: a meta-analysis of published double-blind, placebo-controlled clinical trials. *Clinical Therapeutics* 2000;22:209–221.

11. Majima Y, Inagaki M, Hirata K, et al. The effect of an orally ad- ministered proteolytic enzyme on the elasticity and viscosity of nasal mucus. *Archives of Oto-rhino-laryngology* 1988;244: 355–359.

12. Nakamura S, Hashimoto Y, Mikami M, et al. Effect of the proteolytic enzyme serrapeptase in patients with chronic airway disease. *Respirology* 2003;8: 316–320.

13. Mazzone A, Catalani M, Costanzo M, et al. Evaluation of *Serratia* peptidase in acute or chronic inflammation of otorhinolaryngology pathology: a multicentre, double-blind, randomized trial versus placebo. *Journal of International Medical Research* 1990;18:379–388.

14. Ryan RE. A double-blind clinical evaluation of bromelains in the treatment of acute sinusitis. *Headache* 1967;7:13–17.

15. Brendler T, van Wyk BE. A historical, scientific and commercial perspective on the medicinal use of *Pelargonium sidoides* (Geraniaceae). *Journal of Ethnopharmacology* 2008 Oct 28;119(3):420–433.

16. Bachert C, Schapowal A, Funk P, Kieser M. Treatment of acute rhinosinusitis with the preparation from *Pelargonium sidoides* EPs 7630: a randomized, double-blind, placebo-controlled trial. *Rhinology* 2009 Mar;47(1):51–58.

Sports Injuries, Tendinitis, and Bursitis

1. Miller MJ. Injuries to athletes. *Medical Times* 1960;88:313–314.

2. Cragin RB. The use of bioflavonoids in the prevention and treatment of athletic injuries. *Medical Times* 1962;90:529–530.

3. Taussig S, Batkin S. Bromelain, the enzyme complex of pineapple (*Ananas comosus*) and its clinical application. An update. *Journal of Ethnopharmacology* 1988;22:191–203.

4. Blonstein J. Control of swelling in boxing injuries. *Practitioner* 203:206, 1960.

5. Kerkhoffs GM, Struijs PA, de Wit C, et al. A double blind, randomised, parallel group study on the efficacy and safety of treating acute lateral ankle sprain with oral hydrolytic enzymes. *British Journal of Sports Medicine* 2004 Aug;38(4):431–435.

6. Szczurko O, Cooley K, Mills EJ, et al. Naturopathic treatment of rotator cuff tendinitis among Canadian postal workers: a randomized controlled trial. *Arthritis & Rheumatism* 2009 Aug 15;61(8):1037–1045.

7. Jurenka JS. Anti-inflammatory properties of curcumin, a major constituent of *Curcuma longa*: a review of preclinical and clinical research. *Alternative Medicine Review* 2009 Jun;14(2):141–153.

8. Marczylo TH, Verschoyle RD, Cooke DN, et al. Comparison of systemic availability of curcumin with that of curcumin formulated with phosphatidylcholine. *Cancer Chemotherapy and Pharmacology* 2007 Jul; 60(2):171–177.

9. Sasaki H, Sunagawa Y, Takahashi K, et al. Innovative preparation of curcumin for improved oral bioavailability. *Biological and Pharmaceutical Bulletin* 2011;34(5):660–665.

Strep Throat (Streptococcal Pharyngitis)

1. Corneli HM. Rapid detection and diagnosis of group A streptococcal pharyngitis. *Current Infectious Disease Reports* 2004;6:181–186.

2. Zwart S, Rovers MM, de Melker RA, et al. Penicillin for acute sore throat in children: randomised, double blind trial. *BMJ* 2003;327:1324.

3. Dagnelie CF, van der Graaf Y, De Melker RA. Do patients with sore throat benefit from penicillin? A randomized double-blind placebo-controlled clinical trial with penicillin V in

general practice. *British Journal of General Practice* 1996;46: 589–593.

4. McIsaac WJ, Goel V, Slaughter PM, et al. Reconsidering sore throats. Part I. Problems with current clinical practice. *Canadian Family Physician* 1997;43: 485–493.

5. Stollerman GH. Rheumatic fever in the 21st century. *Clinical Infectious Diseases* 2001 Sep 15;33(6):806–814.

6. Zoppi G, Deganello A, Benoni G, Saccomani F. Oral bacteriotherapy in clinical practice. I. The use of different preparations in infants treated with antibiotics. *European Journal of Pediatrics* 1982;139:18–21.

7. Gotz VP, Romankiewics JA, Moss J, Murray HW. Prophylaxis against ampicillin-induced diarrhea with a lactobacillus preparation. *American Journal of Hospital Pharmacy* 1979;36: 754–757.

8. Rinehart JF. Studies relating vitamin C deficiency to rheumatic fever and rheumatoid arthritis: experimental, clinical, and general considerations. I. Rheumatic fever. *Annals of Internal Medicine* 1935;9:586–599.

9. Rinehart JF. Studies relating vitamin C deficiency to rheumatic fever and rheumatoid arthritis: experimental, clinical, and general considerations. II. Rheumatoid (atrophic) arthritis. *Annals of Internal Medicine* 1935;9: 671–689.

10. Sharma SM, Anderson M, Schoop SR, Hudson JB. Bactericidal and anti-inflammatory properties of a standardized echinacea extract (Echinaforce): dual actions against respiratory bacteria. *Phytomedicine* 2010 Jul;17(8–9):563–568.

11. Brendler T, van Wyk BE. A historical, scientific and commercial perspective on the medicinal use of *Pelargonium sidoides* (Geraniaceae). *Journal of Ethnopharmacology* 2008 Oct 28;119(3):420–433.

12. Bereznoy VV, Riley DS, Wassmer G, Heger M. Efficacy of extract of *Pelargonium sidoides* in children with acute non–group A beta-hemolytic streptococcus tonsillopharyngitis: a randomized, double-blind, placebo-controlled trial. *Alternative Therapies in Health and Medicine* 2003 Sep–Oct;9(5):68–79.

Stroke (Recovery From)

1. Anadere I, Chmiel H, Witte S. Hemorrheological findings in patients with completed stroke and the influence of *Ginkgo biloba* extract. *Clinical Hemorheology and Microcirculation* 1985;4:411–420.

2. Larson MK, Ashmore JH, Harris KA, et al. Effects of omega-3 acid ethyl esters and aspirin, alone and in combination, on platelet function in healthy subjects. *Thrombosis and Haemostasis* 2008 Oct;100(4):634–641.

3. Chang YY, Liu JS, Lai SL, et al. Cerebellar hemorrhage provoked by combined use of nattokinase and aspirin in a patient with cerebral microbleeds. *Internal Medicine* 2008;47(5): 467–469.

4. Kidd PM. Integrated brain restoration after ischemic stroke—medical management, risk factors, nutrients, and other interventions for managing inflammation and enhancing brain plasticity. *Alternative Medicine Review* 2009 Mar; 14(1):14–35.

5. Dávalos A, Castillo J, Alvarez-Sabin J, et al. Oral citicoline in acute ischemic stroke: an individual patient data pooling analysis of clinical trials. *Stroke* 2002;33:2850–2857.

6. Bolland K, Whitehead J, Cobo E, Secades JJ. Evaluation of a sequential global test of improved recovery following stroke as applied to the ICTUS trial of citicoline. *Pharmaceutical Statistics* 2009 Apr–Jun; 8(2):136–149.

7. Aguglia E, Ban TA, Panzarasa RM, et al. Choline alphoscerate in the treatment of mental pathology following acute cerebrovascular accident. *Functional Neurology* 1993;8:S5–S24.

8. Barbagallo Sangiorgi G, Barbagallo M, Giordano M, et al. Alpha-glycerophosphocholine in the mental recovery of cerebral ischemic attacks. An Italian multicenter clinical trial. *Annals of the New York Academy of Sciences* 1994;717:253–269.

9. Consoli D, Giunta V, Grillo G, et al. [Alpha-GPC in the treatment of acute cerebrovascular accident patients.] *Archives Medicina Interna* 1993;45:13–23.

10. Gambi D, Onofrj M. Multicenter clinical study of efficacy and tolerability of choline alfoscerate in patients with deficits in higher mental function arising after an acute ischemic cerebrovascular attack. *Geriatria* 1994;6:91–98.

11. Tomasina C, Manzino M, Novello P, et al. Clinical study of the therapeutic effectiveness and tolerability of choline alfoscerate in 15 subjects with compromised cognitive functions subsequent to acute focal cerebral ischemia. *Rivista di Neuropsichiatrica e Scienze Affini* 1996;37:21–28.

12. Mathew NT, Rivera VM, Meyer JS, et al. Double-blind evaluation of glycerol therapy in acute cerebral infarction. *The Lancet* 1972;2:1327–1329.

13. Parnetti L, Amenta F, Gallai V. Choline alfoscerate in cognitive decline and in acute cerebrovascular disease: an analysis of published clinical data. *Mechanisms of Ageing and Development* 2001;122:2041–2055.

14. Kim MK, Choi TY, Lee MS, et al. Contralateral acupuncture versus ipsilateral acupuncture in the rehabilitation of post-stroke hemiplegic patients: a systematic review. *BMC Complementary and Alternative Medicine* 2010 Jul 30;10:41.

15. Wu P, Mills E, Moher D,

Seely D. Acupuncture in post-stroke rehabilitation: a systematic review and meta-analysis of randomized trials. *Stroke* 2010 Apr;41(4):e171–e179.

Systemic Lupus Erythematosus

1. Petri M. Sex hormones and systemic lupus erythematosus. *Lupus* 2008 May;17(5):412–415.
2. Haija AJ, Schulz SW. The role and effect of complementary and alternative medicine in systemic lupus erythematosus. *Rheumatic Disease Clinics of North America* 2011 Feb;37(1): 47–62.
3. Duffy EM, Meenagh GK, Mc-Millan SA, et al. The clinical effect of dietary supplementation with omega-3 fish oils and/or copper in systemic lupus erythematosus. *The Journal of Rheumatology* 2004;31:1551–1556.
4. Wright SA, O'Prey FM, McHenry MT, et al. A randomised interventional trial of omega-3-polyunsaturated fatty acids on endothelial function and disease activity in systemic lupus erythematosus. *Annals of the Rheumatic Diseases* 2008; 67:841–848.
5. Van Vollenhoven RF, Engleman EG, McGuire JL. An open study of dehydroepiandrosterone in systemic lupus erythematosus. *Arthritis & Rheumatism* 1994; 37:1305–1310.
6. van Vollenhoven RF, Engleman EG, McGuire JL. Dehydroepiandrosterone in systemic lupus erythematosus. Results of a double-blind, placebo-controlled, randomized clinical trial. *Arthritis & Rheumatism* 1995; 38(12):1826–1831.
7. Petri MA, Lahita RG, Van Vollenhoven RF, et al. Effects of prasterone on corticosteroid requirements of women with systemic lupus erythematosus: a double-blind, randomized, placebo-controlled trial. *Arthritis & Rheumatism* 2002;46: 1820–1829.

8. Nordmark G, Bengtsson C, Larsson A, et al. Effects of dehydroepiandrosterone supplement on health-related quality of life in glucocorticoid treated female patients with systemic lupus erythematosus. *Autoimmunity* 2005;38:531–540.
9. Hartkamp A, Geenen R, Godaert GL, et al. Effects of dehydroepiandrosterone on fatigue and wellbeing in women with quiescent systemic lupus erythematosus: a randomised controlled trial. *Annals of the Rheumatic Diseases* 2010;69: 1144–1147.

Uterine Fibroids

1. Woods MN, Gorbach SL, Longcope C, et al. Low-fat, high-fiber diet and serum estrone sulfate in premenopausal women. *The American Journal of Clinical Nutrition* 1989;49: 1179–1183.
2. Goodman MT, Wilkens LR, Hankin JH, et al. Association of soy and fiber consumption with the risk of endometrial cancer. *American Journal of Epidemiology* 1997;146:294–306.
3. Goldin B, Allercreutz H, Gorbach SL, et al. Estrogen excretion patterns and plasma levels in vegetarian and omnivorous women. *The New England Journal of Medicine* 1982;307:1542–1547.
4. Michnovicz JJ, Bradlow HL. Altered estrogen metabolism and excretion in humans following consumption of indole-3-carbinol. *Nutrition and Cancer* 1991; 16(1):59–66.
5. Stoewsand GS. Bioactive organosulfur phytochemicals in *Brassica oleracea* vegetables—a review. *Food and Chemical Toxicology* 1995;33(6):537–543.
6. Rajoria S, Suriano R, Parmar PS, et al. 3,3'-diindolylmethane modulates estrogen metabolism in patients with thyroid proliferative disease: a pilot study. *Thyroid* 2011 Mar;21(3):299–304.

Vaginitis

1. Heidrich F, Berg A, Gergman F, et al. Clothing factors and vaginitis. *The Journal of Family Practice* 1984;19:491–494.
2. Meeker CI. Candidiasis—an obstinate problem. *Medical Times* 1978;106:26–32.
3. Fidel P, Sobel J. Immunopathogenesis of recurrent vulvovaginal candidiasis. *Clinical Microbiology Reviews* 1996;9: 335–348.
4. Erickson K, Hubbard N. Probiotic immunomodulation in health and disease. *Journal of Nutrition* 2000;130(25 suppl): S403–S409.
5. Reid G, Cook R, Bruce A. Examination of strains of lactobacilli for properties that may influence bacterial interference in the urinary tract. *Journal of Urology* 1987;138:330–335.
6. Hawes S, Hillier S, Benedetti J, et al. Hydrogen-peroxide-producing lactobacilli and acquisition of vaginal infections. *Journal of Infectious Diseases* 1996;174:1058–1063.
7. Hilton E, Rindos P, Isenberg H. *Lactobacillus* GG vaginal suppositories and vaginitis. *Journal of Clinical Microbiology* 1995; 33:1433.
8. Williams A, Yu C, Tashima K, et al. Evaluation of two self care treatments for prevention of vaginal candidiasis in women with HIV. *Journal of the Association of Nurses in AIDS Care* 2001;12:51–57.
9. Reid G, Beueman D, Heinemann C, et al. Probiotic *Lactobacillus* dose required to restore and maintain a normal vaginal flora. *FEMS Immunology & Medical Microbiology* 2001;32: 37–41.
10. Reid G, Charbonneau D, Erb J, et al. Oral use of *Lactobacillus rhamnosus* GR01 and *L. fermentum* RC-14 significantly alters vaginal flora: randomized, placebo-controlled trial in 64 healthy women. *FEMS Immu-*

nology & Medical Microbiology 2003;35:131–134.

11. Reid G, Bruce A, Fraser N, et al. Oral probiotics can resolve urogenital infections. *FEMS Immunology & Medical Microbiology* 2001;30:49–52.

12. Petersen E, Magnani P. Efficacy and safety of vitamin C vaginal tablets in the treatment of non-specific vaginitis. *European Journal of Obstetrics & Gynecology & Reproductive Biology* 2004;117(1):70–75.

13. Ratzen J. Monilial and trichomonal vaginitis—topical treatment with povidone iodine treatments. *California Medicine* 1969;110:24–27.

14. Shook D. A clinical study of a povidone-iodine regimen for resistant vaginitis. *Current Therapeutic Research* 1963;5:256–263.

15. Maneksha S. Comparison of povidone-iodine (Betadine) vaginal pessaries and lactic acid pessaries in the treatment of vaginitis. *Journal of International Medical Research* 1974;2:236–239.

16. Reeve P. The inactivation of *Chlamydia trachomatis* by povidone iodine. *Journal of Antimicrobial Chemotherapy* 1976;2:77–80.

17. Mayhew S. Vaginitis. A study of the efficacy of povidone iodine in unselected cases. *Journal of International Medical Research* 1981;9:157–159.

18. Gershenfeld L. Povidone iodine as a trichomoniacide. *American Journal of Pharmacy* 1962;134:324–331.

19. Gershenfeld L. Povidone iodine as a vaginal microbicide. *American Journal of Pharmacy* 1962;134:278–291.

20. Singha H. The use of a vaginal cleansing kit in non-specific vaginitis. *Practitioner* 1979;223:403–404.

21. Jovanovic R, Congema E, Nguyen H. Antifungal agents vs boric acid for treating chronic mycotic vulvovaginitis. *The Journal of Reproductive Medicine* 1991;36:593–597.

22. Swate T, Weed J. Boric acid treatment of vulvovaginal candidiasis. *Obstetrics & Gynecology* 1974;43:894–895.

23. Keller Van Slyke K. Treatment of vulvovaginal candidiasis with boric acid powder. *American Journal of Obstetrics & Gynecology* 1981;141:145–148.

24. Pena EF. *Melaleuca alternifolia* oil. Its use for trichomonal vaginitis and other vaginal infections. *Obstetrics & Gynecology* 1962;19:793–795.

Varicose Veins

1. Lim CS, Davies AH. Pathogenesis of primary varicose veins. *British Journal of Surgery* 2009 Nov;96(11):1231–1242.

2. Raffetto JD, Khalil RA. Mechanisms of varicose vein formation: valve dysfunction and wall dilation. *Phlebology* 2008;23(2):85–98.

3. Trowell H, Burkitt D, Heaton K. *Dietary fibre, fibre-depleted foods and disease.* London: Academic Press, 1985.

4. Vahouny G, Kritchevsky D. *Dietary fiber in health and disease.* New York: Plenum Press, 1982.

5. Latto C, Wilkinson RW, Gilmore OJ. Diverticular disease and varicose veins. *The Lancet* 1973;1:1089–1090.

6. Gabor M. Pharmacologic effects of flavonoids on blood vessels. *Angiologica* 1972;9:355–374.

7. Kuhnau J. The flavonoids. A class of semi-essential food components: their role in human nutrition. *World Review of Nutrition and Dietetics* 1976;24:117–191.

8. Pourrat H. Anthocyanidin drugs in vascular disease. *Plant Medicine and Phytotherapy* 1977;11:143–151.

9. Ihme N, Kieswetter H, Jung F, et al. Leg edema protection from buckwheat herb tea in patients with chronic venous insufficiency: a single-center, randomized, double-blind, placebo-controlled clinical trial. *European Journal of Clinical Pharmacology* 1996;50:443–447.

10. Nuzum DS, Gebru TT, Kouzi SA.Pycnogenol for chronic venous insufficiency. *American Journal of Health Systems and Pharmacy.* 2011 Sep 1;68(17):1589–90, 1599–1601.

11. Belcaro G, Cesarone MR, Errichi BM, et al. Venous ulcers: microcirculatory improvement and faster healing with local use of Pycnogenol. *Angiology* 2005 Nov–Dec;56(6):699–705.

12. Belcaro G, Cesarone MR, Rohdewald P, et al. Prevention of venous thrombosis and thrombophlebitis in long-haul flights with pycnogenol. *Clinical and Applied Thrombosis/Hemostasis* 2004 Oct;10(4):373–377.

13. Cesarone MR, Belcaro G, Nicolaides AN, et al. Prevention of venous thrombosis in long-haul flights with Flite Tabs: the LONFLIT-FLITE randomized, controlled trial. *Angiology* 2003 Sep–Oct;54(5):531–539.

14. Cesarone MR, Belcaro G, Rohdewald P, et al. Improvement of signs and symptoms of chronic venous insufficiency and microangiopathy with Pycnogenol: a prospective, controlled study. *Phytomedicine* 2010 Sep;17(11):835–839.

15. Cesarone MR, Belcaro G, Rohdewald P, et al. Rapid relief of signs/symptoms in chronic venous microangiopathy with Pycnogenol: a prospective, controlled study. *Angiology* 2006 Oct–Nov;57(5):569–576.

16. Belcaro G, Cesarone MR, Ricci A, et al. Control of edema in hypertensive subjects treated with calcium antagonist (nifedipine) or angiotensin-converting enzyme inhibitors with Pycnogenol. *Clinical and Applied Thrombosis/Hemostasis* 2006 Oct;12(4):440–444.

17. Cesarone MR, Belcaro G, Rohdewald P, et al. Comparison of Pycnogenol and Daflon in treating chronic venous insufficiency: a prospective, controlled study. *Clinical and Applied Thrombosis/Hemostasis* 2006 Apr;12(2):205–212.

18. Nicolaides AN. From symptoms to leg edema: efficacy of Daflon 500 mg. *Angiology* 2003;54 suppl 1:S33–S44.

19. Lyseng-Williamson KA, Perry CM. Micronised purified flavonoid fraction: a review of its use in chronic venous insufficiency, venous ulcers and haemorrhoids. *Drugs* 2003;63:71–100.

20. Kreysel HW, Nissen HP, Enghofer E. A possible role of lysosomal enzymes in the pathogenesis of varicosis and the reduction in their serum activity by Venostasin. *VASA* 1983;12: 377–382.

21. Pittler MH, Ernst E. Horse-chestnut seed extract for chronic venous insufficiency: a criteria-based systematic review. *Archives of Dermatology* 1998;134;1356–1360.

22. Incandela L, De Sanctis MT, Cesarone MR, et al. Treatment of superficial vein thrombosis: clinical evaluation of Essaven gel—a placebo-controlled, 8-week, randomized study. *Angiology* 2001;52 suppl 3:S69–S72.

23. Annoni F, Mauri A, Marincola F, Resele LF. Venotonic activity of escin on the human saphenous vein. *Arzneimittelforschung* 1979;29:672–675.

24. Diehm C, Trampisch HJ, Lange S, Schmidt C. Comparison of leg compression stocking and oral horse-chestnut seed extract therapy in patients with chronic venous insufficiency. *The Lancet* 1996;347:292–294.

25. Cospite M, Ferrara F, Milio G, Meli F. [Study about pharmacologic and clinical activity of *Centella asiatica* titrated extract in the chronic venous deficiency of the lower limbs: valuation with strain gauge plethysmography.] *Giornale Italiano di Angiologie* 1984;4:200–205.

26. Brinkhaus B, Lindner M, Schuppan D, Hahn EG. Chemical, pharmacological and clinical profile of the East Asian medical plant *Centella asiatica*. *Phytomedicine* 2000;7:427–448.

27. Cesarone MR, Belcaro G, Rulo A, et al. Microcirculatory effects of total triterpenic fraction of *Centella asiatica* in chronic venous hypertension: measurement by laser Doppler, TcPO2-CO2, and leg volumetry. *Angiology* 2001;52 suppl 2:S45–S48.

28. Pointel JP, Boccalon H, Cloarec M, et al. Titrated extract of *Centella asiatica* (TECA) in the treatment of venous insufficiency of the lower limbs. *Angiology* 1987;38:46–50.

29. Boccalon H, Causse C, Yubero L. Comparative efficacy of a single daily dose of two capsules of Cyclo 3 Fort in the morning versus a repeated dose of one capsule morning and noon. A one month study. *International Journal of Angiology* 1998;17:155–160.

30. Cappelli R, Nicora M, Di Perri T. Use of extract of *Ruscus aculeatus* in venous disease in the lower limbs. *Drugs Under Experimental and Clinical Research* 1988;14:277–283.

31. Beltramino R, Penenory A, Buceta AM. An open-label, randomized multicenter study comparing the efficacy and safety of Cyclo 3 Fort® versus hydroxyethyl rutoside in chronic venous lymphatic insufficiency. *Angiology* 2000;51:535–544.

32. Visudhiphan S, Poolsuppasit S, Piboonnukarintr O, Tumliang S. The relationship between high fibrinolytic activity and daily capsicum ingestion in Thais. *The American Journal of Clinical Nutrition* 1982;35: 1452–1458.

33. Bordia A, Sharma KD, Parmar YK, Verma SK. Protective effect of garlic oil on the changes produced by 3 weeks of fatty diet on serum cholesterol, serum triglycerides, fibrinolytic activity and platelet adhesiveness in man. *Indian Heart Journal* 1982;34:86–88.

34. Baghurst KI, Raj MJ, Truswell AS. Onions and platelet aggregation. *The Lancet* 1977;1:101.

35. Srivas KC. Effects of aqueous extracts of onion, garlic and ginger on the platelet aggregation and metabolism of arachidonic acid in the blood vascular system. In vitro study. *Prostaglandins, Leukotrienes, and Medicine* 1984;13:227–235.

36. Ako H, Cheung AH, Matsuura PK. Isolation of a fibrinolysis enzyme activator from commercial bromelain. *Archives Internationales de Pharmacodynamie et de Thérapie* 1981;254:157–167.

37. Hsia CH, Shen MC, Lin JS, et al. Nattokinase decreases plasma levels of fibrinogen, factor VII, and factor VIII in human subjects. *Nutrition Research* 2009 Mar;29(3):190–196.

INDEX

acarbose (Precose), 534
acemannan, 467
acetaminophen, 830, 837
acetylation, 114, 120–21, 123–24
acetylcholine, 282, 284–86, 288
Achilles reflex, 719
acid, acidity:
    -base values, 92–93, 1021–27
    -blocking drugs, 134–35, 137, 856
    urine and, 473–74
    see also pH
acne, 245–52
    causes of, 245–47
    conventional therapies for, 248
    diet and, 246, 248–49, 251–52
    nutritional supplements and,
        247–50, 252
    rosacea and, 948, 951
    selenium for, 250
    therapeutic considerations for,
        247–51
    topical treatments for, 250–51
    vitamin A and, 249
    vitamin E for, 250
    zinc for, 249–50
acquired immunodeficiency syndrome
    (AIDS), 253–64
    antioxidants for, 258–60
    botanical medicines for, 260–62,
        264
    carnitine for, 259–60
    causes of, 253–54
    diagnosis of, 253–54
    nutritional supplements for,
        257–60, 264
    nutrition and, 255–57
    progression of HIV to, 254–58, 260
    therapeutic considerations for,
        254–62
acrodermatitis enteropathica (AE),
    178
acupressure, 336–37
acupuncture:
    angina and, 309
    asthma and, 336–37
    CTS and, 394
    diabetes and, 541–42
    migraine headaches and, 809
    in naturopathic medicine, 6, 14, 17

osteoarthritis and, 839
    smoking and, 39
    stroke and, 975
adaptogens, 216
adipokines, 224, 226–27
adiponectin, 512
adrenal glands:
    asthma and, 324
    CFS and, 424–25
    depression and, 483–84
    hypothyroidism and, 717–18
    stress and, 204–5, 208, 213–14
adrogens, decreased levels of, 936
advanced glycation end products
    (AGEs), 187–88
adventitia, 147
Aerobics Center Longitudinal Study,
    42
aesthetic needs, 31
affirmations, positive, 35–37
age, aging, 12, 183–90, 475
    acne and, 248
    AD and, 276–77, 281–88
    anemia and, 293–94, 296
    angina and, 301, 307
    BMD testing and, 849
    and bronchitis and pneumonia, 372
    cancer and, 97, 356–57, 362, 785,
        904–6, 910, 916
    cataracts and, 396–97, 400
    causes of, 185
    cells and, 87–88, 185–87
    CHF and, 444–45
    CoQ_{10} and, 90
    CTS and, 392
    CVD and, 166
    CVI and, 408
    depression and, 277, 282, 285, 486,
        488, 498–99
    detoxification and, 119
    DHEA and, 194
    diabetes and, 504, 507–13, 516–17,
        523
    diet and, 48, 186–89
    digestion and, 136, 138, 142
    ED and, 570, 572, 578
    endometriosis and, 565–66
    exercise and, 42, 44
    free radicals and, 186–88, 190, 192

gallstones and, 607
glaucoma and, 615
glucosamine and, 829
glycosylation and, 187–88
hair loss and, 630–31
health care statistics and, 12
heart disease and, 30
hemorrhoids and, 647
high BP and, 666, 672, 674–75,
    678
hypercholesterolemia and, 682, 687
hypothyroidism and, 716
IBD and, 456–57
immune system and, 177–79, 192
infertility and, 724, 726, 731
insomnia and, 749
macular degeneration and, 774–79
menopause and, 781, 783–84, 788,
    848
MS and, 812–13
and myths and reality of longevity,
    184
obesity and, 231
oldest living people and, 184
osteoarthritis and, 827, 829, 835
osteoporosis and, 844, 855–56,
    859–60
Parkinson's disease and, 868, 872
periodontal disease and, 883–84,
    886
positive mental attitude and, 29
prostate enlargement and, 915
sarcopenia and, 188
seborrheic dermatitis and, 954
sleep and, 45–46, 195
slowing process of, 188–89, 193–94
theories on, 185–88, 190
treatment summary for, 196–97
vitamin D deficiency and, 78
see also life extension
Age-Related Eye Disease Study
    (AREDS) Research Group, 397,
    777
age-related macular degeneration
    (ARMD), 774–79
aggression, 709–10
aggression-turned-inward construct,
    478
agoraphobia, 313, 316

Agriculture Department, U.S. (USDA), 53–54, 69, 712
airborne allergens, 329
alcohol, 58, 65
  anemia and, 295
  cancer and, 98–100, 103, 357
  in cholestasis, 126
  CVD and, 153
  depression and, 265, 268–72, 484–85
  detoxification and, 121, 268
  ED and, 573
  gout and, 622, 624–26
  hives and, 694, 699
  hypoglycemia and, 267–68, 713–14
  immune system and, 176
  infertility and, 726, 737
  liver and, 126, 267–70, 273
  metabolic effects of, 267–68
  osteoporosis and, 846–47, 854
  prostate enlargement and, 917–18
  psoriasis and, 925, 927
  and signs of intoxication, 266–67
  stress management and, 213
alcohol dependence, 265–75
  amino acids and, 269, 272
  antioxidants for, 269
  botanical medicines for, 272–73, 275
  carnitine for, 269
  causes of, 266
  consequences of, 265–66
  definition of, 265
  depression and, 265, 268–72
  EFAs for, 271
  exercise for, 272
  fatty liver and, 267, 269
  glutamine for, 271
  health effects of, 265–66
  hypoglycemia and, 267–68
  intestinal flora and, 272
  kudzu for, 272
  magnesium for, 270–71
  metabolic effects of, 267–68
  milk thistle for, 272–73
  psychosocial aspects of, 271
  selenium for, 269–70
  signs and symptoms of, 265–66
  therapeutic considerations for, 268–73
  vitamin A for, 268–69
  vitamin B$_1$ and, 270–71
  vitamin B$_6$ and, 270
  vitamin C for, 269–70
  zinc for, 268
Alexander technique, 82

alkaloids, alkalinity:
  -acidity of foods, 92–93, 1021–27
  diets and, 625
  osteoarthritis and, 829
  urine and, 473
  see also pH
allergens, airborne, 327
allergies:
  asthma and, 322–29, 331, 334
  canker sores and, 389–90
  chronic candidiasis and, 383
  common cold and, 435
  constipation and, 453
  diet and, 64, 596–98
  ear infections and, 557–58
  eczema and, 582–84
  to food, *see* food allergies
  glaucoma and, 617
  hay fever and, 635–37
  hives and, 692, 695–96, 698–99
  immune system and, 139, 171, 173, 592, 594–95
  nutritional supplements and, 77, 594, 602–4
  sinus infections and, 957–58
allicin, *see* garlic
allopathy, *see* conventional medicine
allopurinol, 625
aloe vera, 772
  asthma and, 336
  diabetes and, 542
  peptic ulcer and, 881
  psoriasis and, 928
  seborrheic dermatitis and, 955
  UC and, 467
alpha-linolenic acid (ALA):
  cancers and, 357, 360–61, 908
  CVD and, 155–56, 166
alpha-lipoic acid (ALA):
  diabetes and, 539, 541
  hepatitis and, 655
  HIV/AIDS and, 259
  male infertility and, 741
  MS and, 817
alpha-tocopherol, 909–11
aluminum, 111, 277, 280–81
Alzheimer's disease (AD), 276–91, 869
  aluminum and, 277, 280–81
  antioxidants and, 278, 281–82
  arrest of, 281, 287
  causes of, 276–77, 785
  curcumin for, 289
  definition of, 276
  DHEA for, 286
  diagnosis and, 276–79, 285

diet and, 277–80, 290–91
  estrogen for, 280
  fingerprint patterns in, 278–79
  GBE for, 287–88
  huperzine A for, 288–89
  LAC for, 285–86
  melatonin for, 286–87
  phosphatidylcholine for, 284–85
  prevention of, 277–78, 280–81
  PS for, 285
  risk factors for, 281–82
  signs and symptoms of, 276
  therapeutic considerations for, 278–87
  vitamin B$_1$ for, 282
  vitamin B$_{12}$ for, 282–83, 285
  zinc for, 282, 284
amalgam restorations, 885
American Academy of Otolaryngology-Head and Neck Surgery, 558–59
American Association of Naturopathic Physicians (AANP), 16
American Cancer Society, 56, 62, 107, 754
American College of Chest Physicians, 369
American ginseng (*Panax quinquefolium*), 536
American Heart Association (AHA), 154, 165–66
Amerigel, 542
amines, 140–41, 479, 695, 801–2, 804–5
amino acids:
  alcohol dependence and, 269, 272
  conjugation of, 114, 120–23, 125
  prostate enlargement and, 918
Amish, Old Order, 514
amputations, 503, 524
Amsler grids, 776
amylase, 132
anaerobic metabolism, 314
analytical (adaptive) rumination hypothesis, 479
androgens, 936
anemia, 292–300
  causes of, 292–95
  classifications of, 292–95
  folic acid and, 294–95, 299
  iron and, 293–97, 344
  signs and symptoms of, 292, 294–95
  therapeutic considerations for, 295–299
  vitamin B$_{12}$ and, 294–95, 297–99

angina, 301–12
  acupuncture for, 309
  antioxidants for, 305–6, 308
  arginine for, 308
  carnitine for, 306–7
  causes of, 301
  CoQ$_{10}$ for, 307
  hawthorn for, 308
  hypoglycemia and, 711
  intravenous EDTA therapy for,
    309–11
  khella for, 308–9
  magnesium for, 307–8
  pantethine for, 306–7
  Prinzmetal's variant, 301, 307
  relaxation and breathing for, 309
  signs and symptoms of, 301
  therapeutic considerations for,
    301–10
angioedema, 692, 700
angiograms, angiography, 166, 409
  angina and, 301–5
  supplements for, 304–5
angioplasty, 166
  angina and, 302–4
  CVI and, 409
  supplements for, 304–5
angiotensin-converting enzyme (ACE)
    inhibitors, 542, 675–76
anthocyanosides, 778–79
antibiotics:
  acne and, 247–50
  asthma and, 325
  bladder infections and, 472, 474–75
  bronchitis and, 369
  CD and, 458
  for chlamydia, 735
  chronic candidiasis and, 377, 382,
    385
  detoxification and, 123
  diarrhea and, 552–54
  digestion and, 137–38, 141–42,
    144
  ear infections and, 557–59, 561
  hives and, 695
  IBD and, 458
  overuse of, 9, 377, 558–59, 957,
    967–68
  pneumonia and, 368–69
  side effects of, 247, 377, 382, 385,
    986
  sinus infections and, 957, 959
  strep throat and, 967–69
  vaginitis and, 986, 988
antibodies, 380, 633–34, 814, 934–35
  sperm and, 734–35, 739–40
  see also specific immunoglobulins

antidepressants, 479–83, 486, 491,
    493–99
  effectiveness of, 481
  folic acid and, 489
  GBE and, 498
  5-HTP and, 493–97
  PMS and, 892, 895
  serotonin and, 481–82
  tricyclic, 489, 493, 495
antifungals, 989
antigens:
  C. albicans and, 380
  food allergies and, 592, 594–95,
    597–98
  hives and, 692–95, 698
  see also prostate-specific antigen
antioxidants:
  AD and, 278, 281–82
  alcohol dependence and, 269
  angina and, 305–6, 308
  asthma and, 328–33
  cancers and, 96, 357, 361–63,
    909–10
  cataracts and, 396–399
  and cellular approach to health,
    85–90
  cervical dysplasia and, 416–17
  CoQ$_{10}$ and, 90–91
  CVD and, 154, 156–60
  detoxification and, 117, 121,
    127–28
  diabetes and, 510, 516, 525–26,
    529, 535, 538–39, 542
  health-promoting diet and, 56–57,
    60, 62
  hepatitis and, 654–55
  high BP and, 669, 677
  HIV/AIDS and, 258–60
  IBD and, 464–65
  immune system and, 176, 179
  infertility and, 727, 738–43
  life extension and, 190–92, 195
  macular degeneration and,
    775–78
  Parkinson's disease and, 870
  periodontal disease and, 885–86
  during pregnancy, 79–80
  RA and, 933–34, 939–41
  recommendations on, 71–75
  sleep and, 45
antirheumatic drugs, 936–38
antiseptics, 989–90
anxiety, 313–21
  causes of, 313–15
  kava for, 316–19
  lactic acid and, 313, 315
  omega-3 fatty acids for, 316

signs and symptoms of, 313, 315,
    318
  therapeutic considerations for,
    315–18
appetite:
  dreaming and, 46
  exercise and, 41
  obesity and, 224–28
  weight management and, 233–34,
    238
apple polyphenols (AP), 602, 637
aqueous humor, 615–16, 618
arachidonic acid, 796–98
Arctic root (Rhodiola rosea), 216,
    427–28
arginine:
  angina and, 308
  CHF and, 447–48
  CVD and, 155–56
  ED and, 575–76
  herpes and, 661–63
  high BP and, 675
  infertility and, 727–28, 742–43
  in selected foods, 662–63
arjun tree (Terminalia arjuna), 449
arrhythmias, 643–46
  CoQ$_{10}$ for, 645
  diagnostic considerations for, 644
  diet and, 644
  hawthorn for, 645
  magnesium for, 645
  symptoms of, 643
  therapeutic considerations for,
    644–45
arsenic, 111
arteries:
  CVD and, 146–48, 151
  CVI and, 408–11
  structure of, 146–47
  see also coronary arteries; coronary
    artery disease
arthritis:
  gout and, 622
  IBD and, 462
  nutritional supplements and, 76
  psoriasis and, 923
  statistics on, 11–12
  see also osteoarthritis
ascorbic acid, see vitamin C
ashwagandha (Withania somnifera),
    216, 745
Asperger syndrome, 348
aspirin:
  asthma and, 64, 324, 329
  CVD and, 164–65
  dietary alternatives to, 165–66
  hives and, 64, 695–96, 699

aspirin (*cont.*)
  peptic ulcer and, 876–77
  side effects of, 165–66, 178, 876–77
  tension headaches and, 640–41
asthma, 12, 64, 322–39
  acupuncture and acupressure for, 336–37
  adrenal glands and, 324
  airborne allergens in, 327
  aloe vera for, 336
  antioxidants and, 328–33
  autonomic nervous system and, 324
  boswellia for, 336
  capsaicin for, 335
  carotenes for, 332–33
  causes of, 322–25
  C. forskohlii for, 336
  clinical classification of severity of, 323
  diagnostic considerations in, 323
  flavonoids for, 332
  food and, 327–29
  GBE for, 335–36
  influenza vaccine and, 325
  ivy for, 334
  jujube plum for, 335
  licorice for, 334–35
  magnesium for, 333
  major categories of, 322
  mechanisms of, 326
  omega-3 fatty acids for, 329–30
  pertussis vaccine and, 324–25
  salt in, 328
  signs and symptoms of, 322–24, 330–31, 336
  therapeutic considerations for, 325–37
  tylophora for, 335
  vegan diet for, 329
  vitamin B_6 for, 330
  vitamin B_{12} for, 333
  vitamin C for, 330–32
  vitamin D for, 333–34
Astragalus membranaceus, 180
atherosclerosis, 165
  angina and, 301, 305, 309–10
  CHF and, 446
  CVI and, 408–9
  diabetes and, 512, 517, 523
  diet and, 278–79, 775–76
  ED and, 572–73, 575
  hypercholesterolemia and, 680–81, 687
  hypoglycemia and, 711
  obesity and, 220–21, 227
  prevention of, 156–57, 159
  process of, 147

  psoriasis and, 926–27
  risk factors for, 147–49, 152–53, 159–61, 163, 278, 304, 530
  understanding of, 146–49
Atkins Diet, 231–33
atomoxetine (Strattera), 341
atopic dermatitis, *see* eczema
atorvastatin (Lipitor), 687
atrial fibrillation, 643, 645, 971
atrioventricular (AV) node, 643
attention-deficit/hyperactivity disorder (ADHD), 340–47
  biofeedback for, 345
  causes of, 340–42
  characteristics of, 340
  EFAs and, 343
  environment and, 341–42
  Feingold hypothesis and, 342–43
  food additives and, 342–43
  food allergies and, 344
  GBE for, 345
  grape seed extract for, 344–45
  iron for, 344
  L-theanine for, 345
  magnesium for, 344
  nutrients and, 341, 343–44
  pine bark extract for, 344–45
  sugar and, 343
  therapeutic considerations for, 341–45
  zinc for, 344
autism spectrum disorder (ASD), 348–52
  cause of, 349
  characteristics of, 348
  early and later signs of, 348–49
  forms of, 348
  nutritional supplements and, 350–52
  therapeutic considerations for, 349–51
autoantibodies, 934–35
autoimmune disorders, 503–4, 508–9, 933
azelaic acid (AzA), 251, 952
AZT, 257–59

bacteria, 9
  acne and, 246–48, 250
  detoxification and, 114–16
  digestion and, 132–34, 136–38, 140–45
  hives and, 698
  periodontal disease and, 884–85, 887–88
  probiotics and, 143–44
  RA and, 933–37

  sinus infections and, 957, 959
  strep throat and, 967–70
  see also intestinal flora; *specific bacteria*
bacterial vaginosis (BV), 985–86, 988–89
Bacteroides vulgatus, 461–62
baker's yeast, 180–81
balloon angioplasty, 302–3, 409
basal body temperature, 716, 719–20
basal metabolic rate (BMR), 40–41
basophils, 171, 635, 692
  food allergies and, 592, 602
Bastyr University, 5, 15
B cells, 171, 178
Beecher, H. K., 20
behaviors, behaviorial issues, 424
  ADHD and, 340–41, 343
  ASD and, 348–49, 351
  depression and, 479–80, 487
  hypoglycemia and, 709–10
  obesity and, 230
  Parkinson's disease and, 868, 872
  smoking and, 39
belonging, 31, 33
Benedetti, Fabrizio, 19
benfotiamine, 541
benign prostatic hyperplasia, *see* prostate enlargement
benign tumors, 95–96
Benson, Herbert, 20–21, 23, 209
benzoates, benzoic acid, 697
benzodiazepines, 317, 319
benzoyl peroxide, 248, 250–51
berberine, 141, 552
  chronic candidiasis and, 380, 385–86
  diarrhea and, 553–55
  plants containing, 380, 385–86
  sinus infections and, 958–59
Bernard, Claude, 8–9
berries, 912, 994
beta-amyloid, 276–77, 279–80, 282, 284, 286, 289
beta-carotene, 157
  AD and, 281–82
  cataracts and, 399
  cervical dysplasia and, 415–16
  HIV/AIDS and, 257
  macular degeneration and, 776–77
  male infertility and, 740
beta cells, 504, 507–8, 510–12, 532, 536
beta-glucans, 180–81
betaine, 824
beta-sitosterol, 918, 921
Bethesda System, 412–13

beverages, 856–57, 1021–22
bicycle seats, 575
bilberry (*Vaccinium myrtillus*), 74, 80
    diabetes and, 538–39
    glaucoma and, 617–18
    macular degeneration and, 778–79
bile, bile acids:
    detoxification and, 114–16, 121,
        125–28
    digestion and, 132, 140
    gallstones and, 605–12
    importance of flow of, 125–27
    NAFLD and, 823–24
    NASH and, 825
    psoriasis and, 925–26
biofeedback, 345, 809–10
bioflavonoids, *see* flavonoids
biogenic amine hypothesis, 479
bioidentical hormone therapy, 786
biological needs, 31
biopsies:
    cervical dysplasia and, 413–14, 417
    prostate cancer and, 905, 908
biotin:
    depression and, 487
    diabetes and, 532
    seborrheic dermatitis and, 954
Biskind, Morton, 892
bismuth subcitrate, 137–38, 879
bisphosphonates, 852–55
bitter melon (*Momordica charantia*),
    536
black cohosh (*Cimicifuga racemosa*),
    790–91
bladder:
    detoxification and, 115
    prostate enlargement and, 915–16,
        918–20
bladder infections, 471–77
    chronic interstitial, 471–73
    cranberry for, 473–75
    diagnostic considerations for,
        471–72
    goldenseal for, 475–76
    menopause and, 783
    signs and symptoms of, 471–73
    therapeutic considerations for, 472–73
    uva ursi for, 475
blood, bleeding:
    anemia and, 292–96
    aspirin side effects and, 165, 178
    detoxification and, 114–16
    endometriosis and, 565
    GBE and, 410
    hemoglobin and, 293, 506–7, 535
    hemorrhoids and, 647–49
    hepatitis and, 652–54

nutritional supplements and, 69
    peptic ulcer and, 876–77, 881
    periodontal disease and, 883, 888
    uterine fibroids and, 980
    see also menorrhagia; red blood
        cells; white blood cells
blood glucose, 45, 129, 213
    acne and, 248–49
    aging and, 187–89
    alcohol and, 267
    and cellular approach to health,
        85–86, 88
    charts on, 235
    chromium and, 528–29, 531
    depression and, 485, 487
    diabetes and, 503–7, 510, 512–22,
        524–37, 539–41
    digestion and, 141
    GI and, 712
    health-promoting diet and, 49,
        54–55, 60
    hypercholesterolemia and, 680–81,
        687
    hypoglycemia and, 521–22, 707–13,
        715
    IBS and, 759
    immune system and, 175
    influence of mulberry and
        glyburide treatments on, 535
    insomnia and, 750
    ketoacidosis and, 519–23
    lactic acid and, 314–15
    monitoring of, 517–23
    niacinamide and, 531
    obesity and, 220, 226–27, 234–36
    poor control of, 525
    prediabetes and, 505–6, 514, 517
    reducing after-meal elevations in,
        533–35
    SSRIs and, 482
    stabilizing levels of, 487
    urine ketone testing and, 520–21
    vitamin C and, 530
blood pressure:
    classification of, 666–67
    see also high blood pressure
bloodroot (*Sanguinaria canadensis*),
    888
blood vessels:
    angina and, 301–3, 307–10
    CHF and, 442, 447–48
    diabetes and, 526
    ED and, 572
    hemorrhoids and, 647–48
    migraine headaches and, 800–801,
        806, 808–9
    see also arteries; varicose veins

bodily processes, 41
body, calming mind and, 208–9
body mass index (BMI):
    chart on, 223
    obesity and, 222–25, 231–32, 236,
        238–39
    risk of disease according to, 223
bodywork, 427, 640
    physical care and, 78, 81–82
boils, 353–55
    causes of, 353
    characteristics of, 353
    therapeutic considerations for,
        353–54
bone mineral density (BMD) testing,
    844, 849–52
bones, bone:
    brittle, 853
    exercise and, 41
    metabolism of, 851, 858
    periodontal disease and, 883–85
    prunes in formation of, 858
    secondary causes of loss of, 848–49
    see also osteoporosis
bonito, 675–76
boric acid, 989–90
boron:
    osteoarthritis and, 836
    osteoporosis and, 846, 857–58
boswellia (*Boswellia serrata*):
    asthma and, 336
    IBD and, 467
    osteoarthritis and, 837
botanical medicines:
    AD and, 287–89, 291
    alcohol dependence and, 272–73,
        275
    angina and, 304, 308–9, 312
    anxiety and, 316–21
    arrhythmias and, 645–46
    asthma and, 334–36, 338
    bladder infections and, 473–77
    boils and, 353–55
    breast cancer and, 365–66
    bronchitis and, 369–71
    canker sores and, 390–91
    cataracts and, 399, 401
    cervical dysplasia and, 418–19
    CFS and, 427–28, 430
    CHF and, 449–50
    common cold and, 437–41
    constipation and, 453–55
    CVI and, 409–10
    depression and, 482, 496–499, 502
    detoxification and, 128–29
    diabetes and, 511–12, 534–39, 541,
        545–47

botanical medicines (*cont.*)
   diarrhea and, 553–56
   ear infections and, 561–64
   eczema and, 584–86
   ED and, 576–78, 581
   endometriosis and, 568–69
   FBD and, 590–91
   gallstones and, 611, 614
   glaucoma and, 617–18, 621
   gout and, 624, 627–29
   hemorrhoids and, 650–51
   hepatitis and, 654–57, 659
   high BP and, 676–79
   HIV/AIDS and, 260–62, 264
   hypercholesterolemia and, 690–91
   hyperthyroidism and, 705
   IBD and, 466–67, 470
   IBS and, 760–61, 763
   immune system and, 172, 180–82
   infertility and, 728–30, 743–47
   insomnia and, 754, 756
   kidney stones and, 772–73
   macular degeneration and, 778–80
   menopause and, 789–95
   menorrhagia and, 798–99
   migraine headaches and, 807–9,
     811
   MS and, 819–20
   NAFLD and, 825–26
   in naturopathic medicine, 6, 14
   obesity and, 240
   osteoarthritis and, 836–38,
     842–43
   osteoporosis and, 864, 867
   Parkinson's disease and, 873, 875
   peptic ulcer and, 880–82
   periodontal disease and, 888–89
   PMS and, 899–900, 902
   pneumonia and, 369–71
   prostate cancer and, 913–14
   prostate enlargement and,
     918–22
   psoriasis and, 928–29, 931
   RA and, 943–46
   seborrheic dermatitis and, 955
   silent inflammation and, 201, 203
   sinus infections and, 958–59, 961
   SLE and, 979
   sports injuries and, 964–66
   strep throat and, 969–70
   stress management and, 215–16,
     218
   stroke and, 973, 975
   uterine fibroids and, 982
   vaginitis and, 990
   varicose veins and, 994–97
bottle blowing, 373

bottle-feeding, 559–60
bowels, bowel:
   constipation and, 453–54
   detoxification and, 115
   prunes and, 454
   psoriasis and, 924–25
   see also inflammatory bowel
     disease; irritable bowel syndrome
bradycardias, 643
brain:
   AD and, 276–80, 282–88
   ADHD and, 340–41, 343–45
   ASD and, 349–51
   and calming mind and body, 208–9
   CoQ$_{10}$ and, 90–92
   CVD and, 146
   CVI and, 408–11
   depression and, 479–82, 484,
     488–91, 493–96, 498–99
   detoxification and, 117
   diabetes and, 524
   exercise and, 41–42
   health-promoting diet and, 49, 65
   hypoglycemia and, 707, 709
   insomnia and, 749–51
   menopause and, 782–83
   migraine headaches and, 800
   MS and, 814–15
   in normal menstrual cycle, 891.
   Parkinson's disease and, 868–73
   placebo response and, 19–20
   PMS and, 892–93, 895
   positive mental attitude and,
     29–30, 34
   sleep and, 44–46
   stroke and, 971–73
bran, 452
BRAT diet, 550–51
breads, 53–54, 62, 1016, 1026
breast cancer, 59, 77, 97–100, 587–89
   causes of, 356–57, 784–85
   comparisons between prostate and,
     903–4, 906–8
   detection of, 97, 107, 356–58
   diet and, 356–57, 359–61, 364–66,
     588
   exercise and, 357, 359
   FBD and, 587
   flaxseed and, 361
   HRT and, 784–85
   melatonin and, 365
   menopause and, 784–85, 787–88
   nutrition and, 360–61
   prevention of, 356–66, 588, 785,
     790, 864
   risk factors and, 98–100, 103–6,
     356–60, 362–65, 587

soy products and, 361–62, 864
   therapeutic considerations for,
     358–64
breast-feeding:
   asthma and, 327
   breast cancer and, 357–59
   diabetes and, 508
   ear infections and, 559–60
   eczema and, 583
   vitamin D deficiency and, 78
breasts:
   density of, 357
   PMS and, 890–91, 893–94, 897–99
   self-examination of, 357–58
   see also fibrocystic breast disease
breathing, *see* respiration, respiratory
   tract
bright light therapy, 287
bromelain:
   and bronchitis and pneumonia, 371
   PD and, 573–74
   RA and, 943
   sports injuries and, 963–64
   varicose veins and, 996
bronchitis, 12, 367–75, 431
   differentiating between pneumonia
     and, 367–68
   expectorants for, 369–71, 374–75
   mucolytics for, 371, 375
   postural draining for, 373–74
   signs and symptoms of, 367
   therapeutic considerations for,
     369–74
brown fat, 228
buckwheat (*Fagopyrum esculentum*),
   609, 994
bulimia, 229
bulking agents, 649
Burkitt, Denis, 50
bursitis, 962–63
   see also sports, sports injuries
buspirone, 317
butcher's broom (*Ruscus aculeatus*),
   650, 996
butterbur (*Petasides hybridus*), 809
butylated hydroxyanisol (BHA), 697
butylated hydroxytoluene (BHT), 697
3-n-butylphthalide (3nB), 279–80,
   628, 669

cabbage, 878–79
cadmium, 111
caffeine:
   anxiety and, 313, 315
   CFS and, 425–26
   depression and, 485
   detoxification and, 117, 125

endometriosis and, 567
FBD and, 587
female infertility and, 726
glaucoma and, 619–20
high BP and, 667, 672
insomnia and, 750
stress management and, 212–13
cakes, 1015
calcidiol, 846, 848
calcitonin, 848, 852, 854
calcitriol, 846, 848, 857
calcium:
high BP and, 666–67, 669, 674
kidney stones and, 764–69, 771–73
osteoporosis and, 845–46, 855–61, 864
PMS and, 897
calcium D-glucarate, 365
Calment, Jeanne Louise, 184
calories, 102, 189, 200
Atkins Diet and, 231–33
gallstones and, 610
health-promoting diet and, 48–49, 51–52, 54, 62, 67
obesity and, 226–34, 236, 238–41
restriction of, 188, 193, 238, 610
calprotectin, 467
Canadian College of Naturopathic Medicine, 15, 964
Canadian National Breast Screening Study 2, 358
cancer, 608–10
AIDS and, 253
celiac disease and, 403
cells and, 87, 95–96, 412–13
cervical dysplasia and, 412–17
in children, 61, 97
detection of, 97, 101–7, 356–58
detoxification and, 115–19, 121
diet and, 48–50, 52–54, 56–64, 95–97, 99–105, 356–57, 359–61, 364–66, 588, 904, 906–8, 911
gallstones and, 608, 610
immune system and, 96, 100, 169–72
liver and, 652, 654–56
nutritional supplements and, 73–78, 102–6, 361–66, 906, 908–13
obesity and, 98–99, 102, 221–22
placebo response and, 18–19
positive mental attitude and, 30, 37
prevention of, 30, 57, 95–108, 119, 159, 190–91, 193, 356–66, 588, 785, 790, 864, 903–14
risk factors and, 30, 39, 95–106, 176, 190, 221, 356–60, 362–65, 587

sleeping pills and, 754–55
smoking and, 39, 96–97, 99, 101, 106, 117, 357
statistics on, 11–12, 95–106
toxins and, 107, 112
see also specific cancers
Cancer Causes and Control, 56
Cancer Prevention Studies, 754–55
Candida albicans, 376–88
diarrhea and, 552–53
digestion and, 132, 136, 140–41, 143–44
eczema and, 583
hives and, 698
laboratory confirmation of presence of, 380–81
liver injury and, 384
natural agents for, 385–87
nutrients for, 381
predisposing factors to overgrowth by, 377
psoriasis and, 924
vaginitis and, 984–85, 987–90
candidiasis, chronic, 9, 376–88
causes of, 377
detoxification and, 383–85
diagnostic considerations for, 380
diet for, 381
elimination and, 384–85
enteric-coated volatile oils for, 386
garlic for, 386
immune system and, 376–77, 381–82, 384–85, 387
lipotropic agents for, 384
natural antiyeast agents for, 385–87
probiotics for, 385
profile of patient with, 376–77
propolis for, 387
signs and symptoms of, 376–80, 382
tea tree oil for, 386–87
therapeutic considerations for, 380–87
vicious cycle of, 383
candidiasis questionnaire, 378–80
canker sores:
causes of, 389–90
characteristics of, 389
nutrition and, 389–90
therapeutic considerations for, 390–91
capsaicin:
asthma and, 335
diabetes and, 541
psoriasis and, 928–29
caraway oil, 138

carbohydrates:
acne and, 248–49
Atkins Diet and, 231–33
complex, 52, 712
diabetes and, 503, 514–15, 527, 534
gout and, 626
health-promoting diet and, 52–53, 60
high BP and, 669
hypoglycemia and, 523, 709–12
IBS and, 759
kidney stones and, 767
obesity and, 228–29, 231–33, 236, 238
PMS and, 893–94, 898
prediabetes and, 505
refined, 53, 190, 213, 514–15, 709, 711–12
of selected food, 1013–20
simple, 60, 711–12
stress management and, 213
cardiovascular disease (CVD), 146–68
alcohol dependence and, 270–71
antioxidants and, 154, 156–60
atherosclerosis and, 146–49
cholesterol and, 146, 148–62
coping strategies and, 162–63
diabetes and, 152–53, 503–4, 533
diet and, 153–57, 159, 161, 163, 165–68
fibrinogen and, 150–51, 153, 156, 161–62
grape seed extract and, 160
homocysteine and, 155, 160–62
hypercholesterolemia and, 682, 687
and magnesium and potassium deficiency, 163–64
and nuts and seeds, 155–56
obesity and, 221–22
olive oil and, 154
pine bark extract and, 160
platelet aggregation and, 151, 155, 158, 160–61
prediabetes and, 505
prevention of, 153–61, 163–66
red wine and, 154, 156
risk factors for, 147–53, 155–57, 159–64, 188, 198–99, 224, 688
silent inflammation and, 198–99
type A personality and, 162
vitamin C and, 157–60
vitamin D deficiency in, 164
vitamin E and, 157–60
cardiovascular health:
clinical evaluation of, 149
exercise and, 40–43
positive mental attitude and, 30, 37

cardiovascular system:
  attitude and, 30
  hypothyroidism and, 717
  parts and functions of, 146
  stress and, 204–5
carnitine, 91
  alcohol dependence and, 269
  angina and, 306–7
  CFS and, 427
  CHF and, 443, 445
  HIV/AIDS and, 259–60
  hyperthyroidism and, 704–5
  immune system and, 176
  infertility and, 727, 741–42
  NAFLD and, 824–25
carnosine, 351, 879–80
carob powder, 551
carotenes:
  asthma and, 332–33
  food sources of, 57, 777
  immune system and, 176, 179, 192
  life extension and, 191–92
  macular degeneration and, 776–78
  see also beta-carotene
carotid endarterectomy, 409
carpal tunnel, cross section of, 393
carpal tunnel syndrome (CTS),
    392–95
  alternating hot and cold water
    treatment for, 393
  causes of, 392
  signs and symptoms of, 392–93
  therapeutic considerations for,
    392–94
carrageenan, 461–62
Carrel, Alexis, 185
cartilage:
  glucosamine and, 829–32, 835
  osteoarthritis and, 9–10, 827–28,
    830–31, 834–36
  RA and, 932–33, 936–37
cascara sagrada (*Rhamnus
    purshiana*), 453–54
cataracts, 396–401
  antioxidants and, 396–99
  beta-carotene for, 399
  BH4 for, 399
  causes of, 396
  cysteine for, 399
  flavonoids and, 399, 540
  glutathione and, 396, 398–99
  heavy metals and, 400
  lutein and, 396–97
  selenium and, 396, 398
  signs and symptoms of, 396
  SOD and, 396, 398
  vitamin A and, 396–97, 399

vitamin B$_2$ for, 399
vitamin C and, 396–98
vitamin E and, 396–99
zinc and, 398–99
Cathcart, Robert, 654
cayenne pepper, *see* capsaicin
CD4 counts, 253–55, 257–62
Celadrin, 394, 838–39
celery, celery seed extract, 279, 628,
    669
celiac disease, 402–7
  causes of, 402–3
  diabetes and, 508
  diet and, 402–6
  hair loss and, 634
  mortality risk and, 402–3
  pancreatic enzymes for, 405–6
  symptoms of, 402, 405, 549, 634
  therapeutic considerations for,
    403–5
cell membranes:
  CVD and, 153–54
  homeostasis and, 85–86
cells:
  aging and, 87–88, 185–87
  and approaches to health, 85–94
  cancer and, 87, 95–96, 412–13
  immune system and, 170–71, 177,
    179–81
  life extension and, 186, 190, 193
  see also specific types of cells
Centers for Disease Control and
    Prevention (CDC), 64, 341–42,
    905
  on CFS, 420–21
  on EMS, 492–93
central sleep apnea, 749
ceramides, 929
cereals, 53–54, 1014–15
cerebral vascular insufficiency (CVI),
    408–11
  botanical medicines for, 409–10
  carotid endarterectomy for, 409
  diagnostic considerations for,
    408–9
  signs and symptoms of, 408–9
  therapeutic considerations for,
    409–10
Cernilton, 918, 920–21
cervical dysplasia, 412–19
  beta-carotene for, 415–16
  causes of, 413–14
  diagnosis of, 412
  diet and, 415–16, 419
  DIM for, 417–18
  folic acid for, 416–17
  green tea extract for, 418

I3C for, 417
Pap smears and, 412–18
risk factors for, 413–15, 417
selenium for, 416
therapeutic considerations for,
    414–18
vitamin A for, 415–16
vitamin C and, 414–16
cervical intraepithelial neoplasia
    (CIN), 413, 415–17
chasteberry (*Vitex agnus-castus*):
  endometriosis and, 568
  FBD and, 590
  female infertility and, 728–29
  menorrhagia and, 798
  PMS and, 899
chemicals:
  chronic candidiasis and, 383–84
  detoxification and, 113–14, 116–17,
    121, 123–25, 128–29
  digestion and, 131
  gallstones and, 611–12
  immune system and, 171–72
  infertility and, 726, 736
  MCS and, 422
  toxic, 110, 112–13, 116, 121,
    128–29
cherries, 627–28
childbearing, later, 357
Childers, Norman, 829
children, childhood:
  acne and, 245–46, 250
  ADHD and, 340–45
  ASD and, 348–51
  asthma and, 322–28, 330–31,
    333–34
  bone growth and, 856–57, 861
  bronchitis and, 370
  cancer and, 61, 97
  celiac disease and, 402, 508
  constipation and, 452–53
  decline in exercise among, 152
  diabetes and, 504, 507–13, 527
  diarrhea and, 548–51, 553
  ear infections and, 557–62
  eczema and, 583–84
  food allergies and, 593
  health-promoting diet and, 59,
    61, 64
  hives and, 694, 696, 698
  IBD and, 467–68
  nutritional supplements and, 71–75,
    77
  obesity and, 220, 225
  playing with, 37
  pneumonia and, 368, 372
  progeria and, 186, 194

soft drink consumption of, 856–57
strep throat and, 967–68
toxins and, 111
Chinese ginseng (*Panax ginseng*):
  diabetes and, 537
  ED and, 577
  male infertility and, 743
  stress management and, 215–16
chiropractic, 640
chlamydia (*Chlamydia trachomatis*):
  infertility and, 735
  vaginitis and, 985–89
chlorophyll, 295, 797
cholera, 8, 554
choleretics, 611
cholestasis, 125–27, 892
cholesterol, 24, 269, 301
  aging and, 187
  angina and, 306–8
  and cellular approach to health, 86
  chromium and, 529
  CoQ$_{10}$ and, 88–90
  CVD and, 146, 148–62
  detoxification and, 114–15
  diabetes and, 525–29, 533–35, 537, 539–40
  dietary, 683–84
  ED and, 572
  elevated levels of, 151–52, 539–40, 971
  exercise and, 41
  gallstones and, 605–11
  health-promoting diet and, 62–63, 67
  high-density lipoprotein (HDL), 149–52, 154–55, 159–60, 162, 680–81, 685, 687–88, 690–91
  immune system and, 176
  low-density lipoprotein (LDL), 149–59, 162, 680–83, 680–83, 685–91
  lowering levels of, 157
  manufacture of, 89
  obesity and, 232–34, 237, 239
  prostate enlargement and, 918
  recommendations on, 539–40, 681
  in selected foods, 684
  very low-density lipoprotein (VLDL), 680, 682
  see also hypercholesterolemia
cholinergic urticaria, 694
choline-stabilized orthosilicic acid (BioSil), 633, 861–62
chondroitin, 832–34
chromium:
  acne and, 249
  depression and, 489

diabetes and, 528–29, 531
  glaucoma and, 619
  hypoglycemia and, 713, 715
  obesity and, 236–37
chronic candidiasis, *see* candidiasis, chronic
chronic diseases, statistics on, 11–12
chronic fatigue syndrome (CFS), 35, 213–14, 420–30
  adrenal function and, 424–25
  Arctic root for, 427–28
  breathing, posture, and bodywork for, 427
  carnitine for, 427
  causes of, 421–24
  CDC on, 420–21
  CoQ$_{10}$ for, 427
  depression and, 420, 424–25
  diagnosis of, 420–21, 423
  environmental toxin overload and, 425
  exercise for, 427
  FM and, 422–23
  immune system and, 421–22, 424, 428
  impaired liver function and, 425
  magnesium for, 426–27
  NK cells and, 422, 424, 428
  other names for, 420, 422
  Siberian ginseng for, 427–29
  sleep and, 44, 420–21
  stress and, 424, 428
  symptoms of, 420–22
  therapeutic considerations for, 423–28
chronic obstructive pulmonary disease (COPD), 431–34
  causes of, 431
  magnesium for, 432–33
  NAC for, 432
  symptoms of, 431
  therapeutic considerations for, 431–32
cisapride (Propulsid), 138
citicoline, 974
citrate, 768
Clarke, Norman, 309
Clinical Global Impressions scale, 287
clinical nutrition, 6
Clinical Outcomes Utilizing Revascularization and Aggressive Drug Evaluation (COURAGE) trial, 303–4
Clinical Psychopharmacology Research Group, 494
Clostridium difficile, 551, 553
cobalamin, 283, 298

cod liver oil, 509–10
coenzyme Q10 (CoQ$_{10}$), 644–45
  angina and, 307
  angiograms and, 304–5
  arrhythmias and, 645
  and cellular approach to health, 88–92
  CFS and, 427
  CHF and, 443, 445–47
  CVD and, 157–59
  dosages for, 91
  high BP and, 88, 90, 676
  HIV/AIDS and, 259
  hypercholesterolemia and, 683
  male infertility and, 741–42
  Parkinson's disease and, 90, 92, 870–71
  PD and, 573–74
  periodontal disease and, 886–87
  specific clinical uses of, 90
  stroke and, 973
coenzymes, 68–69
cofactor therapy, 751
cognitive issues, 31, 524, 972
cognitive therapy, 424, 483, 498
colchicine, 624
cold urticaria, 694
coleus (*Coleus forskohlii*), 336
collagen, collagen matrix, 69
  glaucoma, 615–17
  osteoarthritis and, 827–29, 836
  periodontal disease and, 884–87
  sports injuries and, 963
colon:
  CD and, 456–57
  digestion and, 132–33, 140–42
  diverticular disease and, 142
  function of, 141–42
  health-promoting diet and, 50
  IBD and, 457–58, 461–62, 465–66
  IBS and, 138, 142
  UC and, 457, 461, 467
colon cancer, 609
  early detection of, 107
  risk factors and, 99–100, 102–4
  UC and, 457, 461
colposcopy, 414–15, 417–18
common cold, 435–41
  causes of, 435
  echinacea for, 437–40
  immune system and, 169, 177–80, 435–37, 439
  liquids for, 436
  P. sidoides for, 440
  recommendations for, 435–40
  rest for, 436
  sugar and, 436

common cold (*cont.*)
symptoms of, 435–39
therapeutic considerations for, 435–40
vitamin C for, 436–37
zinc lozenges for, 437
communication, keys to, 211–12
complementary practitioners, 12–13
complement system, 884
comprehensive digestive stool analysis (CDSA), 380–81
concentration, 783
conditionally essential nutrients, 71, 91
congestive heart failure (CHF), 442–450
arginine for, 447–48
arjun tree and, 449
carnitine and, 443, 445
and complementary aspects of naturopathic medicine, 10–11
CoQ_{10} and, 443, 445–47
factors that precipitate or worsen, 442
hawthorn for, 449
magnesium and, 443–44
signs and symptoms of, 442, 446
stages of, 443, 445–47, 449
therapeutic considerations for, 443–48
vitamin B_1 and, 443–45
constipation, 142, 451–55
bowel retraining for, 453–54
causes of, 451–52
in children, 452–53
laxatives and, 451–55
signs and symptoms of, 451–52
therapeutic considerations for, 452–54
Consumers Union, 342
continuous glucose monitoring, 708
continuous positive airway pressure (CPAP), 749
contraceptives:
cervical dysplasia and, 413, 416–17
gallstones and, 607
conventional medicine:
comparisons between naturopathic and, 8–9, 12–13
hemorrhoids and, 648
naturopathic medicine as complementary approach to, 10
placebo response and, 21
conventional physicians, 12–14
bias against natural medicine on part of, 13–14

complementary practitioners vs., 12–13
exercise and, 42–43
coping, 162–63, 208
copper:
HIV/AIDS and, 258
osteoarthritis and, 836
osteoporosis and, 861
RA and, 941–42
coronary arteries:
angina and, 301–5, 307–10
bypass surgery and, 166, 302–5
coronary artery disease (CAD), 146, 153
niacin for, 687–88
omega-3 fatty acids for, 491
risk factors for, 159
Coronary Artery Surgery Study (CASS), 303
coronary blood vessels, illustration of, 302
Coronary Drug Project, 685
corticosteroids, 815
IBD and, 463
psoriasis and, 928
RA and, 937, 941
rosacea and, 950–51
cortisol:
depression and, 484, 486
female infertility and, 726
insomnia and, 749–50
stress and, 208, 213, 217
Council on Naturopathic Medical Education (CNME), 15
counseling, *see* psychological factors
Cousins, Norman, 172–73
C-peptides:
blood glucose monitoring and, 519–20
diabetes and, 511, 519–20, 525, 528, 530
niacinamide and, 531
crackers, 1016
cranberry (*Vaccinium macrocarpon*), 473–75
cranberry juice, 767
C-reactive protein (CRP):
high-sensitivity (hsCRP), 147–49, 153–56, 158–59, 161–62, 164
hypercholesterolemia and, 682, 684–85
silent inflammation and, 198–203
Cretans, 155
criminal behavior, 709–10
Crohn's disease (CD), 456–61
boswellia for, 467
causes of, 457–58

children and, 467
curcumin for, 466
diet and, 458–59
features shared by UC and, 457
fiber and, 464
signs and symptoms of, 456, 467
therapeutic considerations for, 459–61, 464–68
vitamin B_{12} for, 465
vitamin D for, 465
zinc for, 465
see also inflammatory bowel disease
cryotherapy, 415
curcumin, 119
AD and, 289
gallstones and, 611
HIV/AIDS and, 260–61
IBD and, 466
osteoarthritis and, 836–37
psoriasis and, 929
RA and, 943
silent inflammation and, 201
sports injuries and, 964–65
cures, removing obstacles to, 25
cutaneous hemorrhoids, 647
cyanocobalamin, 297–99
cyclical allergies, 596
cysteine, 121–23, 127, 129
cataracts and, 399
life extension and, 190
cystic fibrosis, 138
cystine, 765–66, 773
cystitis, *see* bladder infections
cytokines, 510
anxiety and, 316
endometriosis and, 565–66
HIV/AIDS and, 257
MS and, 817
psoriasis and, 923, 925–26
cytotoxic reactions, 595, 597

daidzein, 858, 864
dairy products, 1025–26
acne and, 248
avoidance of, 551
cancer and, 103, 904, 906–7
celiac disease and, 403, 405, 508
chronic candidiasis and, 381
constipation and, 453
CVD and, 154, 165
diabetes and, 508
diarrhea and, 549, 551
digestion and, 145
endometriosis and, 567
health-promoting diet and, 51, 53–55, 59, 61–62, 65

IBD and, 464
PMS and, 893
sperm counts and, 736
damage theories, 185–88
death, 10, 24, 30
  AD and, 278
  aging and, 186
  alcohol dependence and, 265, 273
  angina and, 302–4, 307
  asthma and, 322
  cancer and, 95, 99, 101, 104, 106,
    356, 358–59, 361, 903, 905, 909,
    911
  celiac disease and, 402–3
  CHF and, 445
  CVD and, 146, 149–53, 155,
    158–59, 161, 163–65
  depression and, 478
  diabetes and, 503, 520, 523
  diarrhea and, 549, 552
  exercise and, 42
  health-promoting diet and, 53
  HIV/AIDS and, 253–55
  hypercholesterolemia and, 680
  nutritional supplements and, 77
  obesity and, 220–21
  premature, 39, 183, 188, 193,
    220–21
  sleeping pills and, 755
  stroke and, 971
  top ten causes of, 183
deep tissue work, 81
dehydrocholic acid, 925–26
dehydroepiandrosterone (DHEA):
  AD and, 286
  hypothyroidism and, 721–22
  life extension and, 193–94
  SLE and, 977–78
  stress and, 208, 216–17
Dement, William C., 46
dementia, see Alzheimer's disease
Demodex folliculorum, 950
demyelination, 812–13
deoxycholic acid, 608
deoxyribonucleic acid (DNA):
  aging and, 185–87
  cancer and, 95–97, 99
  and cellular approach to health,
    87–88
  HIV/AIDS and, 254, 260
  male infertility and, 736–41
  RA and, 933–35
depression, 478–503
  AD and, 277, 285, 288
  age and, 277, 282, 285, 486, 488,
    498–99
  alcohol and, 265, 268–72, 484–85

bipolar (manic), 491, 494
  caffeine and, 485
  cancer and, 102
  causes of, 482–83
  CFS and, 424–25
  chromium for, 489
  counseling for, 483, 486, 496, 498,
    500
  diabetes and, 503, 524
  diagnosis of, 478
  diet and, 64, 481–82, 484, 486–88,
    501
  dreaming and, 46
  exercise and, 41, 485–86
  folic acid for, 487–89
  food allergies and, 491
  GBE for, 496–99
  hormonal factors in, 483–84
  5-HTP for, 272, 482, 493–97
  hypoglycemia and, 484–85, 487,
    709
  kava for, 317
  lavender for, 482, 499
  lifestyle and, 482, 484–86, 501
  low thyroid function in, 483
  monoamines and, 479–80, 488–90
  nutritional supplements and, 68, 76,
    482, 485, 488–91, 501–2
  omega-3 fatty acids for, 316, 487,
    490–91
  Parkinson's disease and, 868, 872
  PMS and, 890, 893, 895–96, 898,
    900
  positive mental attitude and,
    29–30, 35
  saffron for, 482, 499
  St.-John's-wort for, 482, 496–498
  SAM-e and, 488, 491
  selenium for, 485, 489
  serotonin and, 272, 480–82, 484,
    488–91, 493–96, 498–99
  sleep and, 44–45
  stress and adrenal function in,
    483–84
  stroke and, 972
  symptoms of, 478, 486, 491, 495
  theoretical models of, 478–80
  therapeutic considerations for,
    481–99
  toxins and, 484
  tryptophan and, 481–82, 484,
    492–93
  vitamin B$_6$ for, 487, 489
  vitamin B$_{12}$ for, 487–89
  vitamin D for, 487, 490
  zinc for, 489
dermographism, 692–94

detoxification, 109–10
  alcohol and, 121, 268
  CFS and, 425
  chronic candidiasis and, 383–85
  fasting in, 128–30
  how it works, 113–26
  indications of need for, 384
  inducers of, 118, 120
  inhibitors of, 118–19, 121
  liver and, 110, 112–16, 118–21, 123,
    125–28, 383, 425, 567
  in naturopathic medicine, 4
  Phase I, 114–20, 125
  Phase II, 114–17, 119–25
  practical applications and, 125
  promotion of, 383–84
  RA and, 935
devil's claw (*Harpagophytum
  procumbens*), 838
diabetes, 503–47
  acupuncture for, 541–42
  AD and, 277
  ALA for, 539, 541
  American ginseng for, 536
  antioxidants and, 510, 516, 525–26,
    529, 535, 538–39, 542
  atherosclerosis and, 512, 517, 523
  benfotiamine for, 541
  biotin for, 532
  bitter melon for, 536
  blood glucose and, 503–7, 510,
    512–22, 524–37, 539–41
  capsaicin for, 541
  causes of, 507–10, 512–17
  and cellular approach to health, 86
  changes in blood vessel linings in,
    526
  Chinese ginseng for, 537
  chromium for, 528–29, 531
  clinical monitoring and
    management of patients with,
    517–22
  cognitive difficulties in, 524
  complications of, 503–4, 521–26,
    530, 537, 539–42
  CVD and, 152–53, 503–4, 533
  depression and, 503, 524
  diagnostic considerations for, 505–7
  diet and, 50, 52, 54, 60, 62–63,
    232, 507–8, 510, 513–15, 518–19,
    521, 526–28, 532, 535–36, 542,
    544
  dietary fat and, 503, 514–16
  early treatment and possible
    reversal of, 510–12
  ED and, 573, 575
  enteroviruses and, 508–9, 512

diabetes (*cont.*)
environment and, 507, 517
epicatechin for, 510–12
exercise and, 513–15, 518, 528, 714–15
fenugreek for, 537
fiber and, 515–16, 527–28, 533–34, 542
flavonoids for, 538–40
foot ulcers in, 524, 542
free radicals and, 516, 525–26, 538
garlic for, 537
genetics and, 507, 513
gestational, 504–5, 531
GI and, 514–16, 534, 712
GLA for, 541
glycosylated hemoglobin and, 506–7, 525, 535
G. sylvestre for, 535–36
high BP and, 503, 526, 529–30
homocysteine and, 526
hypercholesterolemia and, 687, 690
hypoglycemia and, 521–24, 707, 712–14
immune system and, 503–4, 507–11, 524, 527–29, 539
insulin and, 68, 503–4, 507–8, 510–12, 515–16, 518–20, 524–32, 534–37
ketoacidosis and, 519–23
kidney disease and, 503, 524, 533, 542
lifestyle and, 513–15, 517–19, 521, 527–28, 535
magnesium for, 531–32
manganese for, 532
metabolic syndrome and, 505
natural glucosidase inhibitors for, 534–35
neuropathy and, 503, 523–24, 526, 531–33, 539, 541–42
niacinamide for, 510–11, 530–31
niacin for, 530–31, 539–40, 687
nitrates and, 510
nutritional supplements and, 68, 76–77, 509–11, 518–19, 526, 528–42, 544–47
obesity and, 220–21, 224–27, 232, 234, 237, 504–5, 512–14, 516–17
omega-3 fatty acids and, 509–10, 515–16, 532–33
onions for, 537
oxidative stress in, 525–26, 537–39
in Pima Indians, 513
poor wound healing in, 524, 532, 542
proposed triggers of, 509

psychological support for, 527
retinopathy and, 503, 523, 526, 531, 533, 539–40
risk factors for, 220, 224–26, 507–9, 511–14, 516–18, 521
sorbitol and, 525, 530, 538, 541
SSRIs and, 482
statistics on, 11–12
stress and, 519, 527
stroke and, 503, 971
symptoms of, 503, 505, 541
therapeutic considerations for, 526–42
toxins and, 112, 504, 517
type 1, 504–5, 507–12, 518–23, 527–28, 530–34, 536–37, 541, 544–45
type 2, 503–5, 512–20, 524, 527–37, 545–46, 687, 714–15
vitamin B$_6$ for, 531–32
vitamin C for, 529–30, 538–40, 542
vitamin D and, 507, 509
vitamin E for, 516, 530, 542
zinc for, 532, 542
Diabetes Control and Complications Trial, 518
Diabetes Prevention Program, 514
diamine oxidase, 804–5
diarrhea, 293–96, 548–56
anemia and, 293–95
berberine for, 553–55
carob powder or pectin for, 551
causes of, 548–50
dairy products and, 549, 551
exudative, 548–49
HIV/AIDS and, 256, 261
inadequate-contact, 548–49
liquids and BRAT diet for, 550–51
osmotic, 548
parasitic infections and, 144, 552–54
probiotics for, 551–53
replacing electrolytes and, 551
secretory, 548
symptoms of, 548–49, 554
therapeutic considerations for, 549–54
tormentil root for, 555
travelers, 551, 554–55
diazepam (Valium), 214–15
dichlorodiphenyltrichloroethane (DDT), 736
Dietary and Reinfarction Trial (DART), 166
Dietary Approaches to Stop Hypertension (DASH) Diet, 669–71

diethylstilbestrol (DES), 735–36
diets, diet, 851–53
acne and, 246, 248–49, 251–52
AD and, 277–80, 290–91
aging and, 48, 186–90
alcohol and, 267, 274
allergies and, 64, 596–98
anemia and, 293–94, 296–97, 299–300
angina and, 311
anxiety and, 315, 320
arrhythmias and, 644
ASD and, 349–50
aspirin alternatives in, 165–66
asthma and, 328–29, 332, 337–38
blood glucose monitoring and, 518–19
Burkitt and Trowell on, 50
cancer and, 48–50, 52–54, 56–64, 95–97, 99–105, 356–57, 359–61, 364–66, 588, 904, 906–8, 911
canker sores and, 389
celiac disease and, 402–6
and cellular approach to health, 85, 87
cervical dysplasia and, 415–16, 419
CFS and, 425–26, 429
CHF and, 443
chronic candidiasis and, 381
constipation and, 451–55
CVD and, 153–57, 159, 161, 163, 165–68
depression and, 64, 481–82, 484, 486–88, 501
detoxification and, 115–17, 121–23, 126, 425
diabetes and, 50, 52, 54, 60, 62–63, 232, 507–8, 510, 513–15, 518–19, 521, 526–28, 532, 535–36, 542, 544
diarrhea and, 550–51
digestion and, 132–33, 142, 145
diseases strongly associated with low-fiber, 50
eczema and, 583
ED and, 574–75, 580–81
endometriosis and, 567
FBD and, 588, 591
gallstones and, 605–11, 613
gout and, 622–26
and hair loss in women, 633
health-promoting, 25, 28, 48–67
hemorrhoids and, 647–49, 651
hepatitis and, 654, 658
herpes simplex and, 661–65
high BP and, 63, 666–73, 679

high in refined carbohydrates,
514–15
HIV/AIDS and, 256, 263–64
hives and, 696, 698–99
hypercholesterolemia and, 682–84,
689
hyperthyroidism and, 704
hypoglycemia and, 709–13, 715
IBD and, 458–59, 464, 469
IBS and, 758–59
immune system and, 58, 100, 172,
174–75
-induced thermogenesis, 226–28,
241
infertility and, 726–27, 732, 738,
746
kidney stones and, 764–69, 772–73
liver function and, 126–27
macular degeneration and, 775–76,
779
menopause and, 787–88
migraine headaches and, 804–5
MS and, 812–16
NAFLD and, 823–24, 826
nutritional supplements and,
66–68, 73, 76–77
obesity and, 100, 224, 226–33,
238–41
Optimal Health Food Pyramid and,
55–66
osteoarthritis and, 828–29, 835,
841–42
osteoporosis and, 846, 851, 853,
855–59, 862, 866
Parkinson's disease and, 869–70,
874
peptic ulcer and, 878–79
periodontal disease and, 885
pH balance and, 92
plant-based, 48–50
PMS and, 893–94, 897
prediabetes and, 505
prostate enlargement and, 917–18
psoriasis and, 924–26, 930
RA and, 933–36, 938–41, 946
sarcopenia prevention and, 189–90,
855
silent inflammation and, 199–202
SLE and, 976–78
for stress management, 212–14
stroke and, 971
toxins and, 58–60, 64–66, 112
uterine fibroids and, 981–82
vaginitis and, 988
varicose veins and, 992–94
see also foods, food; *specific diets*
diffuse hair loss, 630–31

digestion, 131–45, 552, 924
anxiety and, 313, 317
chronic candidiasis and, 380–81
colon and, 132–33, 140–42
diabetes and, 515
diagram on, 133
diverticular disease and, 142
dreams and, 47
dysbiosis and, 142–43
ear infections and, 560
elimination and, 133, 141–42
exercise and, 41
food allergies and, 139–41,
598–602
GERD and, 134–35, 138
health-promoting diet and, 49
H. pylori overgrowth and, 134,
136–38
IBS and, 138, 142
indigestion and, 134–40
lactose intolerance and, 145
pancreas and, 131–32, 134,
138–39
pancreatic enzymes and, 132,
138–41, 144
peptic ulcer and, 876
prebiotics and, 145
probiotics and, 143–45
process of, 131–32
small intestine and, 131–32, 137,
139–41, 145
stress and, 133–34, 141, 213
digitalis, 443–44, 446
digital rectal exams, 904, 910
digoxin, 645
dihydrotestosterone (DHT), 915, 917,
919, 921
diindolylmethane (DIM), 363–64,
417–18
Diogenes Study, 230–31
dipeptidyl peptidase IV (DPP-IV),
406
disease-modifying antirheumatic
drugs (DMARDs), 936–38
diseases, causes of, 5
diuretics, 443–44
glucosamine and, 831–32
diverticular disease, 142
docosahexaenoic acid (DHA), 86
CVD and, 154–55
CVI and, 409
hypertriglyceridemia and, 685
IBD and, 460
MS and, 816–17
nutritional supplements and, 76–77,
79
prostate cancer and, 907–8

psoriasis and, 926
RA and, 939, 943
dong quai (*Angelica sinensis*), 792
Dossey, Larry, 22
double-blind, placebo-controlled
trials, 20–21
dreams, 46–47
drug-induced lupus erythematosus
(DILE), 976
drugs, illicit:
hepatitis and, 652–53
HIV/AIDS and, 254
male infertility and, 737
drusen, 775
dual energy X-ray absorptiometry
(DEXA), 849–51
duodenal ulcers, 876–78, 881
dysbiosis, 142–43, 461
RA and, 935–37
dysthymia, 478

ear infections (otitis media), 557–64
acute, 557–58
ADHD and, 344
bottle-feeding and, 559–60
causes of, 559
chronic or serous, 557
diagnostic considerations for,
559–61
food allergies and, 560–61
humidifiers for, 562–63
naturopathic ear drops for, 561
spontaneous resolution of, 559
standard medical treatment for,
557–59
symptoms of, 557–58
therapeutic considerations for,
561–62
xylitol for, 561–62
earlobe crease, 166
Eating Right Pyramid, 53–54
echinacea:
common cold and, 437–40
strep throat and, 969
echocardiography, 443, 447, 449
eczema (atopic dermatitis), 582–86
asthma and, 323, 325
C. albicans in, 583
causes of, 582–83
EFAs for, 584
licorice for, 584–86
probiotics and, 583–84
signs and symptoms of, 582
therapeutic considerations for,
583–84
Edible Plant and Animal Kingdoms
Taxonomic List, 599–600

eggs, 600, 1026
  health-promoting diet and, 51,
    58–59, 61–62, 65
  infertility and, 724–27, 731, 734,
    738, 742
  normal menstrual cycle and, 890–91
eicosapentaenoic acid (EPA), 85–86
  CVD and, 154–55
  CVI and, 409
  depression and, 490–91
  hypertriglyceridemia and, 685
  IBD and, 460
  MS and, 816–17
  nutritional supplements and, 76–77,
    79
  prostate cancer and, 907–8
  psoriasis and, 926
  RA and, 939, 943
ejaculation:
  ED and, 575
  male infertility and, 724–25,
    731–32, 740, 742
  in sex act for men, 570–71
ejection fraction, 303, 445–47
electroacupuncture, 839–40
electrolytes, 551
elemental diets, 464
elimination, 131
  chronic candidiasis and, 384–85
  detoxification and, 113–16, 119–25,
    127–29
  digestion and, 133, 141–42
  toxins and, 112–13
elimination diets:
  food allergies and, 596–97
  hives and, 699
  IBD and, 464
emollients, 929
emotions:
  depression and, 478, 481, 484, 486,
    488–90, 498
  diabetes and, 527
  exercise and, 41, 212
  immune system and, 172–73, 181
  peptic ulcer and, 877–78
  physical care and, 81
  placebo response and, 19
  PMS and, 890, 893, 895–99
  positive mental attitude and, 29–30
  of self-actualized people, 32
  stress and, 204–5, 214, 246
  stroke and, 972
emphysema, 431–32
endometrial cancer, 981
endometriosis, 565–69, 725
  causes of, 565–66
  grape seed extract for, 567–68

lipotropic supplements for, 567
pine bark extract for, 567–68
risk factors for, 565–67
symptoms of, 565–67
therapeutic considerations for,
  566–68
endorphins:
  depression and, 486
  exercise and, 41
  hot flashes and, 782, 789
  placebo response and, 19
  PMS and, 893, 895
  positive mental attitude and, 37
endothelium, 146–48
energy:
  angina and, 305–8
  and cellular approach to health,
    85–88
  CHF and, 443–45
  obesity and, 227–29
  physical care and, 80–81
  stress and, 205
  see also chronic fatigue syndrome
enteroviruses, 508–9, 512
environment:
  ADHD and, 341–42
  aging and, 185, 187
  cancer and, 96, 98–99, 102, 107,
    357
  CVD and, 151
  depression and, 479–80, 484
  detoxification and, 115, 117–18, 125
  diabetes and, 507, 517
  endometriosis and, 565–66
  of gingival sulcus, 884
  infertility and, 726, 732, 735–37
  kidney stones and, 764
  MS and, 812–14
  Parkinson's disease and, 869
  RA and, 933–34
  sinus infections and, 958
  toxins and, 110, 115, 117–18, 125,
    425
Environmental Protection Agency
  (EPA), 59, 99, 567
enzyme-linked immunosorbent assay
  (ELISA) test, 597
enzymes:
  CVD and, 159
  detoxification and, 115–18, 120,
    123–24
  digestion and, 131–32, 134,
    138–40, 145
  nutritional supplements and, 68–69
  toxins and, 111, 113
  see also pancreatic enzymes;
    proteolytic enzymes

eosinophilia-myalgia syndrome
  (EMS), 492–93
eosinophils, 171
epicatechin, 510–12
epididymis, 735, 742
epigallocatechin-3-gallate (EGCG),
  418, 913
EPs, 370
equol, 787–88
erectile dysfunction (ED), 570–81
  alcohol and, 573
  arginine for, 575–76
  atherosclerosis and, 572–73, 575
  bicycle seats and, 575
  causes of, 571–73, 575
  Chinese ginseng for, 577
  diabetes and, 573, 575
  diet and, 574–75, 580–81
  diseases in, 573–74
  fenugreek for, 578
  GBE for, 578
  hormonal disorders in, 573
  longjack for, 577
  medications and, 573, 576, 578–79
  penile prosthesis for, 579
  potency wood for, 577
  procedures used in evaluation of, 572
  procyanidolic oligomers for, 575–76
  psychotherapy for, 578
  smoking and, 572–73
  symptoms of, 570
  therapeutic considerations for,
    574–79
  tribulus for, 577–78
  vacuum-constrictive devices for,
    580
  yohimbe for, 576–77
Escherichia coli, 65, 471–72
escin, 995
esophagus, 131, 134–35, 138
essential fatty acids (EFAs):
  ADHD and, 343
  alcohol dependence and, 271
  diabetes and, 509–10, 516
  eczema and, 584
  and hair loss in women, 632
  PMS and, 898
  see also specific essential fatty
    acids
esteem needs, 31
EstroG, 794
estrogen, 126, 846, 864
  AD and, 280
  breast cancer and, 357, 361–64, 785
  cervical dysplasia and, 417
  detoxification and, 123
  endometriosis and, 565–68

FBD and, 587–89
gallstones and, 607
in HRT, 781, 784–85, 791, 852
male infertility and, 735–37
menopause and, 781–82, 784–85,
    788, 790–91, 848
menorrhagia and, 798
metabolism of, 892–93
in normal menstrual cycle, 891
osteoporosis and, 848, 852–54, 857
PMS and, 891–94, 899
prostate enlargement and, 915, 917
RA and, 936
uterine fibroids and, 980–82
ethylenediaminetetraacetic acid
    chelation (EDTA) therapy,
    intravenous, 309–11
European Cooperative Crohn's
    Disease Study (ECCDS), 460
eustachian tube, 557, 559–61, 563
evening primrose oil, 589, 898
exercise, 25, 126, 129
    alcohol dependence and, 272
    cancer and, 99–100, 104, 357, 359
    CFS and, 427
    constipation and, 454
    CVD and, 152–53, 161, 188
    depression and, 41, 485–86
    diabetes and, 513–15, 518, 528,
        714–15
    diet and, 55, 232
    ED and, 572, 574–75
    glaucoma and, 620
    healthful lifestyle and, 28, 39–44
    high BP and, 666–68
    HIV and, 262
    hives and, 694
    hypoglycemia and, 708, 714–15
    hypothyroidism and, 722
    immune system and, 41, 172
    insomnia and, 750
    lactic acid and, 314
    life extension and, 186, 188–89
    menopause and, 786–87
    MS and, 819
    in naturopathic medicine, 4, 6–7,
        13
    nutritional supplements and, 70
    obesity and, 40, 225–26, 228–29,
        232, 237
    osteoarthritis and, 828–29
    osteoporosis and, 847, 854–55
    physical care and, 78–80
    PMS and, 895
    positive mental attitude and, 38
    prediabetes and, 505
    prostate enlargement and, 916–17

RA and, 945
    sarcopenia prevention and, 189
    silent inflammation and, 200
    stress and, 40–41, 212, 217
expectations, power of, 21–22
expectorants:
    for bronchitis and pneumonia,
        369–71, 374–75
    for COPD, 432–34
experimenter effect, 22
extraintestinal lesions (EILs), 462
exudative diarrhea, 548–49
eyes, eye:
    anatomy of, 616, 774
    diabetes and, 503, 523, 526, 531,
        533, 539–40
    hyperthyroidism and, 702–3
    see also glaucoma; macular
        degeneration

fasting:
    in detoxification, 128–30
    immune system and, 175
    psoriasis and, 926
    RA and, 938–39
fat, body, 45
    body weight vs., 224
    brown and white, 228
    diabetes and, 512
    diets and, 59, 62, 232
    exercise and, 40–41, 44
    female infertility and, 725–26
    measurement of, 224–25
    obesity and, 222–24, 228, 232,
        237–41
    positive mental attitude and, 36
fat, dietary, 189, 1022
    acne and, 248–49
    alcohol and, 267, 269
    cancer and, 359–60, 904, 906–8
    and cellular approach to health,
        85–86
    diabetes and, 503, 514–16
    diet and, 49–53, 55, 60–63, 231–33
    endometriosis and, 566–67
    exercise and, 41
    FBD and, 588
    gout and, 626
    high BP and, 666–67, 669, 675
    hydrogenated, 62
    hypercholesterolemia and, 680,
        682–83
    male infertility and, 738–39, 742
    monounsaturated, 62, 85–86,
        153–54, 156, 160, 200, 515–16,
        684, 817
    MS and, 814–17

nutritional supplements and, 75–76
    obesity and, 231–33, 236, 238–39
    PMS and, 893–94
    polyunsaturated, 49–50, 61, 103,
        154, 516, 566, 684
    prediabetes and, 505
    prostate enlargement and, 917
    sarcopenia prevention and, 189
    saturated, 60–62, 85–86, 153, 160,
        239, 359, 505, 514–16, 666–67,
        675, 682–84, 815–16, 904, 917
    in selected foods, 684
    silent inflammation and, 199–200
    wrong types of, 515–16
fatigue, see chronic fatigue syndrome
fatty acids, 189
    angina and, 306–7
    prunes and, 454
    see also specific fatty acids
fatty liver disease, 540
    alcohol dependence and, 267,
        269
    see also nonalcoholic fatty liver
        disease
fava bean (Vicia faba), 873
febuxostat (Uloric), 625
fecal straining, 647–49
feet:
    diabetes and, 524, 542
    menopause and, 783
Feingold hypothesis, 342–43
Feldenkrais technique, 81–82
female infertility, 724–30
    alcohol and, 726
    arginine for, 727–28
    caffeine and, 726
    carnitine for, 727
    causes of, 724
    chasteberry for, 728–29
    chlamydia in, 735
    probiotics for, 728
    smoking and, 726–27
    symptoms of, 724
    therapeutic considerations for,
        724–28
females:
    BMD testing and, 849
    hyperthyroidism and, 702
    osteoporosis and, 844–45, 847–48,
        852–57, 859–64
    SLE and, 976
    varicose veins and, 992
    see also gender; specific female
        disorders
Feminine Forever (Wilson), 784
fenugreek (Trigonella foenigracum),
    537, 578

fermentable oligosaccharides, disaccharides, monosaccharides, and polyols (FODMAP), 759–60
feverfew (*Tanacetum parthenium*), 807–9
fiber:
    Atkins Diet and, 232
    breast cancer and, 588
    chronic candidiasis and, 384–85
    constipation and, 451–54
    detoxification and, 116, 121, 126–27, 129
    diabetes and, 515–16, 527–28, 533–34, 542
    diarrhea and, 551
    dietary, 713, 758
    digestion and, 132–33, 135, 142, 145
    diseases associated with lack of, 50
    endometriosis and, 567
    FBD and, 588
    gallstones and, 608–9
    health-promoting diet and, 60
    hemorrhoids and, 647–49
    high BP and, 666–67, 669
    hypercholesterolemia and, 683–85
    hypoglycemia and, 712–13
    IBD and, 458–59, 464
    IBS and, 758
    impact on cholesterol levels of various sources of, 685
    obesity and, 227, 232–36
    peptic ulcer and, 878
    PMS and, 894
    prunes and, 454
    psoriasis and, 924
    in selected food, 1013–20
    soluble, 713
    toxins and, 112
    uterine fibroids and, 981
    varicose veins and, 992–94
fibrinogen, 150–51, 153, 156, 161–62
fibrinolytic compounds, 973, 996
fibrocystic breast disease (FBD), 587–91
    caffeine and, 587
    causes of, 587
    chasteberry for, 590
    evening primrose for, 589
    fat and, 588
    fiber and, 588
    iodine for, 589–90
    methylxanthines and, 587–88
    signs and symptoms of, 587
    therapeutic considerations for, 587–90
    vegetarian diet and, 588
    vitamin E for, 589

fibromyalgia (FM), 422–23
fight-or-flight reaction, 23, 204–5
finasteride (Proscar), 919, 921
fingerprint patterns, 278–79
fish, 1022–23
    cancer and, 102, 104, 360
    and Edible Plant and Animal Kingdoms Taxonomic List, 600
    health-promoting diet and, 51, 53, 55, 60–62, 65
    MS and, 814, 816
    RA and, 939
fish oil, 102
    diabetes and, 76, 532–33
    gallstones and, 611
    glaucoma and, 619
    gout and, 626
    hives and, 699
    hypertriglyceridemia and, 685
    menopause and, 76, 788
    MS and, 815–17
    pregnancy and, 79
    recommendations on, 71–73, 75–77
fixed allergies, 596
flavokawain B, 319
flavonoids, 57
    asthma and, 332
    cataracts and, 399
    diabetes and, 538–40
    glaucoma and, 617–18
    hemorrhoids and, 650
    H. pylori overgrowth and, 137
    life extension and, 192
    macular degeneration and, 776, 778–79
    menopause and, 788–89
    menorrhagia and, 797
    periodontal disease and, 887–88
    recommendations on, 71–73
    selection of, 74
    sports injuries and, 963
    varicose veins and, 994
flaxseeds, flaxseed oil, 77
    anxiety and, 316
    cancer and, 361, 908
    menopause and, 788
flour, 103, 1023–24
fluids:
    bladder infections and, 473
    cancer and, 104
    common colds and, 436
    constipation and, 454–55
    diarrhea and, 550–51
    gout and, 626
    see also water
fluoxetine (Prozac), 499, 892, 899
    5-HTP and, 494, 496–97

fluvoxamine (Luvox), 496–97
focal hair loss, 630–31
folic acid:
    AD and, 283–85
    anemia and, 294–95, 299
    ASD and, 351
    cataracts and, 399
    cervical dysplasia and, 416–17
    CVD and, 161–62
    depression and, 487–89
    gout and, 626
    high BP and, 674
    HIV/AIDS and, 257
    IBD and, 465
    immune system and, 178
    insomnia and, 752–53
    male infertility and, 741
    osteoporosis and, 862
    periodontal disease and, 888
    pregnancy and, 14
    psoriasis and, 926–27
    seborrheic dermatitis and, 955
follicle-stimulating hormone (FSH), 891–92
    male infertility and, 736–38
    menopause and, 781–82, 791
    in normal menstrual cycle, 891
food additives, 67
    ADHD and, 342–43
    asthma and, 328
    detoxification and, 123–25
    health-promoting diet and, 55, 58–60, 63–64
    hives and, 696–97, 699
    toxins and, 112
food allergies, 592–604
    ADHD and, 344
    AP for, 602
    ASD and, 349–50
    asthma and, 327–29
    bladder infections and, 472
    boils and, 353
    canker sores and, 389–90
    causes of, 593–96
    CFS and, 425
    chronic candidiasis and, 381
    cyclical vs. fixed, 596
    cytotoxic reaction in, 595, 597
    depression and, 491
    diagnostic considerations for, 596–602
    digestion and, 139–41, 598–602
    diseases associated with, 593
    ear infections and, 560–61
    eczema and, 583
    elimination diet and, 596–97
    gallstones and, 609

hives and, 695–96, 698
hypersensitivity reactions in, 595
IBD and, 459
IBS and, 758–59
immune system and, 139, 592, 594–95
migraine headaches and, 803–4
pancreatic enzymes and, 139, 598–602
peptic ulcer and, 878
psoriasis and, 926
quercetin for, 602
RA and, 935, 938–39
rotation diversified diet for, 598, 600–602
scope of, 593
seborrheic dermatitis and, 954
signs and symptoms of, 592–93, 595–97, 602
stress and, 213–14, 594
testing for, 596–97
therapeutic considerations for, 598–602
Food and Drug Administration (FDA), 64, 162, 248, 318, 377, 473, 576, 625, 672, 682, 720, 752
foodborne illnesses, 55, 64–65
food challenge, 596–97
food labels, 63
foods, food, 200
    acid-base values of, 92–93, 1021–27
    arginine and lysine content of, 662–63
    asthma and, 327–29
    carotenes in, 57, 777
    cholesterol and fat content of, 684
    CVD and, 154
    in DASH diet, 669–70
    detoxification and, 114, 118–20, 122–25
    digestion and, 131–33, 140, 142–43
    emulsifiers in, 697
    flavorings in, 696–97
    GI, carbohydrates, fiber, and GL of, 1013–20
    gluten and gliadin in, 404
    hives and, 695–99
    hypoglycemia and, 708–10, 712–13
    IBS and, 759–61
    to increase or reduce, 54, 61
    intolerance of, 803–4
    life extension and, 191
    mold- and yeast-containing, 381
    obesity and, 227
    oxalate content of, 769–71
    preservatives in, 697
    purine and, 625–26

salicylates in, 696–97
in Simplified Four-Day Rotation Diet Plan, 600–602
sleep and, 45
stabilizers in, 697
trends in U.S. consumption of, 51–52
vitamins and minerals in, 70–71
whole, 48, 64, 68
see also diets, diet
forgetfulness, 783
Fosamax, 852–53
fractures:
    assessing risk of, 848, 852
    BMD testing and, 849, 852
    osteoporosis and, 844–45, 847–48, 852–54, 856–57, 859–60, 862–63
Framingham studies, 21, 835
free radicals:
    aging and, 186–88, 190, 192
    cancer and, 96, 99
    and cellular approach to health, 87
    detoxification and, 117–18, 121
    diabetes and, 516, 525–26, 538
    nutritional supplements and, 73
    see also antioxidants
Freud, Sigmund, 46
fructose, 712, 759–60
fruits, 127, 1016–17
    acid-base values and, 92, 1023
    AD and, 282
    asthma and, 328–29
    cancer and, 102, 105
    carbohydrates and, 711–12, 1016–17
    cervical dysplasia and, 415
    CVD and, 153–54, 156, 165
    detoxification and, 118–19, 122, 124, 126, 129
    diabetes and, 516
    in Edible Plant and Animal Kingdoms Taxonomic List, 599
    five-a-day goal for, 58
    gout and, 627–28
    health-promoting diet and, 48–49, 51–56, 58–63, 65
    high BP and, 669, 671
    IBS and, 758
    kidney stones and, 765
    macular degeneration and, 775–76
    nutritional supplements and, 73
    organic, 59
    osteoporosis and, 857–58
    oxalate content of, 769–71
    rainbow assortment of, 56–57
    red and blue, 627–28

fumaric acid, 927
furosemide (Lasix), 444–45

galactans, 759
gallbladder, 131–32
gallstones, 125–26, 605–14
    age in, 607
    bile and, 605–12
    botanical choleretics for, 611
    buckwheat for, 609
    caloric restriction and, 610
    categories of, 605
    causes of, 606–7, 610
    chemical dissolution of, 611–12
    coffee and, 610
    diagnosis of, 605, 609
    diet and, 605–11, 613
    fiber and, 608–9
    food allergies and, 609
    formation of, 605
    gender in, 607
    genetic and ethnic factors in, 607–8
    GI tract diseases and, 607
    lipotropic factors and, 608, 611
    medications and, 607–8
    obesity and, 606, 610
    olive oil liver flush for, 610–11
    phosphatidylcholine and, 605–6, 610–11
    risk factors for pigmented, 607
    silent, 608
    sugar and, 610
    symptoms of, 605–6, 608–10
    therapeutic considerations for, 607–12
    vitamin C for, 610
    vitamin E for, 610
gamma-aminobutyric acid (GABA), 214–15
gamma-glutamyltransferase (GGTP), 517
gamma-linolenic acid (GLA), 541, 898
gamma-oryzanol (ferulic acid), 789
gamma-tocopherol, 909
Gardnerella vaginalis, 984–86, 989
Garland, Frank and Cedric, 106
garlic (Allium sativum):
    cancer and, 104
    chronic candidiasis and, 386
    CVD and, 161
    diabetes and, 537
    high BP and, 669
    hypercholesterolemia and, 690–91
    warfarin precautions and, 973
gastric acid, 856, 876
    see also hypochlorhydria

gastroesophageal reflux disorder (GERD), 134–35, 138
gastrointestinal (GI) tract, 553
  acne and, 246
  aspirin intake and, 165
  asthma and, 325–28, 335
  celiac disease and, 402–3, 405–6
  CFS and, 425
  chronic candidiasis and, 376–82, 385–86
  diabetes and, 508–9, 524
  digestion and, 131–32, 138–42, 144
  gallstones and, 607
  glucosamine and, 833
  health-promoting diet and, 48, 60, 64–65
  HIV/AIDS and, 255–57
  IBD and, 457, 463
  IBS and, 757, 759–61
  immune system and, 176, 178
  laxatives and, 455
  obesity and, 222
  Parkinson's disease and, 868
  peptic ulcer and, 876–81
  permeability of, 200
  PMS and, 890
  psoriasis and, 924
  RA and, 935–37
  silent inflammation and, 200
  stress and, 204
  UC and, 457
  vaginitis and, 986
gemfibrozil, 687
gender:
  gallstones and, 607
  hypothyroidism and, 716–18
  osteoarthritis and, 827
  see also erectile dysfunction; female infertility; females; male infertility
general adaptation syndrome, 204–5, 215
genetics, genes:
  acne and, 246
  AD and, 276
  aging and, 185–87
  alcohol dependence and, 266
  cancer and, 96–97, 356
  celiac disease and, 402–3
  detoxification and, 125
  diabetes and, 507, 513
  eczema and, 583
  food allergies and, 593
  gallstones and, 607–8
  gout and, 623
  hypercholesterolemia and, 681
  hyperthyroidism and, 703

IBD and, 457
MS and, 812–13
obesity and, 226, 237
osteoporosis and, 845–46, 851
psoriasis and, 923–24
RA and, 933–35
testing and, 97, 113
UC and, 457
genistein, 363, 858, 864, 907
geography, 812–14
germ theory, 8–9
ghrelin, 227
giardia, 553–54
Gilbert's syndrome, 124–26
ginger (*Zingiber officinalis*):
  migraine headaches and, 809
  osteoarthritis and, 837–38
  RA and, 943–45
gingival sulcus, 884
ginkgo biloba extract (GBE), 74
  AD and, 287–88
  ADHD and, 345
  asthma and, 335–36
  CVI and, 409–10
  depression and, 496–99
  diabetes and, 538
  ED and, 578
  glaucoma and, 618
  life extension and, 192
  MS and, 819
  Parkinson's disease and, 873
  PMS and, 899–900
  stroke and, 973
GLA Multicenter Trial, 541
glandular cell abnormalities, 412–13
glaucoma, 615–21
  acute, 615, 617
  allergies and, 617
  caffeine and, 619–20
  causes of, 615–16
  chromium for, 619
  chronic, 615, 620
  collagen in, 615–17
  exercise and, 620
  fish oil for, 619
  flavonoid-rich extracts for, 617–18
  intraocular pressure in, 615–20
  magnesium for, 619
  normotensive, 615, 618–20
  symptoms of, 615
  therapeutic considerations for, 616–19
  vitamin C for, 617, 619
gliadin:
  celiac disease and, 402, 404, 406
  hair loss and, 633–34
glucomannan, 533–34

glucosamine, 91
  chondroitin and, 832–34
  NSAIDs vs., 830–32
  osteoarthritis and, 10, 829–35
  side effects of, 831, 833
  sulfate vs. hydrochloride form of, 832–33
glucose, *see* blood glucose
glucose tolerance tests, 506, 707–8
glucosidase inhibitors, 534–35
glucosinolates, 57, 363
glucuronidase, 364–65
glucuronidation, 114–15, 120–21, 124–25
glutamine, 271, 878–79
glutathione, 189–90
  detoxification and, 114, 117, 120–22, 125, 127–28
  hair loss and, 631–32
  HIV/AIDS and, 256, 258–59
  life span extension and, 190
  Parkinson's disease and, 869, 872
glutathione peroxidase, 159, 333
  cataracts and, 396, 398–99
  psoriasis and, 927
gluten:
  canker sores and, 389–90
  celiac disease and, 402–6, 634
  diabetes and, 508
  in selected foods, 404
glyburide, 535
glycemic index (GI):
  diabetes and, 514–16, 534, 712
  health-promoting diet and, 54
  hypoglycemia and, 712–13
  obesity and, 234
  of selected foods, 1013–20
glycemic load (GL):
  acne and, 249
  chromium and, 529
  diabetes and, 514–15, 527, 529, 533
  health-promoting diet and, 60
  heart disease and, 515
  obesity and, 236
  of selected food, 1013–20
  silent inflammation and, 199
glycemic volatility, 213
glycerophosphocholine (GPC), 284–85
  stroke and, 974–75
glycine, 122
glycosaminoglycans (GAGs), 10, 147–48, 829, 833–34, 837
glycosylation:
  aging and, 187–88
  diabetes and, 506–7, 525, 535
glycyrrhizin, 261–62

goal setting, 36, 44

God, Faith and Health (Levin), 24

Goethe, Johann Wolfgang von, 34

goiters, goitrogens, 702–4, 718

goldenseal *(Hydrastis canadensis):*
  bladder infections and, 475–76
  chronic candidiasis and, 380, 385–86
  sinus infections and, 958–59
  strep throat and, 969

gonorrhea, 985, 987–88

gossypol, 738

gotu kola *(Centella asiatica):*
  bladder infections and, 473
  periodontal disease and, 888
  varicose veins and, 995–96

gout, 622–29
  alcohol and, 622, 624–26
  carbohydrates, fats, and protein
    in, 626
  causes of, 623–24
  celery seed extract for, 628
  cherries and other dark red and
    blue fruits for, 627–28
  diet and, 622–26
  fish oils for, 626
  fluid intake for, 626
  folic acid for, 626
  from lead toxicity, 625
  niacin for, 627
  obesity and, 624, 626
  primary, 623
  quercetin for, 627
  secondary, 623, 625
  symptoms of, 622, 624
  therapeutic considerations for,
    624–27
  vitamin C for, 627

grains, 1017, 1023–24
  cancer and, 105
  celiac disease and, 402–5
  health-promoting diet and, 48,
    52–55, 60
  oxalate content of, 769–71
  refined, 54, 60
  whole, 48, 51, 54–55, 105, 126

granules, 884, 886–87

grapefruits, 119–20

grape seed extract, 74–75, 80
  ADHD and, 344–45
  benefits of, 75
  CVD and, 160
  diabetes and, 538
  endometriosis and, 567–68

Graves' disease, 702–3, 705

green foods:
  pH balance and, 92
  recommendations on, 71–75, 80

green tea, green tea extract *(Camellia
  sinensis)*, 74, 80
  cancer and, 104, 365, 913
  cervical dysplasia and, 418
  diabetes and, 511–12, 538
  osteoporosis and, 864
  Parkinson's disease and, 873
  periodontal disease and, 887–88

growth hormone (GH), 45

guaifenesin (glycerol guiacolate), 371

guar gum, 233–34, 758

guided imagery, 23

gut-derived hormone alterations, 227

Gymnema sylvestre, 535–36

habits, 4–5, 28, 39, 95

hair loss:
  antigliadin antibodies and, 633–34
  causes of, 631–33
  drug-induced, 632
  hypothyroidism in, 633, 717
  nutritional deficiencies in, 632–33
  and physiology of hair cycle, 630
  saw palmetto for, 631–32
  therapeutic considerations for,
    631–33
  types of, 630–31
  in women, 630–34

halo effect, 22

Hamilton Anxiety Scale, 316–17

Hamilton Depression Scale (HDS),
  488, 495

hands, 783

Hashimoto's thyroiditis, 718–20

hawthorn *(Crataegus oxyacantha)*, 74
  angina and, 308
  arrhythmias and, 645
  CHF and, 449
  diabetes and, 538
  high BP and, 676

Hawthorne effect, 22

hay fever, 635–38
  AP for, 602, 637
  causes of, 635
  immunotherapy for, 636
  quercetin for, 636–37
  symptoms of, 635–38
  therapeutic considerations for,
    635–37

Hayflick limit, 185

headaches:
  bodywork for, 640
  causes of, 639
  hives and, 694
  menopause and, 782
  migraine, *see* migraine headaches
  nonmigraine tension type, 639–42

PMS and, 890, 898–900
  relaxation training for, 640–41
  symptoms of, 639–40
  therapeutic considerations for,
    639–41
  trigger points of, 639

healing:
  poor, 542
  from within, 18–25

health:
  cellular approach to, 85–94
  cornerstones of, 27–28
  definitions of, 27
  diabetes and, 220–22
  establishing of, 5
  steps to, 24–25

health care:
  cancer and, 98
  costs of, 11, 53
  evolution of, 16–17
  positive mental attitude and, 29
  statistics on, 11–13

health span, 183, 194

heart, 146
  angina and, 301–10
  anxiety and, 313, 317
  CHF and, 442–450
  illustrations of, 302, 447
  spirituality and, 24

heart arrhythmias, *see* arrhythmias

heart attacks, 30, 146, 308, 442, 444,
  784
  angina and, 303–5, 307
  hypercholesterolemia and, 680
  prevention of, 153, 155–56, 164–66
  risk factors for, 148–52, 158–61,
    163–64, 188, 198–99
  second, 164–66
  treatment of, 163–65

heart disease, 86–91, 523
  atherosclerosis and, 146
  and cellular approach to health,
    86–87
  CoQ_{10} and, 88, 90–91
  diabetes and, 503
  ED and, 572
  exercise and, 41–43
  garlic for, 690–91
  health-promoting diet and, 48–50,
    52–53, 60, 62
  hypercholesterolemia and, 680–81,
    683–88
  nutritional supplements and, 73–77
  obesity and, 220–21
  positive mental attitude and, 30
  and power of expectations, 21
  prediction of, 155, 166

heart disease (*cont.*)
prevention of, 153–55, 158–61, 163–66
risk factors for, 24, 30, 39, 42, 99, 150–52, 155, 160–64, 166, 190, 515
statistics on, 11–12
treatment of, 163–64
heart rate, 41–43
heavy metals, 110–12
cataracts and, 400
determining toxicity of, 111–12
detoxification and, 114–15, 121–22, 127
health-promoting diet and, 55, 58–60
high BP and, 666, 674
infertility and, 726, 736, 741
nutritional supplements and, 75, 77
Heidelberg gastric analysis, 136
Helicobacter pylori, 949–50
overgrowth and, 134, 136–38
peptic ulcer and, 876–77, 879–81
Hellerwork, 81
helminths, 552
hemoglobin:
anemia and, 293
diabetes and, 506–7, 525, 535
hemorrhoids, 647–51
bulking agents for, 649
causes of, 647
classification of, 647–48
conventional medical treatment for, 648
diagnostic considerations for, 648
diet and, 647–49, 651
flavonoids for, 650
hydrotherapy for, 649
illustration of, 649
signs and symptoms of, 647–48
therapeutic considerations for, 648–49
topical treatments for, 649–50
hepatitis, 652–59
A, 652–53
ALA for, 655
B, 652–55
C, 652–56
causes of, 652
diagnostic considerations for, 652–53
diet and, 654, 658
licorice root for, 655–56
milk thistle for, 656–57
prevention strategies for, 653–54
selenium for, 654–55
symptoms of, 652–53, 656

therapeutic considerations for, 654–57
vitamin C for, 654
vitamin D for, 655
herbs, 126–27, 1027
comparisons between spices and, 201
detoxification and, 118
health-promoting diet and, 63
in naturopathic medicine, 3–4, 6, 9, 17
oxalate content of, 770–71
recommendations on, 73
herpes, 660–65
arginine for, 661–63
lemon balm for, 664
licorice for, 664
lysine for, 661–63
recurrences of, 660–61
symptoms of, 660–61
therapeutic considerations for, 660–63
vaginitis and, 984–87
vitamin C for, 661
zinc for, 661
Herxheimer reaction, 385
hesperidin, 788–89
hiatal hernia, 135
hibiscus (*Hibiscus sabdariffa*), 678
hierarchy of needs, 31, 33
high blood pressure (high BP), 24, 42, 666–79
anti-ACE peptides for, 675–76
arginine for, 675
caffeine and, 667, 672
calcium and, 666–67, 669, 674
causes of, 666–67
CHF and, 442–43, 446, 449
CoQ_{10} and, 88, 90, 676
CVD and, 149, 152
diabetes and, 503, 526, 529–30
diet and, 63, 666–73, 679
exercise and, 666–68
folic acid for, 674
hawthorn for, 676
hibiscus for, 678
lifestyle and, 666–67
magnesium and, 666–67, 669, 673–74
nutritional supplements and, 76–77, 667, 671–76, 679
obesity and, 220–21, 224
olive for, 676–78
omega-3 fatty acids and, 666, 675
potassium and, 667–69, 671–74
salt and, 666–69, 671, 673–75
statistics on, 12

stress and, 667–68
stroke and, 971
symptoms of, 666
therapeutic considerations for, 667–77
types of, 666–67
vitamin B_6 for, 674–75
vitamin C and, 529, 666–67, 669, 674
vitamin E and, 530
high-fructose corn syrup (HFCS), 709, 712
high-grade squamous intraepithelial lesion (HSIL), 413–17
highly active anti-retroviral therapy (HAART), 254–56, 258, 260–61
Hippocrates, 48, 592
hips:
BMD testing and, 849
osteoarthritis and, 827–28, 836, 838
osteoporosis and, 844–45, 847, 852–54, 856–57, 859–60, 862, 864
-to-waist ratios, 224
histamine:
asthma and, 322, 324, 328, 331, 335
food allergies and, 592, 595–96, 602
hay fever and, 635
hives and, 692, 695, 698–99
migraine headaches and, 801–2, 804–5, 807
hives (urticaria), 64, 692–701
acute, 692, 699
allergies and, 692, 695–96, 698–99
antibiotics and, 695
aspirin and, 695–96, 699
causes of, 692–699
cholinergic urticaria and, 694
chronic, 692, 695–96, 698–700
clinical aspects of, 693
cold urticaria and, 694
dermographism and, 692–94
fish oils for, 699
food additives and, 696–97, 699
inflammation and, 692–94, 698–99
quercetin for, 699
stress and, 694, 698
symptoms of, 692–94, 696, 698–99
therapeutic considerations for, 698–700
thyroid hormone for, 700
ultraviolet light therapy for, 699
vitamin B_{12} for, 699
vitamin C for, 699

holism, 5
homeopathy, 4, 6, 14, 17
homeostasis, 85–86
homocysteine, 123, 674
    CVD and, 155, 160–62
    diabetes and, 526
    osteoporosis and, 862
Honolulu Heart Study, 673
hope, 1011
hormone replacement therapy (HRT):
    AD and, 280
    menopause and, 781, 784–86, 791
    menorrhagia and, 796–97
    natural, 786
    osteoporosis and, 785, 852
    tapering off, 786
hormones, 227
    cancer and, 98, 903–4, 906
    depression and, 483–84
    detoxification and, 123
    ED and, 573
    immune system and, 170
    normal menstrual cycle and,
        890–91
    osteoporosis and, 846–48, 851–52,
        854
    PMS and, 891–92, 897
    see also specific hormones
horse chestnut (Aesculus
        hippocastanum), 995
hot and cold water treatment, 393
hot flashes:
    botanical medicines for, 790–93
    menopause and, 782–84, 786–93
    nutritional supplements for, 788–89
human immunodeficiency virus
        (HIV), 253–64
    advanced stages of, 253
    avoiding contracting of, 254
    diagnosis of, 253
    exercise for, 262
    onset symptoms of, 253
    progression to AIDS of, 254–58,
        260
    risk factors for, 253
    see also acquired immunodeficiency
        syndrome
human papillomavirus (HPV),
        412–15, 417–18
humidifiers, 562–63
humor, 33, 37–38, 173
huperzine A, 288–89
hyaluronic acid (HA), 473, 834
hydrochloric acid:
    anemia and, 293–95
    digestion and, 131, 134, 136–37,
        140

RA and, 942
    rosacea and, 950
hydrotherapy:
    hemorrhoids and, 649
    in naturopathic medicine, 4, 6–7
    RA and, 945
hydroxycitrate (HCA), 238–39
hydroxyethylrutoside (HER), 650
5-hydroxyindoleacetic acid (5-HIAA),
        496, 801
5-hydroxytryptophan (5-HTP):
    depression and, 272, 482, 493–97
    insomnia and, 751–52
    migraine headaches and, 801–2,
        805–6
    obesity and, 237–38
    Parkinson's disease and, 872
    PMS and, 898–99
hyperbaric oxygen, 819
hypercholesterolemia, 680–91
    determining risk of, 680–82, 686
    fiber and, 683–85
    garlic for, 690–91
    inherited, 681–82
    niacin for, 685–89
    onion for, 690
    pantethine for, 689–90
    sterols and stanols for, 689
    therapeutic considerations for,
        682–90
hypersensitivity reactions, 595
hypertension, see high blood pressure
hyperthyroidism, 702–6
    carnitine for, 704–5
    causes of, 702–3
    dietary goitrogens for, 704
    naturopathic care for, 703–4
    signs and symptoms of, 702–3, 705
    therapeutic considerations for,
        703–5
hypertriglyceridemia, 680–83
    fish oils for, 685
    inherited, 681–82
    niacin for, 687
    therapeutic considerations for,
        682–83, 685, 687, 690
    vitamin B₅ for, 690
hypnosis, 39
hypochlorhydria, 135–39
    chronic candidiasis and, 381
    common signs and symptoms of,
        135–36
    diagnoses of, 136
    diseases associated with, 136
    food allergies and, 139
    H. pylori overgrowth and, 136–37
    rosacea and, 950

hypoglycemia, 514, 707–15
    aggressive or criminal behavior in,
        709–10
    alcohol and, 267–68, 713–14
    angina and, 711
    atherosclerosis and, 711
    brain and, 707, 709
    chromium and, 713, 715
    consequences of, 709–11
    depression and, 484–85, 487,
        709
    diabetes and, 521–24, 707,
        712–14
    diagnosis of, 707–8
    diet and, 709–13, 715
    exercise and, 708, 714–15
    fiber for, 712–13
    general considerations for, 709
    GI and, 712–13
    intermittent claudication and, 711
    migraine headaches and, 711
    PGX for, 713
    PMS and, 710–11
    questionnaire on, 708
    reactive, 707, 709–11, 713–14
    stress and, 213, 702–4
    symptoms of, 521–23, 707–9
    therapeutic considerations for,
        711–14
hypothalamus, 782, 789, 891
hypothyroidism, 716–23
    causes of, 717–18
    DHEA for, 721–22
    diagnostic considerations for,
        719–20
    exercise for, 722
    hair loss and, 633, 717
    iodine and, 717–18, 720–21
    PMS and, 891–92, 894
    primary, 716
    secondary, 716
    signs and symptoms of, 716,
        719
    subclinical, 716, 718
    therapeutic considerations for,
        720–21
    tyrosine for, 720
    vitamins and minerals for, 721
hypothyroid syndrome, 717–19

ibuprofen, 831–32, 835
ICAPS Plus, 777
ice cream, 1018
idiopathic oligospermia, 731
ileocecal valve, 140–41
immune-complex-mediated reactions,
        595

immune system, immunity, 127,
 169–82, 192
 AD and, 276
 allergies and, 139, 171, 173, 592,
 594–95
 boils and, 353–54
 botanical medicines and, 172,
 180–82
 bronchitis and, 370
 cancer and, 96, 100, 169–72
 celiac disease and, 508
 CFS and, 421–22, 424, 428
 chronic candidiasis and, 376–77,
 381–82, 384–85, 387
 common cold and, 169, 177–80,
 435–37, 439
 components of, 169–72
 determination of, 169
 detoxification and, 115–16, 567
 diabetes and, 503–4, 507–11, 524,
 527–29, 539
 diet and, 58, 100, 172, 174–75
 digestion and, 139–41
 ear infections and, 559, 561
 endometriosis and, 565–67
 exercise and, 41, 172
 hepatitis and, 654–55
 herpes and, 661
 hives and, 695–96
 IBD and, 458
 in naturopathic medicine, 8–9
 nutritional supplements and, 172,
 174, 176–80, 182
 periodontal disease and,
 883–86
 pneumonia and, 367–68
 positive mental attitude and,
 29–30, 36–37, 172–73
 psoriasis and, 923–24, 926–28
 RA and, 933, 935–36, 942
 sinus infections and, 959
 SLE and, 976
 strep throat and, 967–68
 stress and, 172–73, 176–77, 192
 support for, 172–82
 toxins and, 112
immunoglobulin A (IgA):
 asthma and, 325
 digestion and, 140–41
 food allergies and, 594, 597
 male infertility and, 743
immunoglobulin E (IgE):
 asthma and, 322, 325
 food allergies and, 592–95, 597
 hay fever and, 635
 hives and, 692, 695
 periodontal disease and, 884

immunoglobulin G (IgG), 592,
 594–95, 597
immunoglobulin M (IgM), 592,
 594–95, 597
immunotherapy, 636
impotence, 570–72, 577
inadequate-contact diarrhea, 548–49
Indian frankincense, *see* boswellia
indigestion, 134–35, 138, 140
 see also hypochlorhydria
Individuals with Disabilities
 Education Act (IDEA), 349
indole-3-carbinol (I3C), 118, 363–64,
 417
infection equation, 8
infections, 413–14, 417
 boils and, 353
 bronchitis and, 370, 372
 CD4 counts and, 255
 cervical dysplasia and, 414
 CFS and, 421–22
 chronic candidiasis and, 381–82,
 385–86
 common cold and, 436, 438–40
 diabetes and, 508, 523–24, 532
 diarrhea and, 144, 548–49, 551–54
 food allergies and, 594
 hepatitis and, 652–54
 herpes simplex and, 660–61, 664
 hives and, 698
 IBD and, 457–58, 463
 immune system and, 169–71, 173,
 175–81
 male infertility and, 734–35, 740
 pneumonia and, 367–68, 372–73
 RA and, 934, 942
 silent inflammation and, 198
 vaginitis and, 984–87
 see also bladder infections; ear
 infections; sinus infections
infertility, *see* female infertility; male
 infertility
inflammation:
 acne and, 245–46, 248, 250
 AD and, 276–77
 asthma and, 324–25, 329, 331–34
 boils and, 353
 and bronchitis and pneumonia, 367
 bursitis and, 962–63
 CD and, 456
 and cellular approach to health,
 85–86, 88
 COPD and, 432
 CVD and, 147–49, 153–54, 156
 diabetes and, 521, 525
 ear infections and, 560
 endometriosis and, 566–68

 gout and, 622, 624, 626
 hives and, 692–94, 698–99
 hypothyroidism and, 719
 MS and, 815–17
 and NAFLD and NASH, 822
 nutritional supplements and,
 76–77
 osteoarthritis and, 827–28, 830,
 835–38
 periodontal disease and, 883–85,
 887–88
 placebo response and, 19
 psoriasis and, 923, 925–26, 928–29
 RA and, 932–37, 939–43
 rosacea and, 948–49, 951–52
 sinus infections and, 957–58
 SLE and, 976–77
 sports injuries and, 963–64
 UC and, 457
 see also silent inflammation
inflammatory bowel disease (IBD),
 456–70
 antibiotics and, 458
 boswellia for, 467
 calprotectin and, 467
 causes of, 457–58
 causes of malnutrition in, 463–64
 complications of, 462
 curcumin for, 466
 diet and, 458–59, 464, 469
 eicosanoid metabolism in, 460
 folic acid for, 465
 genetics in, 457
 immune system and, 458
 intestinal microflora in, 461–62
 multiple vitamin and mineral
 formulas for, 464–65
 nutritional considerations for,
 462–64
 pediatric patients with, 467–68
 prebiotics for, 465–66
 probiotics for, 466
 psychological support for, 466
 symptoms of, 549
 therapeutic considerations for,
 459–68
 vitamin B_{12} for, 465
 vitamin D for, 465
 zinc for, 465
 see also Crohn's disease; ulcerative
 colitis
influenza, 370
 common cold and, 435–36
 immune system and, 169, 173
 vaccine for, 325
inositol hexaniacinate, 540, 688–89
inositol hexaphosphate, 771

insomnia, 45, 748–56
  blood glucose and, 750
  causes of, 748–49, 752
  cofactor therapy for, 751
  exercise and, 750
  5-HTP for, 751–52
  melatonin and, 751–52
  nocturnal myoclonus and, 752
  progressive relaxation and, 750
  restless legs syndrome and, 752–53
  serotonin and, 750–51
  sleep apnea and, 748–49
  sleep-maintenance, 748–49, 751
  sleep-onset, 748–49, 751
  stimulants and, 750
  symptoms of, 748, 753
  therapeutic considerations for,
    749–53
  tryptophan for, 750–51
insulin, 213
  acne and, 248
  AD and, 277, 279
  blood glucose monitoring and,
    518–19
  and cellular approach to health, 86
  C-peptide determination and,
    519–20
  CVD and, 147–49, 152–53
  diabetes and, 68, 503–4, 507–8,
    510–12, 515–16, 518–20,
    524–32, 534–37
  glucosamine and, 833
  health-promoting diet and, 60, 62
  hypoglycemia and, 521, 707–8,
    710–14
  improving function and sensitivity
    of, 535–37
  ketoacidosis and, 519–20, 523
  Lantus, 519
  life extension and, 190, 193–94
  NAFLD and, 822–23
  niacinamide and, 531
  obesity and, 220, 222–24, 226–27,
    234, 236–37
  osteoarthritis and, 828
  prediabetes and, 505
  psoriasis and, 926
  silent inflammation and, 198–99
  vitamin C and, 529
  vitamin E and, 530
insulin-like growth factor 1 (IGF-1),
    248
interferon:
  CFS and, 422
  common cold and, 435–36
  hepatitis and, 654–56
intermittent claudication, 711

internal cleansing, *see* detoxification
internal hemorrhoids, 647–48
internal terrain, 8–9
International Index of Erectile
    Function (IIEF-5), 576
interpersonal relationships, 37, 479
  of self-actualized people, 32
  stress management and, 211
intestinal flora, 140–43, 377, 553, 583
  alcohol dependence and, 272
  digestion and, 134, 136–38
  IBD and, 461–62
  RA and, 934–37, 939, 942
intestines:
  acne and, 246–48
  alcohol and, 268, 272
  detoxification and, 114, 116, 125
  diabetes and, 508–9
  diarrhea and, 551
  digestion and, 131–32, 137, 139–41,
    145
  IBD and, 456–58, 461–62, 465–66
  see also bowels, bowel; colon;
    gastrointestinal tract
intima, 146–48
intraocular pressure, 615–20
intravenous
    ethylenediaminetetraacetic
    acid chelation (EDTA) therapy,
    309–11
intrinsic factor, 294
in vitro fertilization, 724, 733, 739–41
iodine:
  FBD and, 589–90
  hyperthyroidism and, 703–4
  hypothyroidism and, 717–18,
    720–21
  vaginitis and, 989
ipriflavone, 858, 863–64
iron:
  ADHD and, 344
  anemia and, 293–97, 344
  dietary sources of, 296–97
  female infertility and, 727
  and hair loss in women, 632–33
  immune system and, 178
  menorrhagia and, 797
  NAFLD and, 824
  during pregnancy, 79
irritable bowel syndrome (IBS),
    757–63
  causes of, 142, 757–60
  conditions that mimic, 757
  dietary fiber and, 758
  FODMAPs and, 759–60
  food allergies and, 758–59
  peppermint oil for, 138, 760–61

probiotics for, 760
psychological factors and, 761–62
sugar and, 759–60
symptoms of, 757–61
therapeutic considerations for,
    758–62
isoflavones, isoflavonoids:
  cancer and, 57, 864, 906–7
  endometriosis and, 567
  menopause and, 787–88, 791–92
  osteoporosis and, 858, 863
  in soy products, 362–63, 567,
    787–88, 858, 863–64, 906–7, 981
  uterine fibroids and, 981
isolated systolic hypertension, 666
isotretinoin (Accutane), 248, 251
Italian Study Group on Carnitine and
    Male Infertility, 742
ivy *(Hedera helix),* 334, 371

jam, 1018
Jastrow effect, 22
John Henry effect, 22
joints:
  bursitis and, 962
  glucosamine and, 829–31
  gout and, 622
  hypothyroidism and, 717
  obesity and, 221
  osteoarthritis and, 827–37, 839–40
  RA and, 932–36, 938, 940–45
  SLE and, 976
  sports injuries and, 963
juices, 129, 156–57, 767, 1016
jujube plum *(Zizyphi fructus),* 335

Kaufman, William, 834–35
kava *(Piper methysticum),* 316–19
Kellogg, John and Will, 4
keratin, 245–46
ketoacidosis, 519–23
ketone testing, 520–23
khella *(Ammi visnaga),* 308–9
kidneys, 442, 444
  bladder infections and, 471
  detoxification and, 114, 117, 121–22
  diabetes and, 503, 524, 533,
    541–42
  gout and, 622, 625–26
  high BP and, 666, 675
  prostate enlargement and, 916
kidney stones, 764–73
  citrate for, 768
  composition of, 764–67
  diagnostic considerations for,
    764–65
  gout and, 622–24, 626

kidney stones (*cont.*)
  inositol hexaphosphate for, 771
  magnesium and, 767
  oxalates and, 766–69
  symptoms of, 764
  therapeutic considerations for,
    765–72
  uric acid and, 764–68
  vitamin B$_6$ and, 767–68
  vitamin C for, 771
  vitamin K for, 768
  and weight control and sugar
    intake, 767
Klopfer, Bruno, 18
knees, 827, 829–34, 837–41
Kohamans, 155
Krebiozen, 18–19
Kripke, Daniel F., 754–55
kudzu (*Pueraria lobata*), 272
Kupperman menopause index (KMI),
  794
kynurenine, 493

laboratory tests:
  on BMD, 844, 849–52
  for dementia, 278
  diabetes and, 520–23
  in evaluating cardiovascular health,
    149
  food allergies and, 597
  for hypoglycemia, 707–8
  IBD and, 468
  on presence of *C. albicans*,
    380–81
  PSA and, 904, 916
  see also biopsies; X-rays
L-acetylcarnitine (LAC), 285–86
lactic acid, 313–15
Lactobacillus acidophilus, 968
  diarrhea and, 551–53
  vaginitis and, 984, 988–89
lactose, lactose intolerance, 145
  diarrhea and, 549
  HIV/AIDS and, 256
  IBS and, 759–60
Lantus, 519
large intestine, *see* colon
laser therapy, 415, 540
lavender (*Lavender officinalis*), 482,
  499
laxatives, laxative effect:
  cautions and warnings on, 454
  constipation and, 451–55
  side effects of, 453, 455–56
  types of, 453
L-carnosine, 351
L-citrulline, 576

lead, 111
  ADHD and, 342
  gout and, 625
  high BP and, 666, 674
leaky gut syndrome, 140
learned helplessness model, 479–80
lecithin, *see* phosphatidylcholine
legs:
  insomnia and, 752–53
  varicose veins and, 992–94
legumes, 1013, 1024
  cancer and, 104
  gallstones and, 608–9
  health-promoting diet and, 48,
    52–53, 55, 62
  oxalate content of, 769–71
lemon balm (*Melissa officinalis*), 664
leptin, 267
leukotrienes:
  asthma and, 324, 329, 332, 334
  food allergies and, 595–96
leuprorelin, 568
levadopa (L-dopa), 869–70, 873
Levin, Jeff, 24
licorice (*Glycyrrhiza glabra*):
  asthma and, 334–35
  canker sores and, 390–91
  deglycyrrhizinated (DGL), 137,
    390–91, 880–81
  eczema and, 584–86
  hepatitis and, 655–56
  HIV/AIDS and, 261–62
  peptic ulcer and, 880–81
life expectancy, 183, 186, 195
  alcohol dependence and, 265
  obesity and, 221
life extension, 186–97
  antioxidants and, 190–92, 195
  carotenes and, 191–92
  DHEA and, 193–94
  flavonoids and, 192
  melatonin and, 194–95
  sarcopenia and, 188–90
  vitamin D and, 186, 193
life spans, 183, 186–87, 190–91
lifestyle, 126, 851–55
  angina and, 311–12
  anxiety and, 320
  cancer and, 95–97, 99, 105, 905–6
  CFS and, 424, 427
  CVD and, 153, 167
  depression and, 482, 484–86, 501
  diabetes and, 513–15, 517–19, 521,
    527–28, 535
  exercise and, 28, 39–44
  healthful, 5, 9, 11, 25, 28, 39–47,
    105

high BP and, 666–67
  HIV/AIDS and, 262
  hypercholesterolemia and, 682
  hyperthyroidism and, 704
  hypoglycemia and, 713–15
  immune system and, 172–74
  infertility and, 726–27, 732
  life extension and, 186
  in naturopathic medicine, 3–7, 9,
    11
  nutritional supplements and, 68
  obesity and, 224, 226, 229
  osteoarthritis and, 829
  osteoporosis and, 846, 851, 853–55,
    865
  periodontal disease and, 883
  prediabetes and, 505
  sleep and, 28, 39, 44–47
  in stress management, 210–12
Lifestyle Heart Trial, 165
light touch therapy, 81–82
lignans, 57, 361, 788
limonenes, limonoids, 57
  detoxification and, 118, 122, 124
  for GERD, 135
lipases, 132, 139
lipids, 683, 685–90
  immunosuppression and, 176
  influence of mulberry and
    glyburide treatments on, 535
  niacin and, 686–89
  peroxidation of, 739–40
  vitamin B$_5$ and, 689–90
lipofuscin, 774–75
lipoproteins:
  atherosclerosis and, 148
  CVD and, 149–52
  see also under cholesterol
lipotropic factors, 127, 129
  chronic candidiasis and, 384
  endometriosis and, 567
  FBD and, 589
  gallstones and, 608, 611
  NAFLD and, 824
  uterine fibroids and, 982
listening, 211
liver, 45, 511
  alcohol and, 126–28, 267–70, 273
  CFS and, 425
  cholestasis and, 892
  cholesterol manufacture in, 89
  chronic candidiasis and, 383–84
  detoxification and, 110, 112–16,
    118–21, 123, 125–28, 383, 425,
    567
  diet and, 126–27
  digestion and, 131–32

gallstones and, 607, 610–11
hypercholesterolemia and, 681–83
IBD and, 462–63
kava and, 318–19
niacin and, 540, 688–89
plant-based medicines and, 128–29
prunes and, 454
psoriasis and, 924–25
see also specific liver disorders
Lobelia infata, 370
long-chain triglycerides (LCTs),
    239–41
longevity, 42, 184
longjack (*Eurycoma longifolia Jack*),
    577
loop electrosurgical excision
    procedure (LEEP), 414–15, 417
loss model, 479
lovastatin, 682, 686–87
love, 31, 33, 35
low back pain, 92
low-glycemic diet, 154
low-oxalate diet, 768–69
low-protein diet, 870
low-purine alkaline-ash diet, 625
low serotonin theory, 229–29
L-theanine, 345
lung cancer, 39, 96–97, 99, 101, 104,
    117
Lust, Benedict, 4
lutein:
    cataracts and, 396–97
    CVD and, 157–58
    macular degeneration and, 776–78
luteinizing hormone (LH), 725
    menopause and, 781–82, 791
    in normal menstrual cycle, 891
lycopene:
    asthma and, 332–33
    CVD and, 156
    macular degeneration and, 776
    male infertility and, 740
    prostate cancer and, 904, 906, 908,
        911
lymphatic system, 170–71, 177–78
lymphocytes, 171, 175, 179, 864
lymphosarcoma, 18
Lyon, Michael R., 234, 708, 713
Lyon Diet Heart Study, 166
lysine, 661–63

maca (*Lepidium meyenii*), 791
macrophages, 171
macular degeneration, 774–80
    appearance of Amsler grid in, 776
    diet and, 775–76, 779
    flavonoids and, 776, 778–79

lutein and, 776–78
risk factors for, 774–77
symptoms of, 774–75
therapeutic considerations for,
    775–78
types of, 774–75
zinc and, 776–78
magnesium, 644–45
    ADHD and, 344
    alcohol dependence and, 270–71
    angina and, 307–8
    arrhythmias and, 645
    ASD and, 350
    asthma and, 333
    CFS and, 426–27
    CHF and, 443
    COPD and, 432–33
    CVD and, 163–64
    diabetes and, 531–32
    glaucoma and, 619
    high BP and, 666–67, 669, 673–74
    HIV/AIDS and, 258
    kidney stones and, 767
    migraine headaches and, 806–7
    osteoporosis and, 846, 861
    PMS and, 896–98
    tension headaches and, 639, 641
magnesium ammonium phosphate,
    764–65, 767, 773
magnetic therapy, 840–41
ma huang (*Ephedra sinensis*), 334
malabsorption, 462–63
male infertility, 724–26, 731–47
    ALA for, 741
    arginine for, 742–43
    ashwagandha for, 745
    beta-carotene for, 740
    carnitine for, 741–42
    causes of, 731–32
    Chinese ginseng for, 743
    CoQ$_{10}$ for, 741–42
    diagnostic considerations for,
        732–34
    diet and, 732, 738, 746
    estrogen and, 735–37
    folic acid for, 741
    infections and, 734–35, 740
    lycopene for, 740
    pygeum for, 743
    selenium for, 741
    symptoms of, 731
    therapeutic considerations for,
        734–44
    tribulus for, 743–44
    velvet bean for, 745
    vitamin A for, 740–41
    vitamin B$_{12}$ for, 741

vitamin C for, 739, 741
vitamin E for, 739–41
zinc for, 740–41
male-pattern baldness, 906
males, *see* erectile dysfunction;
    gender; male infertility
malignant tumors, 95–96
malnutrition, 463–64
mammograms, 107, 356–58
manganese:
    diabetes and, 532
    osteoporosis and, 861
    RA and, 941
Maslow, Abraham, 30–33
mast cells, 64, 171
    asthma and, 322, 324, 335
    food allergies and, 592, 595–96,
        602
    hay fever and, 635
    hives and, 692, 696, 699
    periodontal disease and, 884, 886
mastic (*Pistacia lentiscus*), 881
Mayans, 784
meal planning, 213
meal replacement (MR) formulas, 236
meats, meat, 1025
    cancer and, 102, 360, 904, 906–7
    in Edible Plant and Animal
        Kingdoms Taxonomic List, 600
    health-promoting diet and, 49, 51,
        53–54, 59–62, 65
    MS and, 814, 816
    nutritional supplements and, 76
    preparations of, 360, 510
    prostate enlargement and, 917
    reducing intake of, 60–62
media, 147
medications, 23, 25, 41, 64
    acne and, 247–49, 251
    AD and, 288
    ADHD and, 341, 345
    AIDS and, 254–56
    anemia and, 295
    arrhythmias and, 644–45
    cancer and, 96
    and cellular approach to health, 88
    constipation and, 451, 455
    COPD and, 432
    CVD and, 163
    depression and, 479–83, 486,
        488–89, 491, 493–99
    detoxification and, 114, 118–19,
        123–25, 128
    diabetes and, 517–19, 521, 524,
        527–28, 530, 534–36, 542
    digestion and, 134–35, 137–38,
        141–42, 144

medications (*cont.*)
  ear infections and, 557–59, 561
  ED and, 573, 576, 578–79
  gallstones and, 607–8
  glaucoma and, 617
  gout and, 622, 624–25
  hair loss and, 630, 632
  hepatitis and, 652, 655
  high BP and, 667–68, 672, 676, 678
  hives and, 694–95, 699
  hypercholesterolemia and, 682–83, 686–89
  hyperthyroidism and, 703–4
  hypertriglyceridemia and, 687
  hypoglycemia and, 707–8
  hypothyroidism and, 718, 720
  IBD and, 458–59, 463
  IBS and, 758
  insomnia and, 748, 754–55
  interactions of, 319
  macular degeneration and, 775
  male infertility and, 735
  migraine headaches and, 803–6, 809–10
  MS and, 815
  NAFLD and, 822–23
  naturopathic medicine and, 3–6, 9–10, 12, 17
  nutritional supplements and, 68
  osteoarthritis and, 9–10, 828, 830–32, 835, 837, 840
  osteoporosis and, 852–54, 856, 864
  Parkinson's disease and, 869–70, 872–73
  peptic ulcer and, 876–77
  pH balance and, 92
  placebo response and, 18–21
  pneumonia and, 368–69
  prostate enlargement and, 917–21
  psoriasis and, 923, 928
  RA and, 934–38, 940, 943
  rosacea and, 949–51
  side effects of, 10, 21, 88–90, 134, 138, 165–66, 178, 247–48, 288, 330, 341, 377, 382, 385, 481–82, 497, 517, 534, 579, 624, 632, 639–40, 683, 754, 805–6, 828, 853–54, 869–70, 876–77, 928, 936–38, 986
  sinus infections and, 957–59
  sleep and, 45, 748, 754–55
  stroke and, 972
  tension headaches and, 639–41
  vaginitis and, 986–88
  see also specific medications
medicinal mushrooms, 180
Medifast, 236

meditation, 23, 209, 217
Mediterranean diet, 359
  AD and, 278–79
  CVD and, 154, 156, 161, 165
  depression and, 486
  osteoarthritis and, 829
  RA and, 939–41
medium-chain triglycerides (MCTS), 239–41
melatonin:
  AD and, 286–87
  ASD and, 351
  breast cancer and, 365
  insomnia and, 751–52
  life extension and, 194–95
memory, 276, 279–80, 282, 284–86, 288
menopause, 781–95, 845–48
  anxiety and, 317
  bioidentical hormone therapy and, 786
  black cohosh for, 790–91
  causes of, 781–82
  description of, 781
  diet and, 787–88
  dong quai for, 792
  EstroG for, 794
  exercise and, 786–87
  fish oils for, 76, 788
  flavonoids for, 788–89
  flaxseeds for, 788
  gamma-oryzanol for, 789
  maca for, 791
  natural approaches to, 786–93
  osteoporosis and, 845, 847–48, 852, 854, 857–58, 862–63
  red clover for, 791–92
  St.-John's-wort and, 791–93
  as social construct, 783–84
  soy products and, 787–88
  symptoms of, 781–93
  therapeutic considerations for, 784–93
  vitamin C for, 788–89
  vitamin E for, 789, 791
menorrhagia, 796–99
  bioflavonoids for, 797
  causes of, 796–97
  chasteberry for, 798
  chlorophyll for, 797
  omega-3 fatty acids for, 798
  symptoms of, 796
  therapeutic considerations for, 797–98
  vitamin B complex for, 798
  vitamin C for, 797
  vitamin K for, 797

menstruation, menstrual cycle, 724
  endometriosis and, 565–66, 568
  female infertility and, 725–27, 729
  hypoglycemia and, 710
  menorrhagia and, 796
  normal, 890–91
  osteoporosis and, 848
  see also premenstrual syndrome
mental processes, 41–42
Mentastics, 82
Merck, 853
mercury, 111
Meriva, 201, 261, 943, 965
  AD and, 289
  osteoarthritis and, 836–37
metabolic issues, 717
metabolic syndrome, 153, 505, 709
Metchnikoff, Elie, 8, 142–43
metformin, 517
methionine, 121, 123–24, 127, 129, 190
methotrexate, 937–38
methylation, 114, 120–21, 123
methylcobalamin, *see* vitamin B_{12}
methylxanthines, 587–88
methysergide, 805–6
metronidazole, 553, 952
microbial compounds, 112
micronized diosmin, 994
migraine headaches, 800–811
  acupuncture for, 809
  amines and, 801–2, 804–5
  analgesic rebound, 803–4
  biofeedback for, 809–10
  butter bur for, 809
  causes of, 800–803
  as drug reaction, 803
  feverfew for, 807–9
  food allergies and, 803–4
  ginger for, 809
  5-HTP and, 801–2, 805–6
  hypoglycemia and, 711
  magnesium for, 806–7
  menopause and, 782
  as nervous system disorder, 801
  platelets and, 800–801, 807–9
  relaxation therapy for, 809–10
  serotonin and, 800–802, 807
  symptoms of, 800, 808
  therapeutic considerations for, 803–5
  treatment considerations for, 805–10
  triggers of, 802–4
  unified hypothesis on, 802
  vitamin B_2 for, 806

milk, 600, 1016, 1025–26
    osteoporosis and, 860
    penicillin in, 695
    peptic ulcer and, 878
    prostate cancer and, 906–7
    see also dairy products
milk thistle (*Silybum marianum*), 74,
    128–29
    alcohol dependence and, 272–73
    diabetes and, 538
    hepatitis and, 656–57
    HIV/AIDS and, 260–61
    IBD and, 462
    NAFLD and, 825
    psoriasis and, 925
minerals:
    celiac disease and, 402, 405
    chart on, 72
    deficiencies in, 69–71, 79
    digestion and, 131–32
    health-promoting diet and, 49
    hypothyroidism and, 721
    pH balance and, 92
    see also multiple vitamin and
        mineral formulas; *specific
        minerals*
mitochondria:
    angina and, 306–7
    and cellular approach to health,
        87–92
    CoQ$_{10}$ and, 89–90
    energy production and, 87–88
    optimization strategies for, 88–89
mitoxantrone (Novantrone), 815
mitral valve prolapse, 807
molybdenum, 124, 328, 697
monoamines, 479–80, 488–90, 496
monocytes, 171
moods, *see* emotions
mucin, 461, 876, 879–80
mucolytics:
    and bronchitis and pneumonia,
        371, 375
    COPD and, 432, 434
    sinus infections and, 958
muffins, 1018
mulberry (*Morus indica*), 534–35
multiple chemical sensitivities (MCS),
    422
multiple sclerosis (MS), 812–21
    ALA for, 817
    causes of, 812–15, 817
    diet and, 812–16
    exercise for, 819
    fish oils and, 815–17
    genetics and, 812–13
    hyperbaric oxygen and, 819

proteolytic enzymes for, 818–19
    stress and, 819
    symptoms of, 812–13, 815, 818–19
    therapeutic considerations for,
        815–18
    viruses and, 813–14
    vitamin D and, 814, 817
multiple vitamin and mineral
    formulas:
    and cancer, 103
    and celiac disease, 402, 405
    and CVD, 158
    and detoxification, 126, 129
    and diabetes, 526, 528, 535, 542
    and ED, 575
    and hair loss in women, 633
    and HIV/AIDS, 256
    and IBD, 464–65
    and immune system, 174
    and PMS, 897–98
    recommendations on, 71–73, 79
muscles, muscle, 45
    exercise and, 40–41, 44, 229
    health-promoting diet and, 65
    HIV/AIDS and, 259
    hypothyroidism and, 717
    lactic acid and, 314–15
    life extension and, 188–89
    obesity and, 237
    osteoarthritis and, 828–29, 839
    Parkinson's disease and, 868
    physical care and, 80
    prunes and, 454
    sarcopenia and, 188–90, 855
    stress management and, 210
    tension headaches and, 639–40
musculoskeletal system, 41
mutations, 95–97
mycoplasmal pneumonia, 368
myocardial infarction, *see* heart
    attacks
myoclonus (nocturnal leg cramps),
    752
MyPlate, 54
myringotomies, 557–58
myxedema, 716–17

N-acetylcysteine (NAC), 122, 258–59
    bronchitis and, 371
    COPD and, 432
    Parkinson's disease and, 872–73
    sinus infections and, 958
nails, 717, 923
nasal irrigation, 959–60
National Asthma Education and
    Prevention Program (NAEPP),
    323

National Cancer Institute, 62, 102,
    357, 908
National Cooperative Crohn's Disease
    Study (NCCDS), 459–60
National Health and Nutrition
    Examination surveys
    (NHANES), 69, 505, 514
National Institute of Neurological
    Diseases and Strokes, 871
nattokinase, 161, 996
natural antiplatelet and fibrinolytic
    therapy, 973
natural antiyeast agents, 385–87
natural glucosidase inhibitors, 534–35
natural killer (NK) cells:
    CFS and, 422, 424, 427–28
    immune system and, 171, 173–74,
        179–80
    lifestyle and, 174, 424
nature, healing power of, 5, 9–10, 18
"Nature's Rx," 498
naturopathic ear drops, 561
naturopathic medicine:
    bias against, 13–14
    brief history of, 3–5
    comparisons between conventional
        and, 8–9, 12–13
    complementary aspects of, 10–11
    future of, 16–17
    for hyperthyroidism, 703–4
    need for, 11–12
    philosophy of, 5–6, 17
    prevention and, 5–6, 11
    primary care in, 7–8
    program of cure in, 4
    therapies in, 3, 6–7, 13–14, 17
    as treatment, 9–10
    as wellness-oriented, 12
    what it is, 3–17
naturopathic physicians (N.D.s), 3
    accredited schools for, 15
    curriculum studied by, 14–15
    primary goals of, 7
    professional licensure for, 15–16
    professional organizations of, 15–16
    as teachers, 5
    training of, 6–7, 11, 14–15
negative coping patterns, 208
Neisseria gonorrhea, 984–87
neovascular (wet) macular
    degeneration, 774–75
nephropathy, 503, 524, 533, 541–42
nervous system:
    anemia and, 294
    asthma and, 324
    chronic candidiasis and, 377
    digestion and, 133–34

nervous system (*cont.*)
  migraine headaches and, 801
  prostate enlargement and, 916–17
  in sex act for men, 570–71
  stress management and, 209
  toxins and, 112
neti pots, 959–60
neuropathy, 503, 523–24, 526,
    531–33, 539, 541–42
neutrophils:
  immune system and, 170, 174–75,
    180–81
  periodontal disease and, 884–85
  sugars and, 174–75
New York Heart Association (NYHA),
    443, 445–47, 449
niacin:
  comparisons between atorvastatin
    and, 687
  comparisons between lovastatin
    and, 686
  depression and, 487
  diabetes and, 530–31, 539–40, 687
  gout and, 627
  health-promoting diet and, 66
  hypercholesterolemia and, 685–89
  insomnia and, 751
  side effects of, 511, 540, 686,
    688–89
niacinamide:
  diabetes and, 510–11, 530–31
  osteoarthritis and, 834–35
Niaspan, 540, 686
nickel, 111
nicotinamide adenine dinucleotide
    (NADH), 871
nitrates, 61, 510
nocebo effect, 21
nocturnal leg cramps (myoclonus), 752
nonalcoholic fatty liver disease
    (NAFLD), 822–26
  betaine for, 824
  carnitine for, 824–25
  causes of, 822–23
  diet and, 823–24, 826
  lipotropic agents for, 824
  milk thistle for, 825
  progression of, 823
  therapeutic considerations for,
    823–24
nonalcoholic steatohepatitis (NASH),
    822–23
  bile acids for, 825
  causes of, 822
  progression of, 823
nonspecific vaginitis (NSV), 985–86,
    988–89

nonsteroidal anti-inflammatory drugs
    (NSAIDs), 324
  gout and, 624
  osteoarthritis and, 10, 828, 830–32,
    835, 837, 840
  peptic ulcer and, 876–77
  RA and, 936–37, 942
  side effects of, 165, 828, 876–77,
    937
nontoxic therapies, 3, 5
non-ulcer dyspepsia (NUD), 134,
    138
Northwick Park Heart Study, 161
Nurses Health Studies, 155, 158, 515,
    566, 814–15, 857, 860
  female infertility and, 726–27
nutrition, nutrients, 109, 381
  AD and, 281
  ADHD and, 341, 343–44
  alcohol dependence and, 268
  anemia and, 295
  canker sores and, 389–90
  chronic candidiasis and, 382
  conditionally essential, 71, 91
  CoQ$_{10}$ and, 89–90
  depression and, 487–91
  detoxification and, 118, 120
  diabetes and, 526, 528–33, 537–39
  digestion and, 131–32, 134
  government and education on,
    52–54
  and hair loss in women, 632–33
  HIV/AIDS and, 255–57
  IBD and, 462–63
  immune system and, 174, 180
  in naturopathic medicine, 3–7, 9,
    11, 13–14, 17
  periodontal disease and, 883
  positive mental attitude and, 36
  psoriasis and, 926–27
  sleep and, 45
  see also diets, diet; foods, food
*Nutritional Influences on Mental
    Illness* (Werbach), 487–88
nutritional supplements, 25, 28,
    68–80, 82
  acne and, 247–50, 252
  AD and, 281–84, 289, 291
  ADHD and, 343–47
  alcohol dependence and, 268–71,
    274
  allergies and, 77, 594, 602–4
  anemia and, 293–300
  angina and, 301, 304–8, 312
  anxiety and, 316, 320
  arrhythmias and, 645–46
  ASD and, 350–52

asthma and, 325, 329–34, 338
  bladder infections and, 472–73,
    476–77
  boils and, 355
  and bronchitis and pneumonia,
    372–73, 375
  cancer and, 73–78, 102–6, 361–66,
    906, 908–13
  canker sores and, 389–91
  cataracts and, 396–401
  celiac disease and, 403, 405–7
  and cellular approach to health, 85,
    87–88, 90–92
  cervical dysplasia and, 415–19
  CFS and, 426–27, 429–30
  CHF and, 443–48, 450
  chronic candidiasis and, 386
  common cold and, 436–37, 441
  constipation and, 451–55
  COPD and, 433
  CoQ$_{10}$ and, 88, 90–92
  coronary artery bypass surgery and,
    304–5
  CTS and, 394–95
  CVD and, 154–55, 157–59,
    161–63, 168
  CVI and, 409
  depression and, 68, 76, 482, 485,
    488–91, 501–2
  detoxification and, 122–23, 126–27,
    129
  diabetes and, 68, 76–77, 509–11,
    518–19, 526, 528–42, 544–47
  diarrhea and, 551–53, 556
  diet and, 66–68, 73, 76–77
  digestion and, 136, 143–45
  ear infections and, 563
  eczema and, 583–85
  ED and, 575–76, 581
  endometriosis and, 567–69
  FBD and, 588, 591
  gallstones and, 610–11, 613
  glaucoma and, 617–21
  gout and, 626–27, 629
  growing popularity of, 69–70
  and hair loss in women, 632–34
  hay fever and, 636–38
  hemorrhoids and, 649–51
  hepatitis and, 654–55, 658
  herpes and, 661–63, 665
  high BP and, 76–77, 667, 671–76,
    679
  HIV/AIDS and, 257–60, 264
  hives and, 697, 699–701
  hypercholesterolemia and, 682–83,
    685–91
  hyperthyroidism and, 704–6

hypertriglyceridemia and, 685, 687, 690
hypoglycemia and, 713, 715
hypothyroidism and, 720–22
IBD and, 464–66, 470
IBS and, 750–60, 763
immune system and, 172, 174, 176–80, 182
infertility and, 727–30, 738–43, 746
insomnia and, 750–53, 756
kidney stones and, 767–68, 771–73
lifespan extension and, 190–95, 197
macular degeneration and, 775–80
menopause and, 76, 787–89, 794–95
menorrhagia and, 797–99
migraine headaches and, 802, 805–7, 810–11
MS and, 814–20
NAFLD and, 823–26
in naturopathic medicine, 6, 9, 13–14, 17
obesity and, 226, 233–34, 240
osteoarthritis and, 829–36, 842
osteoporosis and, 851–52, 856, 858–64, 867
Parkinson's disease and, 870–74
peptic ulcer and, 878–80, 882
periodontal disease and, 885–89
PMS and, 896–99, 902
probiotics and, 143–44
prostate enlargement and, 917–18, 922
psoriasis and, 925–27, 930–31
RA and, 940–43, 946
recommendations for, 69–78, 127
rosacea and, 950–53
seborrheic dermatitis and, 955–56
silent inflammation and, 200, 203
sinus infections and, 958, 960
SLE and, 977–79
sports injuries and, 963, 965–66
strep throat and, 968–70
stress management and, 214–18
stroke and, 973–75
tension headaches and, 641–42
uterine fibroids and, 982–83
vaginitis and, 789, 988, 991
varicose veins and, 996–97
when to take them, 73
nuts and seeds, 1022
    and CVD, 155–56
    and diabetes, 516
    and health-promoting diet, 48, 53, 58, 62
    oxalate content of, 769–71

and sarcopenia prevention, 189
    see also flaxseeds, flaxseed oil

oats, 404–5, 684
obesity, 25, 220–41
    abdominal, 199, 222–24, 226, 229, 512, 916–17
    and adipokine and gut-derived hormone alterations, 227
    behavioral therapy and, 230
    cancer and, 99–100, 102, 221–22, 359
    causes of, 224–29
    chromium for, 236–37
    definition of, 222
    depression and, 524
    diabetes and, 220–21, 224–27, 232, 234, 237, 504–5, 512–14, 516–17
    diet and, 100, 224, 226–33, 238–41
    exercise and, 40, 225–26, 228–29, 232, 237
    fiber and, 227, 232–36
    gallstones and, 606, 610
    glucosamine and, 831–32
    gout and, 624, 626
    HCA for, 238–39
    health and, 220–22
    health-promoting diet and, 52, 54
    5-HTP for, 237–38
    immune system and, 175–76
    infertility and, 725–26, 737–38
    low serotonin theory on, 228–29
    MCTs for, 239–41
    MR formulas and, 236
    physiological factors in, 226–29
    in premature death, 183
    psychological factors in, 224–26
    set point theory on, 226–27
    silent inflammation and, 199
    statistics on, 11, 220
    therapeutic considerations for, 229–39
    vitamin D deficiency and, 78
    weight loss and, 229–41
obstructive sleep apnea, 749
oldest living people, 184
oleuropein, 677
olive (Olea europaea), 676–78
olive oil, 62–63
    cancer and, 105
    CVD and, 154
    MS and, 816–17
    RA and, 939–40
olive oil liver flush, 610–11
omega-3 fatty acids, 49–50, 85–86, 91, 189
    ADHD and, 343

anxiety and, 316
ASD and, 350
asthma and, 329–30
cancer and, 357, 359–61, 926–27
CVD and, 153–55, 160–61, 165–66
depression and, 316, 487, 490–91
diabetes and, 509–10, 515–16, 532–33
endometriosis and, 566–67
health-promoting diet and, 60–62
high BP and, 666, 675
hypertriglyceridemia and, 685
IBD and, 459–60
male infertility and, 738
menorrhagia and, 798
MS and, 815–17
nutritional supplements and, 75–77, 79
psoriasis and, 926–27
RA and, 942–43
silent inflammation and, 199–200
omega-6 fatty acids:
    breast cancer and, 360
    endometriosis and, 566–67
    IBD and, 459–60
    male infertility and, 738
    MS and, 816–17
    silent inflammation and, 199–200
onions (Allium cepa):
    diabetes and, 537
    high BP and, 669
    hypercholesterolemia and, 690
opipramol, 317
Optimal Health Food Diet, 55–66
optimism:
    positive mental attitude and, 29–30, 34, 38
    testing your level of, 1007–11
oral allergy syndrome, 595
oral glucose tolerance tests, 707–8
organizing, 210
osteoarthritis, 827–43
    acupuncture for, 839
    boron for, 836
    boswellia for, 837
    chondroitin for, 833–34
    contributors to, 827–28
    conventional drug treatment for, 828
    copper for, 836
    curcumin for, 836–37
    devil's claw for, 838
    diet and, 828–29, 835, 841–42
    electroacupuncture and, 839–40
    exercise and, 828–29
    ginger for, 837–38
    glucosamine for, 10, 829–35

osteoarthritis (*cont.*)
    HA and, 834
    magnetic therapy for, 840–41
    natural vs. drug approach to, 9–10
    niacinamide for, 834–35
    obesity and, 221
    physical therapy for, 839–41
    primary, 827
    procyanidolic oligomers for, 837
    relaxation techniques for, 841
    SAM-e for, 835
    secondary, 827
    symptoms of, 827, 830–31, 834–37, 840
    therapeutic considerations for, 828–40
    topical analgesics for, 838–39
    vitamin A for, 836
    vitamin B₆ for, 836
    vitamin C for, 835–36
    vitamin D for, 836
    vitamin E for, 836
    vitamin K for, 836
    zinc for, 836
osteopenia, 844, 853, 862, 864
    BMD testing and, 849–51
osteoporosis, 41, 783–85, 844–67
    BMD testing and, 844, 849–51
    calcium and, 845–46, 855–61, 864
    causes of, 844–45, 861
    copper and, 861
    diagnostic considerations for, 845–51
    diet and, 846, 851, 853, 855–59, 862, 866
    folic acid and, 862
    green tea and, 864
    HRT and, 785, 852
    ipriflavone and, 858, 863–64
    lifestyle and, 846, 851, 853–55, 865
    magnesium and, 846, 861
    manganese and, 861
    pH and, 92, 855–56
    risk factors and, 785, 845–48, 850–51
    silicon and, 861–62
    strontium and, 863
    symptoms of, 844
    therapeutic considerations for, 851–64
    vitamin B₆ and, 862
    vitamin B₁₂ and, 862
    vitamin C and, 862
    vitamin D and, 845–46, 857, 859–61, 863
    vitamin K and, 846, 857, 859, 862–64
    zinc and, 861

otitis media, *see* ear infections
ovulation disorders, 725
oxalates, 766–71
    kidney stones and, 766–69
    in selected foods, 769–71
oxidative stress:
    detoxification and, 122, 128
    diabetes and, 525–26, 537–39
    hepatitis and, 655
    RA and, 934, 940
oxygen radical absorbance capacity
        (ORAC) values, 75

pancakes, 1018
pancreas:
    blood glucose monitoring and, 518–19
    C-peptide determination and, 519–20
    diabetes and, 504, 507, 510–12, 518–20, 528, 536
    digestion and, 131–32, 134, 138–39
pancreatic enzymes:
    celiac disease and, 405–6
    digestion and, 132, 138–41, 144
    food allergies and, 139, 598–602
    parasitic infections and, 552
    RA and, 942
pancreatic insufficiency, 138–40
pancreatin, 138–39
panic attacks, *see* anxiety
pantethine, 306–7
pantothenic acid, *see* vitamin B₅
Pap smears, 412–18
parasites, 144, 552
parathyroid hormone, 846, 848, 852, 854
parietal cells, 876
Parkinson's disease, 868–75
    antioxidants for, 870
    causes of, 869
    CoQ₁₀ and, 90, 92, 870–71
    diet and, 869–70, 874
    fava bean for, 873
    GBE for, 873
    green tea for, 873
    5-HTP for, 872
    kava and, 319
    NAC for, 872–73
    NADH for, 871
    placebo response and, 19
    PS for, 872
    symptoms of, 868–73
    therapeutic considerations for, 869–73
    velvet bean for, 873
partially hydrolyzed guar gum
        (PHGG), 758
passion fruit peel (PFP), 332

pasta, 1018, 1024
Pasteur, Louis, 8–9
patient-physician relationship, 3, 7
Pauling, Linus, 66, 436
pectin, 551
penicillin, 695
penile prosthesis, 579
pentosan polysulfate sodium (PPS), 473
peppermint oil (*Mentha piperita*):
    digestion and, 134–35, 138, 142
    IBS and, 138, 760–61
peptic ulcer, 831, 876–82
    aloe vera for, 881
    bismuth subcitrate for, 879
    cabbage for, 878–79
    causes of, 876–77
    fiber for, 878
    licorice for, 880–81
    mastic for, 881
    nutritional supplements and, 878–80, 882
    rhubarb for, 881
    symptoms of, 876, 881
    therapeutic considerations for, 878–81
    vitamin A for, 879
    vitamin E for, 879
    zinc for, 879–80
perfectionism, 211
perimenopause, 781, 789, 791–93
periodontal disease, 883–89
    bloodroot for, 888
    causes of, 883–86
    CoQ₁₀ for, 886–87
    diabetes and, 503, 505
    flavonoids for, 887–88
    folic acid for, 888
    gotu kola for, 888
    selenium for, 886
    sugar and, 886
    symptoms of, 883, 885
    therapeutic considerations for, 885–88
    vitamin A for, 885–86
    vitamin C and, 885–86
    vitamin E for, 886
    zinc for, 885–86
permanence, 1010
pernicious anemia, 294, 297–299
persistent organic pollutants (POPs), 112, 504, 517
personality, 29–31
    attitude and, 29–30
    and hierarchy of needs, 31
    type A, 162
    type C, 99–100

personalization, 1011

pertussis vaccine, 324–25

pervasive developmental disorder, not
otherwise specified (PDD-NOS),
348

pervasiveness, 1010–11

pesticides:
ADHD and, 342–43
cancer and, 98
and cellular approach to health, 88
detoxification and, 129
health-promoting diet and, 55,
58–60, 66
nutritional supplements and, 77

Petadolex, 809

Peyronie's disease (PD), 573–74

pH:
bladder infections and, 472–73
and cellular approach to health, 92
digestion and, 134, 136–37, 139
H. pylori overgrowth and, 137
kidney stones and, 764–67
osteoporosis and, 92, 855–56
see also acid, acidity; alkaloids,
alkalinity

PharmaGABA, 214–15

phenolsulfotransferase, 804

phenylbutazone, 943

Phlogenzym, 964

phosphates, tricalcium, 859–60

phosphatidylcholine:
AD and, 284–85
gallstones and, 605–6, 610–11

phosphatidylserine (PS), 285, 872

phthalates, 566

physical care, 78–82

physical examinations, 468, 522

physical medicine:
acne and, 252
ear infections and, 564
hives and, 699
in naturopathic medicine, 7, 14

physical therapy, 7
osteoarthritis and, 839–41
sports injuries and, 965
tension headaches and, 640

Physicians Health Study, 155, 158, 164

physiological factors, 31, 33
in obesity, 226–29

phytochemicals, 93
CVD and, 157
examples of anticancer, 57
health-promoting diet and, 57, 60
nutritional supplements and, 75

phytoestrogens:
menopause and, 787, 790–91
uterine fibroids and, 981

phytosterols, 918

Pillsbury, Donald M., 246–47

Pima Indians, 513

pineal gland, 194–95

pine bark extract (Pycnogenol), 74, 80
ADHD and, 344–45
asthma and, 332
benefits of, 75
CVD and, 160
diabetes and, 538
ED and, 576
endometriosis and, 567–68
male infertility and, 743
osteoarthritis and, 837
silent inflammation and, 200
varicose veins and, 994

pituitary gland, 716, 721, 891

placebo response, 18–22
holy trinity of, 20–21
mechanisms of, 19
in medical research, 19–20
opposite of, 21
and power of expectations, 21–22

plaques, plaque:
AD and, 276, 284
angina and, 301
atherosclerosis and, 148, 153, 409
CVD and, 160–61
ED and, 572, 574
MS and, 812
periodontal disease and, 884–86, 888
psoriasis and, 923, 925, 928–29
seborrheic dermatitis and, 954

platelets, 973
CVD and, 151, 155, 158, 160–61
migraine headaches and, 800–801,
807–9

pneumonia, 367–75
differentiating between bronchitis
and, 367–68
expectorants for, 369–71, 374–75
mucolytics for, 371, 375
mycoplasmal, 368
pneumococcal, 369
postural draining for, 373–74
risk factors for, 367–68
signs and symptoms of, 367–68
special considerations with, 368–69
therapeutic considerations for,
369–74
viral, 368

polyamines, 924, 926

polychlorinated biphenyls (PCBs), 128

PolyGlycoPlex (PGX):
diabetes and, 533–34
hypoglycemia and, 713
obesity and, 234–36

polyphenols:
AD and, 279–80, 282
apple (AP), 602, 637
cancer and, 57, 913
osteoporosis and, 864

polysorbate, 697

pomegranate juice, 156–57

Portfolio Diet, 682–83

positive affirmations, 35–36

positive mental attitude, 28–38, 105
cardiovascular health and, 30, 37
in healthful lifestyle, 28
HIV/AIDS and, 256
immune system and, 29–30, 36–37,
172–73
in naturopathic medicine, 5, 11
nutritional supplements and, 68
pessimism and, 29–30
self-actualization and, 30–34
seven steps to, 34–38
and steps to living with vibrant
health, 25

postmenopause, 361, 781–82, 784, 897
osteoarthritis and, 830
osteoporosis and, 844–45, 852,
854–64

postural draining, 373–74

posture:
CFS and, 427
Parkinson's disease and, 868
physical care and, 78–81

potassium, 213
CVD and, 163–64
health-promoting diet and, 55, 63
high BP and, 667–69, 671–74
senna and, 454–55
-to-sodium (K:Na) ratio, 63, 213

potatoes, 52

potency wood, 577

poultices, 354

poultry, 51, 53, 55, 62, 65

"Powerful Placebo, The" (Beecher),
20

prayer, 22–23

prebiotics, 145, 465–66

prediabetes, 505–6, 514, 517

pregnancy:
diabetes and, 504–5, 509, 520–23,
527, 531
ear infections and, 560
folic acid and, 14
hypothyroidism and, 717, 720
infertility and, 724–28, 733, 738,
741
iron and, 293, 297
nutritional supplements during,
76, 79–80, 297, 860–61

Premarin, 785
premenstrual syndrome (PMS),
    890–902
    -C, 710–11
    calcium for, 897
    causes of, 890–92, 898
    chasteberry for, 899
    diet and, 893–94, 897
    EFAs for, 898
    estrogen and, 891–94, 899
    exercise and, 895
    FBD and, 587–90
    GBE for, 899–900
    hormones and, 891–92, 897
    hypoglycemia and, 710–11
    hypothyroidism and, 891–92, 894
    magnesium for, 896–898
    and multiple vitamin and mineral
        formulas, 897–98
    saffron for, 900
    St.-John's-wort for, 899–900
    signs and symptoms of, 890,
        893–900
    stress and, 895
    therapeutic considerations for,
        892–900
    tryptophan for, 898–99
    vitamin B$_6$ and, 893, 896–98
    vitamin E for, 897–98
    zinc for, 897
prevention, 3
    of cancer, 30, 57, 95–108, 119, 159,
        190–91, 193, 356–66, 588, 785,
        790, 864, 903–14
    definitions of, 11
    exercise and, 42
    in naturopathic medicine, 5–6, 11
    positive mental attitude and, 30
    of stroke, 153, 158–59, 163–65
Prevent Recurrence of Osteoporotic
    Fractures trial, 854
Price, Weston A., 50
"Principles, Aim and Program of the
    Nature Cure, The" (Lust), 4
Prinzmetal's variant angina, 301, 307
priority setting, 210–11
proanthocyanidins, 74–75
    bladder infections and, 474
    prostate cancer and, 912
probiotics, 344, 968
    acne and, 247
    asthma and, 325
    benefits of supplementation with,
        143–45
    chronic candidiasis and, 385
    diarrhea and, 551–53
    eczema and, 583–84

female infertility and, 728
    IBD and, 466
    IBS and, 760
    RA and, 942
problem-solving orientation, 32
procyanidolic oligomers (PCOs), 160
    ED and, 575–76
    menopause and, 789
    osteoarthritis and, 837
progeria (Hutchinson-Gilford
    syndrome), 186, 194
progesterone:
    endometriosis and, 566
    menopause and, 781, 784–86
    PMS and, 891–93, 899
prolactin:
    FBD and, 587
    female infertility and, 726, 729
    PMS and, 891–92, 897, 899
    prostate enlargement and, 915, 917
propolis, 387
propranolol (Inderal), 809–10
propylthiouracil, 704
prostaglandins, 76
    asthma and, 329, 334
    menorrhagia and, 796–97
prostate cancer, 77
    berries for, 912
    causes of, 903–4, 906
    diagnostic considerations for,
        904–5, 910, 916
    early detection of, 107
    flaxseed and, 908
    green tea for, 913
    lycopene and, 904, 906, 908, 911
    male-pattern baldness and, 906
    omega-3 fatty acids and, 906–8
    prevention of, 104, 903–14
    proanthocyanidins for, 912
    pygeum for, 913
    risk factors and, 98, 103–4, 106
    selenium and, 906, 909–11
    soy products and, 906–7
    symptoms of, 903
    therapeutic considerations for,
        905–13
    vitamin D and, 911–12
    vitamin E and, 904, 906, 908–11
prostate enlargement, 913, 915–22
    alcohol and, 917–18
    amino acids and, 918
    causes of, 915
    Cernilton and, 918, 920–21
    cholesterol and, 918
    diagnostic considerations for, 915–16
    exercise and, 916–17
    pygeum and, 918, 921

saw palmetto and, 918–21
    soy products and, 918
    stinging nettle and, 918, 921
    symptoms of, 915–16, 918–21
    therapeutic considerations for,
        916–21
    zinc and, 917
prostate-specific antigen (PSA):
    age-adjusted, 904
    blood tests for, 904, 916
    density of, 905
    free vs. attached, 905
    nutritional supplements and, 910–11
    prostate cancer and, 904–5, 910–11
    prostate enlargement and, 913, 916
    and screening pros and cons, 905
    velocity of, 904–5
proteins, protein:
    acne and, 249
    aging and, 187–88
    alcohol dependence and, 268
    Atkins Diet and, 231–33
    biological value of selected, 257
    breakdown products of metabolism
        of, 112
    detoxification and, 122–23
    diabetes and, 506–9, 512, 525
    digestion and, 131–32, 134,
        139–41, 924
    ED and, 575
    food allergies and, 594–95, 602
    gout and, 626
    HIV/AIDS and, 256–58
    IBD and, 462–63
    obesity and, 230–33, 236
    osteoporosis and, 846, 855
    Parkinson's disease and, 870
    psoriasis and, 924
    sarcopenia prevention and, 189
    whey, 189–90, 256–57
    see also C-reactive protein
proteolytic enzymes (proteases), 132,
    139, 141, 973
    MS and, 818–19
    sinus infections and, 958
    sports injuries and, 963–64
protodioscin, 743
protozoa, 552
prunes, 452, 454, 858
pseudomelanosis coli, 454–55
pseudomembranous enterocolitis, 553
psoralen, 928
psoriasis, 923–31
    aloe vera for, 928
    bile acid deficiency in, 925–26
    capsaicin for, 928–29
    causes of, 923–24

curcumin for, 929
emollients for, 929
fumaric acid for, 927
liver and, 924–25
protein digestion and, 924
sunlight and ultraviolet light for,
   927–28
symptoms of, 923, 926
therapeutic considerations for,
   924–29
topical treatments for, 928–29
toxins and, 924–26
vitamin D and, 927–28
psychological factors:
   alcohol dependence and, 271
   cancer and, 99–100
   depression and, 483, 486, 496, 498,
      501
   diabetes and, 527
   dreams and, 47
   ED and, 578
   high BP and, 666
   hives and, 698
   hypothyroidism and, 717
   IBD and, 466
   IBS and, 761–62
   insomnia and, 748
   menopause and, 788
   naturopathic medicine and, 3, 6–7,
      11, 14
   obesity and, 224–26
   peptic ulcer and, 877–78
   PMS and, 890, 894–95
   psoriasis and, 927
   RA and, 934, 945
   rosacea and, 950
psychoneuroimmunology (PNI), 172
psychosocial factors, 221, 271
psyllium, 452, 758
Pterocarpus marsupium, 511–12
purines:
   gout and, 623–26
   kidney stones and, 768
putting things off, 211
Pycnogenol, *see* pine bark extract
pygeum (*Pygeum africanum*):
   male infertility and, 743
   prostate cancer and, 913
   prostate enlargement and, 918, 921
Pygmalion effect, 22
pyridoxal-5-phosphate (P5P), 896
pyridoxine, *see* vitamin B$_6$
pyruvic acid, 314–15

quercetin:
   asthma and, 332
   food allergies and, 602

gout and, 627
hay fever and, 636–37
hives and, 699
questions, asking better, 34–35

race:
   alcohol dependence and, 265
   cancer and, 98, 356, 366, 904–5,
      908, 910
   diabetes and, 505, 507, 513
   gallstones and, 607–8
   high BP and, 666, 674
   HIV/AIDS and, 254, 260
   hypothyroidism and, 716
   IBD and, 456–57
   lactose intolerance and, 145
   MS and, 812
   psoriasis and, 923
radiation, 736–37
radioactive iodine ablation (RIA),
   703
raloxifene (Evista), 852–54, 858
RAND Corporation, 100, 640
rapid eye movement (REM) sleep,
   45–46
Recommended Daily Intakes (RDIs),
   69–70
Recommended Dietary Intakes
   (RDIs), 297
recurrent aphthous ulcers (RAUs),
   389–90
red blood cells (RBCs):
   anemia and, 292–95
   cervical dysplasia and, 416–17
   diabetes and, 506–7, 510, 530–31,
      535
   glycosylation of, 506
   magnesium and, 896–97
red clover (*Trifolium praetense*),
   791–92
red wine, 193
   CVD and, 154, 156
   macular degeneration and, 776
   migraine headaches and, 804
relationships, *see* interpersonal
   relationships
relative risk (RR), 96
relaxation, 23
   angina and, 309
   high BP and, 667–68
   insomnia and, 750
   migraine headaches and, 809–10
   osteoarthritis and, 841
   progressive, 210, 750
   stress and, 208–10
   tension headaches and, 640–41
RESPeRATE, 668

respiration, respiratory tract, 12
   angina and, 309
   asthma and, 322–23, 325, 328–29,
      331–33, 335–37
   in bronchitis, 367, 370–71
   CFS and, 427
   CHF and, 443
   common cold and, 435–36, 439
   COPD and, 431–32
   diaphragmatic, 209–10, 668
   ear infections and, 557, 560
   high BP and, 668
   immune system and, 176–78, 181
   obesity and, 221–22
   physical care and, 78–81
   pneumonia and, 367–69, 372–73
   sinus infections and, 957, 959
   sleep apnea and, 748–49
   strep throat and, 968
   toxins and, 112
rest, 129–30, 436
rest, ice, compression, elevation
   (RICE), 962–63
restless legs syndrome, 752–53
resveratrol, 193
retinal pigmented epithelium (RPE),
   774–75, 778–79
retinol, *see* vitamin A
retinopathy, 503, 523, 526, 531, 533,
   539–40
rheumatoid arthritis (RA), 932–47
   antioxidants and, 933–34, 939–41
   autoantibodies and, 934–35
   bromelain for, 943
   causes of, 933–36
   copper for, 941–42
   corticosteroids and, 937, 941
   curcumin for, 943
   diagnostic considerations for,
      932–33
   diet and, 933–36, 938–41, 946
   DMARDs and, 936–38
   exercise for, 945
   food allergies and, 935, 938–39
   ginger for, 943–45
   hydrochloric acid for, 942
   hydrotherapy for, 945
   manganese for, 941
   NSAIDs and, 936–37, 942
   omega-3 fatty acids for, 942–43
   other autoimmune diseases and,
      933
   oxidative stress and, 934, 940
   pancreatic enzymes for, 942
   probiotics for, 942
   psychological factors and, 934, 945
   selenium for, 940–41

rheumatoid arthritis (RA) (*cont.*)
SOD and, 941–42
symptoms of, 932–38, 941–42
therapeutic considerations for, 936–45
vitamin B₅ for, 941
vitamin B₆ for, 940–41
vitamin C for, 940–41
vitamin D for, 942
vitamin E for, 940–41
zinc for, 940–41
rhubarb (*Rheum rhabarbarum*), 881
riboflavin, *see* vitamin B₂
Robbins, Anthony, 34
Rolfing, 81
rosacea, 948–53
causes of, 949
stages of, 948
symptoms of, 948–49
therapeutic considerations for, 949–52
topical treatments and, 949–52
vitamin B and, 950–51
zinc for, 951–52
rotation diversified diet, 598, 600–602
rutin, 618

Saccharomyces boulardi, 553
S-adenosyl-methionine (SAM-e), 91, 269
depression and, 488, 491
detoxification and, 123–24, 127, 129
NAFLD and, 824
osteoarthritis and, 835
safety, 31, 33
saffron (*Crocus sativus*), 482, 499, 900
St.-John's-wort (*Hypericum perforatum*), 68
depression and, 482, 496–98
menopause and, 791–93
PMS and, 899–900
salicylates, 696–97
salivary cortisol levels, 208, 217
salt:
asthma and, 328
CHF and, 442–43
health-promoting diet and, 54–55, 61, 63
high BP and, 666–69, 671, 673–75
kidney stones and, 767
stress management and, 213
salt pipes, 373
sanguinarine, 888
sarcopenia, 188–90, 855

sarsaparilla (*Smilax sarsaparilla*), 924–25
saturnine gout, 625
saw palmetto (*Serenoa repens*):
and hair loss in women, 631–32
prostate enlargement and, 918–21
scrotal temperature, 734
seasons, 814
sebaceous glands, sebum, 245–48
seborrheic dermatitis, 954–56
botanical medicines for, 955
causes of, 954
symptoms of, 954
therapeutic considerations for, 954–55
vitamin B₆ and, 954–55
secretin, 352
seeds, *see* nuts and seeds
selective estrogen-receptor modulators (SERMs), 853–54
selective serotonin reuptake inhibitors (SSRIs), 481–82, 489, 496–98, 892
5-HTP and, 493, 496–97
SELECT Prostate Cancer Prevention Trial, 910
selenium:
acne and, 250
alcohol dependence and, 269–70
asthma and, 330, 334
cataracts and, 396, 398
cervical dysplasia and, 416
CVD and, 157, 159
depression and, 485, 489
hepatitis and, 654–55
HIV/AIDS and, 258–59
hypothyroidism and, 721
immune system and, 179
male infertility and, 741
periodontal disease and, 886
prostate cancer and, 104, 906, 909–11
RA and, 940–41
self-actualization, 30–34
self-talk, 34
Seligman, Martin, 29, 34, 479–80, 1007, 1011
Selye, Hans, 204–6, 212
senna (*Cassia senna*), 453–55, 772
sense antibody theory, 814
Sensoril, 216
serotonin:
alcohol dependence and, 269, 271–72
depression and, 272, 480–82, 484, 488–91, 493–96, 498–99
GBE and, 498–99

5-HTP and, 272, 494–95, 872
insomnia and, 750–51
migraine headaches and, 800–802, 807
obesity and, 226, 228–29, 237
PMS and, 892, 895, 898, 900
serotonin deficiency syndrome, 801–2
Serratia peptidase, 958
Sertoli cells, 736
set point theory, 226–27
sex, sexuality, 732
antidepressants and, 481–82
cervical dysplasia and, 413–14
ED and, 570–78
endometriosis and, 565
hepatitis and, 652–54
herpes and, 660
HIV/AIDS and, 254, 260
infertility and, 724–25, 731, 733, 740, 743–45
menopause and, 782, 784, 791
and stages of male sexual act, 570–71
vaginitis and, 984–87
shellfish, 600, 1023
Showa Denko, 492–93
Siberian ginseng (*Eleutherococcus senticosus*), 215–16, 427–28
signatures, doctrine of, 192
silences, 211–12
silent inflammation, 198–204
botanical medicines for, 201, 203
markers of, 198–200
nutritional supplements for, 200, 203
therapeutic considerations for, 199–201
silicon, 861–62
silymarin, *see* milk thistle
Simplified Four-Day Rotation Diet Plan, 600–602
Sinemet, 869, 872–73
sinus infections, 957–61
goldenseal for, 958–59
mucolytics for, 958
nasal irrigation for, 959–60
South African geranium for, 959
symptoms of, 957–58
therapeutic considerations for, 957–59
sinus node, 643
skin:
cross section of, 247
detoxification and, 114
hypothyroidism and, 717
IBD and, 462
obesity and, 221

vitamin D deficiency and, 78
see also specific skin disorders
skin-prick test, 597
sleep:
  AD and, 277, 287–88
  ADHD and, 344–45
  aging and, 45–46, 195
  ASD and, 351
  common cold and, 436
  dreams in, 46–47
  exercise and, 42
  GBE and, 498
  healthful lifestyle and, 28, 39,
    44–47
  how much you need, 45
  IBS and, 761
  immune system and, 173–74
  importance of, 44–47
  normal patterns of, 45–46
  see also insomnia
sleep apnea, 221, 748–49
sleeping pills, 45, 748, 754–55
smoke, smoking, 42, 58
  ADHD and, 341
  cancer and, 39, 96–97, 99, 101, 106,
    117, 357
  and cellular approach to health, 88
  cervical dysplasia and, 414
  COPD and, 431
  CVD and, 149–51, 153, 159
  deadliness of, 39, 183
  detoxification and, 117, 119, 121
  ED and, 572–73
  free radicals and, 187
  healthful lifestyle and, 39–40
  high BP and, 666–67
  hyperthyroidism and, 703
  infertility and, 726–27, 737, 739
  macular degeneration and, 774–75
  osteoporosis and, 845–46, 854
  peptic ulcer and, 877–78
  periodontal disease and, 885
  quitting of, 39–40, 151
  RA and, 933
  stroke and, 971
snacks, 1019
social issues, 271
socialization effect, 22
social readjustment rating scale,
  206–7
sodium:
  -potassium pump, 86
  -to-potassium (Na:K) ratio, 63, 213
  see also salt
sorbitol, 525, 530, 538, 541
sore throat, *see* strep throat
soups, 1019

South African geranium *(Pelargonium
  sidoides)*, 370, 440, 959, 969
soy products, 1016
  calcium in, 858–59
  cancer and, 104, 361–63, 864,
    906–7
  endometriosis and, 567–68
  hypercholesterolemia and, 683
  isoflavone content of, 362–63, 567,
    787–88, 858, 863–64, 906–7, 981
  menopause and, 787–88
  osteoporosis and, 858, 863
  prostate enlargement and, 918
  uterine fibroids and, 981
sperm:
  agglutination of, 739
  anatomy of, 734, 738, 742
  antibodies attacking of, 733–35
  deficient production of, 731–33,
    735–37, 739–40, 742
  male infertility and, 725, 731–45
  normal, 732–33
  scrotal temperature and, 734
spices, 201
spine, spinal cord, 496, 814, 852
  birth defects of, 14
  BMD testing and, 849
  osteoporosis and, 844, 848,
    853–55, 858–59, 863–64
spirituality, 21–25
  in medicine, 5, 8, 22–24
spleen, 170
spontaneity, 32
sports, sports injuries, 962–66
  botanical medicines for, 964–66
  causes of, 962
  glucosamine and, 831–32
  nutritional supplements and, 963,
    965–66
  therapeutic considerations for,
    962–64
squamous cell abnormalities, 412–13
stanols, 689
Staphylococcus aureus, 353–54
statins, 88–89, 682–83, 686–89
sterols, 57, 689
stinging nettle *(Urtica dioica)*, 918,
  921
Stokes, John H., 246–47
stomach, 131–32, 134, 136–37, 139
  see also gastrointestinal tract
stools, 380–81, 451–52
strength training, 44, 78–80, 189
strep throat (streptococcal
  pharyngitis), 967–70
  diagnostic considerations for, 967
  South African geranium for, 969

symptoms of, 967
therapeutic considerations for,
  967–69
vitamin C for, 968–69
stress, 23, 204–19
  acne and, 246–47
  anxiety and, 315, 317
  cancer and, 100
  CFS and, 424, 428
  CVD and, 165
  definition of, 204
  depression and, 483–84
  diabetes and, 519, 527
  digestion and, 133–34, 141, 213
  diseases strongly linked to, 205
  exercise and, 40–41, 212, 217
  food allergies and, 213–14, 594
  in general adaptation syndrome,
    204–5, 215
  hair loss and, 630
  healthy view of, 205–6
  high BP and, 667–68
  hives and, 694, 698
  hyperthyroidism and, 213, 702–4
  IBS and, 761–62
  immune system and, 172–73,
    176–77, 192
  life extension and, 186
  male infertility and, 742–45
  migraine headaches and, 806
  MS and, 819
  peptic ulcer and, 877–78
  physical care and, 81
  PMS and, 895
  positive mental attitude and, 30
  RA and, 934, 940
  salivary cortisol levels in, 208,
    217
  sleep and, 45
  social readjustment rating scale on,
    206–7
  therapeutic considerations for,
    208–17
  see also oxidative stress
stress management, 208–19
  botanical medicines for, 215–16,
    218
  breathing in, 209–10
  calming mind and body in, 208–9
  diet for, 212–14
  exercise for, 212, 217
  lifestyle modification in, 210–12
  nutritional supplements for,
    214–18
  programs for, 217
  progressive relaxation in, 210
Stress of Life, The (Selye), 205–6

stroke, 146, 304, 784, 971–75
  acupuncture for, 975
  CDP-choline for, 974
  CVI and, 408–9
  diabetes and, 503, 971
  GPC for, 974–75
  hypercholesterolemia and, 680, 683
  natural antiplatelet and fibrinolytic
    therapy for, 973
  prevention of, 153, 158–59, 163–65
  recovery from, 972–75
  risk factors for, 150–52, 160–61,
    188, 198–99
  signs of, 971
  therapeutic considerations for,
    972–74
Stronger Neominophagen C (SNMC),
  655–56
strontium, 863
Study of Women's Health Across the
  Nation, 894
substance P, 335, 801–2, 928
sugars, sugar, 129, 145, 1018–19, 1026
  ADHD and, 343
  cancer and, 102
  chronic candidiasis and, 381
  common cold and, 436
  CVD and, 154
  depression and, 484–85
  gallstones and, 610
  health-promoting diet and, 49,
    52–55, 62
  high BP and, 666–67
  hypoglycemia and, 709–14
  IBS and, 759–60
  immune system and, 174–75
  kidney stones and, 767
  neutrophil activity and, 174–75
  osteoporosis and, 856
  periodontal disease and, 886
  PMS and, 893–94
  see also blood glucose
sulfasalazine, 463
sulfation, 114–15, 120–21, 123, 125
sulfites:
  asthma and, 328, 333
  detoxification and, 124–25
  hives and, 697
sulfoxidation, 114, 124–25
sulfur-containing compounds, 190
sumatriptan (Imitrex), 801–2
sunlight:
  AD and, 287
  cancer and, 106
  MS and, 814
  psoriasis and, 927–28
  vitamin D and, 78, 845–46

superoxide, 305–6
superoxide dismutase (SOD):
  cataracts and, 396, 398
  RA and, 941–42
surgery, 23, 409
  cataracts and, 396–97
  CD and, 459
  coronary artery bypass and, 166,
    302–5
  CTS and, 392–93
  ear infections and, 557–59, 561
  ED and, 572
  endometriosis and, 566–67
  hemorrhoids and, 648
  macular degeneration and, 775
  prostate and, 913, 916
  sleep apnea and, 749
  stroke and, 971
  uterine fibroids and, 980
  varicose veins and, 993
  see also angioplasty
Swank Diet, 815–16
Sydenham, Thomas, 622–23
systemic lupus erythematosus (SLE),
  976–79
  causes of, 976
  description of, 976
  DHEA for, 977–78
  diet and, 976–78
  therapeutic considerations for,
    976–78

tachycardia, 643, 645
tai chi, 427
tamoxifen, 363, 607
tartrazine, 64, 324, 696
T cells:
  food allergies and, 593–95
  HIV and, 253–54, 259
  immune system and, 171, 177–80
tea tree (Melaleuca alternifolia) oil:
  acne and, 250–51
  boils and, 353–54
  chronic candidiasis and, 386–87
  seborrheic dermatitis and, 955
  vaginitis and, 990
teeth, 883–85, 887–88
telomeres, 185–88, 193
tendinitis, 962–64
  see also sports, sports injuries
terpenes, 612
testicles, 734, 738, 740–41, 743
testosterone:
  acne and, 245–46, 249
  ED and, 573, 576–78
  male infertility and, 736–38,
    740–41, 743–45

prostate cancer and, 904, 906–8
prostate enlargement and, 915, 917
tetrahydrobiopterin (BH4), 350–51,
  399, 488
Theracurmin, 201, 261, 289
thermogenesis, 227–28, 239–41
thiamine, see vitamin B$_1$
thrombotic hemorrhoids, 647–48
thymus gland:
  enhancing function of, 179–80,
    192, 382
  immune system and, 169–70, 173,
    176–80, 192
thyroid gland:
  depression and, 483
  iodine and, 589–90, 703, 718, 720
  PMS and, 894
  see also hyperthyroidism;
    hypothyroidism
thyroid hormone, 700, 720
thyroid-stimulating hormone (TSH):
  hyperthyroidism and, 702
  hypothyroidism and, 716, 718–21
thyroxine (T4), 702, 704–5
time management, 210–11
tissue plasminogen activator (rtPA),
  972
tocopherols, mixed, see vitamin E
topical treatments:
  acne and, 250–51
  eczema and, 584–86
  hemorrhoids and, 649–50
  herpes and, 664–65
  osteoarthritis and, 838–39
  psoriasis and, 928–29
  rosacea and, 949–52
  vaginitis and, 988–89, 991
tormentil root (Potentilla tormentilla),
  555
touchi, 534
toxins, toxicity, 109–13
  acne and, 246
  ADHD and, 342
  aging and, 187
  avoidance of, 59–60
  cancer and, 107, 112
  and cellular approach to health,
    85, 88
  CFS and, 425
  chemicals and, 110, 112–13, 116,
    121, 128–29
  definition of, 109
  depression and, 484
  diabetes and, 112, 517
  diagnosis of, 113, 122
  diet and, 58–60, 64–66, 112
  endometriosis and, 565–66

gout and, 625
infertility and, 726, 732, 736–37
life extension and, 190
Parkinson's disease and, 869
psoriasis and, 924–26
RA and, 933, 935–36
signs and symptoms of, 109, 111–12
types of, 110–12
see also detoxification
Tragerwork, 81–82
training zone, 43
transcutaneous electrical nerve
    stimulation (TENS), 840, 965
trans-fatty acids, 85–86, 153
acne and, 248
diabetes and, 515–16
endometriosis and, 566
health-promoting diet and, 62
transient ischemic attacks (TIAs),
    408–9, 971
tretinoin (Retin-A), 248, 251
tribulus (*Tribulus terrestris*):
ED and, 577–78
male infertility and, 743–44
tricalcium phosphate, 859–60
Trichomonas vaginalis, 984–85, 987,
    989
triglycerides:
exercise and, 41
health-promoting diet and, 63
in heart disease, 24
medium-chain (MCTs), 239–41
recommended levels for, 681
see also hypertriglyceridemia
Trowell, Hugh, 50
tryptophan:
alcohol dependence and, 269, 272
asthma and, 330
depression and, 481–82, 484,
    492–93, 495
insomnia and, 750–51
metabolism of, 330, 493–94
obesity and, 228, 237–38
PMS and, 898–99
turmeric, *see* curcumin
tylophora (*Tylophora asthmatica*),
    335
tyrosine, 720

ubiquinol, ubiquinone, *see* coenzyme
    Q10
UDP-glucuronyl transferase
    (UDPGT), 124
ulcerative colitis (UC), 456–57
aloe vera for, 467
causes of, 457
children and, 467

curcumin for, 466
features shared by CD and, 457
fiber and, 464
intestinal microflora in, 461
mucin defects in, 461
prebiotics for, 466
signs and symptoms of, 456, 466
therapeutic considerations for,
    460–61, 464–67
vitamin D for, 465
see also inflammatory bowel disease
ultrasound, 965
ultraviolet light, 699, 927–28
United Kingdom Prospective
    Diabetes Study, 518
uric acid:
gout and, 622–27
kidney stones and, 764–68
urinary tract infections, *see* bladder
    infections
urine:
acidifying of, 473–74
alkanizing of, 473
bladder infections and, 471–75
increasing flow of, 473
ketone testing and, 520–23
kidney stones and, 764–68, 771
ursodeoxycholic acid, 825
urticaria, *see* hives
uterine cancer, 107
uterine fibroids, 980–83
causes of, 980
diet and, 981–82
signs and symptoms of, 980
therapeutic considerations for,
    980–82
uva ursi (*Arctostaphylos uva ursi*),
    475

vaccinations:
hepatitis and, 653
immune system and, 173
influenza and, 325
pertussis and, 324–25
pneumococcal and viral, 559
vacuum-constrictive devices, 580
vaginitis, 984–91
atrophic, 782–83, 789
causes of, 984–87, 989
L. acidophilus and, 984, 988–89
local antiseptics for, 989–90
nutritional supplements for, 789,
    988, 991
symptoms of, 984–87, 989
therapeutic considerations for,
    987–90
vitamin C for, 988–89

value effect, 22
varicoceles, 734
varicose veins, 992–97
butcher's broom for, 996
causes of, 992–93
fibrinolytic compounds for, 996
flavonoids for, 994
gotu kola for, 995–96
horse chestnut for, 995
signs and symptoms of, 992, 996
therapeutic considerations for,
    993–95
vein function in normal and, 993
vasoactive amines, 140–41, 695
vegetables, 127, 1019–20, 1026–27
AD and, 282
asthma and, 329
in brassica family, 362–64
cancer and, 101–2, 104, 362–64
carbohydrates and, 711–12
cervical dysplasia and, 415
CVD and, 153, 156, 165
detoxification and, 118–20, 122,
    126, 129
diabetes and, 516
in Edible Plant and Animal
    Kingdoms Taxonomic List, 599
five-a-day goal for, 58
health-promoting diet and, 48,
    53–56, 58–63, 65
high BP and, 669, 671
IBS and, 758
kidney stones and, 765, 768
macular degeneration and,
    775–76
NAFLD and, 823–24
nutritional supplements and, 73,
    75–76
organic, 59
osteoporosis and, 857–58
oxalate content of, 769–71
rainbow assortment of, 56–57
vegetarians, vegetarian diet:
anemia and, 293–94, 297
asthma and, 329
endometriosis and, 567
FBD and, 588
gallstones and, 609
health-promoting diet and, 61–62
high BP and, 668–69
hypothyroidism and, 720
kidney stones and, 765, 768
osteoporosis and, 855, 857
PMS and, 894
psoriasis and, 926
RA and, 939–40
SLE and, 976–77

velvet bean (*Mucuna pruriens*), 745, 873
ventricular ejection fraction, 445–47
Veterans Affairs Normative Aging Study, 30
vinegar, 1027
viruses:
    diarrhea and, 549
    ear infections and, 560
    hepatitis and, 652–53, 655–57
    herpes and, 660–61, 664
    HIV and, 253–64
    hives and, 694, 698
    HPV and, 412–15, 417–18
    MS and, 813–14
    pneumonia and, 368
    sinus infections and, 957, 959
    vaccines and, 559
visualization, 36–37, 40
vitamin A (retinol), 69, 860
    acne and, 249–50
    alcohol dependence and, 268–69
    cataracts and, 396–97, 399
    cervical dysplasia and, 415–16
    and hair loss in women, 632
    HIV/AIDS and, 257
    immune system and, 176, 178–79
    male infertility and, 740–41
    osteoarthritis and, 836
    peptic ulcer and, 879
    periodontal disease and, 885–86
    pneumonia and, 372–73
vitamin B$_1$ (thiamine):
    AD and, 282
    alcohol dependence and, 270–71
    canker sores and, 390
    CHF and, 443–45
    depression and, 487
    diabetes and, 541
    HIV/AIDS and, 257
vitamin B$_2$ (riboflavin):
    cataracts and, 399
    depression and, 487
    migraine headaches and, 806
vitamin B$_3$, *see* niacin; niacinamide
vitamin B$_5$ (pantothenic acid):
    depression and, 487
    hypercholesterolemia and, 689–90
    RA and, 941
    stress management and, 214
vitamin B$_6$ (pyridoxine):
    alcohol dependence and, 270
    ASD and, 350
    asthma and, 330
    CTS and, 392, 394
    CVD and, 160–62
    depression and, 487, 489

diabetes and, 531–32
high BP and, 674–75
HIV/AIDS and, 257–58
immune system and, 178, 180
kidney stones and, 767–68
migraine headaches and, 804–5, 807
osteoarthritis and, 836
osteoporosis and, 862
PMS and, 893, 896–98
RA and, 940–41
seborrheic dermatitis and, 954–55
tryptophan and, 493
vitamin B$_{12}$ (methylcobalamin):
    AD and, 282–83, 285
    anemia and, 294–95, 297–99
    ASD and, 351
    asthma and, 333
    cervical dysplasia and, 417
    CVD and, 161–62
    depression and, 487–89
    diabetes and, 526
    HIV/AIDS and, 258
    hives and, 699
    IBD and, 465
    immune system and, 178
    male infertility and, 741
    osteoporosis and, 862
    seborrheic dermatitis and, 955
vitamin B complex:
    menorrhagia and, 798
    rosacea and, 950–51
    seborrheic dermatitis and, 954–55
    see also biotin; folic acid
vitamin C (ascorbic acid), 69–70, 488, 963
    AD and, 281–82
    alcohol dependence and, 269–70
    angiograms and, 304
    ASD and, 351
    asthma and, 330–32
    and bronchitis and pneumonia, 372
    cataracts and, 396–98
    cervical dysplasia and, 414–16
    common cold and, 436–37
    CVD and, 157–60
    depression and, 487
    detoxification and, 121–22, 129
    diabetes and, 529–30, 538–40, 542
    gallstones and, 610
    glaucoma and, 617, 619
    gout and, 627
    hepatitis and, 654
    herpes and, 661
    high BP and, 529, 666–67, 669, 674
    HIV/AIDS and, 258–59
    hives and, 699

immune system and, 175–77, 180
kidney stones and, 771
macular degeneration and, 776–78
male infertility and, 739, 741
menopause and, 788–89
menorrhagia and, 797
osteoarthritis and, 835–36
osteoporosis and, 862
Parkinson's disease and, 870
periodontal disease and, 885–86
RA and, 940–41
strep throat and, 968–69
stress management and, 214
vaginitis and, 988–89
vitamin D:
    asthma and, 333–34
    cancer and, 103, 105–6, 193, 911–12
    CVD and, 164
    depression and, 487, 490
    diabetes and, 507, 509
    hepatitis and, 655
    HIV/AIDS and, 258
    IBD and, 465
    immune system and, 177
    life extension and, 186, 193
    metabolism of, 847
    MS and, 814, 817
    osteoarthritis and, 836
    osteoporosis and, 845–46, 857, 859–61, 863
    pregnancy and, 79–80, 860–61
    psoriasis and, 927–28
    RA and, 942
    recommendations on, 71–73, 77–78
vitamin D deficiency syndrome (VDDS), 77–78
vitamin E (mixed tocopherols):
    acne and, 250
    AD and, 281–82
    angiograms and, 304
    asthma and, 330–31
    cancer and, 104, 904, 906, 908–11
    cataracts and, 396–99
    CVD and, 157–60
    diabetes and, 516, 530, 542
    FBD and, 589
    gallstones and, 610
    HIV/AIDS and, 258–60
    immune system and, 177–79
    macular degeneration and, 776–78
    male infertility and, 739–41
    menopause and, 789, 791
    natural vs. synthetic, 909–10
    osteoarthritis and, 836
    Parkinson's disease and, 870–71
    peptic ulcer and, 879

periodontal disease and, 886
PMS and, 897–98
RA and, 940–41
vitamin K:
  kidney stones and, 768
  menorrhagia and, 797
  osteoarthritis and, 836
  osteoporosis and, 846, 857, 859,
    862–64
vitamins:
  behavioral effects and, 487
  deficiencies in, 9, 69–71, 77–79,
    487
  in foods, 70–71
  health-promoting diet and, 49
  hypothyroidism and, 721
  recommendations on, 71–73,
    77–78
volatile oils, enteric-coated, 386

waist, 223–24
walking, 43
walnuts, 155–56
warfarin (Coumadin), 410
  arrhythmias and, 644
  glucosamine and, 833
  stroke and, 972–74
wasting syndrome, 256–57
water:
  alternating hot and cold, 393
  detoxification and, 127
  diabetes and, 510, 513
  health-promoting diet and, 54–55,
    65–66
  kidney stones and, 764, 767
  obesity and, 231
Waynberg, Jacques, 577
weight, weight control, 224, 482, 767
  see also obesity
weight lifting, 43–44

weight loss:
  exercise and, 40–41, 43
  obesity and, 229–41
  osteoarthritis and, 828–29
weight loss aids, natural, 233–41
  chromium, 236–37
  fiber supplements, 233–34
  HCA, 238–39
  5-HTP, 237–38
  MCTs, 238–41
  MR formulas, 236
Wellmune WGP, 181
wellness, promotion of, 5–7, 9–12, 17
wellness-oriented medicine, 12
Werbach, Melvin, 487–88
white blood cells (WBCs):
  asthma and, 322, 324, 331
  and bronchitis and pneumonia, 372
  CFS and, 422
  CHF and, 444
  common cold and, 435–36
  diabetes and, 508
  food allergies and, 592–96
  HIV and, 253–54, 257–61
  immune system and, 170–73,
    175–80
  see also specific white blood cells
white coat hypertension, 667
white fat, 228
wild primates, diets of, 48–49, 60–61
Williams, Roger, 66, 71
Wilson, Robert A., 784
wine, 62, 105
  see also red wine
Women's Health Initiative (WHI),
    280, 784–85, 859
World Health Organization (WHO),
    9, 27, 319, 559, 833, 849, 854
wound healing, 524, 532, 542
Wright, Jonathan, 124, 333

xenoestrogens, 980–81
X-rays, 827–30
  DEXA and, 849–51
  osteoarthritis and, 827–30
xylitol, 561–62

yeast, see Candida albicans
yogurt, 1020
yohimbe (Pausinystalia johimbe),
    576–77

zeaxanthin, 776–78
zinc, 69, 104
  acne and, 249–50
  AD and, 282, 284
  ADHD and, 344
  alcohol dependence and, 268
  canker sores and, 390
  cataracts and, 398–99
  common cold and, 437
  depression and, 489
  diabetes and, 532, 542
  ED and, 575
  and hair loss in women, 632
  herpes and, 661
  HIV/AIDS and, 258
  hypothyroidism and, 721
  IBD and, 465
  immune system and, 178–80
  macular degeneration and, 776–78
  male infertility and, 740–41
  osteoarthritis and, 836
  osteoporosis and, 861
  peptic ulcer and, 879–80
  periodontal disease and, 885–86
  PMS and, 897
  pneumonia and, 372
  prostate and, 908, 917
  RA and, 940–41
  rosacea and, 951–52